Public/Community Health and Nursing Practice

CARING FOR POPULATIONS

SECOND EDITION

Christine L. Savage, PhD, RN, FAAN
Professor Emerita
Johns Hopkins University School of Nursing
Baltimore, Maryland

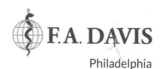

F.A. DAVIS

Philadelphia

F. A. Davis Company
1915 Arch Street
Philadelphia, PA 19103
www.fadavis.com

Copyright © 2020 by F. A. Davis Company

Printed in the United States of America

Last digit indicates print number: 10 9 8 7 6 5 4 3 2 1

Publisher, Nursing: Terri Wood Allen
Senior Content Project Manager: Elizabeth Hart
Digital Project Manager: Kate Crowley
Design and Illustration Manager: Carolyn O'Brien

As new scientific information becomes available through basic and clinical research, recommended treatments and drug therapies undergo changes. The author(s) and publisher have done everything possible to make this book accurate, up to date, and in accord with accepted standards at the time of publication. The author(s), editors, and publisher are not responsible for errors or omissions or for consequences from application of the book, and make no warranty, expressed or implied, in regard to the contents of the book. Any practice described in this book should be applied by the reader in accordance with professional standards of care used in regard to the unique circumstances that may apply in each situation. The reader is advised always to check product information (package inserts) for changes and new information regarding dose and contraindications before administering any drug. Caution is especially urged when using new or infrequently ordered drugs.

Library of Congress Cataloging-in-Publication Data

Names: Savage, Christine L., author.
Title: Public/community health and nursing practice : caring for populations
  / Christine L. Savage.
Other titles: Public health science and nursing practice
Description: 2nd edition. | Philadelphia : F.A. Davis Company, [2020] |
  Preceded by: Public health science and nursing practice / Christine L.
  Savage, Joan E. Kub, Sara L. Groves, 2016. | Includes bibliographical
  references and index.
Identifiers: LCCN 2019007149 (print) | LCCN 2019008721 (ebook) | ISBN
  9780803699878 (ebook) | ISBN 9780803677111 (pbk.)
Subjects: | MESH: Public Health Nursing | Community Health Nursing | Health
  Planning | Population Characteristics
Classification: LCC RT97 (ebook) | LCC RT97 (print) | NLM WY 108 | DDC
  610.73/4—dc23
LC record available at https://lccn.loc.gov/2019007149

To my husband, Joe, for all his love and support.

Preface

The World Health Organization (WHO) partnered with the International Council of Nursing and began the Nursing Now campaign that "… aims to improve health by raising the profile and status of nursing worldwide" (WHO, 2018). They recognized that nurses provide care essential to the optimizing of health for individuals, families and communities. Health occurs from the cellular to the global level; thus nurses must have knowledge related to health across this continuum. Nursing education often begins with understanding health at the cellular level through courses related to pathophysiology and physical assessment. Building on this knowledge, this text covers health, disease, and injury within the context of the world we live in. No matter what settings nurses work in, they apply public health science on a daily basis to prevent disease, reduce mortality and morbidity in those who are ill, and contribute to the health of the communities we serve. Our goal with this book is to lead you on the journey of discovering how the public health sciences are an integral part of nursing practice and how nurses implement effective public health interventions.

About This Book

This book presents public health in a way that captures the adventure of tackling health from a community- and population-based perspective. Public health helps us to answer the question, "Why is this happening?" and to implement interventions that improve the health of populations. Public health issues are usually messy real-world problems that do not always have obvious solutions. You will learn through the examples provided how to gather the needed information to understand important health issues, especially those included in *Healthy People*. You will have an opportunity to explore population-level, evidence-based interventions and learn how to evaluate the effectiveness of those interventions. We aim to provide you with the knowledge to achieve the competencies in public health you increasingly need as a professional nurse across multiple settings. You will be provided with numerous examples of how public health nurses integrate nursing and public health, with a focus on promoting the health of populations.

The application of public health knowledge in the provision of care and the prevention of disease is not new to the nursing profession. Florence Nightingale is often viewed as the first nurse epidemiologist because of her work in the Crimean War. She applied public health science to nursing practice in a way that saved lives and improved outcomes, both in the context of war and back in England, with the development of professional nursing in hospital and home settings. As nurses practicing in the 21st century, we follow in her footsteps. Consider nurses working in primary care with mothers and children or those working in low-income countries facing epidemics of tuberculosis and HIV/AIDS. How does knowledge of public health science enhance our ability to address these complex health issues? Before we can improve health outcomes, we must understand the natural history of disease, the social context in which these health issues arise, and the resources critical to addressing all of the barriers to care. Knowledge of public health and how it applies to nursing practice has taken on increased importance as we move from a fee-for-service model of care to a health-care system that rewards prevention of disease.

Nurses must know how to apply the basics of the public health sciences such as epidemiology, social and behavioral sciences, and environmental health. They must also meet the Quad Council generalist core competencies such as community assessment, health planning, and health policy. To help you to do that, we have employed a problem-based learning approach to the presentation of the material in this book so that you can apply the principles of public health to real-life nursing settings.

Throughout the book, case studies demonstrate how the application of the public health sciences and public health practice to nursing practice is essential to the promotion of health and the prevention of disease. At times, the focus will be on solving health-related mysteries and how that leads to the implementation of interventions to address the health problems at the population level. At other times, the focus will be on the application of the public health sciences to the development and implementation of evidence-based, population-level interventions aimed at addressing the health issue.

Although there have been significant improvements in health during the past 100 years, achieving our stated health goals, whether it be *Healthy People* goals and objectives or global goals, continues to be a challenge. The ability of each individual, family, and community to lead a healthy and productive life involves an interaction among ourselves, our environment, and the communities in which we live. Understanding the multiple determinants of health, including social determinants that significantly influence health disparities and health inequities, is an essential skill for nurses. The public health sciences help us understand the complexity of the interaction of external and internal forces that shape our health. The premise of this book is that all nurses require adequate knowledge of the public health sciences and how to apply it to nursing practice across all settings and populations. With this knowledge, we can truly contribute to the building of a healthy world.

Organization of the Text

The philosophical approach to this text is that all professional nurses incorporate population-level interventions no matter what the setting. We include not only chapters on the traditional public health settings such as the public health department and school health, but also chapters on acute and primary care settings. The book uses a constructivist learning approach by which the learner constructs her or his own knowledge. Thus, the content is delivered by applying the information within the context of the real world.

This text uses a problem-based learning approach so that the student can apply the content to nursing practice. It is organized into three units. Unit I, Basis for Public Health Nursing Knowledge and Skills, covers the essential knowledge based in the public health sciences and core public health nursing competencies needed to solve health problems and implement evidenced-based interventions at the population level. This unit provides the basic public health knowledge needed by all generalist nurses. The content covered in these chapters is applied across the next two units of the book. Unit II, Community Health Across Populations: Public Health Issues, covers health issues that span populations and settings including communicable and noncommunicable disease, health disparity, behavioral health, and global health. Unit III, Public Health Planning, covers the settings in which nurses practice, public health policy, and disaster management.

Understanding health within the context of community includes understanding the role of culture. To help underscore the importance of culture, it has been integrated across each of the chapters rather than have a stand-alone chapter dedicated to culture. In each chapter there is a callout box related to the role of culture specific to the subject of that chapter.

Global health is the other concept now integrated across all of the chapters. In earlier public health textbooks, the term most often used was 'international health'. As it became clearer that the health of one nation does not occur in a vacuum, but rather contributes to the health of the globe, global health became the accepted term. To truly adhere to the concept that health is global across all settings, we have included a cellular to global box in every chapter relevant to the content in that chapter. As nurses dedicated to optimizing health for all, visualizing health within a global context will help us join with the WHO in promoting nursing as a true force in health.

Key Features

▼ CASE STUDIES

Throughout the book, the student will find case studies embedded in the chapters that provide essential content within the context of actual nursing practice. This approach begins with the issue and walks the reader through the process of deciding how best to address the problem presented. In some of the cases presented, the object is to solve the mystery (**Solving the Mystery**), such as the case in Chapter 8 that walks through how to solve the mystery of why people are presenting at the emergency department with severe gastrointestinal symptoms. Other cases (**Applying Public Health Science**) describe how nurses apply the public health sciences, such as epidemiology, to help develop and implement evidence-based interventions at the population level. There is a standard case study at the end of selected chapters. For instructors, there is online access on the Davis*Plus* website for the book to a problem-based learning exercise that can be used to further apply the content presented in the chapter.

■ HEALTHY PEOPLE

Healthy People is referenced throughout, including *Healthy People 2020* and information on *Healthy People 2030* available prior to publication. Boxes are included that present the *Healthy People 2020* objectives and the midcourse reviews on progress towards meeting those objectives.

■ EVIDENCE-BASED PRACTICE BOXES

Evidence-Based Practice (EBP) boxes illustrate how research and its resulting evidence can support and inform public health nursing practice. Cutting-edge EBP is a strong underpinning of the book as a whole.

LEARNING OUTCOMES AND KEY TERMS

Each chapter begins with Learning Outcomes and a list of Key Terms that appear in boldface and color at first mention in a chapter.

Teaching/Learning Package

Instructor Resources

Instructor Resources on Davis*Plus* include the following:

- NCLEX-Style Test Bank
- PowerPoint Presentations
- Instructor's Guide with PBL exercises

- Problem-Based Learning PowerPoint Presentation
- Case Study Instructor's Guides for end-of-chapter case studies
- QSEN Crosswalk
- Quad Council Competencies
- Simulation Experiences

Student Resources

Student Resources on Davis*Plus* include the following:

- Student Quiz Bank
- Student Guide to Problem-Based Learning
- List of Web Resources
- QSEN Crosswalk
- Quad Council Competencies

We hope you will enjoy this book and, most of all, we hope as nurses you will always care for the health of populations no matter the setting, thus increasing the contribution of nursing to the goal of optimal health for all.

Contributors

Laurie Abbott, PhD, RN, PHNA-BC
Assistant Professor
Florida State University College of Nursing
Tallahassee, Florida
Chapter 13

Kathleen Ballman, DNP, APRN, ACNP-BC, CEN
*Associate Professor of Clinical Nursing, Coordinator,
Coordinator of Adult-Gerontology Acute Care
Programs*
University of Cincinnati, College of Nursing
Cincinnati, Ohio
Chapter 14

Derryl E. Block, PhD, MPH, MSN, RN
Dean, College of Health and Human Sciences
Northern Illinois University
DeKalb, Illinois
Chapter 21

Susan Bulecza, DNP, RN, PHCNS-BC
State Public Health Nursing Director
Florida Department of Health
Tallahassee, Florida
Chapter 13

Deborah Busch, DNP, RN, CPNP-PC, IBCLC
Assistant Professor
Johns Hopkins School of Nursing
Baltimore, Maryland
Chapter 17

Amanda Choflet, DNP, RN, OCN
*Director of Nursing, Johns Hopkins Medicine
Department of Radiation Oncology & Molecular
Radiation Sciences*
Baltimore, Maryland
Chapter 11

Christine Colella, DNP, APRN-CNP, FAANP
Professor, Executive Director of Graduate Programs
University of Cincinnati, College of Nursing
Cincinnati, Ohio
Chapter 15

Joanne Flagg, DNP, CRNP, IBCLC, FAAN
Assistant Professor, Director MSN Programs
Johns Hopkins School of Nursing
Baltimore, Maryland
Chapter 17

Gordon Gillespie, PhD, DNP, RN, PHCNS-BC, CEN,
CPEN, FAEN, FAAN
*Professor, Associate Dean for Research, Deputy
Director Occupational Health Nursing Program*
University of Cincinnati
Cincinnati, Ohio
Chapters 5, 20, & 22

Bryan R. Hansen, PhD, RN, APRN-CNS, ACNS-BC
Assistant Professor
Johns Hopkins School of Nursing
Baltimore, Maryland
Chapter 10

Barbara B. Little, DNP, MPH, RN, PHNA-BC, CNE
Senior Teaching Faculty
Florida State University
Tallahassee, Florida
Chapter 13

Minhui Liu, RN, PhD
Post-doctoral
Johns Hopkins University School of Nursing
Baltimore, Maryland
Chapter 19

Donna Mazyck, MS, RN, NCSN, CAE
Executive Director
National Association of School Nurse
Silver Spring, Maryland
Chapter 18

Paula V. Nersesian, RN, MPH, PhD
Assistant Professor
Johns Hopkins University School of Nursing
Baltimore, Maryland
Chapter 16

Michael Sanchez, DNP, ARNP, NP-C, FNP-BC,
AAHIVS
Assistant Professor
Johns Hopkins School of Nursing
Baltimore, Maryland
  Chapters 8 & 11

Phyllis Sharps, RN, PhD, FAAN
Professor
Associate Dean for Community Programs
and Initiatives
Johns Hopkins University School of Nursing
Baltimore, Maryland
  Chapter 17

Christine Vandenhouten, PhD, RN, APHN-BC
Associate Professor (Nursing & MSHWM Programs
Chair of Nursing and Health Studies, Director
of BSN-LINC
University of Wisconsin, Green Bay Professional
Program in Nursing
Green Bay, Wisconsin
  Chapter 21

Erin Rachel Whitehouse, RN, MPH, PhD
Epidemic Intelligence Service Officer at Centers
for Disease Control and Prevention
Atlanta, Georgia
  Chapter 3

Erin M. Wright, DNP, CNM, APHN-BC
Assistant Professor
Johns Hopkins School of Nursing
Baltimore, Maryland
  Chapter 17

Contributors to Previous Edition

Sheila Fitzgerald, PhD

Sara Groves, RN, MPH, MSN, PhD

Joan Kub, PhD, MA, PHCNS-BC, FAAN

William A. Mase, Dr.PH, MPH, MA

Mary R. Nicholson, RN, BSN, MSN CIC

Reviewers

Kathleen Keough Adee, MSN, DNP, RN
Associate Professor
Salem State University
Salem, Massachusetts

Lynn P. Blanchette, RN, PhD, PHNA-BC
Associate Dean, Assistant Professor
Rhode Island College School of Nursing
Providence, Rhode Island

Dia Campbell-Detrixhe, PhD, RN, FNGNA, CNE,
FCN
Associate Professor of Nursing
Oklahoma City University Kramer School of Nursing
Oklahoma City, Oklahoma

Kathie DeMuth, MSN, RN
Assistant Professor
Bellin College
Green Bay, Wisconsin

Bonnie Jerome-D'Emilia, RN, MPH, PhD
Associate Professor
Rutgers University School of Nursing-Camden
Camden, New Jersey

Vicky P. Kent, PhD, RN, CNE
Clinical Associate Professor
Towson University
Towson, Maryland

Kimberly Lacey, DNSc, RN, MSN, CNE
Assistant Professor
Southern Connecticut State University
New Haven, Connecticut

Charlene Niemi, PhD, RN, PHN, CNE
Assistant Professor
California State University Channel Islands
Camarillo, California

Phoebe Ann Pollitt, PhD, RN, MA
Associate Professor of Nursing
Appalachian State University
Boone, North Carolina

Lisa Quinn, PhD, CRNP, MSN
Associate Professor of Nursing
Gannon University
Erie, Pennsylvania

Delbert Martin Raymond III, BSN, MS, PhD
Professor
Eastern Michigan University
Ypsilanti, Michigan

Meredith Scannell, PhD, MSN, MPH, CNM,
SANE, CEN
Nursing Faculty
Institute of Health Professions
Charlestown, Massachusetts

Elizabeth Stallings, RN, BSN, MA, DmH
Assistant Professor
Felician University
Lodi, New Jersey

Acknowledgments

This book exists because of the wonderful students I have had over the years and their dedication to improving the health of individuals, families, and communities. Their thirst for knowledge fed my own. I am grateful to my colleagues who I have had the privilege to work with over my nursing career, with a very special thanks to those who contributed to the writing of this book. I would also like to thank Jeannine Carrado, Elizabeth Hart, and Terri Allen at F. A. Davis for their support and guidance throughout the writing of this book. Improving the health of communities thrives on respectful and thoughtful collaboration between many different people, and so does the writing of a text book.

Table of Contents

Basis for Public Health Nursing Knowledge and Skills

Chapter 1

Public Health and Nursing Practice

Christine Savage, Joan Kub, and Sara Groves

LEARNING OUTCOMES

After reading the chapter, the student will be able to:

1. Identify how public health plays a central role in the practice of nursing across settings and specialties.
2. Describe public health in terms of current frameworks, community partnerships, and the concept of population health.
3. Investigate determinants of health within the context of culture.

4. Explore the connection between environment, resource availability, and health.
5. Identify the key roles and responsibilities of public health nurses (PHNs).
6. Identify the formal organization of public health services from a global to local level.

KEY TERMS

Aggregate	Determinants of	Life expectancy	Public health
Assessment	health	Low-income countries	Public health nursing
Assurance	Diversity	(LICs)	Public health science
Community	Ethnicity	Lower middle-income	Race
Core functions	Global health	countries (LMICs)	Upper middle-income
Cultural competency	Globalization	Policy development	countries (UMICs)
Cultural humility	Health	Population health	
Cultural lenses	High-income countries	Population-focused	
Culture	(HICs)	care	

■ Introduction

Every day the media presents us with riveting stories: "The flu season—the worst in a decade," "Flint's water supply contaminated with high levels of lead," "School shooting leaves 17 dead," "Hurricane Maria leaves 80% of Puerto Rico without power and water," "Zika virus results in congenital brain damage," "The homicide rate in Chicago rises," "More than 80 dead from the Camp Fire in California." All of these stories reflect the connections among the health of individuals and families, the communities they live in, the

quality of the public health infrastructure, and population-level events such as disasters (natural and manmade), communicable diseases (CDs), and violence. As nurses, we provide care directly to individuals and families within the context of the communities we serve. That context encompasses diverse and unifying cultures, demographics, geography, infrastructure, resources, and the vulnerability of certain members of the community. That is why understanding health from a cellular to global level requires a sound grounding in public health science, a central component of nursing science and practice.

■ CELLULAR TO GLOBAL
Health Across the Continuum

The health of individuals occurs across a continuum from the cellular level to the global level. When we care for individuals and their families, understanding the context of their health is vital to the promotion of optimum health. For example, a person with type 2 diabetes who is seeking care may or may not have access to the needed resources depending on what exists in their community as well as their own financial status. Providing care to that person requires use of prescribed medication, encouragement to exercise, and encouragement to maintain a healthy diet. As you learned in pathophysiology, type 2 diabetes occurs at the cellular-level, but external factors may increase the risk for being diagnosed with the disease. In addition, the community in which a person lives, both locally and at the state level, has an impact on their ability to pay for medications, to have access to safe areas for exercise, and to obtain affordable fresh food.

Likewise, individual health at the cellular level depends on the health of the Earth from a global level. Optimal health requires access to basic resources such as potable water, a secure food supply, sanitation, and adequate shelter. Events at the global level such as climate change can result in the inability to obtain these needed resources. For example, following the 2018 Camp Fire in California, which was associated with climate change, many people lost their homes. Outbreaks of communicable diseases (see Chapter 8) in one part of the world can spread and affect many other parts of the world, such as the Zika virus outbreak in the summer of 2016. Natural disasters often have far-reaching effects such as the tsunami of 2004 that resulted in deaths and injury across multiple countries including Indonesia, India, Malaysia, Myanmar, Thailand, Sri Lanka, and the Maldives. Thus, all disease and injury occur within the context of the health of the community and the globe.

As nurses, we apply public health science daily. Obvious examples include infection control nurses, school nurses, and nurses in the public health department. Nurses working in an acute care setting also apply public health science when using protective equipment and caring for a patient in isolation to prevent transmission of a CD. Public health science applies to every setting where nurses work; understanding public health and the science behind it is a core competency of professional nursing. It is expected that upon graduation an entry-level nurse will be able to integrate knowledge from public health into their nursing practice. Nurses must apply the nursing process and incorporate knowledge of the ecological and social determinants of health as they care for individuals and families, and by extension communities and populations. Finally, they are expected to be able to evaluate health within a global context and demonstrate cultural humility in the care of individuals, families, communities, and populations.[1] According to the American Nurses Association's (ANA) Scope and Standards, the importance of public health is clear.[2] Other competencies grounded in public health include infection control (Chapter 8), emergency preparedness and disaster management (Chapter 22), environmental health (Chapter 6), and a basic understanding of epidemiology (Chapter 3).

Public Health Science and Practice

What exactly is public health science? **Public health science** is the scientific foundation of public health practice and brings together other sciences including environmental science, epidemiology, biostatistics, biomedical sciences, and the social and behavioral sciences.[3,4]

Thus, public health science, as a combination of several other sciences, allows us to tackle health problems using a wide range of knowledge. We apply the results of public health science to deal with health problems on a regular basis. For example, the evidence that underlies the reliability and validity of screening and diagnostic test results comes from the analysis of population-level data using the science of epidemiology. Public health science also provides the tools needed to try and solve a problem in the community or in a geographical area.

When confronted with a health problem, health care providers begin with the question "What can we do about it?" This requires an examination of the underlying risks and protective factors related to the health problem, both individual and population based. Based on this type of examination, lead experts in nursing used a population health framework to develop a conceptual model of nursing that reflects the shift from a concentration on individual health alone to an understanding that health occurs within the context of a population and factors that support or undermine the health of the population as a whole.[5] Understanding the factors that contribute to health, both negative and positive, from both a population and an individual/family perspective allows us to develop nursing interventions that incorporate the full continuum of health from individuals to populations, and, it is hoped, to contribute with each intervention to the goal of the World Health Organization (WHO), the public health arm of the United Nations (UN): "… to build a better, healthier future for people all over the world."[6]

According to Issel,[7] individuals do not achieve health through uninformed, individualistic actions. Instead, individual health occurs within the surrounding context of the population and the environment. Therefore, all nurses need skills and knowledge related to their patients' informed actions within the context of the health of their community. During the last century and into the 21st century, public health science has been the backbone of the nursing interventions we provide to individuals, families, and communities. Standard care, such as flu vaccinations, lead poisoning screening, and prevention programs, comes from work done using the principles of public health science. As nurses, we must be sufficiently competent to understand the basics of this science and apply it daily in our care. After all, it is our heritage. The modern founder of our profession, Florence Nightingale, was an early pioneer in epidemiology and public health science.

Although **public health** has contributed significantly to the health of the nation over the past century, it is often difficult to define. In 1920, a respected public health figure, C.E.A. Winslow, defined public health as:

> … the science and art of preventing disease, prolonging life and promoting health and efficiency through organized community effort for the sanitation of the environment, the control of communicable infections, the education of the individual in personal hygiene, the organization of medical and nursing services for the early diagnosis and preventive treatment of disease, and for the development of the social machinery to insure everyone a standard of living adequate for the maintenance of health, so organizing these benefits as to enable every citizen to realize his birth right of health and longevity.[3]

Winslow's definition reflects what public health is, the scientific basis of public health, and what it does, and it remains relevant to this day.[4]

In 1988, the Institute of Medicine (IOM), now known as the Health and Medicine Division (HMD) of the National Academies of Sciences, Engineering, and Medicine, in its report *The Future of Public Health,* added clarity to the term by defining public health as what society does collectively to assure the conditions for people to be healthy.[8] It identified three **core functions** that encompass the purpose of public health: (1) assessment, (2) policy development, and (3) assurance. **Assessment** focuses on the systematic collection, analysis, and monitoring of health problems and needs. **Policy development** refers to using scientific knowledge to develop comprehensive public health policies. **Assurance** relates to assuring constituents that public health agencies provide services necessary to achieve agreed-upon goals.

In 1994, the Public Health Functions Steering Committee, a group of public and private partners, added further clarification to the definition by establishing a list of essential services (Chapter 13). The committee developed the list of essential services through a consensus process with federal agencies and major national public health agencies (see Box 1-1). [9]

Although the government is likely to play a leadership role in ensuring that essential services are provided, public, private, and voluntary organizations are also needed to provide a healthy environment and are a part of the public health system. In a 2012 report by the IOM, experts concluded that "… funding for governmental

---

BOX 1–1 ■ Ten Essential Public Health Services

The 10 essential public health services provide the framework for the National Public Health Performance Standards Program (NPHPSP). Because the strength of a public health system rests on its capacity to effectively deliver the 10 Essential Public Health Services, the NPHPSP instruments for health systems assess how well they perform the following:

1. Monitor health status to identify community health problems.
2. Diagnose and investigate health problems and health hazards in the community.
3. Inform, educate, and empower people about health issues.
4. Mobilize community partnerships to identify and solve health problems.
5. Develop policies and plans that support individual and community health efforts.
6. Enforce laws and regulations that protect health and ensure safety.
7. Link people to needed personal health services and assure the provision of health care when otherwise unavailable.
8. Assure a competent public health and personal health-care workforce.
9. Evaluate effectiveness, accessibility, and quality of personal and population-based health services.
10. Research for new insights and innovative solutions to health problems.

Source: (9)

public health is inadequate, unstable, and unsustainable."[10] Thus the promotion of population level health requires a comprehensive public health infrastructure. According to Healthy People 2020 (HP 2020) the three essential infrastructure components include a capable and qualified workforce, up-to-date data and information systems, and public health agencies capable of assessing and responding to public health needs (see Box 1-2). [11]

Public Health Frameworks: Challenges and Trends

Public health in the 21st century is facing new challenges and trends that are likely to demand different frameworks for its practice. Over the past 2 decades, numerous events both here in the U.S, and globally have brought this fact to the forefront including the attacks of September 11, 2001; numerous hurricanes; mass shootings; emerging CDs such as Ebola and the Zika virus; and massive migrations of populations due to war. These events have brought recognition to alarming public health concerns related to both manmade and natural disasters. These events result in disease, death, displacement of communities, and serious damage to essential public health infrastructures.

To better understand the impact of both natural and manmade disasters, it is helpful to revisit Hurricane Katrina, which savaged the Gulf Coast of the United States in the summer of 2005. A horrified TV audience watched news stories detailing the collapse of the emergency systems in New Orleans. This collapse left people to suffer and die, not only from the destruction of the hurricane, but also from a lack of water, food, sanitation, and medical attention. The aftermath of Katrina and the attacks of September 11, 2001, highlighted the need to strengthen the public health infrastructure, with an increasing emphasis on disaster preparedness and emergency response. Unfortunately, responses to natural disasters continue to challenge the United States as exemplified by Hurricane Maria and the devastation to Puerto Rico, and Hurricane Harvey in Houston, Texas, both in 2017. Full restoration of power and access to food and potable water remained a challenge in Puerto Rico long after the hurricane was over. Individual health requires essential services at the population level including adequate sanitation, potable water, and power. Understanding the interaction among cultural considerations, the economy of a country, and public health infrastructure is essential to promotion of health and adequate response to disasters and subsequent threats to health.

Any disaster can quickly escalate from direct injuries and deaths to indirect illness and risk of mortality because of the destruction of the public health infrastructure and the lack of public health resources especially for vulnerable populations. CD outbreaks challenge communities to respond in a way that provides care for those with the disease as well as protection for those who are in danger of getting the disease. Care for those with long term noncommunicable disease (NCD) requires access to care and to environments that support healthy living. Across the continuum from cellular to global, public health systems are a key component in the promotion of health and adequate care for those with disease. However, much of the emerging threats to population health are tied to increasing globalization.

Globalization is "the process of increasing economic, political, and social independence and integration as capital, goods, persons, concepts, images, ideas, and values cross state boundaries."[12] It is associated with increased travel, trade, economic growth, and diffusion of technology, resulting sometimes in greater disparities between rich and poor, environmental degradation, and food security issues. It has also resulted in greater distribution of products such as tobacco or alcohol. With globalization, there is also an emergence and re-emergence of CDs, including Zika, human immunodeficiency virus (HIV), acquired immunodeficiency syndrome (AIDS),

---

BOX 1–2 ■ *Healthy People 2020*: Public Health Infrastructure

Public health infrastructure is fundamental to the provision and execution of public health services at all levels. A strong infrastructure provides the capacity to prepare for and respond to both acute (emergency) and chronic (ongoing) threats to the nation's health. Infrastructure is the foundation for planning, delivering, and evaluating public health. Public health infrastructure includes three key components that enable a public health organization at the federal, tribal, state, or local level to deliver public health services. These components are:

A capable and qualified workforce
Up-to-date data and information systems
Public health agencies capable of assessing and responding to public health needs

These components are necessary to fulfill the previously discussed 10 Essential Public Health Services.

Source: (11)

severe acute respiratory syndrome (SARS), hepatitis, malaria, diphtheria, cholera, measles, and Ebola virus. Planning for CD outbreaks, including pandemics, may require new ethical frameworks to guide decision making regarding appropriate action with limited resources.[13]

Despite climate change, wars, terrorism, and other challenges, population health at the global level is improving. Infrastructure, educational opportunities, and a growing global economy are some of the factors that contribute to this improvement. According to global data made available through the "Our World in Data" Web site, run by Oxford University economist Max Weber, fewer people are experiencing poverty, life expectancy is up, and more people have access to electricity and drinking water.[14] Some interesting statistics using these data demonstrate the positive news related to global improvements in indicators of a healthy life. In the 1950s, more than 60% of the world's population was illiterate; today, only 14.7% are illiterate.[15] In 1980, 44% of the world's population lived in extreme poverty, which is living with less than $1.90 USD per day. The 2015 projections bring that down to just 9.6%.[16] Another common indicator of the health of a community is access to potable water. According to Richie and Roser, access to potable water also rose from 76% in 1990 to 91% in 2015.[17] A key measure of the health of populations is **life expectancy**, which is the average number of years a person born in a given country would live if mortality rates at each age were to remain constant in the future. The WHO reported a 5-year rise in the global average life expectancy to 71.4 years (73.8 years for females and 69.1 years for males) between 2000 and 2015. According to the WHO this was the fastest increase since the 1960s.[18]

Another challenge facing public health is the advancement of scientific and medical technologies that pose ethical questions.[13] The increasing use of genomics, for example, raises questions of how to protect against discrimination. Another challenge is aging and increasing diversity within populations. With aging, comes an increase in persons living with NCDs and CDs that require long-term care. Examples of disease that require long-term care include diabetes and HIV. In addition, some long-term diseases and health concerns relate to lifestyle choices such as smoking and poor nutrition. In 1926, Winslow discussed the need for new methods to address heart disease, respiratory diseases, and cancer.[19] We still need frameworks to help improve NCD and CD outcomes and, from a global perspective, to address how international collective action becomes essential to combating preventable risk factors associated with development of disease such as the tobacco epidemic.[20,21]

Emerging Public Health Frameworks

In 2003, the IOM (now HMD) produced *The Future of the Public's Health in the Twenty-First Century* as an update of the 1988 IOM report.[22] The new report presented the ecological model as the basis not only for understanding health in populations but also for assuring conditions in which populations can be healthy. The committee built on an ecological model created by Dahlgren and Whitehead,[23] and based its model on the assumption that health is influenced at several levels: individuals, families, communities, organizations, and social systems (Fig. 1-1). The model is also based on the assumptions that:

- There are multiple determinants of health.
- A population and environmental approach is critical.
- Linkages and relationships among the levels are important.
- Multiple strategies by multiple sectors are needed to achieve desired outcomes.[24]

Conventional public health models such as the epidemiological model of the agent, host, and environment (Chapter 3) are grounded in the ecological model. However, the ecological model reflects a deeper understanding of the role not only of the physical environment but also of the conditions in the social environment creating poor health, referred to as an "upstream" approach.[10,21,24]

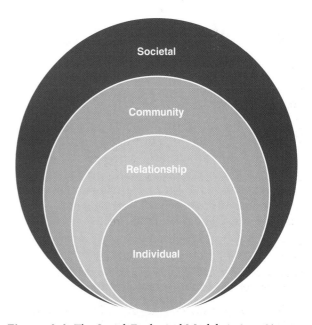

Figure 1-1 The Social-Ecological Model. *(Adapted by CTLT by Dahlgren and Whitehead, 1991; Worthman, 1999)*

Upstream refers to determinants of health that are somewhat removed from the more "downstream" biological and behavioral bases for disease. These upstream determinants include social relations, neighborhoods and communities, institutions, and social and economic policies (see Chapter 2).[24]

Community Partnerships

One of the recommendations of the 2003 IOM report was to increase multisectored engagement in partnerships with the community. In 2016, the National Academy of Sciences published a detailed report *Communities in Action: Pathways to Health Equity* that addresses the importance of community-level efforts aimed at improving health.[25] In the past, the community's role in health programs had often been that of a passive recipient, beneficiary, or research subject, with the active work carried out by public health experts. There is now a growing commitment to collaboration in promoting the health of communities and populations. Evidence shows that such efforts increase effectiveness and productivity, empower the participants, strengthen social engagement, and ensure accountability.[25, 26]

Population Health and Population-Focused Care

According to Caldwell,[27] a **population** is a mass of people that make up a definable unit to which measurements pertain. The WHO defined **health** as "the state of complete physical, mental, and social well-being, and not merely the absence of disease or infirmity."[28] However, **population health** is more than just a combination of these two terms, because it requires an understanding of all the factors listed in the ecological model that contribute to the health of a population.

Much of the curricular content in nursing programs pertains to acquiring the knowledge and skill the nurse needs to deliver nursing care to individuals. When nurses deliver care to an individual, the outcomes of interest are at the individual level. The goal is to implement nursing interventions that contribute to the individual's ability to achieve a maximum health state. However, achieving a complete state of health and well-being usually extends beyond the interventions that nurses and other health-care professionals provide on an individual level during a single episode of care. A state of health and well-being requires meeting an individual's mental, social, and economic needs as well as their immediate health needs. To take in this wider scope of influences on the person's health, the nurse must consider the individual as a part

of a greater whole, which includes the individual's interactions with other individuals and groups. This requires placing the individual within his or her socioecological context.

With individuals, nurses always start their care with an assessment. This requires knowledge of the biomedical, social, and psychological sciences. When providing **population-focused care**, nurses need a basic knowledge of the different scientific disciplines that make up public health science. When nurses assess a community and/or a population, they use their knowledge of epidemiology and biostatistics to help identify priority health issues at the population level. Some terms relevant to a discussion of public health—*aggregate, population,* and *community*—are sometimes used interchangeably, but there are differences among them (see Box 1-3 for

---

BOX 1-3 ■ Definitions for *Aggregate, Population,* and *Community*

For this book, these terms are defined within the context of public health building on standard dictionary definitions and definitions used in the literature.

Aggregate: In public health, this term represents individual units brought together into a whole or a sum of those individuals. In public health science, the term aggregate often refers to the unit of analysis, that is, at what level the health-care provider analyzes and reports data.

Population: Refers to a larger group whose members may or may not interact with one another but who share at least one characteristic such as age, gender, ethnicity, residence, or a shared health issue such as HIV/AIDS or breast cancer. The common denominator or shared characteristic may or may not be a shared geography or other link recognized by the individuals within that population. For example, people with type 2 diabetes admitted to a hospital form a population but do not share a specific culture or place of residence and may not recognize themselves as part of this population. In many situations, the terms *aggregate* and *population* are used interchangeably.

Community: Refers to a group of individuals living within the same geographical area, such as a town or a neighborhood, or a group of individuals who share some other common denominator, such as ethnicity or religious orientation. In contrast to aggregates and population, individuals within the community recognize their membership in the community based on social interaction and establishment of ties to other members in the community, and often join collective decision making.

detailed definitions).[29,30] All of these interventions, grounded in public health science, when framed beyond the individual ultimately improve the health of **aggregates**, **populations**, and **communities**.

Determinants of Health and Cultural Context

Determinants of health include a range of personal, social, economic, and environmental factors.[31] Before developing an intervention to improve health outcomes in a population, a nurse must first identify these determinants of health. MacDonald explained that earlier models related to population health were built on the assumption that patterns of disease and health occur through a complex interrelationship between risk and protective factors.[32] This resulted in a focus on biological and behavioral risk factors that require changes at the individual level. Multiple examples exist of health promotion activities that focus on changing individual behavior to reduce risk, such as smoking cessation, healthy eating, and increased exercise. Some success has occurred with this approach. However, there have also been successful efforts at the macrosocioecological level. These interventions focus on population behavioral change that then trickles down to the individual. Population behavioral change addresses risk factors that affect the whole population, such as provision of potable water to prevent cholera. The underlying assumption is that the population level of risk affects health outcomes independent of individual/family-level risk factors.

Take, for example, lung cancer. One of the well-documented determinants of this disease is the use of tobacco. Efforts to reduce this risk factor focus on changing individual behavior. Theories have emerged that help to explain behavior, such as the Transtheoretical Model of Change.[33] This model theory helps a health-care provider determine in what stage of change a person is and helps the provider put together a plan of care that fits the individual's readiness to quit smoking. Many of the inroads made in tobacco use cessation in this country began with a broader population health approach, including media campaigns related to smoking cessation and governmental nonsmoking policies that resulted in a cultural shift within our society. Once researchers made the case for the hazards of secondary smoke, tolerance of smoking within the community dramatically decreased. The population's exposure to tobacco smoke has decreased because the cultural view of tobacco use has changed. An increasingly negative perception of smoking has also increased the willingness of communities to implement policies that reduce the community's risk. A cultural shift reducing tolerance of smoking in public places and increasing the ostracism experienced by smokers has reduced the prevalence of smoking. Healthy behaviors remain a key issue in the health of populations. Taking a population approach allows for elevation of behavioral changes from the individual/family level to the population level.

Serious disparities in health exist at the global level, which can be seen by comparing life expectancies between high-income countries and low-income countries. For example, the estimated life expectancy in 2017 in Monaco was 89.4 years, whereas in Chad it was 50.6 years. The U.S. was ranked 43 with a life expectancy of 80.0 years.[34] To address these disparities, public health as a science has shifted from focusing on dramatic cases to focusing on existing disparities and addressing the underlying social determinants of health, such as poverty.[35]

Cultural Context, Diversity, and Health

Understanding the determinants of health begins with the cultural context and the diversity of populations across the globe. **Diversity** reflects the fact that groups and individuals are not all the same but differ in relation to culture, ethnicity, and race. **Culture** as defined in the Merriam Webster Dictionary as "… the customary beliefs, social forms, and material traits of a racial, religious, or social group; also: the characteristic features of everyday existence (such as diversions or a way of life) shared by people in a place or time."[36]

■ CULTURAL CONTEXT AND NURSING CARE

Knowledge and understanding of the cultural context of persons constitutes a key aspect in the development of effective nursing interventions. This context includes many aspects of life that affect the health of individuals, such as food preferences, gender roles, birthing practices, language, and spiritual beliefs to name a few. Spector equated culture to a set of luggage that a person carries that contains such things as beliefs, habits, norms, customs, and rituals that are handed down from one generation to the next through both verbal and nonverbal communication. Spector goes on to state, "All facets of human behavior can be interpreted through the lens of culture."[37] Thus, nurses must have an appreciation for cultures represented within the population they are caring for while acknowledging and understanding their own cultural views of the world, also known as cultural lenses.

Ethnicity, Race, and Culture

Having clear definitions of race and ethnicity helps in the understanding of what is meant by cultural context. Race and ethnicity are often used interchangeably but are actually different constructs. Multiple definitions exist for **ethnicity**. Commonalities across definitions include shared geographical origin, language or dialect, religious faith, folklore, food preferences, and culture. O'Neill[38] included physical characteristics as well and suggested that we use ethnicity in two distinct ways: to classify people who may have no specific cultural traditions in common into a loose group, and to classify groups that have a shared language and cultural traditions. For example, to classify an ethnic group under the name Native American results in grouping together people who are actually diverse in both culture and language. However, if the ethnic group is a specific Native American tribe, such as the Navajo, then the group does share specific cultural traditions, beliefs, and language that may not be shared with other Native American tribes such as the Inuit. Therefore, care is required when using the term ethnicity because of the variation in its use. Identifying the ethnicity of a group of people, which only considers broad shared characteristics, may miss key cultural differences within the group.

Geographical differences also play a part in diversity across groups and can result in shared cultural traditions that extend across ethnic groups within that geographical region. In the United States, cultural differences exist among specific regions, such as New England, the South, and the West Coast. These three regions differ in dialect, accepted protocol for social interactions, and food preferences.

Race categorizes groups of people based on superficial criteria such as skin color, physical characteristics, and parentage. In the United States, we continue to use racial categories; these are increasingly less accurate as ethnic groups become less defined. The U.S. Census Bureau acknowledges that the use of racial categories is limited, especially because some people may classify themselves as belonging to more than one category.[39,40] As the field of genetics grows, so does the evidence that there is no scientific basis for placing an individual into one racial group. In a classic article in *Newsweek*, "What Color Is Black?" Morganthau challenged the myth of race and concluded that it is not a legitimate method for classifying groups of people. Scientists found that people with very dissimilar racial characteristics such as skin color and facial features were in some cases more closely related genetically than groups with similar skin color.[41] However, race continues to be used to identify groups.

Traditionally, scientists report epidemiological data using racial categories as a means of identifying disparity between racial groups, especially in relation to health outcomes and access to care. The U.S. 2010 Census shows that the ability to group people using racial categories is increasingly difficult as these categories expand to include individuals who identify themselves as biracial and multiracial.

Understanding diversity in a population enhances the process of partnering with communities and improves the likelihood of the potential success of an intervention. By contrast, if a nurse plans an intervention without taking into account the cultural and ethnic diversity within the population, violation of ethnic and cultural values or beliefs can lead to failure to achieve the goals of the intervention. If the nurse only views an intervention through his or her cultural lens, and if that lens differs from those who will receive the intervention, then a key piece is missing. Does the population view the intervention as culturally relevant? Is the desired health outcome valued? For example, if a nurse develops an intervention aimed at increasing the number of women who breastfeed their infants, the first step is to evaluate the cultural view of breastfeeding. If the target population includes all the women giving birth at a large urban hospital, the population is probably diverse and may include cultures with different practices related to breastfeeding. If the nurse fails to acknowledge this fact and incorporate possible cultural differences into the assessment and planning stage (Chapters 4 and 5), the intervention may not succeed with women who have specific cultural beliefs surrounding breastfeeding.

Respecting culture and diversity when planning population level interventions requires the inclusion of the community members as partners in the process. Interventions planned *for* communities rather than *with* communities ignore the point made by Murphy that communities interpret their own health. In addition, Murphy stated that communities themselves can come up with ways to improve their health. From a population health perspective, collaboration and community participation are essential when developing interventions.[42] Engagement with the community can occur only within the context of culture and ethnic heritage and the community's own perception of what constitutes optimal health.

Cultural Competency and Cultural Humility

Cultural competency is a core aspect of care for healthcare providers. It is traditionally defined as the attitudes, knowledge, and skills the health-care provider uses to provide quality care to culturally diverse populations. It requires an understanding and capacity to provide care in a diverse environment. This implies an endpoint of acquired knowledge related to the culture of others. **Cultural humility**, conversely, acknowledges that the understanding of the multitude of diverse cultures in the world today may be too big a task. Cultural humility is an understanding that self-awareness about one's own culture is an ongoing process, and an acknowledgment that we must approach others as equals, with respect for their prevailing beliefs and cultural norms.[43] One is not exclusive of the other. Cultural competence is the standard to help guide the delivery of health care to individuals and to populations, whereas cultural humility is the underlying quality needed to truly implement interventions to improve health in partnership with communities and populations.

Developing cultural humility takes self-reflection. This provides an essential beginning point for nurses to develop the insight and knowledge needed to provide care to those who differ culturally from themselves. How do nurses create health-care environments that are safe and welcoming for clients and patients from all backgrounds? The first step in this process for individual nurses should be a cultural self-assessment. Cultural self-assessment involves a critical reflection of one's own viewpoints, experiences, attitudes, values, and beliefs. When one can honestly identify learned stereotypes and ethnocentric attitudes, enlightenment can occur. Nurses cannot begin to effectively consider the cultural context while providing care without first exploring their own cultures using basic questions (Box 1-4).

Creating a culturally welcoming health-care environment requires purposeful action by health-care providers. This necessitates commitment to principles and practices on all levels that support inclusion. These principles and practices should be a part of the systemic workings of health-care organizations. There should be visible and tangible signs of culturally welcoming health-care environments. However, more important are nurses who provide care that is inclusionary and culturally appropriate.

Environment and Resource Availability

The environment is another factor that affects health (see Chapter 6). Availability of clean air, abundant and potable water, and adequate food supplies all affect the health of an environment. For much of humankind's existence, the health of a population was concerned with the short-term survival of that population and centered on food sources, predators, and pestilence. This changed dramatically during the industrial revolution

---

> **BOX 1–4 ■ Personal Cultural Assessment**
>
> The following questions can be used to guide cultural self-reflection:
>
> - Where did I grow up? How did this environment influence my worldview (country, region, rural, urban)?
> - What values were emphasized in my family of origin?
> - Who were the people most influential to me in shaping my worldview?
> - Who were the people within my circle of friends and acquaintances during my years of growing up? How did they differ from me?
> - What privileges did I enjoy while growing up?
> - What are some of the key experiences that have shaped my view of the world and the people in it?
> - What are my religious beliefs, if any?
> - What are the values and morals that I adhere to?
> - What does "good health" mean to me? How do I obtain and maintain good health?
> - How do I view those individuals whose values differ from my own?

---

as populations moved from rural communities to urban areas. As large groups of people congregated in these urban areas, new issues arose related to sanitation, food supplies, and water. Communities with fewer resources and inadequate infrastructure to provide these essential components of a healthy life are at greater risk for disease. Poor sanitation and lack of potable water significantly increase the possibility of the spread of CDs. For example, in April of 2015, Uganda experienced a typhoid epidemic. As you can see in Figure 1-2, there are serious environmental risks to children and an increased risk for contaminated water sources.

Epidemiology, the study of the occurrence of disease in humans, identifies environment as a key factor contributing to morbidity and mortality (see Chapter 3). Epidemiology emerged in the 19th century in response to these new challenges brought by the industrial revolution. Though early epidemiologists did not understand that microscopic pathogens caused disease (the germ theory), they firmly established the role that environment plays in the health of humans. Efforts during the last half of the 19th century and into the 20th century focused on the introduction of sanitary measures, including management of sewage and providing clean water and adequate ventilation.[32]

John Snow was an epidemiologist who first studied aspects of the environment related to sanitation (see Chapter 3). He conducted a classic investigation of a cholera

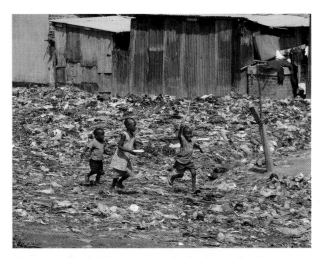

Figure 1-2 Children in Uganda during typhoid outbreak. *(Courtesy of the CDC/Jennifer Murphy)*

outbreak in the Soho area of London in 1854.[44] Snow mapped out cholera deaths block by block and found that they clustered around the Broad Street pump, leading him to conclude that the pump was the source of the contamination. He even examined the water under a microscope and identified "white, flocculent particles" that he thought were the causative agents. Though other authorities dismissed his evidence of a microscopic agent, he convinced others of the link between the disease and the water pump. He was successful in getting the water company to change the pump handle.[55] Snow's work brought attention to the importance of safe water. The measures taken did not require a change in individual behavior but rather a change in how the water company delivered water to the populace.

Initial public health efforts focused on the development of a public health infrastructure related to sanitation and delivery of safe water supplies. In the late 19th and early 20th centuries, large metropolitan municipalities initiated the development of underground sewerage systems and water pipes that are still in service today. The implementation of similar systems in smaller towns and rural areas occurred later, with outhouses still in use in the 1950s. In the United States, long before antibiotics were available, addressing these sanitation and safe water issues directly reduced the spread of CDs such as infantile diarrhea and cholera. In undeveloped countries without this public health infrastructure, these two diseases continue to contribute to the morbidity and mortality of their populations.

To survive, humans need adequate water and food supplies, shelter from the elements, and protection from pestilence and disease. In modern developed societies, geopolitical groups come together to supply adequate potable water and sewerage. Agricultural businesses provide food. In most developed societies, most individuals and families have the means to purchase adequate shelter and the health care needed to protect them from both CDs and NCDs. In some societies, government-based programs provide the means for obtaining health-care resources aimed at protection from pestilence and disease, and in other societies individuals purchase the health care either directly or indirectly through health insurance. Governments and individuals need adequate money to provide these resources; thus, obtaining adequate resources to promote the health of a population depends on that population's economic health. When the economy is healthy, the majority of the population generally has access to adequate water, food, and shelter. However, an economy in jeopardy may result in a reduced ability to meet these basic needs. In all societies, nurses must be aware of the environment in which the patient resides. Does the patient live in a community with a healthful environment? Is there adequate, safe, and usable water? Is food available, affordable, and nutritionally beneficial? Is the economy strong enough to provide access to health-care resources? Environment is one of the main determinants of health for individuals, populations, and the communities they live in.

Public Health as a Component of Nursing Practice Across Settings and Specialties

Nursing practice requires the application of knowledge from multiple sciences, including public health. Health is not just a result of individual factors such as biology, genetics, and behavior; it is also a product of an individual's social, cultural, and ecological environment. To meet our obligation to maximize health on all levels, we must incorporate public health science into our nursing care.

Public Health Science and Nursing Practice

In 2010, the IOM (now HMD) published a report on the future of nursing.[45] The stated goal was to have 80% of all registered nurses prepared at the baccalaureate of science in nursing (BSN) level or higher. The rationale for this goal was that BSN programs emphasize liberal arts, advanced sciences, and nursing coursework across a wide range of settings, along with leadership development and exposure to community and public health competencies. In addition, the authors emphasized that entry-level nurses need to be able to transition smoothly from their academic preparation to a range of practice environments, with an increased emphasis on community and public health settings.[45]

Population-Focused Care Across Settings and Nursing Specialties

Nurses provide population-focused care every day, in every setting. For a staff nurse working in an urban hospital, the population of interest is the patients who come to that hospital for care. The population may include various subpopulations based on shared geographical residence, age group, primary diagnosis, culture, and ethnic group. Staff nurses in an acute or community-based setting take care of patients on an individual level, often serving as the member of the health-care team that delivers the interventions and evaluates the effectiveness of those interventions. Nurses actively participate in reviewing how well the team is delivering care to the patient population as a whole. Over time, the health-care team begins to group patients based on diagnosis or other identifying characteristics to provide better care. This may occur when nurses are engaged in performance improvement activities, the development of a care map, or in response to changes in the population.

Across settings and specialties, nurses work to successfully answer the "who, what, when, where, why, and how" of health problems within the context of populations. Providing individual care alone after disease has occurred is an essential part of what nurses do. In a sense, all nurses are Public Health Nurses (PHN) because our mandate is not only to provide state-of-the-art care to individuals but also to safeguard the public's health and actively participate in optimizing health for all populations.

Public Health Nursing as a Specialty

Public health nursing is the practice of promoting and protecting the health of populations using knowledge from nursing, social, and public health sciences. Public health nursing is a specialty practice within nursing and public health. It focuses on improving population health by emphasizing prevention and attending to multiple determinants of health. Often used interchangeably with community health nursing, this nursing practice includes advocacy, policy development, and planning, which addresses issues of social justice. With a multi-level view of health, public health nursing action occurs through community applications of theory, evidence, and a commitment to health equity. In addition to what is put forward in this definition, public health nursing practice is guided by the ANA Public Health Nursing: Scope and Standards of Practice and the Quad Council of Public Health Nursing Organizations' Core Competencies for Public Health Nurses.[46]

Public health nursing is different from other nursing specialties because of its focus on eight principles outlined in an unpublished white paper by the Quad Council in 1997[47] and cited in the *Public Health Nursing: Scope and Standards of Practice.*[48] (See Box 1-5.) These principles define the client of public health nursing as the population and further delineate processes and strategies used by PHNs.

Public Health Nursing as a Core Component of Nursing History

The roots of public health nursing lie in the work of women who provided comfort, care, and healing to individuals during the Middle Ages. During that time, nuns, deaconesses, and women of religious orders provided comfort and care to the sick in their homes.[49] The immediate precursor to public health nursing was district nursing, which began in England. William Rathbone employed a nurse to care for his wife during her terminal illness and after this experience realized that home visiting to the sick poor could benefit society. This resulted in the

---

BOX 1–5 ■ The Eight Principles of Public Health Nursing

1. The client or unit of care is the population.
2. The primary obligation is to achieve the greatest good for the greatest number of people or population as a whole.
3. The processes used by PHNs include working with the client as an equal partner.
4. PRIMARY prevention is the priority in selecting appropriate activities.
5. Public health nursing focuses on strategies that create healthy environmental, social, and economic conditions in which populations may thrive.
6. A PHN is obligated to actively identify and reach out to all who might benefit from a specific activity or service.
7. Use of available resources must be optimal to assure the best overall improvement in the health of the population.
8. Collaboration with a variety of other professions, populations, organizations, and other stakeholder groups is the most effective way to promote and protect the health of the people.

Source: (1)

development of district nursing, under which towns were divided into districts, and health visitors provided nursing care and education to the sick poor within those districts. In 1861, Rathbone wrote Florence Nightingale to request the development of a training school for both infirmary and district nursing, which eventually resulted in trained nurses in 18 districts of Liverpool.[53] Public health nursing owes much of its early development to Florence Nightingale. She was concerned about the care of the sick poor and the quality of their homes and workhouses. She is also widely known for her work during the Crimean War, during which she kept impeccable statistical records on the living conditions of the soldiers and on the presence of disease. She is also known for her promotion of health reform.[50,51]

Beginnings of Public Health Nursing in the United States

Public health nursing in the United States evolved from district nursing in England. In 1877, the New York City Mission hired Francis Root to make home visits to the sick. Other sites followed suit, and visiting nurse associations were set up in Buffalo (1885), Boston (1886), and Philadelphia (1886). Trained nurses cared for the sick poor and provided instruction on improving the cleanliness of their homes. Originally these associations bore the name District Nursing Services, with the Boston association referred to as the Boston Instructive District Nursing Association. Eventually they all changed their names to Visiting Nurse Associations.[52]

In 1893, Lillian Wald and Mary Brewster established a district nursing service called the Henry Street Settlement on the Lower East Side of New York and coined the term *public health nurse*.[53] In her work, Wald emphasized the role that social and economic problems played in illness and developed unique programs to address the health needs of the immigrant population. During the early part of the 20th century, poverty was increasingly seen as a cause of social problems and poor health in communities. Wald believed that environmental and social conditions were the causes of ill health and poverty.[54,55] For Lillian Wald and her colleagues, efforts of social reform were focused on civil rights for minorities, voting rights for women, the prevention of war, child labor laws, and improving unsafe working conditions.[55]

Public Health Nursing in the 20th Century

Wald's accomplishments were the background for the development of the public health nursing specialty. Public health efforts in the early part of the 20th century made great strides in reducing disease, especially due to advances related to the provision of potable water, regulations around food and milk supply, removal of garbage, and disposal of sewage. However, authorities realized that they needed to implement other programs to work on improving health education among those most at risk, especially the poor. PHNs filled this need and provided care to the sick while educating families on personal hygiene and healthy practices.[55] The visiting nurse movement, with a focus on caring for the sick poor, joined forces with public health to focus on prevention. According to Buhler-Wilkerson, "By 1910, the majority of the large urban visiting nurse associations had initiated preventive programs for school children, infants, mothers, and patients with tuberculosis."[56]

Public health nursing continued to grow with the expansion of the federal government. The Social Security Act of 1935 provided funding for expanded opportunities in health protection and promotion, resulting in the employment of PHNs, increased education for nurses in public health, the establishment of health services, and research. World War II increased the need for nurses both for the war effort and at home. PHNs also played a role in surveillance and treatment of CDs such as tuberculosis and Hanson's disease, also known as leprosy. As seen in the photo in Figure 1-3, taken in 1950, PHNs worked with other nurses caring for the patients receiving care for CDs.

The 1960s and 1970s saw the implementation of neighborhood health centers, maternal-child health programs, and Head Start programs. By the 1980s, however, there was another shift in funding to more acute services, medical procedures, and long-term care. The use of health maintenance organizations (HMOs) was encouraged. By

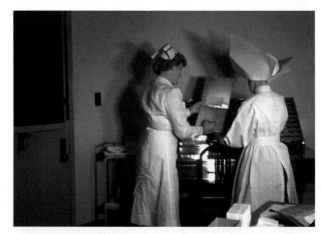

Figure 1-3 Public Health Nurses in the 1950s. *(Courtesy of the CDC/Elizabeth Schexnyder, National Hansen's Disease Museum, Curator)*

the latter part of the 1980s, public health as a focus had declined and the percentage of PHNs working as government employees had dropped.

Public Health Nursing in the 21st Century

In this century, the move toward population health and the need for more services to communities outside of traditional hospital settings has the potential to increase the demand for PHNs. Currently, PHNs work in a wide variety of settings. Some are based in schools, community clinics, local health departments, and visiting nurse associations. PHNs also work at the national level in the United States Public Health Service, a branch of the armed services in the U.S. (Fig. 1-4).

Based on a report completed by the Health Resources and Services Administration on the registered nurse population in the United States, in 2017, 61% of nurses work in hospital settings, 18% work in primary care, 5% work in government, 7% in extended care facilities, and 3% in education.[57] If the predictions of Ezekiel J. Emanuel, vice provost of the University of Pennsylvania Hospital, are correct, hospitals will continue to downsize as health care moves out into the community and individual homes.[58] This may require an increase in the number of practicing PHNs. This will also increase the need for all nurses to have sufficient knowledge and skills to provide care across the continuum from individuals to populations within the context of community.

Public Health Nursing Scope and Standards of Practice

The *Public Health Nursing: Scope and Standards of Practice* outlines the expectations of the professional role of the PHN and sets the framework for public health nursing practice in the 21st century.[1] As with the other nursing specialties' scope and standards, these are based on the nursing scope and standards established by the ANA.[1,2]

Public Health Nursing Standards

Included in the 11 Standards of Professional Performance for Public Health Nursing (see Box 1-6)[1] are six standards of practice that describe a competent level of care using the nursing process: (1) Assessment, (2) Population Diagnosis and Priorities, (3) Outcomes Identification, (4) Planning, (5) Implementation, and (6) Evaluation. Specific standards related to implementation include the coordination of care, health teaching, and health promotion, consultation, and regulatory activities. These standards of practice are differentiated for the PHN and the advanced PHN.

Public Health Nursing Competencies

The *Scope and Standards of Practice* delineates competencies for practice based on the ANA nursing framework assuring that public health nursing fits as a recognized nursing specialty. In addition, the Council of Linkages Between Academia and Public Health Practice, a coalition of organizations concerned with the public health workforce, produced a document in 2001 that has been used as a framework for the development of additional public health nursing competencies. The 2018 revised version of the PHN Core Competencies includes eight domains (Box 1-7) and incorporates three tiers of practice: Basic or generalist (Tier 1); Specialist or mid-level (Tier 2); and Executive and/or multisystem level (Tier 3).[59] These tiers reflect the different levels of responsibility for those working in public health.[60]

Public Health Nursing Roles and Responsibilities

There are roles and responsibilities specific to public health nursing practice built on nursing practice for all

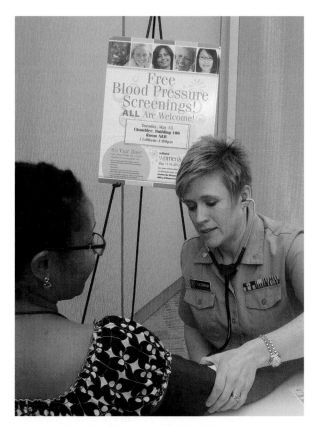

Figure 1-4 United States Public Health Service Nurse at a blood pressure clinic. *(Courtesy of the CDC/Nasheka Powell)*

BOX 1–6 ■ Standards of Public Health Nursing Practice

Standard 1. ASSESSMENT

The PHN collects comprehensive data pertinent to the health status of populations.

Standard 2. DIAGNOSIS

The PHN analyzes the assessment data to determine the diagnoses or issues.

Standard 3. OUTCOMES IDENTIFICATION

The PHN identifies expected outcomes for a plan specific to the population or situation.

Standard 4. PLANNING

The PHN develops a plan that prescribes strategies and alternatives to attain expected outcomes.

Standard 5. IMPLEMENTATION

The PHN implements the identified plan.

Standard 5A. COORDINATION OF CARE

The PHN coordinates care delivery.

Standard 5B. HEALTH TEACHING AND HEALTH PROMOTION

The PHN employs multiple strategies to promote health and a safe environment.

Standard 5C. CONSULTATION

The PHN provides consultation to influence the identified plan, enhance the abilities of others, and effect change.

Standard 5D. PRESCRIPTIVE AUTHORITY

The advanced practice registered nurse *practicing in the public health setting* uses prescriptive authority, procedures, referrals, treatments, and therapies in accordance with state and federal laws and regulations.

Standard 5E. REGULATORY ACTIVITIES

The PHN participates in applications of public health laws, regulations, and policies.

Standard 6. EVALUATION

The PHN evaluates progress toward attainment of outcomes.

Standard 7. ETHICS

The PHN practices ethically.

Standard 8. EDUCATION

The PHN attains knowledge and competence that reflect current nursing practice.

Standard 9. EVIDENCE-BASED PRACTICE AND RESEARCH

The PHN integrates evidence and research findings into practice.

Standard 10. QUALITY OF PRACTICE

The PHN contributes to quality nursing practice.

Standard 11. COMMUNICATION

The PHN communicates effectively in a variety of formats in all areas of practice.

Standard 12. LEADERSHIP

The PHN demonstrates leadership in the professional practice setting and the profession.

Standard 13. COLLABORATION

The PHN collaborates with the population, and others in the conduct of nursing practice.

Standard 14. PROFESSIONAL PRACTICE EVALUATION

The PHN evaluates her or his own nursing practice in relation to professional practice standards and guidelines, relevant statutes, rules, and regulations.

Standard 15. RESOURCE UTILIZATION

The PHN utilizes appropriate resources to plan and provide nursing and public health services that are safe, effective, and financially responsible.

Standard 16. ENVIRONMENTAL HEALTH

The PHN practices in an environmentally safe, fair, and just manner.

Standard 17. ADVOCACY

The PHN advocates for the protection of the health, safety, and rights of the population.

Source: (1)

BOX 1–7 ■ PHN Core Competencies includes Eight Domains

1. Assessment and analytical skills
2. Policy development/program planning skills
3. Communication skills
4. Cultural competency skills
5. Community dimensions of practice skills
6. Public health science skills
7. Financial planning, evaluation and management skills
8. Leadership and systems thinking skills

Source: (60)

---

specialties. They are in alignment with the Scope and Standards of Nursing Practice in general and build in the care of communities and populations.

Coordination, Consultation, and Leadership: A PHN is responsible for coordinating programs, services, and other activities to implement an identified plan.[46] A PHN acts as a consultant when he or she works with community organizations or groups to develop a local health fair or provide the latest information about a CD outbreak to the community. At a more complex level, Advanced Public Health Nurses (APHN) act as consultants when providing expert testimony to the federal or state governments about a health promotion program. As leaders, PHNs can serve in coalition-building efforts around a health issue such as teen smoking prevention or opioid overdose prevention.

Advocacy: Advocacy refers to the responsibility of PHNs to speak for populations and communities that lack the resources to be heard.[1] Assisting families living in poverty to access appropriate services is one example of an important role of PHNs. Another example of advocacy is engaging in strategies to affect policy at the local, state, or national level.

Health Education and Health Promotion: The PHN selects teaching and learning methods to help communities address health issues, presenting the information in a culturally competent manner, implementing the health education program in partnership with the community, and evaluating the effectiveness of the program by collecting feedback from participants.

Regulatory Activities: Since the beginning of public health nursing, health policy has been an important aspect of practice. Responsibilities include identifying, interpreting, and implementing public health laws, regulations, and policies.[1] Activities include monitoring and inspecting regulated entities such as nursing homes. It also includes educating the public on relevant laws, regulations, and policies.

Ongoing Education and Practice Evaluation: PHNs are responsible for maintaining and enhancing their knowledge and skills necessary to promote population health. This requires PHNs to take the initiative to seek experiences that develop and maintain their competence as PHNs. Thus, as with nurses in other settings, PHNs must engage in self-evaluation, seek feedback about performance, and implement plans for accomplishing their own goals and work plans.

Professional Relationships and Collaboration: Effective partnerships with communities and stakeholders provide the mechanism for moving the public health agenda forward.[1] For example, nurses working in health departments often join with other human service providers to develop effective programs aimed at addressing a health issue of mutual concern such as the opioid epidemic. PHNs seek collegial partnerships with peers, students, and colleagues as a means of enhancing public health interventions.

Public Health Nursing Ethics

The principles guiding any ethical discourse in nursing include autonomy, dignity, and rights of individuals. The same is true for public health nursing. Assuring confidentiality and applying ethical standards are critical in advocating for health and social policy.[60,61] Equally important to any discussion of public health ethics is the fact that public health is concerned with the public good, which can override individual rights.[62] This is evident in the enforcement of laws that are aimed at the whole population (e.g., immunizations, disease reporting, or quarantines). Underlying public health ethics is the concept of social justice defined as: "… acting in accordance with fair treatment regardless of economic status, race, ethnicity, citizenship, disability, or sexual orientation."[1] This includes the eradication of poverty and illiteracy, the establishment of sound environmental policy, and equality of opportunity for healthy personal and social development.[1]

Global Health

Global health is "the collaborative transnational research and action for promoting health for all."[63] This definition aligns with the WHO classic definition of health: "a state of complete physical, mental, and social well-being and not merely the absence of disease or infirmity."[64] The constitution of the WHO further recognizes "the enjoyment of the highest attainable standard of health … as one of the fundamental rights of every human being."[65] The WHO recognizes that nurses play a large role in the promotion of global health. In February of 2018, the WHO launched a new global campaign, called Nursing Now, to "… empower and support nurses in meeting 21st century health challenges."[66]

One of the variables associated with differences among countries is their economic well-being. The terms most often used to differentiate countries based on country-level income data are **high-income countries (HICs)**, **upper middle-income countries (UMICs)**, **lower middle income countries (LMICs)**, and **low-income countries (LICs)**. These terms replace the earlier terms of *developed* and *developing* countries. The World Bank classifies countries based on current economic ranges of the annual per capita gross national income (GNI). In 2016, a LIC was a country with a per capita GNI equal to or less than U.S. $1,005; LMIC's per capita GNI ranged from U.S. $1,006 to $3,955; UMIC's per capita GNI ranged from $3,956 to $12,235; and an HIC's per capita GNI was equal to or greater than U.S. $12,236.[67] From a global health perspective, a major concern is the growing disparity between the two lower groups (LIC and LMIC) and the two higher groups (HIC and UMIC). Previously, international health-care workers in LICs and LMICs looked for solutions to health care within the country or collaborated with one other country. The key conceptual change in global health over the past 2 decades is the recognition of the interdependence of countries; the interdependence of the health of people in all countries; and the interdependence of the policies, economics, and values that arise related to health.[68] The 2018 WHO launch of "Nursing Now" with the stated purpose "… to empower and support nurses in meeting 21st century health challenges" showcases this conceptual change.[66]

An example of global efforts to assist countries with fewer resources to improve health is the effort to improve access to vaccines for common childhood illnesses. For example, in 2008 the Cairo M/R Catch-Up Campaign was initiated (Fig. 1-5), a national supplemental immunization activity in Egypt. Another example, in 2018, is the plan by the Bill and Melinda Gates Foundation to pay off the $76 million debt that Nigeria owes Japan for their program to eradicate polio. These efforts demonstrate the importance of health of children as a primary focus of health at the global level. Worldwide in 2016, the number of children under the age of 5 who died was 5.6 million, down from 6.6 million children in 2012 and a sharp decrease from 1990 when

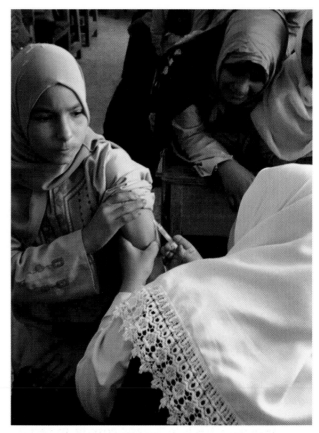

Figure I-5 Vaccinating children for measles and rubella in Egypt. *(Courtesy of the CDC/Carlos Alonso)*

the total number of deaths was 12.4 million.[69] Despite these gains, efforts continue to help lower the number as most of the deaths are preventable.

Public Health Organizations and Management: Global to Local

Public health organizations constitute an essential part of improving health from the cellular to the global level. These organizations provide essential public health services such as conducting surveillance, responding to CD outbreaks and disasters, and evaluating the evidence to make recommendations for action. In addition, these organizations set goals related to the improvement of health such as the UN's Sustainable Development Goals (SDGs).[70]

World Health Organization

The WHO, established in 1948, is the world health authority under the auspices of the UN. Their "… primary role is to direct and coordinate international health within the United Nations' system."[64] Their stated areas of work include health systems, promoting health through the life-course, NCD, CD, and corporate services.[76] Based in Geneva, the WHO employs 7,000 people working in 150 country offices, 6 regional offices, and at the central headquarters.[64]

In 1978, the WHO held a conference in Alma-Ata (now Almaty), Kazakhstan, that supported the resolution that primary health care was the means for attaining health for all. At the beginning of the first decade in the 21st century, a new model emerged of integrated services that respond to multiple threats to health. The WHO has expanded to include emergency response and disaster preparedness initiatives (see Chapter 22). Another key initiative was the institution of International Health Regulations (IHRs) that countries must follow in response to disease outbreaks and to increase the ability of the WHO to respond to public health emergencies brought on by natural or manmade disasters.[64] The WHO continues to set global population heath goals and tracks the attainment of these goals. The current SDGs built on the Millennial Development Goals (MDGs) that ended in 2015. There are 17 goals with a target date of 2030 and, unlike the MDGs, the goals apply to all countries, and there is no distinction between LIC and other countries (Box 1-8). The stated purpose of the SDGs is to "… end poverty, protect the planet, and ensure prosperity for all."[70]

National Health Organizations

Individual countries have their own national organizations dedicated to the promotion of health and the protection of their populations. They coordinate with the WHO and, as evidenced by the new interdependency framework mentioned earlier, often work together to address threats to heath. Some countries, including the U.S., have public health departments, also known as boards of public health. Even though these governmental bodies do not encompass the entirety of the field of public health, they are key to providing infrastructure as well as oversight of the health of populations.

The U.S. Constitution provides for a two-layer public health system composed of the federal level and the state level. However, the Constitution did not make any specific provisions for the management of public health issues at the federal level, therefore, public health management now comes under state authority.[30] After ratification of the 14th Amendment, states were required to provide protections to their own citizens, which helped to legalize activities of local health departments to take such actions as imposing quarantines.

BOX I–8 ■ United Nations' Sustainable Development Goals

According to the United Nations, "The SDGs build on the success of the Millennium Development Goals (MDGs) and aim to go further to end all forms of poverty. The new Goals are unique in that they call for action by all countries, poor, rich and middle-income to promote prosperity while protecting the planet. They recognize that ending poverty must go hand-in-hand with strategies that build economic growth and addresses a range of social needs including education, health, social protection, and job opportunities, while tackling climate change and environmental protection."[70]

The 17 sustainable goals include:

1. No poverty
2. Zero hunger
3. Good health and well-being
4. Quality education
5. Gender equality
6. Clean water and sanitation
7. Affordable and clean energy
8. Decent work and economic growth
9. Industry, innovation, and infrastructure
10. Reduced inequalities
11. Sustainable cities and communities
12. Responsible production and consumption
13. Climate action
14. Life below water
15. Life on land
16. Peace, justice, and strong institutions
17. Partnerships for the goals

Source: (70)

Centers for Disease Control and Prevention

The CDC, founded in 1946, grew out of the wartime effort related to malaria control. In the beginning, the CDC employed approximately 400 people, including engineers and entomologists (scientists who study insects). Only seven employees functioned as medical officers.[71] The work of the CDC contributed to the 10 great public health achievements over the past century (Box 1-9).[72] These included immunizations, fluoridation of water, and workplace safety. The implementation of childhood vaccination programs resulted in the eradication of smallpox and the banishment of mumps and chickenpox from schools in the United States.[79] Without an active public health infrastructure, the marked increases in life expectancy in the 20th century would not have occurred.

Activities of the CDC: From this humble beginning, the CDC has grown into one of the major operating components of the Department of Health and Human

---

BOX 1–9 ■ Top 10 Public Health Achievements

1. Immunizations
2. Motor vehicle safety
3. Workplace safety
4. Control of communicable diseases
5. Declines in deaths from health disease and stroke
6. Safer and healthier foods
7. Healthier mothers and babies
8. Family planning
9. Fluoridation of drinking water
10. Tobacco as a health hazard

Source: (79)

Services (DHHS). The scope of the agency's efforts includes the prevention and control of CDs and NCDs, injuries, workplace hazards, disabilities, and environmental health threats. In addition to health promotion and protection, the agency also conducts research and maintains a national surveillance system. It also responds to health emergencies and provides support for outbreak investigations.[73] According to the CDC, it is distinguished from its peer agencies for two reasons: the application of research findings to people's daily lives and its response to health emergencies.[74]

The CDC collaborates with state and local health departments in relation to disease and injury surveillance and outbreak investigations, including bioterrorism. It sets standards for the implementation of disease prevention strategies and is the repository for health statistics. Health statistics are available to health providers, health departments, and the public.[74] Web sites of interest to nurses needing population level information include CDC WONDER, FASTSTATS, and VITALSTATS (see Box 1-10 for details).

Healthy People: Every decade Healthy People releases a set of goals and health topics with specific objectives aimed at improving health across the life span. As the target date of 2020 approached, the CDC and the USDHHS worked on the development of the next iteration of Healthy People, HP 2030 (see Box 1-11).[73]

■ HEALTHY PEOPLE 2030
Proposed Framework

For 2030, there are five overreaching goals and a plan of action for reaching those goals.

Vision: "Where we are headed"

A society in which all people achieve their full potential for health and well-being across the life span.

Mission: "Why we are here"

To promote and evaluate the Nation's efforts to improve the health and well-being of its people.

Overarching Goals: "What we plan to achieve"

- Attain healthy, purposeful lives and well-being.
- Attain health literacy, achieve health equity, eliminate disparities, and improve the health and well-being of all populations.
- Create social and physical environments that promote attaining full potential for health and well-being for all.
- Promote healthy development, healthy behaviors, and well-being across all life stages.
- Engage with stakeholders and key constituents across multiple sectors to act and design policies that improve the health and well-being of all populations.[65]

Public health systems are commonly defined as "all public, private, and voluntary entities that contribute to the delivery of essential public health services within a jurisdiction." This means that all entities' contributions to the health and well-being of the community or state are recognized in assessing the provision of public health services.[72] As noted earlier, the CDC laid out 10 essential public health services (see Box 1-1) that help guide all public health organizations in the United States.[9] These

---

BOX 1–10 ■ Centers for Disease Control and Prevention Web Resources

CDC WONDER provides online data sources (AIDS public use data, births, cancer statistics); environment (daily air temperature, land service temperatures, fine particulate matter, sunlight, and precipitation); mortality (detailed mortality, infant deaths, online tuberculosis information systems); population (bridged population, census); sexually transmitted morbidity; and vaccine adverse event reporting.
Source: http://wonder.cdc.gov/.
FASTSTATS provides statistics on topics of public health importance.
Source: http://www.cdc.gov/nchs/fastats/.
VITAL STATISTICS ONLINE DATA PORTAL is a Web site that provides users with the ability to access vital statistics, specifically birth and mortality data.
Source: https://www.cdc.gov/nchs/data_access/vitalstatsonline.htm.

BOX 1–11 ■ Healthy People 2030 Goals and Action Plan

Overarching Goals

- Attain healthy, thriving lives and well-being, free of preventable disease, disability, injury, and premature death.
- Eliminate health disparities, achieve health equity, and attain health literacy to improve the health and well-being of all.
- Create social, physical, and economic environments that promote attaining full potential for health and well-being for all.
- Promote healthy development, healthy behaviors, and well-being across all life stages.
- Engage leadership, key constituents, and the public across multiple sectors to take action and design policies that improve the health and well-being of all.

Plan of Action

- Set national goals and measurable objectives to guide evidence-based policies, programs, and other actions to improve health and well-being.
- Provide data that is accurate, timely, accessible, and can drive targeted actions to address regions and

populations with poor health or at high risk for poor health in the future.
- Foster impact through public and private efforts to improve health and well-being for people of all ages and the communities in which they live.
- Provide tools for the public, programs, policy makers, and others to evaluate progress toward improving health and well-being.
- Share and support the implementation of evidence-based programs and policies that are replicable, scalable, and sustainable.
- Report biennially on progress throughout the decade from 2020 to 2030.
- Stimulate research and innovation toward meeting Healthy People 2030 goals and highlight critical research, data, and evaluation needs.
- Facilitate development and availability of affordable means of health promotion, disease prevention, and treatment.

functions and services directly relate to the ability of a public health department to address CDs, eliminate environmental hazards, prevent injuries, promote healthy behaviors, respond to disasters, and assure quality and accessibility of health services.[72] The CDC collaborates with state and local health departments, as well as public health entities across the world, especially the WHO. Globally it has personnel stationed in 25 foreign countries.

State Public Health Departments

States independently decide how they will structure their local and state health departments (see Chapter 13). Variations exist across states in relation to the organization and management of formal public health systems. The variation stems, in part, from how the state government has directed the establishment of public health boards or departments and from the variation in state jurisdictional structure. For example, some states such as Pennsylvania use a town/city (municipality), township, or county system, and other states such as Massachusetts divide their entire state into municipalities. Finally, some states such as Alaska have territories as well as municipalities because they have smaller populations spread across a larger land

mass. States with sovereign Native American nations within their borders add an additional layer to the structuring of their state level public health department.

Local Public Health Departments

The basic mandate of the local public health department is to protect the health of the citizens residing in their county, municipality, township, or territory. However, how public health departments implement this protection varies across states (see Chapter 13). This results in variability in the services offered and the public health activities of the local health departments. As a result of federal mandates, public health departments uniformly perform certain activities. These include surveillance, outbreak investigation, and quarantine as well as mandated reporting of specific diseases and cause of death to state health departments and the CDC. This allows the federal government to track the incidence and prevalence of disease from a national perspective. Local health departments are essential to the health of communities and provide the day-to-day services required to assure safe environments and the provision of essential public health services (see Chapter 13) with state departments and federal health organizations.

▨ Summary Points

- Public health is a core component of nursing knowledge and competency across settings and specialties.
- The goal of nursing is to help people achieve optimal health, which ultimately requires understanding the health of populations and communities due to the intricate interplay between individuals, families, and the communities in which they live.
- Public health science encompasses efforts to improve the health of populations from the cellular to the global level.
- Public health provides us with the means to build a healthy environment and respond to threats to our health from nature and from humans.
- Public Health Nursing is a recognized specialty at the generalist and advanced level with specific scope and standards of practice.
- Formal structures from the global to local level exist to promote health, reduce risk, and protect populations from threats to health.

▼ THE CASE OF THE PARASITE ON THE PLAYGROUND

In 2018, the New York Times published an article related to roundworms, genus Toxocara, found in the intestines of cats and dogs that are shed in the feces.[1] The CDC estimated that about 5% of the U.S. population has been exposed based on positive blood tests for Toxocara antibodies. The rate is higher in those who live below the poverty line (10%) and for African Americans (7%).[1,2] The difference in prevalence appears to be based on economic status due to the higher number of strays in poorer neighborhoods versus pets with regular veterinary care. Based on a recent survey of pediatricians conducted by the CDC, a little less than half of the doctors correctly diagnosed it.[3] Cognitive development is one of the long-term consequences associated with exposure to the worm.[4]

Suggested prompts for discussion:

1. Review the CDC Web site on Toxocara. What interventions are needed at the individual level versus the community level?
2. What knowledge does a nurse need to set up interventions to prevent this disease?
3. What is the role of individual health care providers, health care organizations, and public health departments. Who else might play a role?
4. How does this issue depict the role of the social determinants of health in the spread of disease?

References

1. Beil, L. (2018, January 16). The parasite on the playground. *New York Times*. Retrieved from https://nyti.ms/2ELVbmS.
2. Centers for Disease Control and Prevention. (2013). *Toxocariasis: epidemiology & risk factors.* Retrieved from https://www.cdc.gov/parasites/toxocariasis/epi.html.
3. Woodhal, D.M., Garcia, A.P., Shapiro, C.A., Wray, S., Montgomery, S.P., et al. (2017). Assessment of U.S. pediatrician knowledge of toxocariasis. *The American Journal of Tropical Medicine and Hygiene, 97*(4), 1243-1247. DOI: https://doi.org/10.4269/ajtmh.17-0232.
4. Walsh, M.G., & Haseeb, M.A. (2012). Reduced cognitive function in children with toxocariasis in a nationally representative sample of the United States. *International Journal for Parasitology, 42*(13-14), 1159-1163. https://doi.org/10.1016/j.ijpara.2012.10.002.

REFERENCES

1. American Association of Colleges of Nursing. (2008). *The essentials of baccalaureate education for professional nursing practice*. Washington DC: AACN.
2. American Nurses Association. (2015). *Nursing: scope and standards of practice* (3rd ed.). Silver Spring, MD: ANA.
3. Winslow, C.E.A. (1920). The untilled field of public health. *Modern Medicine, 2,* 183-191.
4. Turnock, B.J. (2016). *Public health: What it is and how it works* (6th ed.). Sudbury, MA: Jones & Bartlett.
5. Fawcett, J., & Ellenbecker, C. H. (2015). A proposed conceptual model of nursing and population health. *Nursing Outlook, 63*(3), 288-298. http://dx.doi.org/10.1016/j.outlook.2015.01.009.
6. World Health Organization. (2018). *About WHO*. Retrieved from http://www.who.int/about/en/.
7. Issel, L.M. (2018). *Health program and evaluation: A practical, systematic approach for community health* (4th ed.). Sudbury, MA: Jones & Bartlett.
8. Institute of Medicine. (1988). *The future of public health*. Washington, DC: National Academies Press.
9. Centers for Disease Control and Prevention, National Public Health Performance Standards Program (NPHPSP). (2017). *The public health system and ten essential public health services*. Retrieved from https://www.cdc.gov/stltpublichealth/publichealthservices/essentialhealthservices.html.
10. Institute of Medicine. (2012). *For the public's health: investing in a healthier future*. Washington, DC: The National Academies Press.
11. U.S. Department of Health and Human Services, Healthy People 2020. (2018). *Public health infrastructure*. Retrieved from http://www.healthypeople.gov/2020/topicsobjectives2020/overview.aspx?topicId=35.

12. Yach, D., & Bettcher, D. (1998). The globalization of public health, I. Threats and opportunities. *American Journal of Public Health, 88*(5), 735-738.

13. Smith, M.J., & Silva, D.S. (2015). Ethics for pandemics beyond influenza: Ebola, drug-resistant tuberculosis, and anticipating future ethical challenges in pandemic preparedness and response. *Monash Bioethics Review, 33*(2-3), 130-47. doi: 10.1007/s40592-015-0038-7.

14. Weber, M. (2018). *Our world in data.* Published online at OurWorldInData.org. Retrieved from https://ourworldindata.org/.

15. Roser, M., & Ortiz-Ospina, E. (2017). *Global rise of education.* Published online at OurWorldInData.org. Retrieved from https://ourworldindata.org/global-rise-of-education.

16. Roser, M., & Ortiz-Ospina, E. (2018). *Global extreme poverty.* Published online at OurWorldInData.org. Retrieved from https://ourworldindata.org/extreme-poverty.

17. Ritchie, H., & Roser, M. (2018). *Water access, resources, and sanitation.* Published online at OurWorldInData.org. Retrieved from https://ourworldindata.org/water-access-resources-sanitation.

18. World Health Organization, Global Health Observatory (GHO) data. (2018). *Life expectancy.* Retrieved from http://www.who.int/gho/mortality_burden_disease/life_tables/situation_trends_text/en/.

19. Winslow, C.E. (1926). Public health at the crossroads. *American Journal of Public Health, 89*(11), 1075-1085. Reprinted in *American Journal of Public Health, 89*(11), 1645-1648.

20. World Health Organization. (2018). *Tobacco.* Retrieved from http://www.who.int/topics/tobacco/en/.

21. Institute of Medicine. (2003). *The future of the public's health in the twenty-first century.* Washington, DC: National Academies Press.

22. Institute of Medicine. (2012). *For the public's health: investing in a healthier future.* Washington, DC: The National Academies Press. https://doi.org/10.17226/13268.

23. Dahlgren, G., & Whitehead, M. (1991). *Policies and strategies to promote social equity in health.* Stockholm, Sweden: Institute for the Futures Studies.

24. Bauer, G., Davies, J.K., Pelikan, J., Noack, H., Broesskamp, U., & Hill, C. (2003). Advancing a theoretical model for public health and health promotion indicator development: Proposal from the EUHPID consortium. *European Journal of Public Health, 13*(3s), 107-113.

25. National Academies of Sciences, Engineering, and Medicine. (2017). *Communities in action: Pathways to health equity.* Washington, DC: The National Academies Press. doi:10.17226/24624.

26. Sullivan, B.J., & Bettger, J.P. (2018). Community-informed health promotion to improve health behaviors in Honduras. *Journal of Transcultural Nursing, 29*(1), 14-20. doi:10.1177/1043659616670214.

27. Caldwell, J. (1996). Demography and social science. *Population Studies, 50*, 1-34.

28. World Health Organization. (1948). *The WHO definition of health. Preamble to the constitution of the World Health Organization.* Retrieved from http://who.int/about/definition/en/print.html.

29. MacQueen, K.M., McLellan, E. Metzger, D.S., Kegeles, S., Strauss, R.P., & Trotter, R.T. (2001). What is community? An evidence-based definition for participatory public health. *American Journal of Public Health, 91*(12), 1929-1938.

30. Fallon, L.F., & Zgodzinski, E.J. (2012). *Essentials of public health management* (3rd ed.). Sudbury, MA: Jones & Bartlett.

31. Jackson, S.F. (2017). How can health promotion address the ecological determinants of health? *Global Health Promotion, 24*(4), 3-4. https://doi.org/10.1177/1757975917747448.

32. MacDonald, M.A. (2004). From miasma to fractals: The epidemiology revolution and public health nursing. *Public Health Nursing, 21*(4), 380-381.

33. Prochaska, J.O., & Velicer, W.F. (1997). The transtheoretical model of health behavior change. *American Journal of Health Promotion, 12*, 38-48.

34. Central Intelligence Agency. (2017). *The world factbook.* Retrieved from https://www.cia.gov/library/publications/the-world-factbook/rankorder/2102rank.html.

35. Have, T.H. (2016). *Global bioethics: an introduction.* Routledge: London.

36. Merriam Webster Dictionary. (2018). Definition of culture. Retrieved from https://www.merriam-webster.com/dictionary/culture.

37. Spector, R.E. (2017). *Cultural diversity in health and illness* (8th ed.). Upper Saddle River, NJ: Pearson.

38. O'Neill, D. (2006). *The nature of ethnicity.* Retrieved from http://anthro.palomar.edu/ethnicity/ethnic_2.htm.

39. Humes, K.R., Jones, N.R., & Ramirez, R.R. (2011). *Overview of race and Hispanic origin: 2010. 2010 Census Briefs.* Retrieved from http://www.census.gov/prod/cen2010/briefs/c2010br-02.pdf.

40. U.S. Census Bureau. (2017). *Race: FAQ.* Retrieved from https://www.census.gov/topics/population/race/about/faq.html.

41. Morganthau, T. (1995, February 13). What color is black? *Newsweek,* 62-69.

42. Murphy, N. (2008). An agenda for health promotion. *Nursing Ethics, 15*(5), 697-699.

43. Foronda, C., Baptiste, D., Reinholdt, M.M., & Ousman, K. (2016). Cultural humility. *Journal of Transcultural Nursing, 27*(3), 210-217. http://dx.doi.org.ezp.welch.jhmi.edu/10.1177/1043659615592677.

44. Sommers, J. (1989). *Soho—a history of London's most colorful neighborhood* (pp. 113-117). London, England: Bloomsbury.

45. The Institute of Medicine. (2010). *The future of nursing: Leading change, advancing health.* Retrieved from http://www.iom.edu/Reports/2010/The-Future-of-Nursing-Leading-Change-Advancing-Health.aspx#.

46. American Public Health Association, Public Health Nursing Section. (2013). *The definition and practice of public health nursing: A statement of the public health nursing section.* Washington, DC: American Public Health Association. Retrieved from https://www.apha.org/~/media/files/pdf/membergroups/phn/nursingdefinition.ashx.

47. Quad Council of Public Health Nursing Organizations. (1997). *The tenets of public health nursing.* Unpublished white paper.

48. American Nursing Association. (2013). *Public health nursing: Scope and standards of practice.* Silver Spring, MD: Nursesbooks.org.

49. Bekemeier, B. (2008). A history of public health and public health nursing. In L. Ivanov & C. Blue (Eds.), *Public health*

nursing: Leadership, policy, and practice (pp. 2-26). Clifton Park, NY: Thomson Delmar Learning.

50. Brainard, A.M. (1922). *The evolution of public health nursing.* New York, NY: Garland.

51. Monteiro, L.A. (1985). Florence Nightingale on public health nursing. *American Journal of Nursing, 75*(2), 181-186.

52. Florence Nightingale Museum. (2018). *Florence Nightingale biography.* Retrieved from http://www.florence-nightingale.co.uk/resources/biography/?v=7516fd43adaa.

53. Doona, M.E. (1994). Gertrude Weld Peabody: Unsung patron of public health nursing education. *Nursing & Health Care, 15*(2), 88-94.

54. Buhler-Wilkerson, K. (1985). Public health nursing: In sickness or in health? *American Journal of Public Health, 75,* 1155-1161.

55. Jewish Women's Archive. (2009). *JWA—Lillian Wald—introduction.* Retrieved from http://jwa.org/womenofvalor/wald/.

56. Buhler-Wilkerson, K. (1993). Bringing care to the people: Lillian Wald's legacy to public health nursing. *American Journal of Public Health, 83*(12), 1778-1786.

57. U.S. Department of Health and Human Services, Health Resources and Services Administration, Bureau of Health Professions. (2018). *Registered nurses: Work environment.* Retrieved from https://www.bls.gov/ooh/healthcare/registered-nurses.htm#tab-3.

58. Emanuel, E.J. (2018, February 25). Are hospitals becoming obsolete? *New York Times.* Retrieved from https://nyti.ms/2sWY9nc.

59. Quad Council Coalition Competency Review Task Force. (2018). *Community/public health nursing competencies.* Retrieved from http://www.quadcouncilphn.org/wp-content/uploads/2018/05/QCC-C-PHN-COMPETENCIES-Approved_2018.05.04_Final-002.pdf.

60. Council on Linkages. (2014). *Core competencies for public health professionals.* Retrieved from http://www.phf.org/resourcestools/Documents/Core_Competencies_for_Public_Health_Professionals_2014June.pdf.

61. American Nurses Association. (2015). *Code of ethics for nursing with interpretive statements.* Silver Spring, MD: ANA.

62. Public Health Leadership Society. (2002). *Principles of ethical practice in public health.* Retrieved from https://www.apha.org/~/media/files/pdf/membergroups/ethics_brochure.ashx.

63. Beaglehole, R., & Bonita, R. (2010). What is global health? *Global Health Action.* Published online. doi:10.3402/gha.v3i0.5142.

64. World Health Organization. (2018). *About the WHO.* Retrieved from www.who.int/about/en/.

65. United States Department of Health and Human Services, Healthy People 2030. (2018). *Leading health indicators.* Retrieved from http://www.healthypeople.gov/2020/LHI/default.aspx.

66. World Health Organization. (2018). *Constitution of WHO: Principles.* Retrieved from http://www.who.int/about/mission/en/.

67. World Health Organization. (2018). *Nursing now.* Retrieved from http://www.who.int/mediacentre/events/2018/nursing-now/en/.

68. World Bank. (2018). *How we classify countries.* Retrieved from data.worldbank.org/about/country-classifications.

69. World Health Organization. (2018). *Global health observatory: Under five mortality.* Retrieved from www.who.int/gho/child_health/mortality/mortality_under_five/en/index.html.

70. United Nations. (2018). *The sustainable development goals.* Retrieved from http://www.un.org/sustainabledevelopment/sustainable-development-goals/.

71. Centers for Disease Control and Prevention. (2015). *CDC 24-7: Our history, our story.* Retrieved from https://www.cdc.gov/about/history/ourstory.htm.

72. Centers for Disease Control and Prevention. (1999). Ten great public health achievements in the 20th century. *Morbidity and Mortality Weekly Report, 48,* 241-243.

73. Centers for Disease Control and Prevention, Office of Public Health Preparedness and Response. (2013). *Funding and guidance for state and local health departments.* Retrieved from http://www.cdc.gov/phpr/coopagreement.htm.

74. Centers for Disease Control and Prevention. (2014). *About CDC: Mission goal and pledge.* Retrieved from http://www.cdc.gov/about/organization/mission.htm.

Chapter 2

Optimizing Population Health

Christine Savage and Sara Groves

LEARNING OUTCOMES

After reading the chapter, the student will be able to:

1. Apply the concept of population health to nursing practice.
2. Describe current public health frameworks that guide prevention efforts from a local to a global perspective.
3. Apply public health prevention frameworks to specific diseases.
4. Compare and contrast different levels of health promotion, protection, and risk reduction interventions.
5. Identify health education strategies and chronic disease self-management within the context of prevention frameworks.
6. Describe components of screening from a population and individual perspective.
7. Identify public health methods used to evaluate the outcome and impact of population-based prevention interventions.

KEY TERMS

Attributable risk	Health prevention	Prevalence	Sensitivity
Behavioral prevention	Health promotion	Prevalence pot	Social determinants of health
Clinical prevention	Health protection	Prevented fraction	
Downstream approach	Indicated prevention	Prevention	Specificity
Ecological determinants of health	Intervention Wheel	Primary prevention	Tertiary prevention
	Multiphasic screening	Reliability	Universal prevention
Environmental prevention	Natural history of disease	Risk reduction	Upstream approach
Health education	Population attributable risk (PAR)	Secondary prevention	Validity
Health literacy		Selective prevention	Yield

Introduction

The proposed vision of *Healthy People 2030 (HP 2030)* is that of "A society in which all people achieve their full potential for health and well-being across the life span." The mission is "To promote and evaluate the nation's efforts to improve the health and well-being of its people."[1] Thus, the health of populations takes center stage in the effort to achieve the vision of reaching the full health potential for all. The major objective of nursing practice is to provide interventions to individuals, families, communities, and populations aimed at addressing disease and optimizing health. This requires implementing multiple levels of prevention along the entire spectrum of health and disease. To provide the best possible care requires not only an understanding of the pathophysiology of disease but also of the concepts of health promotion, risk reduction, and the underlying frameworks of prevention that help guide nursing interventions. These frameworks are not unique to nursing and, for the most part, come from the public health sciences.

In 2018, the New York Times published an op-ed article by Pagan Kennedy who explained that, although there are things individuals can do to improve their health, there are things that remain outside of our control such as bad genes, unintentional injuries, and environmental risk factors. She stated that, "It's the decisions that we make as a collective that matter more than any choice we make on our own."[2] In other words, the effects of the environment and genes can override what we do at the individual behavioral level. Making our collective decisions as a society about our environment is perhaps more important than our individual decisions about our behavior. Kennedy uses examples of experts in healthy living who nevertheless died early despite adherence to a healthy diet and exercise. It is often factors outside our individual control that contribute to early death.

To be effective as nurses, with the understanding that our collective decisions as a society impact our health, we need basic knowledge and skills at the population health level as well as at the individual level to provide expert care to individuals and their families. As evidenced by the launch of the Nursing Now campaign in February of 2018, nurses are key to reaching the goals set by the World Health Organization (WHO) as well as the proposed HP 2030 goals. Nursing Now represents a collaborative effort by the WHO and the International Council of Nurses "… to improve health globally by raising the profile and status of nurses worldwide – influencing policymakers and supporting nurses themselves to lead, learn, and build a global movement."[3]

As a profession, nursing contributes substantially to the health of populations. In turn, healthier populations lead to more robust communities and societies. To achieve the proposed HP 2030 overarching goals (see Chapter 1), HP published the proposed framework for these goals that includes foundational principles that clearly link the health of populations to a well-functioning society.

■ HEALTHY PEOPLE 2030
Foundational Principles: "What Guides Our Actions"

Note: Foundational Principles explain the thinking that guides decisions about Healthy People 2030.

- Health and well-being of the population and communities are essential to a *fully functioning, equitable society.*
- Achieving the full potential for health and well-being for all provides *valuable benefits to society*, including lower health-care costs and more prosperous and engaged individuals and communities.
- Achieving health and well-being requires eliminating health disparities, achieving health equity, and attaining health literacy.
- *Healthy physical, social, and economic environments* strengthen the potential to achieve health and well-being.
- Promoting and achieving the nation's health and well-being is a *shared responsibility* distributed among all stakeholders at the national, state, and local levels, including the public, profit, and not-for-profit sectors.
- Working to attain the full potential for health and well-being of the population is a component of decision making and policy formulation across all sectors.
- Investing to maximize health and well-being for the nation is a critical and efficient use of resources.[1]

The proposed goals and foundational framework for HP 2030 align well with those of the United Nations' (UN) Sustainable Development Goals (SDGs) (Box 2-1) that focus on sustaining and developing healthy environments. In particular, goal three of the SDGs is to "… ensure healthy lives and promote well-being for all at all ages."[4] All of this requires a population level perspective and encompasses more than treating or preventing disease. It requires promotion of a healthy

BOX 2–1 ■ Sustainable Developmental Goals

Goal 1. End poverty in all its forms everywhere.

Goal 2. End hunger, achieve food security and improved nutrition, and promote sustainable agriculture.

Goal 3. Ensure healthy lives and promote well-being for all at all ages.

Goal 4. Ensure inclusive and equitable quality education and promote lifelong learning opportunities for all.

Goal 5. Achieve gender equality and empower all women and girls.

Goal 6. Ensure availability and sustainable management of water and sanitation for all.

Goal 7. Ensure access to affordable, reliable, sustainable, and modern energy for all.

Goal 8. Promote sustained, inclusive, and sustainable economic growth, full and productive employment, and decent work for all.

Goal 9. Build resilient infrastructure, promote inclusive and sustainable industrialization, and foster innovation.

Goal 10. Reduce inequality within and among countries.

Goal 11. Make cities and human settlements inclusive, safe, resilient, and sustainable.

Goal 12. Ensure sustainable consumption and production patterns.

Goal 13. Take urgent action to combat climate change and its impacts.*

Goal 14. Conserve and sustainably use the oceans, seas, and marine resources for sustainable development.

Goal 15. Protect, restore and promote sustainable use of terrestrial ecosystems, sustainably manage forests, combat desertification, and halt and reverse land degradation and biodiversity loss.

Goal 16. Promote peaceful and inclusive societies for sustainable development, provide access to justice for all, and build effective, accountable, and inclusive institutions at all levels.

Goal 17. Strengthen the means of implementation and revitalize the Global Partnership for Sustainable Development.

Source: (4)

*Acknowledging that the UN's Framework Convention on Climate Change is the primary international, intergovernmental forum for negotiating the global response to climate change.

environment, ending poverty and hunger, and increasing access to education.[4] It also requires development of partnerships within nations and across the globe to promote a healthy world.

In the U.S., over the past 2 decades, health care has taken on a central role at the federal policy level. Following the passage of the Affordable Care Act (ACA), the National Prevention Council released a comprehensive plan, the purpose of which was to increase the number of Americans who are healthy at every stage of life.[5] It included four broad strategic directions fundamental to this prevention strategy: (1) building healthy and safe community efforts; (2) expanding quality preventive services in both clinical and community settings; (3) empowering people to make healthy choices; and (4) eliminating health disparities (Fig. 2-1). There were seven priorities: (1) tobacco-free living, (2) preventing drug abuse and excessive alcohol abuse, (3) healthy eating, (4) active living, (5) injury- and violence-free living, (6) reproductive and sexual health, and (7) mental and emotional well-being.[5] The National Prevention Council, per the ACA, was required to provide the president with an annual report until 2015. The last report covered advances made including increasing the number of colleges with tobacco-free campuses, improving school nutrition, increasing supports for breast feeding, and increasing

access to healthier foods in 2014.[6] Although this initiative is not currently active, the framework provides a way to visualize the interaction between the elements that contribute to the health of populations.

Increasing the number of healthy persons at all stages of their life across the globe requires purposeful and well-planned prevention on the part of nurses across the continuum of prevention. The full scope of interventions includes those aimed at health promotion, risk reduction, and disease prevention. Specific population health interventions done routinely by nurses include screening, health education, and evaluation of the effectiveness of disease and injury prevention programs.

Population Health Promotion, Health Protection, and Risk Reduction

The social ecological model of health has been used in the public health field for the last 3 decades and clearly demonstrates that health occurs from the cellular to global level (Chapter 1, Fig. 1-1). It provides a basis for understanding health promotion and prevention efforts key to the achievement of the HP Goals and the SDGs through an inclusion of both the physical and social environments as key components of health.[7,8] More recently some authors have suggested turning the model inside out, "… placing health-related and other social policies and environments at the center."[9] Turning it inside out places the focus on community context as a means for fostering health policy and environmental development.[9] Either way, the model emphasizes the interaction among communities, policy, and environment and their role in the health of individuals and their families.

The social environmental determinants of health are different from the individual-level biological and behavioral determinants of health that are the usual focus of health prevention interventions. The use of the ecological model within the context of health promotion, health protection, and risk reduction requires the inclusion of social relations, neighborhoods and communities, institutions, and social and economic policies in the development of prevention strategies.

Health Promotion, Risk Reduction, and Health Protection

Health promotion-related interventions are an essential component of nursing practice and occur from the individual to the population level. Authors use various terms in relation to reducing the occurrence or severity of disease in a population and enhancing the capacity of

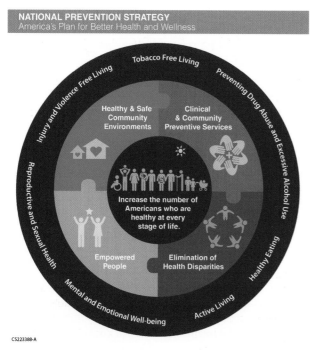

Figure 2-1 National Prevention Strategy Priorities. *(From National Prevention Council, 2012.)*

a population to achieve optimal health. These terms include health promotion, risk reduction, and health protection. The WHO's definition of **health promotion** is: "… the process of enabling people to increase control over, and to improve, their health. It moves beyond a focus on individual behaviour towards a wide range of social and environmental interventions."[10] **Risk reduction** refers to actions taken to reduce adverse outcomes such as the use of a condom to reduce the risk of transmission of a communicable disease (CD). Another term used in conjunction with risk reduction is **health protection**, which puts the emphasis on increasing the person's ability to protect against disease. An example of a health promotion intervention is the institution of an exercise program in an elementary school; an example of a health protection, risk reduction program is a vaccination outreach program. The first intervention promotes a healthy behavior and the second increases the ability of the immune system to protect against a communicable agent, thus reducing risk.

Health promotion often focuses on interventions aimed at helping patients increase healthy behaviors, such as a healthy diet and exercise, and reduce unhealthy behaviors, such as tobacco use or at-risk alcohol use. In 2008, Michael O'Donnell, editor-in-chief emeritus of the Journal of Health Promotion, stated that health promotion is both a science and an art that helps people change their lifestyles to achieve optimal health.[11] From O'Donnell's perspective, health promotion remains rooted in individual behavioral change. However, examined from a broader perspective and following the WHO definition, health promotion encompasses activities taken to promote health that require changes other than behavioral changes, such as facilitating the individuals' ability to improve the health of their environment and increase their access to resources needed to promote health, such as good nutrition or a safe place to exercise.

The socioecological model provides the basis of ecological health promotion that expands on O'Donnell's individual approach to health promotion by taking into account social and ecological determinants of health using an upstream approach. **Ecological determinants of health** include "… potable water and sanitation, affordable and clean energy, climate action, life below water, and life on land."[12] **Social determinants of health**, according to the WHO "… are the conditions in which people are born, grow, live, work, and age. These circumstances are shaped by the distribution of money, power, and resources at global, national, and local levels. The social determinants of health are mostly responsible for

health inequities—the unfair and avoidable differences in health status seen within and between countries."[13] To achieve optimal health for all, educational, policy, economic, and environmental strategies are used to increase access to needed resources as well as interventions aimed at health promotion and protection.[14] Nurses support this goal of achieving optimal health for all not only through the delivery of care to individuals, families, and communities but also through advocacy and active involvement in policy development, implementation, and evaluation (see Chapter 21).

Health Promotion

Health promotion at the individual and family level helps people make lifestyle changes aimed at achieving optimal health. These prevention interventions are implemented in various ways and often focus on behavioral change. In relation to obesity, health promotion activities focus on diet and exercise. Health-care providers deliver these interventions to individuals in their care. These interventions are also delivered to populations via health education programs, media campaigns, or in the workplace. The goal of these health promotion programs is to achieve change at the individual level based on the biological and behavioral issues related to developing disease due to obesity. The assumption is that the promotion of healthy behaviors will reduce risk and thereby reduce the prevalence of morbidity and mortality related to obesity.

The ecological model allows us to expand on this approach to health promotion by incorporating what is referred to as an upstream approach in contrast to a downstream approach to these efforts.[14] An **upstream approach** focuses on eliminating the factors that increase risk to a population's health. In contrast, a **downstream approach** represents actions taken after disease or injury has occurred. These two terms are important in understanding health promotion efforts today. Upstream represents a macro approach to addressing health whereas downstream takes a more micro approach with a focus on illness care. Both are needed to adequately address health issues in the population.[15] Take obesity as an example. With a downstream approach, a health-care provider may focus primarily on nutritional health teaching based on nutritional patterns, portions, and choices without taking into consideration the environmental factors influencing choices within a community. If there are no supermarkets within a community, it is difficult to make healthy choices. In contrast to a downstream approach, an upstream approach to obesity might include interventions focused on agriculture subsidies, transportation policies, and urban zoning. It might also involve interventions restricting television advertising of food to children, creating national nutrition standards for meals served in childcare settings, or working with the private sector to introduce healthier options in restaurants and local markets

An upstream approach to health promotion related to the obesity epidemic examines the environmental factors that contribute to the epidemic and institutes prevention interventions that target environmental change. Using the first and third strategic directions of the National Prevention Strategy as examples, this can occur through empowering community members to initiate and implement the changes to create a healthy community. For example, to promote healthy eating behaviors in children, a school system in Kentucky took action and eliminated all fried foods that had been offered on the school menu. Other communities have eliminated all vending machines in schools that offer unhealthy beverages and food. The National School Lunch Program supports including larger portions of fruits and vegetables, less sodium, and no *trans* fats. It also places a cap on the number of calories for the school lunch at 650 for grades K through 5, 700 calories for grades 6 through 8, and 850 calories for grades 9 through 12. Milk can be at most 1% fat, and flavored milk must be fat-free although there are flexibilities allowed to help provide more local control.[16,17] Such an approach to health promotion requires that the planners for the health promotion intervention take into account the context of the healthy behavior they hope the population will adopt. If the focus is only on having the schoolchildren change their eating habits without taking into account the food available to them in their total environment, then that kind of health promotion program will likely fail.

Health Protection and Risk Reduction

In contrast to health promotion, which focuses on the promotion of a healthy lifestyle and environment, health protection/risk reduction interventions protect the individual from disease by reducing risk. These terms are often used interchangeably, but are in actuality distinct. A good example of health protection is the use of vaccines. When an individual is vaccinated, the body develops immunity to the infectious agent and is therefore protected from the disease. The use of a vaccine has reduced the risk of developing disease. Risk reduction, conversely, encompasses more than biological protection. It can involve removing risk from the environment or reducing the level of risk, for example, by reducing hazardous chemical emissions produced at

industrial plants. Health protection and risk reduction activities are an important component of our national effort to prevent disease.

Much of the health protection and risk reduction activities currently used in our health-care system focus on influencing behavioral change at the individual level. The focus is to have individuals adopt protective health activities, even if the prevention program is offered to groups or populations. For example, policies related to the recommended childhood vaccines are population based and aimed at reducing risk for the development of childhood CDs. However, the actual delivery of the vaccine requires an individual response.

Risk reduction and health promotion must take into account the broader concept of risk for development of disease by incorporating environmental and social risk factors associated with the development of disease that may not be amenable through individual-level interventions. For example, protection from lead poisoning requires an environmental approach aimed at eradicating lead paint in the environment. The risk factor, lead paint, cannot be eliminated solely at the individual level and often requires a system or community approach related to allocation of funds, development of public policy, and follow-through with the removal of lead paint from older buildings in the community.

Prevention Frameworks

Prevention is a word used often in health care, but what does it mean and how does it work? From a simplistic standpoint, *prevention* refers to stopping something from happening. From a health perspective, **health prevention** refers to the prevention not only of disease and injury but also to the slowing of the progression of the disease. It also refers to the prevention of the sequelae of diseases and injury, such as the prevention of blindness related to type 1 diabetes. Health prevention is accomplished through the institution of public health policies, health programs, and practices with the goal of improving the health of populations, thus reducing the risk for disease, injury, and subsequent disability and/or premature death.

Health promotion and protection are fundamental concepts for nursing practice and are based on prevention frameworks in use in the public health field.[18,19] Prevention frameworks help nurses shape prevention interventions within a particular context. In the summer of 2016, a major public health issue was the Zika virus epidemic. Preventing the spread of the disease was the main focus of the public health interventions taken by the Centers for Disease Control and Prevention (CDC) and the WHO. These activities included behavioral, environmental, and clinical interventions. People were asked to modify their behavior by utilizing insect repellent and avoiding unprotected sexual intercourse with a person who had been exposed. Governments worked to reduce the mosquito population through sprays, and travel alerts were put in place. How do these interventions relate to the natural history of disease, and how do they fit into current public health prevention frameworks?

Natural History of Disease

An understanding of the natural history of disease is an essential basis for the discussion of current prevention frameworks that follows. The **natural history of disease** provides the foundation for the public health frameworks currently in use, especially the most widely used framework of primary, secondary, and tertiary prevention. The natural history of disease depicts the continuum of disease from the disease-free state to resolution. The four stages are (1) susceptibility; (2) the subclinical phase after exposure when pathological changes are occurring without the person being aware of them; (3) clinical disease with the development of symptoms; and (4) the resolution phase in which the final outcomes are cure, disability, or death.[20,21] The subclinical phase is also sometimes referred to as the incubation period for CDs and latency period for noncommunicable illness (Fig. 2-2).

This traditional presentation of the natural history of disease with four stages initially appears linear. For some diseases such as influenza, this linear model works well. In some disease processes, an individual may go from a subclinical stage to a clinical stage and then back to a subclinical stage. For example, in human immunodeficiency virus (HIV) infection, during the initial subclinical stage an infected individual has no clinical symptoms that meet the criteria for a diagnosis of acquired immunodeficiency syndrome (AIDS). As the infection progresses, the person may develop one or more clinical diagnoses, thus placing the individual in the clinical stage of the disease. However, with the treatments now available for treating AIDS, an individual may recover from a clinical episode and return to being asymptomatic, but there has been no resolution of the disease; instead, that individual has reverted to a subclinical stage.

Figure 2-2 also depicts the outcome of a particular disease. Following the development of clinical disease, an individual recovers completely (cure), is disabled by the disease (disability), or dies. Some diseases, both communicable and noncommunicable, have no endpoint except death. HIV/AIDS is an example of a CD with no cure. Those who become infected will remain infected for the rest of their lives. An example of a noncommunicable disease (NCD) without a cure is type 1 diabetes. A person diagnosed with this type of diabetes does not at some point in time revert to producing insulin at normal levels.

To further illustrate, examine the prevalence of a disease and the prevalence pot. **Prevalence** is basically the number of total cases of disease (numerator) divided by the total number of people in the population (denominator) and reflects the total number of cases of a disease in a given population. A **prevalence pot** is a way of depicting the total number of cases of the disease in the population that takes into account issues related to duration of the disease and the incidence of the disease (Fig. 2-3). For some CDs with a short incubation period such as influenza, cases rapidly move in and out of the prevalence pot, but for long-term chronic diseases with no known cure, the prevalence pot can grow over time (e.g., HIV infection). If the definition of a case is infection with the HIV virus, then individuals who are subclinical and those who have evidence of clinical illness that meets the criteria for an AIDS diagnosis would all be in the

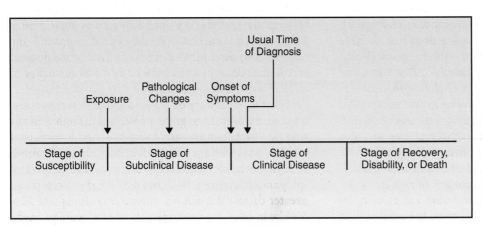

Figure 2-2 The natural history of disease timeline. *(From Centers for Disease Control and Prevention. (1992). Principles of epidemiology (2nd ed.). Atlanta, GA: U.S. Department of Health and Human Services. Retrieved from http://www.cdc.gov/osels/scientific_edu/ss1978/lesson1/Section9.html.)*

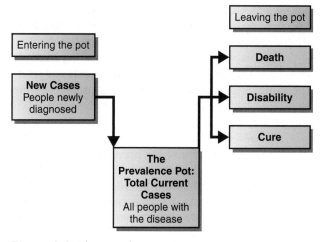

Figure 2-3 The prevalence pot.

prevalence pot. During the early years of the AIDS epidemic, there were few treatment options. Once diagnosed, an individual often died within a short period of time. As treatment has improved and the survival rate for those infected with HIV has greatly increased, the number of AIDS-associated deaths has declined. However, the HIV/AIDS prevalence pot has grown, because the only way out of the prevalence pot is through death. In developing countries where treatment for HIV/AIDS is less available, the prevalence pot has not grown as rapidly, even with a higher number of cases, because the life span of those with HIV/AIDS remains short.

Mapping out a disease using the natural history of disease model helps to identify where on the continuum prevention efforts are needed. The prevalence pot helps identify those health conditions that may have an increasing number of cases over time if the development of new cases is not prevented. In the case of seasonal flu, laying out the natural history of the strain of flu appearing in a given year helps to determine where the primary focus should be. In the beginning of the fall in most years, the majority of the U.S. population does not have influenza. As the next few months progress, more and more people usually become infected, and some die. Based on the severity of the flu epidemic nationwide, large-scale prevention efforts may be instituted. In 2009, during the H1N1 flu outbreak, efforts focused on vaccinating populations at greatest risk, in that case pregnant women, children, and older adults, resulting in a focus on those without disease at highest risk for mortality.[22] This was important due to the shortage of vaccines available. Those who were most vulnerable got priority for receiving the vaccine. The H1N1 virus is now a regular

human flu virus. Based on the 2009 pandemic and data from subsequent years, the CDC updated its warnings related to populations that were most vulnerable. The most vulnerable populations now include children under the age of 5, pregnant women, older adults, Native Americans, and Native Alaskans. [23]

How does the natural history of the disease and the prevalence pot help public health officials focus on interventions? In the case of flu epidemics, the incubation period, that is, the time interval between infection and the first clinical signs of disease (Chapter 8), is short, with those infected rapidly developing symptoms. In addition, the course of the disease is also short. People with influenza are able to infect others from 1 day before getting sick to 5 to 7 days after getting sick. Those who become infected with a flu virus rapidly develop clinical symptoms including fever, cough, and in some cases gastrointestinal symptoms. New cases that enter the prevalence pot usually leave the pot within 7 days. Most recover completely, some experience long-term effects such as coma and/or respiratory problems, and some die.

Using the natural history of disease model, the nurse can lay out the progression of influenza (see Fig. 2-2). The preclinical phase is very short (1 to 2 days), and there are no interventions available that would prevent the progression from this phase to clinical disease. Once the patient is in the clinical phase, there are limited options for intervention because the causative agent, the flu virus, does not respond to antibiotics. However, early recognition in vulnerable patients, such as older adults, and treatment with antiviral medication may help to reduce the risk of complications and adverse consequences.

Because of the limited ability of antiviral medication to prevent adverse consequences in at-risk populations and the short period of time between phases, the best approach is to focus on preventing disease from occurring in the first place. The natural history of influenza provides the basis for the nationwide public focus on primary prevention through the development, distribution, and administration of flu vaccines with the hope of keeping the majority of the population disease-free because of the limited ability to provide effective secondary or tertiary prevention interventions.

The natural history of a disease also allows the nurse to identify who is at greatest risk for developing the disease. For influenza, early evaluation of the prevalence of the disease by age groups helps to establish who is most likely to become ill. In the case of the 2009 H1N1 flu pandemic, the CDC concluded that there was a greater disease burden on those under the age of 25.[22] Unlike in other flu outbreaks, those who were younger, immune compromised, or pregnant were at increased risk of death. This led to the speculation that the virus was related to earlier strains, and those in late adulthood had immunity due to earlier exposure. Thus, the older members of the population had natural biological protection, whereas those under the age of 60 did not. With limited vaccine available in the fall of 2009, decisions were made to provide the vaccine to those at highest risk. This included pregnant women, household and caregiver contacts of children younger than 6 months of age, health-care and emergency medical services personnel, people from 6 months through 24 years of age, and people aged 25 through 64 years who had medical conditions associated with a higher risk of influenza complications.

The natural history of disease for type 1 diabetes is quite different from H1N1 flu. The etiology, or cause, of type 1 diabetes is genetic rather than infectious. Although there is no known prevention for type 1 diabetes, early detection during stage one can lead to early diagnosis and treatment. However, identifying the disease early will not prevent the development of clinical disease, which lasts for a lifetime because the body is unable to produce insulin. There is no cure. This puts the majority of the focus on treatment of the patient in the clinical stage to prevent premature death and disability. Another key distinction between the natural history of these two diseases is that influenza is population based, that is, the disease spreads from one person to another. Interventions are required to protect the entire population at risk. By contrast, a disease such as type 1 diabetes is individual based, and the risk is usually tied to a genetic trait passed down in families.

Public Health Prevention Frameworks

The natural history of a disease and the difference between population-based risks and individual-based risks form the basis for two main prevention frameworks used in public health science. The first framework is the traditional public health prevention model of primary, secondary, and tertiary prevention.[21] The second is the framework of universal, selected, and indicated prevention based on work done by Gordon and put forth by the Health and Medicine Division (HMD) of the National Academies of Sciences, Engineering, and Medicine (formerly known as the IOM).[24] Both use a health promotion and health protection approach, and employ the three types of interventions—clinical, behavioral, and environmental. The best place to start is with the traditional primary, secondary, and tertiary prevention model, because it has been in use since the 1950s, and the newer IOM framework was not used widely until it was mandated by

the Centers for Substance Abuse Prevention (CSAP), a branch of the U.S. Federal Substance Abuse and Mental Health Service Administration (SAMHSA), in 2004.[25]

Levels of Prevention

The traditional public health approach to prevention focuses on health prevention based on the natural history of disease and includes three levels of prevention—primary, secondary, and tertiary. **Primary prevention** interventions are conducted to prevent development of disease or injury in those who are currently healthy.[21] The focus is usually on people at risk for developing the disease or injury but may take a population approach such as recommendations that all persons be vaccinated against the flu. Activities include promoting healthy behaviors and building the ability of populations and individuals within that population to protect themselves against disease. Many health policies are aimed at primary prevention such as banning smoking in public places, which is aimed at reducing the development of diseases secondary to exposure to second-hand smoke. The goal is to reduce risk factors for a health problem. If the risk for developing disease or sustaining an injury can be reduced, then the incidence (occurrence of new cases) of a disease will be reduced. **Secondary prevention** interventions include those aimed at early detection and initiation of treatment for disease, thus reducing disease-associated morbidity and mortality.[21] If early intervention results in cure from the disease, with or without disability, screening can contribute to the reduction of the prevalence of a disease (total number of new and old cases), thereby reducing the size of the prevalence pot. Secondary prevention can include screening or case finding in CD outbreaks by seeking contacts of people already ill. The focus of **tertiary prevention** is the prevention of disability and premature death and, when indicated, the initiation of rehabilitation for those diagnosed with disease.[21] It includes interventions aimed at preventing secondary complications related to disease such as the prevention of bedsores.

Primary Prevention: Primary prevention is a central part of nursing practice. Nurses engage in the delivery of primary prevention across settings, including the acute care setting where, on first glance, it looks as though the nurse is only providing tertiary prevention interventions. Because this approach is based on the natural history of disease, what types of primary prevention does a nurse provide in an acute care setting when every patient admitted has a diagnosis of clinical disease? A prime example is the activities nurses do to prevent hospital-acquired infections. All nurses must follow hospital policy related to the use of personal protective equipment, isolation precautions, and personal hygiene. These activities prevent the spread of infection from a patient with disease to patients or health-care workers without disease. Nurses also participate in primary prevention from a health protection perspective. All nurses must comply with hospital policy related to vaccinations. In this way the members of the health-care workforce who are free of disease take steps to build their immunity to disease, thus preventing the spread of disease to patients and fellow workers who are free of disease. All these activities are population based.

Nurses also apply the principles of primary prevention on an individual level through health education, vaccination, and other activities aimed at promoting and protecting the health of their patients and increasing the patients' ability to protect themselves from disease. Patients receiving nursing care in acute care settings who are receiving care for one clinical disease may be at increased risk for other disease or injury. Nurses often include primary prevention in their plan of care, such as altering the environment to prevent falls and teaching basic fall prevention strategies to patients and their families that can be implemented on discharge. Health education begins with primary prevention, teaching patients to reduce risk for disease (e.g., teaching patients to increase exercise, reduce caloric intake, and perform proper hand hygiene). Nurses working in the community provide primary prevention by providing health education, promoting breastfeeding, and working with communities to reduce hazards such as lead paint.

During epidemics and pandemics, countries depend on nurses as frontline workers in nationwide primary prevention efforts to reduce the incidence of the disease and prevent premature death. Public health departments across the country often mobilize nurses and student nurses to administer the vaccines at schools, health clinics, and other community settings. Because of the need for nurses to deliver the vaccine to large groups of at-risk individuals, nurses and other health-care providers are often the first to receive the vaccine when it becomes available. Primary prevention is an essential part of providing nursing care to individuals and populations across all settings.

Secondary Prevention: Nurses also regularly participate in secondary prevention interventions in all settings. Screening is one aspect of secondary prevention and is an essential component of the nursing assessment focused on early detection of problems in asymptomatic individuals who already have certain risk factors. Screening also targets conditions that are not yet clinically

apparent for purposes of earlier detection. Early treatment reduces risk for further morbidity and for mortality. In acute, community, and long-term care settings, nurses regularly screen patients of all ages for the possible existence of a number of conditions. Screening for developmental delays is an example of secondary prevention in children, whereas encouraging mammograms is an example of a secondary prevention intervention for adults. The goal of mammograms is to detect early stage breast cancer. Some activities done by nurses can serve as both secondary prevention and tertiary prevention. For example, the simple taking of blood pressures at a blood pressure clinic held in a local senior center is a type of screening when conducted with older adults who have not been identified previously as having hypertension. At the same clinic, taking an individual's blood pressure reading may function as a method for monitoring the health status of an older person who has already been diagnosed with hypertension.

Through early detection, nurses can implement interventions that will alter the natural history of the disease. For example, on admission to long-term care facilities, elderly patients are routinely screened for skin integrity. If there is any evidence of skin breakdown, nursing interventions are immediately put in place to halt the progression of a stage 1 pressure ulcer (bed sore) to a stage 2. In stage 1, the skin is reddened, but there is no break in the skin. Without intervention, the patient is at greatly increased risk for skin breakdown and rapid development of a stage 2 to a stage 3 pressure ulcer.

There are many circumstances when early detection and initiation of treatment prior to the development of clinical disease can improve outcomes. Public health efforts to prevent premature death due to cancer include media campaigns for mammography screening, colonoscopies, and prostate screening. Screening is also conducted for behavioral health issues such as at-risk alcohol use (see Chapter 11). Screening for syphilis and early treatment can prevent serious disability, reduce the incidence of syphilis infection in newborns, and prevent premature death. Nurses participate in these efforts by conducting screenings and by educating patients to encourage their participation in screening.

Health education is done with a secondary prevention focus. For example, a nurse participating in a blood pressure screening health fair will include secondary prevention health education for adults with a blood pressure reading greater than or equal to 130/80. Adults with a blood pressure reading between 130/80 and 139/89 are considered to have stage 1 hypertension, and those with a blood pressure reading greater than 140/90 have stage

2 hypertension. It is recommended that the diagnosis of hypertension be based on the average of ≥2 readings obtained on ≥2 occasions.[26] Thus, it is important to refer persons with blood pressures greater than 130/80 to a primary care physician for follow-up. Early intervention through lifestyle changes and medical intervention can reduce the development of life-threatening conditions such as stroke or myocardial infarction.

Tertiary Prevention: The primary focus of nursing interventions in most acute care settings is tertiary prevention. Once an individual has been diagnosed with clinical disease, prevention aims at reducing disability, promoting the possibility of cure when possible, and preventing death. Efforts are made to interrupt the natural progression of the disease or to reduce the impact of the injury through multiple strategies including medical, environmental, and psychosocial.

Health education is a key tertiary prevention activity for the nurse. For those with chronic diseases, a disease self-management approach is often used. This approach puts the individual in charge of managing his or her disease with the goal of reducing disability and preventing premature death. The nurse serves as the teacher/facilitator by helping the individual to identify the key strategies needed to manage disease, such as regular foot care and blood sugar monitoring in patients with diabetes. The use of chronic disease self-management is effective in reducing health-care utilization in general populations, improving perceived self-efficacy, and improving perception of health status for various noncommunicable chronic diseases.[27,28,29]

Universal, Selected, and Indicated Prevention Models

The traditional public health framework consisting of levels of prevention was introduced in the 1950s and still has utility today, especially for diseases in which the natural history and causal pathways for development of the disease are well understood. It is also useful when the early clinical and subclinical signs of the disease are known and the disease is actually preventable. On the flip side, the framework has limitations because of the underlying linear approach to diseases with a clear etiology. The framework is difficult to adapt to diseases or disorders (see Chapters 10 and 11) with complex risk factors; a curvilinear progression; and broad health outcomes that encompass not only physical outcomes but also psychological, social, and economic outcomes. It also limits the majority of the prevention efforts to interventions conducted by health-care providers and is not as readily applicable to the broader interdisciplinary field of public health.

An alternate approach using a continuum-of-health framework was proposed by the IOM in the 1990s and has been adopted by the Substance Abuse and Mental Health Services Administration (SAMHSA).[25] This model divides the continuum of care into three parts: prevention, treatment, and maintenance (Fig. 2-4). Under prevention there are three categories: universal, selected, and indicated. This model was first adopted by the behavioral health field because there is less distinction in mental disorders and substance use disorders between the traditional levels of prevention that were developed based on the natural history of disease—primary (stage of susceptibility), secondary (subclinical stage), and tertiary (clinical stage).[24]

A **universal prevention** intervention is one that is applicable to the whole population and is not based on individual risk. The intervention is aimed at the general population. The purpose is to deter the onset of a health issue within the population. Public health media campaigns use a universal approach by targeting everyone

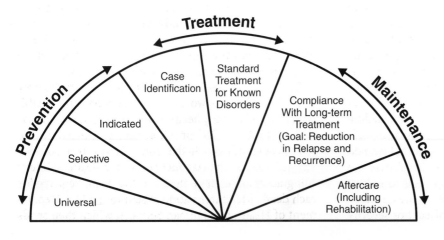

Figure 2-4 Continuum-of-Care Prevention Model. *(From the Substance Abuse and Mental Health Services Administration. [2004]. Clinical preventive services in substance abuse and mental health update: From science to services [DHHS Publication No. (SMA) 04-3906].)*

in the population with such things as a billboard anti-smoking campaign or TV ads aimed at preventing drunk driving. All individuals in the population are provided with the information and/or skills necessary to prevent disease regardless of risk. Often the intervention is passive, as in media campaigns, in that nearly all of the population is exposed to the intervention. The intervention often does not include participation on an individual level. However, universal vaccination programs are not passive and require active participation by individuals. This is an appropriate approach when the entire population is at risk and would benefit from prevention programs.

Selective prevention interventions are aimed at a subset of the population that has an increased level of risk for developing disease. This can be based on demographic variables such as age, gender, or race, or it can be based on other risk factors such as genetic, environmental, or socioeconomic risk factors. Examples of selective prevention interventions include: efforts to screen women for breast cancer who have a known family history of breast cancer, or providing community education programs to prevent lead poisoning in older urban neighborhoods. This level of prevention targets everyone in the subgroup regardless of risk. For example, everyone in a neighborhood with older buildings is included in the selective lead poisoning intervention whether or not they have already removed the lead from their own residence. Once again, a selective intervention can be passive or have an active component on the individual level.

Indicated prevention interventions are provided to populations with a high probability of developing disease. Like secondary prevention, the purpose of indicated interventions is to intervene with individuals with early signs of disease or subclinical disease to prevent the development of a more severe disease. The difference is that the individuals included in the intervention have already been identified as being at greater risk for the disease whereas in secondary prevention the effort is to identify those with the disease among an apparently healthy population. The indicated prevention approach is used in the substance abuse field to develop programs for individuals with early warning signs of increased potential for developing a substance use disorder, such as falling grades or at-risk alcohol use. Only those individuals with specific risk factors for developing the disease but who do not yet meet the diagnostic criteria for the disease are included in the intervention. The purpose is to reduce behavioral risk factors that contribute to the development of disease and to delay onset of disease or severity of disease. The level of intervention provided is more intensive and often multilevel. It always requires individual participation. An example of an indicated prevention program is that of a weight-loss program for adolescents who are obese and are showing signs of hyperglycemia but who have not been diagnosed with type 2 diabetes. Such an intervention would probably include case management, health education, nutritional counseling, and an individualized exercise plan. If the program is effective, participants may not only delay the onset of type 2 diabetes but may also reverse the hyperglycemia and not develop the disease.

Delivery of Public Health Prevention Strategies

The delivery of prevention services includes the use of three basic strategies—clinical, behavioral, and environmental. **Clinical prevention** strategies are those that use a one-to-one delivery method between the health-care provider and the patient, and usually occur in traditional health-care settings. These can include health protection activities such as vaccinations, as well as screening, and early detection of disease. **Behavioral prevention**, often focused on health promotion strategies, is aimed at changing individual behavior such as exercise promotion, smoking cessation, or responsible drinking. **Environmental prevention** focuses on health protection by improving the safety of the environment such as fluoridating water, banning smoking in public places, enacting laws against drunk driving, enforcing clean air acts, and building green spaces for recreation.[21]

In an effort to standardize clinical prevention strategies through the application of evidence-based prevention practices, the Agency for Healthcare Research and Quality (AHRQ) created the U.S. Preventive Services Task Force.[30] This task force is made up of a panel of experts in primary care and prevention. These experts systematically review the evidence found in published research related to the effectiveness of prevention strategies and then develop recommendations for clinical interventions. These recommendations are helpful in the development of a clinical prevention program.

The earlier example of type 2 diabetes illustrates how to apply both frameworks to a serious national health issue. Globally, many health issues contribute to premature death. The CDC provides yearly updates on the top 10 causes of death in the United States (Box 2-2).[31,32] This is based on the classification of the death or injury using accepted codes entered in the death registry for each death. This information is sent to the U.S. Department of Health and Human Services, which then sends

BOX 2–2 ■ Number of Deaths for Top 10 Leading Causes of Death, 2017

- Heart disease: 635,260
- Cancer: 598,038
- Accidents (unintentional injuries): 161,374
- Chronic lower respiratory diseases: 154,596
- Stroke (cerebrovascular diseases): 142,142
- Alzheimer's disease: 116,103
- Diabetes: 80,058
- Influenza and pneumonia: 51,537
- Nephritis, nephrotic syndrome, and nephrosis: 50,046
- Intentional self-harm (suicide): 44,965

Source: (31)

the information to the CDC. The cause of death listed on the death certificates at the local level is the basis for the aggregate statistics related to mortality rates at the state and national levels. Though this provides important information, the underlying risk factors provide the information needed to build health promotion, protection, and risk-reduction interventions.

Not only is cause of death classified by disease or injury, it is also further classified by risk factor, that is, the underlying cause of death. Four health at-risk behaviors—lack of exercise or physical activity, poor nutrition, tobacco use, and drinking too much alcohol—are underlying causes for illness and premature death.[33] In other words, it is important not only to track the causes of actual deaths but also to track the occurrence of preventable risk factors to help predict whether efforts to prevent these deaths are working. This information helps to guide major prevention efforts aimed at reducing both morbidity and mortality in populations.

Each death can also be classified in quantitative terms using attributable risk and prevented fraction. **Attributable risk** is the measure of the proportion of the cases or injuries that would be eliminated if a risk factor was not present. Epidemiologists begin by determining the theoretical limit of the impact of prevention aimed at removing the risk factor. That is, if the risk factor did not exist, how many cases would be eliminated? For example, if no one smoked, how many cases of lung cancer would be eliminated, or if no one drove while intoxicated, how many motor vehicle crashes (MVCs) would not occur? It is calculated using the **population attributable risk (PAR)**, which is based on the strength of the risk factor and the prevalence of the risk factor in the population. To determine the strength of the risk factor, epidemiologists calculate what is referred to as the relative risk (RR) (Chapter 3). If these pieces of the equation are known,

that is, the RR and the prevalence, then the PAR can be calculated.[21]

Those who wish to implement a prevention program can use the PAR to calculate the cost benefit and cost effectiveness of the prevention program. However, the PAR is population based and operates on the assumption that the risk factor is removed from the entire population being targeted. The prevented fraction provides the information on what can be accomplished based on the intervention actually being delivered at the community level. The **prevented fraction** is defined as a measure of what can actually be achieved in a community setting. It includes the proportion of the population at risk that actually participates and the number of cases prevented. This approach takes into account the number of participants in a program who will actually succeed in eliminating the risk factor. For example, how many obese children participating in an after-school activity program will actually reduce their weight to a normal body mass index?

Prior to implementing an intervention aimed at prevention, it is important to understand the underlying risk factors. The top four risk factors for preventable death in the United States—tobacco use, improper diet, physical inactivity, and alcohol use—relate to behaviors.[33] At first glance, it appears that a behavioral intervention is the best approach. However, other interventions are also helpful, including environmental and policy-based interventions. For example, alcohol-related MVCs can occur with just one episode of heavy episodic drinking. The teenage driver who has consumed alcohol for the first time at high levels and then drives home may become involved in an MVC that results in the death of people who are not consuming alcohol. The teen did not have an alcohol use disorder but instead had engaged in at-risk alcohol use. The natural history of disease does not fit this health-related issue, yet prevention of alcohol-related MVCs is an important issue. The questions become:

- What types of interventions will work to prevent disease or injuries?
- Is it primary, secondary, or tertiary prevention?
- Can it occur using a clinical, behavioral, or environmental approach?
- In designing this approach, should it be addressed as a universal, selected, or indicated preventive intervention?

In answering these questions, it is important to have a better understanding of some potential public health nursing interventions and a framework that guides public health nursing practice.

A Public Health Nursing Framework

Conceptual frameworks and models guide the practice of public health nurses (PHNs). One of the models implemented by the Minnesota State Department of Health in 2001 is the **Intervention Wheel**, which illustrates how PHNs can improve the health of the individuals, families, communities, and systems[34,35] (Fig. 2-5). The model evolved from the practice of PHNs in Minnesota and consists of several components. The first component is the population basis of all interventions. This component illustrates that the focus of all interventions is population health. The second component consists of the three levels of care: individual/family, community, and systems. Care can be provided at all three levels of working with individuals, the community as a whole, or with systems. Individual level practice focuses on knowledge, attitudes, practices, beliefs, and behaviors of individuals. A PHN's

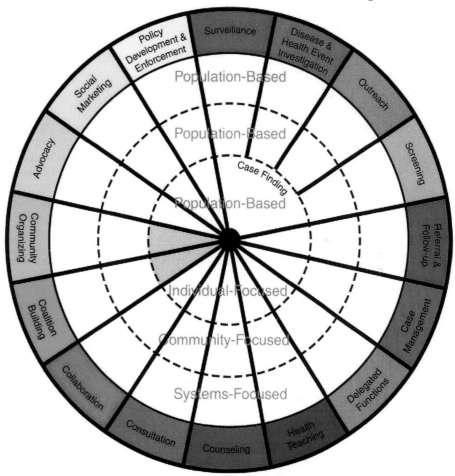

Public Health Interventions
Applications for Public Health Nursing Practice

March 2001

Minnesota Department of Health
Division of Community Health Services
Public Health Nursing Section

Figure 2-5 Components of the Intervention Wheel. *(From Minnesota Department of Health, Division of Community Health Services, Public Health Section. [2001]. Public health interventions: Applications for public health nursing practice.)*

home visit to a new mother is an example of individual-level practice. During the visit, the PHN provides anticipatory guidance about the value of breastfeeding.

Community-level practice is focused on changing norms, attitudes, practices, awareness, and behaviors. An example of community-level practice is the development of a faith-based program focused on smoking cessation. Systems-level practice is concerned with policies, laws, organization, and power structures within communities. For example, a coalition of several senior housing sites could be formed to address pest control and improvement of overall environmental conditions, or a group of parents could come together to build a safe playground for the children.

The third component consists of 17 public health interventions (Box 2-3). Three of these interventions—health education, screening, and case management—are discussed in this chapter as they relate to levels of prevention, and the other interventions are discussed in other chapters.

A Primary Prevention Approach: Health Education

The purpose of health education is to positively change behavior by increasing knowledge about health and disease. Health education is an important nursing intervention,

---

BOX 2–3 ■ Public Health Interventions

Advocacy pleads someone's cause or act on someone's behalf, with a focus on developing the community, system, individual, or family's capacity to plead their own cause or act on their own behalf.

Case finding locates individuals and families with identified risk factors and connects them with resources.

Case management optimizes self-care capabilities of individuals and families and the capacity of systems and communities to coordinate and provide services.

Coalition building promotes and develops alliances among organizations or constituencies for a common purpose. It builds linkages, solves problems, and/or enhances local leadership to address health concerns.

Collaboration commits two or more people or organizations to achieve a common goal through enhancing the capacity of one or more of the members to promote and protect health. (Henneman, Lee, & Cohen. [1995]. Collaboration: A concept analysis. *Journal of Advanced Nursing, 21*, 103-109.)

Community organizing helps community groups to identify common problems or goals, mobilize resources, and develop and implement strategies for reaching the goals they collectively have set. (Minkler, M. [Ed.]. [1997]. *Community organizing and community building for health* [p 30]. New Brunswick, NJ: Rutgers University Press.) Delegated functions are direct care tasks that a registered professional nurse carries out under the authority of a health-care practitioner as allowed by law. Delegated functions also include any direct care tasks that a professional registered nurse entrusts to other appropriate personnel to perform.

Consultation seeks information and generates optional solutions to perceived problems or issues through interactive problem-solving with a community, system, family, or an individual. The community, system, family,

or individual selects and acts on the option best meeting the circumstances.

Counseling establishes an interpersonal relationship with the community, a system, the family, or an individual intended to increase or enhance their capacity for self-care and coping. Counseling engages the community, a system, family, or an individual at an emotional level.

Disease and other health event investigation systematically gathers and analyzes data regarding threats to the health of populations, ascertains the source of the threat, identifies cases and others at risk, and determines control measures.

Health teaching communicates facts, ideas, and skills that change knowledge, attitudes, values, beliefs, behaviors, and practices of individuals, families, systems, and/or communities. (Adapted from American Nurses Association [2010]. *Nursing's social policy statement: The essence of the profession.* [2010]. Silver Springs, MD; American Nurses Publishing.)

Outreach locates populations-of-interest or populations-at-risk and provides information about the nature of the concern, what can be done about it, and how services can be obtained.

Policy development places health issues on decision makers' agendas, acquires a plan of resolution, and determines needed resources. Policy development results in laws, rules and regulations, ordinances, and policies.

Policy enforcement compels others to comply with the laws, rules, regulations, ordinances, and policies created in conjunction with policy development. (Minnesota Department of Health, Division of Community Health Services, Public Health Section. [2001]. *Public health interventions: Applications for public health nursing practice.* Retrieved from http://www.health.state.mn.us/divs/opi/cd/phn/docs/0301wheel_manual.pdf.).

BOX 2–3 ■ Public Health Interventions—cont'd

Referral and follow-up assist individuals, families, groups, organizations, and/or communities to identify and access necessary resources to prevent or resolve problems or concerns.

Screening identifies individuals with unrecognized health risk factors or asymptomatic disease conditions in populations.

Social marketing uses commercial marketing principles and technologies for programs designed to influence the knowledge, attitudes, values, beliefs, behaviors, and practices of the population-of-interest.

Surveillance describes and monitors health events through ongoing and systematic collection, analysis, and interpretation of health data for the purpose of planning, implementing, and evaluating public health interventions (Centers for Disease Control and Prevention. [2012]. CDC's vision for public health surveillance in the 21st century. *Morbidity and Mortality Weekly Report, S61*).

Source: (34)

---

and it is important in changing behavior at all levels of prevention. The Joint Committee on Health Education and Promotion Terminology defined **health education** as learning aimed at acquiring information and skills related to making health decisions.[36] The WHO defines **health education** as "… any combination of learning experiences designed to help individuals and communities improve their health, by increasing their knowledge or influencing their attitudes…"[37] Health education involves not just teaching but also encouraging and giving confidence to people to take the necessary action to improve health, which includes making changes in social, economic, and environmental determinants of health.

Theories of Education

Because health education involves teaching, understanding how people learn is essential to effective teaching. There are a number of learning theories that help us understand how learning occurs from both a physiological and social basis. The main theories come under four categories: behaviorism, cognitivism, constructivism, and humanism.

Behaviorism is the theory of classical conditioning. In this framework, the behavior change is what is important, and it is achieved with an environmental stimulus that results in a response. The focus is only on the observed behavior change and not on the mental activity. Learning is based on reward and punishment by conditioning (e.g., when a monkey learns to push a button for a reward of food).[38]

The cognitive framework focuses more strongly on inner mental activity. It is more rational than it is on reflexively responding to an external stimulus. There is behavior change as a result of knowledge that has changed thought patterns. It frequently occurs as a result of varied sensory inputs with repetition. The social learning theory of Bandura is rooted in both the behavior and cognitive frameworks, emphasizing that understanding, in addition to behavior and environment, are all interrelated. He stresses imitation of a behavior and reinforcement in learning.[39] An example of Bandura's theory of social learning is television commercials. An action is portrayed, eating a certain food or using a certain cleaning product, and the audience, seeing it as desirable, is encouraged to model or imitate that behavior.

Constructivism is a learning theory that reflects on our own experiences.[40] We actively construct our own world as we increase our experience and knowledge. It is a process that builds knowledge within our own unique framework. A good example is problem-solving learning. To learn, students are actively involved in integrating new knowledge in their own frameworks with guidance from the teacher. For example, children can learn about what happens to their heart rate with exercise by experimenting with different types of exercise and counting pulse rates. They experience the concept of a heart rate rather than merely having it verbally explained to them.

Humanism learning uses feelings and relationships, encouraging the development of personal actions to fulfill one's potential and achieve self-actualization.[38] It is self-directed learning, examining personal motivation and goals. This is also a theory of adult learning.[40] As an example, an individual diagnosed with elevated cholesterol purchases books, seeks out articles, talks with knowledgeable people, and in general informs him- or herself about the problem and actions to take to solve the problem then self-initiates these activities to improve health.

All learning theories influence how we teach. The identified teaching methods based on these theories are varied but include the need to be developmentally appropriate with children and with adults with varying levels of education. Many of the more recent theories provide a more balanced learning; encourage experiential learning; and solve real problems in real places by using role playing, visual stimuli, service learning, interpersonal learning, and the promotion of complex higher-order thinking.

Adult Learning

Pedagogy (pedagogical learning) is the correct use of teaching strategies to provide the best learning. **Andragogy** is similar but is specifically the art and science of helping adults learn using the correct strategies.[40] In nursing, we are often teaching adults, as it is adults who generally develop chronic diseases, are in a position to promote health, and care for children. In the 1950s Malcolm Knowles, using humanism learning theory, suggested that adults learn differently from children and that the role of the instructor is quite different. Adults bring a great deal of experience to the learning situation, and this experience influences what education they receive and how they receive it.[41] They are active learners and need to see applications for the new learning. Knowles identified six suppositions for adult learning:

1. The adult needs to know why he or she is learning something.
2. The adult's own experiences are an important part of the learning process.
3. Adults need to participate in the planning and evaluation of their learning.
4. Adults learn better if the information has immediate relevance.
5. Adults like problem-centered approaches to learning.
6. Adults respond better to internal rather than to external motivation.

The role of the teacher in this situation is to direct the learner.[41]

To be an effective educator the nurse needs to be flexible. Nurses organize the learning experience by first assessing the individual's or population's learning needs. They then select the best learning format, create the best possible learning environment, and send a clear message. The learning should be participatory and include evaluation and feedback.

Health Literacy

One of the first considerations before planning health education is to consider the health literacy of the individual client, the group, or the population. In conjunction with literacy, culture and language should also be included. **Health literacy** is defined as "the degree to which individuals have the capacity to obtain, process, and understand basic health information and services needed to make appropriate health decisions."[42] The HMD division of the National Academies of Sciences, Engineering, and Medicine built on this definition and added key issues related to the individual receiving information. They stated that health literacy is something that "emerges when the expectations, preferences, and skills of individuals seeking health information and services meet the expectations, preferences, and skills of those providing information and services. Health literacy arises from a convergence of education, health services, and social and cultural factors."[42]

Assessing literacy levels is currently done based on levels, with levels 4 and 5 representing the top level and level 1 and below representing the lowest literacy level. According to the National Center for Education Statistics, 18% of U.S. adults scored at or below level 1.[43] They reported an association between age and literacy with a greater percentage of those between the ages of 25 and 44 scoring at the top level. For those who were unemployed, 75% had 12 years of education or less and approximately a third scored at level 1 or below.[44] There is evidence of a causal relationship between health literacy and health outcomes. Those individuals with basic health literacy had a higher level of health-care utilization and higher expenditures for prescriptions.[45] To address the problem of health literacy the CDC put together five talking points about health literacy that can be adapted to a specific organization as a means to advocate for promotion of heath literacy (Box 2-4).[46]

Shame and stigma of having low health literacy have been found to be major barriers to seeking care. The IOM committee found that health education occurred in most primary and secondary schools, but there was no universal sequencing, and only about 10% of teachers were qualified health educators. One of the most telling of the IOM findings was that health professionals had limited training in patient/population education and had few opportunities to develop skills to improve a patient's health literacy. The IOM gave multiple suggestions on how to improve health literacy, and points of intervention (Fig. 2-6). Some of the most relevant to nursing included:

- Improve K through 12 basic health education.
- Help individuals learn how to assess the credibility of what they see and read about health.
- Provide clear communication, allow ample time to give this information, and encourage questions from the patient.[42]

BOX 2–4 ■ The CDC's Five Talking Points on Health Literacy

You are a health literacy ambassador. It is up to you to make sure your colleagues, staff, leadership, and community are aware of the issues. Whether to review for yourself, present to others, or convince your leadership, the following resources may help you talk about health literacy.

Five Talking Points on Health Literacy: These brief talking points may be helpful if you need to tell someone quickly what health literacy is and why it is important. Add in talking points relevant to your organization.

1. Nine out of 10 adults struggle to understand and use health information when it is unfamiliar, complex, or jargon-filled.

2. Limited health literacy costs the health-care system money and results in higher than necessary morbidity and mortality.
3. Health literacy can be improved if we practice clear communication strategies and techniques.
4. Clear communication means using familiar concepts, words, numbers, and images presented in ways that make sense to the people who need the information.
5. Testing information with the audience before it is released and asking for feedback are the best ways to know if we are communicating clearly. We need to test and ask for feedback every time information is released to the general public.

Source: (45)

Potential Intervention Points

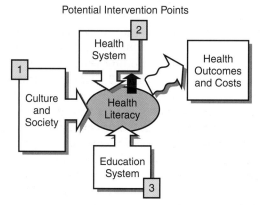

Figure 2-6 Potential points for intervention in the health literacy framework. *(From Nielsen-Bohlman, L., Panzer, A., Kindig, D. [2004]. Health literacy: A prescription to end confusion [IOM Report].)*

BOX 2–5 ■ Health Literacy Universal Precautions

Health literacy universal precautions are the steps that practices take when they assume that all patients may have difficulty comprehending health information and accessing health services. Health literacy universal precautions are aimed at:

• Simplifying communication with and confirming comprehension for all patients, so that the risk of miscommunication is minimized.
• Making the office environment and health-care system easier to navigate.
• Supporting patients' efforts to improve their health.

Source: (47)

In the past few years, considerable research has been done that brings better understanding to the magnitude and consequences of the health literacy problem. One of the issues is how to assess correctly and rapidly the level of health literacy in a patient/population. Though there are tools to screen for health literacy, they were developed primarily for research purposes and are not currently recommended for routine use. Instead the recommendation is to use **universal health literacy precautions**, which translates into providing patients with information both oral and written that is understandable and easily accessible to persons across all education levels.[47] The AHRQ recommends use of universal health literacy precautions and lays out what needs to be done (Box 2-5). The AHRQ developed an evidenced-based toolkit for health-care providers to help implement universal health literacy precautions within a health-care setting. The goal is to increase the health literacy of all patients, not just those that appear to need assistance.[48]

Develop a Teaching Plan

Writing a teaching plan for individuals or populations provides a means to lay out what will be taught, using what methods, as well as a method for evaluating the effectiveness of the teaching plan (Box 2-6). The teaching begins with the assessment of the health education need. What does this individual or population need to learn, or what would they benefit from learning, to promote health, prevent disease, or help manage an identified health problem? Next, the nurse assesses the type of learner or learners who will receive the education. For example, what is their level of health literacy? Also, what is the cultural context for the population? What is their

BOX 2–6 ■ Steps in Developing a Health Education Teaching Plan

1. Identify the health education need in the selected population (individual/family/community).
2. Assess the learner; include health literacy, culture, language, age, and learning style.
3. Write a goal for the teaching intervention.
4. Write specific, measurable objectives for the teaching intervention (consider Bloom's Taxonomy).
5. Identify materials and resources needed for the teaching plan; include the appropriate teaching environment and the length of the lesson.
6. Describe the lesson; include key concepts.
7. Write out the procedure step by step for teaching the lesson using a variety of teaching methods.
8. Have a plan for the evaluation.

age, gender, and level of vulnerability? All of this information will help drive how the information is provided. Inclusion of the recipients in the planning process can be an important strategy as can be the use of peer teachers.

Once the assessment has been completed, the next step is to identify the goal(s) of the health education

■ CULTURAL CONTEXT

National Institutes of Health: Clear Communication

The NIH Office of Communications and Public Liaison (OCPL) established a "Clear Communication" initiative related to health literacy with cultural respect as one of the two foci of the initiative. Specifically:

- *Cultural respect is a strategy that enables organizations to work effectively in cross-cultural situations. Developing and implementing a framework of cultural competence in health systems is an extended process that ultimately serves to reduce health disparities and improve access to high-quality health care.*
- *Cultural respect benefits consumers, stakeholders, and communities. Because a number of elements can influence health communication—including behaviors, language, customs, beliefs, and perspectives—cultural respect is also critical for achieving accuracy in medical research. NIH funds and works with researchers nationwide for the development and dissemination of resources designed to enhance cultural respect in health-care systems.[49]*

Further resources are available through their Web site.

program. Again, inclusion of the recipients in the program will result in shared goals and greater engagement of those receiving the program. For example, if from the nurse's perspective the goal of a proposed health education program is to reduce premature births, including women in the community who are pregnant or who may become pregnant in the development of the program may help shape the articulation of goals. What are the immediate benefits to them for having a full-term baby? What other issues are they concerned about related to pregnancy and birth? This way specific objectives can be written that truly meet the goals of the community.

To help frame learning objectives, Bloom identified three learning domains: cognitive, affective, and psychomotor.[50] Identifying which learning domain is being targeted is important when developing the plan. Within the cognitive domain, Bloom identified six levels of cognitive learning, from simple knowledge recall to more abstract and higher-level synthesis and evaluation. Each level, especially the first three, builds on the next. This is referred to as Bloom's Taxonomy, and this classification is useful in looking at levels of learning, outcomes, and the correct action verbs to be used when writing specific-level learning objectives (Box 2-7). The first level of learning is knowledge, which refers to remembering or recalling specific information that has been taught. Comprehension is the second level and requires some demonstration of really understanding what was learned. Application, the third level, requires using the knowledge in real situations such as problem-solving. The next level is analysis, wherein the acquired knowledge is broken down by its organization and things such as making inferences and looking for motives or causes. The last two are synthesis and evaluation. In synthesis, the acquired knowledge is used creatively to produce something new. Evaluation provides a way to judge the end product. In addition to cognitive learning, Bloom also identified affective and psychomotor learning. The affective domain looks at a growth in feelings, values, and attitudes. Psychomotor learning is the development of manual or physical skills, a domain frequently taught by nurses.

Once the plan is developed, the next step requires identifying materials and resources needed for effective teaching. Factors include the length of the lesson, where it will be taught, what activities will promote the best learning, and how much time will be needed to prepare the lesson. It is helpful to write out a description of the lesson including the key concepts and the learning domain of knowledge, attitude, and/or practice. The final two steps are to write out the detailed procedure for the

---

BOX 2–7 ■ Bloom's Taxonomy of Learning*

Knowledge	Comprehension	Application	Analysis	Synthesis	Evaluation
Define	Discuss	Interpret	Distinguish	Plan	Judge
Repeat	Recognize	Apply	Calculate	Design	Appraise
List	Explain	Use	Test	Assemble	Value
Name	Interpret	Practice	Compare	Invent	Assess
Tell	Outline	Demonstrate	Question	Compose	Estimate
Describe	Distinguish	Solve	Analyze	Predict	Select
Relate	Predict	Show	Examine	Construct	Choose
Locate	Restate	Illustrate	Compare	Imagine	Decide
Write	Translate	Construct	Contrast	Propose	Justify
Find	Compare	Complete	Investigate	Devise	Debate
State	Describe	Examine	Categorize	Formulate	Verify
Arrange	Classify	Classify	Identify	Create	Argue
Duplicate	Express	Choose	Explain	Organize	Recommend
Memorize	Identify	Dramatize	Separate	Arrange	Discuss
Order	Indicate	Employ	Advertise	Prepare	Rate
	Locate	Practice	Appraise	Propose	Prioritize
					Determine

Source: (49)

*Active verbs represent each level.

---

teaching plan, carefully outlining each activity, and, if appropriate, the follow-up for these activities. The final component is to determine how an evaluation will measure whether or not the intended learning took place. The evaluation plan should reflect the learning objectives and be in place before teaching begins to anticipate how to measure the outcomes.

Methods of Instruction

There are many ways to learn the same information, and each of us has a preference for how we like to learn. There are lists of different teaching methods that include formal presentations, small-group work, field trips, role playing, written assignments, and Internet activities, to identify a few. Usually, experiential learning is most effective for adults. Lecture format rarely appeals to an adult who wants guided interactive learning. If people can feel it, handle it, see it, taste it, smell it, and discuss it, they can better integrate it into their own life experiences. A group concerned with nutrition and being overweight may be told that Ritz crackers, potato chips, corn chips, and cheeseburgers are high in fat and also high in calories. The group can be given numbers of calories and grams, but it is not easily integrated into their life experiences. However, if the portion size of four Ritz crackers, 10 potato chips, and 1 ounce of corn chips, all having 8 to 9 grams of fat, are demonstrated, it is easier for people to put it into the context of their own lives.

Using real-life scenarios to teach how to solve health problems has also been quite effective. Giving new mothers a vignette in which a family is having difficulty getting adequate sleep at night because their 4-month-old infant is awake all night allows for group discussion and problem-solving that can be relevant at the moment. This is information these women can take home and apply immediately. Teaching children the importance of exercise by using videos, Internet, and PowerPoint slides can be entertaining and provide basic knowledge. Helping children form walking groups and joining them for their walks can help them apply this knowledge and start to change behavior. Written material can help encourage discussion, but the material must be appropriate for literacy, content, culture, and language.

Regardless of the teaching method, it is always important to emphasize the benefits of the proposed behavior change and to personalize the message. A good strategy is to apply the intended new behavior within the context of the individual's lifestyle and needs. Help clients weigh the cost and benefit of the new health behavior. Key points should be emphasized during teaching and new information provided in small increments. Most people can absorb only one or two new pieces of information in an encounter. Learners are the best source of information about what they want to learn and if the teaching method is meeting their needs. Feedback should be frequently sought from learners.

The environment should not be neglected in a teaching plan. The physical environment is important and should be maximized as much as possible even when many things in a community setting may be outside of one's control. A space should be the right size, have a comfortable temperature, adequate places to sit, the necessary resources for the planned lesson, and a place where, as appropriate, the learners can receive and share confidential information. However, one also needs to create an environment conducive to learning in which the learner has space to be an active learner and to learn from real situations with someone to assist with guidance and direction to master the material. It should be a place in which individuals feel free to voice opinions, experiment with new ideas, and identify what they do not know; a place in which there is enthusiasm for learning in a nonthreatening environment.

Evaluation

Successful learning changes behavior. Deciding how to evaluate whether this learning has occurred requires referring back to the specific objectives for the level of learning that was to take place and the specific outcomes expected. If the first stage of teaching was to increase knowledge, an appropriate method is needed to measure whether the knowledge did increase. If the objective was for the mother to explain how the different childhood immunizations will keep her child healthy and prevent disease, the mothers should be asked to repeat back the information they have just received or play a game in which they have to know the answers to specific factual questions. If the objective was to help individuals apply knowledge, the applied learning should be evaluated in a different way. For application, one can provide a scenario at the end of the teaching session and then note how students solve the problems utilizing the information just taught. A follow-up discussion with the group may be held after they have had time to apply their new knowledge. If the objective was for the mother to practice primary prevention by having her child fully immunized by 2 years of age, the mother's behavior may be observed after the teaching to determine whether the knowledge has been applied and the child has been fully immunized.

There are several tools that can be used to evaluate health education. It is always a good idea to ask for verbal reaction to the teaching at the end of a teaching session. This is useful in planning for future health education sessions. To measure an increase in knowledge, a classic pre- and post-test should be used, or a pre- and post-interview/observation. Using a formal testing method is frequently not well liked by adult learners, especially those who have limited literacy skills. They respond better to the oral interview, but this is more difficult to carry out. To assess change, one can observe and interview over a specific time period, especially to note the sustainability of the change. These tools need to be thoughtfully developed to provide objective, reliable data. Likewise, long-term effects of the teaching may be evaluated using objective predesigned tools (for more complete discussion of evaluation, see Chapter 5).

Health education forms the basis for many health prevention programs aimed at improving the health of individuals as well as of families. Nurses learn this skill first with individuals, then families, and finally with populations and communities. Health education operates under the assumption that improving health literacy is central to improving health. In addition to health education, other activities regularly performed by nurses, such as screening, contribute to building the health of communities. Often these activities require the use of health education as a strategy to improve full participation in the prevention activity.

A Secondary Prevention Approach: Screening and Early Identification

Just as health education is the basis of many primary prevention programs, screening is central to secondary prevention. The classic definition of **screening** is the presumptive identification of unrecognized disease or defect by the application of tests, examinations, or other procedures that can be applied rapidly to sort out those with a high probability of having the disease from a large group of apparently well people.[51] Screening is not diagnostic and only indicates who may or may not have a disease or a risk factor for disease.

Nurses routinely screen for health risks and disease across health-care settings. This type of intervention clearly fits within the secondary prevention phase of the traditional public health prevention model. This allows for early identification and treatment of disease as well as the reduction of risk for those who are at greatest risk for developing disease or sustaining injury. A good example is blood pressure screening. If those with hypertension are identified prior to development of clinical symptoms, the institution of behavioral and clinical interventions such as diet modification and the use of a diuretic can bring the individual's blood pressure back to within the normal range and prevent adverse health consequences associated with hypertension, such as stroke. Screening conducted to detect risk factors in people without disease includes screening for at-risk drinking or fall risk. This type of screening is aimed at distinguishing those with a higher risk for developing disease or injury from those with low risk. For example, screening for at-risk drinking not only identifies those who may have an alcohol use disorder but also identifies those with a current drinking pattern that puts them at risk for developing an alcohol use disorder, developing alcohol-related adverse consequences, or experiencing alcohol-related injury (see Chapter 11).

When using the traditional public health model, screening clearly falls into the category of secondary prevention. The purpose is to identify within a group of apparently well people those who probably have the disease. For those with complex risk factors and a less clear natural history of disease, the traditional model has less utility. This is true with mental health, substance use disorders, and injury. In these cases, screening is done for the purpose of detecting risk for disease or injury prior to the occurrence of disease as well as the detection of disease in those who are apparently well. It can be classified as both primary and secondary prevention.

Using a continuum of health approach to prevention provides a broader context for understanding the role of screening as a prevention intervention. Screening includes identification of those with risk factors for disease or injury as well as those with subclinical disease. In the first case the assumption is that early detection of risk and delivery of risk reduction interventions will reduce disease or injury from occurring. In the second case, the assumption is that early identification and treatment of those with disease will result in reduction of the morbidity and mortality associated with the disease. This allows for screening to prevent disease or injury from occurring in the first place (primary prevention) as well as to prevent adverse health consequences that can be avoided with early detection and treatment of disease (secondary).

Most diseases are associated with a complex set of risk factors and often do not progress in a linear fashion. In addition, the broader continuum health model takes into account not only adverse physical outcomes, but also psychological, social, and economic outcomes. An example of screening that reflects primary prevention is the approach being used to prevent childhood obesity. Screening for risk factors such as inactivity and high caloric intake can help identify children without disease who would most benefit from an intervention. Thus, the screening process is conducted in a population without disease to separate those with a high probability for developing disease or sustaining an injury from those with low or no risk factors for the disease or injury.

Diagnosis, Screening, and Monitoring

The difference between diagnosis, screening, and monitoring is often blurred. For example, taking blood pressure readings at a blood pressure screening event that only includes people who have not been diagnosed with hypertension is clearly screening, detecting probable disease in a population of apparently well people. Taking a blood pressure reading for a patient every 4 hours on a medical-surgical unit in the hospital is done to monitor the patient's vital signs and detect possible changes in the patient's status, and it is not a screening activity. Taking blood pressure readings at a booth at a health fair where many of the participants come to the booth and state that they have hypertension and need to know how they are doing is a combination of screening and monitoring, because many of the participants have already been diagnosed. The nurse practitioner or physician takes a blood pressure reading during a physical work-up to assist in establishing a differential diagnosis for hypertension. The same activity is done to screen, monitor, or assist in obtaining a diagnosis.

For each of these activities, there are set parameters for the measure. In the case of monitoring the patient, the nurse compares the most recent blood pressure reading with the patient's baseline reading and the readings over the admission to determine whether there has been a change in the patient's status. The blood pressure reading is part of a larger nursing assessment and, if the reading reflects a change in the patient's status, the nurse may change the plan of care for either a positive or negative change. When using the blood pressure reading from a diagnostic standpoint, there are specific guidelines for the clinician, and the blood pressure levels are based on the average of two or more readings. These readings are taken during the course of two or more visits.[26] Using the guidelines, the clinician can make a diagnosis of stage 1 or stage 2 hypertension, or classify the patients as prehypertensive. The guidelines have been revised based on growing evidence related to both hypertension and the development of a new category of risk, prehypertension, and are evidence based.[26]

The guidelines state that the process for diagnosing hypertension occurs after an initial screening. So how does the screening differ from the diagnostic stage because the same measurement is taken—a blood pressure reading using standard equipment? In this case, the main difference is that the screening is based on one reading rather than two or more blood pressure readings over a number of visits, and the purpose of taking the blood pressure reading is to identify those who may be hypertensive and are in need of further assessment and possible treatment. The clinician conducting the screening will refer the individual whose blood pressure meets the cutoff for probable hypertension to a clinician who is qualified to conduct the needed assessment and is able to make a differential diagnosis.

Sensitivity and Specificity

For all of these activities—screening, monitoring, and diagnosis—the clinician must have a clear understanding of the reliability and validity of the measure chosen to screen for risk and/or probability of disease. Understanding the reliability and validity of a screening tool provides the clinician conducting the screening with the guidelines for deciding what is a positive screen and what is a negative screen, that is, who most probably has the disease and who most probably does not. Or in the case of screening for risk, it provides the guidelines for deciding what is considered high risk and what is considered low risk. In the case of blood pressure screening, the screening is done for the most part using the same basic instrument used to diagnose disease and monitor physical status, but for other health issues, the screening tool is different from the diagnostic tool. Determining the validity of the instrument for screening uses different criteria than for diagnosis or for monitoring status.

In screening, the reliability and validity of the instrument is crucial. **Reliability** is defined as the ability of the instrument to give consistent results on repeated trials. **Validity** is defined as the degree to which the instrument measures what it is supposed to measure. For screening instruments, the two aspects of validity that are the main concerns are the sensitivity and the specificity of the instrument. **Sensitivity** is defined as the ability of the screening test to give a positive finding when the person truly has the disease, or true positive. **Specificity** is defined as the ability of the screening test to give a negative finding when the person truly does not have the disease, or true negative.

● APPLYING PUBLIC HEALTH SCIENCE

The Case of the Silent Killer

Public Health Science Topics Covered:

- Screening
- Population assessment
- Health planning

Choosing a screening instrument requires understanding the importance of both sensitivity and specificity. For example, in a hypothetical case a team of nurses at a large urban hospital noticed that there had been an increase in admissions of African American men with a diagnosis of cardiovascular disease secondary to hypertension. They wanted to put a large-scale blood pressure screening program in place for the African American men in their city to improve early detection of hypertension and potentially reduce the need for hospitalization. Prior to implementing the program, they wanted to make sure that the method they used to screen for hypertension was valid. This was important for two reasons. First, they did not want to have too many false negatives. In other words, they wanted to identify as many men as possible with hypertension because there was such a high morbidity and mortality rate for untreated hypertension in the male African American population. Second, they did not want too many false positives, because this population had limited resources to pay for care. Unnecessary visits to the physician could result in reduced participation in the program, especially because an accurate diagnosis requires more than one visit to a health-care provider. Too many false positives could result in unnecessary utilization of health-care resources.

Prior to initiating a full-scale screening program, the nurses conducted a pilot with 250 African American men who had not been diagnosed with hypertension, who were not taking antihypertensive (blood pressure–lowering) drugs, and who were not acutely ill. To do the screening, they used a standard blood pressure cuff and stethoscope and measured the blood pressure in millimeters of mercury (mm Hg). The nurses debated over the cutoff point. The 2017 guidelines for a diagnosis of stage one hypertension is a blood pressure reading greater than or equal to 130 systolic (mm Hg) or greater than or equal to 80 diastolic was not yet released.[26] Thus, they chose the then-current diagnostic criteria of a blood pressure reading greater than or equal to 140 systolic (mm Hg) or greater than or equal to 90 diastolic. To evaluate the sensitivity and specificity of the screening, all the participants were asked to complete three follow-up visits with a primary care physician to establish whether or not the participants had hypertension. Because this was a pilot study, the nurses obtained written consent from the participants and followed the Internal Review Board process required by their institution.

Once they had obtained approval, the nurses conducted the pilot study with 250 participants. First, the nurses screened the participants for possible hypertension by obtaining a blood pressure reading. They then obtained follow-up data on all 250 in relation to whether or not they were diagnosed with stage one or stage two hypertension based on the current classification of hypertension for adults age 18 years and older. A diagnosis of hypertension is based on the average of two readings greater than or equal to 130 systolic (mm Hg) or greater than or equal to 80 diastolic.[26] The nurses then calculated basic frequencies on their data and found that 55 of the participants screened positive for hypertension and, on follow-up, 55 were diagnosed with hypertension. On the surface, it looked as though their screening instrument was 100% sensitive as they correctly identified all who had the disease, but that was not the case.

To determine the sensitivity and specificity of the method they used to screen for hypertension, the nurses constructed a two-by-two matrix using screening and diagnostic data (Fig. 2-7). They determined the number of participants that belonged in each box of the matrix. Each box of the matrix corresponds to four different categories of participants: (1) those who were true positives, that is, they screened positive and the physician diagnosed them with hypertension, box A;

(2) those who were false negatives, that is, they screened negative but the physician diagnosed them with hypertension, box C; (3) those who were false positives, that is, they screened positive and the physician did not diagnose them with hypertension, box B; and (4) those who were true negatives, that is, they screened negative and the physician did not diagnose them with hypertension, box D.

Using these numbers, the nurses examined the sensitivity of their instrument. They took the total of all the persons who had positive screens and were subsequently diagnosed with either stage one or stage two hypertension and divided it by the total number of people diagnosed with the hypertension and multiplied this by 100. Another way to express this formula is to use the letters in the lower right-hand corner of two of the boxes in the matrix, boxes A and C. The total number of true positives, or A, is 40, and the total number with disease (true positives plus false negatives) equals 55, or A + C. Thus, the formula for sensitivity is $(A/(A + C)) \times 100$. In this example, the sensitivity is: $(40/55) \times 100$, or 72.7%

They then determined the specificity of their instrument. To do this, they repeated what they had done with sensitivity, but now they were concerned with the relationship between those who were true negatives and the total number who screened negative. Again, the letters in the lower right-hand corner of the boxes are used to construct the formula, but this time the boxes of interest are boxes B and D. The total number of participants who are true negatives, or D, is 180, and the total number without disease equals 195, or D + B. The formula for specificity is $(D/(B + D)) \times 100$. In this example, the specificity is: $(180/(15 + 180)) \times 100 = 92.3\%$

In this example, the specificity of the screening test was higher at 92.3% than the sensitivity that is 72.7%. More than 25% of the participants who had hypertension would have been missed if the participants relied on screening alone, but less than 10% of those without disease were incorrectly identified as possibly having hypertension when they actually did not have the disease (see Fig. 2-5). The nurses had met one of their requirements for the program (high specificity) but not the other requirement of high sensitivity. How could they address these issues?

First, they could look at the reliability of the instrument they were using to obtain the blood pressure reading. Because the method of measurement for screening and diagnosis in this case is the same, the

Screening for stage 1 or 2 hypertension with 250 persons

A = True positives (screened positive and had the disease)

B = False positives (screened positive and did not have the disease)

C = False negatives (screened negative and had the disease)

D = True negatives (screened negative and did not have the disease)

Disease (+ = BP ≥140/90)			
Screening Results	Yes	No	Total
Yes	40	15	55
	A	B	
No	15	180	195
	C	D	
Total	55	195	250

Figure 2-7 Sensitivity and specificity matrix.

reliability could be a concern. There are two possible issues: variation in the method and observer variation. Observer variation has been known to happen when taking blood pressures using the standard method owing to observer variation in hearing acuity and experience in taking blood pressures. The nurses actually addressed this issue prior to conducting the pilot study. They did both inter-rater and intra-rater reliability, testing at baseline for the nurses who would conduct the screening. For the inter-rater reliability, they had different nurses take the blood pressure on the same individual to determine the variation between each rater's blood pressure reading. For intra-rater reliability, they compared one nurse or rater's measure of repeated blood pressures on the same person. They initially found low inter- and intra-rater reliability between the nurses. They then conducted a blood pressure training workshop for all the nurses who participated in the screening. Following training, the reliability of the measure was high.

Because the nurses felt confident that they had been using a reliable instrument, they considered adjusting their cutoff point. As they were working on the project the 2017 Guideline for the Prevention, Detection, Evaluation, and Management of High Blood Pressure in Adults was released. They decided to reexamine the sensitivity and reliability of their screening using the new criteria for stage one hypertension of a blood pressure reading greater than or equal to 130 systolic (mm Hg) or greater than or equal to 80 diastolic. Adjusting the cutoff point to a lower value could improve the sensitivity of the screening process, but would it result in reducing the specificity as they first feared? Making this decision was done not only based on the new guidelines, but also by comparing the consequences of a false negative with the consequences of a false positive. In this case, a false positive would result in extra visits to the physician, whereas a false negative would result in untreated disease. Missing more than a quarter of the population being screened was a serious problem. Hypertension is known as the silent killer, that is, the disease has few if any clinical symptoms until damage has occurred. A person with the disease often does not know he or she has it until damage has already occurred.

The nurses plotted the blood pressure readings on a chart to help determine the cutoff point for 100% sensitivity and 100% specificity to help decide whether a lower cutoff point would increase sensitivity while still maintaining adequate specificity. Plotting out the

normal distribution of the blood pressure values in those with hypertension and those without hypertension helped to illustrate what would happen if they changed the cutoff value (Fig. 2-8). If they changed the value to 130/80, they would have 100% sensitivity, but their specificity would drop to nearly 50%. If they shifted the cutoff point to 145/95, they would achieve 100% specificity but decrease their sensitivity to less than 70%. Choosing a cutoff value is always a compromise. In this case, the nurses decided to use the diagnostic criteria for stage one hypertension as their cutoff point. This increased their sensitivity to over 80% whereas the specificity decreased only a small amount to a little less than 90%.

Armed with the information on the reliability and validity of their screening method, the nurses were ready to present a proposal to their hospital for conducting the hypertension screening program as a citywide outreach program for the hospital. They approached the director of the community outreach department with their information, sure that they would be able to proceed. The director asked them questions to which they could not respond, so they went back to obtain more information.

The first question the director posed was, "What is the expected yield of the screening program?" The nurses were not sure what this meant. They found that the **yield** is defined as the number of previously undiagnosed cases of disease that result in treatment following screening. They already had a crucial piece of information, the sensitivity of the screening program they proposed. The higher the sensitivity is, the greater the potential yield will be. The next issue related to

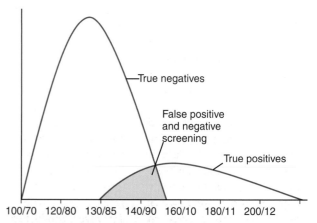

Figure 2-8 Distribution of blood pressure readings in those with and without hypertension.

yield is the prevalence of undetected disease. This depends on the duration of the disease, the duration of the subclinical phase of the disease, and the level of available care. The natural history of disease (see Fig. 2-2) was a helpful guide for the nurses. They went back to their original literature review related to hypertension and once again found clear evidence that the duration of the subclinical phase (stage 1) can be long, and early treatment can have significant effects on reducing morbidity and mortality. They also reviewed the statistics on access to care for the low-income African American population with high levels of poverty in their city. Owing to changes in the cutoff for Medicaid eligibility in their state, access to care was limited and African American males in the immediate area were less likely to have regular physical checkups. The nurses also charted out the current national estimates on the prevalence of undiagnosed hypertension in African American males. They found that more than 40% of African Americans have hypertension, and hypertension was often not diagnosed in this population until individuals became symptomatic.[52,53]

The nurses concluded that, because of the high sensitivity of their screening method and the high prevalence in the target population, the potential yield was high. However, they had not reviewed the availability of medical care. Because they needed to determine whether treatment was available for those who screened positive, they did a review of all the primary care clinics in the area. They also reviewed their pilot data on the resources used by the participants to identify which primary care clinics were most frequently used. They then contacted these clinics to determine whether the clinics would be able to handle a large influx of potentially new clients following the screening. The nurses were able to establish that the existing primary care system was sufficient and that the majority of clinics and primary care offices were willing to put in writing their support for the project.

The second question the director asked had to do with **multiphasic screening**, defined as administering multiple tests to detect multiple conditions during the same screening program. The nurses had not considered this idea, but felt it had merit and reviewed the current information on health and African American males. They found that colorectal cancer (CRC) and high cholesterol were two other serious health problems for African American males. However, conducting CRC screening would require a different approach owing to the complexity of the screening procedure. Although combining blood pressure screening with screening for high cholesterol was promising, it was more invasive and would require purchasing more supplies, possibly using more personnel. The nurses also did not have pilot data to provide information on the sensitivity and specificity of screening with a sample from the target population, so they would have to rely on national data.

The director had also asked about the cost benefit of the program. Because they were asking the hospital to fund this program, the director wanted to know the possible benefits of the program related to cost, simplicity of administration, safety, and acceptability of the population. The nurses mapped out the actual budget of the proposed program. Because no new equipment was needed, the majority of the cost was in staff time. To reduce costs, the nurses collected a pool of nurse volunteers willing to participate in the program. The taking of blood pressures is safe and noninvasive, and takes little time to complete. This helps reduce cost because the time needed to conduct the screening per individual is short.

When reviewing the acceptability of the program, they were careful not to make the assumption that, because blood pressure clinics are common, the population they wished to engage would come to theirs. They had asked the participants in their pilot study for feedback on the best site for conducting the screening and they also enlisted the help of members of the community in identifying the right sites and means of advertising the program. They also reviewed the literature for evidence of other successful screening programs with African American males. Though some of the participants had mentioned schools or churches as good sites, the site that was mentioned most and also supported in the literature was the local barbershop.

The nurses shared their data with the director and reported that the blood pressure screening program they proposed had a potentially high yield and the cost would be low given the availability of volunteers. They suggested that the screening program be conducted in the local barbershops but recommended that further work be done to develop a partnership with the owners of these shops prior to implementing the program. They then discussed the possibility of developing a multiphasic screening program by combining blood pressure screening with other screenings such as cholesterol but cautioned that this would require additional funding and time investment.

The director then challenged them to describe how they would evaluate the success of the program. In response they shared with him the hospital discharge data that had initially sparked their interest in doing the screening. They felt that this would provide sufficient baseline data to help evaluate the outcome of the screening program. The director asked them to clarify what their programmatic outcome would be. They were not sure, so the director asked them to come back when they had a clear idea of how they would evaluate the success of the program (for more on evaluation, see Chapter 5). After reviewing basic models for program evaluation, they decided on a short time span for their evaluation and chose simple measures to evaluate the impact of the program. They chose to measure the number of people who attended the program, the number of positive screens, and the number of positive screens who accepted information related to referral for treatment. They went back to the director and stated that, owing to the limited resources for the targeted population, there were three clinics that were most often used by residents in the targeted community. The nurses felt it would be practical to track individuals postscreening. To do this, they proposed to first keep a record of how many men attended the screening. They then would contact each of the clinics and ask them to track the number of men who said they had been referred by the screening program. Based on all the information provided, the director finally approved their request, and the nurses were able to institute the screening program (Fig. 2-9).

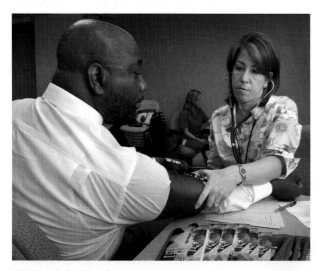

Figure 2-9 Blood pressure screening. *(From Centers for Disease Control and Prevention, James Gathany, 2005.)*

Criteria for Screening Programs and Ethical Dilemmas

Screening is performed on a regular basis across populations and settings, and is often taken for granted as a worthwhile endeavor. Prior to implementing a screening program, it is important to determine whether the screening program meets certain criteria. There are serious ethical considerations that must be addressed. For the majority of screening, the core assumption is that the screening program will reduce disease-associated morbidity and mortality due to early identification and engagement in treatment. The other major assumption is that all those who screen positive for probable disease have access to appropriate assessment and treatment services. These assumptions form the basis of the criteria used to determine whether a screening program should be implemented.

Criteria for Screening Programs

The first criterion is to be certain that the screening test has high specificity and sensitivity. This is complex as demonstrated in the previous case study. There is always a trade-off between specificity and sensitivity. When planning a screening program, it helps to review the impact of missing true cases versus falsely identifying a person with the disease as having the disease. For example, if the disease being screened has a high mortality rate, it may be more important to identify as many individuals with the disease as possible; that is, it should have a high sensitivity. That way there is a good chance of detecting disease, even if the specificity is low and the percentage without disease that ends up going through diagnostic testing is high. However, those who screen positive and do not have disease may unnecessarily experience a high level of stress while waiting to find out whether they do indeed have the disease. On the opposite end, if the mortality for the disease is lower and the cost and inconvenience of diagnostic testing is high, high specificity may be more important than high sensitivity. The best-case scenario is to have a test with both high specificity and high sensitivity. There is always a trade-off.

The next important criterion is that the test needs to be simple to administer, inexpensive, safe, rapid, and acceptable to patients. Screening that can be done quickly with minimal time and effort has a higher likelihood of success. It also needs to be safe. Some screening tests are invasive and may carry some risk. For example, a colonoscopy requires some anesthesia with its associated risk. A paper-and-pencil questionnaire is noninvasive and carries minimal risk. Also, a simple one-page paper-and-pencil screening tool is rapidly administered, whereas a colonoscopy requires a minimum of 24 hours including preparation for the test, the administration of the test, and recovery from the test. Acceptability of the screening test is often dependent on cost, time, safety, and ease of administration, which are reasons that it is harder to get individuals to have the recommended colonoscopy screening than it is other screening tests.

Even paper-and-pencil tests should be reviewed for simplicity. Many screening tests take too long to administer, decreasing the chance that a person will complete a test. Consider the difference between screening for possible depression using a 10-item questionnaire that can be inserted into a regular health assessment versus a 32-item questionnaire. A 10-item test is simpler. It is also easier to learn and perform, and can be delivered by non-medical personnel. A good example of a measurement tool for depression with high sensitivity, specificity, and reliability is the 10-item Center for Epidemiologic Studies Short Depression Scale (CES-D 10).[54,55] The original screening tool was 20 items long and took longer to learn and administer. The shorter form is easier to administer and more acceptable to patients.

The next criterion is that the disease be sufficiently serious to warrant screening. The purpose is to prevent the adverse consequences associated with the disease. In the case of colonoscopy, the screening test does not meet the rapid, simple, inexpensive, and acceptable criteria. However, the severity of the disease outweighs the inconvenience and cost of the screening test. CRC is the third leading cause of cancer-related deaths in the United States.[54] Screening and early detection of CRC increase the chance of a cure in a disease with a high mortality rate when treated in its late stages. Screening often leads to the identification of precancerous lesions (i.e., adenomas), which can be removed, thus preventing CRC.[56]

The next criterion addresses the issue of whether the treatment for disease is easier and more effective when the disease is detected early. This is not the case for all diseases and is the reason that there is ongoing scientific inquiry into the utility of screening tests. If screening is done, will it reduce the disease-associated morbidity and mortality through initiation of early treatment and to what extent? If there was a screening test for Parkinson's disease, what type of early treatment exists? Because there is no known cure and treatment is confined to reducing symptoms, early detection does not serve to reduce the disability associated with the disease. Conversely, mammography has the potential of identifying breast cancer in the early stages, thus increasing the potential survival rate.

This then raises the issue of the acceptability of the available diagnostic services and treatment. If screening is done, will those who screen positive seek further assessment? Will those with a positive diagnosis engage in treatment? This issue was raised over the use of a reliable instrument to screen for at-risk drug use. There is no evidence that screening resulted in subsequent assessment and treatment. Those who screened positive were not likely to follow up with the next steps related to the screening. Based on this, the National Quality Forum's (NQF) publication on evidence-based treatment for substance use disorders does not recommend that health-care providers screen for at-risk drug use as a standard practice in general populations.[54] When screening will not result in the needed follow-up, the screening program will not result in reduced disease-related morbidity and mortality.

Another criterion for implementing a screening program is to determine whether the prevalence of a disease is high in the population to be screened. Despite the NQF's recommendation that screening for at-risk drug abuse not be conducted in the general population, it is applicable in a population in which the prevalence of at-risk drug use is high, such as an inner-city program for adolescent males with failing grades. The prevalence is higher, and the program staff can be trained to provide health education along with the screening, thus improving the acceptability of subsequent referral and possible treatment by the boys in the program who screen positive.

This criterion is also helpful when deciding whom to target when putting together a screening program. The IOM continuum health prevention model referenced earlier[30] provides a framework for deciding whom to include in the screening program. A universal approach would include everyone in the population regardless of age, gender, or other characteristic. A screening program that uses a selected approach would focus on those at higher risk. Making these decisions is based on prevalence and risk for disease. For example, breast cancer screening through mammography is not done using a universal approach. Instead, age, gender, and risk factors are used to determine who should get a mammogram and how often.

The final and ethically the most important criterion is that resources are available for referral for diagnostic evaluation and possible treatment. In our example of putting together a screening program for hypertension in African American men, the team first ascertained whether there were available resources to handle those with a positive screen. The main issues to address are economic access, physical access, and capacity to treat. Economic access refers to the ability to pay for care. Will all those who attend the screening program be able to receive follow-up diagnostic services and possible treatment? If the answer is yes, will they have physical access to the clinics providing the care? For example, what type of transportation is available to get to the clinics providing services, and will everyone who attends the screening have adequate transportation in terms of time, utility, and cost? Finally, if a large-scale screening program is done, does the existing health-care system have the capacity to provide diagnostic and treatment services for the anticipated increase in individuals needing these services? This last criterion is rarely addressed and can result in serious consequences.

Ethical Considerations

The criteria discussed raise serious ethical questions related to screening. It is unethical to conduct screening if treatment is not available. Screening programs are often done without thinking through the consequences. A serious ethical question is, what will be done with the positive screens? Availability of treatment is not just related to the existence of health-care resources that provide the treatment but also to the ability of those participating in the screening to access those resources. What if nurses conducted blood pressure screening with a homeless population in a neighborhood where the nearest hospital was three bus rides away; the nearby clinics required a minimal co-pay of $50.00; there were no pharmacies in the area that provided medications to those without the ability to pay; the soup kitchens in the area served donated food that was high in salt, fat, and sugar; and there were limited public toilets? What would they do with the homeless persons who had a positive screen? Even if they managed to see a physician who then prescribed a salt-free diet and a powerful diuretic, how would they be able to fill the prescription and follow the diet? If they were able to fill the prescription, how would they handle the frequent need to urinate without getting arrested for urinating in public? The primary question is, did the screening program result in reduced morbidity and mortality in this population? Was it ethical to conduct the screening without ensuring first that a system was in place to provide the needed health-care services?

Another example involves the American Cancer Society's eagerness to provide free breast exams and mammography to low-income Hispanic and African American women in a midwestern city. The organization engaged several partners to provide the service (at a time before most states provided free screening to low-income women). The director of one of those clinics agreed to see a specific number per week for free (one criterion was no health insurance). However, the director insisted that the clinic would do this only if the American Cancer Society had a plan in place for diagnosing and treating any woman who screened positive for the cancer. The ethical and moral question that the planners then addressed was what to do if they told a participant in the screening program that she had cancer and then had no way for her to receive treatment. The planners were able to contract with three physicians and two hospitals that agreed to provide care. The screening program began and the first woman screened was positive for breast cancer, requiring major surgery. She had no insurance and no resources to pay for the surgery. To be eligible for Medicaid, she would have had to give up her home, a resource for which she had spent a lifetime saving. Because of the preplanning, this woman and the four other women participating in the program who were diagnosed with cancer all received the needed surgery. Without the generosity of the physicians and hospitals, they would not have been able to have the surgery, and the planners of the screening program would have been left with a serious ethical dilemma.

Another ethical issue has been raised by the possible use of genetic screening as a means of identifying those who are genetically at risk for developing disease. For example, with our increased knowledge related to genetically linked disease, genetic screening can help determine whether a well person without disease is at risk for developing disease. A woman's risk of developing breast and/or ovarian cancer is greatly increased if she inherits a deleterious (harmful) *BRCA1* or *BRCA2* mutation. Men with these mutations also have an increased risk of breast cancer. Both men and women who have harmful *BRCA1* or *BRCA2* mutations may be at increased risk of other cancers. Should genetic screening be done and, if so, what interventions should occur related to positive results? There are no easy answers. Consider the woman who screens positive for a *BRCA1* or *BRCA2* mutation. Should she consider removing her healthy breasts prior to the development of disease?

Tertiary Prevention and Noncommunicable Disease

Secondary prevention attempts to reduce morbidity and mortality through early detection and treatment. Tertiary prevention is another powerful prevention approach that can also reduce the burden of disease. During the past 100 years, as the life span of populations has increased, the prevalence of NCD (Chapter 9), also referred to as chronic diseases, increased, creating a growing burden of **noncommunicable chronic disease** in the United States and across the world.[57] According to the WHO, in contrast to CDs, NCDs are defined as disease that are not passed from person to person, they have a long duration and usually a slow progression. There are four main categories of NCDs: cardiovascular diseases, cancers, chronic respiratory diseases, and diabetes.[55] Almost half of the population in the United States has been diagnosed with at least one noncommunicable chronic disease, and four in every five health-care dollars are spent on the care of NCD. Although the U.S. health system is built on an acute care model, the vast majority of the care provided is for the management of noncommunicable chronic diseases.[56]

Once it has been identified, how do NCDs fit into the prevention frameworks previously presented? Using the traditional public health model, tertiary prevention is the logical choice. The goal of tertiary prevention interventions is to prevent premature mortality and adverse health consequences related to an NCD. For some diseases, such as hypertension, tertiary prevention efforts can result in the person returning to a normal state; that is, a combination of behavioral changes and pharmaceutical interventions can result in the patient's blood pressure returning to normal limits. In other diseases, the prevention strategies are aimed at slowing the progression of the disease and reducing the likelihood of adverse consequences related to the disease. With pharmaceutical interventions, patients with Parkinson's disease can improve their gait and reduce the tremors. This reduces their risk of falls and other injuries while improving their ability to perform ADLs, but they are not returned to a normal state.

Tertiary prevention appears at first glance to be individual based rather than population based. However, the burden of NCDs affects the whole population, and movement toward more population-level interventions is gaining momentum. In 2009, the WHO released a report calling for "urgent action to halt and turn back the growing threat of chronic diseases."[56] In that report, the WHO stressed that population interventions can be done related to reducing the burden of already diagnosed chronic diseases. In the 2014 WHO report on NCDs, the Director General released a statement that: "WHO Member States have agreed on a time-bound set of nine voluntary global targets to be attained by 2025. There are targets to reduce

harmful use of alcohol, increase physical activity, reduce salt/sodium intake, reduce tobacco use and hypertension, halt the rise in diabetes and of obesity, and to improve coverage of treatment for prevention of heart attacks and strokes. There is also a target to improve availability and affordability of technologies and essential medicines to manage NCDs. Countries need to make progress on all these targets to attain the overarching target of a 25% reduction of premature mortality from the four major NCDs by 2025."[57]

Tertiary care also occurs with CDs during both the acute and recovery stages of infection. For many CDs, tertiary care focuses on provision of acute care, that is, treatment of the disease to prevent further morbidity and mortality, such is the case of treatment for influenza or measles. For some CDs such as HIV, there is no cure and the infection requires long term care to prevent and/or treat AIDS. Other CDs require long-term care to bring about a disease-free state such as tuberculosis. Due to the long-term duration of AIDS and other CDs, the preferred term NCD helps to distinguish between diseases based on the ability of a disease to be transmitted from one human to another. In addition, with CDs part of tertiary prevention becomes primary prevention, that is, the prevention of transmission to other persons (see Chapter 8).

■ Summary Points

- Health promotion and protection are major emphases of national and global health organizations.
- The socioecological model of health promotion uses an upstream approach that includes the social, environmental, and economic contexts of healthy populations.
- The health of a population is greater than the sum of the health of each individual in the population.
- Health prevention frameworks provide guidance for the development of prevention interventions.
- Health education and health literacy are keys to improving the health of populations.
- Screening for possible disease has the potential to reduce disease-related morbidity and mortality but has serious ethical issues that must be addressed.
- Tertiary prevention can help to reduce the burden of chronic diseases.

▼ CASE STUDY

The Centers for Disease Control and Prevention Asks the Question: "Should I Get Screened for Prostate Cancer?"

The CDC follows the U.S. Preventive Services Task Force recommendations that the prostate specific antigen (PSA)-based screening should not be done for men who do not have symptoms.[58] Other organizations have made different recommendations. Based on your review, answer the following questions:

1. What is the sensitivity and specificity of PSA tests?
2. The CDC states that one of the reasons is "… the PSA test may have false positive or false negative results. This can mean that men without cancer may have abnormal results and get tests that are not necessary." What is the biggest issue?
3. How well does a PSA differentiate between non-aggressive and aggressive prostate cancer?
4. Review the information on PSA screening and the criteria and ethical guidelines for conducting a screening program on pages 48-50. Of the list of criteria and ethical issues listed in this chapter, which ones are a concern related to PSA screening?

REFERENCES

1. U.S. Department of Health and Human Services, Healthy People. (2018). *Healthy people 2030 draft framework.* Retrieved from https://www.healthypeople.gov/2020/About-Healthy-People/Development-Healthy-People-2030/Draft-Framework.
2. Kennedy, P. (2018, March 9). The secret to a longer life? Don't ask these dead longevity researchers. *The New York Times.* Retrieved from https://nyti.ms/2Gd1NMI.
3. World Health Organization. (2019). Health Work Force: Nursing Now Campaign. Retrieved from https://www.who.int/hrh/news/2018/nursing_now_campaign/en/
4. UN General Assembly. (2015). *Transforming our world: the 2030 Agenda for Sustainable Development.* Retrieved from http://www.un.org/ga/search/view_doc.asp?symbol=A/RES/70/1&Lang=E.
5. U.S. Department of Health and Human Services, Office of the Surgeon General, National Prevention Council. (2011). *National prevention strategy, Washington, DC.* Retrieved from http://www.surgeongeneral.gov/initiatives/prevention/strategy/report.pdf.
6. U.S. Department of Health and Human Services, Office of the Surgeon General, National Prevention Council. (2014). *Annual status report, Washington, DC.* Available at http://www.surgeongeneral.gov/initiatives/prevention/about/annual_status_reports.html.
7. Bauer, G., Davies, J.K., Pelikan, J., Noack, H., Broesskamp, U., & Hill, C. (2003). Advancing a theoretical model for public health and health promotion indicator development: Proposal from the EUHPID consortium. *European Journal of Public Health, 13*(3s), 107-113.
8. Institute of Medicine. (2003). *The future of the public's health in the twenty-first century.* Washington, DC: National Academies Press.
9. Golden, S.D., McLeroy, K.R., Green, L.W., Earp, J.A.L., & Lieberman, L.D. (2015). Upending the social ecological model to guide health promotion efforts toward policy and environmental change. *Health Education & Behavior, 42*(1 suppl), 8S-14S. https://doi.org/10.1177/1090198115575098.
10. World Health Organization. (2018). *Health promotion.* Retrieved from http://www.who.int/topics/health_promotion/en/.
11. O'Donnell, M.P. (2008). Evolving definition of health promotion: What do you think? *American Journal of Health Promotion, 23*(2), iv. doi: 10.4278/ajhp.23.1.iv.
12. Li, A.M. (2017). Ecological determinants of health: food and environment on human health. *Environment Science and Pollution Research International, 24*, 9002-9015. doi: 10.1007/s11356-015-5707-9.
13. World Health Organization. (2018). *Social determinants of health.* Retrieved from http://www.who.int/social_determinants/sdh_definition/en/.
14. Braveman, P., Egerter, S., & Williams, D.R. (2011). The social determinants of health: coming of age. *Annual Review of Public Health, 32*, 381-398.
15. Martins, D.C., & Burbank, P.M. (2011). Critical interactionism: an upstream-downstream approach to health care reform. *Advances In Nursing Science, 34*(4), 315-329. doi:10.1097/ANS.0b013e3182356c19.
16. U.S. Department of Agriculture. (2018). *National school lunch program.* Retrieved from https://www.fns.usda.gov/nslp/national-school-lunch-program-nslp.
17. U.S. Department of Agriculture. (2018). *Interim final rule: child nutrition program flexibilities for milk, whole grains, and sodium requirements.* Retrieved from https://www.fns.usda.gov/school-meals/fr-113017.
18. Morgan I.S., & Marsh, G.W. (1998). Historic and future health promotion contexts for nursing. *Journal of Nursing Scholarship, 30*(4), 379-383.
19. Pender, N., Murdaugh, C.L., & Poarsons, M.A. (2014). *Health promotion in nursing practice* (7th ed.). Upper Saddle River, NJ: Prentice Hall.
20. Dicker, R., Coronado, F., Koo, D., & Parish, G. (2012). *Principles of epidemiology in public health practice* (3rd ed.). Atlanta, GA, Centers for Disease Control and Prevention.
21. Centers for Disease Control and Prevention. (1992). A framework for assessing the effectiveness of disease and injury prevention. *Morbidity and Mortality Weekly Report, 41*(RR-3).
22. Centers for Disease Control and Prevention. (2009). *Novel H1N1 flu facts and figures.* Retrieved from http://www.cdc.gov/h1n1flu/surveillanceqa.htm.
23. Centers for Disease Control and Prevention. (2018). *People at high risk of developing flu complications.* Retrieved from https://www.cdc.gov/flu/about/disease/high_risk.htm.

24. Gordon, R. (1987). An operational classification of disease prevention. In J.A. Steinberg & M.M. Silverman (Eds.), *Preventing mental disorders* (pp. 20-26). Rockville, MD: Department of Health and Human Services.

25. Substance Abuse and Mental Health Services Administration. (2004). Clinical preventive services in substance abuse and mental health update: From *Science to services (DHHS Publication No. [SMA] 04-3906)*. U.S. Department of Health and Human Service, Rockville, MD.

26. Whelton P.K., Carey, R.M., Aronow, W.S., Casey, D.E., Collins, K.J., Dennison Himmelfarb, C.,... Wright, J.K. (2018). ACC/AHA/AAPA/ABC/ACPM/AGS/APhA/ASH/ASPC/NMA/PCNA Guideline for the prevention, detection, evaluation, and management of high blood pressure in adults. *Journal of the American College of Cardiology, 71*(19), 2275-2279. DOI: 10.1016/j.jacc.2017.11.006.

27. Havas, K., Bonner, A., & Douglas, C. (2016). Self-management support for people with chronic kidney disease: Patient perspectives. *Journal Of Renal Care, 42*(1), 7-14. doi:10.1111/jorc.12140.

28. Enworom, C.D., & Tabi, M. (2015). Evaluation of kidney disease education on clinical outcomes and knowledge of self-management behaviors of patients with chronic kidney disease. *Nephrology Nursing Journal, 42*(4), 363-373.

29. Salvatore, A. L., SangNam, A., Luohua, J., Lorig, K., Ory, M. G., Ahn, S., & Jiang, L. (2015). National study of chronic disease self-management: 6-month and 12-month findings among cancer survivors and non-cancer survivors. *Psycho-Oncology, 24*(12), 1714-1722. doi:10.1002/pon.3783.

30. U.S. Preventive Health Services Task Force. (2017). *Home.* Retrieved from https://www.uspreventiveservicestaskforce.org/Page/Name/about-the-uspstf.

31. Centers for Disease Control and Prevention. (2017). *Faststats: leading causes of death.* Retrieved from https://www.cdc.gov/nchs/fastats/leading-causes-of-death.htm.

32. National Center for Health Statistics. (2017). *Health, United States, 2016: With chartbook on long-term trends in health.* Hyattsville, MD: National Center for Health Statistics.

33. Institute of Medicine and National Research Council. (2015). *Measuring the risks and causes of premature death: summary of workshops.* Washington, DC: The National Academies Press. https://doi.org/10.17226/21656.

34. Keller, L.O., Strohschien, S., Lia-Hoagberg, B., & Schaffer, M. (2004). Population-based public health interventions: Practice-based and evidence-supported, part 1. *Public Health Nursing, 21,* 453-468.

35. Minnesota Department of Health, Division of Community Health Services, Public Health Section. (2001). *Public health interventions: Applications for public health nursing practice.* Retrieved from http://www.health.state.mn.us/divs/opi/cd/phn/docs/0301wheel_manual.pdf.

36. Joint Committee on Health Education and Promotion Terminology. (2014). Report of the 2011 Joint Committee on Health Education and Promotion Terminology. *American Journal of Health Education, 43*(sup 2), 1-19. DOI: 10.1080/19325037.2012.11008225.

37. World Health Organization. (2018). *Health education.* Retrieved from http://www.who.int/topics/health_education/en/.

38. Shunk, D.H. (2012). *Learning theories: An educational perspective* (6th ed.). Boston: Pearson.

39. Bandura, A. (1977). *Social learning theory.* New York: General Learning Press.

40. Hughes, N., & Schwab, I. (2010). *Teaching adult health literacy: principles and practice.* Berkshire, England: McGraw Hill.

41. Knowles, M.S. (1990). *The adult learner: A neglected species* (4th ed.). Houston, TX: Gulf.

42. The Institute of Medicine, Committee on Health Literacy, Board on Neuroscience and Behavioral Health. (2004). *Health literacy: A prescription to end confusion.* Washington, DC: The National Academies Press.

43. U.S .Department of Education, National Center for Education Statistics. (2016). *Skills of U.S. unemployed, young, and older adults in sharper focus: results from the program for the international assessment of adult competencies (PIAAC) 2012/2014.* Retrieved from https://nces.ed.gov/pubs2016/2016039rev.pdf.

44. Rasu, R.S., Bawa, W.A., Suminski, R., Snella, K., & Warady, B. (2015). Health literacy impact on national healthcare utilization and expenditure. *International Journal of Health Policy and Management, 4*(11), 747–755. Retrieved from http://doi.org.ezp.welch.jhmi.edu/10.15171/ijhpm.2015.151.

45. Centers for Disease Control and Prevention. (2016). *Talking points about health literacy.* Retrieved from https://www.cdc.gov/healthliteracy/shareinteract/TellOthers.html.

46. Hersh, L., Salzman, B., & Snyderman, D. (2015). Health literacy in primary care practice. *American Family Physician, 92*(2), 118-124.

47. Agency for Health Care Research and Quality. (2015). *AHRQ Health Literacy Universal Precautions Toolkit* (2nd ed.). Rockville, MD: Author.

48. National Institutes of Health. (2017). *Clear communication: cultural respect.* Retrieved from https://www.nih.gov/institutes-nih/nih-office-director/office-communications-public-liaison/clear-communication/cultural-respect.

49. Bloom, B.S. (1956). *Taxonomy of educational objectives: Handbook 1. The cognitive domain.* New York, NY: David McKay.

50. Commission on Chronic Illness. (1951). *Chronic illness in the United States* (Vol. 1, p 45). Cambridge, MA: Harvard University Press, Commonwealth Fund.

51. American Heart Association. (2016). *High blood pressure and African Americans.* Retrieved from http://www.heart.org/HEARTORG/Conditions/HighBloodPressure/UnderstandSymptomsRisks/High-Blood-Pressure-and-African-Americans_UCM_301832_Article.jsp#.Wxly1fZFw2w.

52. Centers for Disease Control and Prevention. (2016). *High blood pressure facts.* Retrieved from https://www.cdc.gov/bloodpressure/facts.htm.

53. Radloff, L.S. (1977). The CES-D scale: A self-report depression scale for research in the general population. *Applied Psychological Measurement, 1,* 385-401.

54. Andresen, E.M., Malmgren, J.A., Carter, W.B., & Patrick, D.L. (1994). Screening for depression in well older

adults: Evaluation of a short form of the CES-D (Center for Epidemiologic Studies Depression Scale). *American Journal of Preventive Medicine, 10,* 77-84.

55. Centers for Disease Control and Prevention. (2017). *Colorectal cancer statistics.* Retrieved from https://www.cdc.gov/cancer/colorectal/statistics/index.htm.

56. Centers for Disease Control and Prevention. (2017). *Chronic disease prevention and health promotion: National Center for Chronic Disease Prevention and Health Promotion.* Retrieved from https://www.cdc.gov/chronicdisease/resources/publications/aag/NCCDPHP.htm.

57. World Health Organization. (2009). *Preventing chronic diseases: A vital investment.* Retrieved from http://www.who.int/chp/chronic_disease_report/en/.

58. World Health Organization. (2014). *Global status report on noncommunicable diseases 2014.* Geneva: Author.

Chapter 3

Epidemiology and Nursing Practice

Erin Rachel Whitehouse and William A. Mase

LEARNING OUTCOMES

After reading the chapter, the student will be able to:

1. Describe aspects of person, place, and time as they relate to epidemiological investigation.
2. Explain the epidemiological triangle.
3. Apply the epidemiological constants to an investigation.
4. Identify sources of epidemiological data.
5. Apply basic biostatistical methods to analyze epidemiological data.
6. Differentiate cohort and case-control study design and select appropriate measures of effect.
7. Explain surveillance and the difference between active and passive surveillance.

KEY TERMS

Active surveillance	Demography	Infectivity	Prevalence
Agent	Descriptive epidemiology	Life expectancy	Prospective
Analytical epidemiology	Environment	Morbidity	Rate
Attack rate	Epidemiology	Mortality	Retrospective
Biostatistics	Host	Passive surveillance	Secondary attack rate
Causality	Incidence	Percent change	Web of causation

◾ Introduction

In 2017, a National Public Radio headline reported "U.S. has the worst rate of maternal deaths in the developed world," based on a recent study of global levels of maternal mortality.[1] Information from the Centers for Disease Control and Prevention (CDC) also confirms that pregnancy-related deaths, defined as the death of a woman during or within 1 year of the end of pregnancy, have been increasing in the United States since 1987 when this information was collected.[2] A headline like this inspires many questions: Why is the mortality rate increasing? What factors are influencing this disparity between the U.S. and other developed countries? Is a particular population affected more by high rates of maternal mortality? How was this information collected? Is this an accurate headline based on the information?

As nurses, if we were to investigate these data further we would discover that there are great disparities in the pregnancy-related mortality within the U.S. According to the CDC, for example, black women have a much higher rate of pregnancy-related deaths compared with white women (12.7 deaths per 100,000 live births for white women vs. 43.5 deaths per 100,000 live births for black women).[2] However, for a public health nurse, this suggests the need for further inquiry into what factors might be driving this difference: poverty, urban/rural differences, racial stigma, or differing access to care. See Chapter 17 for more details specific to maternal child health, and maternal mortality and public health.

Collecting, analyzing, and synthesizing data to understand public health questions such as disparities in maternal mortality is the heart of epidemiology. Epidemiology, the combination of three Greek words: *epi*, translated as "upon"; *demos*, translated as "people"; and *logy*, or "the study of something", is broadly defined as the study of factors that influence health and disease in populations.[3] Epidemiology is a natural fit for the nursing profession because nursing, unlike many of the health-related professions, extends well beyond one-on-one patient-clinician interactions to engaging groups of people where they live, work, and play. Public health nursing has traditionally blended health promotion, disease prevention, health education, and population-based initiatives in an effort to maximize the health and wellness of individuals through population-level strategies. As 21st-century health professionals, nurses are now more than ever required to demonstrate both competency and proficiency in the principles of epidemiology.

■ CELLULAR TO GLOBAL

Epidemiology and biostatistics are critical fields to understand health outcomes from a cellular to global level. *Mycobacterium tuberculosis* (TB), the leading cause of communicable disease deaths globally, is an example of a disease that affects health on a cellular, individual, community, and global level.[4] Diabetes, smoking, and HIV infection are leading risk factors both for the development of TB and for poorer treatment outcomes through mechanisms such as increased inflammation, decreased immunity, and structural lung damage. TB is also related to community factors such as poverty because risk factors like overcrowded housing increase the risk of exposure and subsequent development of TB. Drug-resistant TB, which is resistant to the first-line TB antibiotics, is an increasing challenge in part due to insufficient health systems that do not have the appropriate resources to treat it. Finally, preventing and treating TB is a global challenge given the movement of populations due to migration, war, famine, natural disasters, and even tourism. Epidemiological principles are one tool to understand how risk factors on cellular, local, national, and global levels impact population health outcomes like mortality from TB.

Today the curriculum in accredited colleges of nursing is shifting toward the inclusion of epidemiology as core content. The historical development of epidemiology is replete with references to the same women who carved out the nursing profession. Public health nursing and population-based health and wellness are evident in the pioneering efforts of Florence Nightingale, Lillian Wald, Clara Barton, Mary Breckinridge, and Dorothea Dix. Each of these legendary women initiated public health efforts from a population health perspective toward the reduction of disease and promotion of health within populations.

What Is Epidemiology?

Epidemiology has been defined many ways. Traditionally, it is the study of the distribution of disease and injury in human populations. More recently, broader definitions of the term move beyond the study of disease and include the examination of factors that affect the health and illness of populations, thus providing the basis for interventions aimed at improving the health and well-being of populations. The focus of epidemiology is on populations rather than on individuals. Epidemiology takes an analytical investigative approach to this study of health and disease, and is built on three central elements:

• Person: Which groups of individuals are affected?
• Place: Where does the health issue occur, i.e., what geographically defined region?
• Time: Over what specified period of time does the health issue occur?

These three elements of person, place, and time are the bricks of epidemiology. The mortar cementing these bricks is made up of the methods of quantitative comparison used by epidemiologists when studying patterns of disease and health. The tools used by epidemiologists are best described as comparative, numeric, and analytical. To effectively quantify illness and disease, accurate data are required. Epidemiological data sources vary widely. Some of the more frequently used data sources include hospitals, community-based clinical practices, health departments, workplaces, schools, and health insurance reimbursement claims. The capacity for an epidemiologist to effectively analyze and present data is inextricably linked to the network of health-care–related workers throughout an array of health and human service–related industries. Nurses are pivotal to the accurate assessment and timely reporting of health-related data upon which epidemiology is grounded.

Historical Beginnings

John Snow is celebrated as the founder of modern epidemiology just as Florence Nightingale is recognized as the founder of modern nursing (see Chapter 1). John Snow's watershed work, *Snow on Cholera*, introduced methods of epidemiological investigation and methods upon which contemporary epidemiological methods are founded.[5] His use of the epidemiological strategy, now defined as disease mapping, to study the incidence of cholera deaths reported in London, England, laid the foundation for investigation of disease in populations. The Lambeth Company provided residents of London with drinking water collected from the Thames River.[6] Snow's enumeration and subsequent investigation of cholera deaths reported for residents living near the Lambert Company's Broad Street water pump is heralded as the defining event upon which all future epidemiological methods are based. Snow developed a frequency distribution of the number of human deaths by placing a hash mark on a city street map. Upon visual inspection of the map it became clear to Snow that there were residential patterns of deaths. He demonstrated that greater numbers of cholera deaths were clustered within the vicinity of a specific public water source, the Broad Street water pump. The number of cholera deaths near the Broad Street pump far exceeded the deaths in other areas of London (Fig. 3-1).

Snow's work illustrated the three central elements related to his investigation: person, place, and time. The person variable can be defined as the number of human cholera deaths. Place is visually demonstrated by the street mapping method Snow used to count human deaths by street of residence. Finally, the time variable in Snow's study was the 5-year period between 1849 and 1854 when the Lambeth Company drew community water from the contaminated source, the Thames River. In the 150 years since Snow's community disease mapping, epidemiologists have developed more effective and timely measures for disease investigation using contemporary 21st-century methods. The three elements of person, place, and time are as central to an epidemiological investigation now as they were in the time of Snow, and they form the building blocks for modern-day epidemiological investigations.

Since the time of Snow's work, epidemiology has gone through various phases. The first phase is referred to as the *sanitary phase*. It was based on the miasma theory that illness was related to poisoning by foul emanations from soil, air, and water. During this phase, public health efforts focused on improving sanitation. This approach to illness prevailed until the discovery of microscopic organisms that were linked to disease, which led to the germ theory and the *communicable disease phase* of epidemiology. This phase led to the examination of single causes for a disease and worked well in a world where communicable diseases were the number one killers. With the emergence of antibiotics and the reduction of communicable disease, the life expectancy of populations increased,

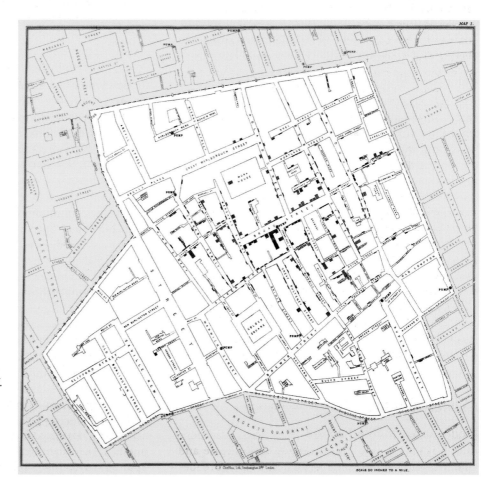

Figure 3-1 Snow map. *(Published by C.F. Cheffins, Lith, Southhampton Buildings, London, England, 1854, in Snow, J. [1885]. On the mode of communication of cholera (2nd Ed.). John Churchill, New Burlington Street, London, England.* http://www.ph.ucla.edu/epi/snow/snowmap1_1854_lge.htm*)*

especially those in developed countries. This resulted in the emergence of noncommunicable diseases and a new phase in epidemiology, the *risk factor phase*. This phase of study is still a mainstay of epidemiological investigations. It relies on the linking of exposures to the occurrence of injury or disease and helps us identify risk factors that, when reduced, may result in a subsequent reduction in morbidity and mortality. The most recent phase in epidemiology is the ecological model as proposed by Susser and Susser in the 1990s.[7,8] This helps move the science of epidemiology to a broader perspective and, as explained in Chapter 1, reflects not only the biological and behavioral influences on health but also a deeper understanding of the role of the physical environment and the underlying conditions in the social environment that create poor health.

Risk Factors

Risk factors are a foundational concept in epidemiology. The World Health Organization (WHO) defines a risk factor as "any attribute, characteristic, or exposure of an individual that increases the likelihood of developing a disease or injury."[9] Although there are several ways to classify risk factors, we will explore three major categories of risk factors: behavioral, environmental, and genetic.

Behavioral Risk Factors

The CDC began the now nationwide Behavioral Risk Factor Surveillance System (BRFSS) in 1984.[10] They intended to study the way that human behavior influences health and wellness, and identify behaviors that might influence health conditions, such as the impact of underage drinking on the risk of unprotected sex. This human health behavioral survey is the largest telephone survey assessment in the world. The BRFSS provides timely health behavior data for policy makers in all 50 states as well as the District of Columbia, Puerto Rico, U.S. Virgin Islands, and Guam. These data are effective in providing health-related trend analysis and serve to guide and direct local, state, and national pro-health initiatives. Figure 3-2 presents national-level trended data on tobacco use.[11] It is exciting to see that the Healthy People 2020 goal for adolescent smoking has been reached! The BRFSS can be used to present population-level trend data related to many behavioral risk factors. For community-based health educators, these data are an effective resource to assist in planning community health interventions.

Environmental Risk Factors

Is it possible that the community in which one lives and/or works puts one at an increased or decreased risk

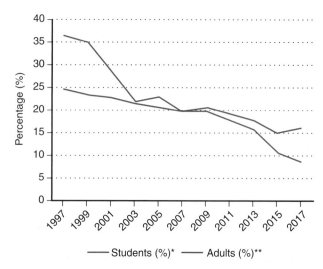

* Percentage of high school students who smoked cigarettes on at least 1 day during the 30 days before the survey (i.e., current cigarette use). (Youth Risk Behavior Survey 1997-2017)

** Percentage of adults who were current past 30-day cigarette smokers (National Health Interview Survey 1997-2017)

Figure 3-2 Trends in Current Cigarette Smoking by High School Students* and Adults** United States 1997 to 2017. (*Source: 11a, 11b.*)

for developing a given illness or disease? Yes, it does. The Agency for Toxic Substances and Disease Registry (ATSDR) Web site provides useful information on adverse health effects linked to health-related environmental risk from exposure ranging from arsenic to zinc and everything in between (see Web Resources on Davis*Plus*). Often, increased environmental risk for residents of communities is related to specific industries located in and around the community. By mapping industries related to hazardous waste, it is possible to identify populations at greater risk for disease at the local and state levels. The federal government has set aside funds referred to as the Superfund to clean up uncontrolled hazardous waste sites across the country through the Environmental Protection Agency (EPA). The states with the greatest number of Superfund clean-up sites include New Jersey, Pennsylvania, and New York, with more than 100 Superfund sites per state. The EPA Web site at http://www.epa.gov/superfund/ provides information on identifying possible industry-related environmental hazards.

Public health professionals working in environmental health often focus on three critical areas in assuring the health of the public: safe air quality conditions, safe water supplies, and safe soils throughout the nation's agricultural industry. The majority of the human health risks are associated with what we breathe and ingest. It is important to keep in mind that the environmental risks affecting humans are indeed vast, including automobile safety, seatbelt use, and safe conditions throughout public recreational facilities. Public health professionals use a combination of education, engineering, and enforcement to achieve our mandated goals and objectives. There are more details about the role of public health science and environmental health in Chapter 6.

Genetic Risk Factors (Genomics)

The field of genetic epidemiology otherwise known as *genomics* seeks to understand and explain heritability of factors that have an impact on the development of illness and disease. The past 2 decades have witnessed the expansion of research into genetic markers for disease. We will likely see a transformation in the evaluation, assessment, and tools surrounding genetically relevant strategies at the population level because of emerging individual-level genetic knowledge.

Application of genomics to population health poses some practical and ethical dilemmas. First, at the population level, the purpose is to develop interventions relevant to the population that will result in a general improvement of health at the population level. Genetic testing is done at the individual level and usually results in individual decision making related to potential risk for development of disease. For diseases such as cystic fibrosis that are related to one gene, genetic testing can help with early identification and treatment for those born with the disease and may assist parents make childbearing decisions prior to conception. However, most diseases occur due to multiple factors and are linked to more than one gene as well as numerous other risk factors. Evidence on the benefit of genetic screening for most diseases is limited. In addition, genetic testing can be costly.

A good example of the controversy over the benefits of genetic testing is the issue of *BRCA1* and *BRCA2*. These human genes are referred to as tumor suppressors. Based on recent research, it is apparent that mutation of these genes is associated with hereditary breast and ovarian cancers.[12] The company that developed the screening test for *BRCA1* and *BRACA2* initiated an advertising campaign encouraging women to have the genetic screen. Though the National Cancer Institute lists possible options for managing cancer risk for those with a positive screen, it acknowledges that the evidence concerning the effectiveness of these strategies is limited. Testing can cost up to $3,000 for those who do not know their family history. The high cost raises the ethical question of taking a

universal approach to screening all women for this genetic risk factor, especially as less than 10% of all breast cancers are genetically related and the direct benefit of the testing in reducing cancer rates is not known. Genomics is a growing field with the potential benefit of better understanding the role individual genetic makeup plays in an individual's health. However, as the *BRCA1* and *BRCA2* screening example illustrates, the applicability of genomics to population-level interventions from a practical and ethical standpoint has still not been determined.

Epidemiological Frameworks

There are several frameworks guiding the field of epidemiology such as the epidemiological triangle, the web of causation, and the ecological model. The latter two frameworks evolved from the epidemiological triangle framework. Public health professionals continue to use these and other frameworks to assist in a better understanding of health phenomena.

The Epidemiological Triangle

The classic model used in epidemiology to explain the occurrence of disease is referred to as the epidemiological triangle. There are three main components to the triangle: agent, host, and environment (Fig. 3-3). In communicable diseases, the model helps the epidemiologist map out the relationship between the agent or the organism responsible for the disease and the host (person) as well as the environmental factors that enhance or impede transmission of the agent to the host.

Although this model is ideally suited for explaining the transmission of an infectious agent to a human host,

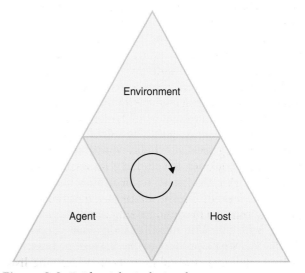

Figure 3-3 Epidemiological triangle.

it is now applied to noncommunicable diseases, such as lung cancer, with a specific exposure, such as cigarette smoke, representing the agent or causative factor. The agent can be viewed as the causative factor contributing to noninfectious health problems or conditions. The **agent** may be biological (organism), chemical (liquids, gases), nutritive (dietary components or lack of dietary components), physical (mechanical force, atmospheric such as an earthquake), or psychological (stress). The **host** is the susceptible human or animal, whereas the **environment** is all of the external factors that can influence the host's vulnerability to the risk factors related to the disease.

The value of this model lies in the fact that it helps in the development of interventions. For example, in the case of the H1N1 outbreak, epidemiologists first worked at isolating the agent. Based on the type of agent, a flu virus, it was clear that the environment needed for transmission was both the breathing in of air droplets that contained the virus and coming in contact with the virus via a *fomite,* that is, an inanimate object such as a water faucet. Based on this information, three prevention interventions were instituted. The initial approach focused on the environment. To reduce exposure of people to the virus in the environment, all those with signs and symptoms of H1N1 were asked to stay home and to cough into their arms rather than their hands. Uninfected individuals were also instructed to use hand sanitizers. The second approach was aimed at protecting the host (person) through the development and distribution of the H1N1 vaccine. The use of a vaccine reduced the susceptibility of hosts to the agent, which, in turn, reduced further introduction of the virus into the environment. In this example, no interventions were aimed at the agent because no viable options were available to directly eradicate the agent.

The Epidemiological Constants of Person, Place, and Time

In addition to the epidemiological triangle, there are three constants that are the foundation for any epidemiological investigation: person, place, and time (Fig. 3-4). The *person* aspect typically includes demographic variables including age, gender, and ethnicity. *Place* considerations include such variables as city resident, office building user, or downhill skier. Finally, the third constant, *time,* is a critical dimension of consideration. Conditions in one location with the same subset of individuals can change substantially as a product of the passage of time. It is important to keep in mind that this model is the foundation upon which our understanding of illness and disease

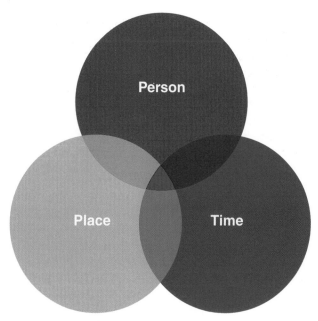

Figure 3-4 Epidemiological constants.

are built and can help guide investigations into a health issue in a population.

Who, What, When, Where, Why, How, and How Long: To further understand the use of the epidemiological triangle and the constants of person, place, and time, seven questions have been used to conduct an epidemiological investigation. These questions have most often been used to examine the epidemiology of communicable diseases. The *who* question relates to the person, the *place* question to where, the *when* and *how long* questions to time, the *what* to the causative agent, and the *why* and *how* to the mechanism for acquiring disease, such as the mode of transmission in communicable diseases. These seven questions provide an effective model by which illness can be analyzed at the population level in order to develop interventions that will improve health and/or prevent disease. This approach is an example of naturalistic experimentation, a study that occurs in the natural world and not in a controlled laboratory environment.

■ CULTURAL CONTEXT

Epidemiology is rooted in asking questions, collecting and analyzing data, and making informed decisions to influence policy or practice. Understanding the cultural context of a given population is critical in all steps of the process. Differences across ethnicity, geography, race, nationality, or religion can potentially affect risk factors or perceptions of health and risk. Are you asking the right questions to understand risk factors that might be particular to the population? Are you using the correct terminology so that the population of people understands the question in the way that it is being asked? One of the best ways to ensure that a survey or outbreak investigation is conducted in a way that respects the cultural context is to involve people from the population in creating and executing the research or investigation. This can provide critical information for access to key informants, asking appropriate and relevant questions, and understanding the data within the perspective of the population. Thus, although epidemiologic principles are broad and apply locally to globally, it is important to always frame epidemiology questions and investigations within the appropriate cultural context.

Causality

Although the seven questions help the investigator learn about the occurrence of disease, that knowledge only begins to provide a broader understanding of the multiple factors that could be related to the occurrence of the disease. Epidemiologists investigate possible causes of disease to better understand how to prevent and treat disease. The term *cause* is traditionally used to indicate that a stimulus or action results in an effect or outcome. For example, if you turn on a light switch, the observed effect is that the light bulb lights up. When it comes to epidemiology, **causality** refers to determining whether a cause-and-effect relationship exists between a risk factor and a health effect. In health, causes can include a number of things related to person, place, and time. Using the light switch example again, it may be first assumed that the singular cause for lighting the bulb is the physical act of flipping the switch. In actuality, there are other factors involved, including the presence of a source of electrical energy, a working electrical connection between the switch and the light, and a light bulb that is not burned out.

As presented throughout this chapter, epidemiological studies typically report measures of associations based on population-based correlations; that is, an increase or decrease in the amount of the risk factor and the frequency of the risk factor are parallel to the increase or decrease of the incidence of the health issue. It is always important to keep in mind that correlation, the fact that two variables are correlated with one another, does not necessarily mean that one factor causes the other. For example, heavy smokers often have a yellow stain on the fingers that hold the cigarette. Although the presence of yellow stains on the fingers may be correlated with lung cancer, the yellow stain is not the cause of lung cancer.

To examine the possibility of causality, the first step is to determine whether there is a statistical relationship between the risk factor and the health issue. In other words, can the association between the two be attributed to chance alone—does the association between the two occur at a frequency higher than what could be attributed to chance? After determining that the relationship does not occur by chance alone, the next step is to determine whether the relationship is causal. In some cases, the relationship between two variables is statistically significant, but the relationship is noncausal. For example, in a group of schoolchildren, height may be statistically correlated with grade level; that is, the higher the grade level, the taller the children, but grade level is not the causal factor for the increase in height.

A causal relationship is present when there is a direct or indirect relationship between the two factors. If it is a direct relationship, then the factor causes the disease. For example, the mumps virus directly causes mumps. A nondirect relationship exists when the factor contributes to the development of the disease through its effect on other variables. Being overweight does not directly cause disease, but it adversely affects the body, thus increasing the risk of cardiovascular disease and diabetes, for example.

Results from studies conducted in the field can be limited because sources of error might be present. These errors most likely relate to assumptions of causality. For example, error can occur when deciding who was actually exposed to a potential risk factor and who was not. There can be errors in how some important variable was measured and errors relating to who received a vaccine and who did not.

● APPLYING PUBLIC HEALTH SCIENCE
Public Health Science Topics Covered:

- Applied Epidemiology
- Health Promotion

Smoking and tobacco use are considered by the WHO to be among the biggest public health threats because they kill up to half of the people who use tobacco.[13] Smoking increases the risk for noncommunicable diseases like cardiovascular disease or lung cancer and also increases the risk for communicable diseases like tuberculosis as described in the cellular to global section of this chapter. However, smoking's influence is not limited to people who use tobacco; it also affects children, families, and communities through second-hand smoke exposure. In addition, 80% of the 1.1 billion smokers globally live in low- and middle-income countries where the burden of disease for tobacco-related conditions and premature death is high.[13]

To think about how to understand the impact of smoking within a specific population, an epidemiologist can explore who is smoking within their community and who might be exposed to smoke (person), where the sources of smoke or tobacco exposure are within a community (place), and how the population of smokers has changed (time). This information is then used to develop community-specific health improvement initiatives that target those populations at greatest risk for harm from smoking or tobacco use. The first step in the investigation of any illness is to begin with inquiry. Ask questions across the seven areas of who, what, when, where, why, how, and how long.

Jane Paterson is a public health nurse employed by the City Health Department of River City, a hypothetical midwestern city with a population of 75,000 and a mix of urban and suburban residents. One of the primary objectives of Jane's job is to develop community-based health promotion and disease prevention initiatives targeting smoking with a focus on youth. According to the most recent U.S. Census data available, there are 3,000 urban and 7,000 suburban River City residents aged birth to 18 years. Of the 3,000 urban residents in this age group, 1,500 have used some form of tobacco product. Of the 7,000 nonurban residents in this age group, 1,000 have used some form of tobacco product.

To understand the smoking data among youth in River City, Jane considers the tools in her epidemiologic toolbox. She needs to ask questions to understand who smokes, why they smoke, what risk factors influence their decision to smoke, how youth are obtaining cigarettes, how much they cost, and what factors might influence their decision to quit. She also needs to look at the data to explore what common risk factors for smoking, such as poverty or parents who are smokers, might be influencing the youth of River City. She needs to understand who already smokes and who is at risk for future smoking to develop an evidence-based intervention that targets these specific populations. The data from the U.S. Census informed Jane that there was a higher percentage of youth who smoked from the urban areas of River City, but do these percentage differences suggest an actual difference in the risk of smoking between urban and nonurban youth? See Box 3-5 later in the chapter to look at the calculation of odds ratio to explore the difference in smokers from urban and nonurban areas and an explanation of odds ratios further in this chapter.

In addition, Jane needs to understand the risk factors within River City and what community factors might influence youth smoking. Jane explored legislation regarding smoking and found that River City has a low tax on cigarettes compared with other cities and counties in the area. She also noted that the public schools were not smoke-free zones and, although restaurants were supposed to be smoke-free, there was minimal enforcement of these regulations especially in places where older adolescents tended to congregate. Thus, on a community level, risk factors for smoking influenced the relatively low cost of tobacco products and the limited bans on public smoking.

Finally, Jane wanted to explore trends over time to understand how smoking had changed over the past 10 years in the community. Jane had previous data from community assessments that documented smoking in River City, and she found that there was an overall decrease in the percentage of adults who smoked, but that the smoking rates for youth remained largely unchanged. Jane realized that, to develop a more thorough understanding of youth smoking, she needed a bit more data about smoking. So, she used the CDC Web site and the Youth Risk Behavioral Survey to understand the specific risk factors related to youth smoking.[14] She was also able to access information from her state to compare the smoking rates in River City to state levels.

Once Jane had looked at the data on smoking, she reported to her supervisor at the Health Department that she felt that a multiprong intervention was needed to prevent smoking, to provide smoking cessation incentive for youths that smoked, and to advocate for policy-level interventions such as proposing an increased tax on tobacco products and extending the smoke-free zones in the community. She was able to advocate for her programming because she had data that demonstrated that River City had higher smoking rates compared with other cities in her region and fewer community-based interventions, such as smoke-free schools and high tobacco taxes. Jane also proposed conducting a survey of high school students in the schools within River City, selecting some urban and some nonurban schools, to better understand why students start smoking and what might motivate them to quit to develop an effective school-based intervention to reduce youth smoking. Jane used her epidemiology skills to understand the existing data and how that might inform smoking reduction efforts but also to help her understand gaps in the data so that she could plan the next steps for developing an effective, tailored public health intervention.

Web of Causation

One difficulty for Jane is determining which risk factors for youth smoking are priority concerns for River City. Multiple factors are correlated with smoking among youth including environmental risk factors both internal and external, parental smoking habits, gender, race, poverty, and educational status of the youth and their parents. Untangling the risk factors to determine what type of intervention should be developed is a challenge. To help understand the multiple factors that contribute to the development of disease, epidemiologists use a framework called the **web of causation**. This framework or model can be used to illustrate the complexity of how illness, injury, and disease are determined by multiple causes and are at the same time affected by a complex interaction of biological and sociobehavioral determinants of health (Fig. 3-5).[15,16,17]

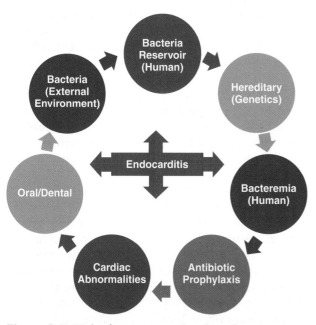

Figure 3-5 Web of causation and endocarditis.

It helps health-care providers develop more comprehensive strategies to reduce disease- and injury-related morbidity and mortality through primary and secondary prevention measures.

The term *web* is used because the model acknowledges the complexity related to occurrence of disease.[15] Simply stated, the spider is the reason the fly is caught in the web. What are the factors that converged, resulting in the ill-fated fly being caught in the web? The fly selected the path that led him to the web, he was ill equipped to extract himself from the web once entangled, the spider selected that specific location to construct his web, etc. The list of predetermining factors is endless. The fact is, for both the fly caught in the spider's web as well as for humans, there is frequently no one single cause for an undesirable outcome but a convergence of circumstances, actions, inactions, and behaviors.

Ecological Model

The ecological model has been used in recent years to design health promotion efforts and understand health behavior. The terms *health promotion* and *health behavior* have been used during the past 25 years to help understand the interventions that can be done to help maintain and improve health (health promotion), and the behaviors that contribute either positively or negatively to overall health (health behaviors). The ecological model provides a formal theoretical foundation on which public health nursing has established a professional identity and knowledge base.

Ecological studies use groups, not individuals, as the unit of analysis.[18] Conclusions from ecological studies should be considered with caution. The classic notion of the stork bringing the baby to new parents is a contemporary manifestation of what one might suggest could have been an ecological study, demonstrating the ecological fallacy discussed later in this chapter. Anchored in the pagan belief that storks brought babies to expecting mothers, the arrival of storks in northern Germany coincided with the storks' spring and the increase in the number of human births. The increased birth rates in spring might have something to do with the 9-month elapsed time between summer and normal human gestation. Analyses of health-related behaviors at the group level are carried out by epidemiologists, providing the evidence by which practice-based health-care providers can begin the development of interventions using the ecological model approach. An effective ecological model defines, understands, changes behavior, and ultimately promotes population-level health and wellness.

Tools of Epidemiology: Demography and Biostatistics

The science of epidemiology requires the use of particular tools to help epidemiologists study health and wellness as well as determine which interventions will help improve the health of populations. Among these tools are demography and biostatistics. Understanding how to apply demography and biostatistics helps nurses in all settings to provide better care and promote the health of the populations they serve.

Demography

Demography is the population-level study of person-related variables or factors. The field of demography has been around since the early 20th century. Warren Thompson, an early pioneer, developed the demographic transition model used today to explain the shift from high birth and death rates to low birth and death rates within populations.[19] Warren Thompson is to the field of demography as Florence Nightingale is to nursing and John Snow is to epidemiology. Establishing methods for tracking populations over time adds to the methods of tracking disease established by John Snow. Public health and health-related disciplines use demography and associated methods to better understand population-level patterns related to health phenomena.

Typically, person-related variables are compared over two or more time periods to establish trends within the population of interest. Comparing demographic data from time 1 to time 2 is fundamental to the promotion and establishment of relevant prohealth environments, policies, and behaviors across time. For example, comparing the percentage of the population below the poverty level in a particular community from 2010 to 2020 can help identify changes in the population that may affect access to health care. Another example is to put together a visual depiction of demographic data using the demographic transition model (Fig. 3-6). This model refers to population change over time, especially in relation to birth and death rates.

One measure of the health of populations used to compare populations from a global perspective is life expectancy. **Life expectancy** is the average number of years a person born in a given country would live if mortality rates at each age were to remain constant in the future.[20] Based on 2015 estimates worldwide, there is a wide range among countries in relation to the average life expectancy at birth (50.1 years in Sierra Leone to 83.7 years in Japan).[20] One of the reasons for lower life expectancy

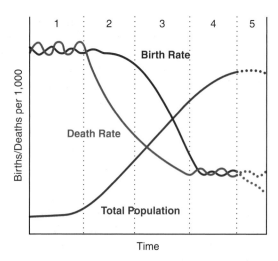

Figure 3-6 Demographic transition.

in low- and middle-income countries is that they experience more difficulty with control and eradication of communicable diseases and the illnesses associated with maternal, child, and women's health. Also, many of these countries lack the health benefits of more stable economies with advanced industrial and technological developments. The study of trends across time results in interventions including policy reform, re-engineering, educational initiatives, and enforcement of standards and laws to assure the health of the public. Public health is a dynamic interdisciplinary field associated with other fields such as political science, sociology, criminology, and psychology. Ultimately, the sociobehavioral determinants of health contributing to the health of individuals are affected substantially by subsystems such as political, social, and environmental factors.[21]

Obtaining Population Data

A challenge for public health professionals is obtaining current and accurate population data. There are various sources of data from the local to the international level. Data are obtained initially through various routes including surveys, mandatory health data reports, independent research, and hospital data, to name a few. Some of the data are available on the Internet, whereas other data are protected and special permission is needed to obtain them.

Census Data: Census data are extremely useful sources of demographic data. These public domain data are available on the official U.S. Census Bureau Web site (see Web Resources on Davis*Plus*) as well as in multiple formats upon special request. It is advised that public health researchers, health promotion planners, and other professionals charged with developing and implementing health promotion and disease prevention initiatives access and review local, regional, and state-level data provided in the U.S. Census. Accessing U.S. Census data related to a population located in a specific geographical area is a very effective starting point when seeking to quantify a health-related phenomenon. Demographic variables include gender, race, housing, economic level, age, and other relevant data. However, census data reflect populations within a specific geographical area. The census data are available from the national level down to the neighborhood or census block level and are useful if the population of interest is defined based on a geographical community. The data can be viewed based on ZIP code, town, county, or state. Accessing the Web site provides a mechanism for exploring a town or county to determine what the population is, how many housing units are rented or owned, and how many people living in the town or county have an income below the poverty level.

Community Data: More typically, public health professionals are asked to address community-level health issues. Community data are valuable resources with both strengths and limitations. Before addressing sources of community data, it would be useful to review the discussion of community in Chapter 1. Which of the following is representative of a community—residents in Portland, Oregon, diabetics in the tri-state area, women above age 65 years, or gay men in Houston, Texas? An answer of "all of the above" would be correct. Community data are not limited to simply a geographical location but can take on additional characteristics such as disease status (diabetes), sexual orientation (gay, lesbian, bisexual), and demographics (race, ethnicity, and age). Examples of typical opportunities for public health nurses and other health-related professionals to use community data include hospital-based initiatives, health plan initiatives, nonprofit agency initiatives, special interest groups, and local/state/federal initiatives.

One example of community data relating to the health of residents in cities, states, and territories is the Behavioral Risk Factor Surveillance Study (BRFSS) found at the CDC Behavioral Risk Factor Surveillance System Frequently Asked Questions section of its Web site. Disease-specific data and health-planning and education resource materials can be found at the American Diabetes Association Web site as well as at local area health-care agencies (see Web Resources on Davis*Plus*). As previously mentioned, if the community is a geographical community, the U.S. Census data can be used to focus on demographic information such as the number of women older than age 65 years. More challenging might be tapping community-level data on variables such as sexual orientation. Challenges in estimating these variables (e.g., number of gay men living in Houston, Texas) are difficult to overcome as there is a lack of accurate and reliable data sources. Data relating to these more complex variables can be, and often are, generated through original data collection at the community level.

The Nurses' Health Study, now more than 30 years old, is of special interest to nursing professionals. Information on this study can be found on a Harvard University Web site (see Web Resources on Davis*Plus*). This study provides community-level data that have been generalized to women's health in the general population. By seeking to better understand community-level data, such as women's health, a more complete understanding of the factors influencing health and appropriate proactive measures toward the improvement of women's health can be successfully achieved. Community data can relate to person, place, and time variables and a myriad of interactions between these three broad categories. Responsible investigators should always take a critical look at the sources of data and remain cognizant that errors likely exist within any data to be used in the development of community health programming. Potential sources of error should not halt efforts to promote the health of the public but should be carefully considered and reported openly.

Biostatistics

Biostatistics reflects the analysis of data related to human organisms and is used in public health science and other biological sciences. It examines variations among biological organisms (people, mice, cells). Thus, it is a core part of public health science.

Mean, Median, and Mode

Demographers use descriptive statistics as well as advanced inferential statistical methods to describe the size, structure, and distribution patterns of populations and subpopulations within geographically defined regions. These measures include the computation of the mean, median, mode, quartiles, and interquartile ranges. Demographers also compute the percent change in populations over time as well as estimate population counts for the future. These come under the umbrella of descriptive data analysis.

Most epidemiologists regard descriptive data analysis as the initial step in analysis of demographic data. However, the analysis of data at the descriptive or inferential level of analysis is only as good as the accuracy of the data being used. Though the accuracy of data and the methods by which data are gathered go beyond the scope of this text, public health scientists should ensure that they develop thoughtful and evidenced-based original data collection protocols and review published science carefully to evaluate whether data were collected in an accurate and meaningful way.

Determining the mean, the median, and the mode uses basic math skills. All three are measures of central tendency. The mean is what is commonly considered the average, as it is the mathematical average of a set of numbers. The *mean* is calculated by summing the total of all values and dividing by the total number of values in the set. The *median* is the middle value in a set of values. For example, if you have 20 individual patient blood pressures, the 10th occurrence in an ordered set from lowest to highest is the median. The *mode* is the value that occurs more times within a data set than any other occurrence. To help you understand these basic concepts, complete the question in Box 3-1.

Percent Change

It is useful to have a time 1 and a time 2 measurement to determine a **percent change** related to a demographic variable or health statistic. The time 1 measure is often referred to as the baseline and can be used to establish the proportion or percentage of illness or disease within the population. This is often used to evaluate changes in a population over time and is calculated by taking the new number (B) and subtracting the original number (A) then dividing the resulting number by the original number A (Box 3-2). This information is quite valuable when completing community assessments (see Chapter 4), because it explains shifts in population that may have an impact on the health of the community or the type of interventions needed. For example, if there has been a positive 20% change in the population who are over the age of 85, then the community may have increased health needs related to aging, but if the opposite has occurred, a 20% decrease in those over the age of 85 and a 20% increase in those aged 1 to 5 years, there may be less need for interventions aimed at the very old and more interventions needed to support infant health.

Rates

To help in understanding the distribution of disease in a population, epidemiologists calculate rates. In understanding the magnitude of a health-related phenomenon, epidemiologists need both a numerator and a denominator. What does this statement mean? Imagine that a health educator in Columbus, Ohio reports that there

---

BOX 3–1 ■ Calculating Population Mean, Median, and Mode

Methods Review

Mean, Median, Mode, Quartiles, and Interquartile Range
Twenty students have been admitted to the dual degree MSN/MPH degree program. You have been asked by the Dean of the College to report the average age of these students.

Data Set [Not real persons]:

Name	Gender	Age in Years
1. Angela Jones	F	23
2. Bill Baker	M	32
3. Connie Clark	F	22
4. Dennis Daniels	M	24
5. Emily Edwards	F	56
6. Frank Fitzgerald	M	23
7. Georgia Grant	F	24
8. Herald Hall	M	22
9. Ingrid Israel	F	22
10. James Jennings	M	24
11. Kelly Karr	F	22
12. Lawrence Lee	M	35
13. Melissa Martin	F	22
14. Nelson Newman	M	21
15. Olivia Owen	F	22
16. Paul Pierce	M	31
17. Quinn Queen	F	27
18. Robert Reynolds	M	23
19. Sarah Salzman	F	22
20. Timothy Tucker	M	22

Q1: The mean, median, and mode are all measures of central tendency—averages. You should report all three.
A: Mean = 25.96
A: Median = 23
A: Mode = 22

BOX 3–2 ■ Calculating Percent Change [Not from an actual data set]

Formula

(Time B–Time A)/Time A × 100 = percent change

Population City A	2010 Time A	2020 Time B	Percent change
Hispanic	1,512	1,955	29.3%
85 years of age or older	215	92	−57.2%

are 12,500 smokers in his city and a health educator in Columbus, Indiana reports that there are 11,800 smokers in his city. Based on these two estimates, it is fair to say that smoking is a greater problem in Columbus, Ohio, than it is in Columbus, Indiana, correct? It is clear that there are 700 more smokers in the Ohio city than there are in the Indiana city. However, the denominator is missing in this equation. By going to the U.S. Census Bureau and learning what the city population estimate was, we can effectively establish a denominator. It is always advisable to use the same source if possible so that comparable population estimates and associated collection methods are assured in establishing estimates. If the estimated population for Columbus, Ohio is 730,657 and for Columbus, Indiana, it is 39,059, then it is possible to calculate the percentage. Now the facts are that 1.7% of the population in Columbus, Ohio, smokes compared with 30.2% in Columbus, Indiana!

Using these data from the two towns, we just calculated the rate of smoking in each population. To further illustrate how a rate is determined, consider being the health commissioner of Petersburg, Oregon, with a population 5,000. Of the total population, 1,250 people report that they are current cigarette smokers. The health department receives a weekly report on the number of influenza cases reported in the city in the month of January (Table 3-1). One should assume that these data are accurate and that no reporting error exists.

Given the data in Table 3-1 and the information on how many people live in the city, we can construct population rates of influenza cases across the two classifications of smoker and nonsmoker. First, using the data in the table, calculate the rate of influenza in smokers during week 1. To do this, divide 50 by 1,250, which illustrates a rate of 4%, or 4 in every 100 smokers came down with the flu in week 1. In comparison, less than 1% of nonsmokers came down with the flu in week 1

(1 in 100). If one considers the total population percentages by week, there was a spike in cases during the third week of January. However, by breaking the data out by smoking status, it is clear that there are variations in the monthly pattern across the two groups. Therefore, a **rate** represents the proportion of a disease or other health-related event, such as mortality, within a population at a certain point in time. It is the basic measure of disease used by epidemiologists and other health professionals to describe the risk of disease in a certain population over a certain period of time.

How to Calculate: Calculating rates is a relatively simple mathematical procedure, if one can secure an accurate estimate of disease or illness in the population to use as the numerator and an accurate total population estimate to serve as the denominator (Box 3-3). Again, using the data in Table 3-1, focus on the first cell corresponding to week 1: smokers with influenza. The numerator is 50 (week 1 influenza cases) and the denominator is 1,250 (smokers residing in Petersburg, Oregon). The number 100 represents a constant, in this case per 100 smokers. The constant could be 1,000 or 10,000 depending on the frequency of the disease in the population. This approach allows for the presentation of rates based on various constants. One may express a rate in terms of 1,000 or 10,000 rather than 100 if the number of cases is small. For example, infant mortality rate is expressed as the number of infant deaths for infants less than age 1 year per 1,000 live births.

Types of Rates: Mortality and morbidity are two commonly used rates in epidemiology as well as within the health-care professions. **Mortality** refers to the number of deaths within a given population. To calculate the mortality rate, take the number of deaths within a specified time-period and divide it by the total number of individuals within the same population during the same time period. A commonly used mortality rate is the

TABLE 3–1 ■ Fabricated Data—Influenza in Anytown, USA

Week	Influenza Smoker	Influenza Nonsmoker	Total Influenza
	Number of New Cases	*Number of New Cases*	*Number of New Cases*
1	50 (4.0%)	20 (0.5%)	70 (1.4%)
2	40 (3.2%)	25 (6.8%)	65 (1.3%)
3	80 (6.4%)	50 (1.35%)	130 (2.6%)
4	700 (56.0%)	100 (2.7%)	800 (16.0%)
	1,250 (Smokers)	3,700 (Nonsmokers)	5,000 (Total Population)

BOX 3–3 ■ Calculating Rates

Using the data in Table 3-1, focus on the first cell corresponding to week 1—smokers with influenza.

The rate of influenza was calculated using the following formula:

(Number of cases [numerator] ÷ population [denominator]) × a constant = rate per 100; 1,000; 10,000; or 100,000.

For this case:

$$(50 \div 1,250) \times 100 = 4.0\%$$

---

infant mortality rate, as this measure is considered an effective metric by which to gauge the health-care "systems" of a nation. To calculate the infant mortality rate, take the number of infant deaths among those ages birth to 365 days and divide by the total number of live births during the same 365-day period. To establish a rate, include a multiplier that represents the previously mentioned constant (e.g., × 1,000). **Morbidity** refers to the number or proportion of individuals experiencing a similar disability, illness, or disease. Examples of conditions and diseases reported using morbidity are the number of infants within a county with pertussis ("whooping" cough), the number of new mothers delivering at St. Ann's in 2020 experiencing postpartum depression, the number of returning service men and women experiencing post-traumatic stress disorder (PTSD), and the number of adults in the United States living with diabetes. Note that the challenge in reporting these conditions as rates is in accurately establishing the denominator or the total number of individuals at risk for the condition in question.

Attack rates are calculated by placing the number of ill or diseased people in the numerator and dividing by the total number of ill plus well people (in the susceptible population) in the population of interest, then multiplying by a given multiplier (e.g., 100,000). The **secondary attack rate** can be calculated by taking the number of new cases of a disease or illness among the contacts of the initial (primary) cases, dividing by the number of people in the population at risk, then multiplying by a given multiplier (e.g., 100,000).

Prevalence, Incidence: Prevalence and incidence rates are used by epidemiologists to demonstrate the burden of disease or illness within the population of interest. However, these practitioners must carefully consider when and how to report these rates, as they can be misleading. What is the difference between prevalence and incidence? **Incidence** can be best understood as the number of new cases of a disease or illness at a specific time or period of time. **Prevalence** is the total number of accumulated cases of a disease or illness both new and pre-existing at a given time.

Imagine that you are a public health official and that you have been serving the people of New York City for the past 25 years. In 1994, the total number of newly diagnosed cases of HIV was 2,500 and the total number of existing or prevalent cases in 1994 was 5,000. In 2014, 20 years later, the number of newly diagnosed cases of HIV is 1,000 and the total number of existing or prevalent cases is 50,000. The change in annualized new HIV cases went from 2,500 to 1,000 and the prevalence went from 5,000 to 50,000 over the 15-year period. This 20-year change shows a decrease in new cases, whereas the prevalence rate comparing the difference across the 20-year period is a 10-fold increase. Given these data, would it be fair for a reporter from the *New York Times* to feature a headline of "HIV in New York City Drastically Increases 10-fold Since the Mid-1990s!" or "HIV in NYC Decreases After 20 Years of Prevention Education"? Both headlines are accurate, yet neither is a fair nor accurate account of the state of HIV in the city.

A prevalence rate is basically the number of existing cases (numerator) divided by the total number of persons in the population (denominator). The rate calculated using the information in Table 3-1 can be understood as a point prevalence or the number of ill people divided by the total number of people in the population "group" at a specific point in time. An associated measure, referred to as the *period prevalence*, is calculated as the number of ill people divided by the estimate of the average number in the population during a specified time period. An application of period prevalence might be the number of people living with a chronic disease within a given population during a specified time, such as a year. Asthma is a chronic disease that might be effectively presented using a period prevalence.

In addition to prevalence, there are other rates reported by epidemiologists that are important to understand and use appropriately (Table 3-2). They are incidence rate, attack rate, and secondary attack rate. An incidence rate can be calculated by placing the number of new cases diagnosed in a given period of time divided by the total number at risk in the population over that same time period and multiplying by a given multiplier (e.g., 100,000). For example, the incidence of H1N1 in a school during a specified period of time would be the number of new cases of H1N1 divided by the denominator, those

TABLE 3–2 ■ Differentiating Rates

Measure	Numerator	Denominator	Multiplier
Point prevalence	Number ill	Population at risk at specific point in time	e.g., 100,000
Incidence rate	Number of new cases over specified time	Total number at risk during time period	e.g., 100,000
Attack rate	Number of new cases during an epidemic period	Total number in population at start of epidemic period	e.g., 1,000
Secondary attack rate	Number of new cases among contacts of known cases	Total number of population at risk	e.g., 1,000

children in the school who had not had H1N1 in the past. Those children who had had H1N1 would be removed from the denominator to indicate those children at risk.

A good way to examine the difference between the incidence and prevalence rate is the *prevalence pot* (Fig. 3-7), defined in Chapter 2. The prevalence pot represents all the current cases of a disease in a population. Entering into the pot are the new cases reflected by the incidence rate. Exit from the prevalence pot occurs by one of three events: death, cure, or disability. For some diseases such as HIV/AIDS the only way a case leaves the prevalence pot is through death. For other diseases such as polio, all three options occur. The size of the prevalence pot depends both on the incidence rate and on the duration of the disease. Over time the prevalence pot for HIV/AIDS in the United States has grown not because of dramatic increases in the incidence of HIV/AIDS but because of the pharmaceutical interventions that have extended life expectancy. For other serious health threats such as the 2017-2018 H3N3 virus, the prevalence pot grew rapidly with the increase in incidence but dropped rapidly once incidence rates dropped because of the short duration of the disease.

The incidence and prevalence rates are affected by factors such as the number of people being screened for the disease and the number of people surviving with a positive HIV status. During the early 1980s and into the 1990s, few people survived a positive diagnosis for more than a few years. Thus, the absence of effective medical treatment options would have resulted in higher death rates and subsequently lower prevalence rates. As screening tests became more widely available and stigmatizing labels began to be reduced, more people became willing to be screened for HIV. What is missing from the presentation is the number of people tested who were not positive for HIV. The lesson to be learned is that data

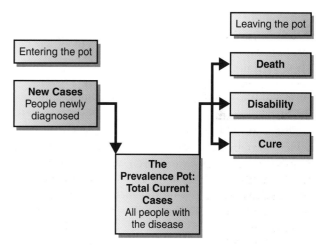

Figure 3-7 Prevalence pot.

reporting does not necessarily result in effective interpretation. Careful, cautious, and intentional epidemiological data reporting is a critical task of the public health information officer.

Comparing Dependent and Independent Rates: Data in Table 3-1 provide a useful illustration of independent and dependent rates. The weekly influenza rates independent of smoking status for the month of January are 15.0, 12.5, 26.0, and 16.0 per 100 persons, respectively. Simply stated, these weekly rates are independent of the smoking status of the individuals within the population. The converse is true for dependent rates where the rates of influenza by smoking status by week range from approximately 40% to 32%, spiking to 64%, and finally dropping to 56%. The week 3 spike pattern is also reflected in the nonsmoking population. However, the proportion of nonsmokers with influenza is consistently 25% to 50% lower than that estimated for smokers. Therefore, a public health official might accurately state that influenza rates (independent of smoking) for Petersburg, Oregon, for January ranged between 12.5% and 26%. In addition, dependent rates adjusted for smoking status for the city and time-period demonstrated a substantially greater proportion of influenza among smokers.

The terms *independent rates* and *dependent rates* are also used to describe rates that are independent or not independent of each other. For example, if you were concerned with the infant mortality rate in city Y compared with the infant mortality rate in city X, the two rates would be independent of each other. By contrast, if you wanted to compare the rates between city Y in state X and the rate in state X, the rates are dependent; that is, all of the cases in city Y are included in the count of cases in state X because the city is in state X.

Descriptive and Analytical Epidemiology

Now that we have examined the basic demographics of the population of interest, what else can be done to learn about the specific health issue? There are three broad categories of epidemiological studies that help to answer questions about the health of populations: descriptive, analytical, and experimental studies. The majority of epidemiological investigations, particularly community-based public health investigations, are defined as either descriptive or analytical. In descriptive or observational case control and cohort studies, the investigator has no control over the exposure or nonexposure status of subjects. By contrast, experimental epidemiology consists of the research methodology whereby the investigator has direct control over the subject's assignment to exposure status. Clinical trials fall into the latter classification. Experimental studies tend to fall under the authority of clinical research scientists and are housed in academic research centers, federal agencies, or private research and development agencies, such as pharmaceutical companies.

Descriptive Epidemiology

Descriptive epidemiology refers to the analysis of population and health data that are already available. It includes the calculation of rates (e.g., mortality) and an examination of how they vary according to demographic variables (e.g., gender, race, socioeconomic status).[22] Similar to demography, descriptive epidemiology provides an understanding of the general features of the population of interest. In contrast to demography, the epidemiologist shifts from a broad population demographic representation to one that illustrates aspects

of health, wellness, and/or disease considerations within the population.

Analytical Epidemiology

Analytical epidemiology involves examining health-related data to determine the association between risk factors and the occurrence of a health phenomenon. In descriptive epidemiology, the epidemiologist can use the findings to formulate a hypothesis about possible causes for the health phenomenon. In analytical epidemiology, the purpose is to test the hypothesis. There are three basic types of studies that use analytical epidemiology methods: the case-control study, the cohort study, and the clinical trial. The study may use a cross-sectional design that reports health-related information for a specific point in time. Or the study may use a prospective, retrospective, or longitudinal design related to data collected in more than one time period.

Cross-Sectional Studies

Cross-sectional studies or surveys examine risk factors and disease using data collected at the same point in time. It is easy to remember that a cross-sectional study provides an estimate of the disease status or frequency at one point in time; thus, it is truly a cross section of the disease or illness within the population of interest at a given moment in time. It is also called a prevalence study. For example, numerous health surveys are conducted by the National Center for Health Statistics as a means of determining the prevalence of disease at a given point in time. They are relatively easy to administer, and the data can be collected in a rather short period of time. However, because they are cross-sectional, they do not provide a temporal, or time-related, sequence of events. For example, if nurse Jane in River City wanted to determine specific risk factors for smoking among adolescents, she might conduct a survey of the students through the school system to ask about specific smoking habits and risk factors. Jane might also ask whether any of the students' parents smoked. However, because Jane collected data at one point in time, she cannot with confidence assert that parental smoking preceded smoking initiation by the student. However, the data can provide valuable information on which risk factors might be related to smoking among the youth in River City.

The cross-sectional design methods are not limited to the study of disease or even illness factors. For example, this research design methodology can be used to evaluate satisfaction with health-care–related services within a community.

Case-Control Studies and Odds Ratio

The case-control study design allows the epidemiologist to compare the ratio of disease in those exposed to a risk factor with those who were not exposed to the same risk factor. Using the case-control method, the epidemiologist has a specified number of people with a disease or illness. These individuals who are defined as diseased or ill are the "cases." The epidemiologist then must seek to establish a representative group of people without the disease or illness as the controls. Then both the cases and controls are measured related to a specific exposure or multiple exposures.

A standard two-by-two table is used to divide individual-level or person-specific data into disease status (yes/no) and exposure status (yes/no). The odds ratio (OR) is defined as the odds of having a disease or condition among the exposed in comparison with the odds of those who were not exposed. The calculation of the OR is a relatively simple mathematical procedure. The OR is mathematically expressed as [OR = AD/BC] (Box 3-4). The epidemiologist then determines whether the OR for those with the disease who have experienced exposure is significantly greater than the controls by calculating confidence intervals and p-values for each OR point estimate. This calculation goes beyond the introductory nature of this text. Intermediate and advanced epidemiology textbooks can and should be consulted to gain depth of understanding of these calculations.

Take, for example, individuals with oral cancer of the gums. The researcher hypothesizes that people who use or have a history of using smokeless tobacco (chewing tobacco) are at greater risk of developing oral cancer. The researcher now needs a group of individuals to serve as the controls. To construct the two-by-two table and establish the risk of oral cancer from chewing tobacco, she needs a group of individuals who have not been exposed to chewing tobacco. The cases are the individuals with oral cancer who are asked to report on exposure variable and use of chewing tobacco. The challenge is to find a fair representative group that fits into the control or "no disease" category. Often studies of this nature are conducted using controls at the same health-care facility with a different disease or illness. In this scenario, skin cancer patients will be used as controls. The biological plausibility of developing skin cancer as a result of using chewing tobacco is unlikely but could indeed be a confounder. A confounder is a studied variable that can cause the disease that is also associated with the exposure of interest. Confounders can make it difficult to establish a clear causal link unless adjustments are made for their effects. Confounders are potential limitations in all epidemiological studies; methods of controlling for confounders are addressed in advanced epidemiological textbooks.

Case-control studies have limitations. There can be effects from multiple determinants of health, the complexity of additive, and/or interactive exposures on health. There are also potential problems related to the representativeness of the cases and the controls, that is, how well they reflect the target population. Another issue is accurately determining exposure. Case-control studies are done **retrospectively**; that is, disease has already occurred in the cases. For both cases and controls, determining whether individuals have been exposed requires obtaining a history from the individuals rather than through direct observation of the exposure. See Box 3-5 for a case-control study of the smoking among youth in River City.

Cohort Studies and Relative Risk

Cohort studies are studies that follow a specific population, subset of the population, or group of people over a specified period of time. Cohort studies can be effective in generating a wealth of data relating to the population

---

BOX 3-4 ■ Calculating Odds Ratio

	Disease Status (Yes)	Disease Status (No)
Exposure status (Yes)	A	B
Exposure status (No)	C	D

BOX 3-5 ■ Case-Control Study for River City

Set up a two-by-two table for children aged birth to 18 years with residency (urban/nonurban) on one axis and smoking status (yes/no) on the other axis.
Answer:

	Smoker (Yes)	Smoker (No)	Totals
Urban	1,500	1,500	3,000
Non-urban	1,000	6,000	7,000
Totals	2,500	7,500	10,000

Calculate the appropriate measure of association. HINT: Either relative risk or odds ratio.
Answer: Odds ratio — AD ÷ BC = 1,500 × 6,000 ÷ 1,500 × 1,000 — [OR = 6.0] Interpretation: River City youth between the ages of birth to 18 years living in the urban district have six times the risk of smoking as compared with nonurban youth.

of interest. The epidemiologist has substantial control over the data collection process; therefore, cohort studies have strong validity. This validity comes with high costs that include actual direct costs in personnel as well as costs in time from data collection to the generation of findings and conclusions. Two types of cohort studies are found in application:

- Prospective
- Retrospective (also called historical)

Two Web links are provided in the following section. The first directs you to the Fels Longitudinal Study established in 1929, the longest-running continuous human life span and development study in the world. This longitudinal study is housed at the Wright State University Boonshoft School of Medicine in Dayton, Ohio, and can be accessed at https://medicine.wright.edu/epidemiology-and-biostatistics/fels-longitudinal-study-collection. The second is to the Framingham study, a commonly referenced cardiovascular health study established in 1948. Both studies are longitudinal and provide useful data to researchers on human populations over time. Information on the Framingham study can be accessed at http://www.framinghamheartstudy.org.[23]

The *relative risk* is the measure of association used for cohort studies. Relative risk is determined by comparing the incidence rate in the exposed group with the incidence rate in the non-exposed group. This measure is calculated by dividing the number of people in the yes/yes (cell A) divided by the row total (cells A+B) divided by the number of people in the yes/no (cell C) divided by that row total (cells C+D) (Box 3-6).

For example, if we were interested in exploring the risks of using oral birth control pills and stroke (these are fabricated data), we could follow 500 women from age 18 to 25 during a specific time period. We would divide these women into two groups: those taking an oral birth control pill (250) and those using alternative birth control or none (250). We find that after following these 500 women during the 32-year study, among those who were taking the pill, 100 suffered a stroke and 150 had no stroke, whereas among those not taking the pill, 24 had

a stroke and 225 had no stroke. How would the relative risk be calculated?

Confounder WARNING

Of the 100 women taking oral contraception, 90 were cigarette smokers. What additional information is needed to establish a confounder effect based on tobacco use? As explained earlier, a confounder is another variable that may actually account in whole or in part for the relationship between the observed variable (taking the pill) and the outcome (stroke).

Most cohort studies use a **prospective** longitudinal approach that requires following a group over a long period of time, which can be 30 years or more. An example is the Nurses' Health Study that began in 1976. The purpose of the study was to examine the long-term effects of oral contraceptives.[24] The researchers have added to this important study with the Nurses' Health Study II in 1989 and the Nurses' Health Study III in 2008. Data are collected from participants every 2 years with a sustained 90% response rate. Clearly, this type of design is limited in application because waiting more than 30 years to establish conclusive results can be problematic. In addition, the notion of confounders, or factors affecting the outcome other than the factor of interest, is a limitation. Despite these challenges, data from large cohort studies have contributed greatly to our understanding of risk factors related to disease. The Framingham heart study is still ongoing today, spanning three generations.[23] Prior to the study, the common belief was that cardiovascular disease was part of the aging process. The information obtained in the study changed the approach to the prevention and treatment of cardiovascular disease and continues to contribute to our understanding of cardiovascular disease today.

There are times when a cohort study is done retrospectively. Imagine a situation in which 500 women today are asked to report on their past 32 years of history. Specifically, data are collected on all 500 women relating to oral contraception usage and stroke. Note: In this retrospective study design, you can add a variable such as cigarette smoking. This design methodology provides the researcher with the opportunity to report findings in the present relating to the variables of interest. Recall is often a problem with any study design that seeks to collect data from the subjects based on their recall regardless of the recall period. Often an individual can't remember what he or she ate for breakfast a week ago, or what his or her last fasting blood sugar was. Imagine how much error might be present in collecting health behavior data from the general population. Sources of error in this design

---

BOX 3–6 ■ Calculating Relative Risk

HINT: $(A \div [A + B]) \div (C \div [C + D])$

	Stroke	No Stroke	Total
Oral pill	100	150	250
No oral pill	25	225	250

also include subject attrition or discontinued participation, a concern known as *right censoring,* which is beyond the scope of this introductory text; confounding; and other issues related to following a large cohort over a long period of time.

Clinical Trials and Causality

Clinical trials represent a special type of epidemiological investigation and the related research methods are a special subset. Clinical trials vary widely in their method, but generally have a control and an experimental group, and require random assignment to one of these groups. The control group is not exposed to a treatment, medication, or therapy, whereas the experimental group is exposed to the treatment or intervention of interest. The two groups are then compared to evaluate whether there are statistically significant differences in outcomes between the two groups. Clinical trials are more likely to result in findings that lend themselves to causal statements of relationships. Cohort and case-control studies can demonstrate an association between two variables, but a clinical trial gets much closer to establishing causality. That said, causality is always a challenging goal to attain and causal assumptions within clinical research trials should be carefully considered.

Outbreak Investigations

Outbreak investigation is fundamental to field epidemiology and pivotal to the role of epidemiologists, public health nurses, and public health workers. As previously confirmed, epidemiology is truly an applied science. Epidemiologists use quantitative data analysis methods at the population level to better understand health-related circumstances within communities. The unit of analysis is groups of people, not the individual. It is critical to remain cognizant of the risk of committing an *ecological fallacy.* The fallacy refers to the erroneous assumption that one can draw conclusions for individuals based on group findings, which occurs when the researcher draws conclusions at the individual level based solely on the observations made at the group level. An example of an ecological fallacy can be illustrated based on a study of obesity in women in two cities. Consider that the women in City A had a higher body mass index (BMI) on average than the women in City B. It would be a fallacy to conclude, just based on these averages, that a randomly selected woman from City A would have a higher BMI than a randomly selected woman from City B. Because the BMI reported in the study reflected an average and not a median, there is no information about the

distribution of BMI values in the two cities, and a randomly selected individual woman from City A may have a lower BMI than a randomly selected woman from City B.

Although much of the work of public health nurses and public health workers is focused on implementing initiatives that prevent disease or illness, the outbreak investigation is in response to elevated levels of a disease or illness within the defined population. The outbreak investigation is one of the more commonly recognized applications of epidemiology by the general public. Examples of commonly recognized outbreak investigations include foodborne illness investigations resulting from salmonella; gastroenteritis illness investigations at community daycare centers resulting from *Shigella*; communities with elevated numbers of pediatric asthma emergency room visits and subsequent hospitalization; health-care providers with unusually high numbers of patients with uncontrolled type 2 diabetes; employees with elevated levels of asbestosis; communities with unexpectedly high numbers of infants with elevated blood lead level; and, on a global level, the Ebola outbreaks in Africa. Outbreak investigations are an important application of epidemiology because of the truly applied nature of the inquiry. The investigation is not simply an academic exercise but an opportunity to initiate disease or illness investigation, analyze data collected within the community or workplace, interpret data, implement health promotion and risk reduction interventions, and evaluate short- and long-term health and the effects of wellness on the population. Precipitating factors relating to person, place, and time are essential as is an awareness of disease or illness etiology. Outbreak investigations can occur in relation to communicable diseases, chronic disease, and exposure to toxic agents.

Investigation strategies are dependent on the type of agent resulting in illness, the communicability of the illness, the virulence of the agent, and the **infectivity** of the agent. The infectivity of the agent is defined as the proportion of persons exposed to an infectious agent who become infected by it and the specific route of infection. As presented earlier in this chapter, three key aspects of tracking disease within a population and developing strategies to reduce the spread and severity of outbreaks are contingent on person, place, and time considerations. The importance of effective surveillance of disease and illness is vital in establishing expected levels of illness within the population. The CDC maintains publicly reportable data on a number of diseases (see Web Resources on Davis*Plus*).

Illnesses such as influenza and pertussis have seasonal variations and can be substantially reduced through preventive vaccination. The number of reported influenza cases typically spikes annually from December through March. Public health community-wide vaccination campaigns are initiated in the autumn each year in an attempt to prevent disease through targeted immunization at the population level. A vaccine for the prevention of pertussis was developed in the 1940s, and aggressive public health childhood immunization initiatives resulted in a low number of reported cases nationally in the mid-1970s. Unfortunately, the number of pertussis cases has increased during the past 30 years with an increasing proportion of cases among the adult and older segments of the U.S. population.[25]

Communicable Disease Outbreaks

Communicable diseases can be the result of a point source or a common source followed by secondary spread within the population. Typically, person-to-person spread is observed as with the case with the Ebola virus. However, communicable diseases such as the West Nile virus are spread through vectors, specifically insect to human. The 21st century has witnessed a substantial reduction of diseases as a result of improved environmental conditions and sanitation systems. Person-to-person spread of communicable disease continues to present substantial challenges to professions charged with promoting health and reducing the burden of disease at the population level. Unlike systems, which can be re-engineered to eliminate risks of exposure, strategies addressing person-to-person transmission of disease can be daunting. Global public health and disease prevention initiatives such as hand hygiene education and safe sex practices are initiatives seeking to address person-to-person spread of communicable diseases. See Chapter 8 for further information on how to investigate a communicable disease outbreak.

Noncommunicable Disease Outbreaks

In the latter decades of the 20th century, chronic diseases have replaced communicable diseases as the most significant disease classification in high-income countries. Simply stated, as a result of aggressive interventions during the past 100 years, the mortality rate from communicable diseases has dramatically declined, contributing to higher life expectancy. With this increased life expectancy, more people are surviving long enough to develop noncommunicable diseases that occur later in life such as cardiovascular disease. Often referred to as lifestyle diseases, illnesses related to poor diet, a lack of exercise, and tobacco and alcohol use have become epidemic. Some typically diagnosed noncommunicable diseases include heart disease, type 2 diabetes, cancer, and chronic obstructive pulmonary disorder (COPD). Initiatives including tobacco cessation programs, balanced nutrition education, and exercise/fitness programs have been and continue to be developed to combat the negative impact of noncommunicable diseases.

Although not necessarily demonstrative of traditional outbreak investigation, noncommunicable diseases can be studied with epidemiological methods comparing risk factors such as tobacco use and BMI, and the presence or absence of disease states. Unlike communicable diseases in which there exists a direct cause-and-effect relationship between the exposure and the onset of disease, noncommunicable diseases are usually connected to multiple risk factors, and it can be harder to demonstrate a direct cause and effect. This presents challenges in both demonstrating direct causes of disease and changing destructive behaviors within the population that compromise health.

Exposure to Toxins

Similar to noncommunicable diseases, exposure to toxins has emerged as a substantial risk to human health and wellness. As with noncommunicable diseases, a direct cause-and-effect relationship is difficult to prove. In fact, toxic substances often have thresholds below which exposures do not present human health risks but above which can prove to have adverse and at times fatal consequences. The movement during the past 40 years has been to advance the study of risk exposure to potentially toxic substances. Organizations including the National Institute for Occupational Safety and Health (NIOSH), CDC, EPA, and ATSDR have made substantial gains in research and policy to reduce toxic risks adversely affecting the health of the public.

Surveillance

James Maxwell, a physician in the 1800s, once said "We owe all the great advances in knowledge to those who endeavor to find out how much there is of anything."[26] This could be a summary of epidemiology but also specifically of surveillance, which focuses on determining and monitoring "how much there is" of diseases, health conditions, environmental disasters, or other risk factors. The CDC defines public surveillance as "the ongoing, systematic collection, analysis, and interpretation of health-related data essential to planning, implementation, and evaluation of public health practice."[27] Surveillance principles are used when universities provide information on interpersonal violence on campus, the CDC reports on communicable disease outbreaks or changes to the rates of tobacco use, or the WHO provides national and global level estimates on the prevalence of tuberculosis infection. All these reports are based on collecting and interpreting data to make practice or policy recommendations.

There are two main types of surveillance: passive and active. **Passive surveillance** is when data are collected based on individuals or institutions that report on health information either voluntarily or by mandate. The onus for collecting and reporting of the data to public health or governmental agencies is on health-care providers or public health professions in the field. For example, day-care centers are often required to report an increase in the number of cases of communicable disease like hand foot and mouth (caused by an enterovirus) to the local or state health departments so that the health departments can report and monitor communicable diseases. One of the challenges in passive surveillance is ensuring that those reporting the data have adequate resources to collect accurate data. If the data is inaccurate or only some agencies are reporting the data then there is a risk that the data will be biased or will not reflect the actual conditions of the population. Surveillance in low- and middle-income countries can be particularly challenging where local and national governments may not have adequate resources to accurately collect morbidity and mortality data. The consequence of poor surveillance data is that it can be difficult to accurately prioritize health-care resources on a national and global level because the true levels of disease are poorly understood.

One example using the results of surveillance to understand the impact of disease is the global burden of disease. As will be discussed in more detail in Chapter 9, the **burden of disease** is defined by the WHO as the difference between a population's actual health status and the "ideal" health status if everyone were to live to their fullest potential and life span. It is measured in the years of life lost to both premature mortality and disability.[28,29] These data include information about the impact of a health problem on a population using indicators such as monetary cost, mortality, and morbidity, and refers to this as the burden of disease. To help measure the burden of disease, statisticians calculate the **disability-adjusted life years (DALY)** that considers not only mortality but also the morbidity and the disability associated with a disease or risk factor. Such reports are compiled by organizations like the WHO based on global surveillance reports and other local and national data sources. These data help researchers evaluate the impact of interventions and identify areas for action (see Chapter 9 for additional information and how to calculate DALY).

A second type of surveillance is **active surveillance**, which involves the deployment of public health professionals including nurses to identify cases of a disease or health condition under surveillance. This could involve reviewing medical records, interviewing health-care providers or hospital administrators, and surveying those exposed to the condition. Active surveillance is typically used in an outbreak where there is a sudden change in the number of cases of a particular disease or condition. The Ebola responses in Sierra Leone and Liberia provide examples of active surveillance where multiple organizations including the CDC and WHO were involved in finding cases, tracking the spread of disease, and deploying staff to prevent further transmission.

▼ CASE STUDY
Investigating Motor Vehicle Crashes using Epidemiology

Learning Outcomes
- Apply epidemiology methods to a public health concern.
- Explore sources of epidemiologic data on a national, state, and local level.

You are a public health nurse at your state's health department tasked with identifying one of the leading causes of mortality and morbidity, and working with a local university to design a study to further explore risk factors related to the identified cause. After comparing state-level surveillance data to national data, you realize that motor vehicle crashes (MVCs) are a leading cause of death and injury in your state.

Discussion Points
- Using the seven questions for epidemiologic investigations, list what type of information you would like to gather about MVCs.
- Identify where you might find additional information regarding MVCs on a local, state, or national level.
- If you were to design an epidemiologic study to gather more data on MVCs in your state, what type of study could you design? What are the pros and cons to your study design?

▮ Summary Points
- Epidemiology provides the scientific basis for understanding the occurrence of health and disease.
- An epidemiological investigation revolves around person, place, and time.

- An understanding of risk factors for disease from an individual and ecological perspective is essential for the development of effective interventions.
- The two-by-two table is a principle pertaining to epidemiological investigation and analysis.
- Epidemiological investigations include descriptive and analytical epidemiology.
- Surveillance, both passive and active, helps to identify and respond to public health concerns such as outbreaks of communicable diseases.

REFERENCES

1. Martin, N., & Montagne, R. (2017, May 12). U.S. has the worst rate of maternal deaths in the developed world. *NPR*. Retrieved from https://www.npr.org/2017/05/12/528098789/u-s-has-the-worst-rate-of-maternal-deaths-in-the-developed-world.
2. Centers for Disease Control and Prevention. (2017). *Pregnancy mortality surveillance system*. Retrieved from https://www.cdc.gov/reproductivehealth/maternalinfanthealth/pmss.html.
3. Friis, R.H., & Sellers, T.A. (2014). *Epidemiology for public health practice* (5th ed.). Boston, MA: Jones & Bartlett.
4. World Health Organization. (2017). *Global tuberculosis report 2017*. Retrieved from http://www.who.int/tb/publications/global_report/en/.
5. Snow, J. (1965). *Snow on cholera*. Cambridge, MA: Harvard University Press.
6. Lilienfeld, A.M., & Lilienfeld, D.E. (1980). *Foundations of epidemiology* (2nd ed.). New York, NY: Oxford University Press.
7. Susser, M., & Susser, E. (1996a). Choosing a future for epidemiology: I. Eras and paradigms. *American Journal of Public Health, 86*(5), 668-673.
8. Susser, M., & Susser, E. (1996b). Choosing a future for epidemiology: II. From black boxes to Chinese boxes and eco-epidemiology. *American Journal of Public Health, 86*(5), 674-677.
9. WHO. (n.d.). *Risk factors*. Retrieved from http://www.who.int/topics/risk_factors/en/.
10. CDC. (2018). *Behavioral risk factor surveillance system*. Retrieved from https://www.cdc.gov/brfss/index.html.
11a. CDC. (2017). *Youth risk behavior survey 1997-2017*. Data retrieved from https://www.cdc.gov/healthyyouth/data/yrbs/.
11b. CDC. (2017). *National health interview survey 1997-2017*. Data retrieved from https://www.cdc.gov/nchs/nhis/index.htm.
12. National Cancer Institute. (2018). *BRCA mutations: cancer risk and genetic testing*. Retrieved from http://www.cancer.gov/about-cancer/causes-prevention/genetics/brca-fact-sheet.
13. WHO. (2018). *Tobacco*. Retrieved from http://www.who.int/mediacentre/factsheets/fs339/en/.
14. CDC. (2018). *Youth and tobacco use*. Retrieved from https://www.cdc.gov/tobacco/data_statistics/fact_sheets/youth_data/tobacco_use/index.htm.
15. Krieger, N. (1994). Epidemiology and the web of causation: Has anyone seen the spider? *Social Science Medicine, 39*(7), 887-903.
16. Diez Roux, A.V. (2007). Integrating social and biological factors in health research: A systems review. *Annals of Epidemiology, 17*(7), 569-574.
17. Shapiro, S. (2008). Causation, bias and confounding: A hitchhiker's guide to the epidemiological galaxy, part 2. Principles of causality in epidemiological research: Confounding, effect modification, and strength of association. *Journal of Family Planning and Reproductive Health Care, 34*(3), 185-190.
18. Reifsnider, E., Gallagher, M., & Forgione, B. (2005). Using ecological models in research on health disparities. *Journal of Professional Nursing, 21*(4), 216-222.
19. Lee, P.R., & Estes. C.L. (2003). *The nation's health* (7th ed.). Burlington, MA: Jones & Bartlett.
20. WHO. (2016). *Life expectancy increased by 5 years since 2000, but health inequalities persist*. Retrieved from http://www.who.int/mediacentre/news/releases/2016/health-inequalities-persist/en/.
21. Szklo, M., & Nieto, F.J. (2012). *Epidemiology: Beyond the basics* (3rd ed.). Boston, MA: Jones & Bartlett.
22. Babbie, E. (2016). *The practice of social research* (14th ed.). New York, NY: Wadsworth.
23. National Heart, Lung and Blood Institute & Boston University. (2018). *Framingham heart study*. Retrieved from http://www.framinghamheartstudy.org/.
24. The Nurses' Health Study. (n.d.). Retrieved from http://www.nurseshealthstudy.org/
25. CDC. (2018). *Pertussis (whooping cough)*. Retrieved from https://www.cdc.gov/pertussis/surv-reporting.html.
26. Gordis, L. (2014). *Epidemiology* (5th ed.). Philadelphia, PA: Elsevier Saunders.
27. Thacker, S.B., & Birkhead, G.S. (2008). Surveillance. In: M.B. Gregg (Ed.), *Field epidemiology*. Oxford, England: Oxford University Press.
28. Murray, C., & Lopez, A. (1996). *The global burden of disease: A comprehensive assessment of mortality and disability from diseases, injuries, and risk factors in 1990 and projected to 2020*. Cambridge, MA: Harvard University Press.
29. Murray, C., & Lopez, A. (2013). Measuring the global burden of disease. *The New England Journal of Medicine, 369*, 448-457.

Chapter 4

Introduction to Community Assessment

Christine Savage and Joan Kub

LEARNING OUTCOMES

After reading the chapter, the student will be able to:

1. Define community health assessment within the context of population health.
2. Describe six approaches to conducting an assessment (comprehensive community assessment, population focused, setting specific, problem focused, health impact, rapid needs assessments).
3. Describe two assessment frameworks (MAPP, CHANGE).
4. Use secondary data to identify health characteristics of a community.
5. Describe qualitative and quantitative methods to collect primary data for conducting an assessment.
6. Describe the use of multiple techniques and tools (geographic information system [GIS], PhotoVoice) to conduct community assessments.
7. Discuss the usefulness of community assessments.
8. Use the frameworks in conducting a hypothetical assessment of a community.
9. Analyze primary and secondary data to identify strengths and needs of a community.

KEY TERMS

Aggregate data
Assets
Census block
Census tract
Community
Community-based participatory research (CBPR)
Community Health Assessment

Community Health Assessment and Group Evaluation (CHANGE)
Comprehensive community assessment
Deidentified data
Focus group
Geographic information system (GIS)

Health impact assessment
Inventory of resources
Kinship/Economics/Education/Political/Religious/Associations (KEEPRA)
Key informant
Mobilizing for Actions Through Planning and Partnerships (MAPP)

PhotoVoice
Population
Population pyramid
Primary data
Qualitative data
Quantitative data
Rapid needs assessment
Secondary data
Windshield survey

▇ Introduction

Assessment, the first step in the nursing process, is focused on determining the health status and needs of an individual. In public health practice, a **community health assessment** is a strategic plan that describes the health of a community by collecting, analyzing, and using data to educate and mobilize communities; develop priorities; obtain resources; and plan actions to improve health.[1,2] Assessment is one of the three core public health functions established by the Institute of Medicine (IOM)[3] in 1988 (see Chapter 1) and is critical to the work of public health, especially as it relates to the other core functions, policy development and assurance.[3]

Nurses conduct community assessments as the first step in the development of health programs and interventions aimed at optimizing the health of a community or population. For example, Dulemba, Glazer, and Gregg (2017) conducted a community assessment prior to developing an action plan for persons with chronic obstructive pulmonary disease (COPD) who were residing in east-central Indiana and west-central Ohio.[4] Other health-care professionals and community partners have come together and used the principles of community health assessment to better understand the health needs of vulnerable groups. For example, a team in Chicago utilized a community participatory method to do an assessment in a Mexican immigrant community.[5] A thorough assessment prior to putting in place community/population health interventions not only provides needed information on risk factors within the community, but also increases the understanding of the complex interactions between multiple aspects of a community that impact health such as culture, environment, infrastructure, and resources. It also provides a method of assessing the resources of the community as well as the perspectives of those who live in the community. Conducting assessments in partnership with the community is an essential component and provides buy-in from the beginning as evidenced by the assessments referenced earlier when conducted in both an urban and a rural community.

Just as an individual nursing assessment requires special skills, a community assessment also requires a unique set of skills to systematically examine the health status, needs, perceptions, and assets or resources of a community. Some of the skills or competencies needed to conduct such an assessment include selecting health indicators, using appropriate methods for collecting data, evaluating data, identifying gaps, and interpreting and using data. Basic community health assessments skills for frontline public health professionals, also referred to as Tier 1 professionals, are set out by the Council on Linkages Between Academia and Public Health Practice (Box 4-1).[6] Note, of the eight competency domains for public health professionals, assessment/analytical competency is the first domain. As with the nursing process, assessment is the first step in the process for achieving optimal health in populations and communities.

Definitions of Community and Community Health

Defining the concepts of community and community health is critical in thinking about a community assessment.

A **community**, as defined in Chapter 1, is a group of individuals living within the same geographical area, such as a town or a neighborhood, or a group of individuals who share some other common denominator, such as ethnicity or religious orientation. In contrast to aggregates and population, individuals within the community recognize their membership in the community based on social interaction and establishment of ties to other members in the community, and often participate in collective decision making.

There is a great deal of media interest in the health of communities. Media outlets often use various indices such as mental wellness, lifestyle behaviors, fitness, health status, and nutrition to identify the healthiest cities in our country. Public health agencies also focus

---

BOX 4-1 ■ Core Assessment Competencies for Public Health Professionals

Analytic/Assessment Skills—Tier I

1. Describes factors affecting the health of a community
2. Identifies quantitative and qualitative data and information
3. Applies ethical principles in accessing, collecting, analyzing, using, maintaining, and disseminating data and information
4. Uses information technology in accessing, collecting, analyzing, using, maintaining, and disseminating data and information
5. Selects valid and reliable data
6. Selects comparable data
7. Identifies gaps in data
8. Collects valid and reliable quantitative and qualitative data
9. Describes public health applications of quantitative and qualitative data
10. Uses quantitative and qualitative data
11. Describes assets and resources that can be used for improving the health of a community
12. Contributes to assessments of community health status and factors influencing health in a community
13. Explains how community health assessments use information about health status, factors influencing health, and assets and resources
14. Describes how evidence is used in decision making

Source: (6)

---

on defining the health of a community. At the national level there are programs with goals to improve the health of communities such as the Centers for Disease Control and Prevention's past program Partnerships to Improve Community Health (PICH).[7]

Three important characteristics help define the health of a community: health status, structure, and competence. Selected biostatistics provide vital information about leading health issues in a community. Statistics commonly used when doing a community assessment related to health and disease are covered in Chapter 3. These statistics include indicators such as mortality rates and morbidity rates (the incidence and prevalence of disease). Mortality is often depicted by crude rates or age-adjusted rates. Next there is the structure of a community, which includes the demographics of the community as well as the services and resources available in the community. The demographic data include such indicators as age, gender, socioeconomic indicators, racial/ethnic distributions, and educational levels. The community health services and resources include information about the resources available in the community as well as service use patterns, treatment data, and provider/client ratios.

Finally, the health of a community may be conceptualized as effective community functioning, a concept developed by Cottrell in the 1970s and expanded by Goeppinger and Baglioni in the 1980s.[8,9] Conditions and select measures of community competence include commitment to the community, conflict containment, accommodation (working together), participant interaction, decision making, management of the relationships with society, participation (use of local services), awareness of self and other, and effective communication. These communities value connections between people in the community as well as those outside of the community. A competent community is able to identify its needs, achieve some goals and priorities, agree on ways to implement those goals, and collaborate effectively.[10,11] The establishment of a Neighborhood Watch program to address growing crime in a community is an example of effective functioning in which the community comes together, works to come up with a solution to a problem, and promotes a higher level of functioning by pulling together to address an issue.

Types of Community Health Assessments

The purpose of assessments is to gather information and identify areas for improving the health of communities and populations. Assessment is the first step in the process of health planning and provides essential data needed to decide where best to allocate community resources. Assessments also provide baseline data. For example, if the community is concerned about the health of infants and mothers, a community assessment can provide the data needed to determine what the actual status of maternal and infant health (MIH) is for the community; whether problems exist for the community as a whole; or whether there is a disparity in MIH based on socioeconomic status, ethnicity, or geographical location in the community. Baseline data on premature births, infant mortality, and vaccination rates help health planners determine whether the intervention had an impact during the evaluation phase of health planning (Chapter 5). The key is to understand what type of assessment is best. There are several types of community health assessments:

- Comprehensive assessment
- Population-focused assessment
- Setting-specific assessment
- Problem- or health-issue-based assessment
- Health impact assessments
- Rapid needs assessment

Comprehensive Assessment

Since the 1988 IOM report, *The Future of Public Health*, improving health in populations or communities has been linked to performing comprehensive assessments.[3] There is a mandate for public health agencies to regularly and systematically collect, assemble, analyze, and make available information on the health of the community, including statistics on health status, community health needs, and epidemiological studies of health problems.[12] In addition, the Affordable Care Act requires that nonprofit hospitals conduct community health assessments.[13] Data regarding demographic and health characteristics of the entire population are collected in these assessments. A **comprehensive community assessment** is the collection of data about the populations living within the community, an assessment of the assets within a community such as the local health department capacity, and identification of problems and issues in the community (unmet needs, health disparity) and opportunities for action.[14]

Since 1992, the CDC has guided communities in conducting assessments, making health decisions, and developing policy. There are a number of tools available for conducting community assessments such as the **Community Health Assessment and Group Evaluation (CHANGE)** tool that includes a process for conducting a comprehensive assessment of a community. Other tools are available such as **Mobilizing for Actions Through Planning and Partnerships (MAPP)** as well as some that are specific to a one aspect of community health such as PACE-EH (Chapter 6), which targets environmental health (Table 4-1).[14]

Population-Focused Assessment

A **population**, as defined in Chapter 1, is a larger group whose members may or may not interact with one another but who share at least one characteristic such as age, gender, ethnicity, residence, or a shared health issue such as HIV/AIDS or breast cancer. The common denominator or shared characteristic may or may not be a shared geography or other link recognized by the individuals within that population. For example, persons with type 2 diabetes admitted to a hospital form a population but do not share a specific culture or place of residence and may not recognize themselves as part of this population. In many situations, the terms *aggregate* and *population* are used interchangeably. An assessment can be focused on a specific population for purposes of planning and developing intervention programs. A population-focused assessment, for example, might focus on pregnant women or immigrants living

TABLE 4–1 ■ Community Assessments Tools

Model	Author, Date Released or Updated	Brief Description
Association for Community Health Improvement, Community Health Assessment toolkit (http://www.assesstoolkit.org/)	American Hospital Association, updated 2011	• Toolkit for planning, leading, and using community health needs assessments • Provides six-step assessment framework and practical guidance • Access to the full toolkit requires paid membership
Catholic Health Association (http://www.chausa.org/ communitybenefit)	Catholic Hospital Association, updated 2012	• For hospital staff who conduct or oversee community health needs assessments and plan community benefit programs • Focus on collaboration, building on existing resources, and using public health data
Mobilizing for Action through Planning and Partnerships (MAPP) (http://www.naccho.org/programs/ public-health-infrastructure/mapp)	National Association of County and City Health Officials and CDC, 2001	• Framework for community health improvement planning at the local level • Strong emphasis on community engagement and collaboration for system-level planning after identifying assets and needs
State Health Improvement Planning (SHIP) Guidance and Resources (http://www.astho.org/WorkArea/ DownloadAsset.aspx?id=6597)	Association of State and Territorial Health Officials and CDC, 2011	• Framework for state health improvement planning • Emphasis on community engagement and collaboration for system-level planning after identifying assets and needs
Community Health Assessment and Group Evaluation (CHANGE) (https://www.cdc.gov/healthy communitiesprogram/tools/ change/pdf/changeactionguide.pdf)	CDC, updated 2010	• Tool for all communities interested in creating social and built environments that support healthy living • Focus on gathering and organizing data on community assets to prioritize needs for policy changes • Users complete an action plan
Protocol for Assessing Community Excellence in Environmental Health (PACE-EH) (http://www.naccho.org/topics/ environmental/PACE-EH)	National Association of County and City Health Officials and CDC, 2000	• Tasks to investigate the relationships among what they value, how their local environment impacts their health, and next steps • For local health agencies to create a community-based environmental health assessment

Source: (14)

within a community. One community assessment was conducted to examine the health needs of Hispanic immigrants, especially in relation to the issue of adolescent pregnancy. The findings provided the information needed for the development of new interventions that would engage adolescents and other stakeholders.[15]

A population-focused assessment can also focus on a certain age range or a population with a specific health characteristic that may put the group at risk (e.g., children or, specifically, children with disabilities). In health departments, nurses are often involved with writing grants to serve the needs of mothers and children (see Chapter 17). Identifying health indicators of interest is a beginning step in the process of conducting this type of assessment. For example, the World Health Organization (WHO) identified 11 maternal-child health indicators (Box 4-2).[16] These indicators provide insight into the health of this population and a mechanism for tracking accomplishment in improving these indicators over time.

Setting-Specific Assessment

Assessments can also be focused on a specific setting. Assessments of this nature may focus on identifying strengths and weaknesses of an organization or policies and programs within an organization. Similar to other assessments, a setting-specific assessment requires a clear understanding of the purpose of the assessment to proceed in an organized manner. An occupational health assessment conducted within a company will

1. Maternal mortality ratio
2. Under-5 child mortality, with the proportion of newborn deaths
3. Children under 5 who are stunted
4. Proportion of demand for family planning satisfied (met need for contraception)
5. Antenatal care coverage (at least four times during pregnancy)
6. Antiretroviral prophylaxis among HIV-positive pregnant women to prevent HIV transmission and antiretroviral therapy for (pregnant) women who are treatment-eligible
7. Skilled attendant at birth
8. Postnatal care for mothers and babies within 2 days of birth
9. Exclusive breastfeeding for 6 months (0–5 months)
10. Three doses of combined diphtheria-tetanus-pertussis immunization coverage (12–23 months)
11. Antibiotic treatment for suspected pneumonia

Source: (16)

most likely consist of a description of the company, the working population, the health programs, and stressors present at the worksite. The same principles apply in assessing a school setting. The PHN must identify indicators relevant to the setting. Health indicators relevant to an industrial setting might include work-related injury or days absent. At a school setting the assessment would most likely begin with a description of the school, the history, policies, support services, the actual school building from an environmental perspective, the population (teachers, staff, and students), and the existing programs with an emphasis on health. There are many additional tools that can be used to assess components of school health. The School Health Index,[17] a tool available through the CDC, addresses physical activity, healthy eating, tobacco use prevention, unintentional injury, violence prevention, and asthma rates within a school system (see Chapter 18).

This type of health assessment treats the setting as the community and considers the population located in the setting. Thus, a setting assessment includes components of a comprehensive assessment and a population assessment. Taking the example of a health assessment conducted at an industrial worksite by an occupational health nurse (see Chapter 20), it would be helpful to collect and analyze data relevant to the environment, the resources available to promote health, and health statistics

specific to the population. According to the CDC, a workplace assessment involves obtaining information related to the health of employees within the workplace setting, including protective and risk factors to identify opportunities to improve the health of the workers.[18]

Problem- or Health-Issue-Based Assessment

Assessments can also focus on a specific problem or health issue. In many cases, assessments and tool kits for specific health issues can be found on the Internet. For example, obesity is a growing problem in the United States, and communities are identifying the need to promote an understanding of the policies, practices, and environmental factors that contribute to the nutrition and physical activity choices within a community. An assessment can help a community identify physical activity and nutrition policies, practices, and environmental conditions within the local community at large, such as worksites, school systems, and the health-care delivery system. Assessments can help identify specific issues related to the health issue and can also be population and/or setting specific. They can also help reach vulnerable populations and identify health needs such as an assessment of the transgender population conducted in Wisconsin. The community assessment helped identify that health-care providers play a key role in facilitating access to care for this population.[19] Often assessments related to a specific health issue include analysis of data to help determine who is at risk for the disease, such as the use of a case control study (see Chapter 3).

Health Impact Assessment

There are two other types of assessments: **health impact assessment (HIA)** and rapid needs assessment. The WHO notes that there are several definitions of a HIA. The main definition it has adopted is based on a 1999 European Centre for Health Policy definition of an HIA. According to the WHO, an HIA "... is a means of assessing the health impacts of policies, plans, and projects in diverse economic sectors using quantitative, qualitative, and participatory techniques."[20] A growing awareness of the multiple determinants of health, with a focus on the environment, has resulted in an increased focus and utilization of HIAs throughout the world. HIA methods are used to evaluate the impact of policies and projects on health, and a successful HIA is one in which its findings are considered by decision makers to inform the development and implementation of policies, programs, or projects. HIAs are often associated with assessments of the environment or assessments focused on the social influences of large projects. Zoning laws, for example, may increase the availability of walking paths that in turn may help to reduce the prevalence of obesity in a community. Examples of these types of assessments include an HIA of urban transport systems[21] or the value of assessing impact of policies on health inequities.[22] An HIA provides advice to a community on how to optimize the health of the community, is conducted prior to implementing a community-level intervention, and includes specific steps (Box 4-3).[20,23]

Rapid Needs Assessment

Another type of assessment is a **rapid needs assessment**, a tool that helps establish the extent and possible evolution of an emergency by measuring the present and potential public health impact of an emergency, determining existing response capacity, and identifying any additional immediate needs.[24,25] This type of assessment was first used in international settings during the 1960s to assess for immunization coverage, morbidity from diarrheal and respiratory diseases, and service coverage. In the 1970s, it was used in the smallpox eradication program in West Africa and was then adapted by the WHO for the Expanded Program of Immunization to assess immunization coverage in the 1980s. At the national level, the CDC, the Federal Emergency Management Agency, and the U.S. Public Health Service (USPHS) have all adopted a rapid needs assessment format when responding to a disaster. A rapid needs assessment is an effective use of limited resources and in general involves a straightforward collection of data. It is undertaken immediately after a disaster or event usually during the first week. The goal is to understand immediate needs, determine possible courses of action, and identify resource requirements.[25]

BOX 4-3 ■ Major Steps in Conducting a Health Impact Assessment (HIA)

- Screening (identifying plans, projects, or policies for which an HIA would be useful)
- Scoping (identifying which health effects to consider)
- Assessing risks and benefits (identifying which people may be affected and how they may be affected)
- Developing recommendations (suggesting changes to proposals to promote positive health effects or to minimize adverse health effects)
- Reporting (presenting the results to decision makers)
- Monitoring and evaluating (determining the effect of the HIA on the decision)

Source: (20)

Concepts of Relevance to Community Assessments

There are important concepts relevant to conducting a community assessment discussion: needs, assets, and the use of community-based participatory research. These reflect the importance of working with a community while maximizing the strengths of the community rather than focusing on deficits within the community. In the past, community assessments were done by outsiders and, for the most part, highlighted where the health gaps were without acknowledging assets within the community or including the community as a partner.

Needs Assessments Versus Asset Mapping

Initially, community assessments were based on the premise that the purpose of a community health assessment was to identify needs. In 1995, Witkin and Altschuld defined a needs assessment as "a systematic set of procedures undertaken for the purpose of setting priorities and making decisions about program or organizational improvement and allocation of resources. The priorities are based on identified needs."[26] A need was considered a discrepancy or a gap between what is and what should be.[26]

In contrast with this view of community health assessments, Kretzmann and McKnight published a landmark book that made the argument that an assessment should focus on the positive **assets** of a community rather than on its deficits. Assets are useful qualities, persons, or things. They combined this concept of assets with the concept of mapping, that is, exploring, planning, and locating, and proposed that community assessments should include asset mapping. Some of their ideas grew out of the plan to rebuild troubled urban communities based on capacity building.[27] According to Kretzmann and McKnight, a needs approach characterizes communities as a list of problems, makes resources available to service providers instead of residents, contributes to a cycle of dependence, and focuses on maintenance and survival strategies instead of development plans. By contrast, an asset mapping approach focuses on effectiveness instead of deficiencies, builds on interdependencies of people, identifies how people can give of their talents, and seeks to empower people.[27]

The assets approach, based on Kretzmann and McKnight's work, is based on constructing a map of assets and capacities. Three aspects of a community can be included in an asset map: (1) people, (2) places, and (3) systems.[27] People include individuals and families living within the community; places include the resources within the community such as schools, businesses, recreational facilities, and health-care resources. Systems include both formal systems such as government and churches as well as informal systems within the community such as neighborhood organizations. These systems are not always discrete and separate but, rather, influence each other.[28] Although these approaches of needs and assets appear diametrically opposed, the reality is that comprehensive community assessments consist of the identification of both weaknesses and strengths. Identifying the strengths as well as the problems is critical in the analysis of data.

Community-Based Participatory Research

The second concept of particular relevance to assessment is community engagement in the process of the assessment. There are various terms used to describe this approach including community engagement, citizen engagement, public engagement, translational science, knowledge translation, campus-community partnerships, and integrated knowledge translation.[34] In this book, we use the term **community-based participatory research (CBPR)**. The definitions related to this approach all include engagement of members of the community as full partners in the process of assessment. The idea is to use a collaborative approach that combines the knowledge and interest of the community members with the expertise of the professionals. The end goal is to achieve change that will work toward improving the health of the community.[29-31]

CBPR emphasizes the essential principles of capacity building, shared vision, ownership, trust, active participation, and mutual benefit.[29] A benefit of this approach is that it is a colearning process wherein the researchers and community members contribute equally and achieve a balance of research and action. In addition, it is a way of providing culturally competent care. For the PHN working with the community, it is important to be aware of the principles of CBPR. One of the first steps in the community assessment is to engage partners in the process and to develop a common vision.[30]

The engagement of communities in the community assessment process using CBPR methods has become an accepted method for not only engaging the community in the process but also engaging the end users in the action that will be taken to improve health.[31] When using CBPR methods, it is important to evaluate the possible ethical issues that can arise. These include issues of power, fairness, appropriate selection of representatives, obtaining consent, upsetting community equilibrium, and issues of dissemination of sensitive data.[29,32]

Assessment Models/Frameworks

Models or frameworks provide the structure and guidance for conducting an assessment. PHNs can choose a model based on what best fits the type of assessment that is being conducted. Examples of models that can help guide a comprehensive community health assessment are the Community Health Assessment and Group Evaluation (CHANGE) tool and the Mobilizing for Actions Through Planning and Partnerships (MAPP) strategic model.

Community Health Assessment and Group Evaluation

The CDC based the CHANGE tool on the socioecological model (see Chapter 2) to help communities build an action plan based on identified assets and areas for improvement. The stated purpose of the CHANGE tool is "to enable local stakeholders and community team members to survey and identify community strengths and areas for improvement regarding current policy, systems, and environmental change strategies."[33] The process provides a community with the foundation for conducting a program evaluation. The idea is to start with the end in mind and include evaluation in the beginning of the assessment process.[33] This tool includes a set of Microsoft Office Excel spreadsheets that communities can use to manage the data they collect. The tool provides a guide to doing a community assessment and helps with prioritizing areas for improvement.

CHANGE uses an eight-step process for conducting the assessment (Table 4-2) and was updated in 2018. The first three steps focus on gathering and educating the team. Steps 4 through 6 involve gathering, inputting, and reviewing data from the assessment. The last two steps are the development of an action plan starting with an analysis of the consolidated data. CHANGE is a tool to help a community complete an assessment that not only provides a diagnosis but also ends with the presentation of an action plan. The idea is to create a living document that the community can use to prioritize the health needs of the community and provide a means for structuring community activities around a common goal.[33]

Mobilizing for Actions Through Planning and Partnerships

The National Association of County and City Health Officials in cooperation with the Public Health Practice Program Office, CDC, developed a planning tool for

TABLE 4–2 ■ Best Practice Approach to Public Health Assessment: Comparison of MAPP With CHANGE

Mapp	Change
Phase 1: Partnership	Action Step 1: Assemble the Community Team.
	Action Step 2: Develop team strategy.
Phase 2: Visioning	Action Step 3: Review all five CHANGE sectors.
Phase 3: Assess residents, public health system, community health, and forces of change	Action Step 4: Gather data.
	Action Step 5: Review data gathered.
	Action Step 6: Enter data.
Phase 4: Identify strategic issues	Action Step 7: Review consolidated data.
	Action Step 7a: Create a CHANGE Summary Statement.
	Action Step 7b: Complete the Sector Data Grid.
	Action Step 7c: Fill Out the CHANGE Strategy Worksheets.
	Action Step 7d: Complete the Community Health Improvement Planning Template.
Phase 5: Formulate goals and strategies	Action Step 8: Build an action plan.
Phase 6: Action cycle	

Source: (33)

improving community health. The tool was developed with input from a variety of organizations, groups, and individuals who made up the local public health system between 1997 and 2000 (Fig. 4-1). The vision for implementing MAPP is for "communities [to achieve] improved health and quality of life (QoL) by mobilizing partnerships and taking strategic action."[34]

The MAPP assessment model was based on earlier models used by public health departments (PHDs) such as the Assessment Protocol for Excellence in Public Health (APEXPH), which was released in 1991.[35] Building on the concepts included in the APEXPH model, MAPP strengthened the community involvement component of assessment and aligned the model with the 10 essential public health services (see Chapter 1).[34] The MAPP tool includes the full scope of health planning including assessing, diagnosing, developing an intervention, implementing the intervention, and evaluating the effectiveness of the intervention. By contrast, CHANGE focuses on assessment and diagnosis with evaluation built in as the goal (see Table 4-2). Communities and PHDs have used MAPP across the country because it includes an action phase, providing a comprehensive approach to improving the health of a community.

The focus of the first five phases of MAPP is the process involved in working with the community on strategic planning and conducting four separate assessments. The MAPP handbook[34] contains access to the tools, resources, and technical assistance needed to conduct the assessment,

including a toolbox to provide an explanation and the many examples of assessments that have been conducted. The MAPP process has six phases: (1) organizing for success and partnership development, (2) visioning, (3) performing the four assessments, (4) identifying strategic issues, (5) formulating goals and strategies, and (6) moving into the action cycle.

Phase 1: Organizing for Success and Partnership Development

This phase is focused on identifying who should be involved in the process and developing the partners who will participate in the process. The recommended partners include the core support team and a steering committee. The core team does the majority of the work including recruiting participants. The steering committee provides guidance and oversight to the core support team and should broadly represent the community. It is important to obtain broad community involvement during this phase that includes inviting persons to serve on the steering committee and informing the community of opportunities for involvement that will occur throughout the planning process.[34]

Phase 2: Visioning

This phase is done at the beginning of the assessment process and is focused on mobilizing and engaging the broader community. An advisory committee guides the effort by conducting visioning sessions, resulting in a vision and values statement. The following are

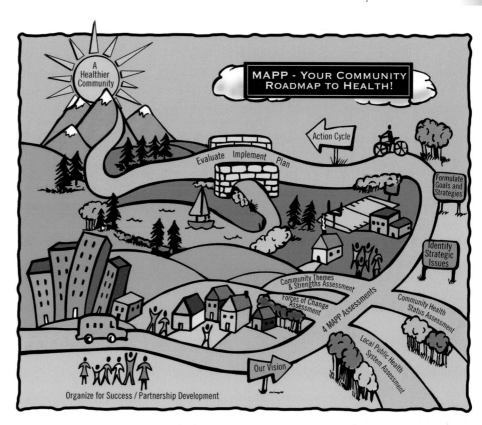

Figure 4-1 Mobilizing for Action Through Planning and Partnerships (MAPP). *(Source: National Association of County and Community Health Officials. [2013]. Retrieved from* http://www.naccho.org/topics/infrastructure/MAPP/index.cfm.*)*

some sample questions that can guide brainstorming during this phase:

- What does a healthy community mean to you?
- What are the important characteristics of a healthy community for all who live, work, and play here?
- How do you envision the local public health system in the next 5 or 10 years?

Phase 3: Performing the Four Assessments

Four assessments form the core of the MAPP process. The assessment phase results in a comprehensive picture of a community by using both quantitative and qualitative methods and consists of the following:

Community Themes and Strengths Assessment: This provides important information about how the residents feel about issues facing the community. It also provides qualitative information about residents' perceptions of their health and QoL concerns. Some questions to guide this assessment include:

- What is important to your community?
- How is QoL perceived in your community?
- What assets do you have that can be used to improve community health?

Local Public Health System Assessment (LPHSA): This focuses on the organizations and entities that contribute to the public's health. It is concerned with how well the public health system collaborates with other public health services. The LPHSA answers the following questions:

- What are the components, activities, competencies, and capacities of your local public health system?
- How are the essential services being provided in your community?

Community Health Status Assessment: The community health status assessment is largely focused on quantitative data about many health indicators. These include the traditional morbidity and mortality indicators, QoL indicators, and behavioral risk factors resulting in a broad view of health.

Forces of Change Assessment: This is an analysis of the external forces, positive and negative, that have an impact on the promotion and protection of the public's health. It is concerned with legislation, technology, and other impending changes that can influence how the public health system can work. It answers questions such as:

- What is occurring or might occur that affects the health of our community or the local public health system?

- What specific threats or opportunities are generated by these occurrences?

Phase 4: Identifying Strategic Issues

During this phase, the assessment data are used to determine the strategic issues the community must address to reach its vision. Some questions to help the community in determining the important strategic issues include the following:

- How large a public health issue is the item?
- Can we do it?
- Is it reasonable, feasible, and financially cost effective?
- What happens if we do nothing about it?

Phase 5: Formulating Goals and Strategies

Goals and strategies are formulated for each of the strategic issues. A community health improvement plan is often created during this phase. Both the steering committee and the core team work together to "… identify broad strategies for addressing issues and achieving goals related to the community's vision."[34]

Phase 6: Moving Into the Action Cycle

This is the phase in which the actual planning, implementing, and evaluating of the strategic plan takes place. Phases 5 and 6 are described in more detail in Chapter 5, which is focused on health planning.[34]

A Comprehensive Community Health Assessment

MAPP and CHANGE are examples of frameworks that provide blueprints for conducting a community health assessment. Regardless of the framework, the first step is engagement of partners in the process. As described in the CHANGE tool, this first action step involves assembling a diverse and representative community team. The team then establishes the purpose of the assessment. This begins with a clarification of how the community is being defined. Is the community being defined in relation to a clear geopolitical community such as a city or a county, or is the community a neighborhood that may not have clear geopolitical boundaries? For example, a group of researchers was conducting a focused assessment of maternal and infant care in subsidized housing in Winton Hills, Ohio, a neighborhood located within the Cincinnati, Ohio, metropolitan area. It had no political standing (it was designated as a town or city but did not have governmental systems in place). Instead, it was a

neighborhood that roughly matched a designated ZIP code, so for the purposes of the assessment the community was defined based on a specific ZIP code.[36]

Once the community has been defined, it is important to identify indicators and the sources of data for those indicators. This step often involves a discussion of the history of the community and the proposed project. Through these efforts, the team can identify sources of data that are already in existence. In some cases, previous surveys have been conducted that can provide good baseline data to help understand trends and changes in the community. Other data can be obtained from national-level surveys; the U.S. Census Bureau; and sources of local data, such as reports on crime, motor vehicle accident, and fire.

Next, the team can develop a timeline to help guide the assessment. A timeline helps the team decide at what point each step in the assessment will take place, the estimated time for completing each of the steps, and who will be responsible for each step. If the team is using the CHANGE model, the members will try to understand the total picture and will include assessment of five sectors of the community: (1) the community-at-large sector, (2) the community institution/organization sector, (3) the health-care sector, (4) the school sector, and (5) the worksite sector. Once this is complete, the team will then begin to gather data for each sector and evaluate the quality of the data. Different methods can be used to collect data, including obtaining secondary data available from other sources and collecting primary data. **Primary data** includes any data collected directly by the assessment team, in contrast to **secondary data**, which is the examination of data already collected for another purpose such as census data. Under step 4 in the CHANGE model, the different primary data collection methods listed that can be used include doing a windshield survey, PhotoVoice, doing a walkability audit, conducting focus groups, and administering a survey to individuals.

Windshield Survey

A **windshield survey** is an example of primary data collection that can help the team get an initial understanding of the community and is sometimes viewed as part of a preassessment phase. The windshield survey is what it sounds like—a drive-through or walk-through the community to observe the community. The idea is to observe the community to help in understanding it prior to conducting a more formal assessment.

A windshield survey is the first step in taking the pulse of the community. The questions a windshield survey can begin to answer include:

- Are there obvious health-related problems?
- What is the perspective of the media in relation to the community?
- What does the community look like?

Just by driving around, key issues related to the environmental health of the community can be observed, such as the number of for-sale signs, the amount of green space, the number of bars, the number of churches, the number of open (or closed) businesses, and the general upkeep of the community. Clean streets, well-kept parks, busy grocery stores, and religious places of worship with multiple services offered are signs of a healthy community. By contrast, trash in the streets, vacant lots, multiple bars, vacant places of worship, boarded-up businesses, and a lack of grocery stores are all visual indicators of a community that may have some serious health challenges.

A windshield survey can also provide information on the demographics of a community. Observations made while driving through (or walking around) can provide a beginning understanding of the age groups in the community simply by observing how many children, older adults, or young people are on the street. This can be time-dependent. For example, in the early morning, young parents and children may be observed as the children walk to the school. Later in the morning, older adults may be observed.

The use of a windshield survey template provides guidance when conducting a windshield survey. A template includes a list of specific aspects of the community to be aware of during the drive/walk through and provides a place to make observations (Table 4-3). It is important to record the observations while conducting the survey rather than filling them in later. Be sure to add observations that stand out even if they are not included in the template. The template should serve as a guide but may not cover all of the information that emerges. For example, in one windshield survey the team was struck by the use of black metal fencing around a neighborhood composed solely of subsidized housing. Later, when conducting interviews with key informants they discovered that the

TABLE 4–3 ■ A Sample Template for Conducting a Windshield Survey

Area	Suggested Prompts for Observation	Findings	Follow Up Needed
Prior to conducting the survey	• Establish geopolitical boundaries that define the community • Access census data for overall information based on census track or ZIP code • Obtain other secondary data as determined by the survey team		
Green space	• Parks • Playgrounds • Trees and other plantings		
Community Organizations	• Churches • Senior citizen centers • Others?		
Health Care	• Pharmacies • Clinics/physician's offices • Hospitals • Dentists		
Transportation	• Bus and trolley lines • Trains • Cars		
Food, beverages and tobacco	• Big chain grocery stores • Corner markets • Farmers' markets • Liquor stores • Bars • Vaping and hookah lounges		

Continued

TABLE 4–3 ■ A Sample Template for Conducting a Windshield Survey—cont'd

Area	Suggested Prompts for Observation	Findings	Follow Up Needed
Entertainment	• Theaters (movie and live) • Concert halls		
Housing	• Types of housing (single family, apartments, subsidized housing • Appearance of houses and lawns • Abandoned houses/apartment buildings		
Business	• Store fronts • Types of businesses (dollar stores, pawn shops, check cashing vs. upper end stores) • Empty store fronts		
Education	• Schools (public/private) • Colleges/universities • School bus routes		
People	• Gender, ethnicity, and age distribution by time of day • Appearance • Interactions		
Environment	• Air quality • Cleanliness of community		
Other observations	• Add other observations that do not fit into the previous categories		

residents felt the fencing further confirmed their perception of being separated from the larger urban community.

One approach to observing the formal institutions within a community is to examine the interrelationship between different aspects of a community, often referred to as **KEEPRA (Kinship/Economics/Education/Political/Religious/Associations)** . It provides a list of categories to consider while collecting observational related data:

• *Kinship*—What observations can you make about family and family life?
• *Economics*—Does the community appear to have a stable economy or are there signs of economic decline or economic growth?
• *Education*—What observations can you make related to schools and other educational institutions such as libraries and museums?
• *Political*—Is there evidence of political activity in the community such as signs supporting someone's candidacy for elected office?
• *Religious*—Are there any mosques, churches, or synagogues in the community?
• *Associations*—What evidence do you see of neighborhood associations? Business associations? What other resources are present such as recreation centers?

Using the CHANGE list of sectors is another possible approach to conducting an observational review of the formal institutions in a community:

• *Community-at-Large Sector* includes community-wide efforts that have an impact on the social and built environments such as improving food access, walkability or bikeability, tobacco use and exposure, or personal safety.
• *Community Institution/Organization Sector* includes entities within the community that provide a broad range of human services and access to facilities such as childcare settings, faith-based organizations, senior centers, boys and girls clubs, YMCAs, and colleges or universities.
• *Health-Care Sector* includes places where people go to receive preventive care or treatment, or emergency health-care services such as hospitals, private doctors' offices, and community clinics.
• *School Sector* includes all primary and secondary learning institutions (e.g., elementary, middle, and high schools, whether private, public, or parochial).

- *Worksite Sector* includes places of employment such as private offices, restaurants, retail establishments, and government offices.[33]

Secondary Community Health Data Collection

Once the windshield survey is complete it is often helpful to review secondary data prior to collecting more primary data. Examples of secondary data sources include census data, crime report data, national health survey data, and health statistics from the state or local department of health. What is usually available is **aggregate data**, data that do not include individual level data, such as infant mortality rate. Many of the sources of aggregate level community data are accessible via the Internet. Obtaining other sources of secondary data, especially data at the individual level, usually requires seeking permission and is usually provided as **deidentified data**, that is, data that does not include individual identifiers.

An essential component of a community health assessment is the review of sociodemographic data. From a geographical perspective, the team can access census data relevant to their community from the U.S. Census Bureau. These data provide the team with information on the number of people in their community; the number of households; and information related to age, gender, marital status, occupation, income, education, and race/ethnicity. The U.S. Census Bureau collects census data in the United States every 10 years. The data are reported at the aggregate level based on geopolitical perspective. Aggregate data are obtainable at the national, state, county, metropolitan area, city, town, census track, or census block. According to the U.S. Census Bureau, a **census tract** is a relatively permanent statistical subdivision of a county that averages between 2,500 and 8,000 inhabitants that is designed to be homogeneous with respect to population characteristics and economic status. A **census block** is an area bounded on all sides by visible features. Examples of boundaries provided by the U.S. Census Bureau include visible boundaries such as roads, streams, and railroad tracks, and by invisible boundaries such as the geographical limits of a city or county. Typically, it is a smaller geographical area, but in some rural areas a census block may be large.[37] The data provide a snapshot of the population every 10 years. In between those years, changes may occur, and local data may be needed to supplement census data especially toward the end of a decade.

Another source of secondary health data at the aggregate level about a community is the PHD. Examples of public health information related to morbidity and mortality, and potentially available at the PHD include the crude mortality rate, the infant mortality rate, motor vehicle crash rate, and the incidence and prevalence rates of communicable and noncommunicable diseases. To get a better understanding of the rates, it helps to obtain age-specific mortality rates for leading causes of death and age-adjusted, race-, or sex-specific mortality rates. An example of Web-based sources of health-related aggregate data at the county level is the Web site maintained by the University of Wisconsin Population Health Institute and sponsored by the Robert Wood Johnson Foundation. It provides information on health indicators at the county level with comparative statistics at the state and national levels.[38] Another source of data is vital statistics. These statistics provide information about births, deaths, adoptions, divorces, and marriages. These data are available through state public health departments.

Information on the health of a community can also be obtained from surveys that are conducted routinely at the national level and often at the regional level. The National Center for Health Statistics (NCHS), a division of the CDC, provides data about the prevalence of health conditions in the United States. The NCHS manages surveillance systems including the National Health Interview Survey (NHIS) and the National Health and Nutrition Examination Survey (NHANES). The NHIS surveys approximately 35,000 households annually. The survey focuses on a core component of health questions including health status and limitations, injuries, health-care access and use, health insurance, and income and assets. In addition, a supplement is used each year to respond to new public health data needs as they arise.[39] The NHANES is an annual survey that began in the 1960s and combines an interview with medical, dental, and lab tests, and physiological measures.[40] The Behavioral Risk Factor Surveillance System (BRFSS), administered by the CDC, is a telephone survey of 350,000 adults in 50 states, the District of Columbia, Puerto Rico, the U.S. Virgin Islands, and Guam. It has been conducted on an annual basis since 1984 and collects information on health risk behaviors, preventive health practices, and health-care access primarily related to chronic disease and injury.[42] The CDC also publishes the *Morbidity and Mortality Weekly Report,* which reports communicable diseases and health concerns by state with each publication providing current state- and city-level incidence data on reportable diseases. Other examples of aggregate health data include the annual report to Congress and other reports to Congress on health-related issues such as alcohol and drug use (see Chapter 11). Other sources of health data include cancer registries and the National Institute of Occupational Safety and Health (NIOSH). The National

Cancer Center of the National Institutes of Health maintains 11 population-based cancer registries. They provide data on the number of individuals diagnosed with cancer during the year. NIOSH monitors exposures to environmental factors in work settings.

Secondary data are also available that are not specific to individuals, that is, data related to the environment. The Environmental Protection Agency (EPA) collects data on environmental pollutants and the Department of Transportation collects data on the number of vehicles using the roads. Another example is information obtained and maintained by the U.S. Department of Agriculture (USDA), which includes information on farmers markets, the Food Access Research Atlas, and the Food Desert Locator, an online map highlighting thousands of areas where, the USDA says, low-income families have little or no access to healthy fresh food.[42] Secondary sources of local data also exist but may not be readily available in aggregate form on the Internet. These include information on the organizations within the community such as hospitals, schools, and police department information. Gathering the data from various local organizations (minutes, reports) may be helpful in relation to the different sectors included in the CHANGE model such as information about the schools. Although these records may be helpful to some extent, there are limitations. Records of any nature often have limitations because they may not be complete, may not be in a usable format, or the keepers of the data may not be willing to provide the information to the community assessment team. The list of available secondary data is long and interesting, and should be reviewed as the first step to avoid the more expensive process of having the team collect the data.

Primary Community Health Data Collection

When the review of the available secondary data is complete, the next step is to determine gaps in the data and decide what further data needs to be collected by the team. The CHANGE model provides a list of possible methods and suggests that multiple methods should be used (two or more).[33] These data are then combined with the secondary data to determine needs and assets.

Inventory of Resources

The agencies and organizations present in a community often have a significant effect on health. The CHANGE handbook has sample organizational questionnaires that can be used for each of the five sectors to help collect data on different organizations such as health-care organizations and schools.[33] The use of these questionnaires can help the team gather essential information about the resources within the community.

Quantitative Data: Surveys

When gaps in data are identified, one method for obtaining the missing data is to conduct a survey to collect community level quantitative data. **Quantitative data** are data that can be assigned numerical values such as the number of new cases of tuberculosis or the assigning of a number to a categorical variable such as ethnic group.

A first step in conducting a community health survey is to outline the purpose of the survey. The team decides on the information needed then decides on the target population and the method for obtaining a representative sample of the population and the survey delivery method. For example, a hypothetical community assessment team in county X found that the members did not have enough information on the health-related quality of life (HRQoL) of older adults living in their community. The county had just completed a telephone health survey, and this population was underrepresented. After careful consideration they decided that their target population was in fact those older than age 65 who were not currently residing in a health-care facility. The use of an e-mailed survey seemed to pose even more problems related to response rate than did a telephone survey. So they decided that a face-to-face approach was best to deliver the survey. The team members decided they needed to reach those living in different areas of the county as well, so they put together a sampling process that would help them include older adults living in different areas of the county. This example demonstrates that conducting a survey can be complex and may include issues related to time, which requires careful planning. The advantages of surveys include their cost-effectiveness and ability to make inferences about a population based on the representativeness of the sample. A survey allows for the collection of a large amount of information from a large number of individuals.

Defining the Sample: There are several approaches to defining the sample. Defining the community or target population is once again the critical step. If the focus of the assessment is on adolescents within a specific school, the sampling will be based on the adolescents in that school; however, if the purpose of the assessment is to say something about adolescents in the city, a different sampling approach is needed.

Sampling Approaches: Once the target population is defined, there are several types of sampling approaches. A simple random sample involves a list of the eligible individuals and then selection is made based on a random selection, possibly based on using a list of random numbers. Convenience sampling is a common approach that takes into consideration the availability of participants. Some different types of convenience sampling include quota sampling, which involves a fixed number of subjects; interval sampling, which is the selection of subjects in a sequence (i.e., every eighth person); or snowball sampling, which starts with a small group of participants and then uses those participants to identify other participants. One other type of sampling used with large numbers is systematic sampling, in which a list of the possible participants is presented, and the number needed for the sample is divided into the total population. For example, from that point, *n,* every *n*th person is chosen.

Methods for Conducting a Survey: There are also several methods for conducting a survey. A survey can be mailed, done by telephone, given in certain settings as a written document or by computer, or conducted through a face-to-face interview. The format for the survey is determined based on consideration of cost, resources, and preference. In some cases, the choice of the format may be determined by the study participants, as noted in the previous example of the survey conducted with the older adults in the county.

Deciding Items to Be Included in a Survey: Choosing and developing the items to be included in a survey is another decision to be made in planning the actual assessment. Most health surveys use a quantitative approach; that is, the questions are closed-ended and can be entered into a database using statistical software to help with analysis. Some surveys also include open-ended questions that allow respondents to provide information not asked in the survey questions.

Evidence-Based Tools for Community Assessment: There are several health status evidenced-based instruments available for conducting a community health assessment. One example is the CDC HRQoL questionnaire, either the 14-item or 4-item set of Healthy Days core questions (CDC HRQoL– 4).[43] The questionnaire is based on the broad concept of QoL as it relates to health. Assessment of QoL includes subjective evaluations of both positive and negative aspects of life. Health is only one aspect of QoL. Other aspects include employment, education, culture, values, and spirituality. The advantage of using the CDC HRQoL questionnaire is that it allows for comparison of the community sample with national benchmarks. The HRQoL has been in the State-based Behavioral Risk Factor Surveillance System (BRFSS) since 1993.

Other reliable and valid tools are available to include in an assessment. The challenge is to find a tool that matches the information needs based on gaps in knowledge related to the health of the community you are assessing and the utilization of the right format for obtaining the data. Most community health assessment surveys include multiple instruments to assess the health of the community. Along with the 4-item HRQoL questionnaire, the team may decide to include a number of other tools within the survey such as a tool that measures satisfaction with available of health care. The key is to use valid and reliable tools whenever possible.

Qualitative Data

Although quantitative data can provide a wealth of information, other approaches to data collection provide an opportunity to gather more in-depth information about the health of a community. One approach to achieving this is to gather **qualitative data**, that is, data that cannot be assigned a value and that represent the viewpoint of the person providing the information. These data are not generalizable to a large population but can provide insight into the how, why, what, and where of the phenomenon being studied, in this case, the health status of a community.

Focus Groups: The most commonly used method for collecting data when conducting a community assessment is the focus group(s). A **focus group** is an interview with a group of people with similar experiences or backgrounds who meet to discuss a topic of interest. It is usually a one-time event that is semistructured and informal, and there is a facilitator and possibly a cofacilitator who guide the discussion.[44] A focus group typically includes six to eight participants. The facilitator(s) use an interview guide that has unstructured open-ended questions for purposes of discovering opinions, problems, and solutions to issues. The interview generally lasts for 1 to 2 hours. Once the focus group has been conducted, an analysis of either the transcribed tape recording or notes from the group session consists of examining the data for patterns that emerge, common themes, new questions that arise, and conclusions that can be reached.[44]

Key Informants: Another approach to gathering more in-depth data is to conduct individual interviews with key informants. A **key informant** is often represented as a gatekeeper, one who comes closest to representing the community. Although interviews can be time consuming, interviews with one or more key informants can provide a wealth of information about the opinions, assumptions, and perceptions of others about the health of a community. The interview can be conducted face-to-face or over the telephone, and the tool to conduct the interview can be structured, semistructured, or unstructured. A structured interview is more formal, with specific identical questions being asked of each person interviewed. A semistructured interview is less structured, with a list of questions that guide the interview but with time for a more relaxed conversation. An unstructured interview is conducted by asking questions that seem appropriate for the person being interviewed.

The next consideration is who to interview. This really depends on the purpose of the assessment and the interview. If a PHN wants to learn more about the resources for adolescents in a community, the nurse will want to interview personnel in health clinics and recreation centers, school nurses, parents, and adolescents about their perceptions of resources and needs in the community. If there is a need to learn about the needs of the older adults living in the community, the sites for identifying key informants may now shift to health clinics, senior citizen centers, nursing homes, long-term care sites, seniors themselves, and organizations representing them. If it is a comprehensive assessment, it is important to make sure that everyone is represented. It is important to include business representatives, government employees, and members of voluntary organizations. Another issue to examine is the makeup of the community based on ethnicity to make sure that each group's members have had a chance to voice their opinions. For example, during a community assessment conducted in Lancaster County, Pennsylvania, the team realized they would have a zero-response rate on the telephone health survey for residents in the county who belonged to the Amish community because they do not use telephones. To address this issue, the team conducted focus groups with both the women and the men in the Amish community.[45]

Determining the type of interview to conduct with a key informant, face-to-face or by telephone, requires some thought about the advantages and disadvantages of both formats. Some of the advantages of face-to-face interviews are flexibility, ability to probe for specific answers, ability to observe nonverbal behavior, control of the physical environment, and use of more complex questions. The telephone interview needs to be shorter but allows for the ability to interview people who do not have the time to meet face-to-face. It is important to summarize the interview immediately, especially if it is not being recorded. An analysis of the interview data is similar to the analysis of focus group data. The community health assessment team reads the notes or transcripts from the interviews and identifies common themes between key informants as well as specific issues for the group they represent. To help verify the information provided by a key informant, it is helpful to use triangulation, a technique that allows the interviewer to verify the information with another source.

PhotoVoice: **PhotoVoice** is another qualitative methodology used to enhance community assessments. It is based on the theoretical literature on education for critical consciousness, feminist theory, and community-based approaches to document photography.[46,47] PhotoVoice involves having community members photograph their everyday lives within the context of their community, participate in group discussions about their photographs, and have an active voice in mobilizing action within the community. When using this technique in a community assessment, residents can be provided with disposable cameras and asked to take pictures that reflect family, maternal, and child health assets and concerns in the community. From these photographs, the participants' concerns will be highlighted, and concerns such as developing safe places for recreation and making improvements in the community environment can emerge.

Additional Tools and Strategies

Community Mapping: Community mapping is another step during the assessment phase that can be used in the initial windshield survey, during the inventory data collection, during interviews, and in more advanced analyses of both assets and problems in a community. The advantages of mapping assets are that the strengths of the community are outlined and can be used then in developing an action plan. Mapping allows the community assessment team to visualize the community and to study concentrations of disease, to identify at-risk populations, to better understand program implementation, to examine risk factors, or to study interactions that affect health. It is a process of collecting data through direct observation and using secondary data sources to describe the physical characteristics of a neighborhood or community, the location of institutions and resources, and the social and demographic characteristics of a community. It has the potential to provide data that can help identify place-based social determinants of health that could then lead to interventions at the individual and the community level to initiate precise risk reduction and mitigation.[48] In the study by Aronson and colleagues, primary data were collected by walking through the community with residents noting categories of interest. Secondary data collected included housing inspection data, liquor license data, crime reports, and birth certificates. The purpose of this assessment was to study the community context and how it might contribute to infant mortality, with an evaluation of Baltimore City Healthy Start, a federally funded infant mortality prevention project. The Healthy Start Program was an initiative whose purpose was to reduce infant mortality by providing comprehensive services to women and their children and partners, and at the same time to contribute toward a neighborhood transformation. The researchers mapped vacant houses, liquor stores, and crime data. The data showed that participation in the prevention program was higher in lower risk census blocks. Changes were made to obtain better penetration of the program based on these findings.[49]

Geographic Information System (GIS): A **geographic information system (GIS)** is a tool that is increasingly used in public health. GIS is a computer-based program that can be used to collect, store, retrieve, and manipulate geographical or location-based information.[50] GIS databases consist of both spatial and nonspatial data. Nonspatial data include demographic or socioeconomic data that can be identified by geographical boundaries, whereas spatial data are assigned by exact geographical location by geocoding or address matching. It is used globally to help identify populations at risk such as maternal and infant populations in Iran and in the U.S.[51,52] In the study conducted in Iran related to maternal health, they were able to identify priority geographical areas.[51] In New Jersey, researchers used GIS to link neighborhood characteristics with maternal infant outcomes.[52] The GIS maps generated demonstrated the associations between adverse birth outcomes, poverty, and crime.[52]

Analysis of the Data

Once the data have been collected, it is important to analyze them. The CHANGE model includes three action steps related to this phase of the assessment: (1) review the data, (2) enter the data, and then (3) review the consolidated data. Reviewing the data refers to having the team brainstorm, debate, and reach consensus on the meaning of the data. Entering the data is the process of transcribing the data into a software program such as Excel to help with the analysis and interpretation of the data. Data are then rated by all researchers. Reviewing the data includes four steps: (1) create a CHANGE summary statement, (2) complete a sector data grid, (3) fill out the CHANGE strategy worksheets, and (4) complete the Community Health Improvement Planning template. Doing so provides the foundation for the final step in CHANGE, building the community action plan.[33]

Making sense of the collected data is done via a variety of ways. One of the most important points to consider is what changes over time or noticeable trends. Sociodemographic comparisons include changes from one census data collection period to another. The time-period for comparing disease trends varies by the prevalence of disease. A communicable disease outbreak may be monitored on a weekly or monthly basis, whereas trends in heart disease might require a trend analysis during a 5-year period. Trends can help identify improvements or declines in health indicators in the community over time, such as the infant mortality rate, or they can be used to determine whether there have been changes in the demographics of the population over time. For example, is the population aging or have there been changes in home ownership?

The health indicators and the demographics of the community can be compared with other populations such as similar local jurisdictions, the state, and ultimately national data. The data can also be compared within the community. Do disparities exist on key health indicators such as prevalence of disease or access to needed resources? These analyses allow the team to interpret the statistics to identify the important health issues for the community. It is a complex process that involves combining the information obtained from all sources and coming to conclusions. The CHANGE handbook provides an excellent guide for a team to use to complete the analysis. It often requires having a member of the team who not only is familiar with software but who also has a background in statistical analysis so that the team can compute rates and complete a meaningful presentation of the data.

Postassessment Phase: Creating, Disseminating, and Developing an Action Plan

In the final action step outlined in the CHANGE model, the community assessment team builds a community action plan.[33] This requires the development of a project period with annual objectives and should reflect the data that were collected. The result of a community health assessment should include a brief narrative describing the adequacy of services currently provided in relation to the overall needs of the community. It should highlight the areas of need in the community that are not met and list any additional resources that could be developed to meet any unmet needs in the community.

Evaluating the Assessment Process

Evaluating assessments is as important as conducting assessments to better understand their impact. It involves including stakeholders in reviewing the findings and having an opportunity for feedback. To use the data to help identify priorities, teams may seek validation from stakeholders or they may engage in a more collaborative process to help come to a final decision on priorities.[53] This is done at the end of the assessment phase and before the beginning of the planning phase (Chapter 5).

● APPLYING PUBLIC HEALTH SCIENCE

The Case of the Sick Little Town

Public Health Science Topics Covered:

- Assessment
- Epidemiology and biostatistics

The director of nurses (DON) at a regional Visiting Nurse Association (VNA) that covered a large regional area including four rural towns noticed that there was an increase in patients being referred for home visiting services from Small Town, a small rural community within their service area. They provided follow-up care for persons following a hospitalization and well-baby visits for mothers and infants deemed to be at risk such as premature infants and teenage mothers. The VNA was part of a large medical center that had just launched its "We are community!" campaign. The DON approached the vice-president responsible for community outreach services, pointed out the increase to him, and suggested that a community assessment might help to identify what was behind the increased admissions. The vice-president stated that this matched the medical center's "We are community!" campaign and asked the DON whether her team would be willing to form a task force to conduct an assessment of the community to uncover the reason for the increase in admissions, better understand the health issues and strengths within the community, and at the same time build a better bridge to the community. He authorized a certain part of the DON's workload to include leading the assessment project and authorized her to designate two of her visiting nurses as members of her initial outreach team.

The next day the DON met with the two of her home health nurses, Sonja and Viki, who covered Small Town. She also invited Donna, the PHN who worked for the county health department, to meet with them and join their assessment team. As they began, Sonja remembered from her public health nursing course that it was important to start with a model to guide the assessment. She also remembered doing a windshield survey for her community health project in school. "I drive around Small Town frequently to see my patients, and I never thought about really looking at the town from a community assessment point of view." Viki agreed and suggested that not only should they do a windshield survey, but they should also invite members of the community to join them.

Donna told them the county PHD was in the planning stages of a county assessment, so the concerns of the visiting nurses were in line with efforts just beginning at the PHD where they were using the CHANGE model[33] to guide the process. She conveyed the health concerns of the visiting nurses to the head of the county PHD who then agreed to support the VNA's work assessing Small Town as a part of their overall comprehensive assessment for the county thus setting up a collaborative effort between the VNA, the regional Medical Center and the county PHD.

For their next step, Sonja, Viki and Donna made a list of those who should be a part of the CHANGE committee and planned how to get broad community involvement. They used the CHANGE guidelines to help develop their process. Sonja and Viki, who had been working in the community and knew some key stakeholders in the community, and the PHN asked the county PHD epidemiologist to assist with the data collection and analysis.

The core team then began building a CHANGE committee that could help broaden community involvement. When completed, the preliminary CHANGE committee consisted of four residents of the community; the school nurse; the director of the community recreation center; a member of the police force; the CEO of the regional medical center; Donna, the PHN from the county PHD; the two visiting nurses, Sonja and Vicki, and their DON; the PHD epidemiologist; and the publisher of the town newspaper.

The CHANGE committee and the core team next began to work on developing the team strategy process included in the CHANGE model. One of the visiting nurses was worried that the project was no longer under the control of the medical center. Donna explained that having the assessment come from the community rather than the medical center would truly support the medical center's "We are community!" campaign. Further, she explained that the CHANGE model would conclude with a community action plan. She explained that having a clear picture of the health of Small Town USA required buy-in from multiple constituents within the community.

The core team expanded to reflect the diversity of the community. The team talked with the town historian to find former community initiatives and built communication strategies for keeping the community informed by writing an article for the weekly newspaper, seeking input and suggestions. After running the article, the editor reported getting many e-mails about the campaign with suggestions for information that the team should include. The committee worked to bring this input together and came up with a final vision statement: "Small Town, the place to be for healthy living."

The next logical step was to map out the borders of Small Town, located in the state of Massachusetts along a small river, using local maps. The town included a total of 75 square miles and was a 35-minute drive from the medical center. Four towns bordered Small Town, three of which had a smaller population than Small Town. The town with the slightly higher population was to the east of the town and could be reached by a main road that went through Small Town. It took 20 to 25 minutes to drive from the center of Small Town to the center of each of the other four towns. Most of the population lived in the center of town. The outskirts of town were wooded and included a small state park.

Collect Secondary Data: Sociodemographic Data

Descendants from the Mayflower and their contemporaries initially settled the town. That gave the team a starting point for the original culture—English and Puritan. These early settlers had moved west to farm. Manufacturing grew over time with the river providing a source of power for mills. The founding families built mills and brought more settlers to the area to work in the mills. Merchants then came to sell goods to the workers. The town developed an informal class system of workers, owners, and merchants. Although the first wave of workers was Irish, eventually most of the workforce came from French Canada. The team found that many of the residents of the town had last names that were French. By World War I, the Irish section of town was small and was considered the lowest rung of the social classes. The church with the largest congregation was the Catholic Church, because this was a town of few owners and many workers, almost all of whom were Catholic. Thus, Small Town had a firm class structure as well as three major ethnic groups—English, French Canadian, and Irish—for most of its history.

In the 1970s, when the town was the recipient of state funds to build subsidized housing for families on welfare, there was an influx of families into the town who were at or below the poverty level, all of whom were white and most of whom were single mothers. They became the new lowest rung on the class ladder. By 2015, a few Hispanic families from Puerto Rico were moving into the town. Despite this modest influx, the majority (89%) of the population still identified themselves as white.

Knowing the history, the team's next step was to complete a demographic assessment of the town beginning with specific demographic indicators that were available from the U.S. Census Bureau including gender, age, race, home ownership, and income. They constructed a **population pyramid** related

to the age of the population from estimates using the 2016 American Community Survey data and the 2010 census data located on the U.S. Census Bureau Web site American Fact Finder for 2010, and compared it with the population of the United States (Fig. 4-2).[54]

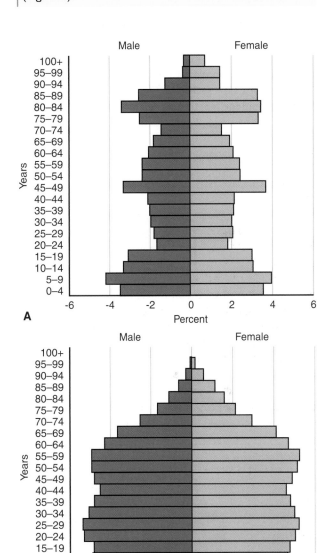

Figure 4-2 Population pyramids: Small Town (top) and the United States (bottom). *(Source: A, Data from Centers for Disease Control and Prevention [2010]. Community Health Assessment and Group Evaluation [CHANGE] action guide: Building a foundation of knowledge to prioritize community needs. Atlanta, GA: U.S. Department of Health and Human Services; B, Data from U.S. Census Bureau, Population Division.)*

A population pyramid can tell you a lot about a population. If the pyramid has a broad base and a small top, it is an example of an expansive pyramid in which there is most likely a rapid rate of population growth. A population pyramid with indentations that even out from top to bottom indicates slow growth. A stationary pyramid has a narrow base, with equal numbers over the rest of the age groups and tapering off in the oldest age groups. A declining pyramid is one that has a high proportion of people in the higher age groups. In 2010, the population pyramid for North America met the definition of a slow growth pyramid. The projected 2050 pyramid for North America is a classic example of a stationary pyramid. By contrast, the population pyramid for Somalia in 2010 demonstrated a clear example of an expansive pyramid, indicative of rapid population growth. However, it also indicated that the longevity of the population was lower than in North America. By 2050 the population pyramid for Somalia is projected to match the 2010 pyramid for North America, indicating that population growth is projected to slow (Fig. 4-3).[55]

The team examined their population pyramid and compared it to the U.S. Data (Fig. 4-2), and made some conclusions about the population in Small Town. What would they be? How does Small Town compare with the United States? Note the larger base and the wide top. This indicates that the population seems to be made up of young families and older adults with a smaller number of in the 45-year to 59-year range. These data provided the team with a starting point for understanding the possible reason for the increase in requests for home health services.

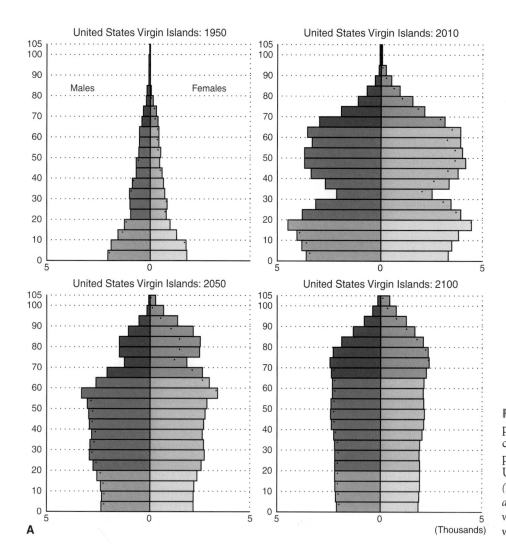

Figure 4-3 United States populations pyramids compared with population pyramids of Somalia. A, United States; B, Somalia. (*Data from Worldlifeexpectancy available at* http://www. worldlifeexpectancy.com/ world-population-pyramid.*)*

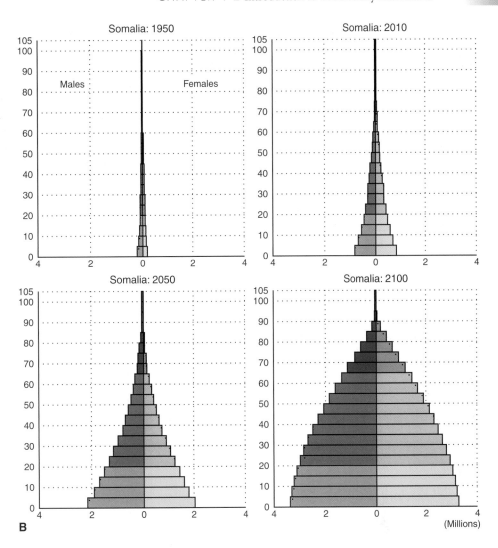

Figure 4-3—cont'd   B

The epidemiologist from the county PHD recommended that they track the population based on age and race, and determine the percent change from 2010 to 2016 using census track data. Percent change (see Chapter 3) represents the change in a variable from one point in time to another. They were surprised at the simplicity of the math required to calculate the percent change. The epidemiologist explained that they should subtract the old value from the new value. They then would divide this by the old value. Then when they multiplied the result by 100, they had the percent change. He showed them how to set it up in an Excel file so that they could enter all the population numbers they were interested in, set up the formula, and then have a table ready for distribution to the committee (Box 4-4, Table 4-4). Percent change can tell a lot

---

BOX 4-4 ■ Percent Change

New value minus the old value divided by the old value times 100 equals the percent change.

Example:

If the town's population in 2000 was 2,000, and in 2010 it grew to 2,520, the percent change is 26%:

$$2,520 - 2,000 = 520$$
$$520/2,000 = 0.26 \times 100 = 26\%$$

---

about a population. In the case of Small Town, the percent change in the Hispanic population showed a shift in the town. In 2010, almost 97% of the population was white. In 2016, 89% of the population was white. This information can also help estimate

TABLE 4–4 ▪ Percent Change for Demographic Characteristics in Small Town USA, 2010–2016

	2010	2016	% Change
Total	9,611	10,164	6%
Male	4,766	5,039	6%
Female	4,845	5,125	6%
White	9,223	9,018	−2%
Black	77	122	58%
American Indian	29	33	14%
Asian	60	45	−25%
Other	98	101	3%
Two or More Races	124	152	23%
Hispanic	195	693	255%
Vacant Housing Units	213	189	−11%
Population 25 Years or Older	6,056	6,591	9%
High School Graduates	4,974		
Bachelor's Degree or Higher	848		
Mean Travel Time to Work	29.5		
Median Household Income	$43,750.00		
Families Below Poverty Level	171		

changes in the population in the future. If the current trend continues with a 2% decline in the white population and a 255% increase in the Hispanic population during the next 6 years, what would the population look like in 2021?

Using Census Bureau data, the team looked at gender, age, race, home ownership, poverty level, crime, and fire safety. As discussed earlier in the section Secondary Community Health Data Collection, secondary data are collected for a different purpose from the current study or assessment. In this case, the federal government collected census data. These data are collected every 10 years, the decennial census, to compile information about the people living in the United States. In addition, the census bureau conducts the American Community survey to provide 5-year estimates. These data provide the federal government with the information needed for the apportionment of seats in the U.S. House of Representatives. The U.S. Census Bureau also conducts many other surveys and is a rich source of secondary population data. The Census Bureau provides these data in aggregate format and by law cannot release data in a way that could identify individuals.[56]

To access the census data, the team went to the American FactFinder section of the U.S. Census Bureau's Web site and were able to print out a sheet that included the estimates for 2016[54] including general, social, economic, and housing characteristics. Under economic characteristics, they found that, in Small Town, 67% of the population older than age 16 were in the workforce, and the median household income was $42,625. The fact sheet also listed comparative percentages for the United States so that they could compare Small Town with the nation. Small Town statistics were comparable to the national statistics on all the economic indicators except poverty. In Small Town, 18.5% of the families lived below the poverty level compared with 15% of the U.S. population. They were also able to print out fact sheets for the county, the state, and the surrounding towns, thus comparing Small Town with its neighbors. The economic indicators between the closest neighboring town and Small Town differed in relation to income, with Small Town having a lower median household income ($38,564 compared with $46,589), although the poverty level statistics were approximately the same. Again, compared with the state, the town had a lower median income ($38,564 compared with $75,297).

The team then reviewed the other demographic categories. A few facts were noted as possibly being important. First, the median value of the houses in Small Town USA was lower than in the rest of the state ($173,600 versus $358,000) and the percentage of the population older than age 25 with a bachelor's degree or higher was lower than in the rest of the state (14% versus 41%). Based on the review of the demographics, a picture was beginning to emerge of the town. What would your impressions be?

What further data would you need if you were on this team?

Health Status Assessment Using Secondary Data

At this point, Sonja wondered about the actual health of the town. She reminded the team that this project was started because of the increased requests for visiting nursing services and suggested that the team look at the Massachusetts Department of Health Community Health Profile that included a health status indicator report for Small Town. This report provided information on health indicators and reduced the need for the team to find these data themselves. This report used secondary sources of data collected by PHDs, referred to as vital records including information on death certificates, reportable diseases, hospital discharges, and infant mortality.

The health status indicators chosen by the Massachusetts Department of Health included perinatal and child health indicators, communicable diseases, injury, chronic disease, substance use and hospital discharge data. The core group brought the published information to the larger community group for discussion. One of the members of the community group noted that at the top of the report was a section on small numbers and wanted to know what that meant. The epidemiologist explained that the numbers of cases for each indicator are placed in a cell in a table. Sometimes the numbers in these cells for smaller towns contain small numbers. The general rule of thumb, he explained, is that if there are fewer than five observations (or cases) then the rates are usually not reported. If they are reported, then rates based on small numbers should be interpreted very cautiously, because there are not enough cases to create a base from which to draw conclusions.

The perinatal and child health indicators included births, infant deaths, and other perinatal and postnatal data from 2016. They found a small numbers problem right away with only one infant death in 2016. However, Small Town had a higher low-birth-weight rate than the state (9.4 per 100 live births versus 7.4 per 100 live births). They also found that the rate of births to teenage mothers was higher than the rate for the state (12.5% versus 9.4%). There were no differences in prenatal care in the first trimester or the percentage of mothers receiving publicly funded prenatal care compared with the rate for the state.

On most of the other indicators, Small Town had lower or similar rates to the state. The rates that were higher than the state rates were those for cardiovascular deaths (397 per 100,000 deaths versus 214 per 100,000 deaths) and for hospital discharges related to bacterial pneumonia (495.3 per 100,000 deaths versus 329.6 per 100,000 deaths). The team also noted that some of the rates were age-adjusted, and they wanted to know more about the process. The county epidemiologist explained that crude rates may not be as good an indicator because populations may differ on a characteristic, in this case age, which accounts for some of the difference between the rates in two populations. For example, if death rates for cardiovascular disease in a city in Florida with a high proportion of retirees in the community were compared with the rates in a town that has a younger population, the crude death rate would most likely be higher in the Florida community. Adjusting the rate based on age allows for comparing rates in such a way that controls for the age variance between the two populations. The **age-adjusted rate** is the total expected number of deaths divided by the total standard population times 100,000, which is why the rate is expressed as per 100,000 deaths.

Comparing Rates

The team concluded that there was a difference between Small Town and the state in relation to low birth weight, teen births, bacterial pneumonia, and cardiovascular disease–related deaths. A member of the team living in the community wanted to know whether these differences should cause concern. The epidemiologist agreed to compare the town's rates with the rates of the state and the four towns adjacent to Small Town to help determine whether the differences were significant, that is, not attributable to chance. He also explained that he would use a different approach to compare the rates between Small Town and Massachusetts than he would when comparing the town with the rates of the other four towns. When comparing the rates between the town and the state, the rates are dependent, that is, the cases in the town are included in the total number of cases for the state. But when comparing the different towns with one another they are independent rates, because the cases in one town are not included in the number of cases in the other town. When he was done, he reported that all the rates were significantly higher than the state rates. However, only three rates—bacterial pneumonia, teen births, and cardiovascular disease–related deaths—were significantly higher than the rates in the adjoining towns.

The team was also interested in gathering secondary data regarding behavioral risk factors. One of the members reminded the group that the Behavioral Risk Factor Surveillance System (BRFSS) was available for the community. Since 1984, the BRFSS has been tracking health conditions and risk behaviors.[41] The assessment committee was interested in lifestyle factors affecting premature mortality. The lifestyle risk factors that they were particularly interested in were tobacco use, alcohol use, exercise, and nutritional patterns. Some of these findings can be seen in Table 4-5. Based on these data, they concluded that nutrition and obesity were important risk factors that might help explain the higher cardiovascular mortality rate.

Health Status Assessment Using Primary Data

At this point, one of the members of the community who regularly attended the meetings stated that this information was good, but it was all just numbers and rates, and did not really capture how the individuals in the town viewed their own health. Others agreed, and they asked whether there was a way to collect data from people living in the town about how healthy they thought they were. They concluded that they could conduct a survey. In addition, the committee members realized they needed to complete an **inventory of resources** first to have a better idea of the resources within the community. They divided the community up and identified common resources in which they were interested. They wanted more information about schools, recreation centers and activities, neighborhood associations, churches, health-related clinics, hospitals, and agencies. They used the CHANGE handbook to help guide their data collection related to these organizations.[33]

TABLE 4-5 ■ BRFSS Adult Data for Small Town

Health Behavior	Prevalence in Small Town USA	Prevalence in Massachusetts
Current smoking (2010-2016)	19%	18%
Binge drinking (2010-2016)	18%	17%
Overweight	67%	54%
Leisure-time activity	68%	74%

Health Status Surveys

When this was complete, it was time to begin the survey. Donna explained that a survey could be constructed to collect health-related information from individuals by using a paper-and-pencil method. Unlike the secondary data they had been reviewing, a survey relies on self-report in which individuals respond to the survey designed for a specific purpose in the assessment. She further explained that a health survey is quite useful when doing a comprehensive community health assessment, because the researchers can decide ahead of time what information they need and provide information missing from the secondary data sets. Donna also told them that they did not have to reinvent the wheel; in other words, different surveys were available for them to review and adapt to their own community. She showed them a survey that included questions related to specific health indictors including HRQoL, protective health practices (see Chapter 3), and behavioral health issues. It also had space at the end for open-ended questions.

The members of the team who were residents of the community began making suggestions on how to improve the survey. The member who worked in the fire department thought that questions should be added about safety, and one of the other community members wanted to know whether people were using the recreation center or the new playground. As the discussion continued, the team built a survey that included key health issues that the team decided were important—safety, recreation, nutrition, and number of hospitalizations in the past year. They also addressed issues related to the cultural relevance of the survey and the language used. The final survey was four pages long and was approved by the members of the committee who lived in the community as being culturally appropriate.

Modifying the survey took some time, but Donna explained that it was better to take the time now rather than rush, then find out they had missed a key piece of information. The team considered how to distribute the survey. They seriously considered the telephone survey approach, but someone pointed out that many households in the town no longer had a landline, especially younger families. The editor of the town newspaper offered to distribute the survey in an issue of the paper (an example of a convenience sample); however, the problem with getting people to return the survey was raised. Another approach for conducting the survey was discussed: taking the survey door to door and having members of the community administer it. This approach seemed the most feasible. Donna explained that they could do a stratified random selection of households. Stratification would allow them to include different types of households based on home ownership. According to the Census Bureau data, Small Town USA had 3,660 housing units, of which 68% were owner occupied, 26% were renter occupied, and 5.8% were vacant. The team members decided they wanted to attempt to get a minimum of 10% of the households to respond to the survey in the two strata. Then someone else spoke up and said that the community was split, with the growing Hispanic population living in one part of town in less expensive housing. They turned to the epidemiologist, who helped them come up with a strategy to include an adequate sample based on both ethnic group and home ownership. Once they identified the strata and their actual representation in the population, random sampling was then used to select the households. The final number of households that needed to be surveyed was approximately 400. The community members of the committee formed a subcommittee to recruit volunteers in the community to administer the survey. Donna agreed to train the volunteers in the administration of the survey.

With the help of the epidemiologist, they analyzed the data and prepared a report on the survey for the community (Box 4-5). The editor of the paper included the report as an insert in the weekly paper. The core

---

BOX 4–5 ■ Sample Report on Findings from a Health Survey

Health Survey Report

Small Town USA, Massachusetts
Vision: "Small Town USA, the place to be for healthy living"

To help provide information about the health of Small Town USA and to obtain recommendations from the community, a health survey was conducted. This report includes the findings from this survey.

Methods
A random sample of households was selected to complete a door-to-door survey. The survey included items designed to measure HRQoL and access to care.

Findings
Of the 400 surveys that were completed, a total of 396 were included in this analysis. Four were not included because they contained incomplete data. The majority (80%) of the respondents were female, 95% identified themselves as white. The mean age was 52 with a range from 27 years of age to 95. Twenty-two percent of the respondents were older than 64. Only 8% of the respondents lived alone, with 56% reporting that there were three or more in their households. Forty-three percent reported that a child younger than 18 years of age lived in their household. Ninety-five percent reported that they had health insurance, and 60% reported having dental insurance.

Health-Related Quality of Life: The majority of respondents reported that their general health was good, very good, or excellent (see the following figure on general health). In relation to the two questions related to physical function, 15% of respondents stated that they were limited physically "a lot" on the first question and 13% on the second. In relation to the two questions related to physical role, 9% responded all or most of the time they accomplished less and/or were limited in the work they could do.

The responses on the next two sections of the SF-12, vitality and pain, had interesting results. Only a little more than half of the respondents (52%) reported having energy (vitality) all or most of the time, and 23% reported that pain at least moderately interfered with their activities. Thirty-two percent reported that their physical and/or emotional health interfered with their social activities.

The last section of the SF-12 relates to emotional health. More than a quarter of the respondents reported that they felt downhearted or depressed at least some of the time (see the following figure on mood) and 8% felt calm only a little or none of the time. In relation to the two questions related to emotional health and their role, 11% responded all or most of the time that they accomplished less than they would like and 6% were limited in the work they could do.

Access to Care and Health Practices: The majority of respondents (84%) reported that they had had a checkup in the past year. However, 30% reported that they did not get care when they needed it, with the majority of these respondents reporting that the reason was lack of money or insurance. The majority of respondents received screening in the past year, with 95% reporting they had had their blood pressure checked, 75% had their cholesterol checked, and 67% had their blood sugar checked. Less than half (48%) had received a flu shot.

Half of the respondents (51%) stated they had a medical condition, and the majority of these (40%) reported a cardiovascular-related diagnosis. Only 7.5% of respondents reported that they were current smokers, and almost half (48%) reported that they did not drink alcohol at all. Of those that reported alcohol use, 25% were daily drinkers.

Continued

BOX 4–5 ■ Sample Report on Findings from a Health Survey—cont'd

Obesity: Of the 94 respondents, height and weight information was available for 89 respondents. Using the standard calculation, a body mass index (BMI) was computed for each respondent. Using the national guidelines, 55% of the respondents were overweight or obese. One quarter of respondents met the criteria for obesity.

Conclusions

There is a match between one of the findings of the health survey and the suggestions given by the respondents. With the majority of the respondents having a BMI greater than 25, the suggestions to develop nutrition and exercise programs would address this issue. However, although respondents rated their general health at the high end, a large percentage reported issues having to do with depression, pain, and the negative impact of both their emotional and physical health on their daily role and ability to function. Suggestions were made to address some of these

issues, but only two respondents mentioned mental health in the open-ended questions. Also, although most respondents indicated that they had health insurance, insurance and access to care were listed in the open-ended questions section. Finally, there were numerous suggestions to include support programs for various health issues. Suggestions ranged from new moms, to seniors, to reaching out to those who were homebound and/or ill.

Recommendations

1. Develop a healthy eating and physical exercise program.
2. Review models for support programs for seniors, new moms, and families experiencing illness and adapt for this community. Include links to existing programs such as Meals on Wheels.
3. Put together an informational packet on existing health services in the community with a focus on helping those with limited or no health insurance.

members of the team met to discuss where they were with the MAPP model that they were using. They decided that they had been mainly focused on the Community Health Status Assessment and they now had data on the traditional morbidity and mortality indicators, QoL indicators, and behavioral risk factors.

The team members then decided to review how to create their CHANGE summary statement as outlined by the CHANGE model. One of the community members suggested that they use the town hall format to have an open town forum on the health of the community. He said that the current town governance structure lent itself to obtaining this more qualitative data from the community and could also reengage the community in the work they had been doing. They enlisted the help of the town moderator and the town selectpersons to help run the meeting. The members of their committee who represented different sections of the community, such as the Hispanic member and the member living in the senior housing complex, agreed to encourage their neighbors and friends to attend.

On the day of the forum more than 900 members of the community attended, more than triple the number that usually attended town hall meetings. The town moderator opened the meeting with one question: "How healthy a community is Small Town?" During the next 2 hours the community engaged in a lively debate over how healthy the community was and what health

problems they thought the town had (Fig. 4-4). The talk began with the lack of health care. The plant in the neighboring town had closed 6 months earlier, and many local people were now signing up for health care through the state health exchange. Some people were now threatened with foreclosure on their homes. The

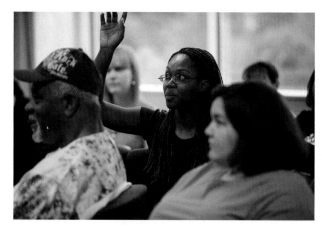

Figure 4-4 Town Hall participation. Raising her hand to pose a question, this African-American woman was one of a number of attendees to a town hall meeting held on behalf of the Agency for Toxic Substances and Disease Registry (ATSDR). The purpose of these meetings is to collect community concerns and share health messages about local environmental issues. *(Source: Centers for Disease Control and Prevention/Dawn Arlotta.)*

cost of gasoline had gone up, making it more problematic to get to the doctor.

One community member brought up the rise in teen births and wanted to know why there was not a family planning clinic in town. This brought opposition from several people. The town moderator demonstrated his skills in working with the community. He carefully brought the discussion back to the vision of healthy living and away from the more polarizing issue of family planning. People then shared opinions about the difficulty of obtaining prenatal care and well-child services because none were available in the town. Even the federally subsidized program for Women, Infants, and Children that provides supplemental foods to women and children at nutritional risk no longer had an office in town. Finally, one person stood up and said that the air seemed to be thicker. Someone else volunteered that there were too many wood stoves burning because of the high cost of heating oil, and that was why the air was hard to breathe. Others chimed in and stated they had to keep their thermostats down because they could not afford the oil, and that their children had more colds in winter.

After the forum ended, committee members compared their notes and concluded that access to care was a major concern for members of the community. They discussed the heated debate that occurred when teen pregnancy was raised. The members of the committee who lived in the community reminded everyone that Small Town has a large population of French Canadians as well as the growing community of Hispanics who had opposed family planning clinics in the past. The committee acknowledged that, for this community to be successful, the issue of teen pregnancy would need to be addressed within the culture of the community. They were also interested in looking into the issue of heating and possible reduction in air quality. They concluded that the town forum had added additional information to their assessment. An interesting finding was the value of the town moderator, and it was suggested that he be added to the committee.

The use of the sector approach to the assessment included in the CHANGE model helped to guide the team in including an examination of the components, activities, capacities, and competencies of the local public health system. By this time, the momentum for the assessment had raised a certain amount of enthusiasm in the community. New members were eager to join the activities. The subcommittee consisted of Donna, the local fire department representative, a local physician in the community, and the vice-president of the hospital who met to discuss how the Ten Essential Public Health Services were being provided in the community. Organizations within the community providing the services were then identified and gaps were noted. The assessment revealed that many organizations in the community were providing more than one of the essential services. The essential services that received the most attention by several agencies were service #1, monitoring health status to identify community health problems; service #3, informing, educating, and empowering people about health issues; and service #7, linking people who needed personal health services and assuring the provision of health care.

Weaknesses of the public health system included a need to develop better use of technology such as GIS (see previous discussion) to better understand vulnerabilities. Another weakness was limited activities and resources for teens, especially those teens who were pregnant. With a recent economic downturn, there was some concern about the adequacy of the workforce. The recent budgetary cuts in public health prevented the public health system from exploring new and innovative solutions to health problems.

The team now came together to reach consensus in relation to the data collected. The broad categories that the committee considered important to consider were: (1) trends or patterns over time; (2) factors that are discrete elements such as a change in a large ethnic population; and (3) events of a one-time occurrence. The core steering committee helped to lead the brainstorming sessions with the final identification of three major trends in the community:

1. Changing demographics
2. Emerging public health issues—teen pregnancy in particular
3. Shifting funding streams within the health department, particularly a loss of a grant that focused on maternal child issues

The core team members next began the final analysis of the data as a means for determining priorities and building the community action plan. They examined trends over time, compared statistics in different jurisdictions, and identified high-risk populations. The primary data corroborated the secondary data in several areas, including cardiovascular health, teen pregnancies, and bacterial pneumonia. Analysis of both the secondary and primary data indicated that access to care was a key issue. The BRFSS data and the survey data supported the need to address some lifestyle behavior issues. The additional assessments supported the need to examine the resources both within the community and the local health department, including the lack of support for young teens in the community and the local health department.

The team used the forms suggested by CHANGE to outline the strengths and problems identified both through secondary data and primary data. The data were presented at another town meeting. This was followed by the core committee and steering committee prioritizing the problems based on the criteria of magnitude of the problem, seriousness of the problem, and feasibility of correcting the problem. In the case of Small Town, the assessment process informed the county of the need for a program to address teen pregnancy. This seemed to be a primary concern of most people in the community. This was followed by the need for additional resources to address the needs of older adults, especially as they related to increased cardiovascular health needs, bacterial pneumonia, and growing problems with being overweight. The downturn in the economy and the changing workforce were important issues. The report highlighted the importance of providing resource information to those experiencing difficulties. Their next steps included completing the final report and the beginning development of an action plan.

Summary Points

- The purpose of an assessment is to provide an accurate portrayal of the health of a community to develop priorities, obtain resources, and plan actions to improve health.
- There are seven different approaches to assessment, varying from comprehensive assessments to more specific narrow assessments focused on a health problem, a specific health issue, or population. Other types of assessments include HIAs and rapid needs assessments.
- Frameworks or models can be used to guide the community assessment process. Two models include MAPP and CHANGE.
- Assessment data consist of both secondary and primary data.
- Qualitative methods of data collection include focus groups and key informant interviews. Quantitative methods often include surveys.
- Newer techniques of collecting data include the use of GIS and PhotoVoice.

- In interpreting the level of health of a community, it is important to join secondary data with the primary data. One needs to consider trends or changes over time, comparison of local data with data from other jurisdictions, and an identification of populations at risk.
- Prioritization of health issues is based on several criteria: magnitude of the problem, seriousness of the consequences, feasibility of correcting, and other criteria as determined by the community assessment team.

▼ CASE STUDY
Exploring Your Town

Many of us think we know a lot about our town, but we do not know the particulars. How many residents own their home and how many are renters? How many vacant homes are in our town? Has the population gotten older, poorer, or richer? The U.S. Census Bureau has already aggregated much of the data that answer these questions and more. It is possible to drill down right to your own neighborhood if you know your census tract. To obtain census tract data, you must first identify the census tract number. This can be identified by a street address or by consulting a census tract map. If you have a street address, use the street address search.

1. Go to American Factfinder at http://factfinder.census.gov.
2. Enter the name of a town in which you are interested. What information can you find about the percentage of families living in poverty? What is the mean income?
3. Identify census tract information.
4. If you have a street address, use the Select Geographies drop-down box to determine in which census tract a family lives in. What does this information tell you about the neighborhood?
5. If you do not have an address, use the reference map feature by selecting Maps from the left menu and then Reference Maps.
6. Select a state from the map and zoom so that you can see census tract boundaries. Determine the correct tract number.
7. Switch to search (on the top menu) and select the Geography tab.
8. Show more selection methods and more geographical types.
9. Change the search boxes with the name of the state, county, and tract number.
10. Search for the map of the census track to determine the population.

REFERENCES

1. National Association of County and City Health Officials. (n.d.). *Community Health Assessment and Improvement Planning*. Retrieved from https://www.naccho.org/programs/public-health-infrastructure/performance-improvement/community-health-assessment.

2. Turnock, B. (2015). *Public health: What it is and how it works* (6th ed.). Boston, MA: Jones & Bartlett.

3. Institute of Medicine. (1988). *The future of public health*. Washington, DC: National Academies Press.

4. Dulemba, L.H., Glazer, G., & Gregg, J.A. (2016). Comprehensive assessment of the needs of chronic obstructive pulmonary disease patients residing in east-central Indiana and west-central Ohio. *Online Journal of Rural Nursing & Health Care*, 16(2), 112-140. doi:10.14574/ojrnhc.v16i2.378.

5. Hebert-Beirne, J., Hernandez, S.G., Felner, J., Schwiesow, J., Mayer, A., Rak, K., Kennelly, J., et al. (2018). Using community-driven, participatory qualitative inquiry to discern nuanced community health needs and assets of Chicago's La Villita, a Mexican immigrant neighborhood. *Journal of Community Health*, 43(4), 775-786. doi:10.1007/s10900-018-0484-2.

6. Council on Linkages Between Academia and Public Health Practice. (2014). *Core competencies for public health professionals*. Retrieved from http://www.phf.org/resourcestools/Documents/Core_Competencies_for_Public_Health_Professionals_2014June.pdf.

7. Centers for Disease Control and Prevention. (2016). *Partnerships to improve community health (PICH)*. Retrieved from https://www.cdc.gov/nccdphp/dch/programs/partnershipstoimprovecommunityhealth/index.html.

8. Cottrell, LS. (1976). The competent community. In B.H Kaplan, R.N Wilson, & A.H. Leighton (Eds.), *Further explorations in social psychiatry*. New York, NY: Basic Books, pp 195-209.

9. Goeppinger, J., & Baglioni, A.J. (1985). Community competence: A positive approach to needs assessment. *American Journal of Community Psychology*, 13(5), 507-523.

10. McKnight, J. & Block, P. (2010). *The abundant community*. San Francisco: Barrett and Koelher.

11. Honoré, P.A., & Scott, W. (2010). *Priority areas for improvement of quality in public health*. Washington, DC: Department of Health and Human Services. Retrieved from http://www.phf.org/resourcestools/Documents/ImproveQuality2010.pdf.

12. Centers for Disease Control and Prevention. (2015). *assessment & planning models, frameworks & tools*. Retrieved from http://www.naccho.org/topics/infrastructure/mapp/chahealthreform.cfm.

13. National Association for State Community Service Programs. (2011). *A community action guide to comprehensive community needs assessments*. Washington DC: Author.

14. Centers for Disease Control and Prevention. (2015). *Assessment & planning models, frameworks & tools*. Retrieved from https://www.cdc.gov/stltpublichealth/cha/assessment.html.

15. Alves, H., Da Silva Brito, I., Rodrigues Da Silva, T., Araújo Viana, A., & Andrade Santos, R.C. (2017). Adolescent pregnancy and local co-planning: a diagnostic approach based on the PRECEDE-PROCEED model. *Revista de Enfermagem Referência*, 4(12), 35–44. https://doi-org.ezp.welch.jhmi.edu/10.12707/RIV16058.

16. World Health Organization. (2018). *Indicators of maternal, newborn and child health*. Retrieved from http://www.who.int/woman_child_accountability/progress_information/recommendation2/en/.

17. Centers for Disease Control and Prevention. (2018). *The school health index*. Retrieved from https://www.cdc.gov/healthyschools/shi/index.htm.

18. Centers for Disease Control and Prevention. (2015). *Workplace health promotion: assessment*. Retrieved from https://www.cdc.gov/workplacehealthpromotion/model/assessment/index.html.

19. Salkas, S., Conniff, J., & Budge, S.L. (2018). Provider quality and barriers to care for transgender people: An analysis of data from the Wisconsin transgender community health assessment. *International Journal of Transgenderism, 19*(1), 59–63. https://doi-org.ezp.welch.jhmi.edu/10.1080/15532739.2017.1369484.

20. World Health Organization. (2018). *Health impact assessments (HIA)*. Retrieved from http://www.who.int/hia/en/.

21. Mueller, N., Rojas-Rueda, D., Basagaña, X., Cirach, M., Cole-Hunter, T., Dadvand, P, Nieuwenhuijsen, M, et al. (2017). Urban and transport planning related exposures and mortality: a health impact assessment for cities. *Environmental Health Perspectives, 125*(1), 89-96.

22. Pennington, A., Dreaves, H., Scott-Samuel, A., Haigh, F., Harrison, A., Verma, A., & Pope, D. (2017). Development of an urban health impact assessment methodology: indicating the health equity impacts of urban policies. *European Journal of Public Health, 27*(suppl_2), 56-61. doi:10.1093/eurpub/ckv114.

23. Centers for Disease Control and Prevention. (2017). *Health impact assessment*. Retrieved from https://ephtracking.cdc.gov/showHealthImpactAssessment.

24. Pan American Health Organization & World Health Organization. (n.d.). *Rapid needs assessment*. Retrieved from http://www.paho.org/disasters/index.php?option=com_content&view=article&id=744:rapid-needs-assessment&Itemid=0&lang=en.

25. International Federation of Red Cross and Red Crescent Societies. (n.d.). *Emergency needs assessment*. Retrieved from http://www.ifrc.org/en/what-we-do/disaster-management/responding/disaster-response-system/emergency-needs-assessment/.

26. Witkin, B., & Altschuld, J.W. (1995). *Planning and conducting needs assessments*. Thousand Oaks, CA: Sage.

27. Kretzmann, J.P., & McKnight, J.L. (1993). *Building communities from the inside out: A path toward finding and mobilizing a community's assets*. Evanston, IL: Institute for Policy Research.

28. McKnight, J.L. & Kretzmann, J.P. (1997). Mapping community capacity. In M. Minkler. *Community organizing & community building for health*. New Brunswick, NJ: Rutgers University Press.

29. Mayan, M.J. & Dum, C.H. (2016). Worth the risk? Muddled relationships in community-based participatory research. *Qualitative Health Research, 26*(1) 69–76.

30. Oetzel, J.G., Wallerstein, N., Duran, B., Sanchez-Youngman, S., Nguyen, T., Woo, K., Alegria, M, et al. (2018). Impact of participatory health research: a test of the community-based participatory research conceptual model. *BioMed Research International, 2018*, 1–12. https://doi-org.ezp.welch.jhmi.edu/10.1155/2018/7281405.

31. Whisenant, D.P., Cortes, C., Ewell, P., & Cuellar, N. (2017). The use of community based participatory research to assess

perceived health status and health education needs of persons in rural and urban Haiti. *Online Journal of Rural Nursing & Health Care, 17*(1), 52-72. http://dx.doi.org/10.14574/ojrnhc.v17i1.427.

32. Flicker, S., Travers, R., Guta, A., McDonald, S., & Meagher, A. (2007). Ethical dilemmas in community-based participatory research: Recommendations for institutional review boards. *Journal of Urban Health, 84*(4), 478-493.

33. Centers for Disease Control and Prevention. (2018). *Community health assessment and group evaluation (CHANGE) tool.* Retrieved from https://www.cdc.gov/nccdphp/dnpao/state-local-programs/change-tool/action-steps.html.

34. National Association of County and Community Health Officials. (2018). *Mobilizing for action through planning and partnerships (MAPP).* Retrieved from https://www.naccho.org/programs/public-health-infrastructure/performance-improvement/community-health-assessment/mapp.

35. National Association of County and Community Health Officials. (n.d.). *APEXPH.* Retrieved from http://www.naccho.org/topics/infrastructure/APEXPH/index.cfm.

36. Savage, C.L., Anthony, J.S., Lee, R., Rose, B., & Kapesser, M. (2007). The culture of pregnancy and infant care African American women: An ethnographic study. *Journal of Transcultural Nursing, 18*(3), 215-223.

37. U.S. Census Bureau. (n.d.). *Geography reference.* Retrieved from https://www.census.gov/geo/reference/.

38. University of Wisconsin Population Health Institute. (2018). *County health ratings.* Retrieved from http://www.countyhealthrankings.org/.

39. Centers for Disease Control and Prevention. (2018). *National health interview survey.* Retrieved from http://www.cdc.gov/nchs/nhis.htm.

40. Centers for Disease Control and Prevention. (2018). *National health and nutrition examination survey.* Retrieved from http://www.cdc.gov/nchs/nhanes.htm.

41. Centers for Disease Control and Prevention. (2018). *Behavioral risk factor surveillance system.* Retrieved https://www.cdc.gov/brfss/index.html.

42. U.S. Department of Agriculture. (2017). *Food access research atlas.* Retrieved from https://www.ers.usda.gov/data-products/food-access-research-atlas.aspx.

43. Centers for Disease Control and Prevention. (2016). *Health-related quality of life: Methods and measures.* Retrieved from http://www.cdc.gov/hrqol/methods.htm.

44. Carey, M.A. & Asbury, J-E. (2016). *Focus group research.* London and New York: Routledge.

45. Savage, C.L. (Ed.). (1996). *Health of Lancaster County.* Lancaster, PA: Lancaster Health Alliance.

46. Valiquette-Tessier, S., Vandette, M., & Gosselin, J. (2015). In her own eyes: PhotoVoice as an innovative methodology to reach disadvantaged single mothers. *Canadian Journal of Community Mental Health, 34*(1), 1-16. doi:10.7870/cjcmh-2014-022.

47. Skovdal, M. (2011). Picturing the coping strategies of caregiving children in western Kenya: From images to action. *American Journal of Public Health, 101*(3), 452-453.

48. Beck, A.F., Sandel, M.T., Ryan, P.H., & Kahn, R.S. (2017). Mapping neighborhood health geomarkers to clinical care decisions to promote equity in child health. *Health Affairs, 36*, 999-1005. doi:10.1377/hlthaff.2016.1425.

49. Aronson, R.E., Wallis, A.B., O'Campo, P., & Schafer, P. (2007). Neighborhood mapping and evaluation: A methodology for participatory community health initiatives. *Maternal Child Health Journal, 11*, 373-383.

50. Croner, C.M., Sperling, J., & Broome, F.R. (1996). Geographic information systems (GIS): New perspectives in understanding human health and environmental relationships. *Statistics in Medicine, 15*, 17-18, 1961-1977.

51. Salehi, F., & Ahmadian, L. (2017). The application of geographic information systems (GIS) in identifying the priority areas for maternal care and services. *BMC Health Services Research, 1*, 482. doi:10.1186/s12913-017-2423-9.

52. Suplee, P.D., Bloch, J.R., Hillier, A., & Herbert, T. (2018). Using geographic information systems to visualize relationships between perinatal outcomes and neighborhood characteristics when planning community interventions. *JOGNN: Journal Of Obstetric, Gynecologic & Neonatal Nursing, 47*, 158-172. doi:10.1016/j.jogn.2018.01.002.

53. Pennel, C.L., Burdine, J.N., Prochaska, J.D., & McLeroy, K.R. (2017). Common and critical components among community health assessment and community health improvement planning models. *Journal of Public Health Management & Practice, 23*, S14-S21. doi:10.1097/PHH.0000000000000588.

54. U.S. Census Bureau. (n.d.). *American FactFinder.* Retrieved from https://factfinder.census.gov/faces/nav/jsf/pages/index.xhtml.

55. World Life Expectancy. (2018). *World population pyramid.* Retrieved from http://www.worldlifeexpectancy.com/world-population-pyramid.

56. U.S. Census Bureau. (2018). Retrieved from https://www.census.gov/.

Chapter 5

Health Program Planning

Gordon Gillespie, Christine Savage, and Sara Groves

LEARNING OUTCOMES

After reading the chapter, the student will be able to:

1. Discuss the use of *Healthy People 2020* in health program planning.
2. Identify components of different health planning models.
3. Describe the steps in writing community diagnoses.
4. Explain the importance of evidence-based practice in program planning.
5. Describe the process of writing goals, objectives, and activities for a health program.
6. Discuss the different types and value of program evaluation.

KEY TERMS

Community capacity
Community diagnosis
Community organizing
Formative evaluation
Goal

Health program planning
Impact
Objective
Outcome
Output

Process evaluation
Program evaluation
Program implementation
Resources
SMART objectives

Social justice
Summative evaluation

Introduction

We all want to live in healthy communities. A healthy community is a place where children are safe to play and learn; a place where there are educational and employment opportunities; a place with safe, affordable housing; and a neighborhood with good communication and support. In a healthy community, if teenagers use alcohol, older adults have difficulty accessing health care, or the percentage of obese adults increases, the community works together with other collaborative partners to solve the problem. Program planning can lead to increased community capacity to solve these problems and create healthier communities.

Community program planning is the process that helps communities understand how to move from where they are to where they would like to be.[1] **Health program planning** is "a multistep process that generally begins with the definition of the problem and development of an evaluation plan. Although specific steps may vary, they usually include a feedback loop, with findings from program evaluation being used for program improvement."[2] Planning occurs at the local level with both public and private agencies, at the state and federal levels, and also as part of strategic planning for the public's health at the global level. Today, public health program planning is one of the

10 essential public health services that should be undertaken in all communities.[3] Program planning is most successful when the community is a collaborative partner, bringing together resources to achieve agreed-upon goals and increasing community capacity. **Community capacity** refers to the ability of community members to work together to organize their assets and resources to improve the health of the community. It is the ability of a community to recognize, evaluate, and address key problems. Building community capacity can increase the quality of the lives of individual community residents; it can promote long-term community health and increase community resilience. The community as a whole can become self-reliant in identifying root causes of health problems and achieving identified outcomes. It can be quite self-sustaining when community members are empowered to make their own decisions about interventions and outcomes. Community capacity building is about working in partnerships and supporting community members in their decision making.[4]

Health program planning is a four-step process that includes assessment, developing of interventions, implementing interventions, and evaluating the effectiveness of interventions. It is the same basic steps of the nursing process applied to populations rather than individuals. It begins with the assessment phase covered in Chapter 4.

Based on the assessment, the collaborative community partners arrive at a community diagnosis. They then decide what action would be most productive to improve the health of the community and begin to plan a program or programs to address the priority health issues identified. Once the plan is in place, they act (implement the plan). The final stages are to evaluate how well the plan addressed the priority issue and, if it works, how best to sustain the program.[4] The program could involve such things as policy change, health education, or the creation of new public health services. Frequently, it means putting in place a program to address the community health diagnosis with the goal of improving health outcomes for the population, reducing the risk of disease, and/or minimizing the impact of disease. Program planning follows the same process for the population level that the nursing process uses with individuals and is similar to the development of a care plan in the nursing process and the evaluation of the effectiveness of the intervention.

National Perspective

Program planning has been an integral part of public health practice since its conception and has received a lot of attention in the past 30 years. In 1988, the Institute of Medicine (IOM) (now the Health and Medicine Division of the National Academies, Engineering, and Medicine) published a landmark report focusing on the future of public health (see Chapter 1). In this document, public health practice was recognized as population focused, not individual focused, health planning was recognized as important at the local level, and the core public health functions of assessment, policy development, and service assurances were identified.[5] The IOM report of 2002 further defined public health practice and the shift from individuals to populations with the essential engagement of the community and diverse partners in the practice of public health.[6] The 2012 IOM report strongly advocated for increased funding of public health and population-level interventions.[7] Public health nurses (PHNs) today embrace this population focus with their community-based assessments, health planning, population-based program designs and interventions, program evaluation, and policy development.[8] Both PHNs and nurses working in other settings need skills related to engaging community partners in these program efforts and how to make successful programs sustainable. Keller and colleagues have been instrumental in identifying the areas of community organizing, coalition building, collaborating, social marketing, and policy development[9,10] within the Intervention Wheel Practice Model (see Chapter 2). All of these perspectives are useful in health planning and program design, implementation, and evaluation.

Healthy People

A key federal effort that provides a tool for community public health planning in the United States is *Healthy People (HP),* a national compilation of disease prevention and health promotion goals and objectives for better health (see Chapter 1). During the past 4 decades, *HP* has become a part of health planning at the local, state, and federal levels. *HP* provides a guide to communities wishing to implement *HP* guidelines.[11] The guide uses MAPIT (Mobilize, Assess, Plan, Intervene, and Track progress) to help communities set targets and identify indicators of success (Box 5-1).

In addition, one of the topics included in *HP 2020* is educational and community-based programs.[12] Thus, *HP* acknowledges the need for health planning at the community level and provides clear objectives and strategies for population-based health programs.

■ HEALTHY PEOPLE 2020
Health Planning and Evaluation

Targeted Topics: Educational and Community-Based Programs

Goal: Increase the quality, availability, and effectiveness of educational and community-based programs designed to prevent disease and injury, improve health, and enhance quality of life.

Overview: Educational and community-based programs play a key role in:

- Preventing disease and injury
- Improving health
- Enhancing quality of life

Health status and related health behaviors are determined by influences at multiple levels: personal, organizational/institutional, environmental, and policy based. Because significant and dynamic interrelationships exist among these different levels of health determinants, educational and community-based programs are most likely to succeed in improving health and wellness when they address influences at all levels and in a variety of environments/settings.

Midcourse Review: Of the original 107 objectives, 10 were archived for *HP 2020*, 7 were developmental, and 90 were measurable. At the midcourse review, 12 objectives had met or exceeded the 2020 targets, 11 were improving, and 16 had demonstrated little or no detectable change. In addition, 17 objectives were getting worse, 31 had baseline data only, and 3 were informational only.

Source: (12)

BOX 5–1 ■ *Healthy People*

Implementing *HP* using MAPIT

Healthy People is based on a simple but powerful model that helps to:

- Establish national health objectives
- Provide data and tools to enable states, cities, communities, and individuals across the country to combine their efforts to achieve them

  Use the MAPIT framework to help:

- Mobilize partners
- Assess the needs of a community
- Create and implement a plan to reach *HP* objectives
- Track a community's progress

Source: U.S. Department of Health and Human Services. (2018). *Program planning.* Retrieved from https://www.healthypeople.gov/2020/tools-and-resources/Program-Planning.

Healthy People goals and objectives were first presented in 1979, and they have continued to influence the nation, not just to assess health status but also to project improved status with outcome measurement (see Chapter 1). The *Healthy People* document in 1979 established national health objectives for the first time and provided the structure for the development of state and community health plans. The first 10-year plan had five goals, each established for distinct age groups, and 226 objectives.[13] The success of the first plan was limited. The reasons may have included too many goals, not enough significant interest generated in the public health and community arenas, and a lack of political support.[14]

The next 10-year plan, *Healthy People 2000* (1990–2000), replaced the first five goals with three new goals, 22 priority areas, and 319 objectives that included specific subobjectives to measure outcomes with special populations experiencing health disparities. The goals were: (1) increase the span of healthy life for Americans, (2) reduce health disparities among Americans, and (3) provide access to preventive health services for all Americans. These goals and objectives were influenced by the first 10-year plan, but they also were influenced by a concern for high-risk populations and the need to increase community organizing to better plan health. In the evaluation of the objectives at the end of the second decade of *HP,* there were some excellent outcomes, but there were situations in which health worsened.

The support for *Healthy People* as a planning tool grew and has now become part of the local, state, and national public health practice.[11] The *Healthy People 2010* (2000–2010) plan continued to build on previous *Healthy People* plans and refined the goals to two: (1) increase quality and years of life and (2) eliminate health disparity. It had more detailed objectives and 28 specific focus areas to help measure outcomes. *HP 2020* built on these previous efforts and included 42 topics (Box 5-2).[15]

All health-related agencies are encouraged to use this document and its indicators, such as a school for its breakfast program and industry in its worksite wellness programs. The proposed *HP 2030* plan is continuing to foster change in health behavior, but it also looks at long-range planning and priority programs for target populations. The intention of *HP* is to continue to guide efforts to plan, implement, and evaluate health promotion and disease prevention interventions for the nation. This is an important document to review and implement when planning health programs. It gives guidance in writing program objectives and identifying appropriate health indicators.

Overview of Health Program Planning

To provide population-focused care, it is necessary to have skill in health program planning and evaluation. Issel states the purpose of health program planning is "to ensure that a program has the best possible likelihood of being successful, defined in terms of being effective with the least possible resources."[16] To design appropriate programs, nurses who are part of a team must contribute to the completion of a reliable community assessment, participate in analyzing the community data, construct the community diagnoses, prioritize needs, and determine resource availability. Using this information, the nurses, other public health staff, community partners, and community members can begin the program planning process.

Health Program Planning Models

A number of models are available to assist with health program planning and evaluation. Program planning begins with a clear statement of the health problem. The assessment helps the team developing health programs to identify the priority health problems for the population and/or community. Following the establishment of the health priority, the team then works to understand the underlying factors contributing to the problem. As explained by Issel, this is the first step in deciding what intervention(s) are the best choice for addressing the

---

BOX 5–2 ■ *HP 2020's 42 Topics*

1. Access to Health Services
2. Adolescent Health
3. Arthritis, Osteoporosis, and Chronic Back Conditions
4. Blood Disorders and Blood Safety
5. Cancer
6. Chronic Kidney Disease
7. Dementias, including Alzheimer's Disease
8. Diabetes
9. Disability and Health
10. Early and Middle Childhood
11. Educational and Community-Based Programs
12. Environmental Health
13. Family Planning
14. Food Safety
15. Genomics
16. Global Health
17. Health Communication and Health Information Technology
18. 30 Health-Care-Associated Infections
19. Health-Related Quality of Life and Well-Being
20. Hearing and Other Sensory or Communication Disorders
21. Heart Disease and Stroke
22. HIV
23. Immunization and Infectious Diseases
24. Injury and Violence Prevention
25. Lesbian, Gay, Bisexual, and Transgender Health
26. Maternal, Infant, and Child Health
27. Medical Product Safety
28. Mental Health and Mental Disorders
29. Nutrition and Weight Status
30. Occupational Safety and Health
31. Older Adults
32. Oral Health
33. Physical Activity
34. Preparedness
35. Public Health Infrastructure
36. Respiratory Diseases
37. Sexually Transmitted Infections
38. Sleep Health
39. Social Determinants of Health
40. Substance Abuse
41. Tobacco Use
42. Vision

Source: https://www.healthypeople.gov/2020/topics-objectives.

---

problem and ultimately improving the health of the population and/or community.[16]

Most program planning models use a systems approach and provide guidance on how to identify the problem and then systematically apply the best solution.

These models all incorporate basic steps, and there are multiple resources that can be used to assist with each step (Table 5-1).

PRECEDE-PROCEED Model

Planning is essential to guarantee appropriate use of resources. One of the oldest models for program planning comes from Lawrence Green's well-researched PRECEDE-PROCEED model. Two other community health planning models in current use that can assist in program planning include Community Health Assessment and Group Evaluation (CHANGE) Action Guide and Mobilizing for Action Through Planning and Partnerships (MAPP) (see Chapter 4). The CHANGE model (see Chapter 4) has eight phases and only the last phase, develop the community action plan, deals with program planning. MAPP's action cycle is the program planning phase.

A model not discussed in Chapter 4 is the PRECEDE-PROCEED model, which gives insight into how to develop an educational program that will positively change health behavior. This model, designed in 1968, has generated evidence-based practice (EBP) in many diverse areas of health education. Green started out with two ideas: (1) health problems and health risks are caused by multiple factors, and (2) efforts to produce change must be multidimensional, multisectoral, and participatory.[17]

The PRECEDE component letters stand for **P**redisposing, **R**einforcing and **E**nabling factors, and **C**auses in **E**ducational **D**iagnosis and **E**valuation. When a community uses the PRECEDE process, it begins with a comprehensive community assessment process as described in Chapter 4. When the assessment phase is complete, the model provides guidance on how to examine the administrative and organizational issues that need to be dealt with before implementing a program aimed at improving the community's health. The final steps of PRECEDE relate to the design, implementation, and evaluation of a program. Evaluation includes examining data related to process, outcome, and impact objectives and indicators established during the development phase of the program planning.

Green believed that the more active and participatory the program interventions were for the recipients of the program, the more likely the recipients were to change behavior. Green also noted that, for behavior change to take place, recipients must be willing to work with the program; the ultimate decision to change behavior remains up to the recipients. The second half of the model is the PROCEED component that was developed from the work with the PRECEDE component. PROCEED goes beyond the recipients of the interventions

TABLE 5–1 ■ Steps in Health Program Planning

The types of steps generally used in program planning are listed here, along with selected resources that may be useful at each step.

Using Evidence-Based Resources for Program Design, Implementation, and Evaluation

Step	Description	Suggested Resources
1	Identify primary health issues in your community.	• Community Health Assessment and Group Evaluation (CHANGE) • County health rankings • National Public Health Performance Standards • MAPP (Mobilizing for Action Through Planning and Partnerships)
2	Develop measurable process and outcome objectives to assess progress in addressing these health issues.	• *HP* Leading Health Indicators • HEDIS (Healthcare Effectiveness Data and Information Set) performance measures
3	Select effective interventions to help achieve these objectives.	• The Guide to Clinical Preventive Services • Health Evidence • National Guideline Clearinghouse
4	Implement selected interventions.	• Partnership for Prevention • CDCynergy
5	Evaluate selected interventions based on objectives; use this information to improve the program.	• Framework for Program Evaluation in Public Health • CDCynergy
1–5	All of the above.	• The Community Health Promotion Handbook: Action Guides to Improve Community Health • Cancer Control P.L.A.N.E.T. (Plan, Link, Act, Network With Evidence-Based Tools) • Community Tool Box • Diffusion of Effective Behavioral Interventions (DEBI)

and reflects an effort to modify social environment and promote healthy lifestyle, which evolved as a clear need. PROCEED involves **P**olicy, **R**egulatory, **O**rganizational Constructs in **E**ducation, and **E**nvironmental **D**esign.[17] This model has served as the basis for other health program planning and assessment models, such as MAPP and CHANGE (see Chapter 4).

Logic Model

Another model used by many program planners is the logic model. A logic model provides the underlying theory that drives the program design. This model guides a team in the careful planning of a well-thought-out program. A logic model approach to program planning can result in a plan that is clear to implement and evaluate; is based on theoretical knowledge; and includes a clear understanding of resources, time, and expected outcomes. Logic models are such useful tools for program

evaluation that many grant agencies now require a logic model in their grant application.[18]

The concept of a logic model is it logically moves like a chain of reasoning from the planned work to the intended results in five steps, starting with input and resources to program activities to outputs to outcomes to impact (Fig. 5-1). The model is read from left to right. The first two components make up the planned work of the health program:[19]

1. **Resources** (inputs) are those items needed and available for the program. This includes human resources, financial resources, equipment, institutional resources, and community resources.
2. Next come the **activities** that produce the program intervention. It can involve processes such as health education, as well as tools, technology, or other types of activities classified as the intended intervention.

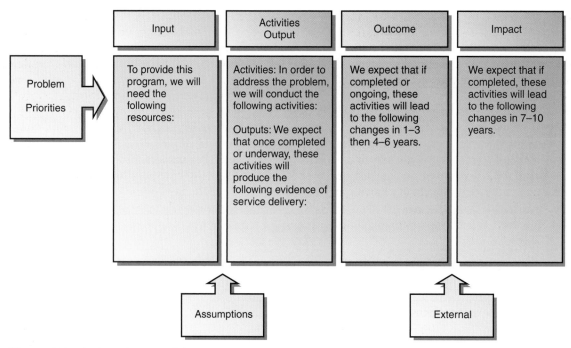

Figure 5-1 The basic logic model.

The next three components of a logic model make up the intended results:

3. **Outputs** are the direct product of the activities of the program, for example, a class completed on family planning, immunization for tetanus, or a service from the dentist. This is the process component of program evaluation. Successful output occurs when the program's intended outcome is achieved.
4. **Outcomes** are the intended results or benefits of the planned intervention and are those items that the team plans to measure. This can include a change in knowledge, skills, behavior, or attitude. The outcomes should be reasonable, realistic, and significant. The short-term and medium-term outcomes are the objectives, which reflect the previously discussed characteristics. In program planning, it is always important to think about potential unexpected or unintended outcomes if a program is implemented.
5. **Impact** is the program goal, producing long-term change in the community. This may often occur only after the program has been in effect for 5 to 8 years and even after the program funding has ended.[19,20]

Although linear reasoning occurs in all logic models, the model can come in all sizes and shapes. Some organizations have added other components and complexities to the model to help with particular clarification of the program design. Two areas can be added and can help in understanding the theory of the logic model. First, the assumptions the program planners have made, such as principles behind the program development; how and why a change in strategies will work; and any research knowledge and clinical experience. Second is a listing of external factors (culture, economics, demographics, policies, priorities) that will affect both resources and the program activities (see Fig. 5-1). A logic model is built on the community assessment, a clear identification of the problem, and best solutions within the context of the community in which the program will take place.

A logic model is a good tool for everyone involved in the program to use to help them organize their thoughts and ideas to work cooperatively for the same outcomes. It helps the program implementers understand why the activities are structured the way they are, helping to maintain the integrity of the program. The model is not static and can be adjusted and improved as the need arises with good, ongoing review and evaluation. If you are entering the program as an implementer after the design has been established, the logic model, read from left to right, offers you an excellent road map of *what* resources are available for implementation, *what* program is to be produced, with *what* results.

If you are entering the program as one of the stakeholders to help with the design, it is often best to start from what you hope the program will have as an impact (goal), move to the left identifying objectives (outcomes), and then determine which activities and output would help the community reach the intended objectives. Then you establish what resources are necessary to implement the intended activities.

In the program planning stage, you read a logic model from right to left. However, as previously noted, there is nothing static in the program planning process. As you complete the different sections you may find that you need to rewrite objectives based on the best practices you have found in the literature about a particular activity you would like to implement. You may find you have fewer resources than what you need to implement a

particular activity, which will change your intended outcomes. You can try various scenarios to determine which one is the best fit for the community and the organization, identifying strengths and weaknesses of the plan.

By the end of the process, the stakeholders will be able to see visually how the program goal(s) relate directly to the objectives that, in turn, relate directly to the program activities and the resources available. An example of a logic model is presented for the Elwood Community incorporating the assessment data, goal, objectives, activities, and output (Table 5-2).

The logic model is not the only tool available for program planning and, like all tools, has its drawbacks. In

TABLE 5–2 ■ Logic Model: Program to Create Social Integration Among Elmwood Residents

Resources	Activities	Outputs	Outcome	Impact
• Space in residential building including heat and electricity • Support (human and material) from the Primary Public School • Support from the community center (staff) at the residential site • PHN time, 8 hours per week for the program and other time for nursing care of the population • Residents of the facility • Support of time and resources from the two local churches • Additional community support	1. A senior outreach program to the public schools for 2 hours twice a week 2. A reading program for young children attending the Primary Public School 3. Creation and maintenance of a resident organization with one of its objectives being the improvement of communication among residents 4. Presentation/ discussion groups twice a month with initial church leadership; suggested first topics include: a. safety in the community b. celebrating differences in culture and ethnicity	• 15 seniors are working with 30 children at the Primary Public School • There is a reading session once a month with 10 seniors and 20 first grade children for 1 hour at the housing site • There is an Elmwood Community Association that has elected leaders and representatives from both buildings that meets regularly • There is a larger community organization that is meeting regularly to unite against crime in the community • The churches are working together to provide twice-monthly interactive programs at Elmwood	1. Establishment of a volunteer school program run by Elmwood residents to work with 50 children at the school and 25 children on site within 6 months 2. Development of consistent monthly programs in each building with a minimum of 40 resident attendees that foster social interaction by October 2023 3. Formation of a resident community organization	• Meaningful communication occurs among the elderly population in the two senior high-rise Elmwood residential buildings • Seniors are integrated into the community, feeling valued

Assumptions: (1) If residents of the Elmwood Buildings work together on programs and reach out to the community, the communication among themselves will increase. (2) If the residents believe their work is meaningful and interesting, they will convey this to other residents, the program will expand, and there will be increased communication. (3) If the residents are offered interesting and appropriate programs in the building, they will attend, have more interaction, and communication will continue to increase.

evaluating the use of the logic model, researchers have found that the emphasis on activities and outcomes has decreased the importance of understanding the rationale for the program choice.[20] Other tools such as concept mapping (a pictorial relation of concepts and relationships), a geographic information system (GIS; a computer-based program that can be used with geographical or location-based information; see Chapter 4), and community mapping (a visual map representation of resources and information corridors) are useful but also are limited. The University of Maryland, like many universities and organizations, created a program plan that can be modeled by others when developing a new program.[21] The tools are comprehensive and interactive, such as the Decision Support System (DSS), which is a step-by-step program planning series that gives on-screen feedback; Empower, which is based on the PRECEDE/PROCEED model; and the Outcome Toolkit, which facilitates planning and data analysis to make community improvement efforts measurable and accountable.

The logic model can serve several functions in addition to the actual program plan. For example, one group of researchers used the logic model to provide ". . . stakeholders with a common framework for the innovation or further development of pharmaceutical care".[22] It also helped the staff to discuss and specify assumptions they all held in common. For example, one assumption within the community was that all families have strengths, and appropriate job training and related activities will prevent homelessness. This then helped them to better define their goal: to prevent homelessness and move families to self-sufficiency. Mulroy and Lauber also were able to limit their activities and more precisely determine immediate and intermediate outcomes. These authors agreed that logic modeling helped provide an analytical structure for better outcome development and better program management and evaluation.

One group developed the ¡Cuídate! Program using the logic model as a means to "... plan, implement, and evaluate a sustainable model of sexual health group programing in a U.S. high school with a large Latinx student population".[23] The nurses believed the logic model was most helpful in providing a visual diagram that could be easily communicated to others. It became the heart of the program development and identified the future direction for the program.

Key Components of Health Program Planning

The important components of health program planning are:

- Active involvement of the community as a partner
- Skill and time to do a competent assessment

- Shared conclusions with the partners of the needed interventions
- Actual program planning, interventions, and evaluation[1]

Nurses at all levels of practice are involved in these processes, and it is critical nurses understand program planning to make significant contributions to the process.

As part of health program planning, nurses need to be involved in community organizing because this plays a pivotal role in successful planning as was recognized in the focus of *HP 2020* and in the Centers for Disease Control and Prevention (CDC) assessment and program model CHANGE (see Chapter 4).[24] **Community organizing** is bringing people together to get things done. It is helping people to act jointly in the best interest of their community. Most frequently, community organizing occurs with poorer communities that are disenfranchised, uniting people to gain power and fight for social justice. The process is inclusive of everyone in the community and is a powerful tool for health planning and program design. The role of the nurse in community organizing is not one of leadership but one of listener, facilitator, and developer of community leadership skills. It is to provide opportunities for the development of new relationships within the community.[1]

Inclusion of the community begins during the assessment phase (see Chapter 4) and continues through the action and evaluation phases. The key is to assemble a representative team from the community to help develop, implement, and evaluate a community health program. The CHANGE manual provides a guide on how to begin to assemble a team (Box 5-3). The public health system described by the CDC (Figure 5-2) also stresses the importance of including the community and provides extensive guidance and examples on how to accomplish this. This includes bringing together a diverse group, actively recruiting members, and developing a plan for engaging the larger community in the process.[1]

Social Justice

Another key construct central to health program planning is **social justice** (see Chapter 7). Improving the health of everyone in the community often requires addressing social injustices. It is also a basic underlying construct of public health. Social justice dictates that society is based on the constructs of human rights and equity. The idea is that those who have plenty will be willing to share with those who do not have enough to provide for equity. In a just health-care system, everyone should have the basic opportunities for a healthy life. Poverty, illness, and premature mortality are a tragic waste of human

BOX 5–3 ■ Assembling the Community Team

Action Step 1: Assemble the Community Team

Assembling a community team starts the commitment phase of the community change process. Representation from diverse sectors is a key component of successful teamwork; enables easy and accurate data collection; and enables data assessment, the next phase of the community change process. All members of the community team should play an active role in the assessment process, from recommending sites within the sectors to identifying the appropriate data collection method. This process also ensures the community team has equitable access to and informed knowledge of the process, thereby solidifying their support. Consider the makeup of the community team (10 to 12 individuals maximum is desirable to ensure the size is manageable and to account for attrition of members). Include key decision makers—the CEO of a worksite or the superintendent of the school board—to diversify the team and use the skill sets of all involved.

Source: Centers for Disease Control and Prevention. (2018). *Community health assessment and group evaluation (CHANGE) tool.* Retrieved from https://www.cdc.gov/nccdphp/dnpao/state-local-programs/change-tool/index.html

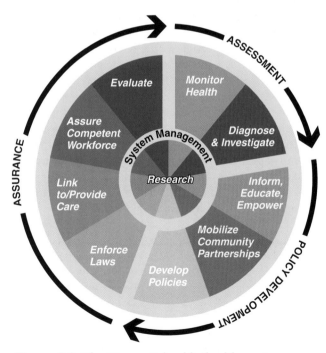

Figure 5-2 The 10 essential public health services. *(From Centers for Disease Control and Prevention. [2018]. The public health system. Retrieved from* https://www.cdc.gov/stltpublichealth/publichealthservices/essentialhealth services.html*)*

resources that defy the dignity and inherent worth of the individual. Social justice dictates everyone should have access to basic health services, economic security, adequate housing and food, satisfactory education, and a lack of discrimination based on race or religion. It is more often the distal social determinants (income, education, housing, racism) that are more impactful to changing the health status of individuals and populations than putting into place programs that change individual behavior in communities with limited resources. Providing adequate education leading to employment with a satisfactory income for housing and food can make a greater impact on health than teaching low-income individuals how to use their minimal income for healthy foods or better housing. Communities with scant resources frequently organize around issues of disparity. As they build their skills in organizing and create change within the community, they build community capacity and work toward social justice. As the community capacity increases, the health of the community improves. Community members learn how to be independent in identifying their problems, the root causes, and the skills to solve these problems.

■ CELLULAR TO GLOBAL

The social determinants of health (see Chapter 7) play an important role in the development of humans and their ability to achieve optimal health. Pregnant women require adequate health and health care to deliver a healthy infant. When access to foods that support healthy eating patterns and access to primary care are limited, fetuses are less likely to develop healthily in utero. The fetuses then have a greater risk for being born premature and/or with long-term physical or cognitive limitations. These limitations can later manifest with decreased educational attainment and increased poverty. Challenges to the social determinants of health are unique to each individual country but occur in all developing and developed nations across the globe. Increased health program planning that directly addresses these determinants will assure the highest likelihood for health for all.

The nurse must always consider social justice in program planning. In making the decision about public health action, there is the consideration of equitable distribution of benefits and burdens based on needs and contribution of the community. The community must decide the minimum goods and services required, how they can be acquired, and what programs will best serve the population with the available resources. In 2008, Buchanan warned against public health paternalism where individual rights are limited for the greater public good. He argued that if communities are given freedom to make choices, including the level of availability of those choices, they will achieve good health.[25] Striking a balance between public health mandates and community freedom of choice continues to present a dilemma for public health today as evidenced by vaccine requirements for attendance at schools.

Working to ensure universal health care has a great impact on health planning in the United States and is a social justice action particularly important to the PHN. It was a major platform promise during President Obama's first campaign and resulted in the establishment of the Patient Protection and Affordable Care Act (ACA). The American Nurses Association has long been a supporter of health-care reform and supported the passing of the ACA.[26] Although the future of the ACA is uncertain, the positive impact of the ACA to date has been documented,[27-29] and it can have a major impact on the health of the entire population. Nurses can also advocate, support, and work for the distal social determinants of a better educational systems, better child welfare, better housing laws, and better occupational and environmental protection. These actions will help the nation achieve the objectives set out in *HP 2030*, with people living longer and leading more active lives with less health disparity.

Community Diagnoses

Community diagnoses have been used in public health by multidisciplinary groups for many years, evolving separately from nursing and medical diagnoses, which tend to focus on individual need. Community diagnoses represent the last phase of the community assessment process and the first phase of the health program planning process. A clear statement of the health problem and the causal reasons or theories for it provide the basis for designing a health program that will actually improve the health issue. A **community diagnosis** is a summary statement resulting from the community assessment and the analysis of the data collected. The diagnosis guides the community team's thinking in how to design the program and what components are necessary. A community-specific diagnosis is needed because each community is unique in how the problems are manifested and solved. There are many types of community diagnoses and most share many parts in common, but the more detailed and complete the diagnoses, the easier it is to tailor them to an appropriate program.

Nursing community diagnoses generally contain four parts:[30] (1) the problem, (2) the population, (3) what the problem is related to (characteristics of the population), and (4) how the problem is demonstrated (indicators of the problem).[16,30]

▶ SOLVING THE MYSTERY
The Case of the Lonely Older Adults
Public Health Science Topics Covered:
- Assessment
- Community diagnosis

The PHN, Meghan, is working with a geriatric population in the Elmwood senior high-rise, composed of publicly funded housing units. Her employer, the city health department, has allocated her one day a week for health programming in these two closely spaced buildings located in the inner city of a moderately large urban area. To determine what kind of programs would be most useful, Meghan enlisted community partners in the Elmwood community and the city housing authority to do an assessment to help identify community strengths and health needs.

During the assessment, residents of the buildings were interviewed, as were both formal and informal leaders. The assessment group toured the Elmwood buildings looking at the apartments and other resources that were part of the units. They spoke with key community informants including the employees in the neighborhood schools and local churches. The group evaluated community safety and resources within walking distance of the Elmwood buildings, which included supermarkets, pharmacies, banks, health-care facilities, social service resources, and local stores. They reviewed demographic data, vital statistics, and other community indicators for the neighborhood, and compared the data with the city and with other areas in the United States. The community partnership, with the help of the PHN as a member of the team, summarized their assessment findings. One of the identified problems, which was at the top of the list for many residents, was the lack of meaningful activities for the residents within their apartment buildings. The residents were justifiably concerned about safety outside their buildings and had many mobility issues, which resulted in boredom and isolation, without an avenue for social communication.

Meghan had initially imagined she would implement an educational program, for example, teaching the residents about the health benefits of eating vegetables, the correct way to take their medications, or the importance of a low-fat diet. This was based on the type of interventions she had already been doing in the buildings one-on-one with individual clients. However, she was more than willing to explore a community-specific program that would facilitate social interaction. To do this, with the help of her community partners she elaborated this problem in a community diagnosis (Box 5-4).

Meghan also decided to include mediating and moderating factors as part of her community diagnosis.[30] This allowed her not only to examine the health problem, the population, indicators, and causal factors but also how the problem was mediated by specific moderating factors and the presence of antecedent factors (those behaviors that existed prior to the health problem).[30] It is frequently important to know that some behaviors may directly cause the problem and others may be more indirect. Moderating factors can make the problem better or worse. Mediating factors occur between the causal factors and the outcomes, and are significant when designing the program because they alter outcome. Increased details of the specific health problem can contribute significantly in determining the best program design.

In reviewing the analysis of the assessment, Meghan noted that in the Elmwood senior buildings the housing authorities mixed two ethnic neighborhood groups that had been hostile to each other for the past 20 years. Also, 15 years ago two of the large churches in this community held different positions on several neighborhood political and religious issues, and each congregation had united against the other with several harsh words spoken in public. The churches had subsequently left the decaying neighborhood, but many of the congregants were still living in the community.

This antecedent information contributed to a better understanding of the current problem of limited communication among Elmwood residents that led to social isolation.

The assessment committee had also spoken with the community center staff 10 blocks from Elmwood. The workers were frustrated at not attracting more senior clients for their multiple programs and expressed concern they might need to discontinue these programs due to lack of participation. They admitted they had done little marketing to the seniors at Elmwood, had no means to transport residents of the apartments to their center, and had little knowledge of the community dynamics, especially in relation to the senior population. They did provide escort services for schoolchildren coming to the community center because of a recent outbreak of gang violence in the area. They had not considered that this might also have an impact on the seniors' decision not to come to the center.

The local churches confirmed that there had been community discord, and many of their current older members were still angry. This had caused some friction in the current churches, but the pastors were working on mediating these factors to create more united congregations and better sharing among the memberships. All of the local churches provided transportation to services on Sunday and Wednesday evenings. They currently had no other outreach to the senior residential buildings.

When visiting the primary school one block from the senior housing, the teachers and principal talked about a lack of resources in the school. They repeatedly mentioned the need for many of the children to have more one-on-one interactions to increase their basic skills of reading and writing. With this additional information, Meghan added to the community diagnosis, and she now had a clearer understanding of some of the origins of the problems and the mediating and moderating factors that could help design a program that not only would provide opportunity for more social interaction among the senior residents but also could enhance the health of the entire community (Fig. 5-3).

Having completed the community diagnosis, Meghan explained to the team it was time to begin the program development phase. She explained they would work together with the stakeholders from all aspects of the identified community to determine how they could solve the problem of the lonely older adults. Meghan said they first must decide who will receive

BOX 5–4 ■ Community Diagnosis

Problem: Lack of meaningful social interaction resulting in social isolation.

Population: Older adult population in the two Elmwood senior residential buildings.

The isolation of the older adults was related to no formal programs in the building, limited social contact among residents, inadequate community safety, and residents' restricted mobility as indicated by residents being able to name only one other person in the building, the fact that no one spoke to others while waiting for the elevator, the neighborhood had the second highest crime rate in the city, 62% of residents complained of loneliness, and 59% of the residents had mobility problems.

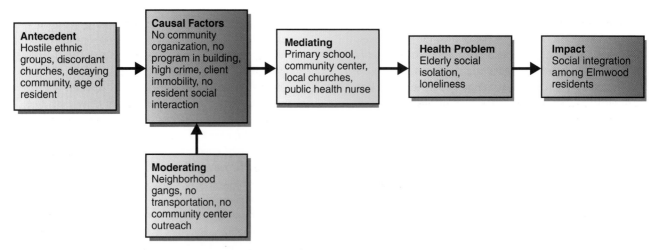

Figure 5-3 Diagram of community diagnosis for Elmwood Senior Housing.

the intervention. They needed to decide whether it would be individuals, families, communities, or a whole system. She cautioned that this was the time to carefully consider what interventions would be most appropriate and effective, and if there was evidence to confirm their decision. The team would together decide what immediate effects they would like this program to have and what long-term effects they might expect. All of this should be reflected from their community diagnosis and would guide the community discussion.

Meghan stressed this approach because she knew the clearer and more rational the explanation for solving the problem, the stronger the program would be. This was the time to discuss what kind of program activities the group would like to implement and what evidence-based practices existed to help guide the development of a program. The team began with a review of the literature, looking not only for established approaches but for new and innovative ones as well. Their discussion was tempered by resources, nature of the community, culture of the community, and other distal variables that influence receptivity to different types of programs. Much of the information gathered during their assessment helped them to think about what might work in their community.

The discussions were somewhat time intensive because of the multiple agendas of the people at the table, different approaches to problem-solving, varied understanding of the process of program planning, different cultural and communication styles, and different expectations. Yet Meghan persevered and helped

guide the discussion, allowing members to voice their opinions, and then bringing them back to the task at hand. Because she had worked in the community for a long time, she was able to help interpret cultural and value differences, facilitate communication, and encourage the planning team to use the community diagnosis statement to guide the design.

Megan carefully considered who should participate in the discussion. Based on the community diagnosis, Meghan specifically invited leadership from the school, churches, and community center. After she reviewed the community diagnosis with the group, the school representative immediately repeated the need for help with more one-on-one activity with the students at the school and mentioned several ways the seniors could participate. The school representative said they could provide on-site orientation at Elmwood for the seniors who would be willing to come to the school. He first suggested a 3-week training program, after which they would provide escorts to the school one block away on Tuesdays and Thursdays for the seniors to work 2 hours each of these days with the children. The Elmwood residents at the meeting asked whether the school also could bring some of the children to the Elmwood buildings once a month for story time with those seniors whose mobility was more limited. Several community members suggested this could be accomplished by creating the Elmwood Community Action Committee, which could meet jointly with school representatives to design the reading program. The community center offered to provide staff to help support these meetings. The community center saw this as an opportunity to get involved with a program the seniors would attend and were happy to do it at the Elmwood site. Other ideas included on-site, church-sponsored discussion groups about ways to decrease crime in the community and participatory cultural presentations (food, music, beliefs) from different ethnic groups in the community. At the end of the brainstorming meeting there were more than eight suggestions, and several people agreed to research programs similar to these for more in-depth applications, successful outcomes, and identification of potential problems when applied to other communities.

Once the planning group reached consensus about the broad aspects of the program design, Meghan explained to them the next step was to write the goals and objectives for the program. She pointed out there were two important points to remember at this stage of program development. The creation of a program is a process, and as a process the planning is fluid. She explained to the group they might decide on an intervention, only to change it later as they start to write goals and objectives and identify indicators, and that this was a normal part of the process. Likewise, the goals and objectives might change as the group more carefully defined the program activities. However, she stressed it was important in the final program design that the activities and outcomes correspond to the goals and objectives agreed on by the team, and this was again reflected in the process and outcome evaluation. She stated members of the group would need to be responsible for monitoring the process and making sure the goals, objectives, activities, and evaluation all worked together. She volunteered to be part of this subgroup.

She then explained to the team the second consideration was how best to write the goals and objectives and determine health indicators. She cautioned that a very large group discussion could be time consuming and result in poorly worded objectives. The team decided to appoint a smaller task force to write these up and present them back to the full group. They asked Meghan to be the facilitator for this task force.

When the task force had its first meeting, Meghan began with an overview of how to write goals and objectives for the program plan and how they formed the framework of the plan. She explained that goals and objectives are different and each has a specific purpose. A **goal** is a broad statement of the impact expected by implementing a program, that is, a short general statement of the overall purpose of a program with a focus on the intention of the program. In most situations, it is a statement of outcome, rather than activity, and frequently projects to a future situation, such as 5 years from program initiation. There are usually only a few goals for a program. There may be only one goal for a simple program and two or three for a more complex program. Because it is a general statement, there are usually no actual outcome measurements in it, but the goal should be realistic and reachable.

Meghan provided the team with examples. One example of a goal she provided was from a colleague of hers who was a high school nurse who developed a program to prevent teen pregnancies. The goal of that program was to prevent all teenage pregnancies at Reed High School. Another example she provided was from a community in Alabama concerned about the increase in obesity in all age groups. They designed a community-based fitness program with the goal of providing opportunities for all community residents to increase or maintain the necessary physical activities for them to be physically fit. After much discussion the task force decided that the goal for the program was the following:

To increase meaningful communication among the older adult population in the two senior high-rise Elmwood residential buildings.

The next step for the task force was to come up with specific objectives for the program. Megan explained that **objectives** clarify the goal, are an outcome measurement, and keep the program focused on the intended intervention. She knew writing objectives was not easy, but she also understood well-written and well-thought-out objectives were components for the success of the program and key in the process of program planning. Objectives include *who* will *achieve what* by *how much* by *when*. They are measurable, time-limited, and action-oriented. She suggested they use an accepted approach to writing objectives first introduced in 1981 called **SMART objectives**. SMART stands for Specific, Measurable, Assignable, Realistic, and Time-related.[31] She explained SMART objectives are action-oriented and specify the goals and the desired results in a concrete, well-defined, and detail-focused statement. A specific objective answers the six "w" questions: who, what, where, when, which, and why. An objective that is measurable tells you the measurement criteria to determine when you have succeeded in meeting the objective, the most essential component of an objective. An objective that is achievable is one that can attain the desired outcome in the prescribed time frame. An objective that is realistic is one in which the resources (economic, human, skills) are available to implement the action. An objective that has defined time parameters indicates when this objective will be achieved and provides a deadline. All of these components working together in one objective can give you the clearest outcome measure.

The task force began to write up their objectives. They made sure there was an objective for every major program activity with a description and desired outcome that was clear to everyone. They hoped this would decrease confusion among stakeholders and the larger team when they presented it to them. They also realized it needed to be clear to those who would implement the program.

As they reviewed each objective, they examined how each would help guide the intended implementation of the program. They asked whether the objectives would work well taken all together and would reflect the goal for the program. Meghan explained this program was somewhat complex. To help provide clarity, the group first added some level objectives that gave more detail. They also added process objectives to measure what the staff would do, how much they would do, and during what time period.

Meghan knew she needed to become very familiar with the objectives and the indicators identified for this program as well as other programs she worked with for the health department. She was particularly concerned with ensuring the integrity of these programs when implemented and ensuring the right data were collected for the program evaluation phase. As the objectives were developed, Meghan identified indicators with which to measure the objectives chosen by the group and helped demonstrate how the program performed. She knew that good indicators are relevant to any health program; are scientifically defensible, when possible; are based on national benchmarks; are feasible to collect; are easy to interpret and analyze; and changes can be tracked over time.[32] The team developed clear and specific objectives and then were able to identify appropriate indicators to measure what was expected to change. The indicators they chose were practical and specific steps were in place to collect the necessary data.

The Elmwood task force presented their final draft of the goals and objectives to the larger community team.

The team accepted the draft and began to move into the implementation of the program.

Goal:
To increase social communication among the older adult population in the two senior high-rise Elmwood residential buildings.

Objectives:
1. *To establish a volunteer school program run by Elmwood residents to work with 50 children at the school and 25 children on-site within 6 months.*
2. *To develop consistent monthly programs in each building with a minimum of 40 resident attendees that foster social interaction by October 2023.*

■ CULTURAL CONTEXT

When assessing communities, analyzing data, and designing programs, the partnership must always consider the culture, ethnicity, and language of the community. It is important for staff and community members to feel secure asking questions and gaining information, so they feel comfortable with the culture of the community the program serves. It also is important that organizations have clearly stated values that endorse cultural competency and sensitivity.

Although cultural competency is always an essential component in program planning, in some programs it takes on a central role. Aitato and colleagues in Hawaii noted in their assessment that cancer is the leading cause of death for Samoans in the United States.[33] They concluded the design of a program aimed at decreasing morbidity and mortality related to cancer for this population required a culturally relevant approach. When designing the program, they linked the Samoan beliefs about health and illness with the need for early cancer detection. They reviewed the sociological and cultural literature to better understand appropriate interventions. Through their examination of the culture they found that most Samoans were fatalistic and passive in response to cancer. This also was observed in clinical settings. Aitato et al. also reported church affiliation was exceptionally important for this immigrant group, especially because it provided them a community where they could practice their traditional lifestyle. Based on this evidence, the program designers used a community-based participatory research method to gather information within the Samoan churches. Through focus groups, the Samoans as a community determined the most appropriate programs, including the need to use the Samoan language, the serving of appropriate Samoan food, and the need to recognize a traditional leader.

Integrating cultural components into program planning is essential. Take, for example, the Discovery Dating program in a western U.S. tribal middle school.[34] The two facilitators of the program were a Native American PHN from the western tribal community and a Native American community health educator from a different tribal community. The use of two facilitators from two different tribal communities showed an understanding that a great deal of diversity exists between tribes in relation to language, spiritual practices, gender roles, and customs among tribal groups.[34]

Evidence-Based Practice in Program Planning

It is important to use EBP in the steps of program planning. The development of a health program begins with a review of the literature for similar problems, the population-based approaches to solving the problem(s), and the evidence that the approach worked. Look at theory and rationales for these other programs and see how they relate to your program. Look for similar programs in similar communities and see whether your strategies are also similar. Note whether the strategies in these other communities produced their expected outcomes. If you want to try something unique, see whether there is anything in the literature that allows you to build your own rationale for the effectiveness of your selected approach. Arguments for using a specific intervention are strongest when there is demonstrated previous success with the method, especially with a similar population.

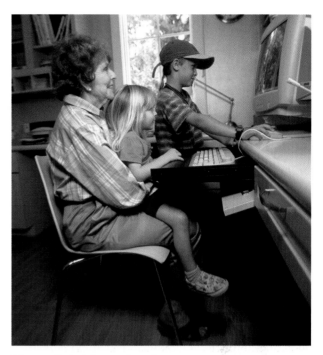

Figure 5-4 Adopt a Grandparent. *(From the Centers for Disease Control and Prevention, Richard Duncan, MRP, Sr. Proj. Mngr, North Carolina State University, the Center for Universal Design, 2000.)*

Another finding was the older adults had a calming effect on the classroom. In one study, the researchers compared two programs, one with a formal design with older adults receiving pretraining and one accepting volunteers and integrating them into the classroom without any training. The final outcome of effectiveness was the same.

Recommend Approaches: Promote an intergenerational program between older adults and school-aged children.

■ EVIDENCE-BASED PRACTICE
Engagement of the Older Adult

Practice Statement: Social isolation poses a significant health risk for older adults.

Targeted Outcome: Engagement with the community

Supporting Evidence: Intergenerational programs at schools that include older adults and young children are shown to have a beneficial impact on both (Fig. 5-4). The children receive additional attention, and the older adults feel needed and appreciated. Specifically, researchers found that older adults had increased self-esteem and better health. Children at risk for failure did much better in these programs, and all the children had a more positive attitude toward older adults.

Sources

1. Kaplan, M.S. (2001). *School-based intergenerational programs.* Retrieved from http://unesdoc.unesco.org/images/0020/002004/200481e.pdf.
2. David, J., Yeung, M., Vu, J., Got, T., MacKinnon, C. (2018). Connecting the young and young at heart: An intergenerational music program: Program profile. *Journal of Interpersonal Relationships, 16*(3), 330-338.
3. Gualano, M.R., Voglino, G., Bert, F., Thomas, R., Camussi, E., & Siliquini, R. (2018). The impact of intergenerational programs on children and older adults: A review. *International Psychogeriatrics, 30*(4), 451-468.

Resources for Evidence-Based Programs

The Community Tool Box, created by the University of Kansas, offers additional suggested resources for information on promising evidence-based programs or programs with interesting new interventions.[1] A central suggestion in the Community Tool Box is networking with local and state agencies, and checking public and private professional organizations or advocacy groups to see whether they have published information on evidence-based programs.

The importance of integrating evidenced-based programs into public health departments was underlined by the National Association of County & City Health Officials' (NACCHO) nationwide support system to disseminate Chronic Disease Self-Management Programs through local health departments (LHD) into communities. With the support of the CDC, NACCHO has provided grants to LHDs with emerging evidence that they are successfully implementing these programs in the communities they serve.[35] They acknowledged that, according to the literature, merely gaining knowledge about nutrition and fitness frequently did not translate into behavior change. Based on their review of the literature, setting goals, strengthening self-efficacy, and using theory of change had more success in actually changing behavior than just providing information. They also found that multifaceted community efforts have increased physical activities. With this evidence, they designed their program.

Determining whether a program has good evidence to support it can be accomplished using a few different approaches. First, examining both the quantitative and qualitative data from studies, as well as from the current program, provides essential information. Even simple statistical analysis can help determine whether a program is thriving, whether participants are reaching their outcomes, and whether positive things are happening in the community. Good indicators that the community likes the program are the continued use of the program by participants and ongoing program growth. However, it is important to know whether there are outside factors contributing to program success that might make it difficult to duplicate the program in other communities or with other groups. Another issue may be that the outcomes are really a measurement of behavior change and not real outcomes. When reviewing program data, it is important to note whether there is a researched theoretical framework to support the intervention, whether the statistical analysis is clear, whether there are enough participants to make conclusions, whether the target outcomes are appropriate, and whether the program

reached these targets. In reviewing the program, it helps to evaluate whether the indicators seemed appropriate and whether the tools were well designed. It also helps to think about the usefulness of the indicators of the program. Did the intervention reach the intended population, and is this population similar to or different from the intended population? It also is important to be aware of what resources were used and to compare the amount of resources available for your program. In the 1990s, Lisbeth Schorr, a well-known social analyst, identified seven characteristics of highly effective programs still relevant today.[36] Although they are focused on programs aimed at improving the health of children, they can also be applied to other populations. Effective programs:

- Are comprehensive, flexible, responsive, and persevering
- See children in the context of their families
- Incorporate families as parts of neighborhoods
- Have a long-term, preventive orientation, a clear mission, and continue to evolve over time
- Are well managed by competent and committed individuals with clearly identifiable skills
- Have staff who are trained and supported to provide high-quality, responsive services
- Operate in settings that encourage practitioners to build strong relationships of mutual trust and respect

Many of these attributes are part of effective program planning, implementation, and evaluation, and include looking at communities and not just individuals, being flexible and persevering, having clear goals, forming partnerships and working collaboratively, and having passion on the part of staff for the work and for social justice. In successful programs, the staff is nurtured and supported, and the program is well managed.

Program Implementation

After the program has been designed and the logic model solidified, it is time to implement the program. **Program implementation** encompasses the resources needed to provide a program as well as the mechanism for putting the program in place. Prior to putting a program in place, it is important to map out exactly how this will be done. For example, when implementing a screening program, it is important to know how many participants are anticipated, how many screening tools/how much equipment will be needed, how many personnel are needed, and what the flow for participants from arrival through the screening and referral process will be. Nurses are frequently part of the implementation team and assist in adding the necessary detail to the actual program activities. Ervin identified five stages related to program implementation:[30]

1. Community accepting the program
2. Specifying tasks and estimating needed resources
3. Developing specific plans for program activity
4. Establishing a mechanism for program management
5. Putting the plan into action

Partnering with the community from the beginning of the planning process facilitates community interest and ownership of the program, which should be culturally and politically specific and acceptable. Although adequate resources to implement the program were identified in the planning, it is important to confirm that the resources are available and adequate, and how these resources are to be used in the program activities and evaluation.

The implementation team needs to make certain the indicators for the outcomes are identified and a mechanism is in place to collect the data. Everyone needs to know the steps of the program. It may be necessary to write protocols and procedures for the intervention. If additional staff members are needed, they need to be hired and undergo orientation. There also may be a need for additional staff training. Several program evaluations have stressed the importance of pilot testing the program or components of the program and the planned evaluation before implementation of the complete program, as was done in one study in China that helped to identify challenges related to the implementation of a community-based stable coronary artery disease management program.[37] The first was the importance of establishing a personal working relationship with the community. They also suggested the program leader strive to build partnerships by listening, observing, and integrating the experiences between the program and the community. They found it was best to be flexible and emphasized simplicity when implementing community activities.

Program Evaluation

Project management and program evaluation are inextricably linked whether in public health programs, a health program, or in an acute care setting.[16,38] **Program evaluation** is the systematic collection of information about the activities, outputs, and outcomes to enhance a program and its effectiveness. Evaluation is defined as the systematic acquirement and analysis of information to provide useful feedback. Evaluation is essential to good management and program design, and evaluation

strategies should be developed prior to the project management and programs being implemented. Evaluation is used to evaluate the effectiveness of the program and provide information to guide any needed improvement of the program. Through evaluation you strengthen the project. Programs need to be evaluated for multiple reasons. You need to know whether objectives and goals are being met. From the evaluation you can determine whether the:

- Activities are implemented as they were designed
- Program is cost effective
- Intervention and program theories are correct
- Time line is appropriate
- Program should be expanded or duplicated in another location

Evaluation helps with program planning, program development, and program accountability. Frequently the PHN works with comprehensive collaborative community interventions that are complex to evaluate, as there may be no clear cause and effect with multiple interventions. Often the program operates within the unique local political issues, and circumstances of the community demand a customized evaluation to really understand what is happening. PHNs and other local providers can help interpret this information for the interior or exterior evaluators or as part of an evaluation team.

Percy provided a good example that underscores the necessity for program evaluation.[39] She described a school health program in one school district that was so busy providing good health care to the schoolchildren that the district failed to design and implement an evaluation plan. Without an evaluation of the program, the district was unable to determine whether the program was effective. Because the program required a registered nurse (RN) in each school, the lack of evaluation data resulted in an inability to demonstrate the need for the added cost of the school health nurses. The city council members had budget constraints and needed to cut programs. Without the evaluation data, the nurses could not show the council members the importance of this nursing intervention. To have a more cost-effective budget, the city council replaced the nurses with nursing assistants. When the city tried to extend this cost savings to another school district, the nurses in the second school district had already been evaluating their program routinely, and they had excellent outcome data to demonstrate the effectiveness of having an RN in each school. Their program did not get cut.

Evaluation of family and individual care, community services, and programs has grown over the past several decades as a response to the stakeholders, especially the funders, who need to know whether the nurse and colleagues from other disciplines are successful in improving health and are doing so in a cost-effective manner. Most grant agencies funding these types of interventions now require evaluation.

Evaluation Models

Formative Evaluation

There are several models for program evaluation. One model is to divide the evaluation into either formative or summative or both. **Formative evaluation** occurs during the development of a program, while the activities are forming and being implemented for the first time. It is an ongoing feedback on the performance of the program, identifying aspects needing improvement and providing opportunities to offer corrective suggestions. Formative evaluation is concerned with the delivery of the program and the organizational context, including structure and procedures. This is an opportunity to examine what happens in the reality of the implementation, and it provides the opportunity to see whether the program outputs can really create the change necessary to meet the objectives and goals. Usually a formative evaluation is internal and ongoing, with the staff constantly assessing the strengths, weaknesses, barriers, and unexpected opportunities of these new program activities. The activities and outputs are the dynamic part of the program and lend themselves to formative evaluation. The program can positively respond to the evaluation and can change interventions, change the way outcome measurements are collected, or change other parts of the program design to better meet the program goals and objectives. It is appropriate to change things if the program is not working as well as possible.

Process Evaluation

Process evaluation is a type of formative evaluation used to investigate the process of delivering the program or technology, including alternative delivery procedures. The main concern with process evaluation is to document to what extent the program has been delivered and whether the delivery was what was defined in the program design. There should be detailed information on how the program actually worked (the program operations), any changes made to the program, and how those changes have had an impact on the program. It is also important for an evaluator to be aware of any outside environmental events or intervening events that may

have influenced the program activities. This type of data can be collected by noting actual numbers related to the interventions, such as the number of people attending a class, the number of pamphlets handed out, or the number of screening tests performed. Qualitative data collection methods can include, among others, direct observations, in-depth interviews, focus groups, and review of documents.

The importance of formative evaluation should not be underestimated. It is a strong tool in helping to improve the activities and output of a program and for determining whether the theoretical understanding of how the program will influence change is accurate and appropriate.

Summative Evaluation

Summative evaluation occurs at the end of the program and is the evaluation of the objectives and the goal. It is judging the worth of the program at the end of the activities and discovering whether the program achieved the intended change. It is an assessment of the outcome and impact of the benefits the selected population has received by participating in the program. It evaluates the causal relationship and the theoretical understanding of the planned intervention. It also can examine program cost, looking at cost-effectiveness and cost benefit.[40] When conducted on well-established programs, it allows funders and policy makers to make major decisions on the continuation of programs and determine how the outcomes could influence policy at the local to the national levels.

As more hospitals strive for magnet status, baccalaureate nurses are being called to initiate health programs in acute care settings and to evaluate their effectiveness. In public health settings, the PHN is often responsible for managing community-based programs in which evaluation is essential to the sustainability of the programs. Several nonprofit funding agencies and the CDC offer suggestions on how to do internal evaluations and when to seek external evaluator assistance.

Nine Steps of Program Evaluation

The W.W. Kellogg Foundation identified essential steps for developing a program evaluation that is useful for both smaller programs and for the complex multiactivity community program interventions that many organizations implement (Box 5-5).[40] The first four steps occur in the program planning stage, the next three in the implementation of the program, and the last two after the program evaluation is complete. Program evaluation is an integral part of the program design, and the program

BOX 5–5 ■ Nine Steps in Developing a Program Evaluation

Program

1. Select the evaluation team.

Planning Stage

2. Develop the evaluation questions.
3. Have a budget in place for the evaluation.
4. Decide whether to use an internal or external evaluator.

Program Implemented

5. Determine data collection methods.
6. Collect the data.
7. Analyze and interpret the results.

Evaluation Complete

8. Communicate findings.
9. Improve the program.

Source: W.K. Kellogg Foundation. (1998). *W.K. Kellogg Foundation evaluation handbook*. Battle Creek, MI: Author. Retrieved from https://www.wkkf.org/resource-directory/resource/2010/w-k-kellogg-foundation-evaluation-handbook.

evaluation plan should be in place before the program is initiated.

Step 1: Step 1 is completed before the program begins. It identifies from among the stakeholders who should be included on the evaluation team, staff representation, and what community representation and participants are needed in the program.

Step 2: In step 2, evaluation questions are created. All participants need to help phrase questions that will be useful in reflecting the program theory, improving the program, and determining effectiveness. These questions can include the following: What data do you need to collect? What kind of information is needed? What do we want to accomplish? What do we need to know about the program? How will we know when we have accomplished our goal? Where do we find the data, and what indicators do we need? The questions also will involve how this information is communicated to others: Who is the audience for the results? What kind of information should we tell them?

Step 3: Step 3 is the creation of a budget. The amount of the budget varies depending on several components such as the size of the program, the number of staff needed to carry out the evaluation, the need for other resources such as software for data entry and analysis, and the length of time needed to complete the evaluation.

Step 4: In step 4, a decision must be made about whether the evaluation will be internal or have an external evaluator. If you decide on an external evaluator, it is good to identify that person, so the evaluator can be a part of the program planning process from the beginning. These are all components of the planning and occur as the program is designed.

Step 5: Steps 5 through 7 occur during the program implementation phase. In step 5, data collection methods are determined.

Step 6: In step 6, data are collected.

Step 7: In step 7, the results are analyzed and interpreted.

Step 8: After the completion of the evaluation, in step 8 the findings and new perceptions of the program are communicated to the stakeholders. It is important that the appropriate information is communicated to the identified audiences.

Step 9: In step 9, evaluation information is used to show evidence for or to improve the program. The better informed we are, the better we are at making good program decisions. This may be sharing with funding agencies to receive more funding for the successful program; it may be to change some of the program activities and outputs to improve outcomes; or it may be to refine the population served, to help change policy, or to discontinue the program (see Box 5-5).

When developing the process for health program evaluation, it is important to be as objective as possible. Some of the ethical dilemmas that can emerge during program evaluation include:

- Pressure to slant the findings in the direction wanted by key stakeholders
- Compromised confidentiality of data sources
- Response on the part of the evaluator to one interest group more than to others
- Misinterpretation or misuse of the findings by the program stakeholders
- Evaluator using a familiar tool to collect data rather than a more appropriate one

The team can use these points to examine the methods chosen to evaluate a program as a means of eliminating as much bias as possible.

Through successful programs, communities can improve their health. These programs can be synergistic in creating positive change and lead to new policies with an even wider influence on health. The purpose of health programs is to strive for a community in which everyone is safe, environments support health, actions are taken to prevent and control acute and chronic disease, and individuals and families can thrive.

Summary Points

- Health planning occurs across health-care settings including public health settings, primary care, acute care, and schools, with the focus on improving the health of the populations served.
- *Healthy People* provides a framework of goals and indicators that can help in creating health programs for our communities.
- All models of program planning include the community as a partner, and it is important that the community is involved in every step of the process.
- Health planning includes community assessment, community diagnoses, program design, program implementation, and program evaluation.
- Using logic modeling can help create a well-structured program with clear indication of how to do both process and outcome evaluation of the program.
- Every program should be evaluated, and evaluation begins when you start designing the program.
- Formative, process, and summative evaluations each provide important information about the program and how to make it more effective.

● APPLYING PUBLIC HEALTH PRACTICE

The Case of Program Evaluation at Elmwood

Public Health Science Topics Covered:

- Assessment
- Community diagnosis

The Elmwood Senior Housing program was designed to increase social integration and has been in place for 9 months. The activities include residents working in the public schools in an intergenerational program, the first and second graders each coming to Elmwood once a month for a 2-hour reading program, the solidification of an Elmwood community organization, and weekly discussion and activity programs at the center with assistance from the community center and the local churches. The PHN and other members of the team have been doing ongoing process evaluation and are now meeting to discuss the implementation of their outcome evaluation plan.

To answer the following questions, use the established goal, outcomes, and output in the logic model (Fig. 5-1) developed by the community group. You also can reference the Community Tool Box from Center for Community Health and Development at the University of Kansas (https://ctb.ku.edu/en/table-of-contents), Evaluating Community Programs and Initiative, Chapters 36–39.

1. What data would you collect as part of the process evaluation? How would these data help you in the formative process of your program? Would you change activities based on these data?
2. What would have been the steps in setting up the evaluation plan? What might be your evaluation questions? What would be your indicators? What kind of data should you collect? How would you specifically know whether your program has been successful?

REFERENCES

1. Center for Community Health and Development at the University of Kansas. (2018). *Community tool box: A model for getting started.* Retrieved from https://ctb.ku.edu/en/get-started#plan.
2. U.S. Department of Health and Human Services. (n.d.). *About the community guide.* Retrieved from https://www.thecommunityguide.org/about/about-community-guide.
3. Centers for Disease Control and Prevention. (2017). *National public health performance standards.* Retrieved from https://www.cdc.gov/stltpublichealth/nphps/index.html.
4. Fawcett, S.B. (2018). *Section 3. Our model of practice: Building capacity for community and system change.* Retrieved from https://ctb.ku.edu/en/table-of-contents/overview/model-for-community-change-and-improvement/building-capacity/main.
5. Institute of Medicine. (1988). *The future of public health.* Washington, DC: National Academies Press.
6. Institute of Medicine. (2002). *The future of the public's health in the 21st century.* Washington, DC: National Academies Press.
7. Institute of Medicine. (2012). *For the public's health: Investing in a healthier future.* Washington, DC: National Academies Press.
8. American Public Health Association: Public Health Nursing Section. (2018). *Public health nursing.* Retrieved from http://apha.org/apha-communities/member-sections/public-health-nursing.
9. Keller, L.O., Schaffer, M., Lia-Hoagberg, B., & Strohschein, S. (2002). Assessment, program planning, and evaluation in population-based public health practice. *Journal of Public Health Management and Practice, 8*, 30-43.
10. Keller, L.O., Strohschein, S., Lia-Hoagberg, B., Schaffer, M. (2004). Population-based public health interventions: Practice-based and evidence-supported. Part I. *Public Health Nursing, 21*(5), 453-468.
11. U.S. Department of Health and Human Services. (2018). *Program planning.* Retrieved from https://www.healthypeople.gov/2020/tools-and-resources/Program-Planning.
12. U.S. Department of Health and Human Services. (2016). *Educational and community-based programs (ECBP).*

Retrieved from https://www.cdc.gov/nchs/data/hpdata2020/CH11_ECBP.pdf.

13. Public Health Service. (1979). *"Healthy People": The Surgeon General's report on health promotion and disease prevention.* Washington, DC: U.S. Government Printing Office, DHEW.

14. Chrvala, C., & Bugar, R. (Eds.). (1999). *IOM report. Leading health indicators for "Healthy People 2010": Final report.* Washington, DC: National Academies Press.

15. U.S. Department of Health and Human Services. (2018). *2020 topics and objectives – objectives A-Z.* Retrieved from https://www.healthypeople.gov/2020/topics-objectives.

16. Issel, L.M. (2018). *Health program planning and evaluation: A practical, systematic approach for community health* (4th ed.). Sudbury, MA: Jones & Bartlett.

17. Green, L.W., & Kreuter, M.W. (2005). *Health program planning: An educational and ecological approach* (4th ed.). New York, NY: McGraw-Hill Higher Education.

18. W.K. Kellogg Foundation. (2004). *Logic model development guide.* Battle Creek, MI: Author. Retrieved from https://www.wkkf.org/resource-directory/resource/2006/02/wk-kellogg-foundation-logic-model-development-guide.

19. Centers for Disease Control and Prevention, Division for Heart Disease and Stroke Prevention (n.d.). *Evaluation guide: Developing and using a logic model.* Retrieved from https://www.cdc.gov/dhdsp/docs/logic_model.pdf.

20. Ball, L., Ball, D., Leveritt, M., Ray, S., Collins, C., Patterson, E., Chaboyer, W., et al. (2017). Using logic models to enhance the methodological quality of primary health-care interventions: guidance from an intervention to promote nutrition care by general practitioners and practice nurses. *Australian Journal of Primary Health, 23*(1), 53–60. https://doi-org.ezp.welch.jhmi.edu/10.1071/PY16038.

21. University of Maryland Extension. (2017). *Guide to 2018 University of Maryland extension program planning.* Retrieved from https://wiki.moo.umd.edu/display/umeanswers/Program+Planning+and+Implementation?preview=%2F84902254%2F121897117%2FUME+Program+Planning+Guide+2018.pdf.

22. Moltó-Puigmarí, C., Vonk, R., van Ommeren, G., & Hegger, I. (2018). A logic model for pharmaceutical care. *Journal of Health Services Research & Policy, 23*(3), 148–157. https://doi-org.ezp.welch.jhmi.edu/10.1177/1355819618768343.

23. Serowoky, M.L., George, N., & Yarandi, H. (2015). Using the program logic model to evaluate ¡Cuídate!: A Sexual health program for latino adolescents in a school-based health center. *Worldviews on Evidence-Based Nursing, 12*(5), 297–305. https://doi-org.ezp.welch.jhmi.edu/10.1111/wvn.12110.

24. Centers for Disease Control and Prevention. (2018). *Community health assessment and group evaluation (CHANGE) tool.* Retrieved from https://www.cdc.gov/nccdphp/dnpao/state-local-programs/change-tool/index.html.

25. Buchanan, D. (2008). Autonomy, paternalism, and justice: Ethical priorities in public health. *American Journal of Public Health, 98*, 15-21.

26. American Nurses Association. (2015). *Health care reform.* Retrieved from https://www.nursingworld.org/practice-policy/health-policy/health-system-reform/.

27. Blewett, L. A., Planalp, C., & Alarcon, G. (2018). Affordable Care Act impact in Kentucky: Increasing access, reducing disparities. *American Journal of Public Health, 108*(7), 924-929.

28. Frean, M., Gruber, J., & Sommers, B. D. (2017). Premium subsidies, the mandate, and Medicaid expansion: Coverage effects of the Affordable Care Act. *Journal of Health Economics, 53*, 72-86.

29. Rice, T., Unruh, L. Y., van Ginneken, E., Rosenau, P., & Barners, A. J. (2018). Universal coverage reforms in the USA: From Obamacare through Trump. *Health Policy, 122*(7), 698-702.

30. Ervin, N., & Kulbok, P.A. (Eds.). (2018). *Advanced public and community health nursing practice: Population assessment, program planning, and evaluation.* New York City, NY: Springer Publishing.

31. Doran, G.T. (1981). There's a S.M.A.R.T. way to write management's goals and objectives. *Management Review, 70*(11), 35-36.

32. United Nations Fund for Population Activities. (2004). *Programme manager's planning monitoring & evaluation toolkit.* Retrieved from https://www.betterevaluation.org/sites/default/files/stakeholder.pdf.

33. Aitato, N., Braun, K., Dang, K., & So'a, T. (2007). Cultural considerations in developing church-based programs to reduce cancer health disparities among Samoans. *Ethnicity and Health, 12*(4), 381-400.

34. Schanen, J.G., Skenandore, A., Scow, B., & Hagen, J. (2017). Assessing the impact of a healthy relationships curriculum on Native American adolescents. *Social Work, 62*(3), 251–258. https://doi-org.ezp.welch.jhmi.edu/10.1093/sw/swx021.

35. National Association of County & City Health Officials (2018). *Chronic disease resources.* Retrieved from https://www.naccho.org/programs/community-health/chronic-disease/resources.

36. Schorr, L. (1997). *Common purpose: Strengthening families and neighborhoods to rebuild America.* New York, NY: Anchor Books.

37. Shen, Z., Jiang, C., & Chen, L. (2018). Evaluation of a train-the-trainer program for stable coronary artery disease management in community settings: A pilot study. *Patient Education & Counseling, 101*(2), 256–265. https://doi-org.ezp.welch.jhmi.edu/10.1016/j.pec.2017.07.025.

38. Ramos Freire, E.M., Rocha Batista, R.C., & Martinez, M.R. (2016). Project management for hospital accreditation: a case study. *Online Brazilian Journal of Nursing, 15*(1), 96–108. Retrieved from http://search.ebscohost.com.ezp.welch.jhmi.edu/login.aspx?direct=true&db=rzh&AN=115736473&site=ehost-live&scope=site.

39. Percy, M. (2007). School health. Quality of care: or why you HAVE to evaluate your program. *Journal for Specialists in Pediatric Nursing, 12*(1), 66-68.

40. W.K. Kellogg Foundation. (2017) *The step-by-step guide to evaluation: How to become savvy evaluation consumers.* Battle Creek, MI: Author. Retrieved from http://ww2.wkkf.org/digital/evaluationguide/view.html#p=10.

Chapter 6

Environmental Health

Christine Savage

LEARNING OUTCOMES

After reading the chapter, the student will be able to:

1. Describe the role of nursing in environmental health.
2. Describe the impact of the built environment on health.
3. Use the principles of home visiting and an environmental health assessment to identify health risk factors at the family and community level.
4. Examine the concept of exposure to hazardous substances from a cellular to global level.
5. Explain the concept of environmental justice.
6. List social, behavioral, cultural, and physical characteristics that increase susceptibility to health effects associated with environmental exposures.
7. Discuss gene-environment interaction.
8. Describe issues related to air and water quality.

KEY TERMS

Air Quality Index (AQI)
Ambient air
Ambient air standard
Area sources
Blood Lead Level (BLL)
Bioaccumulation
Built environment
Community environmental
   health assessment

Criteria air pollutants
Environmental exposure
Environmental health
Environmental justice
Environmental
   sustainability
Exposure
Gene-environment
   interaction

Half-life
Integrated pest
   management
International building
   codes
Latency period
Mobile sources
Point sources
Risk assessment

Routes of entry
Safe Drinking Water Act
Toxicity
Warm handoff

Introduction

Whether tainted water in Flint, Michigan; air pollution on the rise in low income countries;[1] airborne mercury pollution in Victoria, Australia;[2] or natural disasters and climate change,[3] our environment has a direct relationship with our health. The environment affects the air we breathe, the food we eat, the water we drink, and the availability of resources to sustain our economies. The environment also influences our exposure to toxins and infectious agents, and access to resources that support healthy living.

Hardly a day goes by without a report in the media that links environmental conditions to human health. High rates of childhood asthma, industrial explosions, hurricanes and other natural disasters, as well as reports of polluted water and air remind us of the many ways we are affected by the world around us and how the health of individuals and communities strongly depends on environmental determinants. The adverse environmental impact of human-made and natural disasters such as the lack of potable water and lead exposure in Flint, Michigan, and numerous hurricanes as well as the day-to-day aspects of the environment in which we live, work, and play can cause immediate or long-term benefits or harm.

The World Health Organization (WHO) defines **environmental health** as follows:

> *Environmental health addresses all the physical, chemical, and biological factors external to a person, and all the related factors impacting behaviors. It encompasses the assessment and control of those environmental factors that can potentially affect health. It is targeted toward preventing disease and creating health-supportive environments. This definition excludes behavior not related to environment, as well as behavior related to the social and cultural environment, and genetics.[4]*

This perspective of environmental health extends beyond food, air, water, soil, dust, and even consumer products and waste. It includes all aspects of our living conditions, the use and misuse of resources, and the overall design of communities. The ecological models of health promotion (see Chapter 1) encompass the environment in which we live.[5] Using an ecological approach requires an understanding that individuals and populations interact with their environment. In an editorial, one author stressed the need for interventions aimed at protecting the natural environment as an upstream approach to improving our health.[6]

The broad scope of environmental determinants of health is obvious with the inclusion of 68 main and subobjectives under the *Healthy People 2020 (HP 2020)* topic of environmental health.[7] Based on the midcourse review, six of these were archived and four were developmental, which left 58 that were measurable.

■ HEALTHY PEOPLE 2020
Environmental Health

Targeted Topic: Environmental Health
Goal: Promote health for all through a healthy environment.
Overview: Humans constantly interact with the environment. These interactions affect quality of life, years of healthy life lived, and health disparities. The WHO defines *environment,* as it relates to health, as "all the physical, chemical, and biological factors external to a person, and all the related behaviors."[1] Environmental health consists of preventing or controlling disease, injury, and disability related to the interactions between people and their environment.

The *HP 2020* Environmental Health objectives focused on six themes, each of which highlighted an element of environmental health:

1. Outdoor air quality
2. Surface and groundwater quality
3. Toxic substances and hazardous wastes
4. Homes and communities
5. Infrastructure and surveillance
6. Global environmental health[7]

Midcourse Review: Of the 58 measurable objectives in the Environmental Health Topic Area, 10 of them met or exceeded their 2020 targets, 11 were improving, 10 showed little or no detectable change, and 11 objectives were getting worse. Sixteen objectives had baseline data only (Fig. 6-1).[8]

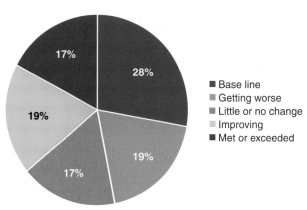

Healthy People 2020 Midcourse Review: Environmental Health

- Base line
- Getting worse
- Little or no change
- Improving
- Met or exceeded

Figure 6-1 Healthy People Midcourse Review for 2020.

Healthy People 2030 Proposed Framework and Environmental Health

There are seven proposed foundational principles for the HP 2030 proposed framework. One pertains specifically to environmental health and reflects the ecological model:

*"What guides our actions … Healthy physical, social, and **economic** environments strengthen the potential to achieve health and well-being."*[9]

The WHO's 10 facts on environmental health published in 2016 illustrated the association between the environment and health.[10] Almost a quarter of all deaths globally were attributable to the environment. Five key factors emerged through an analysis of data related to the global burden of disease attributable to the environment (Table 6-1). Twenty-two percent of the disability-adjusted life years (DALY) (see Chapter 9) were attributable to the environment, and low-income countries (LIC) bore more of the burden of disease associated with the environment. Age and gender play a role in risk for environmental attributable disease with children, older adults, and males at higher risk. Although communicable diseases are the main cause of environmentally attributed deaths in Sub-Sahara Africa, there has been a shift globally to noncommunicable diseases as the main cause of deaths are attributable to the environment. The list of diseases associated with the environment include cardiovascular diseases, diarrheal diseases, and lower respiratory infections. The environmental factors associated with these diseases include ambient and household air pollution, water, sanitation, and hygiene.[10]

TABLE 6–1 ▪ Global Burden of Disease Attributable to the Environment

Five Key Factors	Percent of Deaths Attributable to the Environment	Percent of the DISEASE BURDEN in DALYs Attributable to the Environment
Environmental risks and the global burden of disease	23%	22%
Environmental impacts on health are uneven across life course and gender		Men: 22.8% versus women: 20.6%
Low- and middle-income countries bear the greatest share of environmental disease	The highest number of deaths per capita attributable to the environment occurs in sub-Saharan Africa	
Total environmental deaths are unchanged since 2002, but show a strong shift to noncommunicable diseases		The diseases with the largest environmental risk include cardiovascular diseases, diarrheal diseases, and lower respiratory infections. Ambient and household air pollution, and water, sanitation, and hygiene are the main environmental drivers of those diseases.
The evidence on quantitative links between health and environment has increased		A greater share of the estimates of the burden of disease attributable to the environment can now be determined using more robust methods than previously used.

The Role of Nursing in Environmental Health

Nurses, particularly those in the field of public health, play a significant role in preventing harm from occurring and in restoring well-being to all who face hazardous conditions in their environment. Nurses are among the environmental health professionals with the responsibility to detect and assess the presence of environmental hazards as well as the health risks they pose, and to act to protect the health of populations.[11]

In 2007, the American Nurses Association (ANA) published a report titled *ANA's Principles of Environmental Health for Nursing Practice With Implementation Strategies*.[11] According to the report, registered nurses play a critical role in both assessing environmental health issues and addressing them. The report included 10 principles (Box 6-1) for healthy safe environments that are applicable across settings.

Armed with an appreciation for the complexities of the interaction of environment and health, nurses are leaders in defining and encouraging solutions. As experts in educating individuals and communities, and appreciating the value of leading by example, nurses are catalysts in improving the health of the environment, thus improving health. The environmental health issues in the ANA report specific to nursing practice include: (1) knowledge of the role environment plays in the health of individuals, families, and populations; (2) ability to assess for environmental health hazards and make appropriate referrals; (3) advocacy; (4) utilization of appropriate risk communication strategies; and (5) understanding of policies and legislation related to environmental health. The ANA principles were designed to help support the nurse in the role of environmental health activist.[11]

Approaches to Environmental Health

A useful framework to use in examining human-environment interactions and their potential impact on health of individuals, families, and communities is the well-established epidemiological triangle, which describes the relationship between an agent (exposure), host (human), and environment (the complex setting in which agent and host come together) (see Chapters 3 and 8). In actuality, the epidemiological triangle is a simplistic model and must be placed in the context of the real world to better appreciate the importance of the triangle point—environment—that brings agent and host together in the places we live, that is, housing,

1. Knowledge of environmental health concepts is essential to nursing practice.
2. The Precautionary Principle guides nurses in their practice to use products and practices that do not harm human health or the environment and to take preventive action in the face of uncertainty.
3. Nurses have a right to work in an environment that is safe and healthy.
4. Healthy environments are sustained through multi-disciplinary collaboration.
5. Choices of materials, products, technology, and practices in the environment that impact nursing practice are based on the best evidence available.
6. Approaches to promoting a healthy environment respect the diverse values, beliefs, cultures, and circumstances of patients and their families.
7. Nurses participate in assessing the quality of the environment in which they practice and live.
8. Nurses, other health care workers, patients, and communities have the right to know relevant and timely information about the potentially harmful products, chemicals, pollutants, and hazards to which they are exposed.
9. Nurses participate in research of best practices that promote a safe and healthy environment.
10. Nurses must be supported in advocating for and implementing environmental health principles in nursing practice.

Source: (11)

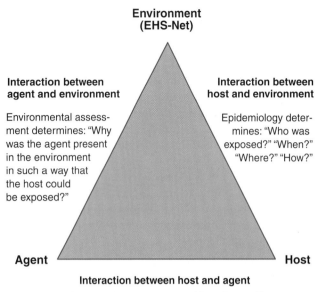

Figure 6-2 Environmental health specialists and the epidemiologic triangle.

schools, workplaces, recreational spaces, communities, and, ultimately, the world (Fig. 6-2).

The approach in the United States for handling environmental health in the past was usually at the state and local health department level rather than at the federal level. Local health departments focused on sanitation and waste management to provide potable (safe, drinkable) water. However, maintaining healthy air and reducing pollutants in water, air, and soil became an issue that crossed state borders. In 1970, the U.S. Environmental Protection Agency (EPA) was formed with the mission to protect human health and to safeguard the natural environment—air, water, and land—by writing and enforcing regulation based on laws passed by Congress.[12] The EPA is a regulatory body that performs environmental assessments, does research, educates, and sets and enforces national environmental standards. Since the early 1970s there have been multiple federal laws passed by Congress. This legislation includes the Clean Air Act;

the Occupational Health and Safety Act; the National Institute of Occupational Safety and Health; the Clean Water Act; and the Comprehensive Environmental Response, Compensation, and Liability Act, also known as the Superfund; among others. The growing concerns among the American people about the environment have created pressure to increasingly monitor and regulate the environment. These concerns have clashed with concerns by industry of overregulation resulting in a relaxing of some of these regulations in 2017 and 2018. Thus, the health benefits of regulating industry and pollution of the environment often conflicts with the economic benefits of relaxed regulations.

In the United States, there is a network of environmental health specialists housed in the Centers for Disease Control and Prevention (CDC) National Center for Environmental Health that, using the epidemiological triangle (Fig. 6-2), works collaboratively with the Environmental Health Services Network to identify and prevent environmental factors that can produce disease. Their stated purpose is to help identify underlying environmental factors, assist with improving prevention efforts, train environmental health specialists, and help strengthen the collaboration among different disciplines and services involved in improving environmental health.[13] Key issues include the built environment, toxic materials, air and water quality, and environmental stability.

The Built Environment

The **built environment**, the human-made surroundings created for the daily activities of humans, reflects the range of physical and social elements that make up a community.[14] Scientists are examining how the structure and infrastructure of a community facilitate or impede health. Poor communities often have a built environment with limited resources, higher pollution, poorer maintenance of buildings, fewer options for outside activities, a smaller selection of goods (including groceries), and limited transportation, all leading to poorer health (e.g., lead poisoning, asthma, cancer). There is considerable interest in examining how communities can modify their built environment to promote the health of the community residents.[14,15]

An example of the relationship between the built environment and health is obesity. There is strong evidence that aspects of the built environment, such as food availability and access to recreational opportunities, are associated with obesity.[10] Many programs have been instituted to help reduce the epidemic of obesity in the United States with growing evidence of the complexity of the built environment including the role not only of walkability but air pollution.[16]

■ EVIDENCE-BASED PRACTICE
Obesity and the Built Environment

Practice Statement: An increasing number of studies have documented that obesity, which has reached epidemic proportions in the United States, is related to several aspects of the built environment.[17-19]
Targeted Outcome: Reduction in prevalence of obesity.
Evidence to Support: The same risk factors that promote weight gain in individuals—increased caloric intake and decreased physical activity—apply on a larger scale to populations. Several measures have been used to describe the risk factors for obesity, but the evidence continues to point to the influence of the built environment on diet and activity.[17] For example, physical activity is associated with community attributes such as road connectivity, presence of sidewalks, availability of safe play areas, and residential density. Dietary influences include the number and proximity of fast-food restaurants, availability of healthy food choices, and the cost of food. Specific risk factors may differ between urban and suburban settings, but the relationship between the built environment and obesity persists in both.[18] Disparity in obesity prevalence based on race and socioeconomic status may in part be associated with the built environment.[19]

There are many resources available to communities to address factors related to diet and the built environment. The recommendations include the following interventions at the community level:

1. Improve availability of affordable healthier food and beverage choices in public service venues
2. Improve geographical availability of supermarkets in underserved areas
3. Improve availability of mechanisms for purchasing foods from farms
4. Provide incentives for the production, distribution, and procurement of foods from local farms
5. Discourage consumption of sugar-sweetened beverages

To address factors related to physical activity and the built environment, communities should:

1. Increase opportunities for extracurricular physical activity
2. Improve access to outdoor recreational facilities
3. Enhance infrastructure that supports walking
4. Support locating schools within easy walking distance of residential areas
5. Improve access to public transportation
6. Enhance traffic safety in areas where people are/could be physically active[20-22]

Hazardous Substances

The probability that individuals will be adversely affected by a hazardous substance depends on three major factors: (1) its inherent **toxicity**, that is, ability to cause harm to humans; (2) whether it enters the body and reaches susceptible organs; and (3) the amount that is present. Toxicologists are fond of summarizing the teaching of Renaissance alchemist Paracelsus with the phrase "the dose makes the poison." In other words, it is very important to recognize that the mere presence of an agent, even if it is known to have toxic properties, does not necessarily mean there is a risk to health. For example, we know that lead can harm several organ systems (as presented in an example later in this chapter). However, it must first be ingested or inhaled, or it will not reach the organs that are sensitive to its effects. When an x-ray technician uses a lead apron for protection from radiation, lead is serving a helpful function and will not cause toxicity to the gastrointestinal, nervous, or hematological system because it is not in a form that allows it to be absorbed. However, if lead is heated and the fumes are inhaled, or if chips of lead paint are ingested, then there is a definite risk of lead poisoning. Many other substances, such as solvents, can enter the body through skin contact. These three pathways or **routes of entry**—ingestion, inhalation, and dermal absorption—differ in their importance according to the specific substance. Also, do not be fooled into thinking a substance is not hazardous just because its effects are not seen immediately. Cancer, for example, often develops many years after an exposure occurs. These time lags, known as **latency periods**, can interfere with our ability to identify cause-and-effect links and hamper our ability to anticipate and prevent negative health effects.[23]

Exposure Risk Assessment

The process used by policy makers and other regulators to evaluate the extent to which a population may suffer health effects from an environmental exposure is called **exposure risk assessment**. Exposure risk assessment involves four steps: (1) *hazard identification* (described in more detail later); (2) *dose-response assessment* (based on experiments that look for a correlation between an increase in harmful effects and an increase in quantity of a substance); (3) *exposure assessment* (consideration of the level, timing, and extent of the exposure); and (4) *risk characterization*. This last step brings together the information from the first three steps to guide a judgment about the risk of health problems to those who are exposed. That judgment is never without its uncertainties.

Types of Exposures

Environmental exposures can be broadly categorized as chemical agents, biological agents, physical hazards, and, perhaps less commonly recognized, psychosocial factors. To identify a hazard, we are interested not only in what agents are present but also whether (and how) they can affect human health.

Chemical Agents

Examples of chemicals are easily named, and many are well known for their dangers to human health. For example, carbon monoxide is produced by combustion and is typically encountered in automobile exhaust and home-heating emissions. Specific metals and pesticides affect many body systems, sometimes accumulating in the body and, because they release over time, perpetuating their effects over a long period of duration. Lead, for example, is stored in the bone, where it can slowly release over time to cause deleterious health effects long after the actual exposure has occurred. As a final example, environmental cigarette smoke contains thousands of chemicals, some of which are associated with cancer.

Although we have knowledge of the actions of some of the chemicals that are in current use, these represent only a minor proportion of those that might be toxic. There are more than 80,000 chemicals in use worldwide, some natural and some made by humans. The Agency for Toxic Substance and Disease Registry (ATSDR) provides detailed information on chemicals. Using their portal, you can search out information on chemicals and how they may affect health.[24]

Biological Agents

The category of biological agents clearly includes infectious agents that are well known to nurses, such as bacteria, viruses, and other organisms such as rickettsia (Chapter 8). However, there are many others. Some molds are known to have effects on the respiratory system and possibly other more systemic outcomes. Also, there are many documented hazards associated with plant and animal contact. Toxic plants and fungi such as poisonous mushrooms and inedible plants are not always thought of as environmental hazards. Likewise, allergens such as dust mites, cockroaches, and pet dander are serious but often unrecognized sources of biological hazards.

Physical Agents

Even more varied are the hazards classified as physical agents, defined as those responsible for the injurious exchange of energy. Examples include heat and cold, all forms of radiation, noise, and vibration. Other physical forms of environmental risk for bodily injury include events such as falls, vehicle crashes, and crush injuries, as well as hazards associated with violence, such as knife or gunshot wounds (see Chapter 12). These are environmental hazards that nurses and the public health system work to prevent and mitigate.

Psychosocial Factors

Finally, psychosocial factors form a category of environmental risk to health that is less frequently included in a formal environmental risk assessment. However, it is important to recognize that communities and individuals that live in fear or experience stress, panic, and anxiety associated with real or perceived threats are subject to psychosocial conditions that affect not only health and safety but also overall well-being. These must be considered in a comprehensive assessment of environmental determinants of health.

Mixed Exposures

Rarely do environmental hazards exist independently. Almost all scenarios that pose environmental risks to health combine more than one threat, and these combinations often act synergistically to raise the level of danger. Chemicals usually exist as mixtures, as is the case with cigarette smoke, which contains at least 70 carcinogens.[25] Interaction and a subsequent increase in hazard may also occur when different agents are combined. For example, noise (a physical hazard) in the presence of some chemicals may result in what is called ototoxicity. **Ototoxicity** is damage to the inner ear, that results due to exposure to pharmaceuticals, chemicals, and/or ionizing radiation.[26] An additional example is the danger related to combining household products. Mixing cleaning agents that contain ammonia with others containing chlorine leads to the production of chloramines, which are much more toxic than ammonia or chlorine alone.

The Environmental Health History

Understanding environmental exposures and the detrimental health effects they can cause is only one step along the way to protecting the health of individuals, families, and communities. That knowledge must then be applied to strategies to effect change. The amount of exposure to an environmental risk varies based on the proximity to the exposure. Those that occur in the workplace are often more concentrated than those in the general environment. This reflects two key components of environmental exposure to hazardous substances: time and location.[28] At the individual level, an environmental exposure assessment begins with time and place. An assessment should include three components: an exposure survey, a work history, and an environmental history.[28] The exposure survey reviews any exposures past and present as well as exposures for members of the household. The work history asks about presence of hazardous substances in the workplace, and the environmental history includes potential exposure within the community. [28]

These questions are only guidelines and should prompt further questions when appropriate. Actions required to address environmental health hazards often raise the ethical question of when to choose the public good over individual rights. For example, in the case of lead poisoning, should homeowners and landlords be required to pay for the cost of lead abatement? Another example is the ban on smoking in public places. The ban reduces the population's exposure to the harmful effects of secondary smoke yet limits the rights of individual smokers.

■ CULTURAL CONTEXT OF OUR ENVIRONMENT

Our culture influences how we live within our environment as well as how we view the importance of that environment. Consider the practice of Fung Shui, based on the concepts of Yin and Yang that influences how objects are placed within a home to help positively affect the energy flow. In a classic article Goodenough addressed the problem of possible conflict between how a professional might perceive a specific environment and how those living in that environment may perceive it. He stated that "...the environment in which people live is a part of their culture."[29] Thus those living in a community may have specific perceptions about their environment that is different from professionals sent in to evaluate the environment from a health perspective. Therefore, as stressed by Goodenough, it is important to account for the cultural perception of the environment through the eyes of those living in the community when conducting an environmental health assessment and to be aware that your cultural perception may differ from that of the community. This opens the opportunity for communication and partnership with a community when working to improve the health of an environment.

● APPLYING PUBLIC HEALTH SCIENCE
The Case of the Peeling Paint
Public Health Science Topics Covered:

- Screening
- Case finding
- Advocacy
- Policy

Jane, a nurse working at a county health department based in a large, urban, midwestern city, was asked to participate in the county lead-screening program to identify families exposed to lead in their environment. The usual method for determining if a child has been exposed to lead is to screen for the amount of lead in blood, which is referred to as the **Blood Lead Level (BLL)**. Measurement of BLLs is done in micrograms of lead per deciliter of blood (µg/dL). Based on recent surveillance data, i.e., the percent of children under the age of 5, it appeared that not all of the children in the high-risk neighborhoods had been tested. Due to the higher percent of children with confirmed BLL of ≥10 µg/dL in the county, the health department felt it was important to once again initiate an outreach program to get children tested. The goal of this secondary prevention screening program was twofold: (1) to identify current cases and initiate medical management if needed and (2) to identify what measures should be taken to prevent further harm to children in these families and other community members.

Jane began her review of the problem with Healthy People (HP) 2020 objective EH-8-1: "To reduce BLL in children aged 1–5 year". She found that the method for measuring BLL in children was revised in 2014. The baseline measure was 5.8 µg/dL with a target of 5.2 µg/dL. The objective was that the concentration level of lead in blood samples would be below the baseline measure for 97.5% of the population aged 1-5 years. This would reflect a 10% improvement.[7]

She then reviewed the HP 2020 midcourse review to determine if the target had been met at the national level. The report stated that: *"The concentration level of lead in blood samples at which 97.5% of children aged 1–5 years were below the measured level (EH-8.1) decreased from 5.8 µg/dL in 2005–2008 to 4.3 µg/dL in 2009–2012, exceeding the 2020 target (Table 12–2)."* [8]

Now that she had information at the national level, she began examining the surveillance data at the county level available on the CDC Web site.[30] She found that, of the 7,031 children tested in 2015, 6% were above the desired level and 1.3% had confirmed BLL 10 µg/dL or higher (see Table 6-1). In comparison to national levels, the county was not meeting the HP 2020 target. She then accessed the current county data and found that the percent of children with a BLL above the desired level had increased to 7.5%, a concerning trend. In addition, 2% of children had confirmed BLLs of 10 µg/dL or higher. She was also surprised to see that, based on the most recent population estimates, the total number of children aged 5 or younger in the county was 56,967. Thus, only about 12% of all children had been tested. If the target population was those living below the poverty level, the county had still come up short in the testing program because 16% of households in the county were living below the poverty level. In addition, she was aware that, with new gentrification of older neighborhoods, the risk for exposure might not be limited based on income. Based on these data she began to develop a lead poisoning outreach screening program for the county.

In the case of lead, a well-known hazard to children, screening in this program consisted of measuring the concentration of lead in the blood to estimate the amount of lead that had been absorbed into the body, and at the same time providing all the parents with health education information about lead. Jane used the current CDC recommendations on childhood lead poisoning prevention guidelines in relation to BLL that would require initiation of prevention measures. The prior BLL that triggered interventions was 10 to 14.9 µg/dL but was changed in 2012 to a BLL value of 5 µg/dL based on evidence that even lower levels of exposure increase the risk for adverse health outcomes in children (Fig. 6-3).[31]

Jane then reviewed the 10 approaches to intervention related to lead poisoning provided by National Center for Healthy Housing (Box 6-2).[32] Many of the recommendations would need action at the county level, but policy items seven and eight matched the use of public health nurses (PHN) in an outreach home visit program. These two items were: (7) Improve blood lead testing among children at high risk of exposure and find and remediate the sources of their exposure; and (8) Ensure access to developmental and neuropsychological assessments and appropriate high-quality programs for children with elevated blood lead levels. For item seven, for children with a BLL value of 5 µg/dL or higher, a home visit would allow for an assessment of the home environment and teaching parents to remediate any sources of exposure as well as connect parents with resources to assist with remediation especially for renters. For item eight, a home visit with children with a BLL value of 10 µg/dL or higher would allow for further assessment of the child and assist parents in obtaining high quality programs for their children. Jane's work to not only research the problem, but also to seek funding for a program for addressing the issue, is an excellent example of nurse advocacy related to environmental health issues as listed in the previously mentioned ANA report.[11]

In the home visiting program Jane designed, parents of children screened with a BLL value at or above 5 µg/dL received a home visit from a PHN and were provided with an environmental assessment of their home, education regarding dietary and environmental actions to reduce the lead poisoning, and help with lead abatement in their homes if needed. The home visit also included providing the parents with information on their legal rights as tenants/homeowners. They were also provided with follow-up BLL monitoring for their child. If a child in the home had a BLL value at or above 10 µg/dL, the PHN would provide the parent with information on how to access the resources they would need for further developmental assessment. The PHN would also provide information about on-going intervention as needed based on the severity of the BLL.

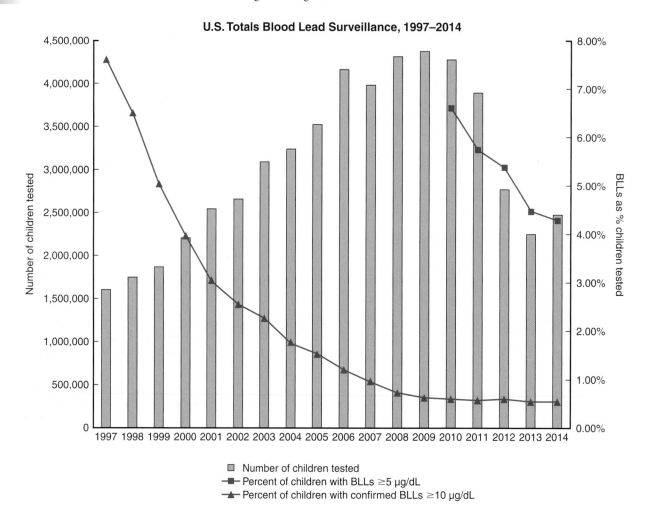

Figure 6-3 U.S. Totals Blood Lead Surveillance, 1997-2014. Comparison of the number tested with the percentage confirmed. *(From the Centers for Disease Control and Prevention. Retrieved from* https://www.cdc.gov/nceh/lead/data/Website_ StateConfirmedByYear_1997_2014_01112016.pdf.*)*

While the health department mounted a screening campaign for lead poisoning, Jane and other PHNs at the health department began conducting the home environmental assessments for all children who had a BLL ≥5 µg/dL. They were all experienced in conducting home visits. They understood that, to achieve the goals of the program, that is, to reduce lead exposure in the home and assist parents in accessing resources for their children, it was important to conduct the home visits using basic principles. First was to understand that they were guests in the family's home. Next, it was important to identify the parent's concerns as a first step toward forming a partnership with the parents. To meet the goals of the program they would explain to the parents changes they could make to reduce exposure and obtain assistance. The best approach is

to use motivational interviewing skills (Chapter 11). The four principles that they routinely employed in their home visits were: (1) expressing empathy for a client or parent's point of view; (2) supporting self-efficacy by highlighting a client's or parent's success at solving problems in the past; (3) remembering to roll with any resistance they may encounter by helping the client or parent define the problem and seek their own solutions; and (4) developing discrepancy, which they knew could be accomplished through helping a parent or client examine the difference between current behavior and future goals.[33]

Based on the findings of their assessments, the PHNs assisted parents who were found to have lead-based paint in their homes or apartments to engage the county level coordinated abatement efforts. The PHNs

BOX 6–2 ■ Policies to Prevent and Respond to Childhood Lead Poisoning

1. Reduce lead in drinking water in homes built before 1986 and other places children frequent.
2. Remove lead paint hazards from low-income housing built before 1960 and other places children spend time.
3. Increase enforcement of the federal Renovation, Repair, and Painting (RRP) rule.
4. Reduce lead in food and consumer products.
5. Reduce air lead emissions.
6. Clean up contaminated soil.
7. Improve blood lead testing among children at high risk of exposure, and find and remediate the sources of their exposure.
8. Ensure access to developmental and neuropsychological assessments and appropriate high-quality programs for children with elevated blood lead levels.
9. Improve public access to local data.
10. Fill gaps in research to better target state and local prevention and response efforts.

also educated parents and others in the home about how to prevent further lead exposure. Together the PHNs developed a community level education program about lead poisoning and how the health department and community could work together to eliminate lead exposure. With extensive interventions the health department hoped to meet the Healthy People targets related to lead poisoning in children aged 5 and under.

Prior to making her first home visit, Jane reviewed the pathophysiology of lead poisoning in children. She found that young children are at greater risk because they are more likely to ingest materials containing lead and absorb more of the lead when it is ingested. A child or fetus is especially vulnerable to the effects of lead and many other toxic substances because their developing organ systems are at high risk of damage. Toddlers are more likely to put items contaminated with lead, such as paint chips, in their mouths, making screening most useful at 1 and 2 years of age. Ingestion of lead, the most common route, can have an irreversible negative effect on the child's developing central nervous and hematopoietic systems. Thus, children exposed to lead can have lifelong health issues. Even with low levels (<5 μg/dL) a child's cognitive and behavioral development can be slowed, resulting in learning disabilities.[33] Children with high levels of lead are at increased risk for serious effects such as encephalopathy

marked by seizures and even coma. These effects can lead to long-term, sometimes irreversible damage. In contrast, the more mature central nervous system of adults is better protected from the effects of lead so that damage to peripheral nerves, rather than the central nervous system, is more likely. Inhalation rather than ingestion is the more common route for lead poisoning in older children and adults.[34]

Jane was assigned to conduct a home visit with the family of a 2-year-old child who had a BLL of 13 μg/dL. Bobby and his family lived in an older building in one of the poorest sections of the city. As Bobby's mother, Sharon, greeted her at the door, Jane noticed that overall the apartment needed major maintenance with older appliances and walls that had not been painted in a while. Due to the initial purpose of the visit, she began her visits with Sharon by letting her know that she was doing the follow-up on Bobby's positive lead screening that Sharon had requested after getting the results of Bobby's BLL test. Remembering the value of using a motivational interviewing approach, Jane began the conversation by asking Sharon what her concerns were and what goals she had. Sharon stated that she was very upset not just about Bobby but her older child. She said that she and her husband were struggling to make ends meet and they took this apartment because they could afford it, but now she found that there were many problems and their landlord was not responsive. Jane repeated back to Sharon what she had heard, that Sharon was worried about her other child, and she was concerned about the condition of the apartment.

Jane encouraged Sharon to tell her a little more about herself and her family so that she could help her address her two concerns, the health of her children and how to correct some of the issues with the apartment. Sharon told Jane that she had rented the apartment for a little more than a year and lived there with her husband and their two children, 2-year-old Bobby and another child in first grade. Sharon held Bobby in her lap for the first half of the interview, but Bobby got restless and slid off of her lap to play on the carpet. Jane built on Sharon's concerns about her children and suggested that Sharon give her a tour of the house to see where the lead might originate.

Jane used her knowledge of environmental risks associated with lead poisoning in children to guide her assessment. In the United States, leaded gasoline and paint were both banned around the same time in the early 1970s. Thanks to these policy interventions, average BLLs in children have been steadily dropping.[34]

However, the threat remains serious especially in communities with a large number of older homes and lead water pipes such as the serious problem in Flint, Michigan.[35, 36] Jane wondered how Bobby became poisoned with lead despite the new regulations. Lead poisoning is a good example of environmental risks in the built environment. Although lead paint has been banned, buildings built before 1978 often contain lead paint. Many cities have initiated lead abatement programs to remove this paint. This population-based policy approach to the problem is one of the best examples of how legislation can improve public and environmental health.[37] However, not all cities have successfully removed all lead paint from city residential buildings, and it is especially problematic in the poorer neighborhoods where older buildings are not well maintained.

Jane learned that Bobby played with his toys on the floor of a room in which the paint was peeling from the windowsills. Suspecting that lead-based paint was largely responsible for the child's elevated levels, she noted the condition of all of the house's painted surfaces and found that many of them were chipping, especially on the baseboards and windowsills, and marred with tooth marks (Fig. 6-4). Paint in older homes is known to be high in lead content, and its availability to a child is a strong indication that the paint is a major source of exposure. Even children who do not directly ingest the peeling paint are at major risk of exposure from lead dust that sloughs from the painted surfaces and contaminates floors and toys that, through the common hand-mouth behavior of children, are ingested or inhaled.

Based on the results of her home environment assessment, Jane explained to Sharon how Bobby probably ingested the lead, primarily through the paint chips. Sharon wondered how the lead paint could be removed. Jane explained that there were steps that could be taken with the landlord to remove the lead-based paint; because precautions are needed when doing any removal or work on painted surfaces in homes built before 1978, it would need to be carefully done. However, there were steps Sharon could take now to reduce paint chips and airborne particulates including keeping the apartment clear of paint chips and dust, and keeping it well ventilated.

Jane asked Sharon if she would like to set up an appointment with technicians from the health department who would come to the home to verify and measure the lead content of the paint and help Sharon

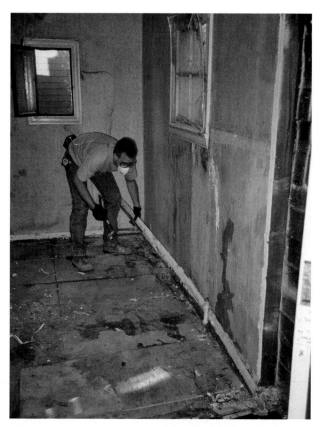

Figure 6-4 Removal of baseboards with lead paint. *(From CDC/Aaron L. Sussell, 1993.)*

identify sources for assistance with the removal of lead from her home. Sharon readily agreed and expressed relief that someone would help her remove the threat to her children. Jane commended Sharon on all the steps she had previously taken to attempt to address the peeling paint in the apartment. Jane further explained that, depending on the state of the home, it might be necessary to physically abate the exposure by entirely removing the paint, which means moving the family either temporarily or permanently to a more suitable, lead-free living environment. Jane explained that there were resources through the county public health department and the housing authority to help the family if this step was necessary.

Remembering Sharon's other goal, Jane asked Sharon about Bobby's health. Sharon reported that he complained occasionally of stomach pain, but she was surprised by the elevated BLL because she had seen no real symptoms of lead poisoning. Jane explained that frequently there are no signs of poisoning and that the results of the poisoning take time to manifest. That is why screening is so important. Jane suggested that Sharon take Bobby for a full checkup at the county's child health clinic or with the child's local provider, and that Sharon and the older child should also be screened for lead poisoning. Pregnant women with high lead levels can transmit lead to their unborn children because it crosses the placental barrier, and lead can also be transmitted in breast milk, affecting both mother and unborn child. Jane also explained that stomach pain can be a sign of lead poisoning and urged Sharon to tell the doctor about Bobby's complaints.

To facilitate the process of setting up an appointment, Jane used what is called a **warm handoff**. This is used in health care as a means for transferring care between two members of the health-care team, in this case the visiting PHN and the primary care provider who would be able to further assess Bobby for lead poisoning and begin treatment if needed. As in this case the warm handoff is done in front of the patient and family. Together Jane and Sharon set up these appointments. In addition, Jane helped Sharon identify the best means for transportation to the appointment. Jane and Sharon then put together a plan that set mutual goals and a timeline for managing the lead poisoning.

At this point, Jane noticed that Sharon still seemed worried. When prompted, Sharon said she had heard about lead poisoning but did not understand what it meant to her and her children. Jane went over the relationship between lead in the home environment and children's health in more detail and explained to Sharon that Bobby's BLL was of concern, and that the trip to the clinic would provide her with more information on Bobby's health status. Jane commended Sharon for having Bobby screened and explained that early intervention can help mitigate the effects of lead poisoning.

Sharon said that she had talked with the landlord about the apartment because of what she had seen on the news about lead poisoning and was assured that there were no problems. She also explained that her sister lived in the same building. Jane knew that finding an elevated BLL in one child had uncovered an environmental hazard that could affect all of the tenants in the building, especially the children. The affordability of the apartments and proximity to the school resulted in the building being home to many young families. Jane was aware that the environmental hazard also extended to mothers in the building who were pregnant or breast-feeding their babies. When questioned, Sharon stated that she had not received any information on the

potential of lead paint in the apartments as required by law.

Jane was concerned about Sharon's story that the landlord had assured her that there were no environmental problems in the apartment. It is against federal law for landlords to withhold information on environmental hazards in their buildings.[38] Specifically, to meet the federal requirements, landlords renting apartments in buildings built prior to 1978 must inform tenants about potential lead paint hazards prior to signing a lease.

Jane was also concerned about the other children living in the building, because this was the only child in the building who had been screened. This resulted in two different levels of action. First, from an advocacy perspective, Jane reported the landlord for failure to disclose the fact the apartment contained lead paint and began to explore alternative housing for the young families living in the building. Second, she implemented her role of case finding. She asked Sharon whether she would introduce Jane to her sister and her neighbor, and help get all the children in the building screened. Thanks to Sharon, a few more of the children in the building were screened, and two of the children had elevated BLLs. Jane recommended further outreach to get all the children in the building screened and helped to put together an on-site screening day at the apartment building. Meanwhile, the health department and the housing authority for the city worked to ensure that the landlord performed lead abatement in the apartment complex and insured that he followed the federal guidelines informing renters before signing a lease of potential lead exposure.

Before ending her visit with Sharon, Jane explained steps that Sharon could take now to protect her family from further lead poisoning. She went over cleaning methods that included mopping hardwood floors with a weak bleach dilution to remove the dust, frequently wiping windowsills with a damp cloth, vacuuming with high-efficiency particulate air (HEPA) filters, and ensuring that the children are kept away from areas with active chipping and peeling paint.[39]

Jane also reviewed a secondary prevention strategy with Sharon that she could use to reduce the amount of lead a child absorbs and increase the amount excreted by providing a calcium-rich, high-iron, vitamin C–containing diet. Jane was aware that this might be more difficult for some families than for others. Impoverished areas, which represent low-income residents and poor social conditions, can be thought of as "food deserts" where access to affordable healthy food is greatly limited. Jane confirmed that Sharon was enrolled in the local Women, Infants, and Children (WIC) supplemental nutrition program and had access to the foods needed to implement this strategy.

Due to her involvement in this lead poisoning outreach program, Jane became very interested in primary prevention for lead poisoning. It was clear that, although screening was important, it would be much better to prevent the problem in the first place. She became interested in the wider issue of the health of the built environment. Jane found that the main primary prevention approach is lead abatement, which is removal of lead-based paint in the home or workplace. As of April 22, 2010, a federal law went into effect that required that all contractors doing renovations, repair, or painting that disturbed more than 6 square feet in homes, schools, and child-care centers be certified in lead abatement.[38] Jane found multiple state and municipal regulations that focused on reducing exposure to lead paint, lead paint dust, and soil contaminated from exterior lead-based paint.

Despite all the regulations, Jane discovered that one of the big stumbling blocks to starting a successful lead abatement program in her county was cost. Because of the seriousness of exposure to lead, the federal government and states have strict lead abatement regulations that result in labor-intensive measures and require the use of specialized equipment. The high cost of abatement raises the question of whether the cost outweighs the benefit, and illustrates a common public health ethical issue of determining whether the benefits of a costly abatement program outweigh the rights of the individual homeowner or landlord to choose not to remove lead paint from a building.

■ CELLULAR TO GLOBAL

Bobby's lead exposure illustrates the fact the lead poisoning and health occur from the cellular level up to the global level. At the individual level, it enters the body through either the oral or respiratory route and ultimately causes permanent harm. However, lead exposure occurs because of the presence of lead in the ambient environment—primarily in paint and dust. In Bobby's case the lead was in a form that resulted in ingestion as the most probable route of exposure, especially given the hand-mouth behavior of a small child. Yet the presence of lead and efforts to eliminate it require interventions that start at the individual level and expand to the global level. Lead poisoning is not confined to the U.S. Globally, in 2015, there were 494,550 lead-exposure associated deaths. In addition, there was a loss of 9.3 million DALYs due to the long-term effects lead has on health. The burden is highest in low- and middle-income countries.[40] In Bobby's case the source of the exposure was the built environment. Globally there are a number of other possible sources of exposure including traditional cosmetics, medicines, and lead-coated dishes and food containers. The WHO is working to eliminate lead poisoning via the global elimination of lead paint to meet Sustainable Development Goal target 3.9: "By 2030 substantially reduce the number of deaths and illnesses from hazardous chemicals and air, water, and soil pollution and contamination"; and target 12.4: "By 2030, achieve the environmentally sound management of chemicals and all wastes throughout their life cycle, in accordance with agreed international frameworks, and significantly reduce their release to air, water, and soil to minimize their adverse impacts on human health and the environment."[40]

Environmental Justice and the Environment

Economically disadvantaged populations and other vulnerable populations (see Chapter 7)—whether as a result of low income, social class, racial or cultural differences, age, health status, or other social indices of susceptibility—are frequently at greatest risk of exposure to environmental hazards. Vulnerable populations face challenges such as substandard housing, lack of access to health care, diminished resources such as nutritious food and safe places to play, poor working conditions, and absence of clean air and water. Those who are employed tend to work in riskier jobs. Disadvantaged communities tend to be located near industrial areas, highways, and rail transportation routes where certain types of cargo and exhaust pose dangers and where hazardous waste disposal sites exist.[41,42] **Environmental justice** refers to fair distribution of environmental burdens.[41] According to the EPA definition, it also refers to fair application of environmental laws, policies, and regulations regardless of race, color, national origin, or income.[42]

Social disadvantage can result in increased exposure to environmental risks as well as an increased susceptibility to the risks.[43] Recognizing the link between environmental health and social determinants of health, the WHO has the Department of Public Health, Environmental and Social Determinants of Health. The goal is to reduce both environmental and social risk factors (Box 6-3). For example, they have worked to promote safe household water storage and to manage toxic substances in both the home and the workplace. They work closely with the United Nations' sectors on energy, transport, and agriculture. They state that reduction in environmental and social risk factors would prevent nearly a quarter of the global burden of disease.[43]

BOX 6–3 ■ World Health Organization: The Department of Public Health, Environmental and Social Determinants of Health

This department advocates at the global and national level for the improvement of environmental health through its influence on policy. It accomplishes this by:

- Assessing and managing risks (such as from outdoor and indoor air pollution, chemicals, unsafe water, lack of sanitation, ionizing and nonionizing radiation) and formulating evidence-based norms and guidance on major environmental and social hazards to health.
- Creating guidance, tools, and initiatives to facilitate the development and implementation of policies that promote human health in priority sectors.

▌ SOLVING THE MYSTERY
The Case of the Hazardous House
Public Health Science Topics Covered:

- Assessment
- Health planning
- Program evaluation

   The work done by Jane and her team on the lead screening outreach program resulted in the nurses identifying other environmental risk factors in the home, especially those associated with an increased risk of asthma. Jane and the other PHNs who worked on the lead poisoning outreach program initiated a county health department safe home program focused on asthma in collaboration with the school nurses (Chapter 18), the local Parent-Teacher Association (PTA), and the county pediatric hospital. The program was initiated because of increased prevalence of

childhood asthma, lost school days for asthmatic children, and increased emergency department (ED) visits for acute asthma attacks. They were able to provide evidence that a home assessment program is a viable intervention that can help address the problem of uncontrolled asthma in children.[44]

   First, the PTA and the school nurses conducted a campaign to promote the benefits of having a PHN from the public health department visit the homes of children with asthma to provide an environmental assessment, additional health education, and links to resources. The program contained three steps: (1) referral, (2) home inspection, and (3) development of a home safety plan. All students with asthma were referred to the health department PHN asthma team, who then contacted the parents of the children. The PHNs offered to provide an environmental assessment for possible pollutants in the home. When invited, the PHN conducted a home visit that focused on residential health.

   The team developed a protocol for conducting these home visits based on the Healthy Homes Manual developed by the CDC in 2006.[45] Each visit began by explaining to family members that the PHN was using an assessment tool that had been adapted by the health department that was specifically designed to identify health hazards in the home in their area. Following the motivational interviewing principle used in the lead screening outreach program previously discussed, the PHN invited them to participate in the review of their home as full partners and began by asking them to share their goals and concerns.

   The team felt it was important to allow time at the beginning of the visit for parents to list the concerns they had as well as commend them for all they were currently doing to address their child's asthma. This helped establish a partnership with the parents and provided the PHN with an understanding of the parents' goals as well as their challenges. From there they could mutually build an intervention specifically targeted to maximize the use of available resources to help improve the health of their home environment and subsequently their child. The PHNs worked to develop a relationship with parents that was nonjudgmental and that would help empower the parents with the knowledge and access to resources they needed to help reduce possible environmental risk factors for childhood asthma and to improve access to adequate care.

   On one visit Jane met a family with a 7-year-old boy, Joshua, who had repeated asthma attacks, multiple absences from school, and an increasing number of

ED visits. The family lived in a three-bedroom apartment in a 300-unit building in an inner-city neighborhood in New York State. There were other children in the home not in school: a 4-year-old, a 2-year-old, and a newborn. The mother, Betsy, reported that the 4-year-old was also being treated for asthma and that the other two children had frequent colds. When Jane asked Betsy about her concerns, Betsy shared that she was very concerned about all the missed school days. She was also exhausted by all the trips to the ED. Although she had been able to sign up for the Children's Health Insurance Program (CHIP) that helped reduce the cost, getting to doctor's appointments was difficult with three other small children. She didn't have a car and her husband worked long shifts. She often had to cancel appointments because she didn't have anyone to watch the other two children. Often when Joshua had an attack it meant she had to rush him to the ED with three other children in tow.

Recognizing that Betsy's focus was on access to care, Jane spent a little more time with Betsy to talk about their environment and the role it played in exacerbating Joshua's asthma. She explained that altering the environment might help reduce the number of attacks severe enough to require a visit to the ED. She also assured Betsy that she would help her find resources such as transportation and childcare to help her keep clinic appointments.

Betsy seemed relieved that Jane understood her main concerns and invited Jane to begin her inspection of the home to help identify environmental risk factors that could be addressed. Beginning with the kitchen, under the sink they found cockroaches and evidence of mice. Jane noted that pesticides and cleaning products were stored in that location and a slow dripping faucet had resulted in an accumulation of a small amount of water in the space under the sink along with some mold. Betsy also kept the kitchen wastebasket under the sink where she disposed of food scraps. Betsy stated that she was constantly trying to deal with the cockroaches and the mice but had not been successful. She had not realized that the black smudges were actually mold.

When Jane asked Betsy about whether anyone smoked in the home, she learned that both parents smoked. Jane also noted that there was worn wall-to-wall carpeting throughout the apartment. When they went into Joshua's room he shared with his 4-year-old brother, Jane noted the large number of stuffed animals. With Betsy, Jane examined Joshua's bed. Betsy explained that there was no money for mattress protectors or

pillow covers. She also stated that, with four children, it was difficult to get to the laundromat to wash the sheets, so she only did them once every 3 to 4 weeks. Jane also asked Betsy about the medications she was using to treat Joshua's asthma. Betsy confirmed that Joshua needed to administer his inhaler frequently and stated that she was careful about giving him his medications on time and regularly.

After completing the overview of the home environment, Jane discussed her findings with Betsy. Jane complimented Betsy on her adherence to the medication plan for Joshua. Jane explained that medications are less effective if there continue to be triggers in the environment such as cigarette smoke, dust mites, and allergens related to vermin.[46] She provided the mother with further information on risk factors for asthma, pulling up the CDC Web site on her tablet so Betsy could see a review of environmental risk factors. The main risk factors mentioned by the CDC were tobacco smoke, dust mites, outdoor air pollution, cockroaches, pets, and mold. The only home environmental risk factor that was not present in this home was pets.

Jane and Betsy discussed actions the family could take to help reduce the risk. Jane began with the problem of secondhand smoke. She explained that this might also explain the frequent colds experienced by the infant.[47] Jane asked Betsy whether either she or her husband would be interested in getting help to quit smoking. Betsy stated that they would consider this if it would improve the health of their children, especially Joshua. Jane gave Betsy information on resources such as local clinics that offer services for smoking cessation. She also encouraged Betsy and her husband to smoke only outside the apartment in a space that was not near where the children played or by an open window.

Jane then discussed with Betsy the issue of cockroaches and mice as serious health risks to families.[46] Aside from producing allergens that can exacerbate asthma, they both carry a host of bacteria and viruses that are dangerous to people, including staphylococcus, streptococcus, *Escherichia coli,* and salmonella. Another hazard associated with pest infestation has to do with the types of chemicals and poisons used to fight them, such as aerosol spray insecticides and poisoned pellets, all of which put children at risk for poisoning. Serious health outcomes associated with pesticides include skin disorders, damage to the nervous system, poisoning, endocrine disruption, respiratory illness, cancer, and death. Jane described methods other than pesticides that Betsy could use for controlling pests within the apartment, beginning with removing food and standing water. Jane described how to use a separate container for food scraps with a tight lid that would provide a barrier to roaches and mice. She also explained how to store food in the pantry in plastic containers with tight lids rather than bags or cardboard containers.

Jane again used her tablet to refer Betsy to the New York State Health Department's Web site on the landlord and tenant's guide to pest control. Together they reviewed steps Betsy could take and what steps her landlord could take to address the rodent and cockroach issue (Box 6-4). Jane also explained to Betsy

---

BOX 6–4 ■ New York State Landlord and Tenant Integrated Pest Control

Proper Pest Management Practices for Landlords and Tenants:

Integrated Pest Management is geared toward long-term prevention or elimination of pests that does not solely rely on pesticides. Integrated Pest Management follows the principles of preventing entry, inspecting, monitoring, and treating pests on an as-needed basis. These principles help manage pests by using the most economical means, and with the least possible hazard to people, property, and the environment. Pests thrive in environments where food, water, and shelter are available. If an undesirable environment is created, pests can be prevented, reduced, or eliminated.

Using Integrated Pest Management:

- Reduce pest problems by keeping the house, yard, and garden free from clutter and garbage. Food should not be left uncovered on counters. Food should be stored in tightly sealed containers or in the refrigerator.
- Keep pests outdoors by blocking points of entry. Quality sealant or knitted copper mesh can be used along baseboards, pipes, drains, and other access points to seal cracks and repair holes.
- If a pest problem arises, identify the pest and the extent of the infestation. Your local branch of Cooperative Extension office can offer assistance.
- Use methods with the least hazard to people and pets, such as setting traps/bait, or using a flyswatter or fly ribbon paper. Bait and traps should be kept out of the reach of children and pets.
- Remove trash on a regular basis and always use trashcans with tight-fitting lids. If pests can get in garbage, they will return repeatedly to get food.
- If a certified pesticide applicator is needed, be sure that (s)he understands and follow Integrated Pest Management principles and practices.

Source: (48)

---

that she could contact her local cooperative extension service for assistance with pest control.

The practice described on the New York State Health Department's Web site is known as **integrated pest management**, a program that includes caulking and sealing cracks and holes larger than a 16th of an inch, eating in one place in the home to consolidate the area that must be cleaned, getting rid of clutter where pests hide, storing food in containers with locking lids, preventing the accumulation of grease, and disposing of the trash nightly.[48,49] Jane also explained about better chemical methods for fighting pests, such as the use of bait stations and gels that do not contaminate surfaces or the air, rather than poisons. She gave Betsy some mice snap traps to be used in place of the poisoned pellets, explaining that mice carry the poison from seemingly safe locations and drop it in places easily accessible to her young children. Jane also handed Betsy a brochure from the local poison control center with a magnet for the refrigerator and a child safety lock for the cabinets under the sink. The lock was for immediate short-term use until chemicals were moved to a safer site. Poisons, solvents, cleaners, and other types of household products should always remain in their original containers, so information contained on the labels will be available to inform emergency care or calls to a poison control center.

Betsy stated that her sink has been leaking for some time, but her landlord was unresponsive to her request for its repair. The same was true of her furnace. Jane pulled up the New York State Tenants' Rights information on the U.S. Department of Housing and Urban Development Web site for Betsy to review.[50] Jane explained to Betsy that she would write up a housing code violation report that should result in the landlord making these repairs.

With Betsy's permission, Jane's assessment of the home expanded to included risk factors beyond those associated with childhood asthma. In the utility room, Jane inspected the furnace and water heater and noted that the water heater was set to 140°F. She told Betsy that she should always make sure the heater is set below 120°F to prevent scalding and demonstrated how to lower the temperature. Jane also observed that the vent connecting the water heater to the furnace was not sealed, thereby allowing the release of combustion products, such as carbon monoxide. Jane explained to Betsy that, just like the gas stove upstairs, water heaters, dryer vents, and furnaces should be regularly maintained, and the level of carbon monoxide should be monitored. She provided Betsy with a carbon monoxide detector with an alarm that emits a warning sound when carbon monoxide levels are too high. Assuring good ventilation, such as turning on the fan when cooking or making sure that a window is open, are other actions that families can take to make sure that the air their families breathe is as healthy as possible.

While still on the topic of alarms, Jane asked whether the family had working smoke alarms, windows that could be opened on each floor, and a fire escape plan. Betsy showed Jane the smoke detector in the living room and then led Jane down the hall to see the other one, which she thought needed new batteries. Jane noticed that there was an extension cord running along the hall floor. While Jane helped Betsy change the batteries in the smoke detector she mentioned to Betsy the hazards associated with extension cords, including fire, tripping, and strangulation. Betsy explained that some of the outlets in the back rooms were not working. Jane went over how Betsy could address this with the landlord.

The final two areas that Jane and Betsy discussed were the problems related to dust mites and mold. Jane suggested that Betsy add repair of the kitchen faucet to her request to the landlord. Meanwhile, Betsy could clean under the sink using a solution of 1/10 bleach to 9/10 water, thus eliminating existing mold. Betsy also explained that there were multiple sources of dust mites in the apartment including the carpets, the stuffed animals, and the bedding. Removal of the carpets should be added to the landlord requests. Removal of stuffed animals might be more difficult if the children were attached to them, but Betsy felt the boys were growing out of the stuffed animal phase and that she would be able to remove most of them and regularly wash the others. Betsy explained that she had limited money to spend on pillow case covers and mattress covers. Together they searched the department store Web sites on Jane's tablet and located stores with reasonably priced mattress protectors and pillow covers that Betsy felt she could afford.

When the visit was complete, Jane and Betsy had developed an action plan that included actions Betsy could take on her own, steps that she would need to take with help from the landlord, and the identification of available resources in the community. Betsy was encouraged by the resources that were available and the assistance that Jane had provided. Jane agreed to follow up with Betsy in 2 weeks to determine whether she needed further assistance.

Over the course of 6 months, word spread among the parents of the school about how helpful the PHN visits were. Prior to starting the home visits, the PHN asthma team and the school nurse, Edward, had developed an evaluation plan for the program (Chapter 5). They had collected baseline data on the key outcome indicators for children with asthma in the school including number of days absent, use of inhalers, number of acute asthma attacks during school, and number of pediatric ED visits related to asthma for children living in the school district. They also kept track of the number of visits Jane made and the time each visit took. Based on these data they found significant improvement for the key outcome indicators and a significant drop in ED use for severe asthma episodes. These data helped them demonstrate that the cost of the PHN home visits were offset by the savings in health-care costs, the reduction in costs related to truancy, and overall improved health outcomes for the children.

Environmental Health and Vulnerable Populations

Vulnerability to health risks varies across populations based on age, gender, geographical location, and socioeconomic status. This also holds true for environmental health risks especially for children and older adults.

Children

Physiological and behavioral characteristics increase vulnerability at each step of early development. Children playing on the ground and floor may spend their time in the most contaminated areas. For example, outdoor soil is often contaminated with heavy metals and pesticides, and hand-to-mouth behavior promotes ingestion of both seen and unseen agents. Children near parents who are washing work clothes may be playing amid toxins that have been carried home as particles from the workplace. Even toys may pose a risk for exposure to toxins including lead and cadmium.[50,51] Children have ingested substances from unlabeled food containers that have been repurposed to hold chemicals or were stored in an easily accessible place such as under the sink.

Compared with adults, children have faster rates of absorption of most toxic substances and, once in the body, the toxic action can be deadlier because children have a higher metabolic rate, a faster rate of cell growth, and less developed immune and neurological systems. There are equally grave concerns for fetuses, which may be affected when a pregnant woman is exposed to toxins. Fetal body systems are selectively more vulnerable according to their stage of development and the timing of exposure. Although women are increasingly aware of the risks associated with alcohol and environmental tobacco smoke during pregnancy, they are often less informed about the dangers of other environmental exposures. In addition, a pregnancy may not be recognized in time to avoid or minimize exposures. This is especially a concern during the first trimester, when the earliest differentiation of organ systems begins. For example, carbon monoxide, which is easily transported across the placental barrier, is potentially devastating to the developing fetus because of its sensitivity to hypoxia. Other substances that cross the placenta may accumulate in fetal tissue, leaving the newborn to begin life with a body burden of a toxin. In addition, breast milk can constitute an ongoing source of ingested toxins because some toxins will transfer from the mother to her milk.

Environmental factors play a role in increasing the risk that children are exposed to toxins and infectious agents as well as risk of injury. In agricultural settings, children and adolescents are at risk of injuries from farm equipment and vehicles with an agriculture-related fatality of someone under the age of 18 occurring every 3 days.[53] In urban settings, there are often limited spaces where children can play, and available play spaces may have faulty playground equipment, as well as exposure to chemical and biological waste or threats of violence (Chapter 12). An example of increased risk in urban playgrounds is the potential for ingestion of canine roundworms, genus Toxocara, found in the intestines of cats and dogs that are shed in the feces.[54] If children get the microscopic eggs on their hands and then swallow them, the eggs soon hatch and the larvae migrate in the body and may reach the brain. The prevalence is higher in poorer urban neighborhoods. For example, in New York City, three quarters of the parks in the Bronx tested positive for Toxocara eggs, but none of the parks in Manhattan did. This is partly due to a higher number of strays in poorer neighborhoods versus pets with regular veterinary care.[55] Exposure to Toxocara may result in long-term damage to the brain.[54,55]

There is clearly a need for community education and assistance in identifying alternative, safer environmental conditions for children. The safety of children is an emotionally charged issue and one that can galvanize a community and spur it to action, whether it is by committing or redistributing resources, enacting policy changes, or seeking other solutions. Nurses who understand the vulnerabilities of children can be partners and change agents in this process.

Older Adults

Older adults are at the other end of the life span, and they face a different set of physical and behavioral characteristics and challenges than children or midlife adults

(Chapter 19). Around the world, based on findings from multiple studies, researchers (e.g., Ralston, 2018; Zhou, 2017) continue to demonstrate the association between both the social and built environment and the psychological, cognitive, and physical health of older adults.[56,57] Not only is access to built resources such as potable water, sanitation, and adequate housing an important factor but so is the social environment. In addition, the movement to help seniors age in place (see Chapter 19) requires not only assuring a safe home environment but also access to community resources to support adequate nutrition and activity.[56-59]

In addition to changes in physical and mental functioning associated with age, older adults also experience increased rates of chronic health conditions, accounting for increased vulnerability to environmental health issues. Some age-related changes that increase risk from environmental hazards include hearing and vision loss, respiratory disease, increased fragility of skin, decreased rates of metabolism, and disorders such as osteoporosis and heart disease. When combined with social stressors in the environment, older adults' vulnerability to environmental hazards appears to increase.[60]

Older adults also have higher body burdens of chemicals that have been absorbed over their lifetimes. Some substances accumulate over time in the body, a process known as **bioaccumulation**. These toxic substances are commonly retained in tissues such as bone or adipose (fat) tissue and can become a long-term cause of poor health outcomes including cancer, organ damage (in particular, to the kidneys, heart, and liver), cardiac disease, increased chance of stroke, and neurological, immunological, and hematopoietic disorders. For example, lead is stored in the bone with a **half-life** (time over which only half of the amount is excreted) of more than 20 years. Its slow release over time is reflected by high BLLs that reach and damage target organs.[61] Those whose organ systems are already compromised are at higher risk. For example, individuals with cardiac disease will be more seriously affected more quickly in oxygen-deprived atmospheres. In addition, many older adults tend to spend a greater amount of their time indoors, where indoor air pollutants and issues related to climate control may be an issue.

In 2013, Gamble and colleagues, based on a review of the literature, called for increased research on the impact of extreme weather on older adults. They found that older adults are more vulnerable and, with the anticipated increase in extreme weather due to climate change, the impact could be greater.[62] To understand how the environment plays a role, consider a hypothetical

Chicagoan, Mr. Roberts, age 78, who lives on the ninth floor of an 18-story high-rise apartment building for low-income older adults and disabled community members during an extreme heat wave. His wife died the year before, and his children live three states away. There are two elevators to serve the 180 occupants, but one of them regularly breaks down. Mr. Roberts had worked most of his life as a carpenter. When he was 62, he fell off a roof, sustaining a hip injury that ended his working career. Following the injury, he began to use a walker and developed failing eyesight. Because of his exercise limitations, he gained weight and developed type 2 diabetes. He tried to be adherent to therapy by checking his blood glucose, but his fixed income, travel distance to the closest supermarket, and solitary cooking situation stood in the way of eating healthy foods. Because of these problems, as well as fear of robbery by strangers who sometimes lurked in his building, he rarely went outdoors. Mr. Roberts mainly kept to himself, did not mix with his neighbors, and simply enjoyed his air-conditioned apartment with its pretty view of the city.

During this hypothetical scenario, the temperatures soar above 110°F. As had occurred in the 1995 heat wave in Chicago,[63] the city begins to experience brownouts, then power outages, resulting in a 3-day loss of power in Mr. Roberts's building. The temperature inside begins to climb, particularly in the afternoon. Two days later, one of Mr. Roberts's neighbors called the building's management concerned that she hadn't seen Mr. Roberts in a few days. When the maintenance person checks, he gets no answer to his knock, and assumes that Mr. Roberts had gone away with family. He leaves a note, the scope of his authorization, because, as in many municipalities, landlords are required to give 24-hour notice to a tenant before they can enter without the owner's permission. Sadly, when the maintenance man enters the apartment the next day, he discovers that Mr. Roberts died during the heat wave.

This scenario is typical of stories that pepper the news each summer in the United States. Mr. Roberts died of heat stroke, a direct result of an environmental hazard amplified by his age, health, and the built environment. Another issue for Mr. Roberts was his social isolation, a factor that may explain why more older men than women died in the 1995 Chicago heat wave.[63] A heat wave is an example of a natural disaster (Chapter 22), but the built environment often increases the risk of morbidity and mortality, especially for the older adult.

One of the contributing environmental factors that increases the vulnerability of older adults is a diminished ability to regulate body temperature; thus, external mechanical methods such as fans and air conditioners are needed to reduce the surrounding temperature. Unfortunately, this susceptibility often combines with other risk factors for heat injuries, particularly in urban settings. Seniors, who are more likely to stay indoors, often live in relative isolation with few social contacts, and those whose incomes cannot support telephones or sophisticated air-conditioning systems are at greater risk for heat-related illnesses. In several extraordinary heat waves, death rates from heat stroke were highest among the oldest age groups. For example, a severe heat wave in France for 3 weeks during August 2003 resulted in 14,800 deaths, mainly among women older than age 75. These deaths, especially when they occur in developed nations, are preventable, and as a result France set up a Heat Health Watch Warning system as well as prevention plans.[64] Thus the environment—adequate cooling, adequate availability of water for hydration, and an effective method of communication—are key components to interventions aimed at reducing environmental issues faced by older adults who are caught in a heat wave.

Many issues also arise in cold climates concerning home heating. In addition to cold injuries and death that can result from lack of heat, many people use space heaters that use fuel such as kerosene. This type of space heater presents a serious fire hazard, as do other makeshift forms of sustaining home heat. Deaths have been caused not only by fire but also from carbon monoxide poisoning when fuels such as charcoal or wood have been burned indoors. There are programs in many locales to assist low-income or older clients. Power companies can provide information about these and, in most locations, cannot abruptly discontinue service before taking certain required steps.

In addition, landlords must also abide by housing codes.[50] For example, when it comes to heating spaces, most housing codes dictate a minimum temperature that must be achievable if the space is to be legally rented. There are many codes that apply to rental properties as illustrated in Solving the Mystery: The Case of the Hazardous House. You should know how to access the code in the community where you work and live and, if it is insufficient, advocate for adoption of the international building codes that are being used increasingly across the United States.[65]

Nurses are often key members of teams that intervene to prevent deaths like that of Mr. Roberts, beginning with those at the office of his primary care provider. Help with contacting the city's social services department can also result in home visiting care. Many older people and others with disabilities are unaware of their eligibility for such services, and many others might be aware of these services but need assistance with applications. PHNs are involved in developing emergency preparedness and disaster management plans, and can help add to the plans' outreach to those most vulnerable such as older adults or the homeless. Such plans include the establishment of warning systems and emergency cooling centers, monitoring of older adults and isolated persons during an extreme heat or cold event, and improving communication and awareness among city officials and emergency medical services. Outreach by PHNs to tenant organizations in buildings such as the one in which Mr. Roberts lived is a means of informing community members about available public health services, fostering better networking and communication among residents, and helping to strategize about safety concerns.

Gene-Environment Interaction

There is growing evidence that genetic factors are responsible for some degree of individual variability in susceptibility to toxic exposures. **Gene-environment interaction** is defined as "an influence on the expression of a trait that results from the interplay between genes and the environment."[66,67] In other words, genes interact with the environment either positively or negatively in a way that influences disease development. Often it involves a complex interaction between multiple genes and the environment. There is a growing body of research that identifies an increased risk for disorders such as diabetes, pulmonary disease, breast cancer, and other diseases when individuals with a specific genetic makeup encounter environmental exposures. In addition, some genes are thought to be protective and thus responsible for a decreased risk of environment-related health outcomes. This knowledge may someday be useful in identifying individuals who are at higher risk and intervening by controlling their exposure. In 2006, the National Institute on Environmental Health Sciences established a 5-year genes and environment initiative in an effort to increase understanding of the interaction between environment and genes with a focus on asthma, diabetes, and cancer. The efforts of this initiative resulted in an increased understanding of the interaction between genes and environment, and helped to develop better ways to measure environmental exposures.[68]

Climate Change and Health

News related to climate change continues to emerge. For example, there is new data that demonstrates that freshwater input from melting ice shelves in the Antarctic in a warming climate is creating a feedback loop and will trigger more melting, which would trigger a rapid sea level rise.[69] Changes in weather patterns, slowing of the ocean currents, rising of sea levels, and melting of glaciers are occurring across the globe.[69-71] According to the WHO, climate change is the result of human activity especially in relation to the burning of fossil fuels.[72] The WHO list of the key facts (Box 6-5) demonstrates that the impact on health is serious, that it includes both social and environmental determinants of health, and that it will have a greater impact on LICs. A good example related to the disparity between high-income and low-income communities is the hurricane season of 2017 with two major hurricanes impacting Houston, Texas, and Puerto Rico. Both areas suffered severe damage from the hurricanes, yet Houston had more resources to restore power and aid persons who suffered losses due to the hurricane. Puerto Rico remained without power over the majority of the island for months, and the devastation and consequent lack of resources resulted in a large exodus of residents from the island to other parts of the United States, especially Florida.

Climate change is associated with numerous extreme weather events including floods, droughts, hurricanes, heat waves, heavy downpours, and blizzards.[73] These events result in increased risk of death, injury, and illness.

BOX 6–5 ■ World Health Organization Key Facts Related to Climate Change

- Climate change affects the social and environmental determinants of health: clean air, safe drinking water, sufficient food, and secure shelter.
- Between 2030 and 2050, climate change is expected to cause approximately 250,000 additional deaths per year, from malnutrition, malaria, diarrhea, and heat stress.
- The direct damage costs to health (i.e., excluding costs in health-determining sectors such as agriculture and water and sanitation), is estimated to be between USD $2-4 billion/year by 2030.
- Areas with weak health infrastructure – mostly in developing countries – will be the least able to cope without assistance to prepare and respond.
- Reducing emissions of greenhouse gases through better transport, food, and energy-use choices can result in improved health, particularly through reduced air pollution.

Source: (72)

For example, heat waves cause direct injury, such as heat exhaustion and heat stroke, which are particularly devastating for older adults and young children. Changes in atmospheric and weather conditions can also increase or exacerbate cardiovascular and pulmonary disease. There are also more indirect effects on health and well-being. Climate-related redistribution of vectors for diseases, such as mosquitoes, allows infections to reach new and broader populations, who are often the least immune. Decreased yield of crops brought about by droughts, floods, or other impacts on the natural environment will add to the current billion people in the world who have inadequate nutrition. In addition, populations are experiencing displacement due to climate change with resulting adverse health consequences.[74]

To help illustrate the complex interaction between climate change and health, the CDC created a figure that depicts the four aspects of climate change: rising temperatures, increased number of extreme weather events, rising CO_2 levels, and rising sea levels (Fig. 6-5). The next level depicts the impact on the climate, and on the outside are the health effects.[75]

The WHO laid out specific actions needed to address climate change. These include: to advocate and raise awareness, to strengthen partnerships, and to enhance scientific evidence.[76] In alignment with the WHO action plan, the Nursing Alliance for Healthy Environments published a report on climate change and nursing. The three areas for action on the part of nursing proposed in this report were research, advocacy, and practice. Their stance is that nurses are in a position ". . .to inform and mobilize society to act on climate change."[77] The issue of **environmental sustainability** reflects the concern of long-term effects on the health of populations related to climate change. Environmental sustainability reflects the rates in which renewable resources are harvested, the depletion of nonrenewable resources, and the creation of pollution that can continue for an indefinite period of time. If the rates of population and diminishing resources continue indefinitely, then the environment is not sustainable. Environmental sustainability was one of the millennium developmental goals of the WHO. The current Sustainable Development Goals (Chapter 1), have integrated the concept of sustainability across all goals related to improving the health of individuals with the environment playing a key role. As the next decades unfold, nursing will have a role in mitigating the impact of our changing climate from the local level to the global level. With the help of organizations around the world, there is optimism that we can make a difference.[76,77]

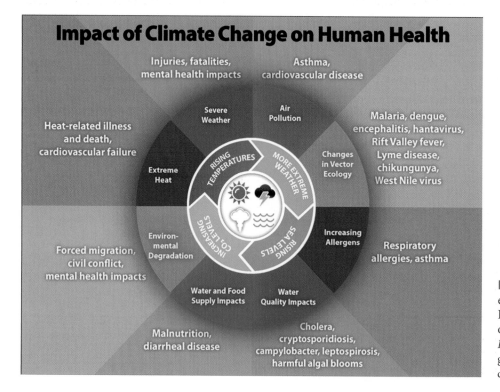

Figure 6-5 Centers for Disease Control and Prevention: Impact of Climate Change on Health. *(From CDC. [2014], Retrieved from* https://www.cdc.gov/climateandhealth/effects/default.htm.*)*

Air

One of the issues related to climate change is the quality of the air we breathe. In 2018, an artist in London, England, Michael Pinsky, set up five geodesic domes (pollution pods) in the city. Each dome replicates the atmosphere of one of five places: Beijing, China; Sao Paulo, Brazil; London, England; New Delhi, India; and Norway's Tautra Island. Many people visiting the pods were unable to remain in them long due to immediate respiratory problems.[78] All animals depend on an adequate supply of oxygen to maintain life. A healthy environment requires not only air with an adequate supply of oxygen but also air that is free from pollutants. Air pollution has long been an issue, but with the arrival of the Industrial Revolution the quality of the air we breathe changed drastically. Industry and the need for energy have resulted in the emission of toxic chemicals into the air. The famous London fog was not a natural weather phenomenon, but rather arrived on the heels of the Industrial Revolution. Cities with high dependence on motor vehicles for transport, such as Los Angeles and London, have struggled with severe smog due to emissions from automobiles. In Pinsky's London geodesic dome, the odor of diesel fuel dominated because it is one of the main pollutants of London air. In the 21st century, the continued emission of CO_2 has resulted not only in the warming of the climate but a reduction in the quality of the air (Fig. 6-5).

Ambient Air

Ambient air is the air surrounding a place or structure and is also referred to as outdoor air. Poor ambient air quality is associated with increased mortality rates from pulmonary and cardiovascular disease.[75,79] Air contamination may occur because of the emission of pollutants into the atmosphere at consistent concentrations over time, such as the emissions from factories. Scientists devised a mechanism to evaluate the current air quality called the **ambient air standard**. This refers to the highest level of a pollutant in a specific place over a specific period of time that is not hazardous to humans. It is the number of parts per million per hour that are considered the safety limit. As evidenced by Pinsky's geodesic domes, the amount of air pollution presents a serious health concern in many urban areas across all income levels.

Variability in air quality often reflects the surrounding built environment. Populations located in the shadow of chemical plants and next to large equipment, railroad tracks, trailer trucks, and dusty access roads are often made up of lower socioeconomic groups, because the property values of homes located next to these sources of pollution are lower. Thus, the population is disproportionately vulnerable to all types of hazardous exposures that come with living in an industrial area. In addition to the risks associated with chemicals emitted in industrial areas, these residents face the social strain brought on by these circumstances.

Many outdoor air contaminants originate from major stationary sources, known as **point sources**, which include chemical plants, power plants, refineries, and incinerators. Alternatively, pollutants may be generated by transportation sources such as buses, trucks, and cars (on-road) and ships, planes, and construction equipment (off-road), all referred to as **mobile sources**. A third type, **area sources**, includes smaller sources of emission such as gas stations, dry cleaners, commercial heating and cooling systems, railways, and waste disposal facilities such as landfills and wastewater treatment operations.[80]

In 1970, the United States promulgated the Clean Air Act, which was reauthorized in 1990. The Clean Air Act, enforced by the EPA, specifies allowable limits, known as the National Ambient Air Quality Standards, for industrial emission of a set of major air pollutants called the **criteria air pollutants** (Box 6-6).[81] These are carbon monoxide, nitrogen dioxide, ozone, particulate matter, lead, and sulfur dioxide. Ground-level ozone and particulate matter are the greatest threats to human health. Because particulate matter varies in size, separate standards are set for all particles less than 10 micrometers (μm) in size (PM_{10}) and for those less than 2.5 μm ($PM_{2.5}$). The size of a particle determines the site of its deposition in the respiratory system. Particles less than 10 μm (less than the width of a human hair) are respirable; they are not removed in the upper airways, as are larger particles. Increased levels of PM_{10} air pollution appear to affect lung function and produce symptoms in asthma patients of all ages.[73] The subset of particles that are less than 2.5 μm enter the alveoli and are associated with lung cancer and cardiovascular death.[82] Vehicle traffic, in particular diesel exhaust, is an important source of particulate matter.

One way to evaluate the degree of air pollution in a specific area is the **Air Quality Index (AQI)** (Box 6-7).[83] The AQI is computed by the EPA based on measures of the five criteria for air pollutants. Although the calculation of the AQI results in values on a scale of 0 to 500, these are generally reported to the public as six category levels: good, moderate, unhealthy for sensitive groups, unhealthy, very unhealthy, and hazardous. They are also denoted by colors that range from green to maroon. A value of 100 or less, corresponding to the levels of "good" and

BOX 6–6 ■ Criteria Air Pollutants

Description of Common Ambient Air Pollutants

Carbon monoxide (CO): An odorless and colorless gas produced by incomplete combustion of fuels in vehicles, heating systems, lawn mowers, and other motorized machinery.
Health effects: Reduces the oxygen carrying capacity of blood, deprives tissues of oxygen to potentially aggravate heart disease, harms fetuses, and damages oxygen-sensitive organs.

Nitrogen oxides (NO_x): Levels are usually low in the United States. Plays a role in the production of ozone. Sources are vehicles, waste disposal systems, power plants, and silage on farms.
Health effects: Lung irritant, aggravates asthma, and lowers resistance to infection; pulmonary edema at high concentrations; pulmonary fibrosis at long-term lower concentrations.

Sulfur oxides (So_x): Sources are metal smelters and processes that burn sulfur-containing coal and oil, such as power plants and industrial boilers. Creates "acid rain" and smog.
Health effects: Bronchoconstriction, aggravates and triggers asthma, long-term exposure pulmonary fibrosis, and possibly lung cancer.

$PM_{2.5}$ and PM_{10}: Sources are vehicles, and wildland and other types of fires.
Health effects: Dangerous to those with heart and lung disease, causing shortness of breath, arrhythmias, angina, and myocardial infarction. Long-term exposures may be related to chronic obstructive lung disease (COPD), lung cancer, and cardiovascular disease.

Lead: A widely used metal present in smelting operations, paint in old housing, water distribution systems, solder, painted items such as some toys, and many others. Organic lead compounds were once used in gasoline, accounting for 81% of transportation emissions in 1985. This quantity has been reduced substantially once lead was banned from this use. Lead often contaminates air, water, food, soil, and bioaccumulates.
Health effects: Damage to renal, gastrointestinal, reproductive, hematopoietic, and nervous system. Affects development and learning ability of children.

Ozone: In the stratosphere, 6 to 30 miles above the earth, ozone is beneficial because it blocks the sun's harmful ultraviolet rays. At ground level, ozone is a dangerous component of urban smog, produced by sources such as power plants, refineries, and chemical plants.
Health effects: Irritates the respiratory system, aggravates and triggers asthma.

Source: (82)

BOX 6–7 ■ Air Quality Index

The features of the AQI include:

- A category that provides specific warnings for sensitive groups, such as children with asthma and others with special respiratory conditions
- Detailed warnings about how all people should protect themselves and their families from harmful levels of air pollution
- Warnings based on the most up-to-date scientific information on the known health effects of air pollution levels

Source: (83)

"moderate" (green and yellow), is the level set by EPA to protect public health. As the index increases, the health hazards associated with air pollution increase, first affecting the most sensitive individuals at levels of 101 to 150, and at higher levels, everyone. As levels above those classified as yellow (index of 100) are reached, individuals should reduce their levels of exertion and outdoor activities accordingly. The EPA provides a daily updated forecast of the AQI and more information about air pollutants on its Web site Air Now. This Web site provides the current AQI for areas around the country and includes information that can be used for teaching clients.[83] Significant advances have been made in reducing ambient air pollution during the past 60 years. Continued efforts to improve the health of ambient air will require collaborative efforts within and across nations.

Indoor Air Pollution

With the exception of laws that ban smoking in public places and Occupational Safety and Health Administration standards for workplace exposures, there is little regulation of indoor air contaminants. Several of these have been mentioned previously in this chapter in the discussion of the home evaluation, including environmental tobacco smoke, animal dander, cockroaches, and the spores of molds that grow in damp environments. Each of these agents can cause allergic reactions, and all are recognized triggers for asthma.

Many pollutants exist in the home in the form of house dust, which may also be composed of heavy metals, pesticides, gram-negative bacteria, and chemicals such as phthalates. The very young are especially at risk because they ingest more dust and are more susceptible to toxins. Home cleaning methods, which PHNs can teach families and reinforce during home visits, significantly reduce dust exposures over time periods as short as 1 week when practiced properly. Effective interventions combine the use of allergy-control bed covers, quality doormats, and vacuum cleaners with dirt finders and HEPA filters. Chemicals associated with the materials used to build homes, such as formaldehyde, are another concern. Buildings that are well insulated, tightly sealed for efficient climate control, and lack windows that can be opened by occupants are more likely to retain indoor air pollutants, especially if the ventilation systems provide infrequent air exchanges per hour.

Potable Water

Just as all animals need oxygen to survive, all living things need water. The availability of potable water has, since ancient times, dictated where humans settle. Humans need water to sustain their own bodies and to sustain their crops and livestock. Water has also played a key role in commerce and the generation of hydroelectrical power. Water has become an important issue in the United States in areas that have limited access to water, especially in the Southwest and in Southern California. The lack of water contributed to the depth of the Depression of the 1930s, creating the dust bowl on the Great Plains and one of the worse environmental disasters in the 20th century. The drought that hit the Midwest economically wiped out farmers and reduced the availability of food, resulting in 3 million leaving their farms and half a million migrating to other states.[84]

The quality of water is a major determinant of the health of a population. Both organic and inorganic contaminates are associated with adverse outcomes. According to the WHO:

> Water is essential for life. The amount of fresh water on Earth is limited, and its quality is under constant pressure. Preserving the quality of fresh water is important for the drinking-water supply, food production, and recreational water use. Water quality can be compromised by the presence of infectious agents, toxic chemicals, and radiological hazards.[85]

Inorganic Water Contaminants

> ▶ SOLVING THE MYSTERY
> ## The Case of the Tainted Water
> Public Health Science Topics Covered:
> - Assessment
> - Epidemiology
> - Rates
> - Surveillance

Flint, Michigan, became front-page news when evidence of lead-contaminated water surfaced. The process of how it happened and how it was discovered provides a special case study not only in the importance of safe drinking water but also the complexity of cultural, political, and monetary influences on decisions related to provision of potable water. In 2014, the city had an estimated population of 100,569 with 58% of the population identifying themselves as African American and 7.6% of the population under the age of 5.[86] In that same year, the city decided to switch the water source for the city from Lake Huron through Detroit Sewer and Water Department to the Flint River. They were in the process of completing a new pipeline to Lake Huron, which would then allow them to join the Karengnondi Water Authority (KWA).[87,88] Part of the reason for taking this course of action was the possible savings to the city of an estimated $200 million over 25 years. The problem was they did not add corrosion control chemicals to the water. Flint River water is more acidic than the water from Lake Huron, and lead as well as other metals in the aging pipes leached into the water.[87]

Within weeks of the switch, problems began to emerge including health problems, the smell and appearance of the water, and water main breaks.[89] The city issued water boil alerts due to the evidence of E. coli and other contaminants in the water. The extent of the lead contamination was not understood at this point, but families began to purchase bottled water due to the boil alert. Due to work by Marc Edwards, a professor at Virginia Polytechnic Institute and State University, and a local pediatrician, Mona Hanna-Attisha, the significant increase of BLLs in children after the switch to the Flint River water source was identified and published. The City of Flint ultimately switched back to using treated Lake Huron water supplied by DWSD, due in part to the study and the subsequent public outcry.[90, 91] Edwards, in his report, issued information to residents on how to reduce their exposure to lead-contaminated water (Box 6-8).[90]

However, understanding the extent of the harm required further evaluation of the data. Zahran and colleagues examined four phases related to the exposure: prior to the switch, after the switch to the Flint River, after the boil advisory, and after the switch back to the original water source. They found that a total of 561 additional children in Flint exceeded a BLL of ≥5 μg/dL following the switch to the Flint River. They found that, after the switch back to the DWSD water system, elevated BLLs returned to the pre-Flint

BOX 6–8 ▪ Recommendations to Flint Residents

Until further notice, we recommend that Flint tap water only be used for cooking or drinking if one of the following steps are implemented:

- Treat Flint tap water with a filter certified to remove lead (look for certification by the National Sanitation Foundation [NSF] that it removes lead on the label).
- Flush your lines continuously at the kitchen tap, for 5 minutes at a high flow rate (i.e., open your faucet all the way), to clean most of the lead out of your pipes and the lead service line, before collecting a volume of water for cooking or drinking. Please note that the water needs to be flushed 5 minutes every time before you collect water for cooking or drinking. For convenience, you can store water in the refrigerator in containers to reduce the need to wait for potable water each time you need it.

Source: (90)

River water period. Zahran concluded that if the city had issued warnings as soon as they had received complaints, much of the increase in BLLs might have been prevented.[89] In 2018, the New York Times reported that the state of Michigan would no longer provide free bottled water because the water had met federal safety guidelines for 2 years. In addition, the City of Flint was on target to replace all of the affected pipelines by 2020 with just over 6,200 replaced so far and 12,000 still to go.[92]

Safe Water from a Global Perspective

The case of Flint, Michigan, demonstrates the importance of a number of standard public health practices such as surveillance, case finding, timely public health alerts, and the need for maintaining adequate infrastructure. Globally, a major issue related to potable water is organic contaminates that increase the risk for communicable diseases (Chapter 8).[93] Improvements have occurred over the last few decades. Currently 71% of the global population has access to safely managed drinking water and 89% have access to at least a basic service. Challenges remain with 50% of the global population projected to live in water-stressed areas by 2025.[93]

The main barriers to the provision of safe drinking water include setting it as a priority, financial capacity, sustainability of the water supply, sanitation, and hygiene behaviors. The main actions recommended by the WHO include increasing the supply of safe water, increasing the number of facilities for the sanitary disposal of excrement, and implementing safe hygiene practices.[93]

Community Environmental Health Assessment

In addition to the environmental assessments discussed thus far that focused on individuals and families, a **community environmental health assessment** can be done as well. It is a means by which public health and environmental health professionals and agencies partner with community members, organizations, and each other to identify, prioritize, and address environmental health issues.[94] One of the most widely used community assessment methodologies is the Protocol for Assessing Community Excellence in Environmental Health (PACE EH), developed in partnership between the National Association of County and City Health Officials (NACCHO) and the CDC.[94] Communities that have implemented PACE EH consider it to be a successful tool for expanding the capacity of health agencies in essential environmental health services; engaging the community in problem-solving; and implementing action plans that use community resources to reduce health risks.[95]

According to the PACE EH guidebook (pp. ix, x), PACE EH is intended for use domestically and internationally, and is being used in numerous locales to take a "collaborative community-based approach to generating an action plan that is based on a set of priorities that reflect both an accurate assessment of local environmental health status and an understanding of public values and priorities."[94] It outlines a series of tasks, shown in Box 6-9, to accomplish this goal. Implementation of the PACE EH process is supported by several resources, including guidebooks in English and Spanish, other

BOX 6–9 ▪ Steps in PACE EH Methodology*

This methodology guides communities and local health officials in conducting community-based environmental health assessments. PACE EH draws on community collaboration and environmental justice principles to involve the public and other stakeholders in:

- Identifying local environmental health issues
- Setting priorities for action
- Targeting populations most at risk
- Addressing identified issues

*PACE EH = Protocol for Assessing Community Excellence in Environmental Health
Source: (94)

publications, a toolbox with a number of materials and resources, and online and regional training. In addition to PACE EH methodologies, there are additional approaches to community assessment in current use, one of which is to conduct a health impact assessment (HIA). These assessments allow communities to examine the impact of city planning related to land use and policy on the health of the community. HIAs are being implemented at a growing rate throughout Europe to effectively gauge the health impacts of land use planning and policy decisions.[96]

■ Summary Points

- The environment plays a role in health from the cellular level to the global level.
- Nurses play a crucial role in the promotion of optimal environmental health and mitigation of the effects of climate change.
- The built environment contributes to the health of individuals, families, and populations.
- Assessment and management of environmental issues are conducted at the individual, family, and community level.
- There is an interaction between genetics and the environment.
- Characteristics of populations, such as age, genetics, health status, and culture play a role in the interactions between health and the environment.
- Climate change is affecting the environment with specific concerns related to air and water quality, an increase in extreme weather events, rising sea levels, and increased risk of communicable diseases.

▼ CASE STUDY
A Contaminated Town

Learning Outcomes

At the end of this case study, the student will be able to:

- Describe the effects of an environmental toxin on the health of a population
- Discuss polices related to environmental hazards
- Apply primary, secondary, and tertiary prevention approaches to an environmental health issue

Since the early 1900s, the major industry in the town of Libby, Montana, was the mining of vermiculite, a material used to insulate buildings. A contaminant of vermiculite is asbestos, which is well known for causing serious lung diseases, including cancer. Concerns about health problems among the town residents, not only the miners, began to surface when a reporter revealed the population's high rate of asbestosis and related diseases. Contaminated soil was the major source of asbestosis around town—near homes, schools, and many public places that included athletic fields—and the dust made its way indoors on vehicles such shoes, pets, and workers' clothes. The mine was closed in 1990, but by then a large proportion of the townspeople had been exposed, with ongoing exposure because the asbestosis remained in the soil. In 2002, the EPA placed Libby on its National Priority List, thereby identifying the town as a site that appeared to warrant remedial action, leading to the testing and inspection of almost 5,000 residential and commercial properties. Cleanup operations began throughout the town. In 2009, the EPA declared the town of Libby a public health emergency. This status mobilizes funds to conduct further home-to-home cleanup and install health-care resources for those with asbestos exposure.

1. What type of hazardous agent is asbestos, what is the typical route of exposure, and what are its major health effects? Are there government standards that regulate the permissible amount of asbestos?
2. List the agencies that would partner to address this extensive environmental disaster.
3. What primary, secondary, and tertiary preventive actions can be applied to protect the public's health?

REFERENCES

1. World Health Organization. (2016). *Air pollution levels rising in many of the world's poorest cities.* Retrieved from http://www.who.int/mediacentre/news/releases/2016/air-pollution-rising/en/.
2. The Guardian. (2018*). Coal-fired power stations caused surge in airborne mercury pollution, study finds.* Retrieved from https://www.theguardian.com/australia-news/2018/apr/03/coal-fired-power-stations-caused-surge-in-airborne-mercury-pollution-study-finds.
3. National Institute of Environmental Health Sciences. (2017). *Climate and human health.* Retrieved from https://www.niehs.nih.gov/research/programs/geh/climatechange/.
4. World Health Organization. (2018). *Environmental health.* Retrieved from http://www.searo.who.int/topics/environmental_health/en/.
5. Richard, L., Gauvin, L., & Raine, K. (2011). Ecological models revisited: Their uses and evolution in health promotion over two decades. *Annual Review Public Health, 3,* 307-326.
6. Coutts, C.J., & Taylor, C. (2011). Putting the capital 'E' environment into ecological models of health. *Journal of Environmental Health, 74*(4), 26-29.

7. U.S. Department of Health and Human Services. (2018). *Healthy People 2020 topics: Environmental health.* Retrieved from http://www.healthypeople.gov/2020/topicsobjectives2020/objectiveslist.aspx?topicId=12.

8. National Center for Health Statistics. (2017). Chapter 12: Environmental health. *Healthy People 2020 Midcourse Review.* Hyattsville, MD: Author.

9. U.S. Department of Health and Human Services. (2018). *Healthy People 2030 framework.* Retrieved from https://www.healthypeople.gov/2020/About-Healthy-People/Development-Healthy-People-2030/Proposed-Framework.

10. Prüss-Ustün, A., Wolf, J., Corvalán, C., Bos, R., & Neira, M. (2016). *10 facts on prevention of disease through healthy environments.* Geneva, Switzerland: World Health Organization. Retrieved from http://www.who.int/features/factfiles/environmental-disease-burden/en/.

11. American Nurses Association. (2007). *ANA's principles of environmental health for nursing practice with implementation strategies.* Retrieved from http://nursingworld.org/MainMenuCategories/WorkplaceSafety/Healthy-Nurse/ANAsPrinciplesofEnvironmentalHealthforNursingPractice.pdf.

12. Environmental Protection Agency (EPA). (n.d.). *Our mission and what we do.* Retrieved from https://www.epa.gov/aboutepa/our-mission-and-what-we-do.

13. Centers for Disease Control and Prevention. (2017). *Environmental health specialists network (EHS-Net).* Retrieved from http://www.cdc.gov/nceh/ehs/EHSNET/.

14. Gunn, L.D., Mavoa, S., Boulangé, C., Hooper, P., Kavanagh, A., & Giles-Corti, B. (2017). Designing healthy communities: creating evidence on metrics for built environment features associated with walkable neighbourhood activity centres. *International Journal Of Behavioral Nutrition & Physical Activity,* 141-12. doi:10.1186/s12966-017-0621-9.

15. Sarkar, C., & Webster, C. (2017). Healthy cities of tomorrow: the case for large scale built environment-health studies. *Journal of Urban Health, 94*(1), 4-19. doi:10.1007/s11524-016-0122-1

16. Hankey, S., Marshall, J.D., & Brauer, M. (2012). Health impacts of the built environment: within-urban variability in physical inactivity, air pollution, and ischemic heart disease mortality. *Environmental Health Perspectives, 120*(2), 247-253. doi:10.1289/ehp.1103806.

17. Garfinkel-Castro, A., Keuntae, K., Hamidi, S., & Ewing, R. (2017). Obesity and the built environment at different urban scales: examining the literature. *Nutrition Reviews,* 7551-61. doi:10.1093/nutrit/nuw037.

18. Huang, R., Moudon, A.V., Cook, A.J., & Drewnowski, A. (2015). The spatial clustering of obesity: does the built environment matter? *Journal of Human Nutrition & Dietetics, 28*(6), 604-612. doi:10.1111/jhn.12279.

19. Sharifi, M., Sequist, T.D., Rifas-Shiman, S.L., Melly, S.J., Duncan, D.T., Horan, C.M., Taveras, E.M., et al. (2016). The role of neighborhood characteristics and the built environment in understanding racial/ethnic disparities in childhood obesity. *Preventive Medicine, 91,* 103-109. doi:10.1016/j.ypmed.2016.07.009.

20. Centers for Disease Control and Prevention. (2015). *Overweight and obesity: Prevention strategies & guidelines.* Retrieved from https://www.cdc.gov/obesity/resources/strategies-guidelines.html.

21. Khan, L.K., Sobush, K., Keener, D., Goodman, K., Lowry, A., Kakietek, J., et al., & Centers for Disease Control and Prevention. (2009). Recommended community strategies and measurements to prevent obesity in the United States. *Morbidity and Mortality Weekly Report, 58*(RR-7), 1-26.

22. Centers for Disease Control and Prevention. (2015). *Physical activity and obesity: Resources and publications.* Retrieved from https://www.cdc.gov/obesity/resources/index.html.

23. Levy, B.S., Wegman, D.M., Baron, S.L., Sokas, R.K. (2011). *Occupational and environmental health: Recognizing and preventing disease and injury* (6th ed.). Philadelphia, PA: Lippincott Williams & Wilkins.

24. Agency for Toxic Substances and Disease Registry. (2017). *ATSDR Toxic Substances Portal.* Retrieved from http://www.atsdr.cdc.gov/substances/index.asp.

25. Centers for Disease Control and Prevention. (2016). *Tobacco and cancer.* Retrieved from https://www.cdc.gov/cancer/tobacco/index.htm.

26. Steyger, P.S., Cunningham, L.L., Esquivel, C.R., Watts, K.L., & Zuo, J. (2018). Editorial: Cellular mechanisms of ototoxicity. *Frontiers in Cellular Neuroscience, 12,* 75. http://doi.org.ezp.welch.jhmi.edu/10.3389/fncel.2018.00075.

27. Nieuwenhuijsen, M.J. (Ed.) (2015). *Exposure assessment in environmental epidemiology* (2nd ed.). New York: Oxford.

28. Agency for Toxic Substances and Disease Registry. (2015). *Taking an exposure history: What are the components of an exposure history?* Retrieved from https://www.atsdr.cdc.gov/csem/csem.asp?csem=33&po=9.

29. Goodenough, W. (1964). Human problems in the conduct of environmental health programs: The role of environment in culture and society. *Journal of Health and Human Behavior, 5*(4), 141-144. doi:10.2307/2948845.

30. Centers for Disease Control and Prevention. (2018). *Lead: CDC's state surveillance data.* Retrieved from https://www.cdc.gov/nceh/lead/data/state.htm.

31. Centers for Disease Control and Prevention. (2016). *Preventing lead poisoning in children.* Retrieved from https://www.cdc.gov/nceh/lead/publications/books/plpyc/contents.htm.

32. National Center for Healthy Housing. (2018). *10 policies to prevent and respond to childhood lead exposure.* Retrieved from www.nchh.org/policy/10 policies.aspx.

33. Miller, W.R. & Rollnick, S. (2013). *Motivational interviewing: helping people change* (3rd ed.). New York: Guilford.

34. American Academy of Pediatrics Committee on Environmental Health. (2018). *Lead exposure in children.* Retrieved from https://www.aap.org/en-us/advocacy-and-policy/aap-health-initiatives/lead-exposure/Pages/Lead-Exposure-in-Children.aspx.

35. Centers for Disease Control and Prevention, National Center for Environmental Health. (2016). *Flint Water Crisis Michigan – 2016.* Retrieved from https://www.cdc.gov/nceh/hsb/disaster/casper/docs/FLINT-H.pdf.

36. Hanna-Attisha, M., LaChance, J., Sadler, R.C., & Schnepp, A.C. (2016). Elevated blood lead levels in children associated with the Flint drinking water crisis: A spatial analysis of risk and public health response. *American Journal of Public Health, 106,* 283-90. doi: 10.2105/AJPH.2015.303003.

37. U.S. Environmental Protection Agency. (n.d.). *America's children and the environment (ACE): Biomonitoring – lead.* Retrieved from https://www.epa.gov/ace/ace-biomonitoring-lead.

38. U.S. Environmental Protection Agency. (n.d.). *Real estate disclosure.* Retrieved from https://www.epa.gov/lead/real-estate-disclosure#renters.

39. U.S. Environmental Protection Agency. (n.d.). *Protect your family from exposures to lead.* Retrieved from https://www.epa.gov/lead/protect-your-family-exposures-lead#homeleadsafe.

40. World Health Organization. (2017). *Lead poisoning and health.* Retrieved from http://www.who.int/mediacentre/factsheets/fs379/en/.

41. Padilla, C.M, Kihal-Talantikit, W., Perez S., & Deguen, S. (2016). Use of geographic indicators of healthcare, environment, and socioeconomic factors to characterize environmental health disparities. *Environmental Health, 15,* 79. https://doi-org.ezp.welch.jhmi.edu/10.1186/s12940-016-0163-7.

42. U.S. Environmental Protection Agency. (2017). *Environmental Justice FY2017 Progress Report.* Retrieved from https://www.epa.gov/sites/production/files/2018-04/documents/4.4.18_environmental_justice_fy2017_progress_report.pdf.

43. World Health Organization. (2018). *Public health, environmental and social determinants of health (PHE): Department of Public Health, Environmental, and Social Determinants of Health.* Retrieved from http://www.who.int/phe/about_us/en/.

44. Krieger, J., Song, L., & Philby, M. (2015). Community health worker home visits for adults with uncontrolled asthma: The HomeBASE trial randomized clinical trial. *JAMA Internal Medicine, 175*(1), 109-117.

45. Centers for Disease Control and Prevention, U.S. Department of Housing and Urban Development. (2006). *Healthy housing reference manual.* Atlanta, GA: U.S. Department of Health and Human Services.

46. Centers for Disease Control and Prevention. (2017). *Asthma: Basic information.* Retrieved from http://www.cdc.gov/asthma/faqs.htm.

47. Centers for Disease Control and Prevention. (2017). *Smoking and tobacco use: Health effects of secondhand smoke.* Retrieved from http://www.cdc.gov/tobacco/data_statistics/fact_sheets/secondhand_smoke/health_effects/.

48. New York State Department of Health. (n.d). *The landlord and tenant guide to pest management—the key to safe pest control is teamwork.* Retrieved from http://www.health.ny.gov/publications/3204/index.htm.

49. U.S. Environmental Protection Agency. (n.d). *Managing pests in schools.* Retrieved from https://www.epa.gov/managing-pests-schools.

50. U.S. Department of Housing and Urban Development. (n.d.). *Tenant rights, laws and protections: New York.* Retrieved from https://www.hud.gov/states/new_york/renting/tenantrights.

51. Centers for Disease Control and Prevention. (2013). *Lead: Toys.* Retrieved from http://www.cdc.gov/nceh/lead/tips/toys.htm.

52. Agency for Toxic Substances and Disease Registry. (2011). *Cadmium.* Retrieved from http://www.atsdr.cdc.gov/substances/toxsubstance.asp?toxid=15.

53. National Children's Center for Rural and Agricultural Health and Safety. (2017). *2017 Fact Sheet: Childhood Agricultural Injuries in the U.S.* Retrieved from https://www.marshfieldresearch.org/Media/Default/NFMC/PDFs/2017%20Child%20Ag%20Injury%20Fact%20Sheet.pdf. doi.org/10.21636/nfmc.nccrahs.fs.2017

54. Liu, E.W., Chastain, H.M., Shin, S.H.Wiegand, R.E., Kruszon-Moran, D., Handali, S., & Jones, J.L. (2018). Seroprevalence of antibodies to toxocara species in the United States and associated risk factors, 2011–2014. *Clinical Infectious Diseases, 66,* 206–212. https://doi.org/10.1093/cid/cix784.

55. Beil, L. (2018, January 16). The parasite on the playground. *The New York Times.* Retrieved from https://nyti.ms/2ELVbmS.

56. Ralston, M. (2018). The role of older persons' environment in aging well: Quality of life, illness, and community context in South Africa. *Gerontologist, 58*(1), 111-120. doi:10.1093/geront/gnx091.

57. Zhou, P., Grady, S.C., & Chen, G. (2017). How the built environment affects change in older people's physical activity: A mixed-methods approach using longitudinal health survey data in urban China. *Social Science & Medicine, 19,* 274-84. doi:10.1016/j.socscimed.2017.09.032.

58. Szanton, S.L., Alfonso, Y.N., Leff, B., Guralnik, J., Wolff, J. L., Stockwell, I., Bishai, D., et al. (2018). Medicaid cost savings of a preventive home visit program for disabled older adults. *Journal of the American Geriatrics Society, 66*(3), 614-620. doi:10.1111/jgs.15143.

59. Szanton, S.L., Samuel, L.J., Cahill, R., Zielinskie, G., Wolff, J.L., Thorpe, R.J., Jr., Thorpe, R.J., et al. (2017). Food assistance is associated with decreased nursing home admissions for Maryland's dually eligible older adults. *BMC Geriatrics,* 171-7. doi:10.1186/s12877-017-0553-x.

60. Ailshire, J., Karraker, A., & Clarke, P. (2017). Neighborhood social stressors, fine particulate matter air pollution, and cognitive function among older U.S. adults. *Social Science & Medicine, 17,* 256-63. doi:10.1016/j.socscimed.2016.11.019.

61. Agency for Toxic Substances and Disease Registry. (2011). *Toxic substances portal: Lead.* Retrieved from https://www.atsdr.cdc.gov/substances/toxsubstance.asp?toxid=22.

62. Gamble, J.L., Hurley, B.J., Schultz, P.A., Jaglom, W.S., Krishnan, N., & Harris, M. (2013). Climate change and older Americans: State of the science. *Environmental Health Perspectives, 121*(1), 15-22. doi:10.1289/ehp.1205223.

63. Kleinberg, E. (2002). *Heat wave: A social autopsy of disaster in Chicago.* Chicago, IL: University of Chicago Press.

64. Pirard, P., Vandentorren, S., Pascal, M., Laaidi, K., Le Tertre, A., Cassadou, S., et al. (2005). Summary of the mortality impact assessment of the 2003 heat wave in France. *Euro Surveillance: Bulletin European sur les Maladies Transmissibles, 10*(7), 153-156.

65. ICC—International Code Council. (2018). Retrieved from http://www.iccsafe.org/Pages/default.aspx.

66. National Institute of Environmental Health Sciences. (2018). *Gene environment interaction.* Retrieved from http://www.niehs.nih.gov/health/topics/science/gene-env/index.cfm.

67. National Human Genome Research Institute. (n.d.). *Talking glossary of genetic terms.* Retrieved from http://www.genome.gov/glossary/index.cfm?id=72.

68. National Institute of Environmental Health Sciences. (2011). *The genes and environmental health initiative.* Retrieved from http://www.genome.gov/19518663.

69. Silvano, A. Rintoul, S.R., Pena-Molino, B., Hobbs, W.R., van Wijk, E., Williams, G.D., et al. (2018). Freshening by glacial meltwater enhances melting of ice shelves and reduces formation of Antarctic bottom water. *Science Advances, 4,* 9467. DOI: 10.1126/sciadv.aap9467.

70. Environmental Protection Agency. (2016). *Climate change indicators: Weather and climate.* Retrieved from https://www.epa.gov/climate-indicators/weather-climate.

71. National Aeronautic and Space Administration. (2018). *Global climate change vital signs of the planet: Sea level.* Retrieved from https://climate.nasa.gov/vital-signs/sea-level/.

72. World Health Organization. (2018). *Fact sheet: Climate change.* Retrieved from http://www.who.int/mediacentre/factsheets/fs266/en/.

73. U.S. Global Change Research Program. (2014). *National climate assessment.* Retrieved from https://nca2014.globalchange.gov/highlights/report-findings/extreme-weather.

74. Schwerdtle, P., Bowen K., & McMichael, C. (2018). The health impacts of climate-related migration. *BMC Medicine, 16,* 1-7. doi: 10.1186/s12916-017-0981-7.

75. Centers for Disease Control and Prevention. (2016). *Climate effects on health.* Retrieved from https://www.cdc.gov/climateandhealth/effects/default.htm.

76. World Health Organization. (2018). *Climate change and human health: What the WHO is doing for climate and health.* Retrieved from http://www.who.int/globalchange/health_policy/who_workplan/en/.

77. Anderko, L., Schenk, E., Huuing, K., & Chalupka, S. (n.d.). *Climate change health and nursing: A call to action.* Retrieved from https://envirn.org/climate-change-health-and-nursing/.

78. Yeginsu, C. (2018, April 22). How is the air in London? 'We should be worried'. *New York Times.* Retrieved from https://nyti.ms/2F8cSNc.

79. World Health Organization. (2018). *Ambient (outdoor) air quality and health.* Retrieved from http://www.who.int/news-room/fact-sheets/detail/ambient-(outdoor)-air-quality-and-health.

80. Environmental Protection Agency. (2016). *Air pollution emissions overview.* Retrieved from https://www3.epa.gov/airquality/emissns.html.

81. Environmental Protection Agency. (n.d.) *National ambient air quality standards table.* Retrieved from https://www.epa.gov/criteria-air-pollutants/naaqs-table.

82. Environmental Protection Agency. (2015). *Consolidated lists under EPCRA/CERCLA/CAA $112(r).* Retrieved from https://www.epa.gov/epcra/consolidated-list-lists-under-epcracerclacaa-ss112r-march-2015-version.

83. Environmental Protection Agency. (2016). *Air now: Air quality index.* Retrieved from https://airnow.gov/index.cfm?action=aqibasics.aqi.

84. Egan, T. (2006). *The worst hard time.* Boston, MA: Houghton Mifflin.

85. World Health Organization. (2018). *Water.* Retrieved from http://www.who.int/topics/water/en/.

86. U.S. Census Bureau. (2018). *Quick facts: Flint Michigan.* Retrieved from https://www.census.gov/quickfacts/fact/table/flintcitymichigan/PST045216.

87. Abuelaish, I., & Russell, K.K. (2017). The Flint water contamination crisis: the corrosion of positive peace and human decency. *Medicine, Conflict and Survival, 33*(4), 242-249. doi:10.1080/13623699.2017.1402902.

88. Lin, J., Rutter, J., & Park, H. (2016, January 21). Events that led to Flint's water crisis. *The New York Times.* Retrieved from https://nyti.ms/2k406rO.

89. Zahrana, S., McElmurryb, S.P., & Sadler, R.C. (2017). Four phases of the Flint Water Crisis: Evidence from blood lead levels in children. *Environmental Research, 157,* 160-172. https://doi.org/10.1016/j.envres.2017.05.028.

90. Edwards, M., (2015). *Our sampling of 252 homes demonstrates a high lead in water risk: Flint should be failing to meet the EPA lead and copper rule. Flint water study: Blacksburg, VA, September 8.* Retrieved from http://flintwaterstudy.org/2015/09/our-sampling-of-252-homes-demonstrates-a-high-lead-in-water-risk-flint-should-be-failing-to-meet-the-epa-lead-and-copper-rule/.

91. Hanna-Attisha, M., et al. (2016). Elevated blood lead levels in children associated with the Flint drinking water crisis: a spatial analysis of risk and public health response. *American Journal of Public Health, 106,* 283-290.

92. Fortin, J. (2018, April 18). Michigan will no longer provide free bottled water to Flint. *The New York Times.* Retrieved from https://nyti.ms/2uW6ubP.

93. World Health Organization. (2018). *Fact sheets: Water.* Retrieved from http://www.who.int/en/news-room/fact-sheets/detail/drinking-water.

94. Centers for Disease Control and Prevention. (2016). *PACE EH—Protocol for assessing community excellence in environmental health.* Retrieved from https://www.cdc.gov/nceh/ehs/ceha/pace_eh.htm.

95. Florida Department of Health. (n.d.). *PACE EH Project: The power of PACE EH.* Retrieved from http://redevelopment.net/wp-content/uploads/2010/11/Thurs11-Role-of-Public-Health-The-Power-of-PACE-EH-Julianne-Price.pdf.

96. World Health Organization. (2018). *Health impact assessment.* Retrieved from http://www.who.int/hia/en/.

Community Health Across Populations: Public Health Issues

Chapter 7

Health Disparities and Vulnerable Populations

Christine Savage, Beverly Baccelli and Sara Groves

LEARNING OUTCOMES

After reading the chapter, the student will be able to:

1. Compare and contrast the concepts of health disparity, equity, and inequality from a local to global perspective.
2. Discuss the magnitude of health disparities both in the United States and internationally.
3. Define and explain the role of the social determinants of health and social justice in the health of populations.
4. Describe the concept of vulnerability from a population perspective.
5. Examine vulnerability of specific populations.
6. Compare and contrast population level strategies for improving health among different vulnerable groups.
7. Understand the role of culture when caring for vulnerable populations.

KEY TERMS

Asylee
Correctional population
Discrimination
Disparity
Equity
Food security
Gene-environment
    interaction
Health disparity
Health gradient

Health inequity
Homelessness
Illegal alien
Immigrant
Incarcerated population
Marginalization
Migrant agricultural
    worker
Migrant worker
Permanent Resident Alien

Point in time estimate
Poverty
Poverty guidelines
Poverty threshold
Primary homelessness
Refugee
Secondary
    homelessness
Social capital
Social gradient

Social determinants of
    health
Social justice
Socioeconomic status
    (SES)
Stigma
Sustainability
Tertiary homelessness
Vulnerability
Vulnerable populations

Introduction

In 2016, the infant mortality rate (IMR) for the World Health Organization (WHO) African Region was 52 per 1,000 live births compared to 8 per 1,000 live births for the WHO European Region with a range of 2 per 1,000 in Iceland and 120 per 1,000 in Mozembique.[1,2] Why is there such a **disparity**, or great difference, between these countries? Is there anything that can be done to reduce this and other gaps in health outcomes between populations? Why

are some populations at greater risk for adverse health outcomes compared to other populations? Answering these questions involves understanding the underlying social determinants of health-realated gaps in health outcomes between populations.

Equity is the underlying concept behind optimum health as a basic human right. To explore this in more detail, consider three people: one tall, one medium height, and one short wanting to watch a ball game over a fence (Fig. 7-1). If all three are provided with a box that

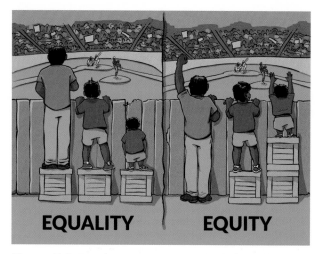

Figure 7-1 Equality versus Equity. (*"Interaction Institute for Social Change | Artist: Angus Maguire." Retrieved from interactioninstitute.org and madewithangus.com.*)

is the same height, this represents the concept of "equality." Although they were all given the same resource to view the game, the shortest person is still not able to see the game. If instead they are provided with boxes at varying heights based on their stature, all of them get to see the game. Then there is "equity" among the three persons.

When health equity does not exist, there are often differences in health outcomes. The terms used to describe gaps in health outcomes include health disparity and health inequity. **Health disparity** exists when "… a health outcome is seen to a greater or lesser extent between populations."[3] The IMR (see Chapter 17) provides a prime example of disparity with higher rates between countries or between ethnic groups within a country. Identifying a disparity is the first step in understanding the underlying risk factors and the development of possible interventions to reduce or eliminate the disparity. **Health inequity** describes *avoidable* gaps in health outcomes.[3] For example, persons with type 2 diabetes who cannot afford the cost of medication and therefore are unable to take it as ordered will experience higher A1C levels and experience more adverse outcomes. The inequity in access to diabetic medications may be a major driver in the disparity in outcomes between lower- and middle-class persons. Drivers of health inequities are linked to the vulnerability experienced by some populations based on the social determinants of health including where they stand in the social hierarchy related to income, education, occupation, gender, race/ethnicity, and other factors.[2]

Addressing health inequity requires providing persons the opportunity for optimal health. This may require more services for those who have noncommunicable chronic diseases and are on a fixed income compared to persons in general good health and who are in higher income brackets. Nurses address health inequity in a variety of ways beginning with advocacy. For example, nurses on the front lines with patients who have difficulty affording their prescriptions advocate for those patients by identifying pharmacies that provide assistance as well as other sources of help to pay for medications. Nurses also advocate for health-care policies aimed at addressing health inequalities at the local, state, and national level. They also actively provide improved care for those in need through nurse-managed clinics or by working as outreach nurses for the public health department.

Vulnerability is the degree to which an individual, population, or organization is unable to anticipate, cope with, resist, and recover from the impact of disease and disasters.[4] An individual or group's vulnerability can be affected by a number of factors, some of which can be changed, and some of which cannot. Vulnerability is especially evident during a natural disaster (see Chapter 22). For example, those with fewer resources have a greater difficulty evacuating during hurricanes due to a lack of transportation and inability to pay for or find alternative shelter. After the hurricane, income level plays a large role in the ability to repair damaged dwellings and obtain needed supplies, as evidenced in Puerto Rico after Hurricane Maria. To understand the increased risk for experiencing health inequities, specific **vulnerable populations** have been identified based on race, ethnicity, age, gender, sexual orientation, history of incarceration, socioeconomic status (SES), exposure to violence and war (Chapter 12), and lack of a permanent residence.[5] Vulnerability is not exclusively tied to social status. For example, frail elderly experience vulnerability related to impaired mobility and difficulty completing activities of daily living. However, when age-related frailty is combined with poverty, the vulnerability of that person increases. Nurses are often confronted with the dilemma of how best to care for a vulnerable person. For example, when discharging a hospitalized patient who has no permanent address or a family member to assist that patient, the nurse must seek resources to help the patient. This requires knowledge of the resources within the hospital, such as the social work department as well as resources within the community.

Comparing life expectancy between countries helps to further demonstrate the health disparity between countries. For example, Monaco's estimated life expectancy in

2017 was 89.4 years whereas the estimated life expectancy in Chad was 50.6 years.[6] For the U.S., in 2016, the estimated life expectancy was 78.6 years, a decline since 2015.[7] There is also health disparity among populations within a country. These disparities are frequently seen as a **health gradient** wherein there is a series of progressively increasing or decreasing differences. The health gradient reflects the relationship between health and income at the population level with health gradually improving as income improves. The WHO uses the term **social gradient**, which refers to "… a gradient in health that runs from top to bottom of the socioeconomic spectrum. This is a global phenomenon, seen in low-, middle-, and high-income countries. The social gradient in health means that health inequities affect everyone."[8] The WHO utilizes the example of maternal mortality to describe social gradient (see Chapter 17). A comparison of the lifetime risk of maternal death during or shortly after pregnancy shows at the top of the gradient, a 1 in 17,400 risk versus 1 in 8 in Afghanistan.[8]

Caution must be taken when interpreting the underlying risk factors contributing to the disparity. On the surface, it might appear that the disparity is due to genetic differences, when in fact, much of the health disparity between groups is driven by socioeconomic factors. Poverty and access to resources such as food, shelter, sanitation, and health care all play a role in improving life expectancy. Other risk factors must also be considered. Since 2015, life expectancy has been declining in high income countries partially due to the rise in opioid overdoses in younger persons (see Chapter 11).[9] Thus, where a person lives, level of vulnerability, and individual health behaviors play a role in increasing or decreasing an individual's risk for premature death.

Disparity and Inequity at the National and Global Level

The WHO stated that "A characteristic common to groups that experience health inequities—such as poor or marginalized persons, racial and ethnic minorities, and women—is lack of political, social, or economic power. Thus, to be effective and sustainable, interventions that aim to redress inequities must typically go beyond remedying a particular health inequality and also help empower the group in question through systemic changes, such as law reform or changes in economic or social relationships."[10] Vulnerable groups with a higher level of risk of experiencing adverse health outcomes are also less apt to have a voice in creating opportunities to reduce health inequity.

■ CELLULAR TO GLOBAL

A 2018 article in the *New York Times* utilized videos and photos to highlight the plight of mothers and newborn infants in South Sudan.[13] The images of mothers and infants accompany the stark facts of limited physicians, electricity, equipment, and medication. Breastfeeding mothers must sleep out in the open. The reality in 2018: 1 in 10 babies brought to the clinic died, most from conditions that were treatable, such as respiratory infections. Because the mothers were unsure if their babies would survive, most were not even named. The lack of resources to treat respiratory infections in newborn infants contributes to the IMR in South Sudan (48.8 per 1,000 births in 2017),[14] which then drives life expectancy (60.6 in 2017)[6].

Health Disparity in the U.S.

Comparing groups based on racial category provides a starting point for illustrating health disparities in the U.S. with the strong caveat that this does not mean that these differences are attributable to genetic differences but rather differences in availability of resources. Again, the IMR illustrates significant differences in birth outcomes. Although the overall IMR for the U.S. in 2016 was 5.9 per 1,000 live births, it was almost double for African Americans (11.4 per 1,000 live births) and much lower for Asians (3.6 per 1,000 live births) (Fig. 7-2).[15] Yet when the data are examined based on geography, differences in IMR by state ranges from less than 1 per 1,000 live births (Vermont) to 9.1 per 1,000 live births (Alabama).[15] Access

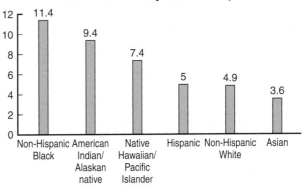

U.S. Infant Mortality Rate 2016 by Race

Non-Hispanic Black: 11.4
American Indian/Alaskan native: 9.4
Native Hawaiian/Pacific Islander: 7.4
Hispanic: 5
Non-Hispanic White: 4.9
Asian: 3.6

Figure 7-2 Comparison of IMR within the United States. (*From Centers for Disease Control and Prevention. [2018]. Infant Mortality. Retrieved from https://www.cdc.gov/reproductivehealth/maternalinfanthealth/infantmortality.htm.*)

to resources and poverty are important risk factors for infant death and help explain the differences seen between racial groups that have a higher percentage living in poverty. Although IMR is just one example of health disparity among groups in the U.S., it underscores the rationale for continuing to keep elimination of health disparities as a priority. HP 2030 continues to include elimination of health disparity as a priority as it has since Healthy People was first initiated.

■ HEALTHY PEOPLE

Disparities: Although the term *disparities* is often interpreted to mean racial or ethnic disparities, many dimensions of disparity exist in the United States, particularly in health. If a health outcome is seen to a greater or lesser extent among populations, there is disparity. Race or ethnicity, sex, sexual identity, age, disability, SES, and geographic location all contribute to an individual's ability to achieve good health. It is important to recognize the impact that social determinants have on health outcomes of specific populations. Healthy People strives to improve the health of all groups.[16]

Healthy People 2030 Framework and Health Disparities

Addressing health disparities in the U.S. continues to be a priority in HP 2030. There are seven foundation principles for HP 2030 that guide the development of HP 2030 topics and objectives including: "Achieving health and well-being requires eliminating health disparities, achieving health equity, and attaining health literacy."[17] There are five overarching goals including: "Eliminate health disparities, achieve health equity, and attain health literacy to improve the health and well-being of all".[17]

Social Determinants of Health, Social Capital, and Social Justice

Health is a complex state that truly reflects a cellular to global model. It reflects a **gene-environment interaction** from the individual to the global level. For example, according to the National Institute of Environmental Sciences, "Nearly all diseases result from a complex interaction between an individual's genetic make-up and the environmental agents that he or she is exposed to."[18] The terms *social determinants of health, social capital,* and *social justice* help to further understand how this gene-environment interaction goes beyond environmental

exposures and incorporates the full context of the communities in which an individual resides and their effect on health.

Social Determinants of Health and Social Capital

The **social determinants of health** are the social and environmental conditions in which people live and work.[19] These social determinants include neighborhood and the built environment (see Chapter 6), economic stability, education, social and community context, and health and health care (Fig. 7-3).[19] These determinants are not only associated with risk for communicable and noncommunicable disease but are also associated with risk for mental health disorders, substance use disorders, injury, and violence. According to the WHO, social determinants of health account for "… the unfair and avoidable differences in health status seen within and between countries".[20] **Social capital**, defined by Lin in 1999 in terms of resources available to individuals and communities based on membership in social networks[21], is another factor to consider when examining underlying factors contributing to disparity in health outcomes.

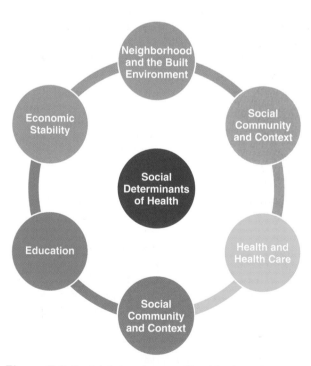

Figure 7-3 Social determinants of health. *(Data from National Institute of Environmental Sciences. [2018]. Gene-environment interaction. Retrieved from https://www.niehs. nih.gov/health/topics/science/gene-env/index.cfm.)*

For all health-care providers, including nurses, understanding social determinants of health and integrating that knowledge into plans of care results in improved outcomes. When patients come to the hospital for care, it is not always easy to understand the context of their daily lives because nurses are not interacting with them in their home environment. Yet with increasingly short hospital stays, nursing care that incorporates this context in the nursing plan of care and discharge instructions becomes even more important. Often patients go home with complex instructions and a need for medical supplies, yet lack the health literacy (see Chapter 2) and/or the resources to implement those instructions. This can result in poor outcomes and a return to the hospital. At the tertiary prevention level, addressing this health inequity may include requesting an order for a home health nurse or home health aide on discharge, thus helping vulnerable patients improve their ability to self-manage the disease. On the secondary prevention level, nurses in public health departments are on the front line with screening programs for vulnerable populations at high risk for disease such as lead poisoning or sexually transmitted infections. On the primary level, nurses provide education to at-risk populations. As explained in Chapter 2, understanding the social determinants of health is essential to help identify persons at risk as well as patterning an intervention at the individual or community level that considers how the social and environmental conditions in which people live affects their ability to achieve optimal health.

Healthy People 2020 highlighted the importance of addressing the social determinants of health by including "Create social and physical environments that promote good health for all" as one of the four overarching goals for the decade. This emphasis is shared by the WHO, whose Commission on Social Determinants of Health (CSDH) in 2008 published the report, *Closing the Gap in a Generation: Health Equity through Action on the Social Determinants of Health.*[2] The emphasis is also shared by other U.S. health initiatives such as the National Partnership for Action to End Health Disparities 3 and the National Prevention and Health Promotion Strategy.[19]

Midcourse Review: For Healthy People 2020, there were eight primary objectives. The midcourse review included 25 related objectives from other topic areas for a total of 33 objectives that were all measurable. Eight were informational. For the other objectives, 10 showed little or no improvement, 9 were improving, and 6 met or exceeded the 2020 targets (Fig. 7-4).[22]

Social Justice

Addressing health disparities comes under the umbrella of **social justice**, defined by the Merriam-Webster dictionary as "a state or doctrine of egalitarianism."[23] In other words, because health disparities represent a lack of equality in health outcomes among groups, it is important to adopt a doctrine of social justice related to

■ HEALTHY PEOPLE
Social Determinants of Health HP 2020

Goal: Create social and physical environments that promote good health for all.

Overview: Health starts in our homes, schools, workplaces, neighborhoods, and communities. We know that taking care of ourselves by eating well and staying active, not smoking, getting the recommended immunizations and screening tests, and seeing a doctor when we are sick all influence our health. Our health is also determined in part by access to social and economic opportunities; the resources and support available in our homes, neighborhoods, and communities; the quality of our schooling; the safety of our workplaces; the cleanliness of our water, food, and air; and the nature of our social interactions and relationships. The conditions in which we live explain in part why some Americans are healthier than others and why Americans more generally are not as healthy as they could be.

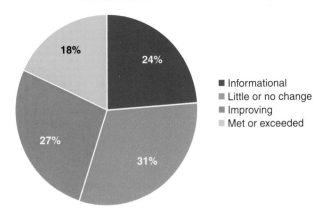

Healthy People 2020 Midcourse Review: Social Determinants of Health

- 24% ■ Informational
- 31% ■ Little or no change
- 27% ■ Improving
- 18% ■ Met or exceeded

Figure 7-4 Social determinants of health midcourse review. *(Data from National Institute of Environmental Sciences. [2018]. Gene-environment interaction. Retrieved from https:// www.niehs.nih.gov/health/topics/science/gene-env/index.cfm.)*

health and to strive to promote equal opportunities to maximize the health of individuals and communities. The CSDH convened by the WHO in 2005 concluded that "… social justice is a matter of life and death".[24] Although this report was completed more than a decade ago, the gaps in life expectancy among countries remain. Social justice continues to be a major issue at the policy level, with the U.S. continuing to debate whether health is a right or a privilege. At the global level, distribution of needed health services, as depicted in the case of newborn care in Southern Sudan earlier, continues to be hampered by poverty, war, and fragile infrastructure in low-income countries.

The Intersection of Race, Poverty, and Place

Although African Americans account for only 13% of the U.S. population, they account for almost 50% of persons infected with HIV when there is no biological or genetic basis for the difference.[26] The driving factors are a "nexus of race, poverty, and place" as demonstrated in 2014 by Gaskin et al.[27] Race is a social construct with no biological foundation and is not a useful clinical marker for disease. Instead, understanding the role of poverty and place should help drive the development of policies aimed at addressing health disparity. Communities with a higher level of poverty are less apt to be able to provide community-level resources, which include grocery stores, parks and recreation facilities, quality schools, and public transportation. There are also fewer employment opportunities and limited access to health care.[27]

Based on the WHO list of 10 facts on health inequities and their causes,[26] addressing health disparity requires more than improving treatments for specific diseases. It requires a more complex approach in which health-care services link with social services.[28] According to the WHO, "The lower an individual's socioeconomic position, the higher their risk of poor health."[26]

● APPLYING PUBLIC HEALTH SCIENCE
The Case of the Doctorless Children
Public Health Science Topics Covered:

• Community assessment
• Health planning

Emily, a school nurse in a large community-based public elementary school, grew concerned due to the increasing diversity among the students. Many first-generation immigrants have moved into the lower-income, working-class community served by the school. Emily found that, among the students, 15 different languages were spoken at home as the primary language, particularly among the 40% of the students whose families came from Asia, Africa, South America, and Central America. The make-up of the rest of the students is: African Americans, 40%; second generation Hispanics, 10%; and whites, 10%.

Emily reviewed the health statistics for the population at her school at the beginning of the school year. In this school, she found disparities in disease/illness rates compared with those in other schools in the district:

• 32% were not completely immunized compared with 3% at other schools.
• 51% had not received the required physical exam.
• There was a higher than average rate of failure for the vision and hearing screening tests.
• There was a higher absenteeism rate.
• 67% had not seen a dentist compared with 31% at the other schools.
• 24% of the children were overweight but not much more than the children in the other community schools.
• Children between 5 and 8 years old had a higher rate of asthma than in other schools in the same district.

Emily wondered if one of the issues facing these families was access to care. To help determine what barriers to health care the families might be experiencing, she examined the children's school records in more detail as well as resources available within the neighborhood. She found that:

• Few children had a primary care physician listed in their school record.
• The nearest pediatric and family practice clinics required that families using the bus system make a minimum of two transfers.

Emily wished to gather more data from the parents but was challenged by the language barriers and by the fact that most of the parents worked. She sought interpreters in the community for the different languages spoken at home and then set up focus groups (see Chapter 4) with parents to help find out more about why the children had received less health care than children in the other schools in the district, especially preventive care.

Although she was unable to conduct a focus group with all of the different groups within the community, she was able to include immigrant groups, Hispanics,

African Americans, and whites. For all of the parents, a central issue was the difficulty of getting to the primary care clinics located outside the neighborhood because it required taking two to three buses with time-consuming transfers, and the offices were only open during working hours. They said the clinics were very crowded and, when they finally got to see someone, they often had less than 10 minutes with the care provider. For the non-English-speaking parents, translators were rarely available. The parents, even those with English as their primary language, reported that going to the clinic had little value because often they did not understand what the health-care provider was telling them, the suggested steps for prevention weren't always possible to carry out ("I can't afford all that fancy fruit!"), and often minimal explanation was provided related to any prescriptions, including where to get them filled. When their children were really sick, most of the parents used the urgent care clinic in the community, but this required up-front payment, so they often delayed going until their child was really sick, which often meant a trip to the emergency room.

The parents mentioned that the department of public health provides free immunization clinics and school physicals for a nominal charge, but they pointed out they cannot afford to miss a day of work without pay to bring the children. They wished the clinics were open on Saturday or in the evenings. Based on the data from these focus groups, Emily identified several factors in the health-care system that contributed to the health-care disparity at her school:

- Limited access to care
- Lack of primary care practitioners in the overburdened clinics
- No primary health care in the immediate neighborhood
- Health department clinics that meet at hours inaccessible to the working population in the community
- Limited public transportation
- Lack of translators at the clinics

She invited parents, teachers, and staff to attend a series of early evening meetings to strategize about how some of these factors could be mitigated to reduce the disparity. Several of the teachers and the school counselor saw this as an important component of school health and also agreed to attend. Emily suggested that the parents who do not speak English find someone who can translate for them and that the translators can also participate. She encouraged the families to bring others from the community. She pointed out that it is

really a community issue and not just a school issue. Emily valued the time of all these stakeholders and tried to be organized to help them arrive at some clear outcomes by the end of the meeting.

The group had three meetings. Participants offered suggestions and concrete plans to be implemented, some to be done at the school and others in the community. These suggested collaborative actions included the following:

- Improve access to care.
- With the partnership of the local public health department, provide an immunization clinic and school physicals one evening a month (or on Saturday) at the school.
- Negotiate with one of the primary care clinics outside the community and the board of education to provide a satellite comprehensive clinic at the school, developing underutilized school space.
- Provide information at the school about the insurance and other health program eligibilities for children of low-income working parents.
- Bridge cultural/literacy gaps.
- Develop evening English as a Second Language (ESL) classes for the parents, coordinated by one teacher at the school, a local social service agency, and volunteers from the local university.
- Start monthly cultural programs organized by the school Parent-Teacher Association to showcase all of the cultures at the school and facilitate more communication among the parents.
- Create information tools that can be used by people with low health literacy to gain information on common childhood illnesses; health promotion and disease prevention actions; and new skills the families can use, even with limited resources, to navigate the U.S. health-care system. Offer to share these information tools with the local primary care clinics.
- Communicate with the clinics about the need to provide required translation services either with trained, certified volunteers including university students, or with a telephone translation service.

With the assistance and support of the community, Emily and the planning group were ready to design actions to implement some of these changes. Emily received two neighborhood development grants to help cover program implementation. The next steps in the process included looking for sustainable funding for an ongoing school health program aimed at reducing the gap in access to care.

Public Health Organizations: Global to Local

Universal Declaration of Human Rights

The Universal Declaration of Human Rights, adopted by the General Assembly of the United Nations in 1948, continues to provide the underlying framework for equity in health at the WHO and down through national- and state-level approaches to improving health equity. The Declaration consists of 30 articles that serve as a standard of achievement for all nations to measure compliance with human rights and fundamental freedoms. Article 25 states, "Everyone has the right to a standard of living adequate for the health and well-being of himself and of his family, including food, clothing, housing, medical care and necessary social services, and the right to security in the event of unemployment, sickness, disability, widowhood, old age, or other lack of livelihood in circumstances beyond his control."[29] Articles 22 to 27 are most specific to equity in health care, examining economic, social, and cultural rights (Box 7-1).

In 1978, at the International Conference on Primary Care, the Alma-Ata Declaration affirmed these human rights (see Chapter 15). The goal was to see the provision of primary health care to every individual by the year 2000, thus achieving the goal of health care for all. The second section of the Alma-Ata Declaration stated, "The existing gross inequality in the health status of the people particularly between developed and developing countries as well as within countries is politically, socially, and economically unacceptable and is, therefore, of common

---

BOX 7–1 ■ *The Universal Declaration of Human Rights, WHO 1948*

Article 22

Everyone, as a member of society, has the right to social security and is entitled to realization, through national effort and international co-operation and in accordance with the organization and resources of each State, of the economic, social, and cultural rights indispensable for his dignity and the free development of his personality.

Article 23

1. Everyone has the right to work, to free choice of employment, to just and favorable conditions of work, and to protection against unemployment.
2. Everyone, without any discrimination, has the right to equal pay for equal work.
3. Everyone who works has the right to just and favorable remuneration ensuring for himself and his family an existence worthy of human dignity, and supplemented, if necessary, by other means of social protection.
4. Everyone has the right to form and to join trade unions for the protection of his interests.

Article 24

Everyone has the right to rest and leisure, including reasonable limitation of working hours and periodic holidays with pay.

Article 25

1. Everyone has the right to a standard of living adequate for the health and well-being of himself and of his family, including food, clothing, housing, and medical care and necessary social services, and the right to security

in the event of unemployment, sickness, disability, widowhood, old age, or other lack of livelihood in circumstances beyond his control.
2. Motherhood and childhood are entitled to special care and assistance. All children, whether born in or out of wedlock, shall enjoy the same social protection.

Article 26

1. Everyone has the right to education. Education shall be free, at least in the elementary and fundamental stages. Elementary education shall be compulsory. Technical and professional education shall be made generally available and higher education shall be equally accessible to all on the basis of merit.
2. Education shall be directed to the full development of the human personality and to the strengthening of respect for human rights and fundamental freedoms. It shall promote understanding, tolerance and friendship among all nations, racial or religious groups, and shall further the activities of the United Nations for the maintenance of peace.
3. Parents have a prior right to choose the kind of education that shall be given to their children.

Article 27

1. Everyone has the right freely to participate in the cultural life of the community, to enjoy the arts, and to share in scientific advancement and its benefits.
2. Everyone has the right to the protection of the moral and material interests resulting from any scientific, literary, or artistic production of which he is the author.

Source: (29)

concern to all countries."[30] In the 21st century, the WHO continues to advocate for reducing health inequity based on the concept that health is a fundamental human right.[10]

United States

Healthy People 2020 stated that the impact of social and physical determinants of health "… determinants affect a wide range of health, functioning, and quality of life outcomes." They provided a number of examples (Box 7-2).[19] As noted earlier, Healthy People 2030's foundational principles include "Achieving health and well-being requires eliminating health disparities, achieving health equity, and attaining health literacy".[17]

Along with Healthy People, a number of U.S. national-level organizations have placed health equity as a priority. The Centers for Disease Control and Prevention (CDC) not only tracks disparity in health outcomes but also provides detailed information on evidenced-based resources to states and local governments. Every few years, they release a report on programs aimed at reducing health disparity.[31] The U.S. Office of Minority Health (OMH) was created to address disparity and inequity in health among racial and ethnic minorities including Native Americans on reservations. The OMH provides funding for assessment, research, education, and intervention with public and private collaborative partners as suggested by the summit.[32] In 2008, the OMH

generated a logic model specific to improving ethnic and minority health that continues to describe what the OMH does (Fig. 7-5) (see Chapter 5).[32,33] The model provides guidance to health-care providers, policy makers, community stakeholders, and researchers to move the process along in a unified way.[32] The goal is to create interventions that change outcomes and decrease racial and ethnic disparities. The five purposes of the model are to:

1. Provide policy makers and others concerned with health disparities a better appreciation of the issues
2. Better understand the interrelationship of all the variables
3. Provide a research format and direction for data input
4. Give building blocks to the community stakeholders so they can contribute input and improve structure
5. Improve the systematic planning of data collection, interventions, and evaluation[33,34]

State and Local Public Health Organizations

At the state and local level, public health departments include minority and ethnic health as part of their mission, and they are often the organizations that implement evidenced-based programs aimed at reducing disparity and promoting health equity as evidenced by the CDC's Racial and Ethnic Approaches to Community Health (REACH) program.[35] The REACH program also funds tribes, universities, and community-based organizations to develop and implement health programs aimed at reducing health disparities. Funded programs have included a wide range of health issues including improving physical activity, increasing access to healthy foods, and increasing breastfeeding.

Vulnerability at the Population Level

Social determinants of health, including economic determinants, environmental determinants, social capital, and health system determinants, are associated with the degree of vulnerability experienced by different populations. Thus, individual risk factors combine with community and population factors to influence the vulnerability of at-risk groups. These at-risk groups who experience vulnerability due to challenges related to the social determinants of health include those experiencing homelessness, migrants, immigrants, asylees, those with a history of incarceration, and members of Lesbian, Gay, Bisexual, Transgender, Queer (LGBTQ+) community. Developmental stages also contribute to vulnerability for older adults (Chapter 19) and children (Chapters 17 and 18)

BOX 7–2 ■ Healthy People: Examples of the Impact of Social and Physical Determinants of Health

- Access to parks and safe sidewalks for walking is associated with physical activity in adults.
- Education is associated with longer life expectancy and improved health and quality of life.
- Health-promoting behaviors like getting regular physical activity, not smoking, and going for routine checkups and recommended screenings can have a positive impact on health.
- Discrimination, stigma, or unfair treatment in the workplace can have a profound impact on health; discrimination can increase blood pressure, heart rate, and stress, as well as undermine self-esteem and self-efficacy.
- Family and community rejection, including bullying, of lesbian, gay, bisexual, and transgender youth can have serious and long-term health impacts including depression, use of illegal drugs, and suicidal behavior.

Source (19)

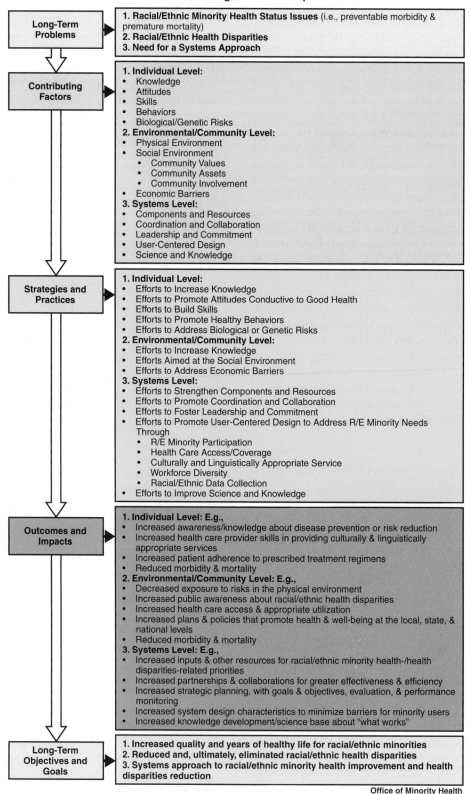

Figure 7-5 Logic Model of a strategic framework for improving health disparities.

especially vulnerable to adverse health consequences such as increased mortality and morbidity due to communicable diseases, injury, environmental exposure to toxins, and during disasters. Experiencing marginalization, stigma, racism, and discrimination increases vulnerability when coupled with the social determinants of health of poverty, education, and place.

Poverty

Economic factors are, perhaps, the most important factor influencing the health status of an individual or group. Lower socioeconomic status is associated with increased vulnerability. **Socioeconomic status (SES)** is a composite measure of the interrelated concepts of income, education, and occupation. With higher levels of education, a person is more likely to secure a better job, which in turn provides a higher rate of pay. By contrast, a person who does not earn a high school diploma has more difficulty finding a job that pays a living wage (a wage that provides access to the means of a healthy living, e.g., housing, food, and health care). Therefore, individuals at a lower SES level have increased vulnerability to poor health because of lack of economic resources.

When household income falls below the economic threshold considered to be adequate to support the number of persons in the household, the members of that household are considered to be living in **poverty**. There are multiple aspects to defining this poverty threshold and the applications of this threshold to determine poverty rates. In the United States, the poverty threshold is the measurement used by the U.S. Bureau of the Census to calculate all official poverty population statistics. The **poverty threshold** is a yearly determination of a standard of living below which a family has the lack of goods and services commonly taken for granted by mainstream society.[36] The census bureau adjusts the threshold based on family size and other demographic variables. For example, in 2017, the threshold for a single person under the age of 65 was $12,752, and for a household of five with three children under the age of 18, the threshold was $29,253.[36] With very few adaptations, the U.S. government's measurement of poverty has remained unchanged for 40 years, although the basis on which the initial calculations were made has shifted. For example, the percentage of income spent on food has decreased, and the percentage spent on such categories as transportation, health care, and childcare have increased.

There are also considerable variances among costs in different parts of the United States and between urban and rural areas (see Chapter 16). These variances are not considered in the current poverty threshold. The poverty threshold is primarily used for statistical purposes, so a consistent method of measurement is used at the national level.

The **poverty guidelines** are another federal measure (see Table 7-1). These guidelines simplify the poverty thresholds and are used for administrative purposes such as determining who is eligible for federal programs aimed at aiding those living in poverty.[37] Both poverty guidelines and poverty thresholds are established on a yearly basis and are issued by the U.S. Department of Health and Human Services.[36,37]

In 2016, the median household income was $59,039, up slightly from 2015. The 2016 U.S. poverty rate remained higher than in 2000 (12.7% versus 11.1%) but had improved from 2012 when it was 15.0%. This translated to 40.6 million people living in poverty in 2016.[38] This is not the highest percentage, as more than 20% lived in poverty in the early 1960s. The War on Poverty, under the Johnson administration, decreased the poverty rate to 11.1% in 1973. Unfortunately, the number rose again in the 1980s and has since fluctuated based on economic growth and recession, even with multiple programs directed at decreasing poverty in the United States. When considering the influence of SES on health, it becomes clear that health-care providers must focus their efforts on improving not just health outcomes but also social determinants of health such as educational and employment opportunities.

TABLE 7–1 ■ The 2018 Poverty Guidelines for the 48 Contiguous States and the District of Columbia	
Persons in Family/Household	Poverty Guideline
For families/households with more than 8 persons, add $4,320 for each additional person.	
1	$12,140
2	$16,460
3	$20,780
4	$25,100
5	$29,420
6	$33,740
7	$38,060
8	$42,380

Source: (38)

Social Capital and Vulnerability

Social capital is a term that has numerous definitions in the literature. The central point of social capital is the benefits that occur through social networks. One example is that persons often secure a job based on whom they know rather than what they know. Social capital usually refers to a person's or a community's capacity to obtain support from the social connections available to the person or community. Social capital resides in the quantity and quality of interpersonal ties among people and communities.[39] These relationships represent a resource (capital) that can be drawn upon during challenging times. Social capital is reflected in the institutions, organizations, and informal practices of giving that people create to share resources and build attachments with others. The values and norms of a community influence the health, well-being, and vulnerability of individuals and populations. Community-level attributes such as social stability, recognition and valuing of diversity, safety, good working relationships, and a cohesive community provide a supportive environment in which to live, thereby reducing a person's potential risk for poor health. These ties may be with family, friends, or colleagues, as well as with various community institutions and agencies. When a person or group has reduced social capital, he or she is at greater risk for vulnerability at all times but especially when faced with a challenge.

A good example of community-level social capital is the case of the community referred to as Little Italy in Baltimore, Maryland. The neighborhood located east of downtown Baltimore experienced a number of assaults and robberies. The community already had a long-standing community committee. The committee called a meeting and invited the Baltimore police and their state representative to attend. Because of the relationships this community had built over time with the city of Baltimore and their state representative, they were able to obtain heightened police presence in the community. The members of the community also banded together and began to pool their resources so that they could obtain further security for the community. As a result, the number of assaults and robberies fell. The community had developed strong social capital over time by building a sense of pride in the community among residents, the support among community businesses, and the ability to gain the attention of lawmakers and the city police department. In addition, the community came together for one assault victim who had sustained serious injuries and raised funds to help cover his hospital expenses.

■ CULTURAL CONTEXT

A person's cultural identity provides a sense of connection to a community of individuals who share a culture. This can lead to an increase in social capital and often improved health. By contrast, those separated from their cultural group may experience increased isolation and thus increased vulnerability. For example, one set of researchers found that the isolation of men who sought same-sex relationships in Indonesia was associated with an increased vulnerability to HIV infections among participants in the study due to prohibitive cultural perspectives and norms with respect to homosexuality.[40] In a 2004 editorial in the *American Journal of Public Health,* Thomas, Fine, and Ibrahim stated: "Efforts to eliminate health disparities must be informed by the influence of culture on the attitudes, beliefs, and practices of not only minority populations but also public health policymakers and the health professionals responsible for the delivery of medical services and public health interventions designed to close the health gap."[41] Addressing disparity in vulnerable populations requires not only understanding the cultural context of the community and the population needing care but also the cultural perspectives of those providing the care.

An individual may have social attachments with other individuals within their community yet remain vulnerable because of a lack of social capital. For example, during Hurricane Maria in Puerto Rico, many of the individuals who were most vulnerable lacked connections with individuals or agencies that could assist them with evacuation during the disaster. Although these individuals and families no doubt had social connections with supportive family and friends, many of those same individuals lacked the capacity to provide needed support for evacuation in the form of money, transportation, and shelter.

Multiple Determinants of Vulnerability

To reduce vulnerability, it is necessary to examine the root causes in a comprehensive manner. Approaches to understanding vulnerability from the lens of individual-level determinants of health can result in a failure to assess the effect that larger social influences have on the individual or population. Conversely, approaches to vulnerability that focus entirely on the social determinants of health at the population level could result in a failure to recognize the manifestation of these influences on individuals and families. Using a multiple determinants of vulnerability approach acknowledges the overlap of risk across many of the determinants of health at the population and individual level that results in increased vulnerability. That is, the more risk factors for poor health that a person or group has distributed across the individual and societal levels, the more likely it is that the person or group will be vulnerable. In particular, marginalization, racism, discrimination, and stigma of a population can result in increased vulnerability.

Marginalization

Marginalization is a social process through which a person or group is on the periphery of society based on identity, associations, experiences, or environment.[42] To marginalize someone is to treat the person as though she is of little or no consequence or is unimportant. The marginalization of certain groups conveys the idea that individuals in those groups do not matter or are of little concern to the rest of society. Often, group differences, such as gender, ethnicity or race, education or income, geographical location, or sexual preference contribute to marginalization. Women, racial and ethnic minorities, and persons living in poverty are examples of groups that have a long history of marginalization within our society. Marginalization limits an individual's or a group's opportunities for establishing beneficial relationships necessary for accessing health-care services. In addition, those who are marginalized can experience heightened levels of stress and despair related to their sense of powerlessness.[43]

Racism and Discrimination

According to the Merriam-Webster online dictionary, **racism** is defined as "A belief that race is the primary determinant of human traits and capacities and that racial differences produce an inherent superiority of a particular race."[44] **Discrimination** occurs when one group gives unjust or prejudicial treatment to another group based on his or her race, ethnicity, gender, SES, or other group membership. Discrimination can occur at the individual, institutional, or structural level (see Box 7-3).[45] Over time, a causal link between racial discrimination and increased risk for morbidity and mortality has emerged demonstrating a negative impact on both mental and physical health.[46,47]

Stigma

Stigma is defined by the online Merriam-Webster dictionary as "a mark of shame or discredit".[48] Stigmatized individuals either possess, or are believed to possess, some attribute that is not valued in a particular social

BOX 7-3 ■ Levels of Discrimination

- **Individual discrimination** refers to the behavior of individual members of one race/ethnic/gender group intended to have a differential and/or harmful effect on the members of another race/ethnic/gender group.
- **Institutional discrimination**, on the other hand, is quite different because it refers to the policies of the dominant race/ethnic/gender institutions and the behavior of individuals who control these institutions and implement policies intended to have a differential and/or harmful effect on minority race/ethnic/gender groups.
- Finally, **structural discrimination** refers to the policies of dominant race/ethnic/gender institutions and the behavior of the individuals who implement these policies and control these institutions, which are race/ethnic/gender neutral in intent but which have a differential and/or harmful effect on minority race/ethnic/gender groups.

Source: (45)

context. For example, being diagnosed with a mental health disorder (see Chapter 10) or a substance use disorder (see Chapter 11) can result in being stigmatized in a demeaning way and seen as less than. Members of vulnerable populations who are stigmatized experience loss of status within society, which can then result in discrimination. This discriminatory treatment leads to further stigma and further loss of status, thus perpetuating a cycle that enhances vulnerability and marginalization that is, once again, beyond the control of the individual.

Ethical Issues

The majority of the literature on ethics and health care with vulnerable populations revolves around the inclusion of vulnerable populations in research. Health-care research focused on vulnerable populations includes participants who are at greatest risk for coercion and may not be able to give informed consent. These groups include prisoners, pregnant women, children, those who are mentally incapacitated, refugees, the poor, older adults, sexual minorities, and persons with a substance use disorder.[49] From a public health perspective, the issue of ethics and vulnerability extends beyond the ethical concerns of including participants in health-care research. Identifying a group as vulnerable must be done in a way that avoids paternalism and stereotyping. Vulnerability does not mean that an individual or group is "less than" but rather acknowledges the increased risk for adverse health outcomes and provides a means to address health inequity.

Nursing care of vulnerable populations uses a framework of cultural competence, social justice, and human rights. The ethical code of nursing states that all individuals, families, groups, and communities will receive equal nursing care.[50] Nurses who demonstrate competence with advocacy for social justice and protection of human rights are better able to address the social inequities of vulnerable populations. There is always a tension between availability of scarce resources and the perceived worthiness of the individual receiving these resources.

Experiencing Homelessness

Although not a disease, homelessness kills. Globally, persons experiencing homelessness often lack the resources needed for basic needs such as shelter, clothing, and food. If they experience a health issue, they may have limited access to health-care insurance, leaving the hospital emergency department (ED) as the primary accessible source of health care for homeless adults.[51] Often health needs are complex and include both mental and physical health issues, and there is limited evidence on the effectiveness of interventions aimed at improving their health.[52,53,54] Persons experiencing homelessness have a shorter life span.[54] Viewed through the lens of social determinants of health, the relationship between homelessness and poorer health in this population is a consequence of adverse social and economic conditions. This situation leads to later diagnosis of disease and fewer resources for treating physical and mental health issues, which in turn leads to higher morbidity and mortality.[54] Thus addressing social issues such as housing and access to primary care could counter the enormous economic costs of hospital care for people who are experiencing homelessness.[54]

Who exactly experiences homelessness? Is it someone who lives on the street or someone who lives in a shelter? What about someone sleeping on the couch of a friend or family member? To answer these questions, the U.S. government has a two-part definition of **homelessness**. According to The McKinney-Vento Homeless Assistance Act of 2009 that was reauthorized in 2015, someone who is homeless meets one or both of the following criteria:[55]

- One who lacks a fixed, regular, and adequate nighttime residence
- One who lives in a supervised shelter or institution designed for temporary residence, or one who lives

in a place that is not normally used as accommodation for people

Using this definition of homelessness, a person who lives on the street, in a shelter, or is couch-surfing is experiencing homelessness. If a person moves from home to home constantly, then that person is lacking a fixed and/or regular nighttime residence and therefore is homeless.

There are then clearly different types or levels of homelessness. Just as we separate prevention into three levels—primary, secondary, and tertiary—the standard for defining the degree of homelessness is to place those experiencing homelessness into three groups:[56]

- **Primary homelessness** includes everyone who is living without adequate shelter—those living in vehicles, surviving on the streets, staying in parks, or squatting in abandoned buildings.
- **Secondary homelessness** includes those who are staying in a temporary form of housing because they have nowhere else to go—those living with friends or family, or in shelters.
- **Tertiary homelessness** includes those who rent single rooms on a long-term basis without security of a fixed or permanent residence.[56]

Time periods provide another way of understanding homelessness. According to the National Coalition on the Homeless, there are three types of homelessness – chronic, transitional, and episodic. Those experiencing chronic homelessness are more likely to require shelter on a long-term basis, are chronically unemployed, older, and more apt to have physical and/or mental health issues. Persons experiencing transitional homelessness require shelter for a shorter period, are younger, and are more likely to experience homelessness due to a catastrophic event. Those experiencing episodic homelessness are also younger, are in and out of the shelter system, are more likely to be chronically unemployed, and have medical and/or mental health issues.[57]

Persons Experiencing Homelessness

Obtaining estimates of the number of persons who experience homelessness is a challenge because of the difficulty in collecting the data. One way to get an estimate of how many people experience homelessness is to determine the number of persons experiencing homelessness on a given night. This is called a **point in time estimate** of homelessness, because a single night, or one point in time, was used to determine prevalence. In 2017, HUD found 553,742 individuals to be homeless on a single night. Less than a fifth were chronically homeless (95,419). According to the report, a little under 112,000 had severe mental illness and little less than 90,000 had chronic substance use issues. About 7% were veterans. Based on racial categories, almost half of those tracked in this report (47%) were African American though only 13.4% of the U.S. population is African American.[58]

Estimating the prevalence is also done by the type of homelessness (primary, secondary, or tertiary) or the different populations experiencing homelessness. Certain segments of the population are at greater risk for experiencing homelessness. For example, families, single youths, and single adults do not experience the same rates of homelessness. There are also differences based on geography, with 50% of persons experiencing homelessness residing in one of five states: California, New York, Florida, Texas, and Washington.[57] Warmer climates make it easier to deal with issues related to weather. In the general population, using data from the 2017 Housing and Urban Development (HUD) report, less than 2% are experiencing homelessness.[58] However, the HUD data does not necessarily include persons doubling up with friends and neighbors.

Single or solitary adults, mostly males, are more likely to experience primary homelessness than those who are either solitary youths or in families. Homeless families are more likely to experience secondary homelessness than primary homelessness, as are solitary youths. Most cities responded that this was likely the result of the policies in place to protect families with children from experiencing homelessness, including policies that made it more difficult to evict families who had fallen behind on their rent.

Homelessness is not just a big city problem; rural homelessness does exist. Estimating how many people experience homelessness in a rural setting is difficult because

estimates such as that reported by HUD (Table 7-2) rely on counts of persons using services. Persons experiencing homelessness in rural areas have access to fewer rural service sites. In addition, there are a limited number of researchers working in rural communities.[57] In comparison with urban homeless populations, the rural homeless are more likely to be white, female, married, homeless for the first time, to have jobs, and to be homeless for a shorter period of time.[57]

Impact on Health

Adults experiencing homelessness are faced with an excess disease burden, a shorter life expectancy, limited access to care, and consumption of significantly more health-care resources when she or he does finally receive care.[59-61] Establishing current prevalence of communicable and noncommunicable disease presents a challenge due to the lack of regular surveillance and the transient nature of the population. Available data underlines the fact that those experiencing homelessness have a higher rate of disease compared with the general U.S. population.[60-62] According to the National Alliance to End Homelessness, those experiencing homelessness are three to six times more likely to have diabetes, HIV/AIDs, cardiovascular disease, and/or a substance use disorder.[61] Between 25% to 33% of homeless persons have mental health issues, including schizophrenia, depression, and bipolar disorder compared with 6% of the general population that experience the same severe mental health issues.[62] A person experiencing homelessness is much more likely to arrive at the hospital in an ambulance, be uninsured, be admitted, and is also more likely to have a longer stay.[60]

The living conditions of those experiencing primary homelessness are not optimal. If a patient who is currently

TABLE 7–2 ■ Prevalence of Homelessness by Race in 2017

	Emergency Shelter	Transitional Housing	Unsheltered	Total
African American	128,721	38,768	57,448	224,937
White	106,543	47,946	106,490	260,979
Asian	2,571	1,132	3,057	6,760
American Indian or Alaska Native	6,228	2,496	8072	16,796
Native Hawaiian or Other Pacific Islander	2,807	1,678	4,040	8,525
Other Race	15,560	6,417	13,768	35,745
TOTAL	262,430	98,437	192,875	553,742

Source: (58)

homeless is admitted to the hospital for surgery, it will be much more difficult for that patient to keep an incision infection-free postdischarge than it will be for someone who is living in a place suitable for human shelter. Second, transportation costs make it difficult for a patient experiencing homelessness to receive follow-up care and testing. Third, the nutritional intake of a homeless patient is irregular and less healthy than that of the general population, making diet instructions hard to follow, which may be further impacted by poor dental care. There are other complicating factors that are easily overlooked. For example, where can a diabetic homeless patient store insulin? How does such a patient keep a medication from being stolen?

● APPLYING PUBLIC HEALTH SCIENCE

The Case of the Rubbermaid Storage Box

Public Health Science Topics Covered:

- Community assessment
- Community diagnosis
- Organization and management
- Community partnerships

While in graduate school pursuing a degree as an advanced public health nurse (APHN), Adele was asked to supervise a group of undergraduate nursing students assigned to take weekly blood pressure readings at a local homeless shelter, the City Gospel Mission. This faith-based nondenominational mission was located in downtown Cincinnati and provided multiple services including meals and shelter beds but did not offer health care. From her first trip to the City Gospel Mission, Adele felt compelled to reach out to this vulnerable population.

Adele recognized that these men had very few options for health care, and she wanted to offer more than blood pressure screenings. As part of her practicum experience, she went to the mission on a weekly basis to provide nursing assessments, health education, and nursing care. She began to interact more with the men when they came to the clinic and worked with them to help identify their health needs and, in some cases, offer referrals. All of her supplies, including her blood pressure cuff and a glucometer, fit into a Rubbermaid storage box, which she left at the shelter. Although she was providing some assistance, she knew these men needed more. When she approached her faculty preceptor, she was encouraged to apply the health planning process, do a focused

assessment that would help her to understand whether there was a need for expanding the care, and consider developing the model of a nurse-managed clinic if there was a need. The faculty member explained that the assessment could provide the data she needed to develop a plan to address the health needs of the men she was seeing.

In conducting part of their assessment, Adele and a fellow APHN student asked key informants, homeless men at the mission, where they sought health care. They all mentioned the ED at a nearby major urban medical center. The students' assessment at the medical center focused on identifying the costs associated with nonurgent ED care for patients experiencing homelessness. The students presented the findings to the hospital performance improvement committee. The committee agreed that an intervention aimed at providing nonurgent care to homeless men outside the ED would result in a cost benefit to the hospital, and that a nurse-managed clinic model had the potential to meet that need.

After Adele graduated, she no longer had time to continue to provide even the small amount of nursing care she had offered at the mission. Having established a need, Adele together with her faculty preceptor sought sources of possible funding for expanding Adele's practicum experience to establish a permanent nurse-managed clinic at the City Gospel Mission. The success of this project depended on the application of public health science and the public health competencies that Adele had acquired. First, a team was formed that included Adele, two faculty members from the University of Cincinnati College of Nursing, the chief nursing officer from the hospital, and the director of the City Gospel Mission. The next step was to flesh out the initial assessment conducted by Adele and her fellow student. Adele's assessment of ED use by the homeless was crucial information for the potential cost/benefit of the clinic. However, to help understand the breadth of the problem, further assessment was done using aggregate data from the City Gospel Mission on the number of potential clients for the clinic as well as secondary analysis of available data on the prevalence of primary homelessness in the city of Cincinnati. These data provided a clear picture of the need for the clinic. The final step was to develop the program expanding on Adele's Rubbermaid container of supplies to include a more comprehensive nurse-managed clinic model.

The team chose a nurse-managed clinic model that would link with other resources in the city. Thus, patients of the clinic would receive nursing assessments, health education, and nursing care under the direction of Adele and be referred to other clinics for more complex medical problems. To do this, the project needed start-up funds to provide supplies, equipment, a method to keep clinic medical records, and to conduct an evaluation.

The first grant application was not funded. The team took the grant reviews, refined the application, and submitted it to another funding agency. They were successful this time in obtaining a 2-year start-up grant. The grant application succeeded based on three key elements: (1) a clear delineation of the need for the clinic; (2) evidence of sustainability of the clinic once the funding was exhausted; and (3) a clear plan to evaluate the effectiveness of the clinic. **Sustainability** refers to the ability of a program to be maintained once the funding period has been completed. In this case, the three organizations that supported the grant—the college, the hospital, and the shelter—all committed to maintaining the clinic if the evaluation demonstrated that it was effective. The college committed to sending students to the clinic for clinical experiences, and the hospital agreed to be the "owner" of the clinic, that is, staff would maintain the medical records and provide salary support for Adele to continue her work at the clinic. City Gospel Mission agreed to continue to provide the space and utilities for the clinic. The homeless men also became partners, offering suggestions about time, location, and some of the health needs they would like to see met. They also saw a role in helping with the running of the clinic.

After 2 years of clinic implementation, the evaluation team demonstrated that the clinic had indeed improved health outcomes. One of the faculty members from the college conducted the evaluation. Attendees at the clinic were asked to complete a survey the first day they used the clinic and at least 2 months after they had begun to use the clinic. Forty-five homeless adults completed both a baseline survey and a survey after starting care at the clinic. There was a significant increase in the percentage of participants who were very satisfied in relation to perceived quality and availability of health care. In addition, there was a significant improvement in health-related quality of life in relation to mental health, physical problems, and vitality.[63]

Adele's story is true. Although the grant ended in 2006, the nurse-managed clinic was still operating in 2018. The City Gospel Mission had built a new facility and included a clinic for the nurses. They continue to see 30 or more persons a night. The clinic is staffed by volunteer nurses, nursing students, and, of course, Adele, who provides nursing care, as well as extra emotional support to her patients. The important issue here is that Adele alone with her Rubbermaid container was not enough. Adele took her enthusiasm and concern for a vulnerable population and built a team. The use of solid public health approaches resulted in organizational commitment. Addressing the health-care challenges for those who are vulnerable requires this approach and can be successfully initiated, implemented, and sustained by nurses.

Interventions and Services for Persons Experiencing Homelessness

Even in the best of circumstances, health-care providers experience problems in an acute care setting in helping any patient manage personal health for the long term. For example, sometimes it is difficult to ensure that, after discharge, patients will follow up on time with their health-care providers. Other times, patients may not take their medicines as prescribed, which makes it even more difficult to ensure that conditions are treated in the best way possible. In primary care, patients might not get recommended testing because of embarrassment (e.g., colonoscopy) or because of costs associated with that testing. Each of these problems is magnified for patients who are also experiencing homelessness.

Shelter

Housing is the biggest need of the homeless. Simply providing housing can improve the health of the homeless and reduce the number of hospital visits and hospital admissions.[59, 60] Homeless shelters provide an immediate and temporary solution, usually for a stipulated and limited amount of time (e.g., 3 months) for an individual or a family. It is a safe and warm place to sleep and, in areas of the United States when the winter weather is more severe, an essential service. Shelters are frequently sponsored by nonprofit organizations that have religious and/or government sponsorship. Most shelters limit their service to certain groups of people, frequently not allowing any alcohol or illegal drugs, and have in place strict rules about there being no violence in the shelter. Many provide separate space or facilities for adolescents and families with children. Most shelters open late in the afternoon and close early in the morning, leaving the person staying at the shelter on the street for the daylight hours. Usually, shelters offer their service free of charge, and some will provide an evening meal for those staying at the shelter. Some communities supplement their night shelters with day shelters where people can go during the time the night shelters are closed. These facilities usually have an array of social services to help with permanent housing, job placements, mental health care and services for those with addictions, and job training. There may also be showers, laundry facilities, used clothing available, as well as other amenities to help individuals and families secure more permanent housing.

A step above the shelters is the more permanent *transitional housing,* which is affordable due to significant subsidies, but again, there is usually a time limit (6 months to 2 years). People who agree to live in transitional housing usually must participate in programs that provide counseling, job searches, and job and educational training. People are taught skills on how to maintain more permanent housing and manage their money.

Permanent affordable housing is the long-term solution. If the rent is subsidized based on the resident's income, the person is usually allowed to stay as long as he or she remains in the low-income bracket. Permanent supportive housing combines this housing assistance with services for homeless persons with disabilities. Usually, they serve individuals and members of that household who have serious mental illnesses, chronic substance abuse problems, physical disabilities, or AIDS and related diseases. People may receive these services either at the housing site or through partnering agencies.

Preventing homelessness is a cost-effective intervention. Funds can be used to pay expenses and resolve situations in certain circumstances so that individuals and households can avoid homelessness, receive support services to help them pay for the cost of their housing, and develop skills and employment to avoid a recurrence of the problem. Moving people rapidly into permanent housing has also been shown to be cost effective and is the goal now of several nongovernmental organizations.

Food

When families and individuals live in poverty, they frequently have to make impossible choices between paying the rent, buying food, or buying essential medications. This can lead to homelessness and decreased ability to provide adequate food. Homelessness and hunger are inseparably linked. Those experiencing homelessness often experience food insecurity. The United Nations World Food Summit in 1996 defined **food security** as existing "when all people at all times have access to sufficient, safe, nutritious food to maintain a healthy and active life."[64] This definition of food security usually includes both physical and economic access to food that meets people's dietary needs as well as their food preferences. In 2017, in the United States, 15.1% of households experienced food insecurity at some time during the year.[65] The rate was higher (18.1%) in households with children.[65] Nonprofit organizations frequently help to provide food security through private donations to food pantries, food banks, and soup kitchens.

Health Care

Steps are being taken to help address some of the barriers the homeless face in trying to attain health care, especially access to health care. In many cities, health-care services are provided at places frequented by those experiencing homelessness, for example, soup kitchens and shelters. Outreach workers often go to the locations where the homeless are and tell them about the availability of different health-care resources. Some communities have mobile medical units that can travel to the patients' locations. Some of these mobile medical units are very specialized (such as only providing dental care), and others provide primary care and referral services.

Policy

The housing-first model promotes providing immediate housing with supportive services and is gaining traction nationally. The underlying premise of housing-first is that obtaining health, security, and wellness is best achieved by first providing housing without other prerequisites.[66] Supportive housing is effective for those who have had a long history of homelessness, for homeless veterans, and for those who are homeless with mental health and addiction problems.[66] Preventing families from becoming homeless, along with very rapid rehousing if the family does become homeless, is also effective policy. Preventing individuals with disabilities from becoming homeless is also effective and requires the collaboration of health-care providers, social workers, and individuals who monitor subsidized supportive housing. Providing more and better mental health services, effective services to individuals who have suffered domestic violence, and creating additional addiction treatment centers also will have an impact on preventing homelessness and will provide the additional support services necessary for individuals to keep their housing.

Immigrants, Migrants, Refugees, and Asylees

In the United States, migrants, immigrants, refugees, and asylees are often grouped together as one population, even though they are distinctly different populations.

They are distinct, though sometimes overlapping, populations with different risk factors for adverse health outcomes and different barriers to achieving optimal health. The recent political debate over whether to admit immigrants or grant asylum highlights the importance of understanding the differences among these populations as well as understanding how membership in one of these groups increases vulnerability in different ways.

Immigrants

Immigrant as defined by the Merriam-Webster dictionary is a person who comes to a country to take up permanent residence.[67] In the glossary of terms on the U.S. Department of Homeland Security (DHS) Web site, a reader looking up the term immigrant is referred to "Permanent Resident Alien." A permanent resident alien is "An alien admitted to the United States as a lawful permanent resident"[68] such as a person who is not a citizen but who entered the country with a valid visa, or obtained a work permit, as well as permission to stay indefinitely. **Illegal alien** is a term sometimes used to describe those who enter a country without proper permission and with the intent of becoming permanent residents. For example, under the definition of permanent resident alien in the DHS glossary of terms is this qualifier: "... however, the Immigration and Nationality Act (INA) broadly defines an immigrant as any alien in the United States, except one legally admitted under specific nonimmigrant categories (INA section 101(a)(15)). An illegal alien who entered the United States without inspection, for example, would be strictly defined as an immigrant under the INA but is not a permanent resident alien."[68] Other terms in use include *undocumented workers* and *undocumented immigrants* based on a concern over possible stigma associated with the use of the term illegal alien. These two terms are not listed in the DHS glossary. (See the DHS Web site for more detail on the different categories of immigrants and different types of visas.)

Migrant Workers

The term **migrant worker** is used to describe those who move from place to place to get work and who often work in another country that is not their own.[69,70] Globally, there are approximately 32 million migrants (3.1% of the global population).[70] Across the globe, migrant workers are at increased risk for exploitation because of limited social protection, inequalities in the labor market, and increased risk for human trafficking.[71]

Migrant workers are at greater risk for experiencing modern slavery. Modern slavery includes the selling of people in public markets; women forced into marriage to provide labor; and forced work inside factories or fishing boats where salaries are withheld, or under threats of violence, that is, labor extracted through force, coercion, or threats.[71] The Walk Free foundation and the International Labour Organization developed the Global Slavery Index to help address the gap in knowledge related to the extent of modern slavery. They reported that, in 2016, there were 40.3 million persons living in modern slavery, 24.9 million were in forced labor, and 15.4 million were living in a forced marriage. Regions with a high level of modern slavery include Africa and Asia. However, data from Arab states in the Middle East were not available, countries that host 17.6 million migrant workers.[72] Modern slavery is also a concern in the U.S., with a particular focus on sex trafficking, forced labor, bonded labor, child labor, and domestic servitude (see Box 7-4).[73]

Migrant Agricultural Workers in the U.S.

In the U.S., migrant agricultural workers provide much of the labor in the agricultural industry, with an estimated 2.5 to 3 million migratory and seasonal agricultural workers in the United States.[73, 74] Not all migrant

---

BOX 7–4 ■ U.S. Department of State's Answer to the Question "What is Modern Slavery?"

"Trafficking in persons," "human trafficking," and "modern slavery" are used as umbrella terms to refer to both sex trafficking and compelled labor. The Trafficking Victims Protection Act of 2000 (Pub. L. 106-386), as amended (TVPA), and the Protocol to Prevent, Suppress, and Punish Trafficking in Persons, Especially Women and Children, supplementing the United Nations Convention against Transnational Organized Crime (the Palermo Protocol) describe this as compelled service using a number of different terms, including involuntary servitude, slavery or practices similar to slavery, debt bondage, and forced labor.

Human trafficking can include, but does not require, movement. People may be considered trafficking victims regardless of whether they were born into a state of servitude, were exploited in their home town, were transported to the exploitative situation, previously consented to work for a trafficker, or participated in a crime as a direct result of being trafficked. At the heart of this phenomenon is the traffickers' aim to exploit and enslave their victims and the myriad coercive and deceptive practices they use to do so.

Source: (73)

agricultural workers are immigrants. In the 2018 report by the National Center for Farm Worker Health, 47% of crop workers were unauthorized, 31% were citizens, 22% had work visas, and 73% were foreign born.[74] Under Title 29 of the U.S. Code, "A **migrant agricultural worker** is a person employed in agricultural work of a seasonal or other temporary nature who is required to be absent overnight from his or her permanent place of residence. Exceptions are immediate family members of an agricultural employer or a farm labor contractor, and temporary H-2A foreign workers. (H-2A temporary foreign workers are nonimmigrant aliens authorized to work in agricultural employment in the United States for a specified time period, normally less than 1 year.)"[75] In 2018, farmers and agricultural businesses that relied heavily on migrant workers blamed severe shortages of labor on the tightening of immigration laws in the U.S.[76,77]

Because migrant workers move around or are frequently away from their permanent place of residence, establishing residency for benefits (e.g., federal assistance through food stamps) is often difficult for this group. Most of these workers have no access to workers' compensation or disability compensation. Many migrant farm workers employed in planting and harvesting follow the crops for jobs. For example, major agricultural work starts in California, Texas, and Florida. These starting points result in three streams of workers: the western stream from California to Washington State, the midwestern stream from Texas to all the midwestern states, and the eastern stream from Florida through Ohio to Maine (Fig. 7-6). These streams represent how migrant workers follow the jobs, especially in agriculture, where the time to harvest crops changes with the seasons. In the past few years, these streams have been less distinct.[74]

Major Migratory Streams for Farmworkers in the United States

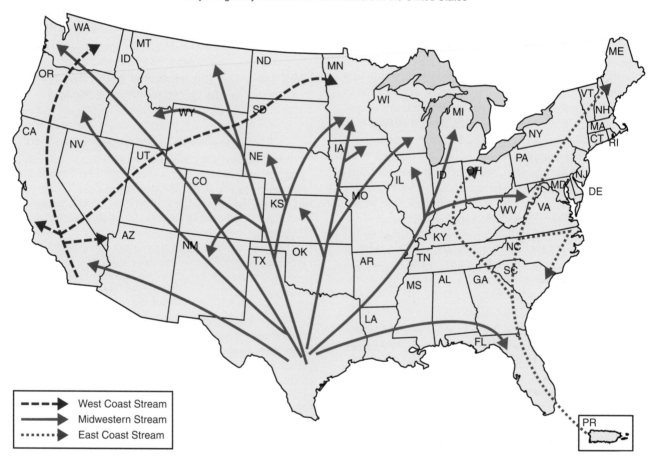

Figure 7-6 Migratory patterns of migrant farm workers. *(Copyright (c) 1985–2002 National Center for Farm Worker Health, Inc. Used with permission. Retrieved from http://www.ncfh.org/)*

This group is particularly vulnerable for multiple reasons. In 2017, only 31% of migrant agricultural workers reported that they could speak English well and 27% could not speak English at all.[74] In relation to health care, more than a third were uninsured (36.3%) and 63.5% lived below the poverty level.[78]

Impact on Health

Poor, substandard housing is frequently a part of the life of a migrant or seasonal farm worker. If a person has to continually move to find work, it is more likely that the person moving will not have long-term or stable housing, putting him or her into one of the groups of tertiary, secondary, or possibly even primary homelessness. The health of migrant workers reflects their poverty and poor living situations, making them vulnerable to conditions no longer thought of as being prevalent in the United States. Most foreign workers are from Mexico[78] and have a higher incidence of tuberculosis, other communicable diseases, and poor nutrition in addition to having daily exposure to the dangerous occupation of farming and to pesticides. The workers live in crowded housing and working conditions, making them six times more likely to develop tuberculosis when compared with other workers.[78]

● APPLYING PUBLIC HEALTH SCIENCE

The Case of the Wandering Diabetic

Public Health Science Topics Covered:

- Focused community assessment
- Partnership building
- Advocacy

Sara, a nurse at the local nurse-managed clinic run by the hospital, met Manuel and listened to his story. He told Sara he had lived in 12 states, following the jobs. He had dropped out of high school to help raise his siblings, and with the tough economy and his lack of education he couldn't find anything except seasonal and other temporary work. This meant he held many different jobs as he traveled from place to place to find work. He worked as a ranch hand, did construction work, and followed the promise of riches to the oil fields of North Dakota. When the oil fields started letting workers go, there were few other jobs available. He returned to his home base in New Mexico and slept on friends' couches for the first few months he was in town. After 4 months, he had worn out his welcome.

Finally, Manuel found a job as an agricultural worker that had a workers' tent city where he could live. Manuel came to the clinic because he was a type 1 diabetic, and with the lack of reliable refrigeration, he was no longer able to store his insulin and hoped that Sara had some ideas about where he could store it. He also had sores on his feet that worried him. He told Sara that many people in the tent city had limited resources, minimal electricity, and only a central water spigot that served as the main source of water for the workers and their children.

After assessing her patient, Sara wondered if the lack of refrigeration and sanitation concerns were part of the underlying health problems being experienced by Manuel and some of her other patients. She started by gathering data about the tent city and its residents. She investigated the unmet health needs of this group of people and examined the impact of the squalid living conditions using a qualitative survey of the residents (see Chapter 4). Many of the respondents to the survey stated that they had recently experienced infections. Others had noncommunicable diseases that they were unable to manage properly.

Based on this preliminary assessment, Sara collaborated with other health partners to come up with solutions. She contacted her colleagues at the hospital, including the diabetes management experts and communicable disease experts. She also contacted the local health department to request assistance in examining options for this group. Next, she formed a coalition with her colleagues and other agencies, and used this coalition to inform policy makers about the situation at the tent city. By doing so, she advocated for the health of her patients. Sara applied for a grant to extend the clinic services to include a weekly outreach clinic at the tent city. She also found a local company to donate a generator so that Steven and other residents would have electricity for refrigeration to safely store their medications.

Sara used a public health approach to the problem. She gathered data to examine the problem and applied her problem-solving skills in helping a population. She worked with the public health department and the hospital to evaluate the outreach program so that they would have evidence to share that would help other free clinics and public health departments that were trying to solve the same problem.

Intervention and Services for Migrant Workers

Despite efforts at the federal level to help with building housing, substandard housing continues to be an issue for migrant workers.[79,80] There is the option of housing located on the farm, but that generally means lower wages because housing rent is removed from the base salary, and there's no guarantee that the housing will be adequate. The off-the-farm option usually consists of very makeshift shelters, not close to any basic infrastructure, and with limited or absent water access and sanitation.

Farm workers, as a vulnerable population (low literacy levels, different culture and language, poverty), have difficulty accessing health care, paying for health care, and participating in prevention activities. Migrant farmers usually work for an hourly wage or per item harvested or planted, and do not have the luxury of sick time or paid time to visit a health-care provider. According to the National Center for Farm Worker Health, migrant workers are faced with numerous barriers related to accessing adequate health care. These include the cost of coverage, lack of health-care providers in the area, and lack of transportation to health-care services.[78] Another issue is the cultural and language barrier that prevents workers from knowing about accessible services.[74, 78]

Children of migrant workers are especially susceptible to unmet health needs. More than half (57%) of migrant workers are parents. In addition, an estimated 300,000 to 500,000 children under the age of 18 are engaged in agricultural work. Not only do children of migrant workers have less access to care, their mothers are often exposed to toxic pesticides during pregnancy. More than one half have unmet medical needs.[81]

Policy

At the global level, goal 10 of the United Nations' Sustainable Development Goals includes as one of the targets: "Facilitate orderly, safe, regular, and responsible migration and mobility of people, including through the implementation of planned and well-managed migration policies".[82] In the U.S., the Immigration and Nationality Act (INA), protects immigrant and workers' against discrimination. The law specifically prohibits "1) citizenship status discrimination in hiring, firing, or recruitment or referral for a fee; 2) national origin discrimination in hiring, firing, or recruitment or referral for a fee; 3) unfair documentary practices during the employment eligibility verification, Form I-9 and E-Verify; and 4) retaliation or intimidation."[83]

The Affordable Care Act (ACA) does not directly benefit migrant workers, especially those who are undocumented. Employers with 50 or more employees are mandated to provide health-care insurance. Because farms use seasonal workers, the ACA uses a different formula. If the farm employs on average more than 50 full-time seasonal workers for fewer than 121 days, then the farm is not required to provide health-care coverage. In addition, workers who are undocumented are not required to purchase individual health-care insurance. This may leave a segment of the workforce uninsured. In some cases, large farms are establishing clinics. Many migrant workers currently pay for health care out of pocket. Thus, further policy may be needed to cover the cost of health care to this population.

Refugees and Asylees

The 1980 Refugee Act in the United States, which is still in effect, defines a **refugee** as "a person outside of his or her country of nationality who is unable or unwilling to return because of persecution or a well-founded fear of persecution."[84] This definition is based on a United Nations 1951 Convention that states, "any person who, owing to a well-founded fear of being persecuted for reasons of race, religion, nationality, membership in a particular social group, or political opinion, is outside the country of his nationality and is unable or, owing to such fear, is unwilling to avail himself of the protection of that country; or who not having a nationality and being outside the country of his former habitual residence as a result of such events, is unable or, owing such fear, is unwilling to return to it."[85]

Refugees and **asylees** seeking resettlement in the United States constitute a special type of immigrant. An asylee is also a person "who is unable or unwilling to return to his or her country of nationality because of persecution or a well-founded fear of persecution on account of race, religion nationality, membership in a particular social group, of political opinion."[86] The distinction between the two is that a person asking to receive refugee status is outside the United States and seeking to enter, whereas an asylee is a person already residing in the United States when applying for asylum.[86] Other terms used to describe forcibly displaced persons include internally displaced persons, stateless persons, and returnees (Box 7-5).[87] The challenges facing refugees are the subsequent political issues around who should and who should not be allowed to seek asylum, with political parties taking sides.

Refugees Seeking Asylum

In 2017, 68.5 million persons worldwide were forced from their homes by disasters, conflict, and persecution, up from 43.3 million in 2010. According to the UN HCR, every 20 minutes "… people leave everything behind to escape war, persecution, or terror."[88] Of these, 25.4 million

BOX 7–5 ■ Types of Forcibly Displaced Persons

Refugees

A refugee is someone who fled his or her home and country owing to "a well-founded fear of persecution because of his/her race, religion, nationality, membership in a particular social group, or political opinion", according to the United Nations 1951 Refugee Convention. Many refugees are in exile to escape the effects of natural or human-made disasters.

Asylum Seekers

Asylum seekers say they are refugees and have fled their homes as refugees do, but their claim to refugee status is not yet definitively evaluated in the country to which they fled.

Internally Displaced Persons

Internally Displaced Persons (IDPs) are people who have not crossed an international border but have moved to a different region than the one they call home within their own country.

Stateless Persons

Stateless persons do not have a recognized nationality and do not belong to any country. Statelessness situations are usually caused by discrimination against certain groups. Their lack of identification—a citizenship certificate—can exclude them from access to important government services, including health care, education, or employment.

Returnees

Returnees are former refugees who return to their own countries or regions of origin after time in exile. Returnees need continuous support and reintegration assistance to ensure that they can rebuild their lives at home.

Source: (87)

TABLE 7–3 ■ Refugees Accepted by Country

Country	Approximate Number of Refugees Hosted
Turkey	3.5 million
Pakistan	1.4 million
Lebanon	998,900
Islamic Republic of Iran	979,000
Germany	970,400
Bangladesh	932,200
Sudan	906,600

Source: (88)

Refugees seeking asylum are often in a position of insecurity and unknown outcomes, many remaining in refugee camps for several years as the problems resolve in their own country. There currently are three suggestions for a permanent solution to the temporary refugee settlements. The preferred solution is for the refugees and asylees to be repatriated, returning to their home country when it is once again safe. However, this must be voluntary and currently is occurring less frequently. If they can't go home, there are two other options—they can stay in the host country, which most host countries do not want, or request resettlement to a third country.[88]

Impact on Health

Refugees victimized by war and/or political repression, famine, or natural disasters frequently experience food insecurity, poor sanitation, exposure to multiple communicable diseases, violence, and mental health issues with limited medical care both while fleeing their country of origin and while in refugee settlement camps in the host country. Many live in refugee camps, some for several years, with a major impact on their health. Those living in refugee camps are at greater risk for a number of health issues including chronic disease[90], intimate partner violence,[91] and poor sanitary conditions.[92] Children in refugee camps are at increased risk for stunted growth due to chronic malnutrition.[93]

Mental health poses a significant health risk for refugees. Post-traumatic stress disorder (PTSD) and depression are common diagnoses among those in the resettlement programs who have had severe exposure to violence.[94-96] Silove, Ventevogel, and Rees presented an ecological model related to the mental health risk factors associated with migration including events prior to migration, the stresses that occur during migration, and

were refugees and 3.1 million were seeking asylum. More than half (57%) were from three countries, South Sudan, Afghanistan, and Syria. Turkey accepted the highest number of refugees (Table 7-3).[88]

In the U.S., the Trump administration announced in September of 2018 that the maximum number of refugees the U.S. would accept in 2019 would be dropped from 45,000 (the cap in 2018) to 30,000, the lowest number in decades. Given the total number of refugees worldwide (25.4 million), this represents only 0.12% of refugees worldwide. Despite the existing cap of 45,000, only 19,899 refugees were admitted into the U.S. between October 2017 and the end of August 2018.[89]

events that occur during the resettlement phase. They state that these events represent a "… dynamic inter-relationship of past traumatic experiences, ongoing daily stressors, and the background disruptions of core psychosocial systems, the scope extending beyond the individual to the conjugal couple and the family."[96]

Intervention and Services

The U.S. Public Health Service requires a health screening for all immigrants and refugees prior to departure from their country of origin or their host countries. Refugees can be kept from immigrating if they have untreated communicable disease, an untreated substance abuse disorder, or a mental illness that causes them to respond violently. If the refugee agrees to treatment, then he or she can be reconsidered for immigration.[97] Upon arrival, refugees are eligible for 8 months of Medicaid or Refugee Medical Assistance (RMA).[98] During this 8-month period, refugees need to complete required health screenings, begin to understand the health-care system, begin to learn English, and seek out and secure paid employment. After the 8-month period is over, many are then eligible for expanded health insurance options under the ACA.[98] They are also encouraged to apply if eligible for other subsidy programs, such as Supplemental Security Income, for which they are entitled in their status as a refugee.

Based on current global trends, the refugee issue constitutes a complex crisis. Politically, countries struggle with whether to accept refugees while millions continue to flee conflict and violence. Unaccompanied children and orphans further complicate the crisis. Central to the crisis is the ongoing short- and long-term consequences on the physical and mental health of the refugees. Health-care professionals continue to provide a central role in addressing the adverse effect of migration on populations seeking work, asylum, and resettlement because it is the nurses, physicians, and other health-care providers who provide health screening and treatment, and contribute to overall planning for the care of these extremely vulnerable populations.

Incarcerated and Correctional Populations

According to the U.S. Department of Justice, the **incarcerated population** includes persons living under the jurisdiction of state or federal prisons, and in the custody of local jails. The **correctional population** includes the incarcerated population as well as persons living in the community while supervised on probation or parole.[99]

According to global data the U.S. has the highest incarceration rate in the world. In 2017, the U.S. incarceration rate was 655 inmates per 100,000 people compared to 77 per 100,000 in Germany.[100] This is an alarming statistic for the sheer numbers, but equally important because once individuals have a history of incarceration, they have limited opportunities for employment, education, housing, and a stable family life. This in turn has significant impact on health.[101]

Persons Experiencing Incarceration

Based on the U.S. Department of Justice data in 2016, a total of 2,162,400 persons were incarcerated in the U.S., out of an estimated 6,613,500 persons supervised by U.S. adult correctional systems or approximately 1 in 38 adults age 18 or older in the United States.[102] Overall the jail incarceration rate in the U.S. was 860 prison or jail inmates for every 100,000 adults ages 18 and older, down from 1,000 per 100,000 in 2006 to 2008.[103]

African Americans were disproportionately represented in this population with an incarceration rate among Non-Hispanic black adults 3.5 times higher than non-Hispanic white adults (599 per 100,000 versus 171 per 100,000, respecively).[103, 104] However, looking at trends over the past decade, there has been a drop in the incarceration rate for African American men (9.8%) and women (30.7%) while at the same time there has been an increase in incarceration rate for white men (8.5%) and women (47.1%). The incarceration rate for Latino men declined 2.2% and rose 23.3% for Latina women.[104]

The U.S., even in states with more progressive approaches to incarceration, has a higher rate of incarceration than almost all other countries.[105] However, many of the issues related to incarceration remain the same across countries. Issues include the debate related to punishment versus rehabilitation and what constitutes progressive reform related to imprisonment.

Impact on Health

Under the 1976 U.S. Supreme Court ruling *Estelle v. Gamble*, states are compelled to provide a constitutionally adequate level of medical care for those who are incarcerated or care that generally meets a "community standard."[106] As the cost of health care increases, the cost to the state prison system increases as well. Not only does incarceration itself increase a person's vulnerability, vulnerable subpopulations are over-represented in prisons and jails. This translates into a greater need for health care. For example, the prevalence of hepatitis C is higher in prisons.[107] In addition there is an increasing prevalence of noncommunicable diseases, and a high prevalence of mental health and substance use disorders.[101] The increase in the number of incarcerated older adults presents an emerging challenge for the correctional system due to a higher prevalence of noncommunicable diseases as well as cognitive disorders such as Alzheimer's disease.[108]

The health needs of the incarcerated and correctional population reflect the health needs of the other populations they represent—in general, a vulnerable population of poverty with limited access to health care, low education levels, at-risk drug and alcohol use, mental health issues, and communicable disease such as hepatitis and HIV. All of these problems are amplified in prison. The stresses of prison life, poor diet, and frequently less than adequate medical care often exacerbate noncommunicable conditions such as diabetes and hypertension.

Men and women who are incarcerated or in the correctional system experience higher rates of comorbidities of substance use and psychiatric disorders. These psychiatric diagnoses include major depressive disorder, antisocial personality disorder, anxiety, PTSD, borderline personality disorders, and eating disorders. In one study, incarcerated women with a history of at-risk drug and alcohol use were nearly twice as likely to have affective disorder, a major depressive disorder, PTSD, or borderline personality disorder as women in the community.[101] With 2.4 million schoolchildren having an incarcerated parent, there is also a collateral impact on families, including both significant economic effects and major mental health effects on the children.[109]

Policy

Approaching the issue of incarceration requires implementing policy across the continuum of upstream, midstream, and downstream. An example of upstream policy is working with high-risk youth at the community level to promote education, provide opportunity for advancement, and prevent incarceration. Examples of midstream policies include providing alternatives to jail and prison for minor offenses, promoting education through these alternative sentencing options, providing treatment for mental health and substance use disorders, and providing opportunities for employment. This requires a cultural shift from zero tolerance to a broader concept of early rehabilitation and remediation efforts outside of the jail or prison to help prevent later, more serious crimes. Downstream interventions provided within the context of rehabilitation rather than punishment have the potential to

help vulnerable populations obtain access to education and behavioral health services with the intention of improving their opportunities of gainful employment on release.

■ EVIDENCE-BASED PRACTICE
Use of Agonist Treatment for Persons Experiencing Incarceration

In the U.S., more than half of persons incarcerated in state prisons and more than 60% of those incarcerated in jails meet the criteria for a substance abuse disorder.[1] Yet few prisons or jails provide treatment for Opioid Use Disorder (OUD) to their inmates.[2]

Practice Statement: During incarceration persons with an OUD should be offered medication-assisted treatment (MAT), the gold standard for treatment of an OUD (Chapter 11).

Targeted Outcome: All persons incarcerated in jails or prisons diagnosed with an OUD will be provided with MAT as well as direct links to providers of MAT in their community on release.

Supporting Evidence: The effectiveness of MAT to treat OUDs in the general population is well documented.[3] There is emerging evidence that MAT delivered to persons while incarcerated can result in better outcomes. In one study conducted in Britain, "... prison-based opioid substitution therapy was associated with a 75% reduction in all-cause mortality and an 85% reduction in fatal drug-related poisoning in the first month after release."[4]

Recommended Approaches: MAT can be delivered using three different medications. Methadone and buprenorphine work as opioid agonists and thus suppress and reduce cravings for the abused drug. Naltrexone is an opioid antagonist that works in the brain to prevent opiate effects (e.g., feelings of well-being, pain relief) as well as the desire to take opiates. Choosing which medication to administer is done on a case-by-case basis (see Chapter 11). In addition to the administration of MAT, during the period of time a person is incarcerated additional psychosocial treatment should be provided, as well as a warm handoff at the time of release. That is, the person should not only be told where to obtain a continuation of MAT but have a firm appointment and evidence that they have any needed transportation assistance to make their first appointment at the clinic, primary care office, or treatment facility.

References

1. Bronson, J., & Stroop, J. (2017, June). Drug use, dependence, and abuse among state prisoners and jail inmates, 2007-2009. *U.S. Department of Justice Special Report*. Retrieved from https://www.bjs.gov/content/pub/pdf/dudaspji0709.pdf
2. Lopez, G. (2018, Mar 26). How America's prisons are fueling the opioid epidemic. *Vox*. Retrieved from https://www.vox.com/policy-and-politics/2018/3/13/17020002/prison-opioid-epidemic-medications-addiction
3. Substance Abuse and Mental Health Services Administration. (2015). *Medication and counseling treatment*. Retrieved from https://www.samhsa.gov/medication-assisted-treatment/treatment#medications-used-in-mat
4. Hedrich, D., Alves, P., Farrell, M., Stöver, H., Møller, L., & Mayet, S. (2012). The effectiveness of opioid maintenance treatment in prison settings: A systematic review. *Addiction, 107*(3), 501–517. https://doi-org.ezp.welch.jhmi.edu/10.1111/j.1360-0443.2011.03676.x

Lesbian, Gay, Bisexual, Transgender, Queer+

According to the WHO, persons who do not conform to established gender norms often face stigma, discriminatory practices, and/or social exclusion. This can adversely affect health through increased susceptibility to diseases as well as their mental and physical health. It can also result in decreased access to health services, all of which can result in poorer health outcomes.[110] In the U.S. and in other high-income countries, LGBTQ+ persons have experienced growing inclusion into the mainstream of society as evidenced by the increasing recognition of LGBTQ+ marriages. Despite this growing acceptance, those who identify as LGBTQ+ continue to experience discrimination from friends, family, and others, with increased risk for adverse health outcomes and becoming victims of violence. From a public health perspective, LGBTQ+ persons' risk for poorer health outcomes requires action at the population level. However, before health-care professionals can address the health-care needs of this population, they must first understand the underlying social constructs associated with the LGBTQ+ community.

The traditional social construct focuses on the characteristics of women and men including the "… norms, roles, and relationships of and between groups of women and men."[110] Moving away from this traditional construct is the presentation of gender identification and sexual orientation occurring across a continuum rather than in the more traditional binary model of female or male. This continuum includes persons who identify as straight (cisgender), gay, lesbian, bisexual, transgender, agender, or other gender-based terms (LGBTQ+) (see Box 7-6).[111] Understanding these terms requires shifting from only a biological approach to a broader understanding of how we view ourselves. As depicted in the graphic, Gender Bread Person, this involves an intricate interplay of our gender identity, our gender expression, and who we wish to be with sexually and romantically (see Fig. 7-7). This not only includes gender identity but also gender expression, our biological sex, as well as who we are sexually attracted to and who we are romantically attached to. For example, a cisgender person identifies

---

BOX 7–6 ■ Gender Identity Terms

Asexual: The lack of a sexual attraction or desire for other people.

Androgynous: Identifying and/or presenting as neither distinguishably masculine nor feminine.

Bisexual: A person emotionally, romantically, or sexually attracted to more than one sex, gender, or gender identity although not necessarily simultaneously, in the same way, or to the same degree.

Cisgender: A term used to describe someone whose gender identity aligns with the sex assigned to them at birth.

Gay: A person who is emotionally, romantically, or sexually attracted to members of the same gender.

Gender fluid: A person who does not identify with a single fixed gender and expresses a fluid or unfixed gender identity.

Genderqueer: A term for people who reject notions of static categories of gender and embrace a fluidity of gender identity and often, although not always, sexual orientation.

Lesbian: A woman who is emotionally, romantically, or sexually attracted to other women.

Queer: A term people often use to express fluid identities and orientations. Often used interchangeably with "LGBTQ."

Transgender: An umbrella term for people whose gender identity and/or expression is different from cultural and social expectations based on the sex they were assigned at birth.

Source: (111)

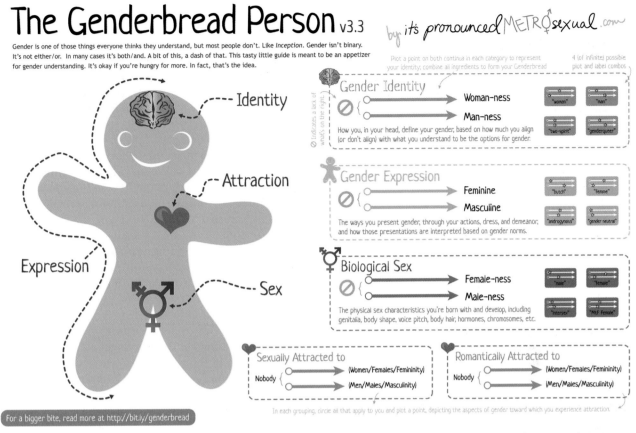

Figure 7-7 Gender Bread Person. (*Artist Sam Killerman, uncopyrighted. Retrieved from http://itspronouncedmetrosexual.com/ genderbread-person/*)

with the gender they were assigned to at birth, they express themselves in that gender, and they are sexually and romantically attracted to cisgender persons assigned to a different gender at birth.

The challenge for health-care providers is to provide an opportunity for patients to share their identity in relation to gender and sexual orientation in a way that is accepting. In 2011, the Joint Commission, the primary accreditation body for health-care facilities, stated that "Admitting, registration, and all other patient forms should provide options that are inclusive of LGBTQ+ patients and families, and should allow LGBTQ+ patients to self-identify if they choose to do so."[112] Yet most health admission and assessment documents continue to use the binary approach of male or female. In addition, few medical schools or nursing schools include essential content related to caring for LGBTQ+ persons in their curriculum.[113]

Another problem is the lack of data on LGBTQ+ persons due to how health surveys ask the gender question.

To address this, HP 2020 included two measurable objectives under the new topic of Lesbian, Gay, Bisexual, and Transgender Health with targets for increasing the number of population-based data systems that include questions related to sexual orientation and gender identity at the state and national level.[114]

■ HEALTHY PEOPLE
Lesbian, Gay, Bisexual, and Transgender Health

Goal: Improve the health, safety, and well-being of lesbian, gay, bisexual, and transgender (LGBT) individuals.

Overview: LGBT individuals encompass all races and ethnicities, religions, and social classes. Sexual orientation and gender identity questions are not asked on most national or state surveys, making it difficult to estimate the number of LGBT individuals and their health needs.[114]

Midcourse Review: Of the two measurable objectives, objective one (Increase the number of population-based data systems used to monitor Healthy People 2020 objectives that include in their core a standardized set of questions that identify lesbian, gay, bisexual, and transgender populations) showed improvement. Objective two (Increase the number of states, territories, and the District of Columbia that include questions that identify sexual orientation and gender identity on state level surveys or data systems) had little or no improvement.[115]

LGBTQ+ and Health

According to a Gallup poll, in 2017, 4.5% of Americans identified as LGBTQ+ with 5.1% of women identifying as LGBTQ+ and 3.9% of men. This reflects an increase mostly in millennials.[116] Persons who identify as LGBTQ+ reflect a diverse population across all racial and ethnic groups.[117] They are also at increased risk for poorer health compared to their heterosexual peers. Some of these differences are attributable to differences in sexual behavior, but the underlying issues for those who identify as LGBTQ+ "… are associated with social and structural inequities, such as the stigma and discrimination that LGBTQ+ populations experience".[117] They are at increased risk for communicable diseases, suicide, mental health issues, and substance use disorders often linked to discrimination and social isolation.[117]

Another health issue for the LGBTQ+ community is the increased risk of being a victim of violence, specifically hate crimes. Persons who identify as LGBTQ+ are more apt to be victims of hate crimes than any other minority group.[118] The Orlando, Florida, mass shooting in 2016 highlighted the violence attached to these hate crimes. Adolescents and adults also experience partner violence.[119,120] Park and Mykhyalyshyn explained that, as LGBTQ+ persons become more an accepted part of American society, those opposed to this community become more radicalized and less tolerant.[118]

Providing appropriate care to persons based on how they identify themselves in relation to gender is an important first step. Health-care delivery to all persons must occur within the context of the person. For nurses, this begins with a clear understanding of the complexity of gender identity, gender expression, and sexual orientation. From a public health perspective, it requires advocating for policies that support a more inclusive approach to health care across the continuum of gender. It also requires policies aimed at reducing hate crimes, stigma, and social isolation, the main drivers of disparity in health for those who identify as LGBTQ+.

At-Risk LGBTQ+ Groups

Civil rights expansions, most notably the U.S. Supreme Court decision in Obergefell vs. Hodges (5/15/15), which established the right to gay marriage in all 50 states, has encouraged more openness and societal acceptance of LGBTQ+ individuals and families. However, despite much research, landmark legal rulings, and the increasing willingness of individuals to publicly identify themselves as LGBTQ+, homophobia and its resulting behaviors of discrimination, violence, and shunning remain prominent in all areas of our society. Three subgroups of the LGBTQ+ community are especially vulnerable and face daunting barriers to leading a physically and emotionally healthy life: transgender youth, LGBTQ+ elders, and gay/bisexual men and women with HIV/AIDS.

Transgender youth include an increasing number of very young children (ages 3 years and older) who are expressing gender nonconforming identities (gender dysphoria). Parents of these young children find themselves searching for medical assistance and support as they navigate uncharted territory. These children are also vulnerable to bullying and societal/familial denial of their expressed gender, circumstances that can lead to depression, anxiety, and other problems that can inhibit a healthy social and physical development. Medical support may not be readily available outside of large metropolitan areas, and local community and educational support are often scarce. Older transgender youth are among our most vulnerable population groups. They are at high risk for family rejection, homelessness, substance use, risky sexual behavior, depression and suicide, as well as targets of sexual violence.[121]

LBGTQ+ elders face a variety of challenges as they grow older. Like their non-gay counterparts, they often feel socially isolated and less able to provide for themselves or live independently. However, having experienced the depths of homophobia in their earlier years, the rejection of family and being "in the closet" at work and in their community, LGBTQ+ elders tend to be mistrustful of mainstream medical and social services. Fearing discrimination and rejection, they are often wary of sharing their sexual orientation with their medical and social service providers, or even seeking out such services when needed. Many have already experienced insensitivity and discrimination by health care and social service providers in their younger years.[122]

Gay/bisexual men and women with HIV/AIDS continue to be marginalized in our society for several reasons.

The stigmas of HIV/AIDS and homophobia have not diminished in many rural areas and among some ethnic, cultural, and religious groups. This reality leads many LGBT+ people with HIV/AIDS to avoid accessing medical and social services for fear that their health status will be discovered and result in family rejection and discrimination in employment and housing.[123,124]

Interventions and Policy

In October 2009, the Matthew Shepard and James Byrd, Jr., Hate Crimes Prevention Act was signed into law and makes hate crimes based on sexual orientation, among other offenses, federal crimes in the United States.[125] For the parents of children who express a nonconforming gender identity, there is often confusion and a sense of being an inadequate parent. Unless the family lives near a large urban area, it is unlikely that parents will have access to the medical care, psychosocial services, and educational resources that they and their child will need. This lack of resources is currently being filled by online groups and Web sites, sites where parents and children can search for information and connect with other families. One potential resource for parents is the school nurse (see Chapter 18).

Fortunately, there is a growing awareness in the medical/academic community to provide accurate information to families and their local health providers, as well as a growing number of clinics and clinicians trained to provide services to transgendered youth and their families. The American Psychological Association has published "Guidelines for Psychological Practice with Transgender and Gender Nonconforming People",[126] a comprehensive guide for those professionals working with transgendered people of all ages. In addition, many urban university medical centers and hospitals are establishing clinics and programs for transgendered and gender nonconforming children and young adults.

Medical issues aligned with transgendered youth and children who express a nonconforming gender identity include pharmacologic therapies to address body image issues, depression, anxiety, and suicidal ideations. Social and psychological therapies can address social functioning, peer issues, school adjustment, and family issues as they arise. The availability of these resources is vital to the healthy development of these children in all areas of functioning.

For LGBTQ+ older adults, their invisibility to mainstream elder service providers and medical personnel in many settings significantly diminishes their quality of life.[127] Additionally, the lack of training for staff and residents in most long-term care settings such as assisted living complexes and nursing homes leave LGBTQ+ older adults open to psychological and physical abuse, which can lead to depression and self-isolation. For LGBTQ+ older adults living at home but in need of assistance in a variety of areas, the same problem arises with home care services. Staff may not be trained to respect the individual's LGBTQ+ identity and her/his relationships with others.[127,128]

Understanding the needs of LGBTQ+ older adults is an essential skill for nurses who provide care and begins with not assuming a patient's sexual orientation is heterosexual, and/or dismissing the relationship between two partners. Nurses in all settings need to be understanding of the discrimination and abuse LGBTQ+ older adults may have encountered in their lives and provide a supportive, affirming environment for the patients.[128]

Gay/bisexual men and women with HIV/AIDS present a variety of serious medical problems and psychological issues. Despite the many advances in medical care for people with HIV, there are significant disparities in how these new therapies are utilized in geographic and racial areas. In 2016, the CDC predicted that, if current rates continue, one in two African American gay and bisexual men will be infected with HIV.[129] These statistics clearly demonstrate the need for more comprehensive measures to address the issues of poverty, race, and class inherent in the health care of gay/bisexual men and women with HIV/AIDS.

Community-based organizations can be supportive of LGBTQ+ people and can influence the general community to provide a more inclusive environment. Public campaigns are a way to reach a large number of people with messages challenging homophobia. Schools also can educate young people, confronting widely accepted prejudices. This might include specific curriculum and action against bullying, creating a school environment wherein all students feel comfortable. Political leaders, police departments, health services, broadcasters, and employers can all positively influence the way that the LGBTQ+ population is treated.

■ Summary Points

- Health disparity and vulnerability reflect a complex intersection of risk factors at the individual, community, national, and global levels.
- Social forces such as discrimination and stigma lead to the marginalization of certain segments of our society, resulting in increased levels of marginalization overall.

- Health disparities disproportionately affect members of racial, ethnic, minority, underserved, and vulnerable groups and affect the overall health of the United States.
- Social determinants of health including poverty, access to care, cultural barriers, and education play a role in increasing the vulnerability of certain populations.
- Nurses are uniquely positioned to provide care for vulnerable populations, functioning in a variety of roles through which they enhance health and reduce vulnerability.
- Certain populations like the homeless, migrant workers, immigrants, refugees, the incarcerated, and LGBTQ+ people are more likely to be vulnerable and benefit from specific interventions and changes in policy.

▼ CASE STUDY

Vulnerability extends from the cellular to the global level and increases the risk of adverse health consequences. Financial factors often drive access to the resources necessary to ensure optimal health. The most vulnerable populations live in poverty and often in a community and/or country that lacks the financial resources to provide needed medical care. For example, low-income countries are often unable to treat strep throat due to lack of funding to do basic throat cultures and provide antibiotics when children present with a sore throat. Untreated strep throat can lead to rheumatic fever, which in turn can result in life-threatening damage to the heart valves. One group, Team Heart, composed of 40 to 60 volunteers, started by an intensive care nurse and her husband, a cardiac surgeon, goes to Rwanda once a year to provide needed surgery to persons with rheumatic health disease.

1. Access their Web site at teamheart.org and review their mission. How does this fit into a population approach to disease?
2. Map out the natural history of disease in relation to strep throat, rheumatic fever, and rheumatic heart disease. What are the appropriate prevention steps over the course of the natural history of the disease?
3. The issue of rheumatic heart disease in Rwanda exemplifies the upstream, midstream, and downstream approach to addressing health at the population level. Discuss this in more detail. With limited resources what should be the main focus when addressing this issue in Rwanda?

REFERENCES

1. World Health Organization. (2018). *Social determinants of health*. Retrieved from http://www.who.int/social_determinants/thecommission/finalreport/key_concepts/en/.
2. World Health Organization. (2018). *Infant Mortality*. Retrieved from http://www.who.int/gho/child_health/mortality/neonatal_infant_text/en/.
3. Healthy People 2020. (2017). Disparities. Retrieved from https://www.healthypeople.gov/2020/about/foundation-health-measures/Disparities.
4. World Health Organization. (2002). *Environmental health in emergencies and disasters: a practical guide*. Geneva, Switzerland: Author.
5. Centers for Disease Control and Prevention. (2016). *Health equity: strategies for reducing health disparities*. Retrieved from https://www.cdc.gov/minorityhealth/strategies2016/index.html.
6. Central Intelligence Agency. (2018). *The world fact book country comparison: Life expectancy*. Retrieved from https://www.cia.gov/library/publications/the-world-factbook/rankorder/2102rank.html.
7. Centers for Disease Control and Prevention. (2017). *Mortality in the U.S.* Retrieved from https://www.cdc.gov/nchs/products/databriefs/db293.htm.
8. World Health Organization. (2018). *Social determinants of health*. Retrieved from http://www.who.int/social_determinants/thecommission/finalreport/key_concepts/en/.
9. Rapaport, L. (2018, August 22). Life expectancy declines seen in U.S. and other high-income countries. *Reuters*. Retrieved from https://www.reuters.com/article/us-health-lifeexpancy/life-expectancy-declines-seen-in-u-s-and-other-high-income-countries-idUSKCN1L723R.
10. World Health Organization. (2018). *Equity*. Retrieved from http://www.who.int/healthsystems/topics/equity/en/.
11. United Nations. (1948). *Universal declaration of human rights*. Retrieved from http://www.un.org/en/universal-declaration-human-rights/index.html.
12. World Health Organization. (1978). Declaration of Alma-Ata, International Conference on Primary Care. Retrieved from http://www.who.int/hpr/NPH/docs/declaration_almaata.pdf.
13. Bracken, K. & Specia, M. (28 Aug, 2018). Born too soon in a country at war. Their only hope? This clinic. *New York Times*. Retrieved from https://nyti.ms/2N32bDL.
14. Central Intelligence Agency. (2018). *The world fact book country comparison: Infant mortality*. Retrieved from https://www.cia.gov/library/publications/the-world-factbook/rankorder/2091rank.html.
15. Centers for Disease Control and Prevention. (2018). *Infant mortality*. Retrieved from https://www.cdc.gov/reproductivehealth/maternalinfanthealth/infantmortality.htm.
16. U.S. Department of Health and Human Services. (2018). *Disparities*. Retrieved from https://www.healthypeople.gov/2020/about/foundation-health-measures/disparities.
17. U.S. Department of Health and Human Services. (2018). *Healthy People 2030 framework*. Retrieved from https://www.healthypeople.gov/2020/About-Healthy-People/Development-Healthy-People-2030/Proposed-Framework.

18. National Institute of Environmental Sciences. (2018). *Gene-environment interaction.* Retrieved from https://www.niehs.nih.gov/health/topics/science/gene-env/index.cfm.

19. U.S. Department of Health and Human Services. (2018). *Healthy People 2020 social determinants of health.* Retrieved from https://www.healthypeople.gov/2020/topics-objectives/topic/social-determinants-of-health.

20. World Health Organization. (2018). *About social determinants of health.* Retrieved from http://www.who.int/social_determinants/sdh_definition/en/.

21. Lin, N. (1999). Building a network theory of social capital. *Connections, 22*(1), 28e51.

22. U.S. Department of Health and Human Services. (2018). *Healthy People 2020 midcourse review: Social determinants of health (SDOH).* Retrieved from https://www.cdc.gov/nchs/data/hpdata2020/HP2020MCR-C39-SDOH.pdf.

23. Merriam Webster. (2018). *Definition of social justice.* Retrieved from https://www.merriam-webster.com/dictionary/social%20justice.

24. World Health Organization. (2008). *Commission on social determinants of health final report.* Retrieved from http://www.who.int/social_determinants/thecommission/finalreport/en/.

25. Centers for Disease Controls and Prevention. (2018). *prevalence of both diagnosed and undiagnosed diabetes.* Retrieved from https://www.cdc.gov/diabetes/data/statistics-report/diagnosed-undiagnosed.html.

26. World Health Association. (2017). *Health inequities.* Retrieved from http://www.who.int/features/factfiles/health_inequities/en/.

27. Gaskin, D.J., Thorpe, R.J., McGinty, E.E., Bower, K., Rohde, C., Young, J.H., Dubay, L., et al. (2014). Disparities in diabetes: The nexus of race, poverty, and place. *American Journal of Public Health, 104*(11), 2147–2155. http://doi.org.ezp.welch.jhmi.edu/10.2105/AJPH.2013.301420.

28. Boozary, A.S., & Shojania, K.G. (2018). Pathology of poverty: the need for quality improvement efforts to address social determinants of health. *BMJ Quality & Safety, 27*(6), 421-424. doi:10.1136/bmjqs-2017-007552.

29. World Health Organization. (1948). *The universal declaration of human rights.* Retrieved from http://www.un.org/en/documents/udhr/.

30. World Health Organization. (1978). *Declaration of Alma-Ata, international conference on primary care.* Retrieved from http://www.who.int/hpr/NPH/docs/declaration_almaata.pdf.

31. U.S. Department of Health and Human Services, Office of Public Health and Science, Office of Minority Health. (2008). *A strategic framework for improving racial/ethnic minority health and eliminating racial/ethnic health disparities.* Rockville, MD: Office of Minority Health.

32. Centers for Disease Control and Prevention. (2019). *Health disparities and strategies reports.* Retrieved from https://www.cdc.gov/minorityhealth/chdir/index.html.

33. Office of Minority Health. (2017). *What we do.* Retrieved from https://minorityhealth.hhs.gov/omh/browse.aspx?lvl=1&lvlid=2.

34. U.S. Department of Health and Human Services, Office of Public Health and Science, Office of Minority Health. (2008). *A strategic framework for improving racial/ethnic minority health and eliminating racial/ethnic health disparities.* Rockville, MD: Office of Minority Health.

35. Centers for Disease Control and Prevention. (2017). *Racial and ethnic approaches to community health.* Retrieved from https://www.cdc.gov/nccdphp/dnpao/state-local-programs/reach/.

36. U.S. Census Bureau. (2018). *Poverty thresholds.* Retrieved from https://www.census.gov/data/tables/time-series/demo/income-poverty/historical-poverty-thresholds.html.

37. U.S. Department of Health and Human Services, Office of The Assistant Secretary for Planning and Evaluation. (2018). *Poverty guidelines.* Retrieved from https://aspe.hhs.gov/poverty-guidelines.

38. Semega, J.L., Fontenot, K.R., & Kollar, M.A. (2017). *Income and poverty in the United States: 2016.* U.S. Census Bureau, Report Number P60-259.

39. World Bank. (2011). *What is social capital?* Retrieved from http://web.worldbank.org/WBSITE/EXTERNAL/TOPICS/EXTSOCIALDEVELOPMENT/EXTTSOCIALCAPITAL/0,,contentMDK:20185164~menuPK:418217~pagePK:148956~piPK:216618~theSitePK:401015,00.html.

40. Fauk, N.K., Merry, M.S., Sigilipoe, M.A., Putra, S., Mwanri, L. (2017). Culture, social networks and HIV vulnerability among men who have sex with men in Indonesia. *PLoS ONE, 12*(6), e0178736. https://doi.org/10.1371/journal.pone.0178736.

41. Thomas, S.P., Fine, M.J., Ibrahim, S.A. (2004). Health disparities: the importance of culture and health communication. *American Journal of Public Health, 94*(12), p. 2050.

42. Hall, J.M., Stevens, P.E., & Meleis, A.I. (1994). Marginalization: A guiding concept for valuing diversity in nursing knowledge development. *Advances in Nursing Science, 16*(4), 23-41.

43. Lynam, M., & Cowley, S. (2007). Understanding marginalization as a social determinant of health. *Critical Public Health, 17*(2), 137-149.

44. Merriam-Webster Dictionary. (2018). *Racism.* Retrieved from https://www.merriam-webster.com/dictionary/racism.

45. Pincus, F.L. (1994). "From Individual to Structural Discrimination." In F.L. Pincus and H.J. Ehrlich, *Race and ethnic conflict: Contending views on prejudice, discrimination, and ethnoviolence.* Boulder, Colo.: Westview.

46. Cobbinah, S.S., Lewis, J. (2018). Racism & health: A public health perspective on racial discrimination. *Journal of Evaluation in Clinical Practice, 2018,* 1-4. https://doi.org/10.1111/jep.128944.

47. Paradies, Y., Ben, J., Denson, N., Elias, A., Priest, N., Pieterse, A., Gee, G., et al. (2015). Racism as a determinant of health: A systematic review and meta-analysis. *PLoS ONE, 10*(9), e0138511. doi:10.1371/journal.pone.0138511.

48. Merriam-Webster Dictionary. (2018). *Stigma.* Retrieved from https://www.merriam-webster.com/dictionary/stigma.

49. National Institutes of Health. (2018). *Research involving vulnerable populations.* Retrieved from https://humansubjects.nih.gov/prisoners.

50. American Nurses Association. (2015). *Code of ethics with interpretative statements.* Silver Spring, MD: Author. Retrieved from http://www.nursingworld.org/MainMenuCategories/EthicsStandards/CodeofEthicsforNurses/Code-ofEthics-For-Nurses.html.

51. Murria, A. (2018). Homelessness: A public health problem. *Access, 32*(3), 13-20.

52. Davies, A. & Wood, L.J. (2018). Homeless health care: Meeting the challenges of providing primary care. *Medical Journal Australia, 209*(5), 230-234. doi: 10.5694/mja17.01264.

53. Nicholas, W.C. & Henwood, B.F. (2018). Applying a prevention framework to address homelessness as a population health issue. *Journal of Public Health Policy, 39*, 283. https://doi-org.ezp.welch.jhmi.edu/10.1057/s41271-018-0137-9.

54. Stafford, A., & Wood, L. (2017). Tackling health disparities for people who are homeless? start with social determinants. *International Journal of Environmental Research and Public Health, 14*(12), 1535. http://doi.org.ezp.welch.jhmi.edu/10.3390/ijerph14121535.

55. U.S. Department of Health and Human Services. (2009). *The McKinney-Vento Homeless Assistance Act as amended by S. 896 The Homeless Emergency Assistance and Rapid Transition to Housing (HEARTH) Act of 2009*. Retrieved from http://portal.hud.gov/hudportal/documents/huddoc?id=HAAA_HEARTH.pdf.

56. Government of Western Australia, Department for Child Protection. (n.d.). *What is homelessness?* Retrieved from http://www.childprotection.wa.gov.au/Resources/Documents/StatisticsForMedia/WAHomelessness.pdf.

57. National Coalition for the Homeless. (2018) *Homelessness in America*. Retrieved from http://nationalhomeless.org/about-homelessness/.

58. Housing and Urban Development. (2017). *The 2017 Annual Homeless Assessment Report (AHAR) to Congress*. Retrieved from https://www.hudexchange.info/resources/documents/2017-AHAR-Part-1.pdf.

59. National Alliance to End Homelessness. (2018). *Health and homelessness*. Retrieved from https://endhomelessness.org/homelessness-in-america/what-causes-homelessness/health/.

60. Amato, S., Nobay, F., Amato, D.P., Abar, B., Adler, D. (2018). Sick and unsheltered: Homelessness as a major risk factor for emergency care utilization. *American Journal of Emergency Medicine*, https://doi.org/10.1016/j.ajem.2018.06.001.

61. Baggett, T.P., Liauw, S.S., Hwang, S.W. (2018). Cardiovascular disease and homelessness. *Journal of the American College of Cardiology, 22*, 2585-2597.

62. Kim, M. (2017). Mental illness and homelessness: Facts and figures. *Students in Mental Health Research*. Retrieved http://www.hcs.harvard.edu/~hcht/blog/homelessness-and-mental-health-facts.

63. Savage, C.L., Gillespie, G.L., Lee, R.J., & Lindsell, C. (2008). The effectiveness of a United States nurse managed clinic for the homeless in improving health status. *Health and Social Care in the Community, 16*, 469-475.

64. World Food Summit. (1996). *Rome declaration on world food security*. Retrieved from http://www.fao.org/docrep/003/w3613e/w3613e00.htm.

65. Food Research and Action Center. (2018). *Food hardship in America: A look at national, regional, state, and metropolitan statistical area data on household struggles with hunger*. Retrieved from http://www.frac.org/wp-content/uploads/food-hardship-july-2018.pdf.

66. Haskins, J. (2018). Housing first model gaining momentum. *American Journal Of Public Health, 108*(5), 584. doi:10.2105/AJPH.2018.304378.

67. Merriam Webster Dictionary Immigrant. (n.d.). *Immigrant*. Retrieved from https://www.merriam-webster.com/dictionary/immigrant.

68. U.S. Department of Homeland Security (n.d.). *Definition of terms*. Retrieved from https://www.dhs.gov/immigration-statistics/data-standards-and-definitions/definition-terms#permanent_resident_alien.

69. Dictionary.com. (n.d.). *Migrant*. Retrieved from http://dictionary.reference.com/browse/migrant.

70. International Labor Organization. (2018). *International labour standards on migrant workers*. Retrieved from http://www.ilo.org/global/standards/subjects-covered-by-international-labour-standards/migrant-workers/lang—en/index.htm.

71. Mideroo Foundation. (2018). *Global slavery index*. Retrieved from https://www.globalslaveryindex.org/2018/findings/global-findings/.

72. International Labour Office & Walk Free Foundation. (2017). *Methodology of the global estimates of modern slavery: Forced labour and forced marriage, ILO*. Retrieved from: http://www.ilo.org/global/topics/forced-labour/publications/WCMS_586127/lang—en/index.htm.

73. U.S. Department of State. (n.d.). *What is modern slavery?* Retrieved from https://www.state.gov/j/tip/what/.

74. National Center for Farm Worker Health. (2018). *Agricultural worker demographics*. Retrieved from http://www.ncfh.org/uploads/3/8/6/8/38685499/fs_demographics_2018.pdf.

75. U.S. Department of Labor (n.d.). *Code of Federal Regulations (CFR) – Title 29 – Labor*. Retrieved from https://www.dol.gov/general/cfr/title_29.

76. Basham, B. (2018, Aug 2). The uncertain fate of migrant workers and their families. *Nashville Scene*. Retrieved from https://www.nashvillescene.com/news/cover-story/article/21015652/the-uncertain-fate-of-migrant-workers-andtheir-families.

77. Pager, T. (2018, Aug 22). Blame Trump's tariffs and the weather. New York's farmers do. *The New York Times*. Retrieved from https://nyti.ms/2nZ50aD.

78. National Center for Farm Worker Health. (2017). *A profile of migrant health: 2016*. Retrieved from http://www.ncfh.org/fact-sheets—research.html.

79. U.S. Department of Agriculture. (2018). *Farm labor housing direct loans & grants*. Retrieved from https://www.rd.usda.gov/programs-services/farm-labor-housing-direct-loans-grants.

80. Wiltz, T. (2016, May 2). States struggle to provide housing for migrant farmworkers. *Stateline*. Retrieved from https://www.pewtrusts.org/en/research-and-analysis/blogs/stateline/2016/05/02/struggle-to-provide-housing-for-migrant-farmworkers.

81. National Center for Farm Worker Health. (2018). *Maternal and child health*. Retrieved from http://www.ncfh.org/uploads/3/8/6/8/38685499/fs-maternal_and_child_health_2018.pdf.

82. United Nations. (n.d). *Sustainable Development Goals (SDSN) Goal 10*. Retrieved from https://www.un.org/sustainabledevelopment/inequality/.

83. U.S. Department of Justice. (2018). *Immigrant and employee rights section*. Retrieved from https://www.justice.gov/crt/immigrant-and-employee-rights-section.

84. Refugee Act of 1980, Pub. L. No. 96-212. (1980). Retrieved from http://www.answers.com/topic/refugee-act-of-1980.

85. United Nations (1951). *Convention and protocol relating to the status of refugees*. Geneva SZ: Author.

86. U.S. Department of Homeland Security. (2018). Refugees and asylees. Retrieved from https://www.dhs.gov/immigration-statistics/refugees-asylees.

87. United Nations. (2018). *World Refugee Day.* Retrieved from https://www.un.org/en/events/refugeeday/background.shtml.

88. United Nations High Commissioner for Refugees. (2018). *Figures at a glance.* Retrieved from http://www.unhcr.org/en-us/figures-at-a-glance.html.

89. International Rescue Committee. (2018). *Breaking down the stats as the U.S. plans to cut refugee arrivals to 30,000.* Retrieved from https://www.rescue.org/article/breaking-down-stats-us-plans-cut-refugee-arrivals-30000.

90. Jonassen, M., Shaheen, A., Duraidi, M., Qalalwa, K., Jeune, B., & Brønnum-Hansen, H. (2018). Socio-economic status and chronic disease in the West Bank and the Gaza Strip: In and outside refugee camps. *International Journal of Public Health, 63*(7), 875–882. https://doi-org.ezp.welch.jhmi.edu/10.1007/s00038-018-1122-6.

91. Wachter, K., Horn, R., Friis, E., Falb, K., Ward, L., Apio, C., Puffer, E., et al. (2018). Drivers of intimate partner violence against women in three refugee camps. *Violence Against Women, 24*(3), 286–306. https://doi-org.ezp.welch.jhmi.edu/10.1177/1077801216689163.

92. Ali, S.I., Ali, S.S., & Fesselet, J.-F. (2015). Effectiveness of emergency water treatment practices in refugee camps in South Sudan. *Bulletin of the World Health Organization, 93*(8), 550–558. https://doi-org.ezp.welch.jhmi.edu/10.2471/BLT.14.147645.

93. Walpole, S.C., Abbara, A., Gunst, M., & Harkensee, C. (2018). Cross-sectional growth assessment of children in four refugee camps in Northern Greece. *Public Health* (Elsevier), *162*, 147–152. https://doi-org.ezp.welch.jhmi.edu/10.1016/j.puhe.2018.05.004.

94. Soykoek, S., Mall, V., Nehring, I., Henningsen, P., & Aberl, S. (2017). Post-traumatic stress disorder in Syrian children of a German refugee camp. *Lancet, 389,* North American Edition (10072), 903–904. https://doi-org.ezp.welch.jhmi.edu/10.1016/S0140-6736(17)30595-0.

95. Schweitzer, R.D., Vromans, L., Brough, M., Asic-Kobe, M., Correa-Velez, I., Murray, K., & Lenette, C. (2018). Recently resettled refugee women-at-risk in Australia evidence high levels of psychiatric symptoms: Individual, trauma and post-migration factors predict outcomes. *BMC Med. 16*(1), 149. doi: 10.1186/s12916-018-1143-2.

96. Silove, D., Ventevogel, P., & Rees, S. (2017). The contemporary refugee crisis: An overview of mental health challenges. *World Psychiatry, 16*(2), 130-139. doi: 10.1002/wps.20438.

97. Centers for Disease Control and Prevention. (2014). *Medical examination of immigrants and refugees.* Retrieved from https://www.cdc.gov/immigrantrefugeehealth/exams/medical-examination.html.

98. U.S. Department of Health and Human Services, Office of Refugee Resettlement. (2015). *Health insurance.* Retrieved from https://www.acf.hhs.gov/orr/health.

99. U.S. Department of Justice Bureau of Justice Statistics (n.d.). Total Correctional Population. Retrieved from https://www.bjs.gov/index.cfm?tid=11&ty=t.

100. Gramlich, J. (2018, May 2). America's incarceration rate is at a two-decade low. Pew Research Center. Retrieved from https://www.pewresearch.org/fact-tank/2018/05/02/americas-incarceration-rate-is-at-a-two-decade-low/.

101. Centers for Disease Control and Prevention. (2014). Correctional Health. Retrieved from https://www.cdc.gov/correctionalhealth/default.htm.

102. Kaeble, D., & Cowhig, M. (2018). Correctional populations in the United States, 2016. *U.S. Department of Justice Office of Justice Programs Bureau of Justice Statistics Bulletin.* Retrieved from https://www.bjs.gov/content/pub/pdf/cpus16.pdf.

103. Zeng, Z., (2018, Feb 22). Jail inmates in 2016. *Office of Justice Program, Justice Bureau of Statistics.* Retrieved from https://www.bjs.gov/index.cfm?ty=pbdetail&iid=6186.

104. Love, D. (2018, Feb 12). Black incarceration rates are dropping while white rates rise, but what's really behind this surprising trend? *Atlantic Black Star.* Retrieved from https://atlantablackstar.com/2018/02/17/black-incarceration-rates-dropping-white-rates-rises-whats-really-behind-surprising-trend/.

105. Wagner, P., & Sawyer, W. (2018). States of Incarceration: The Global Context 2018. *Prison Policy Initiative.* Retrieved from https://www.prisonpolicy.org/global/2018.html.

106. Estelle v. Gambelle, 429 U.S. 97. (1976). Retrieved from http://caselaw.lp.findlaw.com/cgi-bin/getcase.pl?court=US&vol=429&invol=97.

107. Larney, S., Zaller, N.D., Dumont, D.M., Willcock, A., & Degenhardt, L. (2016). A systematic review and meta-analysis of racial and ethnic disparities in hepatitis C antibody prevalence in United States correctional populations. *Annals of Epidemiology, 26*(8), 570–578.e2. https://doi-org.ezp.welch.jhmi.edu/10.1016/j.annepidem.2016.06.013.

108. Skarupski, K.A., Gross, A., Schrack, J.A., Deal, J.A., & Eber, G.B. (2018). The health of America's aging prison population. *Epidemiologic Reviews, 40*(1), 157–165. https://doi-org.ezp.welch.jhmi.edu/10.1093/epirev/mxx020.

109. Turney, K., & Goodsell, R. (2018). Parental incarceration and children's wellbeing. *Future of Children, 28*(1), 147–164. Retrieved from http://search.ebscohost.com.ezp.welch.jhmi.edu/login.aspx?direct=true&db=rzh&AN=129524480&site=ehost-live&scope=site.

110. World Health Organization. (2018). *Gender equity and human rights: Gender.* Retrieved from http://www.who.int/gender-equity-rights/understanding/gender-definition/en/.

111. Human Rights Campaign. (2018). *Glossary of terms.* Retrieved from https://www.hrc.org/resources/glossary-of-terms.

112. The Joint Commission. (2011). *Advancing effective communication, cultural competence, and patient- and family centered care for the lesbian, gay, bisexual, and transgender (LGBT) community: A field guide.* Oak Brook, IL: Author. Retrieved from https://www.jointcommission.org/assets/1/18/LGBTFieldGuide.pdf.

113. Bonvicini, K.A. (2017). LGBT healthcare disparities: What progress have we made? *Patient Education & Counseling, 100*(12), 2357–2361. https://doi-org.ezp.welch.jhmi.edu/10.1016/j.pec.2017.06.003.

114. Healthy People 2020. (2018). *Lesbian, gay, bisexual, and transgender health.* Retrieved from https://www.healthypeople.gov/2020/topics-objectives/topic/lesbian-gay-bisexual-and-transgender-health/objectives.

115. National Center for Health Statistics. (2016). *Chapter 25, Lesbian, gay, bisexual and transgender health: Healthy People 2020 midcourse review.* Hyattsville, MD: Author. Retrieved from https://www.cdc.gov/nchs/data/hpdata2020/HP2020MCR-C25-LGBT.pdf.

116. Newport, F. (2018, May 22). In U.S., estimate of LGBT population rises to 4.5%. *Gallup: Politics.* Retrieved from https://news.gallup.com/poll/234863/estimate-lgbt-population-rises.aspx.

117. Centers for Disease Control and Prevention. (2014). *Lesbian, gay, bisexual, and transgender health.* Retrieved from https://www.cdc.gov/lgbthealth/about.htm.

118. Park, Y., & Mykhyalyshyn, I. (2016, June 16). L.G.B.T. people are more likely to be targets of hate crimes than any other minority group. *New York Times.* Retrieved from https://nyti.ms/2jSzpDG.

119. Langenderfer-Magruder, L., Walls, N.E., Whitfield, D., Brown, S., & Barrett, C. (2016). Partner violence victimization among lesbian, gay, bisexual, transgender, and queer youth: Associations among risk factors. *Child & Adolescent Social Work Journal, 33*(1), 55–68. https://doi-org.ezp.welch.jhmi.edu/10.1007/s10560-015-0402-8.

120. Langenderfer-Magruder, L., Whitfield, D.L., Walls, N.E., Kattari, S.K., & Ramos, D. (2016). Experiences of intimate partner violence and subsequent police reporting among lesbian, gay, bisexual, transgender, and queer adults in Colorado. *Journal of Interpersonal Violence, 31*(5), 855–871. https://doi-org.ezp.welch.jhmi.edu/10.1177/0886260514556767.

121. Heina, L.C., Stokes, F., Smith-Greenberg, C., Saewycd, E.M. (2018). Policy brief: Protecting vulnerable LGBTQ youth and advocating for ethical health care. *Nursing Outlook, 66,* 505–507.

122. Clay, R. (2014). Double-whammy discrimination. *American Psychological Association, Monitor on Psychology, 45*(10), 46.

123. Perez-Brumer, A., Nunn, A., Hsiang, E., Oldenburg, C., Bender, M., Beauchamps, L., Mena, L., MacCarthy, S. (2018). We don't treat your kind: Assessing HIV health needs holistically among transgender people in Jackson, Mississippi. *PLoS One, 1;13*(11), e0202389. doi:10.1371/journal.pone.0202389.

124. Bauermeister, J.A., Muessig, K.E., Flores, D.D., LeGrand, S., Choi, S., Dong, W., Harper G.W., Hightow-Weidman, L.B. (2018). Stigma diminishes the protective effect of social support on psychological distress among young black men who have sex with men. *AIDS Education and Prevention, 30*(5), 406-418. doi: 10.1521/aeap.2018.30.5.406.

125. United States Department of Justice. (2015). *Matthew Shepard and James Byrd, Jr., Hate Crimes Prevention Act.* Retrieved from https://www.justice.gov/crt/matthew-shepard-and-james-byrd-jr-hate-crimes-prevention-act-2009-0.

126. American Psychiatric Association. (2015). Guidelines for psychological practice with transgender and gender nonconforming people. *American Psychologist, 70,* 832–864. http://dx.doi.org/10.1037/a0039906 Retrieved from https://www.apa.org/practice/guidelines/transgender.pdf.

127. Fredriksen-Goldsen, K.I., Kim, H.-J., Shiu, C., & Bryan, A.E.B. (2017). Chronic health conditions and key health indicators among lesbian, gay, and bisexual older U.S. adults, 2013-2014. *American Journal of Public Health, 107*(8), 1332–1338. doi:10.2105/AJPH.2017.303922.

128. Muraco, A., & Fredriksen-Goldsen, K.I. (2014). The highs and lows of caregiving for chronically ill lesbian, gay, and bisexual elders. *Journal of Gerontological Social Work, 57*(2–4), 251–272. doi:10.1080/01634372.2013.860652.

129. Centers for Disease Control and Prevention. (2016). *HIV Surveillance Report, 2015; vol. 27.* Retrieved from http://www.cdc.gov/hiv/library/reports/hiv-surveillance.html.

Chapter 8

Communicable Diseases

Michael Sanchez and Christine Savage

LEARNING OUTCOMES

After reading this chapter, the student will be able to:

1. Apply the cycle of transmission to specific communicable diseases.
2. Describe the steps in an outbreak investigation.
3. Investigate the role of culture and environment in the management of an epidemic.

4. Discuss current issues related to emerging communicable diseases.
5. Describe the role of the nurse in the prevention and treatment of hospital- and community-acquired infections.

KEY TERMS

Active immunity
Agent
Antigenicity
Attack rate
Carrier
Case fatality rate
Cellular immunity
Chronic carrier
Colonization
Common source
Community immunity
Continuous source

Convalescent carrier
Endemic
Environment
Epidemic
Epidemic curve
Epidemic threshold
Generation time
Herd immunity
Host
Humoral immunity
Immunity
Inapparent carrier

Incubating carrier
Index case
Infectivity
Inherent resistance
Intermittent source
Outbreak investigation
Pandemic
Passive immunity
Pathogen
Pathogenic
Pathogenicity
Point source

Reservoir
Resistance
Secondary attack rate
Secondary case
Sexually transmitted disease
Susceptibility
Toxigenicity
Vaccine
Vector
Virulence

Introduction

Communicable diseases (CDs) make national headlines on a regular basis. There was an outbreak of Zika virus that placed fetuses at risk for adverse outcomes. In the U.S., there were 116 live infants with Zika-related birth defects and 9 pregnancy losses due to Zika-related defects.[1] In May 2018, an Ebola outbreak in the Democratic Republic of Congo in a less remote area brought concerns of a wider outbreak.[2] In June of 2018, an outbreak of Salmonella Adelaide infections related to pre-cut melon affected 60 people in 5 states.[3] These headlines demonstrate the very real threat of CDs in today's world as a result of both acute outbreaks and the long-term adverse effects of chronic infection.

CDs have plagued humankind throughout recorded history. As recently as the first part of the last century, CDs were the leading causes of death. In the 1950s and 1960s, chickenpox, measles, and mumps were endemic in school-age children. With the advent of antibiotics and vaccines, CDs were no longer the primary killer of humans with a resulting increase in life expectancy. In the 1980s, the effectiveness of vaccines and antibiotics led some health-care providers to predict that CDs would be eliminated in many sections of the world, especially after the successful eradication of smallpox worldwide.[4] While these pronouncements were being made, a new CD emerged, AIDS caused by HIV. During this period, other diseases emerged such as those caused by the Ebola family of viruses and the Zika virus. At the same time the predicted decline in the incidence of other CDs, such as tuberculosis (TB), did not occur.

In the 21st century, CDs are a main reason for morbidity and mortality in the United States and the world. In the United States, acute respiratory infections, including influenza and pneumonia, are listed in the top 10 leading causes of death.[5] In low-income countries, 5 of the 10 top leading causes of death are related to CD.[6] For lower-middle-income countries, 3 of the top 10 leading causes of death are related to CDs. For upper-middle-income countries and high-income countries, acute respiratory diseases are the only CDs on the list of the top 10 causes of death (Table 8-1).[6]

A major responsibility of public health officials from the local to the global level is to conduct surveillance to determine whether there is a CD epidemic that threatens the health of populations. The surveillance in turn can help determine what if any action will be necessary to stop an epidemic. The term **epidemic** is the combination of two Greek terms, *epi* (upon) and *demos* (people), and has the same roots as the term *epidemiology* (see Chapter 3). At first the term *epidemic* was used to describe a collection of illnesses based on their characteristics such as diarrhea or cough,

but with the arrival of the Black Death (bubonic plague) in Europe, the word was used to describe the increased occurrence of a single disease.[7] In the 21st century, the term *epidemic* is used when there is a significant increase in number of cases than would normally occur. **Endemic** refers to the usual number of cases of a disease that occur within a population. At the other end of the spectrum, **pandemic** describes epidemics occurring across the globe.

Communicable Diseases and Nursing Practice

CDs are a public health issue and an important concern for nurses working in the community and in acute care settings. Nurses are confronted with CDs on a constant

TABLE 8–1 ■ Top 10 Leading Causes of Death by Level of Income

Cause of Death	Low Income	Lower Middle Income	Upper Middle Income	High Income
Lower respiratory disease	Number 1	Number 3	Number 6	Number 6
Diarrheal diseases	Number 2	Number 6		
Ischemic heart diseases	Number 3	Number 1	Number 1	Number 1
HIV/AIDS	Number 4			
Stroke	Number 5	Number 2	Number 2	Number 2
Malaria	Number 6			
Tuberculosis	Number 7	Number 5		
Preterm birth complications	Number 8	Number 8		
Birth asphyxia and birth trauma	Number 9			
Road Injury	Number 10	Number 10	Number 8	
Chronic obstructive pulmonary disease		Number 4	Number 3	Number 5
Diabetes mellitus		Number 7	Number 7	Number 8
Cirrhosis of the liver		Number 9		
Trachea, bronchus, and lung cancers			Number 4	Number 4
Alzheimer's disease and other dementias			Number 5	Number 3
Liver cancer			Number 9	
Stomach cancer			Number 10	
Colon and rectal cancers				Number 7
Kidney diseases				Number 9
Breast Cancer				Number 10

(See WHO; http://www.who.int/news-room/fact-sheets/detail/the-top-10-causes-of-death for updates.)
Source: (6)

basis. Nurses provide care to patients with a CD and also must incorporate preventive measures in their practice, such as the use of personal protective equipment (PPE) and proper cleaning of patient areas to prevent transmission of these diseases to themselves, co-workers, and other patients. These practices protect individuals and populations. For the practicing nurse, an understanding of CDs at both an individual level and a population level is essential. If the nurse only focuses on caring for the patient with a CD without considering the implications for the population, the care falls short and potentially endangers others.

The key to all these activities is to understand the infectious agents that cause disease, the environment relevant to the transmission of disease from one person to another, and who is at risk for becoming infected. Professional nurses back up their interventions related to the prevention and treatment of CDs with knowledge of the public health science behind these interventions. In the same way that nurses do not dispense medications without understanding the pharmacokinetics behind the medications, nurses cannot intervene in relation to CDs without understanding the science behind these diseases.

Public health science provides the basis for understanding how CDs have an impact on the health of humans. Professional nurses armed with scientific knowledge related to infectious agents can intervene in ways that reduce the risk for not only their individual patients and themselves but also for the larger population they serve, with prevention the primary goal.

Communicable Disease and the Burden of Disease

Twenty-first-century improvements in technology and transportation have brought populations closer together and eliminated geographical barriers to transmission of disease. This increases the possibility of spreading CDs that in the past may have been contained in one geographical area. This chapter provides an overview of the CDs that are leading causes of death with a focus on incidence and prevalence in the United States.

Infectious Respiratory Disease

Many agents are associated with respiratory disease (Box 8-1). These diseases are either bacterial or viral. Many of these diseases can be prevented through vaccination. Children are required to receive vaccination for many CDs before attending public schools, such as vaccines for prevention of chickenpox, diphtheria, and rubella. A new policy for most health-care settings is to

---

BOX 8–1 ■ Respiratory Communicable Diseases that Can Infect the Respiratory System

Chickenpox
Diphtheria
Group A *Streptococcus*
Haemophilus influenzae type b
Influenza
Legionnaire's disease
Measles (rubeola)
Mumps
Pneumococcal meningitis
German measles (rubella)
Tuberculosis
Whooping cough (pertussis)
Anthrax
Hantavirus pulmonary syndrome
Plague

---

require that all employees receive an annual flu vaccine. Because of vaccination programs across the United States and other countries, the incidence of many communicable respiratory diseases is declining. Despite these advances, respiratory disease caused by infectious agents continues to be a significant public health issue. Some of these diseases are seasonal, for example, influenza (flu). Many have a higher morbidity and mortality rate in vulnerable populations, such as older adults and children.

Influenza, or flu, is a communicable respiratory disease and is a major public health concern. Flu is seasonal, with a peak in early December and a peak in February. Because of the higher mortality rate in vulnerable populations such as children, older adults, and those who are already ill, many hospitals require that all employees receive a flu vaccination. The CDC publishes a report titled *FluView* that follows trends in flu across the year. Trends in flu vary from year to year. In 2009–2010, there was a pandemic outbreak of H1N1 influenza that peaked earlier in October, which resulted in an estimated midrange of 61 million cases, 240,000 hospitalizations, and 12,470 deaths. Then the following 2011–2012 flu season was the mildest season on record.[8] In 2015-2016 H1N1 reemerged as the predominant virus for the season.[9] Unlike the 2009-2010 season, the peak month for flu activity was January (Fig. 8-1). [10]

Malaria

Malaria is a subtropical disease caused by a parasite, the intraerythrocytic protozoa of the genus *Plasmodium* transmitted through the bite of an infected female

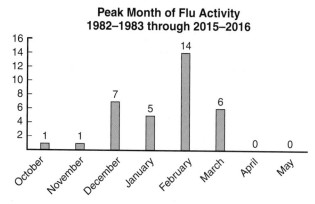

Figure 8-1 Peak flu activity. *(Data source reference 10.)*

Anopheles gambiae mosquito, often referred to as the "malaria **vector**".[11] About half of the world's population is at risk for malaria. According to the World Health Organization (WHO), in 2016, an estimated 445,000 deaths, mostly African children, were caused by malaria.[12] The estimated number of cases in 2016 was 216 million worldwide, an increase of 5 million from the year prior.[12] By comparison, in 2014, in the United States, there were 1,724 cases of malaria with 5 fatalities.[13] Malarial infections in the United States are primarily the result of exposure that occurred during travel abroad. In addition, these travelers had not adhered to recommended malaria prophylaxis. Malaria is a preventable disease, and much is being done globally to eradicate it. Globally, the economic and social burdens affect both individuals and governments including the cost of care, lost work, and burial expenses. Direct costs (for example, illness, treatment, premature death) have been estimated to be at least U.S. $12 billion per year.[14]

Human Immunodeficiency Virus (HIV) and Acquired Immune Deficiency Syndrome (AIDS)

HIV impairs and destroys the immune cells in the infected person's body, affecting the ability to fight off infection. A person infected with HIV may not develop AIDS until 10 to 15 years after the initial infection.[15] HIV/AIDS status is classified across five stages: 0, 1, 2, 3, unknown. A negative HIV test within 6 months of the first HIV infection diagnosis is stage 0 and remains 0 until 6 months after diagnosis. If a stage-3-defining opportunistic illness has been diagnosed, the stage is 3 (Box 8-2). Otherwise, the stage is determined by the CD4 test immunologic criteria based on the CDC case definition guidelines.[15] According to UNAIDS, HIV has killed 35 million people over the past 3 decades, and, in 2016, an estimated 36.7 million people were living with HIV/AIDS worldwide, with 1.8 million new cases in 2016.[16] In the United States, an estimated 1.1 million people are living with HIV/AIDS. In 2016, in the U.S., 39,782 persons were newly diagnosed with HIV/AIDS, and nearly 15% of those infected with HIV are unaware they are infected.[17,18]

In the U.S., the prevalence of HIV and AIDS is higher among persons in the 25- to 44-year-old age group, those who are African American and Hispanic, and in men. Racial disparity is especially apparent in children, with 80% of all pediatric cases being African American or Hispanic.[17,18] HIV infection is also on the rise among older adults because of increased longevity of those living with HIV as well as an increase in risky behaviors in this age group.[19] Certain behaviors increase the risk for transmission of HIV, including men having sex with men, those engaging in injection drug use, and those engaging in unprotected sex. There is also variation in the distribution of cases geographically. The South has the highest number of people living with HIV, whereas the highest rates of new infections occurred in California, Florida, Texas, New York, and Georgia.[20]

Healthy People (HP) has a specific topic related to HIV/AIDS.[21] The objectives related to the topic not only address disparity but also prevention, screening, and treatment.

■ HEALTHY PEOPLE
HIV

Goal: Prevent human immunodeficiency virus (HIV) infection and related illness and death.

Overview: HIV infections in the United States continue to be a major public health crisis. An estimated 1.2 million Americans are living with HIV, and 1 out of 8 people with HIV do not know they have it. Although recent data show that annual HIV infections declined

18% in the U.S. from 2008 to 2014, HIV continues to spread.

In 2010, the White House released a National HIV/AIDS Strategy. The National HIV/AIDS Strategy was updated to 2020 (NHAS 2020) in July 2015. The strategy includes three primary goals:

1. Reducing new HIV infections.
2. Increasing access to care and improving health outcomes for people living with HIV.
3. Reducing HIV-related disparities and health inequities.[22]

Midcourse Review: Of the 27 objectives under the topic of HIV in Heathy People 2020, 11 were measurable. Of these, two exceeded or met targeted goals, five were improving, three had little or no change, and one was baseline only (Fig. 8-2). For persons aged 13 or older, there was no change in the number of new infections.[23]

UNAIDS 909090

Along with the HP goals related to HIV/AIDS are the 2014 UNAIDS goals related to the AIDS epidemic titled *UN AIDS 909090: An ambitious treatment target to help end the AIDS epidemic.* They have since published a midcourse review as well.

The three main goals by 2020 were:

- 90% of all people living with HIV will know their HIV status.
- 90% of all people with diagnosed HIV infection will receive sustained antiretroviral therapy.

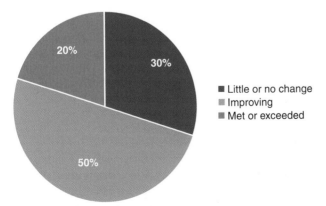

Healthy People 2020 Midcourse Review: HIV

- ■ Little or no change
- ■ Improving
- ■ Met or exceeded

Figure 8-2 Healthy People 2020 Midcourse Review: HIV. *(Data source reference 22.)*

- 90% of all people receiving antiretroviral therapy will have viral suppression.[24]

Midcourse Review 2016:
- 70% of all people living with HIV knew their HIV status.
- 77% of all people with diagnosed HIV infection were on sustained antiretroviral therapy.
- 82% of all persons on treatment were virally suppressed.[25]

Diarrheal Disease

Diarrhea is defined by the WHO as the passage of three or more loose or liquid stools per day. There are approximately 2 billion cases of diarrheal disease worldwide each year.[26] In low-income countries, it is a leading cause of death among children. In 2017, the WHO estimated that 525,000 deaths in children under the age of 5 were caused by diarrhea.[27] The most common route for transmission of diarrheal disease is the fecal-oral route. Good hand hygiene, especially hand washing, and soap alone can reduce the incidence of diarrheal disease by as much as 48%.[28] Efficient sanitary systems and safe drinking water also play a huge role in preventing diarrheal diseases.

Pathogens that cause diarrheal disease include viruses, bacteria, and protozoa. Transmission is usually waterborne (e.g., cholera), foodborne (e.g., *Escherichia coli [E. coli]*), or through person-to-person contact; pathogens can infect the small bowel, the colon, or both.[29] Worldwide, rotavirus is the most common cause of diarrheal disease among children, accounting for almost 40% of all cases of infant diarrhea and is responsible for a half million deaths in children under 5 years old.[26] Until recently, infections with rotavirus among children under the age of 5 resulted in up to 70,000 hospitalizations and 60 deaths annually. In 2006, a vaccine was introduced that has helped reduce the incidence of this disease. There are now two vaccines available for use with infants. Since the introduction of these vaccines, the incidence of rotavirus-associated diarrheal infections in children has declined.[30]

Emerging and Re-emerging Communicable Diseases

The WHO defines an emerging disease as "one that has appeared in a population for the first time, or that may have existed previously but is rapidly increasing in incidence or geographic range."[31] Through public health efforts, some CDs are close to eradication, for example, polio mellitus and dracunculiasis (guinea worm disease), or have been eradicated, as in the case of smallpox. Yet, at the same time, new CDs have emerged such as severe acute respiratory syndrome (SARS), West Nile virus, and the Zika virus. Other diseases, such as malaria, TB, and bacterial pneumonias, are reemerging in forms that are resistant to drug treatments, for example, multidrug-resistant tuberculosis (MDRTB).[33] New diseases are emerging at a rate of one per year. In the 21st century, emerging CDs continue to make global headlines such as the Zika virus. Response to such diseases results in a burden on the economic, social, and health-care systems of countries. Pandemics such as the SARS outbreak and epidemics within countries such as the West Nile virus epidemic in the summer of 2012 required a coordinated early response across political entities such as countries or states.

Tuberculosis

TB is an infectious disease caused by the *Mycobacterium tuberculosis*. It has been called many names, including white death, the great white plague, and consumption. The word *consumption* is even found in the Bible. It wasn't until the end of the 19th century that the disease received the name *tuberculosis* after the agent that caused the disease was identified. In 1889, the National Tuberculosis Association (now the National Lung Association) realized that TB was preventable and not inherited. Since that time, prevention efforts have resulted in a steady downward trend in the incidence and prevalence of TB, so much so that 100 years later, in 1998, a TB elimination project was initiated in the United States with the target date of 2010 for TB elimination. Although this has not occurred, the downward trend in TB incidence and prevalence is encouraging. The WHO End Strategy and the United Nations' Sustainable development goals also have the goal of ending the global TB epidemic. These organizations aim to have a 90% reduction in TB deaths and 80% reduction in TB incidence.[34,35] In the U.S., continued efforts are needed to address the disparity in incidence between U.S.-born and foreign-born individuals as well as between whites and minorities.[35]

Back in 1988, infection control experts were optimistic that the elimination of TB was a realistic goal. Unfortunately, at the same time, reports began to emerge of hospital-acquired MDRTB outbreaks. Between 1988 and 1992, five clusters of TB cases appeared in six hospitals. Four occurred in New York City, one in Florida, and one in New York State. What stood out about these cases was that the agent *M. tuberculosis* had mutated (changed) and was now resistant to drugs used to treat active TB. Surveillance was initiated that identified more patients who met the case definition of MDRTB. Upon investigation,

some issues emerged. First, most of the patients were also infected with HIV. With HIV, TB does not always present in a classic manner, and diagnosis was delayed in these cases. In addition, recognition of drug resistance was hampered by the length of time it took to complete the drug susceptibility tests. The **case fatality rate (CFR)** was high. A CFR is determined by taking the number of fatal cases and dividing it by the total number of cases. Within 16 weeks of diagnosis, 72% to 89% of patients had died.[36] Since that time, dramatic changes have taken place in acute care settings including strict Occupational Health and Safety Administration (OSHA) guidelines.

Globally, in 2015, there were 10.4 million new cases of TB and 1.4 million TB deaths in HIV-negative persons, and an additional 0.4 million deaths due to HIV-associated TB.[34] In 2015, in the United States, there were 9,577 reported cases of TB with an incidence rate of 3.0 per 100,000. Overall, both the prevalence and incidence of TB are decreasing, albeit at a slow rate of 3% per year.[37] It was estimated that the rate of decline would need to accelerate to a 4%-5% annual decline to achieve the End TB Strategy by 2020. The number of new cases in 2015 in the United States was the lowest since 1953. However, the national goal to eliminate TB (less than 0.1 case per 100,000 population) was not met.[37]

The story of TB rates in the United States illustrates the importance of following trends of CDs. As mentioned earlier, many CDs must be reported to the health department. This information is electronically forwarded from all 50 states and the District of Columbia to the CDC. The CDC follows these trends of data over time. On the surface, this is a simple process in that the total number of cases is followed by year. However, just knowing the number of cases does not provide the CDC with additional information needed to protect the health of the public. Through careful surveillance of TB, the CDC can determine who is at greatest risk based on numerous factors including race, age, geographical location, and place of birth. The CDC can then examine whether the goal of eliminating TB is being met, and if not, where it needs to concentrate its efforts to meet the goal.

▶ SOLVING THE MYSTERY
The Case of the Wandering Patient

In February 2002, a 42-year-old man with HIV and schizophrenia was admitted twice to one hospital for fever and unproductive cough. Chest radiographs were read as normal, and a sputum culture was negative for *M. tuberculosis*. In April, he was admitted to another hospital with similar symptoms, treated with antibiotics, and released. Three days later he was readmitted and treated for suspected pneumonia. However, his stool culture came back positive for *M. tuberculosis*. A subsequent acid-fast bacillus (AFB) smear test was 4+, indicating that he was highly infectious. Although he was placed in isolation, he continued to have contact with other patients and hospital personnel because of a lack of vigilance on the part of the staff to observe strict isolation procedures, with serious consequences.[38]

The investigation into this case started with identifying the **index case**, that is, the first case identified in a particular outbreak. Because the normal mode of transmission is airborne from person to person, identifying the index patient provides the investigators with the starting point for their investigation. The investigators working on this case identified this 42-year-old man as the index case.

Their next step was to identify **secondary cases**, that is, patients who were diagnosed with active TB and who had contact with the index patient. Five secondary cases were identified; one had diabetes and HIV, one had diabetes, two had end-stage renal disease, and one was a phlebotomist. The first two steps of the investigation were now complete, identifying the index patient and secondary patients, but the investigation did not stop there. Because the index patient's sputum came back with a 4+ AFB smear, there was a high level of infectivity, that is, anyone who came in contact with the patient was probably exposed to a high level of the *M. tuberculosis* bacillus. If that were the case, then everyone who came in contact with the patient would be at risk.

The next step in the investigation was to identify all contacts. With some agents, once humans are infected the incubation period prior to the occurrence of symptoms is short and can last less than a week. In others, it might be a little longer and last up to 3 months, as with syphilis. With TB, a person can become infected and show no sign of disease for decades. This is known as latent TB. The investigators identified a total of 1,045 contacts, both patients and employees of the hospital. They were able to test close to two-thirds of all these contacts. Eleven percent of the tested employees tested positive, and 23% of the tested patients tested positive. Those who tested positive were provided appropriate interventions to prevent development of the disease.[38]

This case illustrates the challenges faced in identifying the presence of an active infection and the urgency of taking measures to prevent further spread of the infection. The investigation focused on three stages: (1) identification of the index patient; (2) finding secondary cases; and (3) investigation of contacts. The report included recommendations for hospital infection control programs. The patient had been placed in isolation, and the investigators established that the isolation room was in accordance with appropriate isolation procedures. However, the patient came into contact with other patients, so the possibility is raised that the patient did not remain in his room.[38]

This case highlights the issue of isolation procedures in health-care agencies (see Chapter 14). The type of isolation is based on the cycle of transmission. Nurses are required to institute appropriate isolation procedures based on the known or suspected agent. These procedures are public health interventions aimed at preventing the spread of disease in three populations (other patients, employees, and community visitors). For airborne agents such as the bacterium that causes TB, isolation procedures involve preventing the spread of the agent through the hospital ventilation system, thus the need for negative pressure rooms. A negative pressure room is used in hospitals when respiratory isolation is needed. The ventilation system uses negative pressure so that air can come into the room but does not go back out into the building and is instead ventilated to the outside. Choosing the right level of isolation requires knowing how the agent is transmitted to humans (person-to-person, airborne, etc.).

Infectious Agents and the Cycle of Transmission

Public health departments are charged with protecting the population at large from the spread of infection. This requires understanding the cycle of infection. The key components of the cycle of infection begin with the epidemiological triangle, which includes the three main constructs needed for disease to occur in humans: the agent, the environment, and the host (see Chapter 3, Fig. 3-2). In CDs, the epidemiological triangle is expanded to help understand the cycle of transmission of the infectious agent from the reservoir to the host (Fig. 8-3).

Agent Characteristics

The term **agent** or **pathogen** refers to the infectious organism that causes the disease such as a virus or bacteria. Knowledge of agent characteristics begins with a review of the six general categories of pathogens based on the biological properties of the pathogens (Table 8-2). The

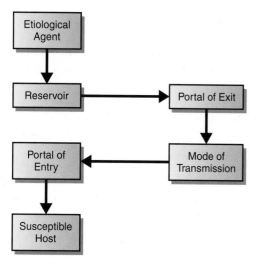

Figure 8-3 The cycle of communicable disease transmission.

categories include bacteria, rickettsia, viruses, mycoses (fungi), protozoa, and helminths. Also grouped with these agents are arthropods, parasitic insects that in themselves do not cause disease but transmit disease (e.g., ticks, fleas, and mosquitoes). This category also includes head, body, and pubic lice, though only body lice are known to transmit disease. The other two types of lice are included, because scratching from lice can result in a secondary bacterial infection of the skin and because lice are transmitted from human to human.

Once the class of the pathogen is known, the specific characteristics of the category provide further necessary information. For example, if the pathogen is a helminth, it is a parasitic worm. This relates directly to the biological characteristics of the group of pathogens. Knowing the class of pathogen can help with the care of the individual patient. For example, because general antibiotics work with bacteria but not with viruses, knowing the

TABLE 8–2 ■ Types of Infectious Agents

Category	Type of Agent	Examples of Diseases
Bacteria	Microorganism, unicellular Either gram-positive or gram-negative	Bacterial meningitis Anthrax Bubonic plague Tuberculosis Streptococcal infections
Rickettsia	Though in a separate class, they are a genus of bacteria that grows in cells. They are structurally similar to gram-negative bacteria	Typhus Rocky Mountain spotted fever
Viruses	A submicroscopic organism with a protein coat that are a piece of genetic material (RNA or DNA) are microorganisms. They are unable to grow or reproduce outside a host cell.	HIV Common cold Influenza
Mycoses	A disease caused by fungi	Candida Histoplasmosis Fungal meningitis
Protozoa	Single-celled animals such as flagellates, amoeboids, sporozoans, and ciliates	Malaria *Giardia* Toxoplasmosis Trichomoniasis
Helminths	Parasitic worm-like organisms that feed off living hosts	Hookworm Pinworm Trichinosis
Anthropods	Insects that act as vectors and transmit the agent from its reservoir to its host.	Malaria Dengue fever Lyme disease Bubonic plague

Source: Friss, R.H., & Sellers, T.A. (2014). *Epidemiology for public health practice,* (5th ed.) Burlington, MA: Jones & Bartlett.

class of the pathogen can help to determine whether the patient should receive an antibiotic or an antiviral.

In addition to the class of the agent, other characteristics of the agent are helpful to understand. The first characteristic is the **infectivity** of the agent. This reflects the capacity of an agent to enter and multiply in the host. Some agents have low infectivity, meaning either they have a decreased capacity to enter a human host and/or they have a decreased capacity to multiply once they are in the human host. The next characteristic of an agent is its **pathogenicity**, which is the capacity of the agent to cause disease in the human host. Not all infectious agents have the same capability to cause disease.

Toxigenicity is another key issue with an infectious agent and reflects the pathogen's ability to release toxins that contribute to disease within the human host. Not all agents release toxins. There is also variability among agents in relation to their resistance to survive environmental conditions. For example, HIV survives for only a short time outside its host (the human body), whereas anthrax can survive for decades in the soil or in warehouses where untreated animal hides have been processed.

Another important characteristic of the agent is **virulence**, which is defined as the ability of the pathogen to cause disease. Finally, agents differ on **antigenicity**, that is the ability of the agent to produce antibodies in the human host. For example, prior to the arrival of vaccines, parents attempted to expose their children to infectious parotitis (mumps). Because a case of mumps usually results in the development of antibodies, the parents hoped their children would develop immunity to mumps during childhood because the disease can cause serious complications in adults. Thus, mumps virus has a high level of antigencity.

Environmental Characteristics

Reservoir

The **environment** refers to the conditions external to the host and the agent associated with the transmission of the agent. The first of these is the **reservoir**, or where the agent resides. For most CDs, the reservoir is a human (the agent resides in an infected human). Another common reservoir is animals, and these CDs are known as zoological diseases (e.g., Lyme disease and anthrax). For Lyme disease, the agent is a spirochete, *Borrelia burgdorferi*, and the reservoir is both animals and humans. For anthrax, the reservoir is also animals, including elephants, hippopotami, cattle, sheep, and goats; in spore form, the reservoir is soil exposed to the feces of these animals. Reservoirs also include water

(waterborne diseases), food (foodborne diseases), and the air (airborne diseases).

The human reservoir can be a person who is acutely ill or someone who is a **carrier**, that is, a human who is infected but who has no outward signs of disease. There are four main types of carriers: an incubating carrier, an inapparent carrier, a convalescent carrier, and a chronic carrier. An **incubating carrier** is someone who has been infected but has not yet shown signs of the disease. An **inapparent carrier** is someone who is infected but does not develop the disease, yet continues to shed the agent, such as Typhoid Mary (Box 8-3). A **convalescent carrier** is a person who is infected but who no longer shows signs of acute disease. The **chronic carrier** remains infected with the agent with no sign of disease for a long period of time.

Mode of Transmission

The next consideration is the mode of transmission, the method through which the agent leaves its reservoir and enters its host. Transmission can occur through water, food, air, vectors, fomites, unprotected sexual contact, or penetrating trauma (Table 8-3). Vectors are usually

---

BOX 8–3 ■ Typhoid Mary

Mary Mallon worked as a cook and had no idea that she was an inapparent carrier of typhus. She was the first identified "healthy carrier" of typhoid fever in the United States. She worked in several households between 1900 and 1907. During that time, members in each household came down with typhus. She even nursed those who were sick, continuing to spread the disease. Although public health officials explained to her the reason she needed to be quarantined, she did not believe that she could spread the disease. Because of her disbelief, she escaped from her quarantine and went back to working as a cook. When she was once again apprehended, she was taken to North Brother Island near New York City and remained there for 3 years. She was released when she promised not to work as a cook. She worked as a laundress for a period of time, but the wages were low, so she changed her name and once again took a job as a cook, this time at New York's Sloane Hospital for Women. She infected 25 people and one died. She was apprehended again by authorities and spent the rest of her life on North Brother Island. Her name has become synonymous with the healthy carrier of disease.

Source: Leavitt, J.W. (1996). *Typhoid Mary: Captive to the public's health*. Boston, MA: Beacon Press.
For more information, watch the PBS special *The Most Dangerous Woman in America*: http://www.pbs.org/wgbh/nova/typhoid/

TABLE 8–3 ■ Types of Transmission

Type of Transmission	Examples	Examples of Breaking the Cycle of Transmission
Fomite transmission: An inanimate object carries the pathogen from the reservoir to the host.	Transferring of viruses on the surface of inanimate objects such as a phone. Transferring of lice through exchange of clothing. Using a cutting board for meat products and then vegetables without cleaning the board in between use.	Decontamination of the fomite through the use of disinfectants or proper cleaning.
Aerosol or airborne transmission: The agent is contained in aerosol droplets and is transferred from one human to another or animal to human.	Transferring of the agent through the air, usually after the human host expels droplets into the air by coughing or sneezing.	Use of negative pressure rooms in hospitals and personal protective equipment such as facemasks.
Oral transmission: The agent is transferred through food or water.	Ingestion of food or water contaminated with the agent such as cholera in untreated water and *E. coli* through the ingestion of contaminated beef	Eradication of the agent through cleaning of the water supply, implementation of food processing regulations, proper cooking of foods, hand hygiene.
Vector borne transmission: An insect acquires the agent from an animal and transmits it to another.	Fleas, ticks, and mosquitoes are common vectors of agents to humans.	Eradication of the vector such as control of mosquito breeding grounds, use of insect repellent, and mosquito netting.
Zoonotic transmission: The agent is transmitted directly from animals to humans.	Dogs, sheep, pigs are common sources of direct transmission from animals to humans such as hookworm or rabies.	Vaccination of the animal.
Person-to-person transmission: The agent is transmitted through direct contact between persons, usually through contact with mucous membranes, blood, or saliva. It also occurs through venereal and in utero routes.		Vaccination such as the hepatitis B vaccine, use of personal protective equipment.

insects that carry the disease from the reservoir to humans without becoming ill themselves. A fomite is an inanimate object. An infected host touches the object and sheds the agent onto the object. The agent is then transmitted to the next person who touches the object. Possible fomite transmission of the cold or the flu virus is used by marketers to sell their disinfecting products.

Life Cycle of an Infectious Agent

The two aspects of the environment, reservoir and mode of transmission, are best illustrated through a review of the life cycle of an infectious agent. The life cycle provides essential information on the environment and how an agent goes from its normal reservoir to the host, known as the mode of transmission. Some agents have complex life cycles, such as the human hookworm (*Ancylostoma duodenale* or *Necator americanus*) (Fig. 8-4).[39] For other agents the life cycle of the vector is more important than the agent's own life cycle, as in the case of the agent responsible for Lyme disease, *B. burgdorferi*. A vector transmits the agent without becoming infected itself. The reservoir for *B. burgdorferi* includes mice, squirrels, and other small animals. This is where the agent resides. The blacklegged tick then transmits the agent among these animals to humans by biting an animal infected with the agent (the reservoir) and then biting a human. The blacklegged tick has a 2-year life cycle. This life cycle, rather than the life cycle of the agent, provides the environmental information needed to develop prevention programs. The tick feeds on small animals in the larval and nymphal

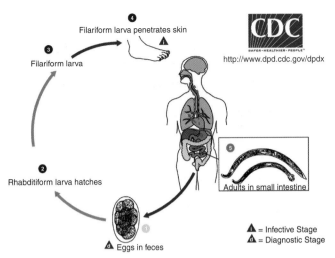

Figure 8-4 Life cycle of the hookworm.

stage and on deer in the adult stage. During the nymphal stage, the tick is most aggressive and more apt to bite the host. The tick's life cycle explains what seasons of the year humans can become infected and clarifies the mode of transmission.

The life cycle of the agent or the vector provides added information on the transmission of an infectious agent, including how the agent exits its reservoir (portal of exit), the mode of transmission (water, vector, fomite, etc.), and how the agent enters the host (the portal of entry). For example, the agent that causes TB, *M. tuberculosis*, primarily infects the lungs; thus, the portal of exit is coughing. The action of coughing expels the agent from the reservoir (human) into the air. The agent has now left its reservoir and is contained in the droplets expelled from the lungs. The mode of transmission is through the air, so TB is considered an airborne disease. The portal of entry for TB is almost always through the host's respiratory system (the host breathes in the droplets that contain the agent and inhales them into the lungs).

Host Characteristics

The final aspect of the cycle of transmission is the host. The **host** is the human who is at risk for disease due to exposure to the agent. The main characteristic is the **susceptibility** of the host, that is, the likelihood of becoming infected with the agent. This is expressed in terms of the host's **immunity**, or **resistance** to the disease.

Immunity

There are two types of immunity, humoral and cellular. **Humoral immunity** means that the host carries antibodies to the agent in the blood, and **cellular immunity** is specific to each type of cell. Immunity is passive or active. When a person has **passive immunity**, immunity is transferred from one individual to another. It can occur naturally or artificially and lasts for only a short time. Passage of immunity from the mother to her infant is an example of natural passive immunity. Artificial passive immunity involves the transfer of antibodies and can be done in various forms. **Active immunity** is acquired through exposure to the agent. It is long-lasting and can last for life, as when a person who had mumps as a child remains immune for the rest of his life.

Inherent Resistance

Another measure of the host's level of susceptibility is **inherent resistance**. This is the ability of the host to resist the disease independent of antibodies. It can be inherited or acquired and is often linked to health status and is temporary rather than permanent. Even if exposed to the agent, the host does not become ill due to her own ability to resist the disease because of other factors that boost the body's ability to resist the disease, such as adequate nutrition.

Colonization

Another host characteristic is **colonization**. In this case, a person is infected with the agent but has no signs of infection. This term is mentioned frequently in acute care settings in relation to multiple drug resistant agents such as methicillin-resistant *Staphylococcus aureus*. Patients are admitted with no signs of infection but are colonized with a serious multidrug-resistant pathogen. Colonized hosts are able to spread the disease despite not being apparently ill.

Breaking the Chain of Infection

When clinical signs and symptoms are present, the host is not only infected, but disease has now occurred. The cycle of transmission is complete. The agent has travelled from the reservoir to the new host and has caused disease. For the nurse, understanding the cycle of transmission for a specific pathogen can guide the type of intervention developed to break the chain of infection. Interventions can be aimed at any point in the cycle of transmission. For example, with the outbreak of the Zika virus in the summer of 2016, Florida attempted to break the cycle of infection by eradicating the vector, the Aedes aegypti mosquito, through application of pesticides. The use of mosquito nets in malaria-prone areas attempts to block the mode of transmission by placing a barrier between the portal of exit and the portal of entry.

One of the key components in breaking the chain of transmission is to reduce the susceptibility of the host.

This is primarily achieved through vaccination. Because of the importance of this approach, the *HP* topic related to CDs includes a strong focus on immunization. The first objective under this topic is to "reduce, eliminate, or maintain elimination of cases of vaccine-preventable disease" and has 10 vaccine-related targets, 4 of which have a target of total elimination (no cases). The four CDs targeted for elimination through vaccination include acute paralytic poliomyelitis, rubella, hepatitis B, and congenital rubella syndrome.[40]

■ **HEALTHY PEOPLE**
Immunization and Communicable Diseases

Goal: Increase immunization rates and reduce preventable CDs.

Overview: The increase in life expectancy during the 20th century is largely a result of improvements in child survival associated with reductions in infectious disease mortality because of immunization.[1] However, CDs remain a major cause of illness, disability, and death. Immunization recommendations in the United States currently target 17 vaccine-preventable diseases across the life span.

HP 2020 goals for immunization and CDs are rooted in evidence-based clinical and community activities and services for the prevention and treatment of CDs. Objectives new to *HP 2020* focused on technological advancements and ensuring that states, local public health departments, and nongovernmental organizations are strong partners in the attempt on the part of the United States to control the spread of CDs. Objectives for 2020 reflected a more mobile society and the fact that diseases do not stop at geopolitical borders. Awareness of disease, and completing prevention and treatment courses remain essential components for reducing infectious disease transmission.[40]

Midcourse Review: Of the 67 measurable objectives, 21 were met or exceeded targets, 26 were improving, 11 had little or no change, and 6 were worse (Fig. 8-5). Among the objectives that were getting worse were the number of U.S.-acquired cases of mumps, pertussis, and measles.[41]

Outbreak Investigation

Despite efforts to prevent transmission of disease, outbreaks of infectious disease continue to occur. When they do, public health departments conduct outbreak investigations. An **outbreak investigation**, related to CDs, involves conducting a systematic epidemiological investigation into

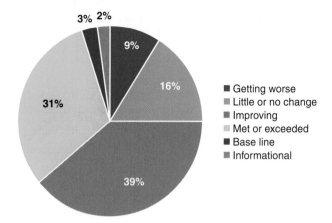

Figure 8-5 Healthy People 2020 Midcourse Review: Immunization and Infectious Disease. (*Data source reference 41.*)

the sudden increase in the incidence of a CD. Conducting an outbreak investigation requires solving the mystery, similar to what a detective does in solving a murder case. With CDs, though, solving the mystery always involves more than knowing "whodunit." In the game Clue, the winning player announces their final conclusion that it was, for example, Mrs. White who did it in the parlor with the lead pipe, based on a process of elimination. Unlike Clue, a CD outbreak investigation requires much more. Investigators seek to identify who got sick, what made them sick, when they got sick, and at what point it happened. The public health team's goal is to gather enough information so that measures can be put in place to halt the spread of disease. These facts are essential to determine what is the best action to take to break the chain of transmission and prevent further spread of the disease to uninfected members of the population. Public health science provides the guide for answering these questions (see Chapter 3). Sometimes the investigation is completed more quickly, as in some foodborne disease outbreaks, but sometimes unravelling the mystery takes much more time and detective work, especially if the disease is an emerging disease, as was the case with HIV in the 1980s.

▶ **SOLVING THE MYSTERY**
The Case of the Halloween Cider
Public Health Science Topics Covered:
• Epidemiology
• Surveillance

In this hypothetical case, Susan and Mary, the infection control nurses in two hospitals located in the same county, noticed an increase in positive laboratory results for *E. coli* 0157:H7 infections in their patients. On Monday, the laboratory informed Mary that there were two patients with positive results for *E. coli* 0157:H7. Mary called Susan to see whether her hospital had any cases. Susan called Mary back on Tuesday to report three cases; Mary had an additional seven cases. As required, they reported their findings to the county public health department. The public health nurse, Joe, asked them to join the investigation team. In any outbreak investigation, identifying the culprit, that is, the infectious agent responsible for causing the disease, is crucial.

Outbreak Investigation

The first thing Joe did was to determine whether there was an epidemic. He accomplished this through a review of the 10 reported cases at the time of Susan and Mary's first call. Most *E. coli* bacteria are harmless and are normal flora living in the intestines. However, Shiga toxin-producing *E. coli* (STEC) such as 0157:H7 are **pathogenic**; that is, they cause disease.[42] There are federal health regulations that require that certain diseases are designated as notifiable. *E. coli* 0157:H7 is one of these diseases. For each notifiable disease, there is a CDC case definition.[37,38] To begin the investigation, they used the CDC guide to define what constituted a case. Case identification provides the investigators with information needed to plot the outbreak and helps to determine whether there is a common source.

Sometimes the agent is not known at the outset, so clinical parameters define a case until the pathogen is identified. When the pathogen is not known, a patient is considered a case if he or she manifests specific clinical symptoms such as fever, diarrhea, and vomiting, which the team determines based on review of the presenting cases. Because Mary and Susan had already identified the agent, a case was defined based on laboratory-confirmed *E. coli* 0157:H7. Much is known about the agent *E. coli* 0157:H7, which was isolated in the early 1980s, and there are specific guidelines for defining a case (Box 8-4).[43] In addition to the guidelines, the team included in the case definition the date on which symptoms first occurred. This helped to confirm that the case occurred within a similar time frame as the other cases. The team members also extended their search outside of the county to determine whether there were any cases that had occurred within the same time frame but diagnosed elsewhere.

BOX 8–4 ■ *Escherichia coli* 0157:H7—CDC Clinical Description

Culture-independent diagnostic testing (CIDT), defined as the detection of antigen or nucleic acid sequences of the pathogen, is rapidly being adopted by clinical laboratories. For Shiga toxin-producing *Escherichia coli* (STEC), these are generally PCR-based testing methods that do not require a stool culture and thus do not yield an isolate. Although concerted efforts are being made to ensure reflexive culture is performed at the clinical laboratory or the state public health laboratory, CIDT-positive reports are not always culture-confirmed. The current STEC case definition classifies a positive CIDT result detecting Shiga toxin, that is not culture-confirmed, as a suspect case.

To prevent an increase in underreporting of STEC infection cases and to make case definitions for enteric bacterial pathogens more consistent, this position statement proposes that: 1. Detection of Shiga toxin, Shiga toxin genes, *E. coli* O157, or STEC/EHEC by CIDT without culture-confirmation in a clinically compatible person be classified as a probable STEC case. 2. Illnesses among persons who are epidemiologically linked to a confirmed or laboratory-diagnosed probable case will be classified as probable epidemiologically-linked cases.

Source: (43)

Because the team members knew the identity of the agent, they also knew the common reservoir and method of transmission. Because *E. coli* normally lives in the intestinal tracts of humans and animals, the usual route for transmission is the fecal-oral route. *E. coli,* therefore, is either water- or food-borne and has been traced in previous outbreaks to various types of produce, such as spinach, as well as meats, such as undercooked hamburger. Thus, the team must determine whether there was a common source of infection and whether it was foodborne or waterborne. A **common source** of infection occurs when the pathogen is transmitted from a single source, such as cantaloupes grown on a particular farm or hamburgers served at a particular restaurant.

To help determine the severity of the outbreak, the team calculated the CFR using the total number of fatal cases divided by the total number of cases. In this outbreak, there was a total of 106 cases including 5 deaths. The CFR was 4.7%. Because of the CFR and the potential that this *E. coli* outbreak could be multistate, the county public health department worked in collaboration with the state health department and the CDC to help locate cases outside the county.

$$CFR = \frac{Number\ of\ fatal\ cases}{Total\ number\ of\ cases}$$

Once the team defined what constituted a case based on laboratory confirmation of infection with the agent, the members used basic epidemiology to help plan the next step. The team began to figure out the essential aspects of this potential outbreak and then plan the prevention efforts based on whether the intervention was aimed at the agent (eradicating the agent), the environment (interrupting transmission), or the host (reducing susceptibility). To do this, they collected further data on each of the cases, such as onset of symptoms, place of residence, and information about where they were and what they ate, starting with the maximum exposure date. Because the range of incubation is 8 to 10 days, the team started with the day of onset of symptoms and worked backward to the maximum date of exposure. For example, for case number one symptoms began on November 7. The team worked backward to October 28 and collected data on where the person was and what he or she ate.

The team used the data to build an epidemic curve. An **epidemic curve** is constructed by plotting on a graph the number of cases (y-axis) based on the date of onset (x-axis). This requires making a graph that includes the number of new cases per day and month (Fig. 8-6). The graph helped determine how much time elapsed between exposure to the pathogen and the beginning of clinical symptoms. Because the incubation ranges from 8 to 10 days, the team could estimate what date(s) the exposure probably occurred.

The epidemic curve also helped determine whether there was a **point source**, that is, the source of the exposure happened at one point in time; a **continuous source**, that is, the exposure is ongoing; or an **intermittent source**, that is, exposure comes and goes. After looking at the epidemic curve (see Fig. 8-5), Joe noted that after day 5 there was a decline in the number of cases, but there was a subsequent increase in cases on days 10 and 11. This represented a bimodal curve that could be a result of two different point sources or of possible household exposure, because E. coli can be transmitted from person to person. When the cases that occurred on the second curve were reviewed, all of them were family members of an earlier case. This led the

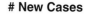

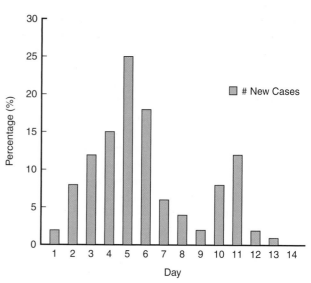

Figure 8-6 Plotting the epidemic curve.

team to conclude that there was a point source for the exposure.

Because it appeared to be a point source, team members then examined all the cases to determine whether there was a common source, that is, something that all of the cases ate, drank, or did that could have been contaminated with E. coli. The team also examined the data on where the patients were and whether there was a common restaurant or a food market where the people purchased food or drink.

The team next needed to determine how the cases come in contact with the agent. To help with this process, the team mapped out the cycle of transmission for E. coli 0157:H7. Mapping out this information helped the team's investigation because members needed to know the most likely places where patients may have come in contact with E. coli. Knowing something about the pathogen helped the team members develop a hypothesis for the source of the infection so they could begin to build an intervention to prevent further cases.

Generating a hypothesis about the sources of infection is a key step in outbreak investigations. The team began by reviewing the sources of infection in prior E. coli 0157:H7 outbreaks. There was an outbreak of E. coli 0157:H7 in Washington State in 1993 that resulted in 700 cases and 4 deaths. All of the fatalities were children. In 1999, there was an outbreak at the Washington State Fair. A total of 781 people were infected, and 2 died.[44] An outbreak in 2007 resulted in only 12 cases but caused the recall of 21.7 million pounds of ground beef and the closing of the Topps Meat Company.[45] E. coli outbreaks continued with one in 2018 linked to romaine lettuce that resulted in a nationwide alert to avoid eating any romaine lettuce.[46] Based on these cases, the team members developed the hypothesis that the outbreak was foodborne and began by examining the data to determine whether there were any commonalities among the cases. The data they examined included their survey of all the patients who met the definition of being a case. The infection control nurses, Susan and Mary, interviewed patients still in the hospital, and Joe conducted phone interviews with those who were discharged or who were cared for at home. Based on information from the CDC, cases were located outside the county and outside the state. The CDC and the state health department helped coordinate data collection for these cases.

Based on the epidemic curve, the team narrowed the possible date of the initial exposure to a 5-day period that extended from October 28 to November 1. During that time, the county held a Halloween festival, and all of the primary cases had attended the festival. At the festival, there were multiple possible sources for exposure, including a petting zoo, the sale of apple cider from a local farm, a fresh fruit and salad stand, and a hamburger stand. With all the information gathered, the team then narrowed down possible sources based on the ones that the cases had in common. About half of the cases had gone to the petting zoo, a quarter of the cases had eaten fresh salads from the fruit and salad stand, and a third had consumed hamburgers. In contrast, all but four of the cases reported drinking cider. The team then calculated relative risk (see Chapter 3) for the disease based on the possible exposure to hamburgers, petting zoo, and cider. Based on their survey, they found that approximately 95% of the cases reported consumption of the apple cider sold at the food stand next to the kiddy rides. They then questioned the vendor and found that the cider came from a local farmer who made the cider just for the fair.

Management of the Epidemic

Now that the team had identified the probable source of the outbreak, the team had to isolate the source. In some of the E. coli 0157:H7 outbreaks,

isolating the source had proved to be problematic. For example, in the 2018 epidemic associated with the consumption of romaine lettuce, cases were distributed across multiple states.[46] In this hypothetical case, to manage the epidemic, the team located the farmer who supplied the cider to the stand at the fair. The cider was homemade and unpasteurized cider thus a possible source of E. coli 0157:H7. If the cider had come from a commercial enterprise, the health department would want to intervene and make sure no further sale of the cider occurred. In this case, the public health department questioned the farmer about further sale of the product and discovered that the farmer had a vegetable stand. The county public health department closed the stand and all of the cider the farmer had was destroyed. The public health department also alerted the public to the threat of infection for those who had consumed the cider so that they could be screened for possible infection and provided with treatment if needed. A public service announcement was released advising the public to destroy any cider that had been purchased from this farm.

Managing an outbreak, especially in the case of a disease known to have an increased risk for mortality, requires prompt action on multiple levels. The key is to know how best to break the cycle of transmission. In this case, the reservoir was the target. The team focused on removal of the cider, the actual reservoir for the E. coli 0157:H7. The team also sought to eliminate further consumption of the Halloween cider. In this hypothetical case, a local intervention would work if the farmer who made the cider sold only to the vendor at the fair who then sold only single servings of the cider at the fair. Instead, the farmer owned a farm stand with cider products; therefore, a broader intervention was warranted.

Infectious Agents and Attack Rates

The hypothetical Case of the Halloween Cider illustrates how humans become infected with an agent that can cause disease. A few other pieces of information are useful to have when conducting an outbreak investigation related to an infectious disease. First, transmission can occur from the reservoir directly or indirectly. Person-to-person contact is an example of direct transmission and occurs with sexually transmitted infections (STIs). Indirect transmission occurs when the agent leaves the reservoir and is transferred to the human host through an indirect means such as a vector or in the case of fomite transmission.

Once transmission has occurred, disease is not necessarily immediately apparent. As mentioned earlier, inapparent infection is the subclinical phase during which there are no apparent clinical symptoms. From a public health perspective, it is often important to identify those with inapparent infection not only to provide early treatment, but also to stop the spread of infection, as you will see in the next case. To help understand how long this inapparent infection phase can last, it is important to know the incubation period. This is the time interval between infection and the first clinical signs of disease. For *E. coli,* the incubation period is short, but for other pathogens, it can be quite long. For example, persons infected with TB during childhood may not develop the disease until later in life.

As discussed in Chapter 3, time is a key issue in epidemiology. With CDs, the incubation period for the pathogen is one example of time that must be considered when investigating an outbreak and planning prevention. Another factor to consider is the **generation time**, which is the interval between infection with the agent and the maximum time that the host is infectious, that is, the communicability of the host. Sometimes the incubation and generation time are the same. If that is the case, then when symptoms appear, the host can no longer transfer the agent to other hosts, but that is not always the case. Generation time helps when dealing with the spread of agents that have a large number of subclinical cases.

Another issue related to infection at the population level is **community or herd immunity**. This refers to the immunity of a population to an agent. If a large portion of the population is immune (by vaccine or past infection), that can prevent the spread of the disease to persons in the population who do not have immunity. There is usually a threshold of immunity that needs to be achieved to establish herd immunity. In other words, a certain percentage of the population must be immune to achieve herd immunity to a specific agent. With herd immunity, even if a few members of the community become infected, the population as a whole is protected from an outbreak.

In the hypothetical Case of the Halloween Cider, the team calculated a CFR. There are other rates that can be helpful in an investigation, including **attack rate** and **secondary attack rate**. An attack rate is actually a type of incidence rate (see Chapter 3 for more in-depth discussion). It is calculated using the number of persons who are ill divided by the total number of the population, which includes persons who are ill plus those who are well. This is multiplied by a constant (usually 100) and expressed over a certain time period. The attack rate can be calculated based on a particular risk factor. For example, suppose the team had narrowed down the possible risk factors at the county fair as the consumption of burgers at the burger stand, the petting zoo, and the cider. For each risk factor, the team would calculate a separate attack rate for those exposed to the risk factor and those not exposed. Group A could be those who drank the cider and group B could be those who did not drink the cider. Once these two attack rates are calculated, the difference between the two attack rates would be determined. This process would then be repeated for the burgers and the petting zoo (Box 8-5). The risk factor with the greatest difference in attack rates may be your common source for the outbreak.

Another calculation useful in an outbreak investigation is the secondary attack rate. This reflects the spread of disease from those who contracted the disease from the initial source to others usually within the same household or other unit where people come in close contact with others. The secondary attack rate is calculated by dividing the number of new cases in a particular group minus the initial case(s) by the number of susceptible persons in the group minus the initial case(s) (see Box 8-5).

Sexually Transmitted and Reproductive Tract Infections

Not all CD outbreaks follow the course described in the Case of the Halloween Cider. In that case, the outbreak required public health officials to take action related to a

---

BOX 8–5 ■ Rate Calculations

$$\text{Attack Rate} = \frac{\text{ill}}{\text{ill} + \text{well}} \times 100 \text{ during a time period}$$

$$\text{Secondary Attack Rate (\%)} = \frac{\text{Number of new cases in group} - \text{initial cases}}{\text{Number of susceptible persons in the group} - \text{initial cases}} \times 100$$

food product and those who became ill were not aware of their risk. On the other hand, Sexually transmitted infections (STIs), also referred to as sexually transmitted diseases, are related to behavior. Much has been done to alert those who are sexually active to the risk involved in unprotected sexual activity.

In *HP*, the topic "sexually transmitted disease" is a separate topic area from the topic "immunization and infectious diseases." Specific diseases targeted in the objectives are chlamydia, pelvic inflammatory disease (PID), gonorrhea, syphilis, and human papillomavirus.

■ HEALTHY PEOPLE
Sexually Transmitted Diseases

Goal: Promote healthy sexual behaviors, strengthen community capacity, and increase access to quality services to prevent STDs and their complications.

Overview: Sexually transmitted diseases (STDs) refer to more than 25 infectious organisms transmitted primarily through sexual activity. STD prevention is an essential primary care strategy for improving reproductive health.

Despite their burdens, costs, and complications, and the fact that they are largely preventable, STDs remain a significant public health problem in the United States. This problem is largely unrecognized by the public, policy makers, and health-care providers. STDs cause many harmful, often irreversible, and costly clinical complications, such as:

- Reproductive health problems
- Fetal and perinatal health problems
- Cancer
- Facilitation of the sexual transmission of HIV infection[47]

Midcourse Review: Of the 14 measurable objectives, 4 were met or exceeded targets, 4 were improving, 3 had little or no change, and 3 were worse (Fig. 8-7). Among the objectives that were getting worse were the number of new cases of primary and secondary syphilis among males and the number of new cases of gonorrhea among males.[48]

Burden of Disease and Sexually Transmitted Infections

STIs are caused by pathogens transmitted from human to human through sexual contact. The reservoir of the agent is the human body. These infections can cause serious illness and disability, and are preventable. There are three notifiable sexual infections that have federally

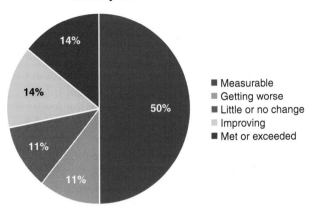

Healthy People 2020 Midcourse Review: Sexually Transmitted Diseases

- Measurable
- Getting worse
- Little or no change
- Improving
- Met or exceeded

Figure 8-7 Healthy People 2020 Midcourse Review: Sexually Transmitted Diseases. (*Data source reference 48.*)

funded control programs: chlamydia, gonorrhea, and syphilis.[49]

The incidence rate of chlamydia (agent: *Chlamydia trachomatis*) has increased from 160.2 per 100,000 in 1990 to 497 per 100,000 in 2016 with the rate in women double the rate in men.[50] Chlamydia is associated with PID and can be passed on to the infant during delivery. The agent *Chlamydia trachomatis* is a bacterium and is treatable with antibiotics. Unfortunately, for many women there are no symptoms, and often the infection goes undiagnosed. If the infection is not treated and PID develops, women can experience complications such as infertility, ectopic pregnancy, and chronic pelvic pain. As this is a treatable infection public health efforts focus on screening and early treatment, as well as education and promotion of condom use during intercourse.

Another serious STI is gonorrhea (*Neisseria gonorrhoeae*). After chlamydia, it is the most commonly reported STI in the United States. At the end of the 20th century, the incidence rate fell 75% from 1975 to 1997 and reached a historic low in 2009 with a national rate of 98.1 cases per 100,000. However, in 2016 there was an 18.5% increase from 2015 with a total of 468,514 cases of gonorrhea (a rate of 145.8 per 100,000).[51] Like chlamydia, it is a major cause of PID, infertility, and ectopic pregnancies. Also, like chlamydia, the infection is treatable, but serious health consequences occur if it is untreated. In addition, there is now widespread resistance to a class of antibiotics used to treat gonorrhea, the fluoroquinolones, resulting in a change in CDC guidelines for the treatment of gonorrhea with cephalosporins.[52]

The third STI under national surveillance is syphilis, a genital ulcerative disease caused by the bacterium *Treponema pallidum*. Syphilis has four stages: primary, secondary, tertiary, and latent. The primary stage occurs between 10 and 90 days following infection, and is evidenced by a sore, or multiple sores, at the site where the bacterium entered the infected person. The sore or chancre often heals without treatment. If there is no treatment, then the infection enters the secondary stage. During the secondary stage, the person develops a skin rash and mucous membrane lesions can occur while the chancre is healing or shortly thereafter. It can be accompanied by various other symptoms such as fever or swollen lymph nodes, or the symptoms may be so mild that they are not noticed. These symptoms will also resolve with or without treatment. However, if no treatment is given it can progress to the latent stage of syphilis, which is a period of time when there are no symptoms of the infection and can last for years. The tertiary stage does not occur in all cases of untreated syphilis, but a person with tertiary syphilis can experience adverse effects on numerous internal organs, including the brain, resulting in paralysis and dementia. Historical examples of people with late-stage syphilis include Al Capone and King George III of England, who was on the throne at the time of the American Revolution.

In 2017 there were a total of 30,644 cases of both primary and secondary syphilis reported in the United States, a rate of 9.5 cases per 100,000 population, up from 8.6 per 100,000 in 2016. In 2017, in the U.S., the rate in men was 10 times higher than in women (16.9 cases per 100,000 males vs. 2.3 cases per 100,000 females) with men accounting for 87.7% of primary and secondary syphilis cases. Men who have sex with men accounted for 57% of the cases. The rate of congenital syphilis increased in 2017 to 23.3 cases per 100,000 live births, a 43.8% increase from 2016 (16.2 cases per 100,000 live births) and a 153.3% increase from to 2013 (9.2 cases per 100,000 live births).[53]

Risk Factors

The main risk factor for STIs is unprotected sexual contact. The pathogens responsible for STIs are transmitted through the exchange of bodily fluids. Some groups are more at risk than others based on gender, ethnicity, and socioeconomic status. As noted earlier, men accounted for almost 90% of all cases, and men who have sex with men accounted for more than half the cases. (Fig. 8-8).[54] There was also a difference in the number of syphilis cases among racial groups. For example, according to the CDC in 2017, the rate of reported primary and secondary syphilis increased across all racial ethnic groups with the highest prevalence rate in blacks with 24.2 cases per 100,000 population, up from 23.1. For whites the rate increased from 4.1 to 5.94 cases per 100,000.[53,55] The disparity in rates of STIs across ethnic and socioeconomic status has been well documented over the past decades.[56,57] For example, although blacks represent only 13% of the population, rates of gonorrhea among blacks was 8.6 times higher than the rates among whites.[51] This may be due in part to socioeconomic factors. For example, those with less health insurance coverage are more apt to seek care at public health clinics. Although STIs are reportable infections, compliance with this law for reporting cases is higher in public clinics than it is in private physicians' offices. Access to care may also prevent early diagnosis and treatment.[56,57]

Syphilis Cases by Gender and Sexual Partner

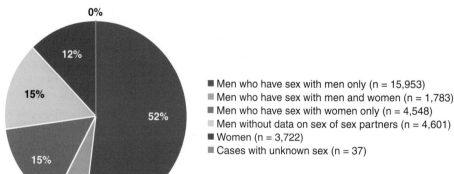

- ■ Men who have sex with men only (n = 15,953)
- ■ Men who have sex with men and women (n = 1,783)
- ■ Men who have sex with women only (n = 4,548)
- ■ Men without data on sex of sex partners (n = 4,601)
- ■ Women (n = 3,722)
- ■ Cases with unknown sex (n = 37)

Figure 8-8 Syphilis cases by gender and sexual partner. *(Data source reference 54.)*

● APPLYING PUBLIC HEALTH SCIENCE

The Case of Syphilis in Baltimore City

Public Health Science Topics Covered:

- Health planning
- Community assessment

The Baltimore Syphilis Elimination Project provides an excellent example of how a collaborative effort between a public health department and health care providers, including nurses, can result in a reduction in disease. The project began due to a 40% increase in prevalence of syphilis in Baltimore City that prompted an assessment of the data related to the new syphilis cases and the implementation of a population-level intervention.[58] Because syphilis is a notifiable disease, all diagnosed cases in Baltimore are reported to the local public health department, which in turn reports the cases to the state health department. This information is then reported to the CDC. The case of syphilis in Baltimore City helps to illustrate the differences between a public health response to a foodborne infectious disease outbreak and an increase in new cases of an STI.

The first step for the team in Baltimore City was to determine whether the increase in cases was an epidemic. An excess of cases above the endemic levels in a specific community or region is considered an epidemic. To decide whether there is a need for action, public health officials examine the increase in cases to determine whether the increase has reached an **epidemic threshold**, that is, the number of cases above the endemic rate associated with an increased risk for spread of the disease. The epidemic threshold is used to make decisions about whether to alert the public about a possible epidemic. Epidemic thresholds differ from disease to disease, and the methods for determining the threshold can also vary. These calculations require a sophisticated approach, but they help guide public health officials in deciding when an epidemic alert is needed.[59,60] The choice of an epidemic threshold usually reflects the number of cases that exceeds a certain number per 100,000 population over a specified time period. Because the term *epidemic* is emotionally charged, public health officials use it with caution. When a general public alert is needed, the epidemic threshold can help the public health officials either assure the public that there is not an epidemic or alert the public to a real risk.

Next, it is important to determine the type of epidemic related to the specific mode of transmission.

The Case of the Halloween Cider fits the description of a common-source epidemic as do other water- and foodborne infections. There can also be a vector-borne epidemic such as the Zika epidemic, which was spread by mosquitos. In the case of syphilis, the disease has been endemic in the human population for thousands of years. Therefore, unlike an *E. coli* outbreak, the increase in syphilis cases in Baltimore City did not reflect a national epidemic or a pandemic but rather a specific increase in one particular geographical area.

In this case, once the public health officials realized there was a dramatic increase in the number of cases, they first defined what constituted a case. They looked at the cases based on demographics and found that the increase was occurring mainly in the Hispanic population. In that population, the incidence rate had increased by 73% compared with a 40% increase for the population in general. Another interesting detail also emerged in their review of cases. They found that the majority of all Hispanic cases were primary cases.[58]

Health Planning

Now the team was ready for action. Instead of a national media campaign and product recall as in the case of an *E. coli* 0157:H7 or *Salmonella* outbreak, a local program was put together, the Syphilis Elimination Project, an excellent example of how to plan a health program (see Chapter 5). It is also a good example of incorporating both a primary and a secondary approach to prevention. In addition, they developed a prevention program that targeted a population at increased risk with a selected level of prevention (see Chapter 2).

The Syphilis Elimination Project had two goals. The first goal focused on knowledge, awareness, and decreasing incidence of syphilis in the Baltimore City Hispanic community, and the second was to get those with syphilis into treatment. Under the first goal, the objective was to increase the number of Hispanics tested for syphilis by 50% from baseline.[58] This is an example of *case finding*. Case finding comes under the umbrella of secondary prevention. The purpose of finding cases is to identify those who are infected and get them into treatment. In STIs, the reservoir is humans. If there is an effective treatment for the disease, it is possible to eliminate the agent in the reservoir. Early treatment for the disease from a population perspective is therefore both a primary and a secondary prevention measure. Through case finding, public health officials can intervene in relation to the agent's reservoir.

For the Baltimore City Syphilis Elimination Project, there were specific challenges related to culture, stigma, and access to the population. Before the team members initiated their project, they had to address these challenges. In addition, skills related to cultural competency were needed to develop a program that would be accepted by the intended recipients. The team members combined their efforts at case finding with a multi-method patient education campaign. Bilingual outreach workers conducted street outreach by providing education on syphilis in bars, stores, and on the street. Because there is no known method of reducing our biological susceptibility to syphilis, the Elimination Project could not reduce biological susceptibility of the host. Instead, they developed a culturally relevant educational program that provided the population at risk, Hispanics living in Baltimore City, with behavioral strategies to reduce their chances of becoming infected.

When there are no means available to reduce the biological susceptibility of the host, the focus of primary prevention in CD becomes both the mode of transmission and the portal of entry. Through education, it is hoped that those who are not infected become educated on how the disease is transmitted and how it enters the body so that they can implement effective strategies to prevent becoming infected. In this case, an additional challenge was to reach the population most at risk, because the project fit the definition of a selective prevention program (see Chapter 2). The Syphilis Elimination Project team members had done their homework on who was getting infected, and they had a good grasp of where this selected population resided. They designed a program that incorporated cultural and geographical issues related to the population. They used bilingual outreach workers who conducted their educational interventions during the evening hours and in the early mornings in high-traffic areas. They chose these times to try to reach the most people by targeting working and partying hours. By the end of 10 weeks they had met their first goal, with 2,825 Hispanics having received patient education and health information materials. Thus, by taking into consideration the role of culture and the importance of engaging the community, the project was successful in primary prevention (providing education to those not yet infected). They were also able to meet their second goal, screening (secondary prevention) and identifying those in need of treatment. Because the cases that were identified through screening were almost all primary infections, few needed tertiary interventions, that is, treatment of clinical disease as seen in secondary and latent syphilis.

Emerging Sexually Transmitted Infections

Gonorrhea and syphilis are mentioned throughout history, whereas other STIs are new arrivals. In 1981, a new STI emerged that grabbed the attention of the world—HIV. Unlike gonorrhea and syphilis, there currently is no cure for this infection. When it was first identified, those with the infection had few treatment options and the CFR was high. Over the years, science has developed successful treatments, and the diagnosis of HIV infection is no longer a death sentence in the United States. At the end of 2015, it was estimated by the CDC that 1.1 million people aged 13 and older were living with HIV infection in the United States. This estimate included more than 162,500 (15%) persons with undiagnosed infection.[61]

The emergence of this STI changed how nurses provide care. Unlike other STIs, this virus could be transmitted through exposure to other bodily fluids, including blood. In the late 1980s, when surveillance data indicated that health-care workers were at increased risk for HIV infection through exposure to blood and other bodily secretions, a legal approach was taken to prevent the spread of this disease in health-care workers. OSHA put into law the requirement that health-care workers use PPE. As always, the prevention measures taken were based on the mode of transmission and targeted a population at risk for becoming infected. Following the institution of this law, the incidence rate of HIV in health-care workers with no other risk factors dropped dramatically. The use of PPEs has become routine in all health-care settings. This dramatic change in hospital-based infections control created as dramatic a shift in care as hand hygiene did after the discovery that germs cause disease (see Chapter 1).

HIV/AIDS is a pandemic and has had a severe impact on certain portions of the globe, especially in developing countries where access to treatment is limited. Once again, disparity exists related to this STI because of socioeconomic status, culture, and governmental support of prevention efforts. This infection is an example of the emerging diseases affecting the United States and world as a whole.

■ CULTURAL CONTEXT
Prevention of Sexually Transmitted Infections

Due to the mode of transmission, STIs bring additional challenges to prevention efforts. Changing risky behaviors in general can be difficult but addressing sexual behaviors may be tied to feelings of shame, guilt, or powerlessness, and that can present barriers to the nurse wishing to intervene. The Syphilis Elimination Project demonstrates that these barriers can be overcome, especially if a population approach is taken that includes consideration of the culture of the target population and that includes that population in the design, implementation, and evaluation of the intervention. However, stigma continues to present a barrier to health-care providers attempting to care for persons with an STI. One group of researchers in Uganda concluded stigma associated with HIV resulted in poor communication between HIV clients and providers about childbearing.[62] In other cases, the loosening of cultural norms around sexual behaviors may actually increase the risk of contracting an STI. For example, a group of nurses working to address the rise in STIs in Thailand noted that the increase in tourism, the adopting of western culture, and the loosening of cultural norms has coincided with the increase in the demand for entertainment and sex business by tourists including sex shows and sexually provocative performances.[63]

Communicable Diseases and Communicability

Not all diseases caused by an infection are communicable. Understanding the difference between an agent that infects humans and causes disease, and the communicability of the agent is based on the transmission of the infection from one person to another. A person may become infected with a pathogen, but no public health response is required to prevent further transmission of the agent to other persons, because the agent is not actually communicable. One example that helps illustrate the difference between the agent and the threat of transmission from one person to another is the Case of the Flesh-Eating Bug.

❭ SOLVING THE MYSTERY
The Case of the Flesh-Eating Bug
Public Health Science Topics Covered:
- Epidemiology
- Surveillance

On June 20, 2006, David Walton, a leading economist in the United Kingdom, was admitted to Cheltenham General Hospital complaining of fever and stomach pain. Within 24 hours, he was dead. According

to one physician, the infection "seemed to spread before our eyes, down the thigh, growing towards the shoulder and chest".[64]

In another case, a 3-year-old girl, Isabel Maude, was brought to the emergency room with high fever, nausea, and vomiting. Her parents explained that their daughter had recently come down with chickenpox. The physician reviewed the care of chickenpox with the parents and sent the child home. The symptoms worsened, and the child was readmitted to the pediatric intensive care unit because of organ failure. The first physician had missed the diagnosis based on the recent history of chickenpox. The child actually had a much more serious infectious disease. She eventually recovered after a 2-month stay at the hospital.[65] The case would have turned out differently if the health-care provider who first saw the little girl had asked more questions. The health-care providers failed to solve the mystery when they first saw the girl. They did not go beyond the obvious clinical conclusion that this was chickenpox and ask what else might be going on.

A third case related to this same infectious disease occurred in Lanarkshire, England. Between December 24, 2008, and January 3, 2008, two persons with a history of intravenous (IV) drug use died of the flesh-eating bug. There was one other confirmed case and one suspected case. These deaths prompted a public health announcement from the public health authorities in Lanarkshire. The first two cases did not result in a public health alert. This third case did, but it was different from the other CD investigations reviewed in this chapter. In the Case of the Halloween Cider and in the syphilis epidemic in Baltimore City among Hispanics, the infection occurred within a population. The hypothetical E. coli outbreak took place at a fair, and anyone who attended that fair and drank the unpasteurized cider was at risk for becoming infected. In Baltimore City, an increase in the incidence rate for an STI occurred within a specific ethnic population with less access to care and less awareness about their risk for infection. In both cases, interventions were aimed at reducing the incidence rates within a population. The cases also differed on the CFR. In the first case, though the CFR is low for many E. coli outbreaks, many of those deaths are in children and older adults, and occur soon after infection. In the second case, the period between infection and death in untreated cases can be as long as 20 years. Therefore, the urgency related to an E. coli outbreak is fueled not only by the need to decrease illness but also by the importance of decreasing the risk of mortality, especially in children. In this case, the case of the flesh-eating bug, although the virulence of the disease was extreme, the disease was not spreading to the general public. One group of persons appeared to be at greater risk.[66]

One of the issues in CDs is separating the agent from the disease or diseases caused by the agent. In the case of the "flesh-eating bug," the agent can cause rapid death in some cases and no illness at all in other cases. In addition, the disease is linked to more than one agent. This is where the cycle of transmission gets interesting. Although the specific agent may differ, the portal of entry is the same; bacteria are introduced through an opening in the skin. In some cases, the introduced bacteria are those that are often found on the skin or in the throat.[67] This was not the case with the men who had a history of IV drug use. Therefore, although the disease was the same and the portal of entry was the same, the reservoir differed. This then has implications for the decision of whether or not to proceed with a public health alert. In relation to *E. coli* 0157:H7, the primary concern was to deal with an outbreak. In the case of the "flesh-eating bug", only one of the scenarios given earlier resulted in a public health initiative similar that in *E. coli* outbreaks.

To answer the question about whether a public health alert is needed, it helps to go back to the lessons learned in the Case of the Halloween Cider. In that case, the team conducted an assessment to determine whether this was a common source of outbreak. Based on the agent, the team members rightly suspected that this was a foodborne outbreak. In the three scenarios presented related to the "flesh-eating bug", the first two cases represented an isolated incident. No new cases were admitted to the hospital. Knowing the usual portal of entry of an agent that causes this disease lowered the public health concern that others were at risk. However, in the third case there were three more cases in rapid succession. The one thing the patients had in common was IV heroin drug use. This raised the potential threat to the health of persons who were IV drug users of heroin, not the public in general.

One reason for the public health response was the virulence of the "flesh-eating bug". When it enters the body through a wound, the agents associated with the "flesh-eating bug" have a very high level of virulence; that is, the severity of the disease produced by the agent and the CFR were high. In the United States, the CFR for this disease ranges from 20 to 30 per 100 cases.[67] However, not all persons exposed to

agents that cause this disease become ill. Bacteria that cause this disease include *S. aureus, Clostridium perfringens, Bacteroides fragilis, Aeromonas hydrophila,* and others. Again, the presence of the agent is not what is important but rather the portal of entry. The agent itself can be present on the skin or in the throat and cause no disease or mild disease with a very low CFR. However, when introduced to the host through a wound, the disease agent causes changes. The formal name for this infectious disease is necrotizing fasciitis (NF). One of the known agents responsible for this disease is group A (-hemolytic streptococci (GABHS). In the throat, GABHS can cause mild illness, but when introduced into the human body through a break in the skin, NF can result.

This leads us back to the issue of the infectivity of the agent. From one perspective, the infectivity is low because there must be an opening in the skin for the agent to enter and cause disease. Therefore, the CDC does not recommend antibiotic prophylaxis in all persons exposed to the patient, unless there are certain other risk factors present. However, from another perspective, the infectivity of the agent is a key issue. Once the agent has entered the host through a break in the skin, it can rapidly multiply in the host, resulting in what is reflected in the quote that the infection "seemed to spread before our eyes, down the thigh, growing towards the shoulder and chest".[64]

For the first two cases, no public health alerts were made, but in the third case there was reason to believe that it was actually a common source outbreak. All of the cases had a history of heroin IV drug use. Although there were only four cases and two deaths, the virulence of the agent prompted action. In addition, a similar outbreak a few years earlier in the United Kingdom had resulted in 43 deaths. What the public health officials discovered was each of the cases had injected heroin that had been contaminated with the causative agent that was in spore form. They had a common source outbreak. This discovery led to a selective prevention effort that targeted those at risk, persons engaged in current IV drug use. Their efforts included alerting emergency departments. This part of their alert focused on case finding and early treatment.

The three examples of NF provided here illustrate that not all CDs require an immediate public health response and that various issues come into play when making these decisions. Key issues include the virulence of the agent or agents causing the disease, whether or not there is a common source for the outbreak, and whether the public health alert will reduce the occurrence of more cases as well as promote early detection and treatment. Of interest in the second case, the disease resulted in the parents of the child developing an organization, Isabel Healthcare, that provides a diagnosis system that prompts health-care providers to reach a timely diagnosis, thus preventing the delay in treatment experienced by their daughter.[65]

Controlling Communicable Diseases

In all the cases presented here, the main focus is to control the spread of disease. There are three main approaches: (1) changing the environment; (2) inactivating the agent; and (3) increasing host resistance. Changing the environment can involve altering or eliminating the reservoir, controlling the vector, applying personal measures of hygiene, and using aseptic technique. Nurses engage in these measures regularly in patient care settings through their own use of proper hygiene and aseptic technique. In this way, they help reduce the occurrence of healthcare-acquired infections. Public health officials actively engage in these measures on a regular basis through general community-level sanitation measures related to water, food, and sewerage. They also actively participate in vector control. Communities at risk for mosquito-borne diseases have mosquito control programs aimed at eliminating the breeding grounds of the insects. This may include the use of insecticides or the draining of swampy areas.

Inactivating the agent includes the use of physical and chemical agents. Pasteurization of cider uses heat to inactivate infectious agents such as *E. coli* 0157:H7. One of the main issues with transmission of *E. coli* 0157:H7 through beef products is the failure to properly cook the beef at a high enough temperature to inactivate the agent. Cold is also used to inactivate agents in food products. The advent of refrigeration greatly reduced the spread of foodborne diseases. There are specific guidelines related to adequate refrigeration of foods to prevent the growth of bacteria that can cause disease. Chemical methods involve the use of chemicals to control agents such as the chlorination of water or the use of disinfects to clean potentially infected areas or items.

Finally, breaking the cycle of transmission can be accomplished through increasing host resistance. As mentioned above, resistance can be active or passive. Eradication of smallpox was accomplished through the use of vaccines. This was a global campaign launched in 1967. At that time, smallpox had a CFR of 24% and left most of the survivors either scarred or blind. Once a person had the disease, there was no known treatment. However, since the late 1700s, it was known that inoculation with cowpox protected against the disease. The global effort to increase host resistance was successful and in 1977 the last documented case occurred. The use of vaccines to increase host resistance has dramatically changed the impact of CDs on populations, especially children. **Vaccine** refers to the immunizing agent used to increase the host's resistance to viral, rickettsial, and bacterial diseases.[68] They can be killed, modified, or changed into a variant form of the agent. In the United States, children routinely receive a series of vaccines that protect against measles, mumps, diphtheria, poliomyelitis, and rubella.[69] Recently, there has been controversy over the potential risk of autism related to childhood vaccinations despite the lack of scientific evidence to support the link. The CDC has put together a guide for parents on the use of vaccines.[70] The use of vaccines is a good example of evidence-based practice, because all vaccines go through a vigorous process to establish safety and effectiveness prior to being used.[69]

■ CELLULAR TO GLOBAL

Using the WHO definition, CDs begin with a pathogen: *Infectious diseases are caused by pathogenic microorganisms, such as bacteria, viruses, parasites, or fungi; the diseases can be spread, directly or indirectly, from one person to another. Zoonotic diseases are infectious diseases of animals that can cause disease when transmitted to humans.*[71]

Addressing CD requires action at the population level, with the WHO providing a central leadership role through their emergency preparedness program. Their stated vision: *An integrated global alert and response system for epidemics and other public health emergencies based on strong national public health systems and capacity and an effective international system for coordinated response.* In the first 6 months of 2018, the WHO responded to the following outbreaks: Ebola in the Democratic Republic of Congo, Measles in Japan, Rift Valley Fever in Kenya, Middle East Respiratory Syndrome Coronavirus in Saudi Arabi, and Cholera in Cameroon. Preventing and responding quickly to CD outbreaks requires the ability to treat at the cellular level and implement actions at the national and global level to reduce the impact of CDs.[72]

■ EVIDENCE-BASED PRACTICE
Vaccination Recommendations During Childhood

Practice Statement: Vaccination is recommended by the CDC for all children as outlined on the CDC's Web site for parents related to vaccination.[70]

Targeted Outcome: Decrease in incidence of vaccine preventable diseases in children.

Evidence to Support: Childhood vaccinations have been part of pediatric care for more than 70 years with a significant reduction of childhood CDs.

Recommended Approaches: Vaccines are held to the highest standard of safety. The United States currently has the safest, most effective vaccine supply in history. Years of testing are required by law before a vaccine can be licensed. Once in use, vaccines are continually monitored for safety and efficacy. Immunizations, like any medication, can cause adverse events. However, a decision not to immunize a child also involves risk. It is a decision to put the child and others who come into contact with him or her at risk of contracting a disease that could be dangerous or deadly. Consider measles. One out of 30 children with measles develops pneumonia. For every 1,000 children who get the disease, 1 or 2 will die of it. Thanks to vaccines, we have fewer cases of measles in the United States today. However, the disease is extremely contagious, and each year dozens of cases are imported from abroad into the United States, threatening the health of people who have not been vaccinated and those for whom the vaccine was not effective.[73] The CDC and the Food and Drug Administration continually work to make already safe vaccines even safer.[69] In the rare event that a child is injured by a vaccine, he or she may be compensated through the National Vaccine Injury Compensation Program (VICP).[74]

Vaccines are used to increase host resistance to other diseases. These include influenza, pneumonia, and tetanus. Health-care workers are immunized for hepatitis B. In some countries, a tuberculosis vaccination program is in effect for all members of the population. Several factors influence the decisions of public health agencies to make vaccines mandatory and how much protection will be provided by vaccines. First, vaccines are given when the risk to the population is high. For example, hepatitis B is not given to the general public because the risk is low. Health-care providers are at higher risk from their exposure to blood and bodily fluids; thus, health-care workers providing direct care to patients are required to be vaccinated for hepatitis B. For most of the childhood diseases, the risk is high for all children, so vaccination is often required prior to enrollment in schools, and health departments have active outreach programs for all the children in the population.

The vaccine for TB is not used universally in all countries. In a country such as India, where the prevalence of TB is high, the vaccine is used to prevent childhood TB. However, in the United States it is not recommended because of the low risk of infection related to receiving the vaccine and the variability of effectiveness of the vaccine against adult pulmonary TB.[75]

Vaccines continue to be a major prevention tool in public health. Science continues to work at developing new vaccines such as a possible vaccine against HIV. In addition to the development and testing of vaccines, continued efforts are needed to implement effective vaccination programs. Not all persons at risk for increased morbidity and mortality related to influenza and pneumonia get vaccinated. There continues to be negative press related to the side effects of vaccines. However, without vaccines, smallpox eradication would not have happened. Altering the environment, inactivating the agent, and increasing the resistance of the host are all powerful tools that nurses can use to decrease the incidence of CDs.

▨ Summary Points

- CDs are significant health issues that place populations at risk for increased morbidity and mortality.
- Preventing the transmission of disease requires an understanding of the cycle of transmission.
- Specific actions taken by nurses and other health-care providers at the population level include:
  - Participating in an outbreak investigation
  - Instituting appropriate isolation within an acute care setting
  - Screening patients or aggregates for an infectious disease
  - Developing and implementing a community outreach program to educate the public on a specific disease
- Vaccination is an important public health intervention aimed at reduction of the transmission of infectious agents.

▼ CASE STUDY
The Measles Epidemic

Learning Outcomes

By the end of this case study, the student will be able to:

• Gain understanding of the investigation of an epidemic.
• Describe appropriate prevention measures.
• Apply the cycle of transmission to individual infectious agents.

In 2016, there were 86 cases; in 2017, there were 118 cases; and from January 1 to April 25, there were 63 confirmed cases of measles reported to the CDC with the majority unvaccinated.[76] Starting with the current year, plot the number of cases of measles for the past decade then answer the following questions:

1. What would represent an endemic incidence rate, and at what point would the CDC decide there was an epidemic that required action?
2. What is the mode of transmission for the agent?
3. In 2018, the CDC identified lack of immunization as the key issue. Using the epidemiological triangle, is the appropriate prevention approach related to the agent, the environment, and/or the host?

REFERENCES

1. Centers for Disease Control and Prevention. (2018). *Outcomes of pregnancies with laboratory evidence of possible Zika virus infection, 2015-2018.* Retrieved from https://www.cdc.gov/pregnancy/zika/data/pregnancy-outcomes.html.
2. Centers for Disease Control and Prevention. (2018). *2018 Democratic Republic of the Congo, Bikoro.* Retrieved from https://www.cdc.gov/vhf/ebola/outbreaks/drc/2018-may.html.
3. Centers for Disease Control and Prevention. (2018). *Multistate outbreak of Salmonella Adelaide infections linked to pre-cut melon.* Retrieved from https://www.cdc.gov/salmonella/adelaide-06-18/index.html.
4. World Health Organization. (2018). *Smallpox.* Retrieved from http://www.who.int/csr/disease/smallpox/en/.
5. Centers for Disease Control and Prevention, National Center for Health Statistics. (2018). *Leading causes of death.* Retrieved from https://www.cdc.gov/nchs/fastats/leading-causes-of-death.htm.
6. World Health Organization. (2018). *The top ten causes of death.* Retrieved from http://www.who.int/mediacentre/factsheets/fs310/en/index1.html.
7. Martin, P.M.V., & Martin-Granel, E. (2006). 2,500-year evolution of the term *epidemic. Emerging Infectious Diseases, 12*(6), 976-980.
8. Centers for Disease Control and Prevention. (2012). *2011–2012 flu season draws to a close.* Retrieved from http://www.cdc.gov/flu/spotlights/2011-2012-flu-season-wrapup.htm.
9. Centers for Disease Control and Prevention. (2017). *Summary of the 2015-2016 influenza season.* Retrieved from https://www.cdc.gov/flu/about/season/flu-season-2015-2016.htm.
10. Centers for Disease Control and Prevention. (2018). *Influenza (Flu): The flu season.* Retrieved from https://www.cdc.gov/flu/about/season/flu-season.htm.
11. World Health Organization. (2017). *Key points: World malaria report 2017.* Retrieved March 21, 2018, from http://www.who.int/malaria/media/world-malaria-report-2017/en/.
12. World Health Organization. (2017). *World malaria report 2017.* Geneva Switzerland: Author.
13. Mace, K.E., & Arguin, P.M. (2017). Malaria surveillance — United States, 2014. *MMWR Surveill Summ, 66*(ss-21) Retrieved from https://www.cdc.gov/mmwr/volumes/66/ss/ss6612a1.htm.
14. Centers for Disease Control and Prevention. (2018). *Malaria's impact worldwide.* Retrieved from https://www.cdc.gov/malaria/malaria_worldwide/impact.html#.
15. Centers for Disease Control and Prevention. (2016). *Terms, definitions, and calculations used in CDC HIV surveillance publications.* Retrieved from https://www.cdc.gov/hiv/statistics/surveillance/terms.html.
16. UNAIDS. (2017). *FACT SHEET – WORLD AIDS DAY 2017.* Retrieved from http://www.unaids.org/sites/default/files/media_asset/UNAIDS_FactSheet_en.pdf.
17. Centers for Disease Control and Prevention. (2017). *HIV/AIDS basic statistics.* Retrieved from https://www.cdc.gov/hiv/basics/statistics.html.
18. Dailey, A.F., Hoots, B.E., Hall, H.I., Song, R., Hayes, D., Fulton, P., Prejean, J., Hernandez, A.L., Koenig, L.J., Valleroy, L.A. (2017). Vital signs: human immunodeficiency virus testing and diagnosis delays — United States. *Morbidity and Mortality Weekly Report, 66,* 1-7.
19. Centers for Disease Control and Prevention. (2018). *HIV/AIDS: HIV among people aged 50 and over.* Retrieved from https://www.cdc.gov/hiv/group/age/olderamericans/index.html.
20. Centers for Disease Control and Prevention. (2018). *HIV in the United States by Geography.* Retrieved from HIV in the United States by Geography at https://www.cdc.gov/hiv/pdf/statistics/cdc-hiv-geographic-distribution.pdf
21. U.S. Department of Health and Human Services. (2018). *Healthy People 2020 topics and objectives—HIV.* Retrieved from http://www.healthypeople.gov/2020/topicsobjectives2020/overview.aspx?topicId=22.
22. U.S. Department of Health and Human Services. (2017). *NATIONAL HIV/AIDS STRATEGY: UPDATED TO 2020 • 2017 PROGRESS REPORT.* Retrieved from https://files.hiv.gov/s3fs-public/NHAS_Progress_Report_2017.pdf.
23. U.S. Department of Health and Human Services. (2017). *Healthy People Midcourse Review Chapter 20: HIV.* Retrieved from https://www.cdc.gov/nchs/data/hpdata2020/HP2020MCR-C22-HIV.pdf.
24. UNAIDS. (2014). *90-90-90 An ambitious treatment target to help end the AIDS epidemic.* Retrieved from http://www.unaids.org/sites/default/files/media_asset/90-90-90_en.pdf.

25. UNAIDS. (2017). *Ending AIDS: Progress towards the 90-90-90 targets.* Retrieved from http://www.unaids.org/sites/default/files/media_asset/Global_AIDS_update_2017_en.pdf.

26. World Health Organization. (2015). *Diarrhoea.* Retrieved from http://www.who.int/topics/diarrhoea/en/.

27. World Health Organization. (2017). *Diarrhoeal disease.* Retrieved March 20, 2018, from http://www.who.int/en/news-room/fact-sheets/detail/diarrhoeal-disease.

28. Centers for Disease Control and Prevention. (2015). *Diarrheal disease in less developed countries.* Retrieved from http://www.cdc.gov/healthywater/hygiene/ldc/diarrheal_diseases.html.

29. Centers for Disease Control and Prevention. (2018). *Rotavirus.* Retrieved from http://www.cdc.gov/rotavirus/index.html.

30. Tate, J.E., Burton, A.H., Boschi-Pinto, C., Parashar, U.D., World Health Organization–Coordinated Global Rotavirus Surveillance Network. (2016). Global, regional, and national estimates of rotavirus mortality in children< 5 years of age, 2000–2013. *Clinical Infectious Diseases, 62*(suppl_2), S96-S105. doi: 10.1093/cid/civ1013.

31. World Health Organization. (2018). *Emerging disease.* Retrieved from http://www.searo.who.int/topics/emerging_diseases/en/.

32. National Center for Emerging and Zoonotic Infectious Diseases. (2018). *About the National Center for Emerging and Zoonotic Infectious Diseases.* Retrieved from http://www.cdc.gov/ncezid/.

33. Centers for Disease Control and Prevention. (2018). *Tuberculosis: Multidrug-Resistant Tuberculosis (MDR TB).* Retrieved from https://www.cdc.gov/tb/publications/factsheets/drtb/mdrtb.htm.

34. World Health Organization. (2016). *Global tuberculosis report 2016.* Retrieved from http://apps.who.int/iris/bitstream/handle/10665/250441/9789241565394-eng.pdf;jsessionid=ACA0E2B6D09D5A5E5E78593A6EE3816A?sequence=1.

35. LoBue, P.A., & Mermin, J.H. (2017). Latent tuberculosis infection: The final frontier of tuberculosis elimination in the USA. *The Lancet Infectious Diseases, 17*(10), e327-e333.

36. Centers for Disease Control and Prevention. (1991). Tuberculosis outbreak among HIV-infected persons. *JAMA, 266*(15), 2058, 2061.

37. Centers for Disease Control and Prevention. (2016). *Reported tuberculosis in the United States, 2015.* Atlanta, GA: U.S. Department of Health and Human Services.

38. Tipple, M.A., Heirendt, W., Metchock, B., Ijaz, K, & McElroy, P.D. (2004). Tuberculosis outbreak in a community hospital—District of Columbia, 2002. *Morbidity and Mortality Weekly Report, 53*(10), 214–216.

39. Centers for Disease Control and Prevention. (2013). *Life cycle of the hookworm.* Retrieved from https://www.cdc.gov/parasites/hookworm/biology.html.

40. Healthy People 2020. (2018). *Immunization and communicable diseases.* Retrieved from http://www.healthypeople.gov/2020/topicsobjectives2020/overview.aspx?topicid=23

41. Healthy People 2020. (2017). *Healthy People 2020 Midcourse Review Chapter 23: Immunization and communicable diseases.* Retrieved from https://www.cdc.gov/nchs/data/hpdata2020/HP2020MCR-C23-IID.pdf.

42. Centers for Disease Control and Prevention. (2018). *Escherichia coli.* Retrieved from http://www.cdc.gov/ecoli/general/index.html.

43. Council of State and Territorial Epidemiologists. (2017). *Public health reporting and national notification for Shiga Toxin-Producing Escherichia coli (STEC).* Retrieved from https://c.ymcdn.com/sites/www.cste.org/resource/resmgr/2017PS/2017PSFinal/17-ID-10.pdf.

44. Rangel, J.M., Sparling, P.H., Crowe, C., Griffin, P.M., & Swerdlow, D.L. (2005). Epidemiology of *Escherichia coli* 0157:H7 outbreaks 1982–2002. *Emerging Infectious Disease, 11*(4), 603–609.

45. Centers for Disease Control and Prevention. (2007). *Multistate outbreak of* E. coli *0157 infections linked to Topp's brand ground beef patties.* Retrieved from http://www.cdc.gov/ecoli/2007/october/100207.html.

46. Centers for Disease Control and Prevention. (2018). *Multistate outbreak of E. coli O157:H7 infections linked to romaine lettuce.* Retrieved from https://www.cdc.gov/ecoli/2018/o157h7-04-18/index.html.

47. U.S. Department of Health and Human Services. (2018). *Healthy People 2020. Topic—sexually transmitted diseases.* Retrieved from http://www.healthypeople.gov/2020/topicsobjectives2020/overview.aspx?topicid=37.

48. U.S. Department of Health and Human Services. (2017). *Healthy People 2020 Midcourse review Chapter 37: sexually transmitted disease.* Retrieved from https://www.cdc.gov/nchs/data/hpdata2020/HP2020MCR-C37-STD.pdf.

49. Centers for Disease Control and Prevention. (2017). *2016 sexually transmitted disease surveillance.* Retrieved from https://www.cdc.gov/std/stats16/natoverview.htm.

50. Centers for Disease Control and Prevention. (2016). *Sexually transmitted disease surveillance: Chlamydia 2016.* Atlanta, GA: U.S. Department of Health and Human Services. Retrieved from https://www.cdc.gov/std/stats16/chlamydia.htm.

51. Centers for Disease Control and Prevention. (2016). *Sexually transmitted disease surveillance: Gonorrhea 2016.* Atlanta, GA: U.S. Department of Health and Human Services. Retrieved from https://www.cdc.gov/std/stats16/gonorrhea.htm.

52. Centers for Disease Control and Prevention. (2017). *Gonorrhea treatment and care.* Retrieved from https://www.cdc.gov/std/gonorrhea/treatment.htm.

53. Centers for Disease Control and Prevention. (2017*). Sexually transmitted diseases surveillance: Syphilis 2017.* Atlanta, GA: U.S. Department of Health and Human Services. Retrieved from https://www.cdc.gov/std/stats17/syphilis.htm.

54. Centers for Disease Control and Prevention. (2017). *Syphilis statistics.* Retrieved from https://www.cdc.gov/std/stats17/figures/39.htm.

55. Centers for Disease Control and Prevention. (2017). *Syphilis.* Retrieved from https://www.cdc.gov/std/stats16/Syphilis.htm.

56. Hogben, M., & Leichliter, J.S. (2008). Social determinants and sexually transmitted disease disparities. *Sexually Transmitted Disease, 35*, S13-S18.

57. Chesson, H.W., Kent, C.K., Owusu-Edusei, K., Jr., et al. (2012). Disparities in sexually transmitted disease rates across the "eight Americas". *Sexually Transmitted Disease, 39*, 458-464.

58. Endyke-Doran, C., Gonzalez, R.M., Trujillo, M., Solera, A., Vigilance, P.N., Edwards, L.A., & Groves, S.L. (2006). The Syphilis Elimination Project: Targeting the Hispanic community of Baltimore City. *Public Health Nursing, 24*(1), 40–47.

59. Martin P.M.V., & Martin-Granel, E. (2006). 2,500-year evolution of the term *epidemic*. *Emerging Infectious Diseases, 12*(6), 976–980.

60. Green, M.S., Swartz, T., Mayshar, E., Lev, E.B., Leventhal, A. Slater, P.E., & Shemer, J. (2002). When is an epidemic an epidemic? *Israel Medical Association Journal, 4*, 3–6.

61. Centers for Disease Control and Prevention. (2017). *HIV/AIDS*. Atlanta, GA: U.S. Department of Health and Human Services Retrieved from https://www.cdc.gov/hiv/basics/statistics.html.

62. Beyeza-Kashesya, J., Wanyenze, R.K., Goggin, K., Finocchario-Kessler, S., Woldetsadik, M.A., Mindry, D., ... Wagner, G.J. (2018). Stigma gets in my way: Factors affecting client-provider communication regarding childbearing among people living with HIV in Uganda. PLoS One, Open Access. https://doi.org/10.1371/journal.pone.0192902.

63. Praditporn, P., & Wilawan, M. (2016). Challenges in the prevention of HIV among Thai homosexual males in the era of diversity and freedom of culture. *Australian Nursing & Midwifery Journal*, 24(5), 41.

64. Koster, O. (2007). Flesh-eating bug killed top economist in 24 hours. *Mail Online*. Retrieved from http://www.dailymail.co.uk/news/article-428234/Flesh-eating-bug-killed-economist-24hours.html.

65. Isabel. (2018). *Isabel's story*. Retrieved from https://symptomchecker.isabelhealthcare.com/about-isabel-symptom-checker.

66. Waldron, C., Solon, J.G., O'Gorman, J., Humphreys, H., Burke, J.P., McNamara, D.A. (2015). Necrotizing fasciitis: The need for urgent surgical intervention and the impact of intravenous drug use. *Surgeon, 13*(4), 194-9. doi: 10.1016/j.surge.2014.01.005.

67. Centers for Disease Control and Prevention. (2017). *Necrotizing fasciitis*. Retrieved from https://www.cdc.gov/features/necrotizingfasciitis/index.html.

68. U.S. Department of Health and Human Services, Vaccines.gov. (n.d.). *Glossary of terms*. Retrieved from http://www.vaccines.gov/more_info/glossary/index.html.

69. Centers for Disease Control and Prevention. (2017). *Vaccine safety*. Retrieved from https://www.cdc.gov/vaccinesafety/index.html.

70. Centers for Disease Control and Prevention. (2017). *For parents: Vaccines for your children*. Retrieved from https://www.cdc.gov/vaccines/parents/vaccine-decision/index.html.

71. World Health Organization. (2018). *Infectious diseases*. Retrieved fromhttp://www.who.int/topics/infectious_diseases/en/.

72. World Health Organization. (2018). *Emergency preparedness, response*. Retrieved from http://www.who.int/csr/en/.

73. Centers for Disease Control and Prevention. (2018). *Measles (rubeola)*. Retrieved from http://www.cdc.gov/measles/.

74. Health Resources and Services Administration. (n.d.). *National Vaccine Injury Compensation Program*. Retrieved from http://www.hrsa.gov/vaccinecompensation/index.html.

75. Centers for Disease Control and Prevention. (2018). *Fact sheet: BCG vaccine*. Retrieved from http://www.cdc.gov/tb/pubs/tbfactsheets/BCG.htm.

76. Centers for Disease Control and Prevention. (2018). *Measles cases and outbreaks*. Retrieved from https://www.cdc.gov/measles/cases-outbreaks.html.

Chapter 9

Noncommunicable Diseases

Christine Savage

LEARNING OUTCOMES

After reading the chapter, the student will be able to:

1. Describe the impact of noncommunicable diseases on the health of a population.
2. Define the burden of noncommunicable diseases using current epidemiological frameworks.
3. Describe the risk factor at the individual and population levels related to development of a noncommunicable disease.
4. Apply current evidence-based population interventions to the prevention of noncommunicable diseases.

KEY TERMS

Burden of disease
Chronic disease
Chronic disease
  self-management
Cultural shift
Disability-adjusted life
  years (DALY)

Health-adjusted
  life expectancy
  (HALE)
Health-related quality
  of life (HRQoL)
Human genome
  epidemiology

Human genomics
Life expectancy
Monogenetic
Noncommunicable
  disease (NCD)
Polygenetic

Premature death
Years of productive life
  lost (YPLL)

Introduction

In contrast with communicable diseases, a **noncommunicable disease (NCD)** is a disease that is not passed from one person to the next through direct or indirect means and is not associated with an infectious agent. The broader term, **chronic disease**, refers to either communicable diseases such as AIDS, or NCDs such as diabetes that have a long duration and usually slow progression, require medical attention over time, and/or limit the ability to perform activities of daily living (ADLs).[1] According to the World Health Organization (WHO) there are four main categories of NCDs: cardiovascular diseases (CVD), cancers, chronic respiratory diseases (CRD), and diabetes.[1]

The news and talk shows constantly reference our risk for NCDs and encourage us to engage in healthy behaviors. We are told to eat healthfully, engage in regular exercise, and avoid unhealthful behaviors such as tobacco use, overeating, and risky use of alcohol and drugs. For those of us who are currently healthy, it is easy to assume that NCDs do not affect us directly. The truth is that the burden of disease associated with NCDs affects us all. NCDs decrease our community's ability to reach optimal productivity and health, and contribute to the increasing cost of health care. If we solely focus on combating NCDs on the individual level after disease has occurred, we are doomed to failure in the long run. Many risk factors that contribute to the development of NCDs, such as exposure to secondary smoke in public places, are beyond the ability of an individual to control or modify. True change requires a population-level approach that encompasses interventions that require action at the individual, family, and community level. Nurses in all settings play an important role in prevention of NCDs across the continuum of prevention through primary-, secondary-, and tertiary-level interventions.

Noncommunicable Chronic Diseases

The majority of NCDs cannot be prevented or cured through vaccination or medication; rather, they require maintaining a healthy lifestyle, early diagnosis and treatment, and long-term management. Annually, a total of 40 million people die from a NCD, approximately 70% of all deaths globally.[2,3] In the United States, preventing NCDs is a major priority as reflected in many of the *Healthy People (HP)* objectives.[4] The majority of NCDs could be prevented through a reduction in behavioral risks such as tobacco use, sedentary lifestyle, harmful alcohol use, and an increase in healthful eating.[2]

Health-care providers, including nurses, typically care for those with NCDs on an individual basis, often during an acute phase of the disease or at the end stages of disease. More recently, especially with the implementation of the Affordable Care Act, the care of NCDs is moving away from an acute care model to a chronic care model in which the disease is managed over time and the focus is decreasing morbidity and mortality associated with NCDs through an integrated care delivery model (Fig. 9-1).[5] This model requires health-care providers to reframe the care provided from the treatment of acute phases of an NCD within an acute care setting to long-term management in the community. Care of an existing NCD should be provided within a secondary and tertiary prevention framework that focuses on early detection and treatment as well as a long-term plan of care aimed at reducing morbidity and mortality (see Chapter 2). To accomplish this, nurses must use not only their knowledge of the pathophysiology of an NCD but an understanding of the public health issues associated with the disease. All nurses have a role to play in reducing the burden of disease related to NCDs in populations they serve. Nurses across settings and specialties become part of national and global efforts aimed at reducing the toll that chronic diseases take on the health of not only individuals but also of populations.

■ CELLULAR TO GLOBAL

Chronic noncommunicable disease occurs at the cellular level for an individual, yet management of a NCD over time requires an understanding not only of the risk factors across the continuum of cellular to global but also of the resources needed to provide care to those with NCDs. There is also a need for community and global level interventions aimed at reducing morbidity and mortality associated with NCDs. Building on the chronic disease care model that focuses on care of individuals and families is the wider scope of factors that contribute to the morbidity and mortality associated with NCDs. The WHO acknowledges that action to reduce the burden of disease associated with NCDs includes "… a comprehensive approach … requiring all sectors, including health, finance, transport, education, agriculture, planning and others, to collaborate to reduce the risks associated with NCDs, and promote interventions to prevent and control them."[2] Prevention of NCDs and care for individuals with NCDs occurs within the context of the community where they live.

The Chronic Care Model

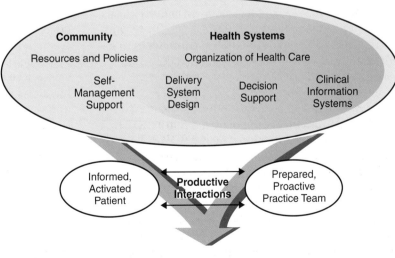

Figure 9-1 The Chronic Care Model.
*(Developed by the MacColl Institute,
°American College of Physicians-ASIM
Journals and Books.)*

Burden of Disease

NCDs add significantly to the overall burden of disease for a population. The **burden of disease** uses the disability-adjusted-life-year (DALY) measure to determine the extent of the burden a disease has on a population (see later).[6] Knowing about the burden of disease associated with a specific disease helps in understanding the impact the disease has on the population or community. Estimating the burden of a disease can help a community prioritize health promotion and prevention efforts by targeting those diseases that account for the greatest burden to the community. Determining the burden of disease involves calculating not only the cost of treatment but also the social and economic impacts. Analysis of the burden of a disease allows for the assessment of the comparative importance of a disease, injury, or risk factor. This assessment takes into account how much the disease, injury, or risk factor contributes to overall disability and premature death in the population.

For example, if in Berryton, a hypothetical U.S. town of 8,000 adults, the prevalence of type 2 diabetes rose from 160 (2%) to 800 (10%) cases, the impact on the town would involve more than the cost to treat the individuals with the disease. Let's add another aspect to this town. It is a rural farming community recently hit with a shortage of migrant farm workers resulting in an inability to harvest all of the tomatoes, the town's main crop. The new cases are occurring for the most part in 35- to 45-year-old males, and the closest medical center is 100 miles from the town. With a depressed economy, rural setting, and reduced access to care, the potential for adverse consequences and premature death associated with diabetes is increased. This could result in a decrease in the number of able-bodied people to work on the farms, further depressing the economy. Thus, the impact of an NCD extends beyond individuals and their families. For this community, the disease contributed to reduced productivity and adversely affected the economic viability of the town.

Life Expectancy

Estimating the health of a population is calculated based on a number of measures. First, mortality rates are used to estimate the life expectancy of a group of people. **Life expectancy** is defined as the number of years a person could be expected to live based on the current mortality rates in a specific setting, usually a country. There is great variability across countries in life expectancy, especially between developed and developing countries. For example, the estimated life expectancy in the United States for 2017 was 80 years and in Afghanistan it was 51.7 years.[7]

Life expectancy is a valuable tool, but it fails to capture the burden of ill health caused by NCDs. To help adjust for these factors, public health officials use the healthy life expectancy measure. **Health-adjusted life expectancy (HALE)** reflects the average number of years that a person can expect to live in good health by adjusting for disease and/or injury. The WHO uses HALEs to measure the average level of health in countries and regions by evaluating population-specific prevalence of disease and injury as well as severity distribution of health states.[8] As a result of problems with comparable health state prevalence data, the WHO uses a four-stage strategy to compute HALE (Box 9-1). This allows the WHO to estimate HALE for countries across the globe. Epidemiologists compute the HALE for a chronic disease using data related to age, the number of survivors, and the number of years lived.

Premature Death

NCDs often lead to **premature death**, that is, a death that occurs earlier than the standard life expectancy. For those who die prior to reaching the age they would be expected to live, their death is defined as premature. Therefore, premature death reflects the number of potential life years lost. Premature death is usually expressed as the

---

BOX 9-1 ■ Application: Health-Adjusted Life Expectancy (HALE): Methods of Estimation

The World Health Organization uses death registration data that are reported annually to estimate HALE. This information is part of the WHO Global Burden of Disease (GBD) study. Other sources of data include the WHO Multi-Country Survey Study (MCSS) and World Health Survey (WHS). Information use includes estimates for the incidence, prevalence, duration, and years lived with disability for 135 major causes. However, comparable health state prevalence data are not available for all countries, so a four-stage strategy is used:

- Data from the WHOGBD study are used to estimate severity-adjusted prevalence by age and sex for all countries.
- Data from the WHOMCSS and WHS are used to make independent estimates of severity-adjusted prevalence by age and sex for survey countries.
- Prevalence for all countries is calculated based on GBD, MCSS, and WHS estimates.
- Life tables constructed by WHO are used to compute HALE for countries.

Source: (8)

years of potential life lost (YPLL). YPLL is calculated by subtracting the age at which a person dies from their expected life expectancy.[10] For example, if a man died of a heart attack in the United States in 2011 at the age of 42, the YPLL would be 36 because the life expectancy in the United States was 78 years that year.[11] By contrast, the YPLL for a man who died in a motor vehicle crash at the age of 21 would be 57.

From a population perspective, premature death is calculated based on the number of potential life years lost prior to the life expectancy of the population per 100,000 persons—in other words, how many total years of useful life were not available to the population because of early death. If you calculated the YPLL for a 50-year-old man who died of a heart attack in Afghanistan in 2011, the YPLL would be 0 because the life expectancy for males was 49.

Disability-Adjusted Life Years

In addition to premature death, most NCDs lead to disability that can affect an individual's quality of life and productivity. For that reason, YPLL does not adequately capture the full burden of disease. A method for quantifying the burden of disease that takes into account both premature death and disability is called the **disability-adjusted life year (DALY)**. This is defined as measurement of the gap that exists between the ideal health status of a disease- and disability-free population that lives to an advanced age.[9] It is calculated using population-level data. One DALY represents 1 lost year of life. It is calculated as a sum of the years of life lost (YLL) related to premature death in the population plus the years lost to disability (YLD) related to the disease.

To calculate the DALY, you start with the YLL. The YLL is the number of deaths multiplied by the standard life expectancy at the age at which death occurs. For this you need the number of deaths attributed to the disease or risk factor and the expectancy at age of death in years. YLL measures lost years of life due to deaths using an incidence perspective (number of new cases or deaths), this perspective is also taken to calculate the YLD. For an estimation of the YLD for a particular cause in a particular time period, you take the incidence (number of new cases) during that time period and multiply it by the average duration of the disease. To account for the variability of the severity of the disease, a weight factor is included that reflects the severity of the disease on a scale from 0 (perfect health) to 1 (dead). The basic formula for YLD requires multiplying the incidence times the disability weight times the average duration of the disease until remission or death (Box 9-2).[9]

BOX 9–2 ■ Application: Disability-Adjusted Life Year (DALY) calculation

DALY = YLL (Years of Life Lost) + YLD (Years of Life Disabled)

The basic formula for YLL is:

$$YLL = N \times L$$

where:
- N = number of deaths
- L = standard life expectancy at age of death in years

The basic formula for YLD is the following (again, without applying social preferences):

$$YLD = I \times DW \times L$$

where:
- I = number of incident cases
- DW = disability weight
- L = average duration of the case until remission or death (years)

Source: (9)

Noncommunicable Diseases in the United States

NCDs are the number one cause of death and disability in the United States. The four common risk factors that account for much of the NCDs in our country are the same as the risk at the global level and are modifiable. These include (1) nutrition, (2) physical activity, (3) tobacco use, and (4) alcohol use. One-fourth of all persons living in the United States with an NCD have one or more limitations in their daily activities.[10] The first proposed goal of *HP 2030* is to "Attain healthy, thriving lives and well-being, free of preventable disease, disability, injury, and premature death."[11] This requires prevention and early treatment of NCD. Healthy People includes multiple topics related to specific NCDs as well as the four common risk factors associated with development of NCDs.

Diabetes is an example of a topic for HP 2020 related to NCD that will continue to be a focus of HP 2030. According to the American Diabetes Association, in 2015 more than 30 million people, almost 10% of the population of the U.S., had diabetes with 7.2 million undiagnosed and was the seventh leading cause of death. The annual cost in 2017 was $327 billion USD. [11]

■ HEALTHY PEOPLE

Noncommunicable Disease: Diabetes

Goal: Reduce the disease burden of diabetes mellitus (DM) and improve the quality of life for all persons who have, or are at risk for, DM.

Overview: DM occurs when the body cannot produce enough insulin or cannot respond appropriately to insulin. Insulin is a hormone that the body needs to absorb and use glucose (sugar) as fuel for the body's cells. Without a properly functioning insulin signaling system, blood glucose levels become elevated and other metabolic abnormalities occur, leading to the development of serious, disabling complications.

Many forms of diabetes exist. The three common types of DM are:

• Type 2 diabetes, which results from a combination of resistance to the action of insulin and insufficient insulin production
• Type 1 diabetes, which results when the body loses its ability to produce insulin
• Gestational diabetes, a common complication of pregnancy. Gestational diabetes can lead to perinatal complications in mother and child, and substantially increases the likelihood of cesarean section. Gestational diabetes is also a risk factor for the mother and, later in life, the child's subsequent development of type 2 diabetes after the affected pregnancy.[12]

Midcourse Review: Of the 20 objectives for this topic area, 2 were developmental and 18 were measurable. For 4 of the measurable objectives, the target was met or exceeded, and 1 was improving. For 10 there was little or no detectable change, and 1 objective was baseline only and 2 were informational (Fig. 9-2).[13]

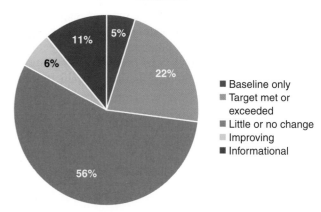

Healthy People 2020 Midcourse Review: Diabetes

- Baseline only
- Target met or exceeded
- Little or no change
- Improving
- Informational

Figure 9-2 Midcourse Review Diabetes.

BOX 9–3 ■ Top 10 Leading Causes of Death, CDC 2017

• Heart disease: 635,260
• Cancer: 598,038
• Accidents (unintentional injuries): 161,374
• Chronic lower respiratory diseases: 154,596
• Stroke (cerebrovascular diseases): 142,142
• Alzheimer's disease: 116,103
• Diabetes: 80,058
• Influenza and pneumonia: 51,537
• Nephritis, nephrotic syndrome, and nephrosis: 50,046
• Intentional self-harm (suicide): 44,965

Source: (14)

Leading Causes of Death and Disability

According to the WHO, NCDs are not only costly but are common and often preventable causes of death and disability.[1] Seven of the top ten leading causes of death in the United States are NCDs including heart disease, cancer, chronic lower respiratory diseases, stroke (cerebrovascular disease), Alzheimer's disease, diabetes, nephritis, nephrotic syndrome, and nephrosis (Box 9-3).[14] Understanding NCDs from a public health perspective allows us to step back and examine the context of these diseases and the causal factors linked to the occurrence of disease.

Heart Disease and Stroke

In the U.S., CVD and stroke are the first and fifth leading causes of death.[14] They are costly and widespread. One in every four deaths in the U.S. is attributable to CVD,[15] and one in every 20 deaths is attributable to stroke.[16] Together they account for close to one-third of all deaths in the United States.[15, 16] Although rates for coronary heart disease have dropped over the last 3 decades, large regional variations in the burden associated with CVD exist across the U.S. with dietary risk exposures being the largest attributable risk factor related to CVD burden of disase.[17,18] Other risk factors include high blood pressure, obesity, tobacco use, high cholesterol, and low levels of physical activity.[18]

Understanding the risk factors for CVD has come from public health science. Before World War II, hypertension was accepted as a part of the normal aging process and little was understood about how to treat it, never mind how to prevent it. As life expectancy improved, the prevalence of CVD grew. Because of this increase in prevalence, the National Heart Institute (now known as the National Heart, Lung, and Blood Institute) initiated a longitudinal cohort study in 1948 (defined in Chapter 3) in Framingham, Massachusetts, which is still going on today.[19] From the data collected over the past 6 decades, we now know a great deal about the risk factors for CVD and stroke. Based on the findings from this study, both individual and population level interventions have been developed aimed at reducing risk and subsequently reducing the prevalence of CVD.

Cancer

Although great strides have been made in the prevention and treatment of cancer, it is the second leading cause of death in the United States and the world.[14,20, 21] In the U.S., cancer mortality rates rose over the 20th century but are now declining mostly due to the drop in tobacco use. In addition, public health efforts to promote increased screening for breast and colorectal cancer have resulted in a decrease in deaths because of early detection and screening, and the length of cancer survival has increased.[20] Globally, cancer accounts for 1 in 6 deaths with 30% to 60% preventable.[21] Tobacco use is the leading risk factor for cancer with Lung cancer the leading cause of cancer death in both men and women; 80% of all lung cancers result from smoking or exposure to secondhand smoke.[21]

Risk for cancer is a combination of behavioral, genetic, and environmental factors. For example, in breast cancer all three levels of risk apply. Family history, diet, exercise, reproductive history, and alcohol use have all been associated with increased risk for breast cancer (Fig. 9-3).[22,23] An example of genetic risk is the harmful mutation of *BRCA1* or *BRCA2,* tumor suppressor genes. Women who test positive for this gene mutation have an increased lifetime risk for developing breast and ovarian cancers.[24]

Chronic Lower Respiratory Disease

According to the WHO, CRD includes chronic obstructive pulmonary disease (COPD), asthma, occupational lung diseases, and pulmonary hypertension. One of the most common is COPD, which includes emphysema and chronic bronchitis. Although treatable, these diseases are not curable and 90% of the deaths attributable to CRD occur in middle-income and low-income countries.[25] The major risk factor for COPD and other CRDs is tobacco use, and the causative link between the two is the abnormal inflammatory response of the lungs to the noxious particles or gases present in tobacco smoke. Other risk factors include exposure to air pollutants, chemical fumes, and dust from the environment or workplace.[25]

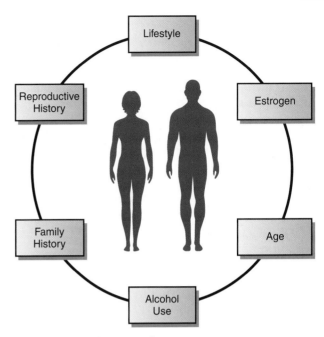

Figure 9-3 Risk Factors for Breast Cancer.

Globally, indoor air quality is thought to play a bigger role in the development of COPD.[26]

Diabetes

Over the past few decades, great improvements have occurred in the management of diabetes and the reduction in complications such as blindness and diabetes-related end-stage renal disease. Despite these advances, diabetes remains a leading cause of death in the U.S. and globally. According to the WHO, 422 million adults worldwide have diabetes, representing an almost quadrupling incidence since 1980.[27]

Although the incidence of diabetes in the U.S. has declined since 2008, the prevalence of diabetes is growing. In 2015, a little over 9.4% of the U.S. population and 12.2% of adults had diabetes.[28] Differences exist in age-adjusted prevalence based on ethnic group with 15.1% of Native Americans and 12.7% of African Americans compared to 7.4% of white non-Hispanic and 8.1% of Asians, which may reflect socioeconomic status rather than an underlying genetic risk factor.[28] Two underlying factors that have contributed to the increase in the incidence of type 2 diabetes globally are changes in lifestyle, especially exercising and diet. In addition, improved treatment has resulted in a longer survival rate. Thus, an increased incidence combined with an increased survival rate has resulted in an overall increase in the prevalence of type 2 diabetes (see Fig. 3-7, Chapter 3).[27]

Public health efforts are in full force in attempting to turn this trend around. The focus has been on behavioral change to reduce individual risk. The prevention or delay of the onset of type 2 diabetes can happen through a healthy lifestyle that includes making healthful changes to diet, increasing the level of physical activity, and maintaining a healthy weight.[27, 29] These recommendations are based on solid epidemiological data related to risk, that is, persons who exercise regularly, eat healthy, and maintain a normal body mass index (BMI) are at a much lower risk for type 2 diabetes. Type 1 diabetes is another story. Less than 10% of persons with diabetes have type 1. It is usually diagnosed in childhood and is associated with genetic risk rather than behavioral risk.

Risk Factors

Risk for NCDs is complex and related to numerous factors, individual behaviors, genetics, and environmental exposure as well as the larger socioeconomic context in which people live. To prevent NCDs, the epidemiologist explores factors that increase the risk of disease occurring. As explained in Chapter 3, two types of studies are often conducted to help determine what leads to development of disease: a case control study and a cohort study. Based on these studies, we can determine the relative risk or the odds ratio of disease that can occur based on exposure to a risk factor. In chronic diseases, there are two major categories of risk that have received a great deal of attention nationally: lifestyle or behavioral risk factors and socioeconomic risk factors.

▶ **SOLVING THE MYSTERY**
Applying Public Health Science: The Case of the Struggling Heart Patients
Public Health Science Topics Covered:

- Assessment
- Program Planning and Evaluation
- Building Partnerships

In the Mississippi Delta, a section of western and northwestern Mississippi bordered by the Mississippi River and the Yazoo River, health-care providers were alarmed by the high rate of CVD in the Delta. According to the Mississippi State Health Department, residents of the Delta have the highest rates of stroke in Mississippi. In addition, the Delta and the state have the highest rates of obesity and CVD in the

United States.[30] This area of Mississippi is faced with serious socioeconomic risk factors including poverty and low educational attainment. The poverty rate for the Delta ranges from 30% to 40% compared to 22% for Mississippi and 15% nationally.[30,31] The challenge, then, was to develop a program to increase access to routine health screenings and improve on disease self-management.

The Mississippi Department of Health, in partnership with the CDC, formed the Mississippi Delta Health Collaborative (MDHC) that included individuals and groups across the community. They currently report progress in attaining their goal of reducing stroke and heart disease through three program areas: clinical, community, and faith-based. The clinical component has involved incorporating community health workers (CHWs) into the health-care team.[30] Evidence has demonstrated the effectiveness of using community workers to address health needs in populations at risk. One of the challenges is to clarify the role of these workers.[32] The most commonly used definition is the one by the American Public Health Association: "A Community Health Worker (CHW) is a front line public health worker who is a trusted member of and/or has an unusually close understanding of the community served. This trusting relationship enables the CHW to serve as a liaison/link/intermediary between health/social services and the community to facilitate access to services and improve the quality and cultural competence of service delivery. A CHW also builds individual and community capacity by increasing health knowledge and self-sufficiency through a range of activities such as outreach, community education, informal counseling, social support, and advocacy."[33]

The MDHC conducted an initial assessment and identified community assets including mayoral health councils, schools, and churches. Building on these assets, they partnered with the CDC and implemented the Clinical-Community Health Worker Initiative (CCHWI). The focus was to improve clinical outcomes for CVD through use of the ABCS—appropriate Aspirin use, A1c (hemoglobin control), Blood pressure control, Cholesterol management, and Smoking cessation.[34]

The CCHWI program uses a system in which referrals are made from multiple sources including health-care providers in federally qualified health centers (FQHCs) and rural clinics as well as referrals based on elevated blood pressure readings obtained during from health screenings conducted in barbershops, churches, and other MDHC partner locations. A MDHC program manager and two registered nurses provide oversight for the CHWs and are available for consultation.[34] According to the CDC, a total of 8 CHWs visit patients throughout 17 of the 18 Delta counties. [34] CHWs follow the ABCS protocol during their visit (Box 9-4).

As noted in Chapter 5, evaluation is a key component of health planning. For this program, evaluation demonstrated the benefits of using CHWs to help reduce the morbidity and mortality associated with CVD. According to the MDHC report they had seen 1,057 patients and found significant mean changes in both diastolic and systolic blood pressure readings indicating better controlled blood pressure. They established relationships with churches and barbershops. Of the 27 barbershops who joined the collaborative, 17 became smoke free. In the 77 churches that partnered with the collaborative, 73 congregational nurses and advocates were trained. They concluded their report with the following: "Every time a local barber identifies someone with high blood pressure, every time a church holds a wellness fair, every time a clinical CHW encourages her clients to get up and move, and every time someone doesn't light up a cigarette in public spaces, the Delta becomes a healthier place."[30]

The Case of the Struggling Heart Patients illustrates the role that socioeconomic status plays in increasing risk for CVD as well as the importance of incorporating community members into population-level programs to assure that the programs are relevant to the community, reflect an understanding of the cultural context of a community, and the power of bringing together multiple groups and individuals to address a serious health issue in the face of limited resources. Using CHWs, the program provided patients with members of their own community to help them self-manage their disease and address behavioral risk factors, specifically smoking and obesity.

Behavioral Risk Factors

The WHO posed a question: "Why treat people's illnesses without changing what made them sick in the first place?"[35] We must strive to understand what contributes to the occurrence of NCDs. In addition to environment, much attention has been given to the role of individual behaviors. The current focus is on healthy nutrition, adequate exercise, and avoidance of substance misuse, especially tobacco and alcohol (see Chapter 11). The evaluation of risk factors has been the dominant paradigm of the late 20th century and through the first decade of the 21st century. Understanding risk factors requires an understanding of public health science, especially epidemiology. Most of the studies that have established the link between a risk factor and a disease are based on case control and cohort studies (see Chapter 3). Often, the exploration of risk factors begins with a basic community/population assessment (see Chapter 4).

Nutrition, Exercise, and Obesity

More than a third of U.S. adults are obese (have a BMI greater than or equal to 30).[36] Differences in prevalence exist in relation to racial/ethnic groups, an age-adjusted obesity rate of 48.1% in African Americans, 42.5% in Hispanic non-blacks, 34.5% of white non-Hispanic, and 11.7% in Asians.[36] About 17% of children and adolescents are obese.[37] It is well-known that obesity and overweight increase the risk for NCDs, especially heart disease, type 2 diabetes, certain cancers, and stroke.

The main risk factors associated with obesity are poor nutrition and lack of exercise, which reflect individual

---

BOX 9–4 ■ ABCS protocol

Once referrals are made, the CHWs follow-up with patients within 48 hours through face-to-face contact, phone calls, or mailings to establish and maintain linkages to health care, promote adherence to treatment protocols, and work toward improvement in the ABCS. Specifically, CHWs conduct home visits that last about 1 hour, where they:

- Offer informal counseling on medication adherence, tobacco cessation, healthy nutrition, and physical activity.
- Encourage patients to use a primary care provider if screenings indicate the need.
- Reduce barriers to health-care access by arranging transportation, assisting patients with scheduling appointments, and helping patients prepare for medical visits.
- Contact clinical systems when patients have elevated blood pressures.
- Use an online web-based portal to collect quantitative and qualitative information during the home visits as part of MDHC's ongoing evaluation.

Source: (30, 34)

behaviors that are thought to be modifiable, that is, they can be changed with intervention. However, using the web of causation (see Chapter 3), these two risk factors are linked to numerous other factors at the population level, including changes in population behaviors, environmental factors, and socioeconomic factors. The risk factor model often fails to establish the complex link between individual behaviors, population-level factors, and the development of NCDs. A good place to start when faced with a growing health problem such as obesity is to do a population-level focused assessment that allows for assessment of both the individual level and community level data. This type of assessment can help identify who is at greatest risk for obesity as well as the population-level factors that contribute to obesity. For example, the prevalence rate for obesity in Mississippi was higher than the national level.[30] A more thorough population-level assessment can help the primary health network (PHN) develop an intervention that is culturally relevant and takes into consideration barriers faced by the population.

Environmental Risk Factors for Noncommunicable Disease

It is also important to remember that environment plays a key role in the development of NCDs (see Chapter 6). Pollutants in the environment increase the risk for asthma, cardiovascular health problems, and cancer.[38,39] These pollutants include those found in the air, the home, the water supply, and the ground. Since 1950, the United States has experienced drastic changes in the food supply, the built environment, increased population, and proliferation of environmental chemicals. The built environment includes the structures that exist in our towns and cities such as buildings, roads, sewage systems, parks, and recreation facilities (see Chapter 6). In 1800, only 3% of the world's population lived in an urban setting. In 2018, 55% of the population was urban, and the United Nations (UN) projected that, by 2050, 68% of the world's population will be urban. The most urbanized region in the world is North America with 82% of the population living in an urban area. By contrast, 48% of the population in Africa lives in a rural setting, but this is changing, with most of the future urban growth projected by the UN to occur in Africa and Asia (see Chapter 16).[40] The growth of cities reflects a growth in commerce, economic opportunities, and opportunities for building social capital. However, it also increases issues related to environmental pollutants. For example, most of us are aware of the potential pollutants in the air. Local news stations report on

the air quality and alert residents when the air quality places a person at risk for health consequences (see Chapter 6). The environment plays a key role in understanding the risk for NCDs and is best understood through the application of public health science methodologies.

● APPLYING PUBLIC HEALTH SCIENCE
The Case of the Growing Children
Public Health Science Topics Covered:

• Assessment
• Program planning

In Marksville County, a hypothetical county located in the state of Florida close to the Everglades, there was a growing concern among the citizens about the prevalence of obesity and overweight among the children as well as county adults. The issue arose at a city council meeting in Yonston, the only major city in the county. The mayor and city council charged the health officer with heading up a task force to address this issue and asked the task force members to concentrate on childhood obesity. The most obvious step in addressing the issue was first to conduct an assessment. The county had a population of 10,576. The ethnic profile of the county was 5% Seminole Indians, 11% African American, 17%, Hispanic, 65% Caucasian, and 2% other races. Seventeen percent of the population was under the age of 18. The health officer knew that the first step would be to mobilize a broad band of stakeholders and community residents. Before doing so, the health officer decided to seek a commitment from a smaller group, the steering committee.

After thinking about this in consultation with other people, the health officer chose the following people for the steering committee: the principal of the local high school, a university professor from the local nursing school, the county political representative, CEO of the local hospital, two businesspeople, and the director of the Head Start program. The CEO talked with the nurse manager of the pediatric unit and asked her to represent him on the committee. Orientation meetings were held, and goals and objectives of the initiative were set. The overall goal was to conduct a community assessment focused on determining the extent of obesity and overweight in Marksville County, to examine trends of the epidemic, to identify resources for addressing the issue, and to develop an action plan.

An assessment related to a specific health issue helps bring about a greater understanding of the factors influencing that health issue for that particular population. This committee conducted a focused assessment (see Chapter 4) related to obesity in children and adolescents. Overweight and obesity, which are determined by using weight and height to calculate a BMI, are growing public health problems for adults and children.[37] An adult who has a BMI that ranges between 25.0 and 29.9 is considered overweight. If the BMI is 30 or higher, then the person is considered obese. For children and adolescents, overweight is often defined as at or above the 95th percentile of the sex-specific BMI for age growth chart. Ranges above a normal weight have different labels: at risk for overweight and overweight.[41]

After establishing the steering committee, a larger coalition was formed to build the structure needed to conduct the assessment. Invitations were sent out to a broader constituency to develop a coalition to address the issue. Initially, the public was invited to a town hall meeting. The goal was to increase awareness about obesity and overweight within the community and to gain a commitment to get involved. They provided the community with the data on obesity in their county based on data from the Florida Department of Health.

The committee then presented the community with the facts about why childhood obesity is an important public health issue for their county. They explained that obesity occurs when more calories are consumed than are expended. They further explained that they were tackling this problem because childhood obesity has both immediate and long-term health impacts. If the community did not act, they would be faced with sicker children as well as the long-term cost of caring for more adults with chronic diseases occurring at an earlier age. According to the CDC, 70% of obese youth have at least one risk factor for CVD, such as high cholesterol or hypertension. Obese children and adolescents are at greater risk for bone and joint problems. They also suffer from psychological problems because of social stigma and low self-esteem. As adults, they are at higher risk for CVD, type 2 diabetes, stroke, cancer, and osteoarthritis.[37]

The committee was able to grab the community's attention when they gave the facts about type 2 diabetes among the children of the county. Based on hospital discharge data from the county hospitals, 50 of their children were already being treated for type 2 diabetes with an overall prevalence rate of 2.8 per 1,000 children and adolescents, higher than the national prevalence of 1.7 per 1,000. The subpopulation most affected in their community was the Seminole Indians, with 14 Seminole children in their county diagnosed with type 2 diabetes, a prevalence rate of 4.9 per 1,000 children under the age of 18. Thus, 28% of the children diagnosed with type 2 diabetes in their county were Seminole Indians.

With the support of the community, the committee added key members suggested by the community to help them complete a more in-depth assessment. They began by reviewing national statistics related to the prevalence of obesity/overweight in children and adolescents and comparing those rates with their own rates. They were able to find national reports on the extent of the problem as well as a national-level concern related to the problem. One of the objectives of *HP* is concerned with reducing the proportion of children and adolescents who are obese.[42]

■ HEALTHY PEOPLE
Nutrition and Weight Status

HP 2020: Objective: Nutrition and weight status (NWS)—children and adolescents

NWS-10: Reduce the proportion of children and adolescents who are considered obese

NWS-10.1	Children aged 2 to 5 years
NWS-10.2	Children aged 6 to 11 years
NWS-10.3	Adolescents aged 12 to 19 years
NWS-10.4	Children and adolescents aged 2 to 19 years

HP 2020 Midcourse Review: Based on the data reported in the Healthy People Midcourse review, there was little or no detectable difference from baseline.

Source: (42, 43)

The team reviewed the National Center for Health Statistics Data Brief and found that the prevalence of obesity among children remained high.[43] After further review they also discovered that, on the national level, the prevalence of obesity is higher in Native American children than the population as a whole.[44] Another source of secondary data came from the Youth Risk Behavioral Surveillance System (YRBSS), which is a state-based health survey that annually collects information on health conditions, behaviors, preventive practices, and access to health care.[45] It is used to monitor health problems in youth as well as healthy and unhealthy behaviors, including the prevalence of obesity among youth and young adults. They also located information on youth behaviors specific to Florida that was helpful in comparing the state statistics with national statistics.[46]

Based on their review of the YRBSS, they noticed that, not only were the health behaviors of individual students assessed, but environmental factors were included as well. The nurse manager of the pediatric unit at the community hospital remembered a discussion in a recent nursing practice committee meeting about the problem of only focusing on individual risk factors when examining a health problem. She went back to the literature and examined new developments in public health science and again reviewed the web of causation (see Chapter 3). She brought back to the committee her concerns about focusing on behavioral risk factors alone. She argued that the risk factor paradigm targets individual change only and ignores the difference between individual risk factors and population risk factors; she encouraged the committee to take a macro-look at risk factors as well.[47] The committee agreed to do this.

Taking this broader view of risk related to healthy diet and exercise in children and adolescents, the committee reviewed the importance of a healthy school environment that should include a focus on health education, healthy food availability, and physical education (PE). On the CDC's Web site they found a model for schools to use to help prevent childhood obesity called the Whole School, Whole Community, Whole Child (WSCC) (Fig. 9-4).[48] The four main components of this model were: (1) Physical education and physical activity; (2) Nutrition environment and services; (3) School

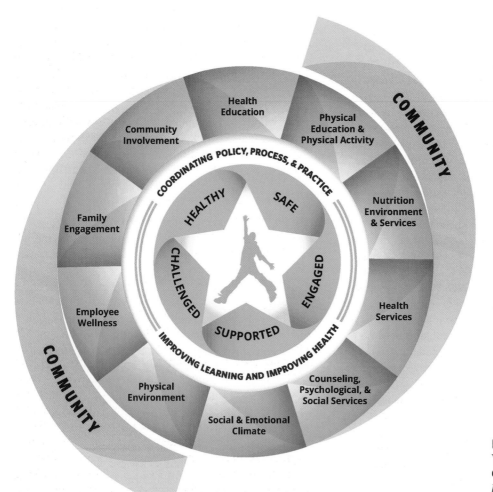

Figure 9-4 Whole School, Whole Community, Whole Child (WSCC). *(From the CDC https://www.cdc.gov/healthyyouth/wscc/)*

health services to support physical, psychological, and emotional health; and (4) Family and community engagement. The committee now had some important data using secondary data sources from the national, state, and county level as well as a framework to help design a prevention program.

They decided they were missing key information, especially the information found in the YRBSS, because their analysis of county data was hampered by a small numbers problem; that is, there were not enough respondents in the national survey to make any conclusions. They decided to do their own survey of school-age children in the county as well as collect institution-level data on the schools in the county to determine what was being offered related to health education, PE, and nutrition. In addition, they collected data from the Head Start and the Women, Infants, and Children (WIC) programs.

In looking at the data, a growing trend in the community was noted from the 2015-2016 program year and the 2016-2017 program year. During the 2015-2016 program year, 22% of children in Head Start and 18% of children in Early Head Start were identified as overweight. In the 2016-2017 program year, the percent for Early Head Start stayed the same but for Head Start it increased to 24%. In the two WIC programs in the county, 18% of children were identified as overweight. These percentages were higher than the population of those under the age of 18 as a whole. These data on the under-5 age group illustrated the need to develop a program that extended beyond school-age children. Also, based on their earlier data, those at greatest risk for adverse consequences related to obesity were the Seminole Indian children.

They also examined the school data and found that the county schools performed similarly to the rest of the state on the CDC indicators. Healthy nutrient and dietary behavior habits were taught at both the elementary and high school levels, but they did not include key physical activity topics in these courses. Because of recent budgetary problems, PE was no longer offered in the schools, though they had an intramural sports program at the high school and middle school levels. The vending machines in the school did not sell healthy foods, and soft drinks were advertised in the school. Notably, the Pepsi Cola Company donated the new school football scoreboard. They also found that the school cafeteria prepared foods using a deep-fat fryer.

Based on these findings, the committee began to put together action steps to address the issues specific to

their community. They wanted to develop a broad program that would include children aged 5 and below as well as children and adolescents attending school. They also felt it was important to engage the Seminole Indian community in the planning to make sure that any intervention developed was culturally relevant. They started with the nine guidelines found on the CDC Web site.[49] In this way, the schools became leaders in the fight against childhood obesity and in the promotion of a healthier lifestyle in their community.

Tobacco Use

In addition to nutrition and exercise, tobacco use is a major behavioral risk factor for chronic disease (see Chapter 11). The use of tobacco is strongly associated with increased risk for adverse health outcomes including cancer, pulmonary disease, and CVD. According to the CDC, approximately 90% of all lung cancer deaths in men and close to 80% of lung cancer deaths in women are directly related to tobacco smoking.[50] Although tobacco use has declined over time, in 2015, 15% of adults in the U.S. were current smokers and 1.1 billion people smoked tobacco worldwide with 80% of users living in low-income countries.[51-53] The single most preventable cause of morbidity and mortality is the use of tobacco.[51] Globally, tobacco use kills half of its users with an estimated 7 million people dying each year prematurely of diseases related to smoking.[53] To address this major health issue, in 2000 *Healthy People 2010* set an objective of reducing tobacco use to 12% of adults aged 18 or older (see Chapters 3 and 11). By 2016 this goal was met in only two states, California and Utah. The percentage of current smokers in the United States in 2016 by state ranged from 8% in Utah to 24.6% in Kentucky and 24.8% in West Virginia.[54]

There is strong evidence to support the benefit of smoking cessation. People who quit smoking have a lower risk of lung cancer than if they had continued to smoke.[55,56] The challenge is that the use of tobacco is more than an individual issue and requires interventions at the population and community level. Both the WHO and the U.S. Department of Health and Human Services have presented population-level strategies aimed at reducing tobacco use. From a global perspective, the WHO initiated an international tobacco treaty in 2005. Based on a recent study, researchers concluded that there was a significant association between the demand-reduction measures included in the treaty and lower smoking prevalence. They concluded that there would be future reductions in tobacco-related morbidity and mortality.

These findings demonstrate the value of implementing population-level interventions.[57]

Alcohol Use

Alcohol use accounts for 5.1% of the global burden of disease and is a component cause of more than 200 diseases and injury conditions (see Chapter 11).[58-60] Reduction in the burden of disease associated with alcohol use requires a health-care workforce capable of implementing evidence-based interventions across the continuum of alcohol use and the life span. If health-care providers understand the continuum of alcohol use across the life span, including adverse alcohol-related health consequences for both the drinker and non-drinker, the scope of prevention and intervention efforts is greatly expanded. Although alcohol consumption is a socially acceptable and normative practice in the United States, it has the potential to adversely affect health across the life span, including but not limited to injury, breast cancer, hypertension, stroke, liver disease, and brain damage.[58,59]

Genomics and Risk for Noncommunicable Disease

Understanding risk for NCDs includes the genetic risk each person or group of genetically related persons has for disease. **Human genomics** is the study of the genetic structure or genome of a living human. Evidence gathered through genomics clearly demonstrates that there is a genetic role in the major NCDs including cancer, diabetes, health disease, and asthma.[61,62] Genetic risk predisposes a person to disease independent of environmental and behavioral risks. Understanding genetic risks and identifying genetic mutations offer hope for both prevention and treatment of chronic disease. An example of genetic risk is the *BRCA1* and *BRCA2* gene mutations, known as tumor suppressors, which increase the risk for breast cancer.[63] Persons who screen positive for *BRCA1* and *BRCA2* mutations can choose either to undergo prophylactic surgery (removal of both breasts) or to avoid known risk factors associated with the development of breast cancer.[63] The WHO has a human genetics research project that is critically evaluating genetic research related to the four NCDs, cancer, asthma, diabetes, and CVDs, in the hopes of identifying strategies to control or prevent these diseases.[61]

The CDC has a dedicated site on human genomics and public health. The organization states that the study of the relationship among genes, environment, and behaviors will help us understand why some people get sick and others do not.[62] The role of family history in the development of disease is not a new concept, but the mapping of the human genome has allowed scientists to identify the actual genes linked to the development of disease and thus increase the ability of researchers to develop and evaluate genetic screening and other interventions that can improve health and prevent disease.

Despite the promise of genomics to help control NCDs, there are potential problems with reliance on genomics to help solve the problem of these diseases. Most chronic diseases are not **monogenetic**; that is, the disease is linked to a single gene mutation such as cystic fibrosis. Only 2% of total diseases are monogenetic. All other diseases result from multifactorial causes and are **polygenetic**, meaning multiple genes act together to cause the disease. Many diseases are experienced in the later years of life rather than early in life when genetic interventions are more apt to be beneficial. To further complicate the understanding of the role of genetics in the development of disease, Strohman pointed out in the early 1990s that slower genetic change fails to compensate for rapid environmental change. He explained that "genes are regulated by cellular responses to the external world and that diseases are initiated by those responses."[64] In other words, our genetic makeup is not static and as we age will adapt to the environment we are exposed to. Thus, genetic risk is not a linear source of complex chronic disease but is rather a dynamic process based on interaction between the gene and the environment. The question Strohman raised was whether genomic research should focus on genetic engineering that would fit the individual human organism to a hostile environment or on environmental engineering that would refit the environment to be consistent with the evolving human genome.[64]

Building on the complexity of the interaction between genetics and the environment described in detail by Strohman[64] a new field is emerging, **human genome epidemiology**. This field provides the scientific basis for the study of the distribution of gene variants, gene-disease associations, and gene-environment and gene-gene interactions within and across populations. This allows public health scientists to estimate the absolute, relative, and attributable risks for disease based on genomic factors (see Chapter 3). Thus, the growing understanding of the human genome from a population perspective offers new essential information on the occurrence of chronic disease based on population-level as well as individual risk.

Disparity and Noncommunicable Disease

Differences in socioeconomic status are a major contributor to health status and risk for development of disease and thus a disparity in life expectancy.[65] As defined in Chapter 7 disparity is a difference or inequality in some aspect of health such as a disparity in the infant mortality rate between two groups. Disparity in morbidity and mortality statistics for NCD persists (see Chapter 7). For example, African Americans and persons living in the southeastern United States bear a statistically greater disease burden related to stroke.[66] The challenge is to understand the upstream determinants of these disparities and to separate out biological causes from those related to the conditions of life, that is, the infrastructure of society and why society is set up as it is.[65]

Socioeconomic Risk for Noncommunicable Disease

As demonstrated previously, the development of an NCD is multifactorial. In addition to the physical environment, behavior, and genetic risk, socioeconomic factors play a role in determining who is at greater risk for developing an NCD. Health is remarkably sensitive to the social environment, and those who are less well-off are at greater risk for experiencing ill health. The term often used to describe these factors is the social determinants of health (see Chapter 7). According to the WHO, multiple factors contribute the differences in health status (Box 9-5) with poverty a major driving factor.[67,68] The premise is that it does not make sense to treat people for disease without addressing the things that make them sick in the first place. Interventions aimed at reducing risk must consider the social determinants of health and the barriers that exist within a socioeconomic context that reduce the ability of individuals, families, and communities to experience a healthy lifestyle.

Disparity in NCD rates between different populations is also linked to socioeconomic and geographical factors (see Chapter 7). As evidenced by regional disparity in the United States relative to prevalence rates of NCDs. For example, West Virginia has the highest prevalence rate of diabetes at 15% in 2016 (Table 9-1).[69] These regional disparities reflect differences in socioeconomic factors and cultural lifestyle. Within states, disparity exists between counties and is often correlated with socioeconomic status, as exemplified by the difference in tobacco use and obesity rates.

There is good news. There has been a narrowing of the gap in premature deaths between African Americans and whites in the United States. Researchers from the University of Pittsburgh reported that between 1990 and 2014 African Americans had a 28% reduction in YLL compared to whites with a 4% reduction. The decline in heart disease and cancer death rates helped to account for the decline in YLL especially in African American adults aged 30 to 40.[70]

BOX 9–5 ■ Social Determinants of Health

Income and social status: Higher income and social status are linked to better health. The greater the gap between the richest and poorest people, the greater the differences in health.

Education: Low education levels are linked with poor health, more stress, and lower self-confidence.

Physical environment: Safe water and clean air, healthy workplaces, safe houses, communities and roads all contribute to good health.

Employment and working conditions: People in employment are healthier, particularly those who have more control over their working conditions

Social support networks: Greater support from families, friends, and communities is linked to better health.

Culture: Customs and traditions, and the beliefs of the family and community all affect health.

Genetics: Inheritance plays a part in determining lifespan, healthiness, and the likelihood of developing certain illnesses.

Personal behavior and coping skills: Balanced eating, keeping active, smoking, drinking, and how we deal with life's stresses and challenges all affect health.

Health services: Access and use of services that prevent and treat disease influences health.

Gender: Men and women suffer from different types of diseases at different ages.

Source: (67, 68)

TABLE 9–1 ■ Top 10 Highest Rates of Type 2 Diabetes (2016)

Rank	State	Diabetes Rate
1	West Virginia	15.0% ±0.9
2	Alabama	14.6% ±1.0
3	Mississippi	13.6% ±1.1
4	Arkansas	13.5% ±1.4
5	Kentucky	13.1% ±0.9
6	South Carolina	13.0% ±0.8
7	Tennessee	12.7% ±1.0
8	Georgia	12.1% ±1.0
9	Louisiana	12.1% ±1.2
10	Oklahoma	12.0% ±0.9

Source: (69)

The relationship between socioeconomic status and prevalence of NCD presents an ethical dilemma for providers of health care (Box 9-6). A central risk factor for increased morbidity and mortality related to NCD is access to health care including preventive screening, early and ongoing treatment, and resources needed to manage care. In the United States, the Affordable Care Act (ACA) was designed to attempt to increase access to care. However, for the most part, U.S. health care is based on a fee-for-service basis, and health-care providers are reimbursed based on the care they provide (see Chapter 21). For those who are unable to obtain adequate insurance or who do not have adequate transportation to services, care is often delayed until the disease has become advanced. For example, an insulin-dependent diabetic single man who is currently homeless faces daily challenges, which may include maintaining an adequate diet when he is dependent on soup kitchens, checking his blood sugar when he does not have his own glucometer, obtaining insulin and insulin supplies, and storing those supplies in a safe place. By contrast, an insulin-dependent diabetic married man currently employed and domiciled has the financial means and the social support needed to meet those challenges. For both men, diabetic care will continue for the rest of their lives. Prevention of morbidity and mortality related to their diagnosis requires careful self-management over time including monitoring of blood sugar, diet and exercise, foot care, adherence to medication regimens, and regular check-ups with their health-care provider. Is it ethical for those who have the financial means to have the resources needed to meet their ongoing daily health-care needs necessary for survival whereas those who do not have the financial means do not?

BOX 9–6 ■ Ethics and Disparity Related to Chronic Diseases

Critical ethical questions related to chronic disease health care include the following:

- Is health care for the management of chronic diseases a right or a privilege?
- Should government pay for medically necessary services when an individual cannot afford those services?
  - If yes, does this approach truly serve the greater good for the greater number?
  - If no, who should be responsible for paying for these services?
- How does failure to provide services to those in need impact the community in general?

Prevention Strategies for Noncommunicable Diseases

Prevention and management of NCDs are global priorities.[1] Prevention strategies extend across the continuum from primary to tertiary prevention (see Chapter 2). Prevention of NCD across all three levels occurs across many settings (see Chapters 13 to 20). Prevention efforts are often focused on reducing the individual risk factors mentioned earlier, but often the success of prevention efforts require multifaceted interventions at the individual, family, community, and policy levels. For the nurse, these efforts can seem overwhelming.

At the individual and family levels, primary prevention focuses on behavioral change with a strong emphasis on healthy eating and exercise. These approaches not only provide information as to what constitutes a healthy lifestyle but also provide participants with strategies for making improvements in nutrition and physical activity and accessing the resources needed. The difficulty is that the populations at greatest risk for NCDs are those with limited access to the resources needed to maintain a healthy lifestyle. Thus, population-level primary prevention programs help to change barriers to a healthy lifestyle. For example, obtaining an adequate level of exercise in an urban setting requires safe streets for walking and/or access to recreational activities. This requires action at the community and policy levels. Nurses, especially those working in a public health role, can help facilitate community engagement in improving the safety of streets and improving access to healthy foods at reasonable prices.

Secondary prevention efforts are also associated with reduced morbidity and mortality related to NCD, especially screening (Chapter 2). Examples of screening programs recommended by the CDC for the prevention of NCDs include mammograms and screening for colorectal cancer.[71,72] Such programs result in the early detection of disease and thus in early treatment.

Often the nurse provides care related to tertiary prevention efforts aimed at reducing the adverse consequences experienced by a person who has already been diagnosed with a disease. The goal is to reduce the morbidity and disability associated with the disease and to prevent premature death. During the course of the disease, there can be periods of acute illness that are usually shorter and often require admission to an acute care facility for care. Chapter 14 provides in-depth coverage of the role of public health science in the nursing care of patients during an acute phase of an NCD that requires interventions to address an acute stage of an illness. Primary care settings provide care to help patients manage a chronic disease as well as care for milder acute phases of the disease (see Chapter 15). Two concepts grounded in public health prevention models and used in both acute care and primary care settings are health-related quality of life and chronic disease self-management.

Health-Related Quality of Life

Health-related quality of life is central to the overarching goals for *HP*. The primary goal is to attain and promote "a high quality of life for all people, across all life stages."[4] **Health-related quality of life (HRQoL)** is a multidimensional construct related to the desired physical and psychological health outcomes for most of the interventions that nurses provide to individuals and families. HRQoL is defined here as the self-perceived impact of physical and emotional health on quality of life, including the effects on general health, physical functioning, physical health and role, bodily pain, vitality, social functioning, emotional health and role, and mental health.[73,74] The CDC has a whole Web site dedicated to HRQoL.[74] Included on the Web page is the four-questions measure it uses for HRQoL that can easily be used in any health-care setting, and the evidence supports it as a reliable and valid measure of HRQoL. This healthy data measure not only can help in measuring an individual's HRQoL, but according to the CDC, it is also being used at the national and state levels to identify health disparities (see Chapter 7), to track population trends, and to build broad coalitions around a measure of population health. This measure is compatible with the WHO's definition of health (see Chapter 1).[75] The CDC uses the Healthy Days measure in the Behavioral Risk Factor Surveillance system.[73,76] Numerous studies have been conducted using HRQoL as a central measure.[77,78]

■ EVIDENCE-BASED PRACTICE
Measuring Health-Related Quality of Life (HRQoL)

Screening for HRQoL

Practice Statement: The use of the HRQoL screening tool can help health-care providers identify persons whose health is negatively impacting their quality of life and can provide a means to measure key health indicators for public health assessments.

Targeted Outcome: Identify those in need of interventions aimed at improving their quality of life and identifying vulnerable populations.

Evidence to Support: The CDC's 14-item HRQoL tool includes the standard four-item set of Healthy Days core questions and the Standard Activity Limitation and Healthy Days Symptoms modules. When used together, these measures make up the full CDC HRQoL-14 Measure. Public health departments have used the tool to identify vulnerable groups when conducting community assessments. The screening tool not only provides a method for assessing an individual's HRQoL but also provides PHNs with a useful indicator of health at the population level.

Recommended Approaches: The CDC HRQoL screening tool is used in community assessments and surveillance. A guide published in the late 1990s described the use of HRQoL as one of the main indicators for monitoring health in populations and evaluating outcomes, and is still recommended by the CDC. According to the CDC, the following are the main reasons for measuring HRQoL:

- HRQoL is related to both self-reported chronic diseases (diabetes, breast cancer, arthritis, and hypertension) and their risk factors (BMI, physical inactivity, and smoking status).
- Measuring HRQoL can help determine the burden of preventable disease, injuries, and disabilities, and can provide valuable new insights into the relationships between HRQoL and risk factors.
- Measuring HRQoL will help monitor progress in achieving the nation's health objectives.

Sources

Linde, L., Sørensen, J., Ostergaard, M., Hørslev-Petersen, K., & Hetland, M. (2008). Health-related quality of life: validity, reliability, and responsiveness of SF-36, EQ-15D, EQ-5D, RAQoL, and HAQ in patients with rheumatoid arthritis. *Journal of Rheumatology, 35*(8), 1528-1537.

Andresen, E.M., Catlin, T.K., Wyrwich, K.W., & Jackson-Thompson, J. (2003). Retest reliability of surveillance questions on health-related quality of life. *Journal of Epidemiology Community Health, 57*(5), 339-343.

Centers for Disease Control and Prevention. (2016). *Health-related quality of life methods and measures.* Retrieved from https://www.cdc.gov/hrqol/measurement.htm.

Ware, J.J., Kosinski, M., & Keller, S.D. (1996). A 12-item short-form health survey: Construction of scales and preliminary tests of reliability and validity. *Medical Care, 34*(3), 220-233.

Chronic Disease Self-Management

An evidence-based approach to improving HRQoL for persons with NCD is **chronic disease self-management (CDSM)**. CDSM is an ongoing process by which individuals with a chronic illness or condition engage in self-management of medications, symptoms, and promotion of their own health, and can be applied to both noncommunicable and communicable chronic disease.[79] CDSM requires implementation of health-promotion and health protection strategies, which are fundamental concepts for nursing practice (Chapter 2). Extensive research exists related to the efficacy of patient education programs for specific chronic diseases such as asthma and diabetes and has now shown effectiveness with diverse populations and diseases.[79-83] Evidence is accumulating that heterogeneous CDSM programs that include persons with different chronic diseases are effective, reduce emergency department usage and health distress, and transcend ethnic boundaries.[81,83] Moreover, they apply to underserved populations who do not have regular health-care providers.[80,84] CDSM has great potential for improving self-management of disease, health behaviors, health-care utilization, and health status.

NCD prevention and reduction of risk factors that lead to NCDs continues as a focus in the development of the Healthy People 2030 framework and objectives.[85] It is an issue across all health-care settings. Strategies for specific NCDs are discussed across the chapters in this text. The key is to remember that prevention efforts require interventions at all levels with the goal of not only reducing the prevalence of NCD but also of improving the overall HRQoL for individuals, families, and populations.

■ CULTURAL CONTEXT
Noncommunicable Diseases

Culture plays a big part in the prevention and treatment of NCDs. For the most part, when culture is mentioned in conjunction with prevention of NCDs, the focus is on its role in relation to individual risk behaviors such as food, nutrition, and exercise. Culture is also important in the development of education materials (Chapter 2). However, another issue in relation to culture and NCDs has to do with the cultural shifts that have occurred at the national level in relation to prevention.

Cultural shifts occur over time because no culture is static. In the past 50 years, there have been cultural shifts in the United States in relation to risk behaviors associated with NCDs. A **cultural shift** is defined as a change in society's dominant views, morals, and behaviors. When applied to health, it represents a shift in how society views that issue and the risk factors associated with development of disease. For example, there has been a cultural shift in how society perceives drinking alcohol and driving; once this was viewed as a normal behavior and now it is one that is not tolerated and results in criminal consequences. Another example is the shift in how we view the foods we eat. Some states have passed laws prohibiting the sale of large, sugary drinks or the use of deep-fat fryers in schools. A cultural shift changes the way organizations are structured, the environment we live in, and the activities we participate in.

Let's examine a major cultural shift in the United States related to a major preventable risk factor associated with the development of NCDs. In the 1950s, no one questioned a person's right to smoke in public. Smoking occurred in all public places, including banks, hospitals, and restaurants. As the evidence grew that secondhand smoke affected the health of the nonsmoker, public health policy initiatives were begun to reduce smoking in public places. In the beginning, science drove the change. Based on the evidence, public health policies were put in place that required restaurants to designate no smoking sections, and employers constructed separate places for their workers to smoke, often referred to as "butt huts." However, what began as evidence-based public health policy shifted to a social reality. As fewer people smoked, tolerance of smoking declined, and the culture shifted from viewing tobacco use in a positive manner to viewing it as a negative and unpleasant behavior. In the 1930s and 1940s, movie stars smoked on screen, and in the 1950s, cigarette ads depicted the male smoker as rugged and manly, as in the Marlboro Man. Today, most public spaces are smoke free. It is hard to determine which comes first, the policy or the cultural shift. Often, one reflects the other. However, to be effective, public polices need the support of the community. When the culture matches the policy, the policy is more apt to bring about change.

Not only does the culture of groups play a role in individual behavior, but also the cultural norms of a population shift over time and can have a significant impact on health. Sometimes there are opposing cultural values in relation to a risk factor. For example, people may have differing views about the appropriateness of using public policy to restrict the ingredients that restaurants put in foods. Understanding that cultural shifts occur over time related to reducing NCD is important for the nurse who wishes to actively engage in prevention efforts. Nursing can play a role in helping the cultural shift along. As the largest segment of the health-care workforce, nurses can be in the forefront of positive cultural shifts related to prevention; the shift can happen at a more rapid pace and populations will get healthier. A world with reduced morbidity and mortality related to NCDs and improved HRQoL can happen, and nurses are major drivers of the shift to healthier living as part of our culture.

■ Summary Points

- NCDs contribute significantly to the overall burden of disease.
- Seven out of the top ten leading causes of death in the United States are NCDs.
- Risk for NCD is a combination of individual behaviors, the environment, genes, and socioeconomic factors.
- Prevention occurs across the continuum, starting with primary prevention during the perinatal period through tertiary prevention measures such as chronic disease self-management programs.

▼ CASE STUDY
Prevention of Chronic Obstructive Respiratory Disease (COPD)

A group of nurses on a medical-surgical unit in a hospital that serves an Appalachian community in Kentucky on the West Virginia border were growing frustrated with the continued readmission of persons with COPD. One of the nurses came across statistics on the age-adjusted death rate of COPD in Kentucky. It was 62.8 per 100,000 compared to other states such as Hawaii at 15.5 per 100,000. She also found that COPD death rates were highest in the states surrounding the Ohio and Mississippi Rivers.[85] The nurses decided to put together a proposal related to the prevention of COPD.

1. Choose a primary, secondary, and/or tertiary prevention approach and support your decision.
2. Choose a target population based on age and level of intervention (primary, secondary, and tertiary).

3. Access information on the Huntington/Ashland area of West Virginia and Kentucky and see what can be learned about:
   a. Cultural considerations
   b. Possible partners for the intervention
   c. Possible barriers
4. Review the literature again for evidence-based interventions relevant to your chosen population and prevention level.
5. Using Chapter 5 as a guide, draft a possible prevention intervention the nurses in the journal club could help initiate.

REFERENCES

1. World Health Organization. (2018). *Noncommunicable diseases*. Retrieved from http://www.who.int/topics/noncommunicable_diseases/en/.
2. World Health Organization. (2017). *Noncommunicable diseases: Key facts*. Retrieved from http://www.who.int/en/news-room/fact-sheets/detail/noncommunicable-diseases.
3. World Health Organization. (2014). *Global status report on noncommunicable diseases 2014*. Geneva, Switzerland: Author. Retrieved from http://www.who.int/nmh/publications/ncd-status-report-2014/en/.
4. U.S. Department of Health and Human Services. (2018). *Healthy People 2020*. Retrieved from https://www.healthypeople.gov/2020/topics-objectives.
5. Davy, C., Bleasel, J., Liu, H., Tchan, M., Ponniah, S. & Brown, A. (2015). Effectiveness of chronic care models: Opportunities for improving healthcare practice and health outcomes: A systematic review. *BMC Health Services Research 2015*, 15, 194. DOI 10.1186/s12913-015-0854-8.
6. World Health Organization. (2018). *Global burden of disease*. Retrieved from http://www.who.int/topics/global_burden_of_disease/en/.
7. Central Intelligence Agency. (2018). *The world fact book*. Retrieved from https://www.cia.gov/library/publications/the-world-factbook/rankorder/2102rank.html.
8. World Health Organization. (2018). *Health statistics: Mortality; health adjusted life expectancy (HALE)*. Retrieved from http://www.who.int/healthinfo/statistics/indhale/en/.
9. World Health Organization. (2018). *Mental health*. Retrieved from http://www.who.int/mental_health/management/depression/daly/en/.
10. Centers for Disease Control and Prevention. (2017). *Chronic disease prevention and health promotion: Chronic disease overview*. Retrieved from https://www.cdc.gov/chronicdisease/overview/index.htm.
11. American Diabetes Association. (2018). *Statistics about diabetes*. Retrieved from http://www.diabetes.org/diabetes-basics/statistics/.
12. U.S. Department of Health and Human Services. (2018). *Healthy People 2020: Topic—diabetes*. Retrieved from http://www.healthypeople.gov/2020/topicsobjectives2020/overview.aspx?topicid=8.

13. U.S. Department of Health and Human Services. (2018). *Healthy People 2020 Midcourse Review Chapter 8: Diabetes.* Retrieved from https://www.cdc.gov/nchs/data/hpdata2020/HP2020MCR-C08-Diabetes.pdf.

14. Kochanek, K.D., Murphy, S.L., Xu, J.Q., & Arias, E. (2017). *Mortality in the United States, 2016. NCHS Data Brief, no 293.* Hyattsville, MD: National Center for Health Statistics.

15. Centers for Disease Control and Prevention. (2017). *Heart disease fact sheet.* Retrieved from https://www.cdc.gov/dhdsp/data_statistics/fact_sheets/fs_heart_disease.htm.

16. Centers for Disease Control and Prevention. (2017). *Stroke fact sheet.* Retrieved from https://www.cdc.gov/dhdsp/data_statistics/fact_sheets/fs_stroke.htm.

17. Roth, G.A., Dwyer-Lindgren, L., Bertozzi-Villa, A., Stubbs, R.W., Morozoff, C., Naghavi, M., ... Murray, C.J.L. (2017). Trends and patterns of geographic variation in cardiovascular mortality among U.S. counties, 1980-2014. *JAMA, 317*(19), 1976-1992.

18. Roth, G.A., Johnson, C.O., Abate, K.H., Abd-Allah, F., Ahmed, M., Alam, K., ... Murray, C.J.L. (2018).The burden of cardiovascular diseases among U.S. states, 1990-2016, *JAMA Cardiology* [epub ahead of print]. doi: 10.1001/jamacardio.2018.0385.

19. The Framingham Heart Study. (2018). Retrieved from https://www.framinghamheartstudy.org/.

20. American Cancer Society. (2018). *Cancer facts and figures.* Retrieved from https://www.cancer.org/content/dam/cancer-org/research/cancer-facts-and-statistics/annual-cancer-facts-and-figures/2018/cancer-facts-and-figures-2018.pdf.

21. World Health Organization. (2018). *Cancer.* Retrieved from http://www.who.int/cancer/en/.

22. Sun, Y., Zhao, Z., Yang, Z., Xu, F., Lu, H., Zhu, Z., ... Zhu, H. (2017). Risk factors and preventions of breast cancer. *International Journal of Biological Sciences, 13*, 1387–1397. doi: 10.7150/ijbs.21635.

23. Centers for Disease Control and Prevention. (2017). *What are the risk factors for breast cancer?* Retrieved from https://www.cdc.gov/cancer/breast/basic_info/risk_factors.htm.

24. Centers for Disease Control and Prevention. (2015). *BRCA gene mutations.* Retrieved from https://www.cdc.gov/cancer/breast/young_women/bringyourbrave/hereditary_breast_cancer/brca_gene_mutations.htm.

25. World Health Organization. (2018). *Chronic respiratory disease.* Retrieved from http://www.who.int/respiratory/en/.

26. Centers for Disease Control and Prevention. (2017). *Chronic obstructive pulmonary disease.* Retrieved from https://www.cdc.gov/copd/index.html.

27. World Health Organization. (2016). *Global report on diabetes.* Geneva, Switzerland: Author.

28. Centers for Disease Control and Prevention. (2018). *Diabetes Report Card 2017.* Atlanta, GA: Author

29. Centers for Disease Control and Prevention. (2017). *Living with diabetes.* Retrieved from https://www.cdc.gov/diabetes/managing/index.html.

30. Mississippi State Department of Health. (n.d.). *Working together for healthy hearts.* Retrieved from https://msdh.ms.gov/msdhsite/_static/resources/4964.pdf.

31. Pettus, E.W. (2017, Aug. 6) Entrenched poverty tough to shake in the Mississippi delta. *U.S. News and World Report.* Retrieved from https://www.usnews.com/news/best-states/mississippi/articles/2017-08-06/entrenched-poverty-tough-to-shake-in-the-mississippi-delta.

32. Sabo, S., Allen, C.G., Sutkowi, K., & Wennerstrom, A. (2017). Community health workers in the United States: Challenges in identifying, surveying, and supporting the workforce. *American Journal of Public Health, 107*(12), 1964-1969. doi:10.2105/AJPH.2017.304096.

33. American Public Health Association. (2018). *Community health workers.* Retrieved from https://www.apha.org/apha-communities/member-sections/community-health-workers.

34. Centers for Disease Control and Prevention. (n.d.). *Field notes: Clinical community health worker initiative.* Retrieved from https://www.cdc.gov/dhdsp/docs/field_notes_clinical_community_health_worker.pdf.

35. World Health Organization. (2018). *Social determinants of health: Posters.* Retrieved from http://www.who.int/social_determinants/tools/multimedia/posters/en/.

36. Centers for Disease Control and Prevention. (2017). *Adult obesity: Facts.* Retrieved from https://www.cdc.gov/obesity/data/adult.html.

37. Centers for Disease Control and Prevention. (2017). *Childhood obesity: Facts.* Retrieved from https://www.cdc.gov/obesity/data/childhood.html.

38. Centers for Disease Control and Prevention. (2017). *Asthma and community health branch.* Retrieved from https://www.cdc.gov/nceh/airpollution/.

39. Centers for Disease Control and Prevention. (2018). *National center for environmental health.* Retrieved from https://www.cdc.gov/nceh/.

40. United Nations. (2018). *World urbanization prospects: The 2018 revision: Key facts.* Retrieved from https://esa.un.org/unpd/wup/Publications/Files/WUP2018-Key-Facts.pdf.

41. Centers for Disease Control and Prevention. (2018). *Healthy weight: About child and teen BMI.* Retrieved from https://www.cdc.gov/healthyweight/assessing/bmi/childrens_bmi/about_childrens_bmi.html.

42. U.S. Department of Health and Human Services. (2018). *Healthy People 2020 topics and objectives: Nutrition and weight status.* Retrieved from http://www.healthypeople.gov/2020/topicsobjectives2020/objectiveslist.aspx?topicId=29.

43. National Center for Health Statistics. (2016). *Chapter 29: Nutrition and weight status. Midcourse review.* Hyattsville, MD: Author.

44. Bullock, A., Sheff, K., Moore, K., & Manson, S. (2017). Obesity and overweight in American Indian and Alaska Native Children, 2006-2015. *American Journal of Public Health, 107*:1502-1507. doi: 10.2105/AJPH.2017.303904.

45. Centers for Disease Control and Prevention. (2018). *Youth risk behavior surveillance system.* Retrieved from https://www.cdc.gov/healthyyouth/data/yrbs/index.htm.

46. Florida Health. (n.d.). *Florida youth survey.* Retrieved from http://www.floridahealth.gov/statistics-and-data/survey-data/florida-youth-survey/index.html.

47. MacDonald, M.A. (2004). From miasma to fractals: The epidemiology revolution and public health nursing. *Public Health Nursing, 21*(4), 380-381.

48. Centers for Disease Control and Prevention. (2018). *Healthy schools: Childhood obesity prevention.* Retrieved from https://www.cdc.gov/healthyschools/obesity/index.htm.

49. Centers for Disease Control and Prevention. (2017). *Healthy schools: School health guidelines.* Retrieved from https://www.cdc.gov/healthyschools/npao/strategies.htm.

50. Centers for Disease Control and Prevention. (2017). *Lung cancer: What are the risk factors?* Retrieved from http://www.cdc.gov/cancer/lung/basic_info/risk_factors.htm.

51. Centers for Disease Control and Prevention. (2018). *Smoking and tobacco use: Fast facts and fact sheets.* Retrieved from https://www.cdc.gov/tobacco/data_statistics/fact_sheets/index.htm?s_cid=osh-stu-home-spotlight-001.

52. World Health Organization. (2018). *Global health observatory (GHO) data: Prevalence of tobacco smoking.* Retrieved from http://www.who.int/gho/tobacco/use/en/.

53. World Health Organization. (2018). *Tobacco: Key facts.* Retrieved from http://www.who.int/en/news-room/fact-sheets/detail/tobacco.

54. Centers for Disease Control and Prevention. (2018). *State tobacco activities tracking and evaluation (STATE) system.* Retrieved from https://www.cdc.gov/statesystem/index.html.

55. World Health Organization. (2018). *Tobacco free initiative (TFI): Fact sheet about health benefits of smoking cessation.* Retrieved from http://www.who.int/tobacco/quitting/benefits/en/.

56. Centers for Disease Control and Prevention. (2017). *Smoking and tobacco use: Quitting smoking.* Retrieved from https://www.cdc.gov/tobacco/data_statistics/fact_sheets/cessation/quitting/index.htm.

57. Gravely, S., Giovino, G.A., Craig, L., Commar, A., D'Espaignet, E.T., Schotte, K., & Fong, G.T. (2017). Implementation of key demand-reduction measures of the WHO Framework Convention on Tobacco Control and change in smoking prevalence in 126 countries: an association study. *The Lancet Public Health, 2*(4), e166-e174. doi.10.1016/S2468-2667(17)30045-2.

58. Shield, K.D., Parry, C., & Rehm, J. (2013). Chronic diseases and conditions related to alcohol use, alcohol research. *Current Reviews, 35*(2), 155-173.

59. World Health Organization. (2018). *Management of substance abuse: Alcohol.* Retrieved from http://www.who.int/substance_abuse/facts/alcohol/en/.

60. Centers for Disease Control and Prevention. (2017). *Alcohol and public health.* Retrieved from https://www.cdc.gov/alcohol/index.htm.

61. World Health Organization. (2018). *Human genomics in global health: WHO's Human Genetics areas of work.* Retrieved from http://www.who.int/genomics/about/commondiseases/en/index.html.

62. Centers for Disease Control and Prevention. (2014). *Public health genomics: Genomics and diseases.* Retrieved from https://www.cdc.gov/genomics/disease/genomic_diseases.htm.

63. National Cancer Institute. (2018). *BRCA mutations: Cancer risk and genetic testing.* Retrieved from http://www.cancer.gov/cancertopics/factsheet/Risk/BRCA.

64. Strohman, R.C. (1993). Ancient genomes, wise bodies, unhealthy people: Limits of a genetic paradigm in biology and medicine. *Perspectives in Biology and Medicine, 37*(1), 112-145.

65. Ratcliff, K.S (2017). *The social determinants of health: looking upstream.* Medford, MA: Polity Press.

66. Benjamin, E.J., Virani, S.S., Callaway, C.W., Chamberlain, A.M., Chang, A.R., Cheng, S., ... Muntner, P. (2018). Heart disease and stroke statistics—2018 update: A report from the American Heart Association. *Circulation, 137*(12): e67-e492. https://doi-org.ezp.welch.jhmi.edu/10.1161/CIR.0000000000000558.

67. World Health Organization. (2018). *Health impact assessment: Determinants of health.* Retrieved from http://www.who.int/hia/evidence/doh/en/.

68. World Health Association. (2018). *Noncommunicable disease.* Retrieved from http://www.who.int/en/news-room/fact-sheets/detail/noncommunicable-diseases.

69. State of Obesity, Robert Wood Johnson, Trust for America's Health. (2018). *States with the highest type 2 diabetes rates.* Retrieved from https://stateofobesity.org/lists/highest-rates-diabetes/.

70. Buchanich, J.M, Doerfler, S.M., Lann, M.F., Marsh, G.M., & Burke, D.S. (2018). Improvement in racial disparities in years of life lost in the USA since 1990. *PLoS ONE 13*(4): e0194308. https://doi.org/.

71. Centers for Disease Control and Prevention. (2018). *Breast cancer.* Retrieved from https://www.cdc.gov/cancer/breast/index.htm.

72. Centers for Disease Control and Prevention. (2018). *Colorectal cancer.* Retrieved from https://www.cdc.gov/cancer/colorectal/index.htm.

73. Centers for Disease Control and Prevention. (2016). *Health-related quality of life methods and measures.* Retrieved from http://www.cdc.gov/hrqol/methods.htm.

74. Centers for Disease Control and Prevention. (2016). *Health-related quality of life.* Retrieved from http://www.cdc.gov/hrqol/index.htm.

75. World Health Organization. (2018). *About WHO: Constitution of WHO: principles.* Retrieved from http://www.who.int/about/mission/en/.

76. Ware, J.J., Kosinski, M., & Keller, S.D. (1996). A 12-item short-form health survey: Construction of scales and preliminary tests of reliability and validity. *Medical Care, 34*(3), 220-233.

77. Havens E., Slabaugh S.L., Helmick C.G., Cordier, T., Zack, M., Gobal, V., Prewitt, T. (2017). Comorbid arthritis is associated with lower health-related quality of life in older adults with other chronic conditions, United States, 2013-2014. *Prevention and Chronic Diseases. 14:E60.* doi: 10.5888/pcd14.160495.

78. Shockey, T.M., Zack, M., Sussell, A. (2017). Health-related quality of life among U.S. workers: variability across occupation groups. *American Journal of Public Health. 107,* 1316-1323. doi: 10.2105/AJPH.2017.303840.

79. Lorig, K. (2014). Chronic disease self-management program: Insights from the eye of the storm. *Frontiers in Public Health, 2,* 253. http://doi.org.ezp.welch.jhmi.edu/10.3389/fpubh.2014.00253.

80. Smith, M.L., Towne, S.D., Herrera-Venson, A., Cameron, K., Kulinski, K.P., Lorig, K., Ory, M.G., et al. (2017). Dissemination of chronic disease self-management education (CDSME) programs in the United States: Intervention delivery by rurality. *International Journal of Environmental Research and Public Health, 14*(6), 638. http://doi.org.ezp.welch.jhmi.edu/10.3390/ijerph14060638.

81. Smith, M.L., Wilson, M.G., Robertson, M.M., Padilla, H.M., Zuercher, H., Vandenberg, R., DeJoy, D.M., et al. (2018). Impact of a translated disease self-management program on employee health and productivity: Six-month findings from a randomized controlled trial. *International Journal of Environmental Research and Public Health, 15*(5), 851; doi:10.3390/ijerph15050851.

82. Groessl, E.J., Sklar, M., Laurent, D.D., Lorig, K., Ganiats, T.G., & Ho, S.B. (2016). Cost-effectiveness of the Hepatitis C self-management program. *Health Education & Behavior, 44*, 113-122. https://doi.org/10.1177/1090198116639239.

83. Salvatore, A.L., Ahn, S., Jiang, L., Lorig, K., & Ory, M.G. (2015). National study of chronic disease self-management: 6-month and 12-month findings among cancer survivors and non-cancer survivors. *Psycho-oncology, 24*, 1714-1722.

http://dx.doi.org/10.1002/pon.3783 Retrieved from https://escholarship.org/uc/item/7zb19131.

84. Savage, C., Xu, Y., Richmond, M.M., Corbin, A., Falciglia, M., Gillespie, G. (2014). A pilot study: Retention of adults experiencing homelessness and feasibility of a CDSM diabetes program. *Journal of Community Health Nursing, 31*, 238-48. doi: 10.1080/07370016.2014.958406.

85. Healthy People. (2018). *Healthy People 2030 Framework.* Retrieved from https://www.healthypeople.gov/2020/About-Healthy-People/Development-Healthy-People-2030/Proposed-Framework.

86. Centers for Disease Control and Prevention. (2016). *Chronic obstructive pulmonary disease (COPD): Data and statistics.* Retrieved from https://www.cdc.gov/copd/data.html.

Chapter 10

Mental Health

Bryan R. Hansen and Christine Savage

LEARNING OUTCOMES

After reading the chapter, the student will be able to:

1. Define the global burden of disease related to mental disorders using current epidemiological frameworks.
2. Apply the National Academy of Medicine framework related to prevention of mental health disorders.
3. Define the difference between behavioral, biological, environmental, and socioeconomic risk factors related to mental health disorders.
4. Apply current evidence-based population-level interventions to the prevention of mental disorders and the promotion of optimal mental health for communities and populations.
5. Describe systems approaches to the promotion of mental health and the prevention and treatment of mental health disorders.

KEY TERMS

Any mental illness (AMI)
Behavioral health
Burden of disease
Deinstitutionalization
Emotional health
Health-related quality of life (HRQoL)
Indicated prevention
Intersectoral strategies
Major depressive disorder (MDD)
Mental disorder
Mental health
Mental illness
Protective factors
Resilience
Selective prevention
Serious mental illness (SMI)
Stigma
Transinsitutionalization
Universal prevention

Introduction

Achieving optimal **mental health** is an essential component of programs aimed at improving the health of populations. Mental health is defined as mental and psychological well-being, which includes our emotional, psychological, and social well-being, and is essential to health overall.[1,2] In 2005, the Institute of Medicine (IOM), now named the National Academy of Medicine, reported that mental or substance-use problems and disorders are the leading cause of combined disability and death for women and the second highest for men.[3] Of the 10 leading health indicator topics of *Healthy People 2020 (HP 2020)*, four topics related directly to behavioral health: mental health, substance abuse, tobacco, and injury/violence.[4] These four topics come under the umbrella of the term **behavioral health**. Each of these interrelated issues has an impact on the health of individuals, families, and communities. Often mental illness, substance abuse, and/or intentional injury and violence co-occur. Thus, there is a logical and empirical connection among these health issues. Taken together, they make up the most serious and prevalent public health problems of our times. So that each aspect of behavioral health can be covered in depth, these four leading health indicator topics of health are covered in three separate chapters. Chapter 10 covers mental health and mental health disorders; Chapter 11 covers substance use including alcohol, tobacco, and other drugs; and Chapter 12 covers injury and violence.

This chapter focuses on promotion of **mental health**, which is best defined by *HP 2020* as "a state of successful performance of mental function, resulting in productive activities, fulfilling relationships with other people, and the ability to adapt to change and to cope with challenges."[4] The term **emotional health** is used interchangeably with *mental health* and is defined the same way. *HP* also includes *mental disorder* and *mental illness* under the topic of mental health. *Mental health* reflects a positive state of health, whereas *mental disorder* refers to the diagnosable disorders that negatively affect the mental health of individuals and affect an individual's ability to cope with everyday life. *Mental illness* is a term that refers to all mental disorders collectively. The terms **mental disorder** and **mental illness** are often used interchangeably and are defined as "clusters of symptoms and signs associated with distress and disability (i.e., impairment of functioning), yet whose pathology and etiology are unknown."[1,4] Mental illnesses are disorders, not diseases. *Disease* is a term used when the pathology is known or can be detected, which is not the case with a mental health disorder. Diagnoses that come under the category of mental disorders include depression, anxiety disorders, bipolar disorder, and schizophrenia. Not all mental health disorders have the same etiology (cause) or require the same population-level interventions.

Mental disorders can vary in severity from mild to severe. The term **any mental illness (AMI)** is defined as a mental, behavioral, or emotional disorder. AMI can vary in impact, ranging from no impairment to mild, moderate, and even severe impairment.[5] The term **serious mental illness (SMI)** is used to refer to a diagnosable mental disorder that severely disrupts a person's ability to function socially, to obtain and maintain employment, to have adequate financial resources, and to access appropriate and adequate support or maintain family supports.[5] SMI does not refer to any particular diagnosis; rather, it implies eligibility for specific kinds of support services. The mental disorders that can lead to SMI include major depression, schizophrenia, bipolar disorder, obsessive-compulsive disorder (OCD), panic disorder, post-traumatic stress disorder (PTSD), and borderline personality disorder.

In contrast with mental disorders, mental health represents a state of emotional well-being. Persons who are emotionally healthy are those who can meet the demands and stresses of everyday life and function in society. Mental health does not merely represent the absence of a mental disorder but rather the cognitive and emotional ability to deal with the ups and downs of life while contributing to society through work and play. Viewed from a population perspective, the health of a population reflects not only the physical well-being of the members of the population or community but also their social and emotional well-being. Because of their overall importance to health, mental health and mental disorders are included in the *HP* list of topics

■ HEALTHY PEOPLE
Mental Health

Goal: Improve mental health through prevention and by ensuring access to appropriate, quality mental health services.

Overview: *Mental health* is a state of successful performance of mental function resulting in productive activities, fulfilling relationships with other people, and the ability to adapt to change and to cope with challenges. Mental health is essential to personal well-being, family and interpersonal relationships, and the ability to contribute to community or society.

Mental disorders are health conditions characterized by alterations in thinking, mood, and/or behavior associated with distress and/or impaired functioning. Mental disorders contribute to a host of problems that may include disability, pain, or death. *Mental illness* is the term that refers collectively to all diagnosable mental disorders.[4]

Optimal mental health is an essential component of healthy communities. The promotion of mental health involves interventions at the individual and community levels. At the individual level, promotion of optimal mental health requires not only the delivery of interventions focused on behavioral change but also the availability of adequate systems for care of those with mental health disorders. At the community level, promotion of mental health requires an environment that encourages strong social networks and a safe place to work and live. Because of the importance of mental health, in 2012, the World Health Organization (WHO) issued a resolution on mental health that aims to reduce the global burden of mental disorders and improve the overall mental health of countries. This resolution includes recognition of "the need for a comprehensive, coordinated response to addressing mental disorders from health and social sectors at the country level. The delegates recognized this includes approaches such as programs to reduce stigma and discrimination, reintegration of patients into workplace and society, support for care providers and families, and investment in mental health from the health budget."[6]

■ HEALTHY PEOPLE

Objectives: Reduce the proportion of persons who experience major depressive episode (MDE)
MHMD-4.1: Adolescents aged 12 to 17 years
Baseline: 8.3% of adolescents aged 12 to 17 years experienced an MDR in 2008.
Target: 7.4%
Target-Setting Method: 10% improvement

Midcourse Review: In the 4 years from 2008 to 2012, the percentage of adolescents aged 12 to 17 reporting having had a major depressive episode (MDE) in the past 12 months increased about 10%, from 8.3% to 9.1%, moving away from the Healthy People 2020 target of 7.5%. See Figure 10-1.
Data Source: National Survey on Drug and Health, SAMHSA

Source: (4)

Epidemiology of Mental Disorders

Tracking the prevalence of mental health disorders at the global level is challenging due to differences in tracking and the reliance on diagnoses that results in an underestimation of disease. It is estimated that globally 1 billion people have a mental health disorder.[7] In the United States, in 2018, an estimated 25% of adults reported having mental disorders within the previous year.[8] The U.S.

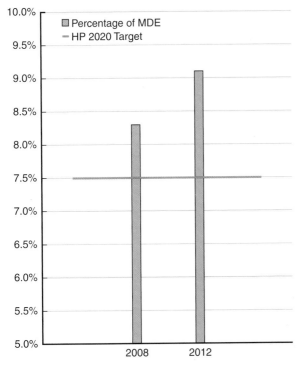

Figure 10-1 Percentage of Adolescents Experiencing Major Depressive Episode in Previous 12 months. *(See reference [4].)*

annual economic burden associated with SMI, including direct costs such as medical care, loss of earnings, and indirect costs such as disability, homelessness, incarceration, and early mortality, have been estimated to exceed $317 billion.[9] As reviewed in Chapter 9, the **burden of disease** is measured in years of life lost related to ill health and reflects the difference between total life expectancy and disability-adjusted life expectancy. Examining the burden of disease related to mental disorders allows us to consider what impact mental disorders have on the population or community. The best place to start is to examine the prevalence of mental disorders across the life span from both a global and an international perspective.

Surveillance of Mental Health Disorders

Estimating the prevalence of mental disorders is challenging because there has been no centralized method for conducting surveillance of mental health disorders in the United States or globally. The Centers for Disease Control and Prevention (CDC) compiles data from eight surveillance systems to identify gaps in surveillance and make recommendations for an improved method for collecting data on mental health disorders. This allows the CDC to address the broad spectrum of mental health using surveillance systems that, in many cases, do not focus specifically on mental health but include important indicators of mental health and mental health disorders. Through this process of examining data from all data sources, they were not only able to provide some estimates of prevalence of different mental disorders but also to help make recommendations about how to address the gaps in mental illness surveillance. The data sources included the Pregnancy Risk Assessment Monitoring System (PRAMS), National Nursing Home Survey, National Health Interview Survey, National Hospital Discharge Survey, National Health and Nutrition Examination Survey, National Ambulatory Medical Care Survey, National Hospital Ambulatory Medical Care Survey, and Behavioral Risk Factor Surveillance System.[10] At the global level, the WHO has developed the World Mental Health Survey to help determine estimates of human capital costs and prevalence of mental disorders in a wide range of countries.[11]

Prevalence of Mental Health Disorders

Mental health is an important part of overall health across the entire life span. Differences exist among age groups in relation to specific disorders. To understand the importance of the issue and to evaluate the effectiveness of interventions from a population perspective requires knowledge of the prevalence of mental disorders within and across communities and populations.

The 12-month prevalence is a measure that estimates the occurrence of a disorder within 1 year prior to assessment. In 2015, the 12-month prevalence of all mental disorders not including substance-use disorders in the U.S. was 4% and most prevalent in those aged 18-44.[12]

There are gender, ethnic, and age differences in the prevalence of SMI (Fig. 10-2).[12] In 2015, the 12-month prevalence of any mental disorder was higher in females than in males.[12] Those reporting two or more races had the highest prevalence of SMI, followed by American Indians/Alaska Natives.[13] American Indians/Alaskan Natives also have a high rate of lifetime PTSD compared to other races.[14] Children also experience mental disorders, with 49.5% of teens diagnosed with AMI between the ages of 13 and 18 years.[12]

Under the umbrella of SMI are specific diagnostic categories that have been the focus of population level prevention efforts, especially **major depressive disorder (MDD)**. MDD is a mood disorder that is diagnosed based on the occurrence of one or more major depressive episodes in the absence of a manic or hypomanic episode. In 2016, about 13%, or 3.1 million, of U.S. teens between 12 and 17 years had at least one episode of MDD in the previous 12 months, as did about 6.7%, or 16.2 million adults.[15,16] For adults, it is most prevalent among those aged 18 to 25 years and is more prevalent in women than in men.[16] Because of the high prevalence and the impact on health, *HP 2020* includes reduction of the number of persons who experience an MDD as one of the mental health objectives.

Over the beginning of this century, the morbidity and mortality rate associated with SMI increased, with 4.2% of all adults in the U.S. experiencing SMI in 2016. Persons diagnosed with an SMI died 10 to 20 years earlier than the general population. Part of this is attributed to suicide and injury. The other contributing factor is the strong association among SMI, chronic disease, and substance use.[17–19] Persons with SMI are less likely to receive preventative screening and interventions, less likely to receive treatment for diagnosed comorbidities, and more likely not to adhere to medical interventions, which exacerbates the disparity in mortality rates.[20]

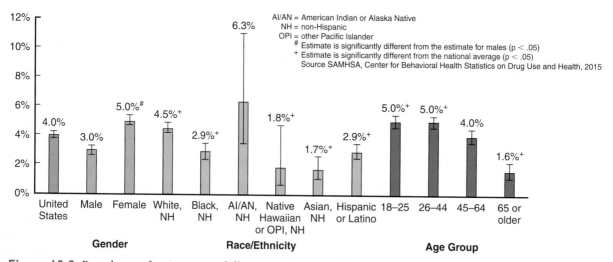

Past Year Serious Mental Illness (SMI) Among Adults Aged 18 or Older in the United States, by Gender, Race/Ethnicity, and Age Group (2015)[11]

In 2015, 4.0% of adults aged 18 or older in the United States (an estimated 9.8 million adults) had a serious mental illness (SMI) in the past year. This percentage was not significantly different from the percentage in 2011 (3.9%).

In 2015, the percentage of adults aged 18 or older in the United States with past year SMI was higher for females than for males. This percentage was higher than the national average for Whites, and for those aged 18–25 or aged 26–44. This percentage was lower than the national average for those who were Black, Native Hawaiian or other Pacific Islander, Asian, or Hispanic or Latino. This percentage was also lower than the national average for adults aged 65 or older.

AI/AN = American Indian or Alaska Native
NH = non-Hispanic
OPI = other Pacific Islander
# Estimate is significantly different from the estimate for males (p < .05)
+ Estimate is significantly different from the national average (p < .05)
Source SAMHSA, Center for Behavioral Health Statistics on Drug Use and Health, 2015

Figure 10-2 Prevalence of serious mental illness among U.S. adults, 2015. *(See reference 12.)*

Behavioral, Biological, Environmental, and Socioeconomic Risk Factors

Numerous factors contribute to the development of mental disorders at both the individual and community levels, and must be considered when attempting to understand the etiology of mental disorders. There is interplay among the individual, the family, and the community environment. From a public health perspective, improving the mental health of a population requires taking all these factors into account when developing interventions.

Individual-Level Risk Factors for Mental Disorders

At the individual level, both nature and nurture play roles; that is, genetics, family environment, and individual behavior are associated with the risk of developing a mental disorder, along with socioeconomic factors and community environment. Therefore, it is difficult to define the exact etiology of most mental disorders; the precise cause is poorly understood. There are, however, specific factors that have been associated with the development of mental disorders (Box 10-1). Recent work has helped demonstrate the link between genotype and mental illness through an environmental pathway. For example, PTSD is moderately heritable, but environmental factors play a large role in whether a person who has a susceptible genotype develops PTSD after severe trauma.[21]

Another issue related to the development of a mental disorder is the relationship between physiology and mental health. Conditions that affect brain chemistry, hormonal imbalances, or exposure in utero to viruses or toxins can increase the risk for development of a mental disorder.[22] Physical trauma such as traumatic brain injury is also associated with an increased risk of developing a mental disorder.[23] Individuals who have experienced malnutrition or low birth weight are also at higher risk for development of a mental disorder.[24] Some medication side effects include depression, anxiety, or suicidal ideation. In addition, an interaction between medications can result in increased risk for depression and other mental health disorders. Also, persons with diseases that reduce their quality of life or terminal diseases such as cancer may experience mental health disorders.[25] Conversely, there is evidence that mental disorders are themselves independent risk factors for cardiovascular disease, type 2 diabetes, and injuries.[26]

BOX 10–1 ■ Risk Factors for Mental Illness

- Family history of mental disorders or history of being diagnosed with a mental disorder in the past
- Traumatic events: military combat, assault, or witness to a violent crime
- In utero exposure to viruses and toxins; poor nutrition
- Cerebral injury: experiencing brain damage as a result of a serious injury such as a violent blow to the head, traumatic brain injury
- Stressful life situations: financial problems, the death of a loved one, or marital problems and/or divorce
- Social isolation: having few friends or few healthy relationships
- Developmental delays
- Substance use: illicit drugs, alcohol, medication side effects, and drug interactions
- Poor health: living with a chronic medical condition such as cancer
- History of being abused or neglected as a child
- Low self-esteem, social isolation, poor social skills
- Lesbian, Gay, Bisexual, Transgender, Queer (LGBTQ+) adolescents
- Anxiety, depression, suicidal tendencies
- Poverty and socioeconomic level
- Rural versus urban populations
- Lower education level
- Dangerous communities, high crime rates

Family instability is a factor in the development of mental disorders, with a higher incidence rate in individuals raised in situations of abuse or neglect, including sexual abuse, or for those who have experienced exposure to traumatic events, including serious loss.[24] In addition, children of parents with mental disorders are at increased risk for developing mental disorders themselves because of the negative impact a mental disorder has on parenting skills.[27] Exposure to family stress because of poor financial situations, death, divorce, or unemployment is also associated with mental disorders.[22] Along with family environment, individual characteristics can increase the risk for development of a mental disorder. For example, individuals with low self-esteem; those who are lonely, isolated, and/or have poor social skills; and those who have unhealthy thinking patterns are at higher risk. Some behaviors also increase the risk of mental disorders, or substance use disorders (Chapter 11).[24]

An emerging issue is the increased incidence of mental disorders in Lesbian, Gay, Bisexual, Transgender, Queer (LGBTQ+) adolescents (see Chapter 7). They are more likely to be depressed and anxious, and attempt and/or commit suicide because of insecurity and difficulty in negotiating their coming out, family disapproval, rejection, victimization, and chronic stress from stigmatization.[28] Thus, the development of a mental disorder is a complex combination of genetics, other physical disorders, and family environment.

Community-Level Risk Factors for Mental Disorders

The determinants of health also play a role in the development of mental disorders because the community environment plays a pivotal role. There is a clear inverse relationship between poverty and prevalence of mental disorders, with a greater prevalence of mental disorders in populations and communities experiencing social and economic disadvantages.[29] Part of this risk is associated with a lower level of education, fewer job opportunities, and lower job satisfaction.[29] Living in dangerous communities (Chapter 12), especially those with high crime rates, is another risk factor.

Protective Factors: Building Resilience

Although a risk-based approach is one strategy for addressing the prevention of mental disorders, an examination of protective factors is equally important. Understanding why some individuals can overcome adversity is a key component in the development of intervention programs focused on prevention of mental disorders. **Protective factors** are processes within individuals, families, or communities that exist, can be strengthened, or can be incorporated into interventions for purposes of building resilience. They are the supports and opportunities that buffer adversity.[30] **Resilience** is an individual's ability to access protective factors that exist at different levels to withstand chronic stress or recover from traumatic life events (Box 10-2).[31] Individual strengths such as social competence, problem-solving ability, autonomy, and a sense of purpose show resilience. Protective factors can reduce risk for mental health disorders and can promote optimal mental health. Understanding what factors help individuals, families, and communities reach optimal health, then, is as important as understanding the factors that increase the risk for developing a mental disorder. Both prevention and treatment interventions can build on these protective factors to help promote optimal mental health.

Research on individual protective factors provides the foundation for supporting protective factors in prevention interventions. According to Harvard University's

---

BOX 10–2 ■ Protective Factors and Resilience

- Environmental capital: structural factors and features of the natural and built environments
- Environment that enhance community capacity for well-being
- Social capital: norms, networks and distribution of resources that enhance community trust, cohesion, influence, and cooperation for mutual benefit
- Emotional and cognitive capital as resources that buffer stress and/or determine outcomes and contribute to individual resilience and capability

Source: (32)

Center on the Developing Child, "… the single most common factor for children who develop resilience is at least one stable and committed relationship with a supportive parent, caregiver, or other adult."[32] The use of resilience building in children exposed to adverse childhoods to reduce the potential of mental health diagnoses holds promise.[33,34]

More than 2 decades ago, the report from the President's New Freedom Commission on Mental Health was published, emphasizing that the transformation of the mental health delivery system depends on a focus on coping with challenges in life and building resilience.[35] Interventions to promote resilience focus on a strengths-building approach. Because strengths recognized in resilience are inherent psychological needs, humans are compelled to meet them throughout their lifetime, and the factors determining whether they do meet them are often dependent on the wider systems in which an individual interacts, including families, schools, and communities.[31]

A community can also be resilient.[31] Similar to how resilience in an individual is defined, a resilient community is characterized by social competence, problem-solving, a sense of identity, and hope for the future. A resilient community has certain resources available that are important for human development. These resources include health care, childcare, housing, education, job training, employment, and recreation.[31] A journal's special edition addressed the factors that are important for communities to promote childhood resilience, including increasing the availability of programs that foster healthy parent-child interactions and increase parental social support.[36]

A community's resilience contributes to an individual's capacity to develop resilience and whether a MHD is present or not. The community develops and nurtures resilience by valuing and providing the means of connectedness, by supporting and nurturing commitment and shared values where everyone participates in meaningful structure and role responsibilities, and by engaging in critical reflection and skill building that feeds back into the community. The ability of a community to build resilience is called *community capacity*.[37]

An example of community-level resilience is that of community members and organizations working in partnership with youths, families, and schools. A sense of connectedness can result when schools work in partnership with students, families, and community groups. An example of this connectedness is a program called Elev8 in Baltimore, Maryland, which is focused on improving educational and social outcomes for middle grade adolescents and their families in East Baltimore.[38,39] "Each Elev8 Baltimore school is assigned a site manager and a family advocate responsible for collaborating with the principal and staff; building relationships with students and families; responding to the needs of students, parents and school staff; promoting the integration of learning, health and family support strategy; and developing a family engagement plan to facilitate connections among families, the school, and the broader community."[39]

School connectedness is an example of a way to build community resilience. Such programs demonstrate that building resilience at the community level not only can improve the mental health of children and youth but also can have a positive impact on children's behavioral and academic outcomes.[40,38] The importance of interdisciplinary programs that work together to build community resilience is also increasingly recognized as an approach to address social determinants of health, inequities in education, and the urban environment overall.[32,41] Some programs operate at the intersection of public health, education, and urban planning. Examples have included the Obama administration's Neighborhood Revitalization Initiative, which focused on standardized test scores and educational inequities, and the Choice Neighborhoods program, which is based on Hope VI, which targets severely distressed public housing developments.[42,43] A focus in these programs is to develop community health centers and full-service community schools, and to pursue community development for purposes of revitalizing neighborhoods.[38]

■ CELLULAR TO GLOBAL

The factors affecting mental health exist on a continuum from the cellular to the global. The interactions among an individual's genetics, epigenetics, and the larger environment are myriad, predicting much of what we know about mental well-being. Although individuals may have a stronger genetic predisposition for certain types of mental illness, factors across the life span heavily influence its expression. Even beginning before birth, factors such as access to nutrients in utero and exposure to maternal trauma contribute to an individual's mental health risk profile. As a person ages, employment opportunities and exposure to disease also cumulatively affect mental health status. Even into older age, factors such as social integration and chronic illness continue to impact mental well-being. Thus, public health interventions to promote mental wellness must address all levels of this continuum.[24]

Cultural Context and Stigma

Culture has tremendous influence on the meaning of mental illness for individuals, families, and communities. A culture's deeply rooted beliefs and attitudes exert considerable influence on how mental illness is viewed by society, the individual with the illness, his family, and the community. It may be viewed as real or imagined, adaptive or maladaptive, or as a valued distinction or intentional deviance from the norm. Beliefs and attitudes determine how likely it is that support will be available and whether a person with a mental health disorder will seek help or accept treatment.[44–47] For example, studies of cross-cultural stigma have suggested that Latino groups may view taking psychoactive medications as a sign of weakness, preferring instead to be self-reliant, whereas some Asian groups may see mental health as emotional weakness that causes one to "lose face," thus jeopardizing family lineage.[47]

■ CULTURAL CONTEXT

Cultural Influences on Mental Health[48]

"People often think of mental health as a very personal matter that has to do only with the individual. However, mental illnesses and mental health in general are affected by the combination of biological and genetic factors, psychology, and society. This intersectionality is important, but the heavy influence of societal factors often goes ignored. An interesting aspect of society is its diversity in cultures and backgrounds that affect an individual's mental health related experiences ... For instance, culture affects the way in which people describe their symptoms, such as whether they choose to describe emotional or physical symptoms. Essentially, it dictates whether people selectively present symptoms in a 'culturally appropriate' way that won't reflect badly on them … Every culture has its own way of making sense of the highly subjective experience that is an understanding of one's mental health. Each has a prevailing attitude about whether mental illness is real or imagined, an illness of the mind or the body or both, who is at risk for it, what might cause it, and perhaps most importantly, the level of stigma surrounding it."

Stigma is one of the barriers to the treatment of mental health problems.[48] Goffman's classic definition views stigma as a combination of personal attributes and societal stereotypes related to human characteristics viewed as unacceptable.[49] Stigma refers to a trait or attribute of a person that results in the discrediting of that person. Stigma occurs when the person, rather than the trait or condition, is held responsible for the inability to perform an action.[50, 51] Cultural belief systems can produce stigma, the form of social disapproval that pervades the attitudes and actions of the community, the family, and even the individual.

Stigma acts as a barrier to achieving health and well-being, and can greatly undermine a community's efforts to capitalize on strengths. There is a growing awareness of disparities in access and use of mental health services among ethnic and racial minority populations. Treatment disparities among African American and Hispanic groups, for example, are especially acute. Although African Americans and Hispanics are more than 20% more likely to report psychological distress than non-Hispanic whites, African Americans are 15% less likely and Hispanics are half as likely as non-Hispanic whites to receive mental health care.[52-55] There are many possible explanations for these disparities, including variations in expression of symptoms, bias or prejudice among providers, experiences of mistreatment, difficulties in accessing treatment, and stigma among various populations.[56] These groups also have the highest numbers of people who lack insurance coverage.[57] Stigma can cause individuals with mental illness to adopt a number of behaviors that serve to protect them from stigma but may result in failure to seek treatment (Box 10-3).[56]

The American Psychiatric Association (APA) has developed strategies to address issues related to culture and stigma. These strategies address challenges related to the complexity of the issue, including illness progression, family history and cultural influences, impenetrable isolation reinforced by stigma, and multiple system failures. An example is the organization's recommendations for

BOX 10–3 ■ Impact of Mental Health Stigma

- Not telling other people about symptoms
- Masking the symptoms
- Normalizing mental health symptoms
- Emphasizing somatic aspects
- Refusing to seek treatment
- Fearing rejection by family and friends
- Concern about difficulty finding housing and employment
- Being socially ostracized

Source: (56)

---

providing culturally competent care for Asian Americans who may have a mental disorder (see Box 10-4).[58] The term *Asian* refers to people whose country of origin is located in the Far East and includes people from Southeast Asia, the Indian subcontinent, and the Pacific Islands. Providing care requires an understanding of the diversity of cultures as well as the possibility that presenting symptoms may represent culture-bound syndromes that can affect Asian American populations.[58]

The importance of understanding culture and stigma is exemplified by the incident that occurred on April 16, 2007. Seung-hui Cho, aged 23 years and a senior at Virginia Polytechnic Institute and State University (Virginia Tech), wounded 25 people and killed 32 and then himself in a shooting rampage that lasted several hours. Cho was only 8 years old when his family arrived in the United States from South Korea. He was a shy child and apparently was bullied. His childhood years had been troubled, and in middle school, he was diagnosed with selective mutism, a severe anxiety disorder, and an MDD. He began to receive treatment and therapy, which continued through his sophomore year in high school. During college, he was hospitalized for mental illness symptoms and offered treatment, which he declined.[59, 60]

The tragic shooting incident led campus police and state government officials to investigate and make recommendations. Due to this incident and others, colleges and universities across the nation have evaluated and revised safety and security plans, and strengthened campus mental health services.[61] This case illustrates that a traumatic experience of this nature has a widespread impact on a community, with lasting psychological distress. Violent acts such as this; the Columbine High School shootings; the movie theater shootings in Aurora, Colorado; the shootings in Newtown, Connecticut; and the shootings in Parkland, Florida, are linked with mental disorders and social-identity threats.[61]

The high-profile case at Virginia Tech is an example of the impact that culture has on understanding the

BOX 10–4 ■ APA Best Practices for Working with Asian American Patients

A Few Best Practices for Working with Asian Patients

- Assess the language barrier. Ascertain whether the patient speaks English or not, their native dialect, and the degree of acculturation.
- Ask about traditional beliefs as part of your cultural formulation. These may influence how the individual expresses mental distress, such as through somatic symptoms. For non-English speaking unacculturated individuals, particularly among the elderly, many hold traditional values and a concept of health and disease (e.g., Yin/Yang) that may influence the individual's expression of mental distress such as through somatic symptoms. They may seek traditional healers such as acupuncturists and herbalists. Their ideas about bodily symptoms may affect drug compliance.
- Many Asian immigrants view physicians and other providers as authority, so encourage patients' participation in their care. Taking blood pressure, checking pulse, and giving advice about diet and foods/use of herbal products can promote rapport.
- Involve the family in health-care decisions. If interdependence among family members is valued, treat the family as a unit.
- Familiarize yourself with ethnopsychopharmacological research. You may, for example, start with a lower prescribed dosage of psychotropic medications for Asians.

- Prescribe cognitive behavioral therapy, where appropriate. Talking therapy is foreign to many Asians. If psychotherapy is indicated and involvement of the family is discouraged to maintain confidentiality, explain the rationale and procedure to both the patient and the family.
- Allow sufficient time for interviews. Translation needs extra time, and it takes time for Asian patients to feel comfortable in sharing very intimate, personal information with outsiders.
- Be attentive to comorbid medical problems.
- Consider traditional interventions in addition to medication and, if indicated, diets, exercises, and other traditional methods (Tai Chi, breathing exercises) of stress-reduction and relaxation.
- Ask detailed clinical history with open-ended questions first, and be attentive to nonverbal clues (facial expression, tearing, etc.).

Please refer to the APA Web site for further information on treating Asian patients and resources to help you provide culturally competent care: https://www.psychiatry.org/psychiatrists/cultural-competency/treating-diverse-patient-populations/working-with-asian-american-patients.

Source: (58)

---

expressions and presentation of mental disorders. Korean Americans make up 9% of the Asian population in America, up 41% from 2000. Of these, a little less than two-thirds are foreign born, but they rank 12th of all U.S. naturalizations since 2012 and fifth among Asians.[62] Han and Pong (2015) reported that Asian American college students are unlikely to present to a health-care provider and complain of mental problems. Rather, their concerns are focused on schooling, and vocational or employment-related problems. Families are likely to insist that a family member suffering with mental problems should keep her or his problems hidden because of the shame it can bring on the family. By the time help is sought, the problems have often become severe.[63]

Prevention of Mental Disorders and Promotion of Mental Health

Because mental health is not simply the absence of a mental disorder, prevention of mental disorders and promotion of mental health are key components of efforts to optimize the mental health of individuals and communities. Promotion focuses on building communities with living conditions and environments that support mental health. Prevention focuses on implementing strategies that prevent mental disorders and providing early intervention and adequate treatment for those with mental disorders.[64]

Measure of Mental Health: Health-Related Quality of Life

One way to assess mental health is to measure **health-related quality of life (HRQoL)**. It is a marker not only of physical health but also of mental health. As noted in Chapter 9, HRQoL is central to the overarching goals for *HP 2020*. HRQoL as defined in Chapter 9 is the self-perceived impact of physical and emotional health on quality of life, including the effects on general health, physical functioning, physical health and role, bodily pain, vitality, social functioning, emotional health and role, and mental health.[65,66] The HRQoL measure used by the CDC includes items specifically aimed at measuring emotional and mental health. It is a useful tool for the nurse who wishes to assess the level of mental health in a patient as well as a tool for assessing the overall mental health in a population. The tool is available on the CDC Web site and can be easily downloaded.

National Academy of Medicine Model of Prevention

In 1997, the IOM, now the National Academy of Medicine, reported that the primary, secondary, and tertiary continuum of prevention was confusing when applied to mental disorders and developed a new model that more clearly separates prevention from treatment.[67] This framework, presented in Chapter 2 and again in Chapter 11, divides the prevention category into three levels developed specifically for behavioral health issues: (1) universal, (2) selective (also referred to as selected), and (3) indicated, with possible interventions at each level. **Universal prevention** refers to prevention interventions provided to the entire population, not just those who might be at risk. The interventions include but are not limited to public service announcements provided to the public at large through billboards, media messages (print and electronic), or general health education programs. **Selective prevention** includes interventions provided to specific subgroups who are known to be at high risk for mental disorders because of biological, psychological, social, or environmental factors but who have not yet been diagnosed with mental disorders. High-risk subgroups include but are not limited to those with a family history of mental disorders, with a history of adverse childhood events, or who are victims of violence. An example is counseling delivered to students at a school where violence has occurred, such as the extensive counseling required following the Parkland, Florida, shootings. Selective interventions include opportunities for learning strategies to prevent the development of a mental disorder as well as early warning signs to help individuals and families seek help early. **Indicated prevention** addresses specific subgroups at highest risk for development of a mental disorder or individuals who are showing early signs of a mental disorder. The purpose of indicated techniques is to delay or reduce the severity of a mental disorder. At this level, there is less concern about community prevention and more emphasis on individuals who demonstrate early signs of mental disorders.[67]

Promotion of Mental Health and Policy

The WHO strongly supports the implementation of strategies that will create healthful living conditions and environments that result in optimal mental health.

The organization stated that mental health promotion depends on **intersectoral strategies**. These are defined as strategies that engage more than one sector of society with a shared interest such as governmental agencies, grass roots citizen groups, nonprofit groups, and/or businesses. Some strategies proposed by the WHO include those that address needs of specific age groups, vulnerable populations, and women. Other strategies focus on the environment, such as the workplace, schools, housing, and community development. The WHO recommended that governments mainstream mental health promotion across policies and programs.[64] The WHO warns against focusing only on mental disorder treatment and stresses that an upstream approach (see Chapter 2) is vital to the health of communities.

To support its efforts related to mental health improvement, the WHO developed a model to guide its activities called the Mental Health Improvements for Nations' Development (MIND) (Fig. 10-3). It includes four components: (1) Action in Countries, (2) Mental Health Policy, Planning & Service, (3) Mental Health, Human Rights & Legislation, and (4) Mental Health, Poverty & Development. This model demonstrates not only the need for intersectoral strategies but also for interrelationships between multiple factors that contribute to mental health.[68]

Secondary Prevention: Screening for Mental Disorders

The focus of the National Academy of Medicine's report *Improving the Quality of Health Care for Mental and Substance-Use Conditions: Quality Chasm Series* is the need for appropriate behavioral health treatment.[69] The report has a strong emphasis on early identification and treatment. The model for secondary intervention in mental health is screening, brief intervention, and referral for treatment (SBIRT), an approach also used in secondary prevention programs related to at-risk alcohol use (Chapter 11). The Substance Abuse and Mental Health Service Administration (SAMHSA) issued a report on the use of screening for behavioral health that includes screening for depression and trauma/anxiety disorders. Although SAMHSA concludes that no evidence exists to support a comprehensive SBIRT program for these disorders, there is evidence that screening is effective.[70]

Reliable screening tools exist that have validity across the life span and across health-care settings. Tools differ based on the specific mental disorder being screened. The screening tools most often used in primary care are

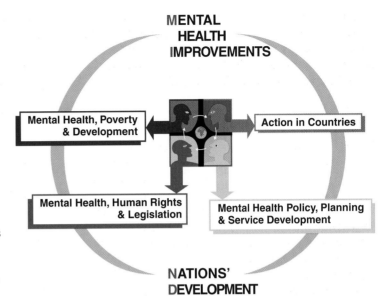

Figure 10-3 WHO Mental Health Improvements for Nations' Development (MIND). *(From World Health Organization. [2012]. Mental Health, MIND— mental health in development. Retrieved from http://www. who.int/mental_health/policy/en/index.html.)*

for depression and anxiety disorders. Tools to screen for depression include the Patient Health Questionnaire 2 and the Center for Epidemiological Studies Depression Scale. Screening tools for anxiety disorders include the Brief Symptom Checklist-18 of the My Mood Monitor.[70] The challenge is not only to screen but also to provide care to those who screen positive. Thus, universal screening for depression is only recommended in situations in which accurate diagnosis and treatment are available.[70]

One approach related to screening and engagement into treatment for disorders is to integrate care for mental disorders within primary care settings. Because most people identified with mental disorders are seen in a primary care setting, integrating care within this setting is a logical approach. Without an integrated system, those who screen positive may not receive the care they need. Kroenke and Unutzer (2017) suggest there are six key components to successfully integrating mental health care into primary care settings (Box 10-5).[71]

BOX 10–5 ■ Six Key Components for Mental Health Care Integration into Primary Care Settings

- *Population-Based Care:* Depends on systematic efforts to identify all patients with disease, provide treatment, and track outcomes. This may be difficult to do with current system of nonintegrated electronic health records.
- *Measurement-Based Care:* Essential for public health surveillance, but most mental disorders depend on patient-reported outcomes (PROs). The ideal PRO is brief, self-reported, public domain, multipurpose, easy to score and interpret, and available in multiple languages. Although a few scales meet these criteria, most do not. One that does meet most of these criteria is the Patient Health Questionnaire family of scales.
- *Treatment to Target:* Requires regular monitoring of disorder severity and adjusting treatment based on monitored outcomes. Interventions must be evidence-based and, if patients are not improving as expected,

there is a systematic protocol to incorporate measurement results in treatment changes.
- *Care Management:* Dedicated clinician who follows patients with particular disorders in (a) practice(s). Also, maintains disease registry, provides disease-related education, tracks treatment adherence, and coordinates care.
- *Psychiatric Consultation:* Accessible and dedicated psychiatrist who can meet frequently with care manager and occasionally will also meet with patients. Can also facilitate referrals and may be integrated by telepsychiatry.
- *Brief Psychological Therapies:* Can be administered in primary care clinics or remotely by trained behavioral health specialists. Approaches include motivational interviewing, behavioral activation, and problem-solving treatment.

Source: (71)

● APPLYING PUBLIC HEALTH SCIENCE

The Case of Sadness Under the Rainbow

Public Health Science Topics Covered:

- Epidemiology
- Surveillance
- Program Planning

Enrico, a nurse for 2 years, recently started working in a pediatric medical-surgical unit in a rural, critical access hospital. Last week, he was involved in the care of Yuichi, a 17-year-old male who was admitted for surgery to remove a ruptured appendix. As Enrico provided care to Yuichi on the third day after surgery, he noticed that Yuichi was withdrawn and quiet, rarely looking at Enrico or even appearing to notice his attempts to start a conversation. However, when Enrico brought in his afternoon pain medicine, Yuichi seemed to notice Enrico's left wrist and brightened visibly. Enrico looked at his left wrist where he had a rainbow band on his wristwatch. Yuichi asked, "Why do you wear the rainbow watch?" Enrico considered carefully for a moment, then decided to disclose personal information because he felt this was the first time there was an opening to develop a therapeutic connection with Yuichi. Enrico disclosed he was gay and wore the wristband in solidarity with the LGBTQ+ community. Immediately, Yuichi, smiling shyly, visibly relaxed. He then told Enrico that he was also gay and had recently come out to his friends at school but was still in the closet to his parents and family. He told Enrico that his parents emigrated to the United States from Japan when he was a baby and are very conservative. He confessed that he has been very worried about how his parents will react to his coming out and has even been feeling like "being dead would be better than living like this, especially if they kick me out."

After Enrico had returned to the nurses' station, he started to review the evidence about LGBTQ+ adolescents, mental health risks, and mental health interventions. Over the next day, Enrico found several journal articles and a book chapter that helped him to better understand the current evidence about the prevalence of and interventions for the mental health challenges of sexual and race/ethnic minority youths.[72-77] Enrico learned that, among the many risk factors for suicide, LGBTQ+ youths have been reported to experience higher odds of sadness, suicidal ideation, self-harm, and suicide attempts than their heterosexual, cisgender counterparts.[72,73] As is recommended, when Enrico considered cultural risk factors as part of his suicide risk assessment, he discovered that one protective factor for Yuichi was that Asian adolescents had lower odds of suicidal ideation, planning, and self-harm when compared to white adolescents, despite the continuing issue of stigma that has not yet been eliminated in Japanese culture.[73-75]

Enrico discussed these findings with his colleagues and nursing supervisor. Given the sensitive nature of Yuichi's disclosure, he cautioned the team that it was especially important they consider how to address Yuichi's suggestion that he was considering suicide, while also not outing him to his parents against his will. Enrico pointed out to his colleagues that social support is critically important to the mental health of LGBTQ+ adolescents.[76] He explained how he is concerned that if Yuichi is outed to his parents, he may lose a key component of his current social support network. The team discussed whether they had a duty to tell Yuichi's parents about his sexual orientation and his thoughts about ending his life. One reference Enrico found provided support and guidance for the team's conclusion.[77] The team decided that they would only tell Yuichi's parents that the team was concerned about Yuichi's mental well-being and had requested a consult with a psychiatrist while he was still inpatient. The team also recommended that Yuichi follow up with counseling once he was discharged from the hospital.

Following Yuichi's discharge with this recommended plan, Enrico worked with the hospital policy committee to develop a new policy outlining the protocol for notification of parents about sensitive issues regarding their children. He also worked with the policy committee to update the suicide risk assessment protocol to include a cultural component.

Four months after Yuichi was discharged, he returned to the hospital to thank Enrico for his help. He told Enrico that the counselor his parents had found had been very helpful to him and that, with the counselor's guidance, he had decided to wait until after his 18th birthday and his high school graduation before coming out to his parents. Yuichi did say, however, that he was feeling much better and more hopeful for the future. Enrico thanked him for coming in to update him and told Yuichi that his experience as a patient had helped the hospital create new policies to make things better for the patients who followed him.

■ EVIDENCE-BASED PRACTICE
Screening for Suicide Risk Among Adolescents in Primary Care

Practice Statement: Adolescents should be screened in primary care for suicide risk using a validated and reliable screening tool if there is reason to believe an adolescent is at elevated risk.

Targeted Outcome: Identification of those at risk, initiation of prevention strategies, and, when indicated, referral to treatment

Evidence to Support: The evidence for the effectiveness of screening for suicide risk in adolescents, as well as in adults and older adults, has been found to be incomplete by the U.S. Preventive Services Task Force (USPSTF).[1] The American Academy of Pediatrics recommends that, if adolescents are screened for suicide risk, they should be asked directly about suicidal ideation.[2] There is some evidence that screening for suicide can detect adolescents who are at increased risk for suicide, but there is insufficient evidence yet to determine whether that identification translates to improved outcomes, such as decreased attempted and completed suicide rates.[3]

Recommended Approaches: Adolescents that have known risk factors for suicide, such as recent mental illness, increased substance use, or withdrawal from social support networks, should be screened by suicide assessment. Direct questioning regarding suicidal ideation should be used, such as asking, "Have you ever had thoughts about taking your own life or wishing you were dead?" Standardized assessments may be helpful, but most have been found to be too sensitive while lacking specificity in this population.[1-3] If adolescents are positive for suicidal ideation, they should be referred for immediate psychiatric evaluation by hospitalization, transfer to an emergency department, or same-day appointment with a mental health provider.[2]

Sources:

1. LeFevre, M.L. (2014). Screening for suicide risk in adolescents, adults, and older adults in primary care: U.S. Preventive Services Task Force recommendation statement. *Annals of Internal Medicine*, *160*(10), 719-726. doi:10.7326/M14-0589.
2. Shain, B.N. (2007). Suicide and suicide attempts in adolescents. *Pediatrics*, *120*(3), 669-676. doi:10.1542/peds.105.4.871.
3. Kennebeck, S., & Bonin, L. (2017). Suicidal ideation and behavior in children and adolescents: Evaluation and management. *UpToDate*. Retrieved from https://www.uptodate.com/contents/suicidal-ideation-and-behavior-in-children-and-adolescents-evaluation-and-management.

Tertiary Prevention: Treatment for Mental Disorders

At the individual level, a person diagnosed with a mental disorder must meet the clinical criteria for the diagnosis. Because there are no definitive diagnostic laboratory tests or scans useful for diagnosing mental disorders, experts in the field developed a manual, the *Diagnostic and Statistical Manual of Mental Disorders* (DSM), to guide diagnostic decision making and provide consistency and accuracy in diagnoses among clinicians. The newest revision of the manual, DSM-5, is organized so the chapters are based on underlying vulnerabilities as well as symptom characteristics. The goal of the DSM is to facilitate a more comprehensive approach to diagnosis and treatment, and the DSM-5 represented a major change from earlier versions of the manual.[78] Thus, at the individual level, experts re-examined diagnostic criteria based on the best evidence in developing the DSM-5. Treatment of mental health usually focuses on the individual and can include many different treatment modalities. At the population level, tertiary treatment and policy are closely related with access to treatment as the central issue.

Mental Health Policy Related to Treatment

Access to treatment and the type of treatment available have been central issues since the end of World War II. Prevention at the population level related to treatment entails reduction of disparity in access to treatment, whereas promotion of mental health requires policies that will strengthen the mental health of populations.[79] Historically, government policy focused on treatment of mental disorders and was influenced by underlying attitudes concerning mental disorders. In the latter half of the 20th century, policy changes were put in place that led to deinstitutionalization. Other events that influenced policy related to treatment include pharmacological advances, for example, the introduction of drugs such as Thorazine, as well as a cultural change from focusing on treatment of those with mental disorders to improving mental health for all.

Supreme Court decisions also affected policy. For example, the "least restrictive alternative" principle in the ruling in *Shelton v. Tucker* (1960), which allowed involuntary admission to a psychiatric facility only if there were no another alternative that would allow more freedom, and the ruling in *O'Connor v. Donaldson* (1975), which stated that mental patients who were not dangerous and involuntarily institutionalized had the right to be treated or discharged.[80] These landmark decisions resulted in **deinstitutionalization** of those diagnosed with mental disorders from psychiatric hospitals to independent living arrangements, thus shifting the burden of treatment to the community. President John F. Kennedy signed the Community Mental Health Centers Act in 1963, which opened the way for a network of community mental health centers to provide comprehensive services and continuity of care.[81]

Unfortunately, community facilities did not develop at the same pace as deinstitutionalization. In addition, insufficient planning for alternative facilities and services (medical and psychiatric care, social services, housing and nutrition, income and employment, and vocational and social rehabilitation) resulted in thousands of vulnerable and severely ill persons left behind to become imprisoned by poverty, neglect, victimization, substance abuse, and homelessness, all conditions that exacerbate psychiatric disorders.[82,83] The term **transinstitutionalization** began to appear in the literature in the 1980s and refers to the growing numbers of mentally ill persons ending up on the streets, in jails and prisons, in nursing homes, boarding houses, and homeless shelters, and not in places of their own or in the hospital. Today, it is estimated that between 30% and 50% of persons in the United States who are homeless are also mentally ill.[80, 83]

The Mental Health Parity Act represents a step forward as the United States grapples with accepting treatment of mental illness as integral to promoting and ensuring a healthy public. The Paul Wellstone and Pete Domenici Mental Health Parity and Addiction Equity Act of 2008 was signed into law October 3, 2008, and mandates that group health plans of 50 or more persons, which cover mental health and substance-use disorders, must provide benefits equivalent to (or better than) those benefits provided for medical or surgical benefits. The Affordable Care Act of 2010 has also helped to fill in some of the gaps by requiring Medicaid and plans purchased by small businesses to include mental health and substance abuse coverage. However, significant gaps remain, and further work is needed to transform the delivery of health care to those with mental disorders.

Attention is needed not only on parity of access but also on the ethics of providing treatment for mental disorders at parity with treatment for physical disorders.

▌ Summary Points

- Behavioral health is essential to overall health.
- Behavioral health disorders will surpass all physical diseases as a major cause of disability worldwide.
- Mental health, substance abuse, and violence are interconnected.
- Mental health is the vehicle for developing meaningful relationships, sound thinking, skills for learning and communication, emotional maturity, resilience, and self-esteem.
- Resilience is an individual's ability to access protective factors.
- Risk factors and protective factors related to mental health outcomes occur at several levels: individual, family, social, and community.
- Interventions occur at all levels, but societal interventions are critical to transforming the mental health system.

▼ CASE STUDY
Promoting Mental Health among Older Adults

Learning Outcomes

At the end of this case study, the student will be able to:

- Apply demographic methods to determine the severity of a problem at the population level.
- Examine the role that members of the community play in addressing a population level health issue.
- Discuss policy approaches to a population-level health problem.
- Examine the evidence to support a population-based intervention.

The nurses working for a primary health clinic were concerned about the increase in suicides among older adults in the clinic's practice population. One of the nurses brought in an article about suicide risk among older adults.[84] The nurses found the risk of suicide among older adults to be startling and decided to investigate what steps they might be able to take to address this type of situation in their own primary care clinic. One of the nurses stated they should not proceed without including members of the local community, including the senior center. How should they begin?

To complete this case study, do the following:

1. Starting with Jahn's article, review the national statistics on suicide among older adults.
2. Determine which stakeholders should be involved in helping to design a community-level intervention.
3. Critique proposed policy initiatives in relation to their utility in reducing suicide among older adults—are there any?
4. Critique the evidence for programs aimed at preventing suicide and evaluate whether they have been tested with older adult populations.
5. Complete a draft plan.

REFERENCES

1. Mental Health.gov. (2017). *What is mental health?* Retrieved from https://www.mentalhealth.gov/basics/what-is-mental-health.
2. World Health Organization. (2018). *Mental health*. Retrieved from http://www.who.int/mental_health/en/.
3. Institute of Medicine. (2005). *Improving the quality of health care for mental and substance-use conditions: Quality chasm series*. Retrieved from http://nationalacademies.org/hmd/Reports/2005/Improving-the-Quality-of-Health-Care-for-Mental-and-Substance-Use-Conditions-Quality-Chasm-Series.aspx.
4. *Healthy People 2020*. (n.d.). Retrieved from http://www.healthypeople.gov/2020/topicsobjectives2020/default.aspx.
5. National Institute of Mental Health. (2017). *Mental illness: Definitions*. Retrieved from https://www.nimh.nih.gov/health/statistics/mental-illness.shtml#part_154784.
6. World Health Organization. (2012). *The 65th World Health Assembly closes with new global health measures*. Retrieved from http://www.who.int/mediacentre/news/releases/2012/wha65_closes_20120526/en/index.html.
7. Ritchie, H. (2018, May 16). *Our World Data Blog: Global mental health: Five key insights which emerge from the data*. Retrieved from https://ourworldindata.org/global-mental-health.
8. Congressional Research Service. (2018). *Prevalence of mental illness in the United States: Data sources and estimates*. Retrieved from https://fas.org/sgp/crs/misc/R43047.pdf.
9. Trautmann, S., Rehm, J., & Wittchen, H. (2016). The economic costs of mental disorders: Do our societies react appropriately to the burden of mental disorders? *Science & Society, 17*(9), 1245-1249.
10. Centers for Disease Control and Prevention. (2018). *Mental health data and publications*. Retrieved from https://www.cdc.gov/mentalhealth/data_publications/index.htm.
11. Harvard School of Medicine. (2018). *The world mental health survey initiative*. Retrieved from http://www.hcp.med.harvard.edu/wmh/.
12. Substance Abuse and Mental Health Services Administration. (2017). *Behavioral health barometer: United States,*
13. National Institute of Mental Health. (2017). *Mental illness: Prevalence of serious mental illness (SMI)*. Retrieved from https://www.nimh.nih.gov/health/statistics/mental-illness.shtml#part_154788.
14. Bassett, D., Buchwald, D., & Manson, S. (2014). Posttraumatic stress disorder and symptoms among American Indians and Alaska Natives: A review of the literature. *Social Psychiatry and Psychiatric Epidemiology, 49*(3), 417-433. doi:10.1007/s00127-013-0759-y.
15. National Institute of Mental Health. (2017). *Major depression: Prevalence of major depressive episode among adolescents*. Retrieved from https://www.nimh.nih.gov/health/statistics/major-depression.shtml#part_155031.
16. National Institute of Mental Health. (2017). *Major depression: Prevalence of major depressive episode among adults*. Retrieved from https://www.nimh.nih.gov/health/statistics/major-depression.shtml#part_155029.
17. Liu, N.H., Daumit, G.L., Dua, T., Aquila, R., Charlson, F., Cuijpers, P., ... Saxena, S. (2017). Excess mortality in persons with severe mental disorders: A multilevel intervention framework and priorities for clinical practice, policy and research agendas. *World Psychiatry, 16*(1), 30-40.
18. National Institute of Mental Health. (2017). *Mental illness*. Retrieved from https://www.nimh.nih.gov/health/statistics/mental-illness.shtml.
19. Gadermann, A.M., Alonso, J., Vilagut, G., Zaslavsky, A.M., & Kessler, R.C. (2012). Comorbidity and disease burden in the National Comorbidity Survey Replication (NCS-R). *Depression and Anxiety, 29*, 797-806. https://doi.org/10.1002/da.21924.
20. Rao, S., Raney, L., & Xiong, G. L. (2015). Reducing medical comorbidity and mortality in severe mental illness: Collaboration with primary and preventive care could improve outcomes. *Current Psychiatry, 14*(7), 14.
21. Yehuda, R., Hoge, C.W., McFarlane, A.C., Vermetten, E., Lanius, R.A., Nievergelt, C.M., ... Hyman, S.E. (2015). Post-traumatic stress disorder. *Nature Reviews Disease Primers, 1*, 1-22. doi:10.1038/nrdp.2015.57.
22. Mayo Clinic. (2015). *Mental illness. Risk factors*. Retrieved from http://www.mayoclinic.org/diseases-conditions/mental-illness/basics/risk-factors/CON-20033813.
23. Perry, D.C., Sturm, V.E., Peterson, M.J., Pieper, C.F., Bullock, T., Boeve, B.F., ... Welsh-Bohmer, K.A. (2016). Association of traumatic brain injury with subsequent neurological and psychiatric disease: A meta-analysis. *Journal of Neurosurgery, 124*(2), 511-526. doi:10.3171/2015.2.jns14503.
24. World Health Organization. (2012). *Risks to mental health: An overview of vulnerabilities and risk factors*. Retrieved from http://www.who.int/mental_health/mhgap/risks_to_mental_health_EN_27_08_12.pdf.
25. McKee, J., & Brahm, N. (2016). Medical mimics: Differential diagnostic considerations for psychiatric symptoms. *Mental Health Clinician, 6*(6), 289-296. doi:10.9740/mhc.2016.11.289.

volume 4: Indicators as measured through the 2015 National Survey on Drug Use and Health and National Survey of Substance Abuse Treatment Services. Retrieved from https://www.samhsa.gov/data/sites/default/files/National_BH-Barometer_Volume_4.pdf.

26. World Health Organization. (2015). *Risk factors of ill health among older people.* Retrieved from http://www.euro. who.int/en/health-topics/Life-stages/healthy-ageing/data-and-statistics/risk-factors-of-ill-health-among-older-people.

27. American Academy of Child and Adolescent Psychiatry. *Children of parents with mental illness, #39.* Retrieved from https://www.aacap.org/aacap/families_and_youth/facts_for_families/Facts_for_Families_Pages/Children_Of_Parents_With_Mental_Illness_39.aspx.

28. Russell, S.T., & Fish, J.N. (2016). Mental health in lesbian, gay, bisexual, and transgender (LGBT) youth. *Annual Review of Clinical Psychology, 12,* 465-487. doi:10.1146/annurev-clinpsy-021815-093153.

29. World Health Organization & Calouste Gulbenkian Foundation. (2014). *Social determinants of mental health.* Retrieved from http://www.who.int/mental_health/publications/gulbenkian_paper_social_determinants_of_mental_health/en/.

30. Masten, A.S., & Cicchetti, D. (2016). Resilience in development: Progress and transformation. *Developmental Psychopathology,* 1-63. doi:10.1002/9781119125556.devpsy406.

31. World Health Organization. (2009). *Mental health resilience and inequalities.* Retrieved from http://www.euro.who.int/__data/assets/pdf_file/0012/100821/E92227.pdf.

32. Harvard University: Center on the Developing Child. (2001). *Resilience.* Retrieved from https://developingchild.harvard.edu/science/key-concepts/resilience/.

33. McAllister, M., Knight, B.A., Hasking, P., Withyman, C., & Dawkins, J. (2018). Building resilience in regional youth: Impacts of a universal mental health promotion programme. *International Journal of Mental Health Nursing 27*(3), 1044-1054. doi:10.1111/inm.12412.

34. Lou, Y., Taylor, E.P., & DiFolco, S. (2018). Resilience and resilience factors in children in residential care: A systematic review. *Children & Youth Services Review, 89,* 83-92. doi:10.1016/j.childyouth.2018.04.010.

35. New Freedom Commission on Mental Health. (2003). *Achieving the promise: Transforming mental health care in America, Final Report.* (DHHS Publication No. SMA-03-3832). Rockville, MD: U.S. Department of Health and Human Services.

36. Luthar, S.S., & Eisenberg, N. (2017). Resilient adaptation among at-risk children: Harnessing science toward maximizing salutary environments. *Child Development, 88*(2), 337-349. doi:10.1111/cdev.12737.

37. Hargreaves, M.B., Verbitsky-Savitz, N., Coffee-Borden, B., Perreras, L., White, C.R., Pecora, P.J., ... Hunter, R. (2017). Advancing the measurement of collective community capacity to address adverse childhood experiences and resilience. *Children and Youth Services Review, 76,* 142-153. doi:10.1016/j.childyouth.2017.02.021.

38. Maier, A., Daniel, J., Oakes, J., & Lam, L. (2017). *Community schools as an effective school improvement strategy: A review of the evidence.* Palo Alto, CA: Learning Policy Institute. Retrieved from https://learningpolicyinstitute.org/sites/default/files/product-files/Community_Schools_Effective_REPORT.pdf.

39. Elev8 Baltimore. (n.d.). Retrieved from http://www.elev8kids.org/local-initiatives/content/baltimore.

40. World Health Organization. (2015). *Child and adolescent mental health.* Retrieved from http://www.who.int/mental_health/maternal-child/child_adolescent/en/.

41. Monahan, K.C., Oesterle, S., & Hawkins, J.D. (2010). Predictors and consequences of school connectedness: The case of prevention. *The Prevention Researcher, 17*(3), 3-6.

42. The White House. (n.d.). *Neighborhood revitalization initiative.* Retrieved from https://obamawhitehouse.archives.gov/administration/eop/oua/initiatives/neighborhood-revitalization.

43. U.S. Department of Housing and Urban Development. (n.d.) *Choice neighborhoods.* Retrieved from https://www.hud.gov/program_offices/public_indian_housing/programs/ph/cn.

44. Mascayano, F., Tapia, T., Schilling, S., Alvarado, R., Tapia, E., Lips, W., & Yang, L.H. (2016). Stigma toward mental illness in Latin America and the Caribbean: A systematic review. *Revista Brasileira de Psiquiatria, 38*(1), 73-85. doi:10.1590/1516-4446-2015-1652.

45. Shannon, P.J., Wieling, E., Simmelink-McCleary, J., & Becher, E. (2015). Beyond stigma: Barriers to discussing mental health in refugee populations. *Journal of Loss and Trauma, 20*(3), 281-296. doi:10.1080/15325024.2014.934629.

46. Angermeyer, M.C., & Schomerus, G. (2017). State of the art of population-based attitude research on mental health: A systematic review. *Epidemiology and Psychiatric Sciences, 26*(3), 252-264. doi:10.1017/S2045796016000627.

47. Andrade, S. (2017). Cultural influences on mental health. *The Public Health Advocate.* Retrieved from https://pha.berkeley.edu/2017/04/16/cultural-influences-on-mental-health/.

48. Yang, L.H., Thornicroft, G., Alvarado, R., Vega, E., & Link, B.G. (2014). Recent advances in cross-cultural measurement in psychiatric epidemiology: Utilizing 'what matters most' to identify culture-specific aspects of stigma. *International Journal of Epidemiology, 43*(2), 494-510. doi:10.1093/ije/dyu039.

49. Goffman, E. (1963). *Notes on the management of spoiled identity.* Englewood Cliffs, NJ: Prentice-Hall.

50. Thornicroft, G. (2006). *Actions speak louder ... Tackling discrimination against people with mental illness.* Mental Health Foundation. Retrieved from https://www.mentalhealth.org.uk/sites/default/files/actions_speak__louder_0.pdf.

51. Mayo Clinic.com. (n.d.). *Mental illness: Mental health; Overcoming the stigma of mental illness.* Retrieved from https://www.mayoclinic.org/diseases-conditions/mental-illness/in-depth/mental-health/art-20046477.

52. U.S. Department of Health and Human Services Office of Minority Health. (2017). *Mental health and African Americans.* Retrieved from https://minorityhealth.hhs.gov/omh/browse.aspx?lvl=4&lvlid=24.

53. U.S. Department of Health and Human Services Office of Minority Health. (2017). *Mental health and Hispanics.* Retrieved from https://minorityhealth.hhs.gov/omh/browse.aspx?lvl=4&lvlid=69.

54. Mental Health America. (n.d.). *Black & African American communities and mental health.* Retrieved from http://www.mentalhealthamerica.net/african-american-mental-health.

55. National Alliance on Mental Illness. (n.d.). *African American mental health.* Retrieved from https://www.nami.org/Find-Support/Diverse-Communities/African-American-Mental-Health.

56. Clement, S., Schauman, O., Graham, T., Maggioni, F., Evans-Lacko, S., Bezborodovs, N., ... Thornicroft, G. (2015). What is the impact of mental health-related stigma on

help-seeking? A systematic review of quantitative and qualitative studies. *Psychological Medicine, 45*(1), 11-27. doi:10.1017/S0033291714000129.

57. National Center for Health Statistics. (2016). *Health, United States, 2015: With special feature on racial and ethnic health disparities.* Retrieved from https://www.cdc.gov/nchs/data/hus/hus15.pdf.

58. Gaw, A. (n.d.). Working with Asian American patients. *Cultural competency: Treating diverse populations.* Retrieved from https://www.psychiatry.org/psychiatrists/cultural-competency/treating-diverse-patient-populations/working-with-asian-american-patients.

59. Biography.com Editors (2014). *Seung-Hui Cho Biography.* Retrieved from https://www.biography.com/crime-figure/seung-hui-cho

60. Virginia Tech Review Panel. (2007). *Mental health history of Seung Hui Cho.* Retrieved from http://wayback.archive-it.org/263/20070904222258/http://www.governor.virginia.gov/TempContent/techPanelReport-docs/8%20CHAPTER%20IV%20LIFE%20AND%20MENTAL%20HEALTH%20HISTORY%20OF%20CHOpdf.pdf.

61. Bonanno, C.M., & Levenson Jr, R.L. (2014). School shooters: History, current theoretical and empirical findings, and strategies for prevention. *Sage Open, 4*(1), 1-11. doi:10.1177/2158244014525425.

62. Asia Matters for America, America Matters for Asia. (n.d.). Korean-American population data. *South Korea Matters for America, America Matters for South Korea.* Retrieved from http://www.asiamattersforamerica.org/southkorea/data/koreanamericanpopulation.

63. Han, M., & Pong, H. (2015). Mental health help-seeking behaviors among Asian American community college students: The effect of stigma, cultural barriers, and acculturation. *Journal of College Student Development, 56*(1), 1-14.

64. World Health Organization. (2018). *Mental Health Atlas: 2017.* Geneva, Switzerland: Author. Retrieved from http://apps.who.int/iris/bitstream/handle/10665/272735/9789241514019-eng.pdf?ua=1&ua=1.

65. Centers for Disease Control and Prevention. (2016). *Health-related quality of life.* Retrieved from http://www.cdc.gov/hrqol.

66. Ware Jr., J.E., & Sherbourne, C.D. (1992). The MOS 36-item short-form health survey (SF-36). I. Conceptual framework and item selection. *Medical Care, 30*(6), 473-483. doi:10.1097/00005650-199206000-00002.

67. Substance Abuse and Mental Health Services Administration. (n.d.). *Mapping interventions to different levels of risk.* Retrieved from https://www.samhsa.gov/capt/tools-learning-resources/mapping-interventions-levels-risk.

68. World Health Organization. (n.d.). *Mental Health, MIND—mental health in development.* Retrieved from http://www.who.int/mental_health/policy/en/.

69. Institute of Medicine. (2005). *Improving the quality of health care for mental and substance-use conditions: Quality Chasm Series.* Retrieved from https://www.nap.edu/catalog/11470/improving-the-quality-of-health-care-for-mental-and-substance-use-conditions.

70. Substance Abuse and Mental Health Services Administration. (2017). *Screening, brief intervention and referral to treatment (SBIRT).* Retrieved from https://www.samhsa.gov/sbirt.

71. Kroenke, K., & Unutzer, J. (2017). Closing the false divide: Sustainable approaches to integrating mental health services into primary care. *Journal of General Internal Medicine, 32*(4), 404-410. doi:10.1007/s11606-016-3967-9.

72. Puckett, J.A., Horne, S.G., Surace, F., Carter, A., Noffsinger-Frazier, N., Shulman, J., ... Mosher, C. (2017). Predictors of sexual minority youth's reported suicide attempts and mental health. *Journal of Homosexuality, 64*(6), 697-715. doi:10.1080/00918369.2016.1196999.

73. Bostwick, W.B., Meyer, I., Aranda, F., Russell, S., Hughes, T., Birkett, M., & Mustanski, B. (2014). Mental health and suicidality among racially/ethnically diverse sexual minority youths. *American Journal of Public Health, 104*(6), 1129-1136. doi:10.2105/ajph.2013.301749.

74. Chu, J., Robinett, E.N., Ma, J.K., Shadish, K.Y., Goldblum, P., & Bongar, B. (2018). Cultural versus classic risk and protective factors for suicide. *Death Studies, 43*(1): 56-61. doi:10.1080/07481187.2018.1430085.

75. Kasai, M. (2017). Sexual and gender minorities and bullying in Japan. In S.T. Russell & S. S. Horn (Eds.), *Sexual orientation, gender identity, and schooling: The nexus of research, practice, and policy* (pp. 185-193). New York: Oxford University Press.

76. McDonald, K. (2018). Social support and mental health in LGBTQ adolescents: A review of the literature. *Issues in Mental Health Nursing, 39*(1), 1-14. doi:10.1080/01612840.2017.1398283.

77. Hyatt, J. (2015). Maintaining the privacy of a minor's sexual orientation and gender identity in the medical environment. *Journal of Healthcare Risk Management, 35*(1), 31-36. doi:10.1002/jhrm.21176.

78. American Psychiatric Association. (2013). *Diagnostic and Statistical Manual of Mental Disorders* (5th ed.). Arlington, VA; American Psychiatric Association.

79. Thompson, J.W. (1994). Trends in the development of psychiatric services, 1844–1994. *Hospital and Community Psychiatry, 45*(10), 987-992. doi:10.1176/ps.45.10.987.

80. Krieg, R.G. (2001). An interdisciplinary look at the deinstitutionalization of the mentally ill. *The Social Science Journal, 38*(3), 367-380. Retrieved from http://www.accessmylibrary.com/article-1G1-78901856/interdisciplinary-look-deinstitutionalization-mentally.html.

81. Talbott, J.A. (1982). Twentieth-century developments in American psychiatry. *Psychiatric Quarterly, 54*(4), 207-219. doi:10.1007/bf01064816.

82. Reddi, V. (2005). *Dorthea Lynde Dix (1802–1887).* Center for Nursing Advocacy. Retrieved from http://www.nursingadvocacy.org/press/pioneers/dix.html.

83. Sisti, D.A., Segal, A.G., & Emanuel, E.J. (2015). Improving long-term psychiatric care: Bring back the asylum. *JAMA, 313*(3), 243-244. doi:10.1001/jama.2014.16088.

84. Jahn, D.R. (2017). Suicide risk in older adults: The role and responsibility of primary care. *JCOM, 24*(4).

Chapter 11

Substance Use and the Health of Communities

Michael Sanchez, Christine Savage, and Amanda Choflet

LEARNING OUTCOMES

After reading the chapter, the student will be able to:

1. Describe the impact of substance use on the health of a population.
2. Define the burden of disease related to substance use using current epidemiological frameworks.
3. Apply current evidence-based population interventions to the prevention of harm associated with substance use across the continuum of use.
4. Describe population-level approaches to the prevention and treatment of substance use disorders.

KEY TERMS

Abstinence
At-risk substance use
Binge drinking
Blood alcohol level
Duration
Environmental tobacco smoke (ETS)
Frequency

Harmful use
Low-risk use
Heavy drinking
Involuntary smoke exposure
Moderate use
Opioid epidemic
Passive smoke exposure

Pattern
Physical dependence
Psychological dependence
Psychoactive substances
Screening and Brief Intervention (SBI)
Secondhand smoke exposure

Stigma
Substance use
Substance use disorder
Tolerance
Quality
Quantity
Withdrawal

Introduction

In 2017, media headlines blared alarming statistics on the opioid overdose epidemic in the U.S. In the fall of 2017, the president declared a national public health emergency, and states scrambled to both prevent at-risk opioid use and provide life-saving treatment for opioid overdoses.[1] The recent opioid epidemic in the U.S. put a spotlight on the dangers associated with the use of psychoactive drugs and brought a media-driven public health response to substance use that had not occurred since perhaps the emergence of cocaine use and the media spotlight on "crack babies" in the 1980s. The number of states that have legalized marijuana for medical and/or recreational use is increasing, with a subsequent increase in current use. At the same time, federal efforts focus on continuing to criminalize the use of marijuana. Current use of marijuana increased from 6.2% in 2004 to 7.9% in 2017.[2] In the past decade, the largest increase occurred among

those 55 years of age or older with 1.1% reporting current use in 2004 and 6.1% reporting current use in 2014.[3]

Despite the recent focus on opioids, tobacco and alcohol, both legal substances, are leading causes of preventable deaths both globally and in the U.S.[4,5,6,7] In 2017, based on the National Survey on Drug Use and Health, 87.1% of Americans aged 26 or older reported lifetime alcohol use. Of those aged 12-17 years old, 21.9% reported alcohol use within the past year, and 5.3% reported binge drinking.[6] Although tobacco use has dropped over the past few decades, in 2017, 22.4% of those aged 18 or older reported past month tobacco use, and 62.7% reported lifetime use.[2] With such a large proportion of the population using tobacco and/or alcohol, which are two leading causes of preventable death[6,8,9], as well as the emerging issues such as the opioid epidemic and the emergence of legalized use of marijuana, it is important for nurses to have evidence-based knowledge and competency related to the prevention and treatment of at-risk substance use at the individual and community level.

At-risk substance use, defined as use linked to adverse health consequences for individuals, families, and communities, occurs across the globe. From a public health perspective, the consequences go beyond the negative impact on the health of the individual using the substance.[8,9] Substance use increases the risk for injury, crime, and adverse health issues, and poses a risk for other individuals through environmental factors. For example, illicit drug use is linked to increased crime in a neighborhood, alcohol use while driving injures and kills drinkers and nondrinkers, and tobacco use pollutes the environment through the release of toxic chemicals. Substance use is a major public health issue affecting all ages, populations, and countries.[6,7,9]

Substance use occurs within the social, cultural, and economic context of the community with different impacts at the national level. These differences can include quantity consumed, the type of substance consumed, and the cultural norms around consumption. In relation to the quantity consumed, the U.S. represents 4.8% of the global population, yet globally, in 2015, the U.S. accounted for 49% of all consumption of morphine, 29.8% of fentanyl consumption, and 69% of oxycodone.[7, 10] Lower socioeconomic status is associated with an increased risk of alcohol-related harm due to increased vulnerability to alcohol based on nutritional and health status, as well as decreased access to care. The other economically associated issue is the quality of the alcohol, with a higher rate of alcohol-related deaths due to consumption of illegal alcohol that contains toxins.[9]

In addition, cultural differences exist around the use of substances. Cultural norms in some countries such as the U.S. and Russia include the acceptance of **binge drinking**, that is, consumption of more than the recommended limits of total alcohol during one episode of drinking. By contrast, in some countries, any consumption of alcohol can result in adverse social consequences. Finally, lack of economic resources within a country or community can reduce the ability to develop and/or enforce policies aimed at preventing at-risk substance use. These policies include ones designed to reduce distribution of illicit substances, control distribution of legal substances, and provide programs aimed at preventing substance use-related harm. Advocating to prevent harm associated with substance use and to provide access to treatment for those with a substance use disorder (SUD) requires an understanding of the context in which substance use occurs, the extent of the burden of disease, and evidence-based approaches that work across the continuum of use and life span.

Substance Use and the Global Burden of Disease

Substance use is a term used across the globe in reference to the use of **psychoactive substances**. These are chemical substances that have a pharmacological effect on the brain and central nervous system (CNS). The effects of these substances on an individual include altered mood, perception, and level of consciousness.[6] The classes of psychoactive substances include stimulants, depressants, inhalants, dissociative anesthetics, narcotics, hallucinogens, and cannabis (Table 11-1).[11] Some are legal, such as alcohol and tobacco, whereas others are illegal (or illicit), such as heroin. Some are legal with a prescription, such as narcotics prescribed for pain. Although cannabis is still illegal at the federal level in the U.S., in a growing number of states, marijuana (cannabis) can be obtained with a prescription. In a growing number of U.S. states and some Western European countries, it is legal for recreational use.

Understanding Substance Use and Risk Across the Continuum of Use and the Life Span

Substance use includes four components: quantity, frequency, pattern, and duration.[12] Assessment of these four components helps to determine the risk of adverse consequences. Consequences range from low to high risk with a diagnosis of an SUD at the high-risk end of the continuum (Fig. 11-1). **Quantity** is defined as the amount consumed, in other words, the dose. **Frequency** refers to how often the substance is consumed: daily, weekly, or monthly. The **pattern** of use refers to whether the use is consistent or occurs in an episodic manner, usually referred to as binging. Finally, **duration** of the use refers to how long over a lifetime the use has occurred.

Another important factor is the **quality** of the substance consumed.[9] Quality reflects the process for the manufacturing of the substance consumed and whether the product might include toxins, other substances such as Fentanyl-laced heroin, or not reflect a consistent dose. This usually occurs when manufacturing of the substance is done through an illegal and/or unregulated process. This is most apt to occur when the substance itself is illegal or when it is legal, but there are inadequate regulations controlling manufacturing.

Risk for harm associated with substance use occurs across the life span from fetal exposure to the last decades

TABLE 11–1 ■ Classes of Drugs

Category	Description	Examples
Stimulants	Overstimulate the CNS resulting in accelerated heart rate, high blood pressure, and other symptoms related to stimulation of the CNS.	Cocaine, amphetamines, methylphenidate, nicotine, methamphetamine, Ritalin, caffeine, and Methadrine
Narcotics	Relieve pain and can result in a state of euphoria and other mood changes.	Vicodin and OxyContin, opium, morphine, heroin, codeine, hydromorphone, meperidine, methadone, Darvon
Dissociative Anesthetics	Inhibit the body's ability to perceive pain.	PCP
Depressants	Depress the CNS thus slowing down the brain and the body.	Alcohol, barbiturates, and anti-anxiety tranquilizers (e.g., Valium, Librium, Xanax, Prozac, and Thorazine)
Inhalants	Come from a wide range of chemicals inhaled producing mind-altering effects.	Butyl nitrite, amyl nitrite gas used in some aerosol cans, gasoline and toluene vapors from correction fluid, glue, marking pens
Hallucinogens	Result in altered perception of reality.	PCP, LSD, mescaline, peyote, psilocybin, ecstasy, PCE, and methamphetamine, and Cannabis
Cannabis	Result in a feeling of euphoria, and can include distorted perceptions, memory impairment, as well as difficulty thinking and solving problems.	Cannabinoids including marijuana, tetrahydrocannabinol, or THC; hashish; hashish oil; and synthetics like Dronabinol

Source: (11)

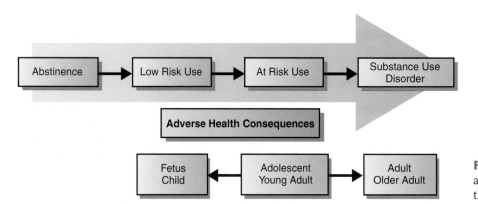

Figure 11-1 Substance use across the continuum of use and the life span.

of life. Life span-associated risk for adverse consequences, both acute and chronic, differs based on human stages of development, ability to metabolize the substance, and peer influence. Fetal exposure to alcohol can result in **fetal alcohol spectrum disorders (FASD)**, which can occur due to fetal exposure to maternal alcohol use, and it can include physical, behavioral, and/or learning problems.[13] Based on findings from multiple studies on heavy alcohol use by adolescents, there is strong evidence of an association between alcohol use and adverse effects on the brain including brain development, brain functioning, and neuropsychological performance.[14-17] For older adults, changes in the ability to metabolize alcohol, frailty, and other health issues increase the risk of alcohol-related acute adverse outcomes such as falls, interactions with other medications, and increased risk of intoxication.[16] Duration of use over the lifetime can increase the risk for other health issues such as liver disease, cancer, and cardiovascular disease even in the absence of an SUD.[8]

Differences exist in the addictive properties of substances, yet all have the potential to result in an SUD. Other factors that play a role in increasing the risk for substance use related adverse outcomes include genetics, the health of an individual, age, psychological issues, environment, cultural norms, exposure to stress, and access to social support.[7,8,18] Prevention of harm associated with substance use requires much more than prevention of an SUD. It requires reframing our approach to substance use from the cellular to the global level. Substance use places persons and communities at risk for adverse consequences that encompasses more than 200 diseases and injuries, as well as economic burdens to populations.[8]

A comparison of substance use across the life span from the cellular to global level helps to illustrate the variability of use. Alcohol is the most prevalent substance used worldwide. Globally, more than 50% of adults reported current use of alcohol. When broken down by gender, 65% of males and 45% of women report current alcohol use.[6] In the U.S., the statistics are similar, with a little more than 50% of adults reporting current alcohol use. The second most prevalent substance is tobacco with 19% of adults in the U.S. reporting current tobacco use.[2] The World Health Organization (WHO) reported that, in 2008, 155 to 250 million people, or 3.5% to 5.7% of the global population used psychoactive substances other than alcohol and tobacco. The most commonly used substance after alcohol and tobacco was cannabis.[18,19] In 2017, the percent of adults 12 or older in the U.S. who reported current drug use was higher, at 11.2% of that portion of the population.[2]

The Global Burden of Disease

Globally, the burden of disease (see Chapter 3) associated with alcohol use has risen over the past decade from 4.2% to 5.1%.[9] A total of 3 million deaths every year are due to the harmful use of alcohol, which represents 5.3 % of all deaths in 2016.[8] For young adults, the mortality risks are higher, with 25% of all deaths in persons aged 20 to 39 attributable to alcohol use.[18] Estimates of the global burden of disease attributable to drug use is 0.8%, with opioid use the largest contributor.[19] Tobacco contributes significantly to the global burden of disease, accounting for 1 in 10 deaths, killing more than 6 million people annually, almost double the number of deaths attributable to alcohol use.[20] Taken together, alcohol, tobacco, and drug use contribute significantly to the burden of disease, with alcohol and tobacco as two of the three top leading causes of preventable death. Substance use is linked to a wide spectrum of adverse health consequences at the individual, family, and community levels (Table 11-2). Worldwide, tobacco and alcohol are among the top 10 risk factors for mortality, with tobacco being the number one risk factor in high-income countries.[18-22]

■ CULTURAL CONTEXT

World Health Organization Report on Alcohol and Health: Culture and Context[9]

"The degree of risk for harm due to use of alcohol ... varies with the physical and socioeconomic context in which a given drinking occasion and the ensuing hours take place. Moreover, the nature and extent of the harm that results from drinking can vary widely depending on the context. In some contexts, drinkers will be vulnerable to alcohol-related social harm, disease, injury, or even death if any volume of alcohol is consumed. This is the case, for instance, if a person drinks before driving a car or piloting an aeroplane [sic], when consuming alcohol can result in serious penalties and harm. Also, in many countries, there can be serious social or legal consequences for drinking at all, due to laws and regulations or cultural and religious norms, which can increase the vulnerability of drinkers to alcohol-related social harm."

Substance Use Disorders

Use of alcohol, tobacco, and other drugs all have the potential to result in an SUD. A **substance use disorder** is "a maladaptive pattern of substance use leading to clinically significant impairment or distress" and can be diagnosed as moderate or severe.[23] The broader term used to refer to SUDs is **addiction**, defined as meeting the criteria for an SUD. In recent years, the professional literature has moved away from the term *addiction* in an effort to view the full continuum of risk rather than dichotomize the problem into categorizing a person as addicted or not addicted, thus negating the full continuum of harm associated with substance use. The gold standard for diagnosing an SUD used by health-care providers in the U.S. is the *Diagnostic and Statistical Manual of Mental Disorders* (DSM). In 2015, new criteria were introduced that represented a radical change from the approach used in earlier editions of the DSM, which included two diagnoses: substance abuse and substance dependence. With the fifth edition of the manual, DSM-V, an SUD is presented as a continuum that utilizes severity, evidence of physiological dependence, and course of treatment to classify the disorder (Box 11-1).[23] An SUD can be established with or without physiological

TABLE 11–2 ■ Adverse Consequences Related to Substance Use

Level	Injury	Environment	Physical Health	Psychosocial Health
Individual	Increased risk for unintentional injury and suicide		Increased risk for adverse health outcomes	Negative impact on: • Mental health • Employment • Social networks
Family	Increased risk for intentional and unintentional injury	Adverse effect on home environment (e.g., secondhand smoke in the home)	Increased risk for adverse health outcomes secondary to impaired family member	Negative impact on: • Mental health • Employment • Social networks
Community	Increased risk for intentional and unintentional injury	• Secondhand smoke • Increased crime • Decreased property values	Increased burden for cost of health care	Negative impact on: • Community Social networks

Source: (7-10)

BOX 11–1 ■ Diagnosis of Substance Use and Addictive Disorders

Severity Specifiers:

Moderate: 2-3 criteria positive
Severe: 4 or more criteria positive

Specify If:

With Physiological Dependence: evidence of tolerance or withdrawal (i.e., either Item 4 or 5 is present)
Without Physiological Dependence: no evidence of tolerance or withdrawal (i.e., neither Item 4 nor 5 is present)

Course Specifiers (see text for definitions):

Early Full Remission
Early Partial Remission
Sustained Full Remission
Sustained Partial Remission
On Agonist Therapy
In a Controlled Environment

Source: (23)

---

dependence. **Physiological dependence** is defined as evidence of tolerance to or withdrawal from a foreign substance. **Tolerance** involves an adaptation of the body to a drug that results in needing more of the drug to achieve a certain effect. If use of the drug is stopped abruptly, drug-specific physical and/or mental symptoms occur, also known as **withdrawal.**[23] Physical dependence alone does not meet the criteria for a diagnosis of an SUD because withdrawal can occur even with chronic use of a

drug as prescribed.[24] Thus, the terms *substance abuse* and *substance dependence* are not legitimate clinical terms. This also shifts the clinical picture away from pejorative language, such as abuser or addict, to a disease-oriented approach of a person with an SUD.

For years, much of the focus related to substance use was on the treatment of those who met the criteria for an SUD. In other words, the focus was a downstream approach (Chapter 2) with a simultaneous policy approach that focused on criminalization of certain substance use and control of access to legal psychoactive substances such as alcohol and tobacco. Over the past few decades, the global focus has shifted to include a broader upstream approach. This new focus attempts to reduce harm at the population level through prevention of harmful substance use, reduction of harms associated with use and early treatment of SUDs, decriminalization of substance use, and broader policy initiatives.[6,9]

■ CELLULAR TO GLOBAL

Alcohol provides an excellent example of the potential adverse outcomes associated with use from the cellular to global level. At the cellular level, continued use of alcohol at higher than recommended levels can result in a toxic effect on cellular DNA, increasing the risk of developing cancer. Harm associated with use affects the family, the community, all the way up to global impacts on population health related to the burden of disease. In 2016, more than 3 million people died globally as a result of alcohol use, more than deaths associated with diseases such as tuberculosis,

HIV/AIDs, and diabetes.[9] The range of harm associated with the use of alcohol extends across the full continuum of risk and requires not only mechanisms to care for individuals and families negatively affected by at-risk alcohol use but public health approaches at the local, state, national, and global level.[8] The WHO's global strategy is currently the most comprehensive international policy document that provides guidance on reducing harmful alcohol use, which impacts many of the health-related targets of the Sustainable Development Goals.[9]

Measurement, Surveillance, and Risk

Before developing interventions to help reduce the harm related to substance use, it is important to understand how surveillance of substance use and associated adverse health outcomes (see Chapter 3) is conducted in the U.S. and across the globe in relation to the prevalence of substance use and adverse health consequences associated with use. The first step in conducting surveillance is defining how substance use is measured. Across all substances, there is a classification of use that reflects the associated level of risk (Fig. 11-1). Because multiple terms are sometimes used, clarity is needed. The first term is **abstinence**, defined as no use of the substance. For alcohol, it is usually measured as two or fewer drinks in the past 12 months, and for tobacco and other drugs, it reflects no use at all in the past 12 months. **Low-risk use** or **moderate use** is use of the substance that places the user at little or no risk. For example, if a healthy person drinks at or below the recommended limits for alcohol consumption of no more than two drinks in one day for adult men (one drink for adult women) and no more than 14 drinks (7 drinks for women) in a week, they are considered low-risk.[24] A number of terms are used to describe the next level of use including risky use, at-risk use, binge/heavy episodic use, harmful use, and nondependent heavy use. For example, at-risk use and harmful use are used interchangeably. For the purpose of this chapter, we will use the term **at-risk use**, defined as use associated with harm to the individual, family, and/or community.[6,12,13] Moderate- or low-risk alcohol use is defined as no more than four drinks in one day for healthy adult men and no more than three in one day for healthy adult women and persons over the age of 65. At-risk alcohol use includes **heavy drinking** and **binge drinking**. Heavy drinking is defined based on the number of drinks consumed during a week. For adult men, heavy drinking is

15 or more drinks in a week, and for women or adults over 65, it is 8 or more in a week. Binge (episodic heavy) drinking is defined as five or more drinks (four or more for women) consumed on a single drinking occasion and is associated with drinking that brings the blood alcohol level up to a **blood alcohol concentration (BAC)** of 0.08 grams percent or above.[24]

For substances other than alcohol, the distinction between low-risk use and risky use is less clearly defined. In general, any use of tobacco or illegal substances is considered at-risk use. Use of psychoactive substances available by prescription is termed risky use when the use is not in alignment with the prescription. At the end of the spectrum of risk is an SUD, as described earlier. For some substances or some situations, all use is seen as at-risk. For example, there is no level of low-risk use of substances during pregnancy including tobacco, alcohol, marijuana, and illegal drugs.

When collecting individual substance use data, it is important to measure the four aspects of consumption of use: quantity, frequency, pattern, and duration. For alcohol use, quantity is measured as a standard drink, so the intake reflects the amount of alcohol (or dose) consumed rather than the amount of beverage consumed (Fig. 11-2). In the United States, a standard drink is 0.6 fluid ounces or 14 grams of pure alcohol. The amount of pure alcohol varies based on the type of beverage. For example, 12 ounces of beer or 5 ounces of wine represent one standard drink because they contain the same amount of pure alcohol.[24] For some substances, especially street drugs like heroin, quantity is hard to determine because there is no standard. Frequency is usually measured as number of times a week. Duration questions reflect how long over the lifetime the substance has been used, and pattern is measured based on whether the use is constant or varying. These terms are important not only when asking an individual about substance use but also when measuring use at the population level.

Surveillance related to substance use is conducted on a regular basis to help measure the prevalence of substance use. How use is measured in these surveys helps public health officials determine the level of risk at the population level. Eleven different national surveillance surveys that involve the collection of data on substance use are listed on the Centers for Disease Control and Prevention (CDC) Web site, including the Behavioral Risk Factor Surveillance System (BRFSS), the National Survey on Drug Use and Health (NSDUH), and the National Epidemiologic Survey on Alcohol and Related Conditions (NESARC). This surveillance process

What Is a Standard Drink?

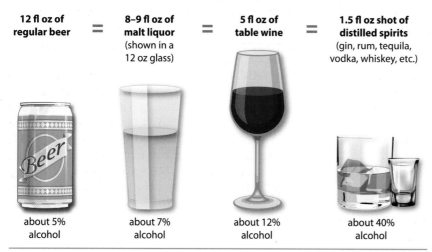

12 fl oz of regular beer = **8–9 fl oz of malt liquor** (shown in a 12 oz glass) = **5 fl oz of table wine** = **1.5 fl oz shot of distilled spirits** (gin, rum, tequila, vodka, whiskey, etc.)

about 5% alcohol   about 7% alcohol   about 12% alcohol   about 40% alcohol

Figure 11-2 Standard drink. *(From NIH, National Institute on Alcohol Abuse and Alcoholism. [2018]. What is a standard drink? Retrieved from https://www. niaaa.nih.gov/alcohol-health/overview-alcohol-consumption/what-standard-drink.)*

Each beverage portrayed above represents one U.S. standard drink (also known as an alcoholic drink-equivalent). The percent of pure alcohol, expressed here as alcohol by volume (alc/vol), varies within and across beverage types.

provides information on the distribution of substance use and SUDs, as well as information on health-related consequences. Understanding the terms helps in the interpretation of the findings. For example, the report on binge drinking in the U.S. released by the CDC requires an understanding of what binge drinking is and is not.[25]

Models for Prevention and Treatment of Substance Use Disorders

Prevention efforts related to substance use and adverse health consequences have shifted over the past 20 years from a narrow focus on the end of the continuum of use, an SUD, to a broader focus that includes the continuum of use across the life span. There are two models that guide prevention efforts: the harm reduction model and the Health and Medicine Division (HMD) of the National Academies of Sciences, Engineering and Medicine's (formerly the Institute of Medicine [IOM]) prevention model presented in Chapter 2.

Health and Medicine Division Prevention Model

Prevention is aimed at promoting resilience. In 1997, the HMD of the National Academies of Sciences, Engineering and Medicine identified the primary, secondary,

and tertiary continuum of prevention as confusing and developed a new, simpler model that more clearly separates prevention from treatment.[26] As explained in Chapter 2, this framework divides the prevention category into three levels—universal, selective, and indicated—and includes possible interventions at each level that can be applied easily to behavioral health issues.

Universal Level of Prevention

The universal level of prevention addresses identified populations regardless of identified risk. In the case of substance abuse prevention, older adults, pregnant women, and teenagers can be offered skills to allow the postponement of use of substances of abuse. Universal prevention techniques include: education regarding the effects of alcohol, tobacco, and other drugs on one's own health, on the health of children, and the danger of fetal alcohol syndrome (FAS)/effects and risk factors; the danger of using substances of abuse when using prescribed medication; and special education for older adults in an age-appropriate manner. It includes appropriate decision-making and social skills to empower participants to make good decisions.

Selective Level of Prevention

With substance abuse, the selective level of prevention addresses specific subgroups known to be at risk for at-risk substance use by virtue of biological, psychological, social, or environmental factors. Whether or not individual members of the specific subgroups are using alcohol, tobacco, or other drugs is not taken into consideration when applying selective interventions. What is important is that the subgroups are at higher risk for at-risk substance use than the general population. The selective interventions are tailored to specific characteristics of the subgroups such as age, gender, reproductive status, availability of drugs in the communities in which the members live, community attitudes toward substance use, substance use by peers, family history of substance use, family attitudes, social problems, history of sexual abuse, and marginal or poor academic achievement in school. Selective interventions include opportunities for learning social skills that might delay initial use of alcohol, tobacco, and other drugs. After-school activities, services and resources available at community centers, classes on how to interview for a job, drug and alcohol education, role-playing, and self-esteem building exercises and opportunities are examples of selective interventions.

Indicated Level of Prevention

The indicated level of prevention addresses specific subgroups at highest risk for development of an SUD or that are showing early signs of an SUD. These groups may appear to be experimenting with substances and, without aggressive preventative action, some members of the group will develop a full-fledged SUD. In addition to delaying initial substance use, the purpose of indicated techniques includes delaying or reducing the severity of an SUD. At this level, there is less concern about community prevention and more emphasis on those demonstrating early SUD. Indicated techniques might include continued alcohol and drug education, with specific attention to the consequences of continued use, and self-tests to determine the level of SUD a person might be experiencing, providing an opportunity for the early user to identify his or her risk factors and any signs or symptoms of SUD that might be present.

Harm Reduction Model

The harm reduction model is another model used in the prevention of adverse consequences associated with alcohol and drug use. Harm reduction refers to any program, policy, and/or intervention that seeks to reduce the harm related to alcohol and drug use or other high-risk behavior, rather than focusing solely on attainment of abstinence of the risky behavior at the individual level.[27] Thus, it includes a wide spectrum of interventions from

safer use (needle exchange programs) to abstinence. Thus, those engaged in at-risk use of substances who are not willing or able to engage in treatment that leads to abstinence are provided with options to minimize the harm associated with substance use. From a public health perspective, harm reduction is used to minimize the physical, emotional, social, and economic harm associated with substance use not only in relation to the individual but also to the larger population and the community. The guiding principles of harm reduction are based on the assumption that interventions aimed at reduction of the adverse consequences associated with substance use should be free of judgment or blame.[27] The Canadian Center for Substance Abuse proposed guiding principles for harm reduction (Box 11-2).[28] The reduction of the harm associated with substance abuse is a goal of Healthy People.[29]

■ HEALTHY PEOPLE AND SUBSTANCE USE

Goal: Reduce substance abuse to protect the health, safety, and quality of life for all, especially children.
Overview: Although progress has been made in substantially lowering rates of abuse of some substances, the use of mind- and behavior-altering substances continues to take a major toll on the health of individuals, families, and communities nationwide. Substance abuse—involving drugs, alcohol, or both—is associated with a range of destructive social conditions, including family disruptions, financial problems, lost productivity, failure in school, injuries, domestic violence, child abuse, and crime. Moreover, both social attitudes and legal responses to the consumption of alcohol and illicit drugs make substance abuse one of the most complex public health issues.
Midcourse Review: Of the 44 objectives for this topic area, 2 were developmental and 42 were measurable. For 10 of the measurable objectives, the target was met or exceeded, and 1 was improving. For 12 there was little or no detectable change and 9 were getting worse. Eight of the objectives were informational (Fig. 11-3).

Source: (30)

Alcohol Use

Alcohol consumption is a socially acceptable and normative practice in the U.S. As noted earlier, more than half (51.7%) of the U.S. population 12 years of age or

BOX 11–2 ■ Guiding Principles on Harm Reduction

- Clients are responsive to culturally competent, non-judgmental services, delivered in a manner that demonstrates respect for individual dignity, personal strength, and self-determination.
- Service providers are responsible to the wider community for delivering interventions that attempt to reduce the economic, social, and physical consequences of drug- and alcohol-related harm and harms associated with other behaviors or practices that put individuals at risk.
- Because those engaged in unsafe health practices are often difficult to reach through traditional service venues, the service continuum must seek creative opportunities and develop new strategies to engage, motivate, and intervene with potential clients.

- Comprehensive treatments need to include strategies that reduce harm for those clients who are unable or unwilling to modify their unsafe behavior.
- Relapse or periods of return to unsafe health practices should not be equated with or conceptualized as "failure of treatment".
- Each program within a system of comprehensive services can be strengthened by working collaboratively with other programs in the system.
- People change in incremental ways and must be offered a range of treatment outcomes in a continuum of care from reducing unsafe practices to abstaining from dangerous behavior.

Source: (28, 29)

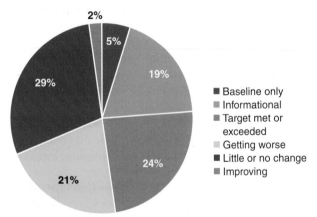

Figure 11-3 HP 2020 Midcourse Status of Objectives; Substance Abuse Objectives. *(Data from National Center for Health Statistics. [2016]. Chapter 40, Substance Abuse in Healthy People 2020 Midcourse Review. Hyattsville, MD: National Center for Health Statistics.)*

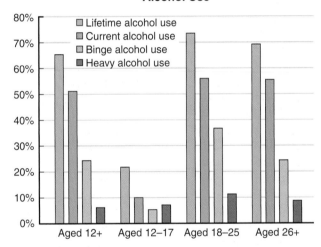

Figure 11-4 Alcohol Use by Age Group. *(Data from World Health Organization. [2017]. Global status report on alcohol and health 2017. Geneva, Switzerland: WHO Press.)*

older reported current use of alcohol. In the U.S., in 2016, nearly a quarter (24.5% up from 23.1% in 2010) of Americans age 12 and over reported binge (heavy episodic) alcohol use (five or more drinks on the same occasion at least once in the past 30 days for men and four or more drinks on the same occasion for women), and 6.1% reported heavy alcohol use (five for men and four for women or more drinks on the same occasion on at least five different days in the past 30 days) as depicted in Figure 11-4.[2]

For those between the ages of 18 and 25, 36.9% reported binge drinking and 9.6% reported heavy drinking.[2] As noted earlier, alcohol accounts for 5.1% of the global burden of disease. According to the WHO, at-risk alcohol use is the third leading risk factor for poor health with approximately 3 million deaths each year associated with the at-risk use of alcohol. Worldwide, binge drinking is highest in middle to high per capita consumption countries and is higher for males than for females.[2]

Until recently, much of the focus in health care was on the person with an alcohol use disorder (AUD). Now, efforts are emerging to address at-risk alcohol use earlier to prevent acute and chronic harm associated with alcohol use. An AUD takes time to develop whereas one episode of heavy/at-risk alcohol use can lead to serious adverse health consequences such as motor vehicle crashes, drowning, and alcohol poisoning. Health issues related to at-risk alcohol use occur across the life span beginning with fetal exposure to alcohol and can affect the nondrinker as well. For example, researchers looked at state data related to pediatric mortality in turn related to motor vehicle crashes and found that in 9% of the cases the operator was under the influence of alcohol.[31] Overall, 16% of all pediatric and 29% of all motor vehicle-related deaths were due to alcohol.[32]

At-risk alcohol use increases the risk for adverse consequences both in the short and long term. Short-term or acute harms include injury, violence, interaction with medications, increased risk for unprotected sex, and other harms. Long-term or chronic harms include an increased risk for a number of cancers, cardiovascular disease, liver disease, dementia, and AUD.[33,34] Thus harm associated with alcohol use as laid out by the WHO is not only due to the actual consumption of alcohol but is also due to societal and individual level vulnerability factors (Fig. 11-5).[9] Timely prevention and early treatment is the key to saving lives, and the professional health-care workforce is the key to meeting national and global objectives related to reducing alcohol-related morbidity and mortality, and increasing the age and proportion of adolescents who remain alcohol-free.

Because of the severity of consequences associated with at-risk alcohol use, prevention of adverse alcohol-related health consequences is a major public health issue across the life span. Since its inception, *Healthy People* has included prevention of adverse alcohol-related consequences related to at-risk use including reduction in motor vehicle crash deaths and injuries, alcohol-related hospital emergency department visits, alcohol-related violence, lost productivity related to alcohol use, and deaths of adolescents riding with a driver who has been using alcohol.[35] Of the 21 main objectives listed under the substance abuse topic in *HP 2020*, 10 were specific to alcohol. The objectives included primary, secondary, and tertiary prevention. The objectives were grouped under three headings: policy and prevention, screening and treatment, and epidemiology and surveillance. *HP 2020* also chose specific objectives under different topic areas as leading health indicators (see Chapter 1). For substance abuse, two leading health indicators were chosen, one related to adolescent use and the other to binge drinking in adults. Although use among adolescents dropped, the target for binge drinking among adults was not met.

■ HEALTHY PEOPLE AND ALCOHOL USE

Healthy People Leading Health Indicator relevant to alcohol use reduction

Targeted Topic: Substance use

Specific Objective: SA 14-3

Objective: Reduce the proportion of persons engaging in binge drinking during the past 30 days – adults aged 18 or older

Baseline: 26.9% of adults aged 18 years and over reported that they engaged in binge drinking during the past 30 days in 2008

Target: 24.4%

Progress: The percentage of adults aged 18 and older who had engaged in binge drinking in the past 30 days has remained the same, measuring 27.1% in 2012 and 26.9% in 2015.[34,36]

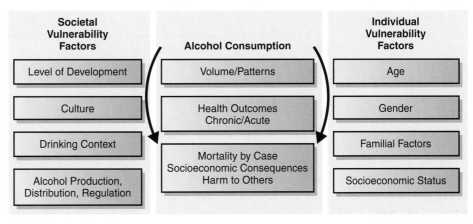

Figure 11-5 WHO Conceptual causal model of alcohol consumption and health outcomes. *(Data from World Health Organization. [2017]. Global status report on alcohol and health 2017. Geneva, Switzerland: WHO Press.)*

Consequences of Alcohol Use

Alcohol is a causal factor in 200 types of diseases and injuries[9] and as noted earlier accounts for 5.1% of all deaths worldwide.[6] The underlying pathophysiology reflects that alcohol use can result in multi-organ toxicity, and toxicity in one organ system affects other systems.[4,8] Damage occurs not only in the liver and brain but also in the gastrointestinal (intestinal mucosa), endocrine (pancreas), and other organ systems, including the immune and cardiovascular systems.[37] Acetaldehyde, the primary metabolic product of ethanol, is thought to be the instrumental toxin in developing alcohol-related disease. For example, long-term exposure to alcohol results in alteration of cellular DNA, thus increasing the risk for cancer.[38,39]

In addition to physical problems, there are many psychosocial consequences associated with alcohol use for individuals and their families.[40] These can include legal problems such as traffic violations, driving while intoxicated, and public intoxication. Early employment problems can include lateness, frequent absences, an inability to concentrate on the job, and decreased competency, which can eventually lead to on-the-job accidents and injury, or loss of employment leading to chronic unemployment. It does not take a great deal of exposure to problem drinking for the family to also manifest dysfunction. Family conflict, erratic child discipline, neglect of responsibilities, and social isolation can progress to divorce, spousal abuse, and child abuse or neglect. Other problems associated with at-risk alcohol use include injury (Chapter 12) and psychiatric illness (Chapter 10).[9,40] Comorbidity of psychiatric illness and alcohol use is also common with evidence that alcohol is a causal factor for depression.[41,42]

Alcohol and Vulnerable Populations Across the Life Span

Alcohol use can affect vulnerable populations interacting with their environment at key points over the life span (see Fig. 11-1). For the fetus exposed to alcohol, there is the risk of FASD, often characterized by prenatal or postnatal growth deficiency, certain facial features, and CNS structure or function changes.[43,44] Alcohol is a leading teratogen, and it is estimated that the ratio of school children who were born with FASD is 1 in 20.[44] Globally, approximately 8 in every 1,000 live births (0.8%) had FASD, and a little under 8% of women who used alcohol during pregnancy delivered a child with FASD.[43]

The vulnerable time periods following pregnancy are those of childhood and early adolescence followed by early adulthood. Adolescence is a time often marked by willingness to take risks and experiment with alcohol, which can extend into early adulthood.[45] In 2017, among young adults aged 18 to 25, the rate of binge drinking was 39% compared to 24.9% for all persons aged 12 and older.[2] This underlines the need to begin primary prevention with children prior to the age of 12. The significance of focusing on children is twofold. First, children who initiate drinking before the age of 15 are five times more likely report a diagnosis of an AUD than persons who first used alcohol after the age of 20.[46] In addition, the brain is developing during adolescence. The lack of executive functioning among this age group may inhibit good decision making, and unique characteristics in the adolescent brain may increase the reaction to the rewarding sensations of alcohol use.[44,45]

To address the issue, the National Institute on Alcohol Abuse and Alcoholism (NIAAA) published a guide to screening and brief intervention for youth. The guide uses an approach to screening that includes asking adolescents about peer use as a marker of at-risk use. It also suggests different questions based on age. The guide stresses that health-care providers are in an ideal position to prevent use as well as to identify those who may be drinking. The age range covered in the guide is 9 to 15.[46] The importance of prevention within this age range is underlined by the fact that those who start drinking before the age of 15 are at greater risk of developing an AUD.[47,48]

Older adults are another group at particular risk of detrimental consequences of alcohol use (Chapter 19). For older adults who continue to drink heavily throughout their life, the cumulative effect of alcohol exposure may result in damage to cells, tissues, and organs.[40,49] In addition, there is the possibility that even low-risk alcohol use may place the older adult at a higher risk because of the increased potential for falls and the interaction of alcohol with prescriptive drugs for comorbid conditions.[45,50]

Screening Brief Intervention and Referral for Treatment

Globally, screening for at-risk alcohol use is an essential component in the fight to prevent the harm related to alcohol use.[51] In the past, screening tools were developed to help identify those who may have an AUD, but screening tools now in use also help the health-care provider identify persons at risk for adverse consequences related to alcohol use across the continuum of use (see Fig. 11-1).[51] More recently, acute care settings are adopting a universal approach to screening for alcohol use.[52-55]

● APPLYING PUBLIC HEALTH SCIENCE

The Case of the Drinking Oncology Patients

Public Health Science Topics Covered:

- Setting Assessment
- Secondary data analysis
- Screening

Jane worked with lung, esophagus, and head and neck cancer patients in the radiation oncology clinic in an urban academic hospital on the east coast. After several alcohol- and drug-related incidents with her cancer patients, she became concerned that the hospital was not doing enough to help cancer patients with risky alcohol and drug use. One patient in particular, who completed chemotherapy and radiation for a large neck tumor and subsequently died from alcohol withdrawal, motivated Jane to try to find some solutions. The doctors, nurses, and social workers were doing everything they knew to do for patients with alcohol- and drug-related problems but commented frequently that the advice they were giving to patients was contradictory and often insufficient. Jane asked around and convened a small team of doctors, nurses, social workers, clinical nurse specialists, and advance practice providers to develop an action plan for these patients.

The first step was to consult the literature. Jane and her team knew there were recommendations for drug screening as it related to cancer pain management and started with big organizations, like the Oncology Nursing Society[56] and the National Cancer Institute,[57] to look for guidelines. She was right—these groups suggested basic practices, like routine urine drug testing and the use of validated instruments designed to screen for substance "abuse" potential. The use of words like "abuse" and "addiction" common in the cancer literature told Jane and her team that the thinking might be out of date. Jane knew it would be difficult to ask the oncology doctors and nurses to use a long, unfamiliar screening tool in routine practice, especially without identifying strategies to cope with substance use issues simultaneously. A PubMed review of the oncology literature wasn't very helpful; beyond the basic recommendations that oncology providers keep the potential for substance abuse and addiction in mind when writing prescriptions for narcotics, there were no prospective trials testing screening tools or interventions specific to the cancer population.

Jane was hopeful that the substance use literature would be more instructive, and she was right. Whereas many chronic pain and substance use studies specifically excluded cancer patients because of the complex nature of their pain issues, there were some important lessons to be gleaned from the literature. First of all, Jane and her team learned about validated screening tools that were easy to apply in the ambulatory clinics to help providers identify patients whose substance use might place them at risk, meaning drug and alcohol use that would place them at higher risk for unintended negative consequences. The team reached out to experts in the area affiliated with the hospital who confirmed that a new approach to the problem, framing it with the context of risk rather than assigning a label such as "addict", would help reframe their approach to prevention of harm in their patients associated with substance use.

The experts explained that nurses and doctors could be taught a quick and relatively easy intervention in the clinic to give practical and meaningful advice called a "brief intervention." The Substance Abuse and Mental Health Services Administration (SAMHSA)[58] recommends using screening, brief intervention, and referral to treatment (SBIRT) in primary care offices, emergency departments, and trauma centers. One example of this strategy was validated by a small study of upper aerodigestive cancer patients. Lopez-Pelayo et al. (2016) noted that patients who received direct feedback about alcohol risk from their head and neck surgeon after a diagnosis of cancer were much more likely to reduce their alcohol intake than those who did not.[59]

Several public health-orientated resources were available to help guide the implementation of this strategy of screening, and then using brief interventions in the clinic; examples include the WHO's SBIRT guide[60] and the CDC guide, *Planning and Implementing Screening and Brief Intervention for Risky Alcohol Use.*[61] For patients who needed more than brief advice to cut back on their drug and alcohol consumption, such as patients who might be at risk for alcohol withdrawal or patients who use illicit drugs daily, a referral to treatment or substance use specialists would be called for.

The team met to review the literature and decided to implement an SBIRT program as a pilot project in one of the oncology clinics. Although there was no evidence that SBIRT had been previously attempted in an oncology clinic, there was good reason to believe it might be a good place to start. The technique had been shown to be effective in reducing alcohol consumption in different groups of primary care and emergency department patients, both of whom are similar to oncology patients.

First, the team met with colleagues from the psychiatry department to discuss the concept of motivational interviewing, an approach to patient care that encourages clinicians to partner with patients to make positive behavioral changes to enhance their health. Jane learned that motivational interviewing techniques were used when delivering an effective brief intervention. Experts from the psychiatry department agreed to work with Jane and her team to develop a short education program to introduce the idea of SBIRT and motivational interviewing to the clinicians in the department.

A training program for nurses, residents, and other allied health professionals combined motivational interviewing skills with specific substance use in oncology patients training. The project team worked with the training facilitators to incorporate oncology-specific considerations into the curriculum. The training included two 2-hour sessions (four sessions total). Confirmation of fidelity to the process of screening, brief intervention, and referral to treatment was obtained using standardized patients and role playing. The project trainers created pre- and post-training assessment tools, which were used to evaluate the effectiveness of the training.

The team next turned their attention to the electronic health record. They understood from their colleagues that the best way to implement valid screening tools would be to incorporate them into the patients' electronic record. Working with the Information Technology (IT) department, they developed an electronic documentation infrastructure using validated instruments for SBIRT and clinical decision support in patients' electronic medical records. Electronic forms were developed for patients' radiation oncology electronic health records (Mosaiq) that incorporated validated and reliable instruments for screening (the three-item Alcohol Use Disorders Identification Test-Consumption [AUDIT-C] and a single question drug screen).[59-66] This approach allowed the population of patient data into patients' medical records and into the data system that facilitated retrospective, aggregate data collection. The forms included a clinical decision support feature that totaled results from screenings and assessments.

Finally, electronic "just in time" toolkits were installed on every computer in the clinic to help clinicians find the information they needed to implement SBIRT at the moment they needed to use it. Toolkits for staff use contained resources for low-, moderate-, and high-risk patients. The low-risk toolkit included oncology-specific substance use handouts, copies of the screening tools, and a list of resources for self-referral. The moderate-risk toolkit included examples of brief intervention language and all resources available in the low-risk folder. The high-risk toolkit included a readiness for change ruler, a brief intervention script, referral resources and instructions, oncology-specific fact sheet, tips for reducing substance use, and follow-up recommendations.

The department tracked screening rates for all new patients, and Jane and her team discovered that clinicians were struggling with the three-question AUDIT-C screening tool. Fortunately, the team found that researchers were validating single-question alcohol and drug screening tools in other settings, which Jane believed would increase the screening rate in her department. After the initial 3-month implementation process using longer screening tools, the department converted to two one-item screening questions. They also knew that an oncology-specific guide or set of recommendations would be helpful in the future. Their experience taught them that specialties do not always communicate and providing specific recommendations for the cancer patient population would be essential.

Policy Level Interventions to Reduce Alcohol-Related Harm

The interest in developing and disseminating both evidence-based practices and policies to minimize the harms associated with alcohol misuse is widespread.[8,9] From a policy perspective, the WHO has brought together member states to come up with policy strategies. They have outlined 10 areas for national action and four at the global level (Box 11-3).[68] In the U.S., alcohol policies focus on five main areas. The first is regulation of the physical availability of alcohol (e.g., minimum age, restrictions on sites). Next is altering the drinking context (e.g., serving intoxicated clients). A third policy approach is limiting alcohol promotion, such as the ban on advertising hard liquor on TV. A fourth policy is deterrence though sanctions on drunk driving. The fifth approach is developing policies related to treatment and early intervention as evidenced by the policy on including Screening and Brief Intervention (SBI) on level one

BOX 11-3 ■ World Health Organization Global Strategy to Reduce Harmful Alcohol Use

The 10 areas for national action are:

1. Leadership, awareness, and commitment
2. Health services' response
3. Community action
4. Drunk-driving policies and countermeasures
5. Availability of alcohol
6. Marketing of alcoholic beverages
7. Pricing policies
8. Reducing the negative consequences of drinking and alcohol intoxication
9. Reducing the public health impact of illicit alcohol and informally produced alcohol
10. Monitoring and surveillance

The four priority areas for global action are:

1. Public health advocacy and partnership
2. Technical support and capacity building
3. Production and dissemination of knowledge
4. Resource mobilization

Source: (9)

and level two trauma units. These policies can be enacted at the national, state, and local level, or may be instituted outside of the government.

Tobacco Use

According to the WHO, tobacco use accounts for more than 7 million deaths each year. Of these deaths, 6 million are linked to direct tobacco use and the rest are due to exposure to secondhand smoke.[69] Tobacco is the number one cause of preventable death in the U.S., causing approximately 480,000 deaths each year attributable to smoking, with 41,000 attributable to secondhand smoke exposure. In the U.S., tobacco use accounts for one out of every five deaths.[70] It is the only legal product that causes the death of half of its regular users. More than one billion people use tobacco products worldwide.[70] According to the U.S. Surgeon General's 2014 report, *The Health Consequences of Smoking—50 Years of Progress: A Report of the Surgeon General*, there is enough evidence to infer a causal relationship between cigarette smoking and a number of diseases and conditions, many of which were not, initially, seen as smoking-attributable diseases or conditions. The report documents the devastating effects and explains how tobacco causes disease.[71]

In addition, those who consume both alcohol and tobacco may be at greater risk for adverse health outcomes.[72]

Tobacco users are directly exposed through three routes: (1) smoking cigarettes, pipes, or cigars; (2) chewing smokeless tobacco; and (3) inhaling snuff. Tobacco use through any of these routes is a major public health issue for the entire community. **Secondhand smoke exposure** occurs when nonsmokers are exposed to a mixture of the smoke produced from the end of the cigarette, cigar, or pipe as well as the smoke exhaled by the smoker. Because exposure to secondhand smoke is an environmental issue, it is also referred to as **environmental tobacco smoke (ETS)** as well as **involuntary or passive smoking**. According to the American Cancer Society, ETS contains more than 7,000 chemicals, 70 of which cause cancer.[73]

Based on data from the National Drug Use and Health Survey for 2016, tobacco use within the previous year was higher among males (35.6%) compared to females (21.8%).[2] Tobacco use was higher in the lesbian, gay, bisexual, transgender population; among those living below the poverty level; and among the disabled.[74] The South and Midwest regions of the country also reported higher tobacco use.[75] Tobacco use is more prevalent in persons with a mental health disorder at 36.5%.[76] Differences exist in the prevalence of current tobacco use across ethnic groups, with American Indians/Alaska Natives having the highest prevalence of 42.6%, up from 35.8% in 2010, followed by Non-Hispanic whites (31.3%), African Americans (27.8%), Nonblack Hispanics (23.8%), Hawaiian/Pacific Islanders (26.1%), and Asians (15%).[2]

Globally, differences in the prevalence of tobacco use also exist among countries. Although tobacco use is declining in the U.S., it is increasing globally, especially in low-income countries. According to the WHO, "The tobacco epidemic is one of the biggest public health threats the world has ever faced." [69] Almost 80% of smokers live in middle- or low-income countries.[69]

Tobacco product use in the U.S, which includes cigarettes, smokeless tobacco, cigars, and pipe tobacco, generally, is on the decline. In 2017, approximately 24% of adults were current consumers of tobacco products (used within the last 30 days). Youth cigarette use has also steadily declined. In 2017, 4.9% of those aged 12-17 were current cigarette smokers, compared with 5.3% in 2016.[2] Tobacco use varies by state and region. The prevalence of tobacco use ranges from 11.3% in Utah to 32% in West Virginia.[75] Despite the decline in use, 44% of the 68 measurable objectives related to tobacco use in HP 2020 showed little or no detectable change and three were getting worse (Fig. 11-6). [77]

■ HEALTHY PEOPLE AND TOBACCO USE

Goal: Reduce illness, disability, and death related to tobacco use and secondhand smoke exposure.

Overview: Scientific knowledge about the health effects of tobacco use has increased greatly since the first Surgeon General's report on tobacco was released in 1964.[78]

Midcourse Review: Of the 77 objectives in the Tobacco Use Topic Area, 9 were developmental and 68 were measurable. Eight objectives had met or exceeded their 2020 targets, 25 objectives were improving, 30 objectives had demonstrated little or no detectable change, 3 objectives were getting worse, and 2 objectives had baseline data only (Fig. 11-6).[77] Adolescent tobacco use continued to decline from 26% in 2009 to 22.4 % in 2016.[77]

Healthy People Leading Health Indicator Relevant to Tobacco Use Reduction

Objective: Reduce tobacco use by adolescents past month TU-2.1.

Target: 21.0%

Baseline: 26.0% of adolescents in grades 9 through 12 used cigarettes, chewing tobacco, snuff, or cigars in the past 30 days in 2009.[30]

Progress: The proportion of students in grades 9–12 who used tobacco products in the past 30 days decreased from 26.0% in 2009 to 22.4% in 2013, moving toward the 2020 target.[77] By 2017, prevalence of tobacco use in high school students dropped to 7.6%.[70] In 2013, there were statistically significant disparities in the rates of adolescent tobacco use by sex, race, and ethnicity.[74] By 2017, the gender gap had narrowed related to any tobacco use.[70]

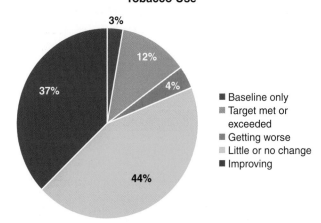

Figure 11-6 HP 2020 Midcourse Status of the Tobacco Use Objectives. *(Data from Source: [75])*

Consequences of Tobacco Use

The adverse health consequences experienced by tobacco users include cardiovascular disease, cancer, chronic obstructive pulmonary disorders, adverse effects on the oral cavity and teeth, and adverse maternal and neonatal outcomes.[70,72] For nonsmokers exposed to ETS, the adverse effects are similar but also include other serious health risks, especially in children, including increased risk for asthma, sudden infant death syndrome (SIDS), middle-ear infections, and lower respiratory tract infections.[71,72]

Vulnerable Populations Across the Life Span

Those who are most vulnerable to the adverse effects of tobacco use are in many cases children of smokers. From conception, children of smokers are at higher risk. Mothers who smoke during pregnancy are more apt to have children who are small for their gestational age. In addition, fetal exposure to tobacco increases the risk for SIDS. Children exposed to ETS in their home have higher rates of asthma and upper respiratory infections.[73] This fact has resulted in a public service announcement campaign from the CDC to inform the public of the risk.

Another concern is that youth are the most vulnerable population for initiation of tobacco use. According to the National Cancer Institute, initiation of tobacco use begins for most smokers prior to the age of 18.[79] Based on this, of the six objectives in *HP 2020* related to tobacco, three were focused on adolescents. The tobacco use objective aimed at the reduction of the initiation of tobacco use among children, adolescents, and young adults has eight targets. For objectives centered around initiation of use of tobacco products in those aged 12 to 17, by 2017 there was a decline across all products exceeding the 2020 target.[70]

Screening and Treatment for Tobacco Use

Like other substance use, screening for tobacco use includes assessment of quantity and frequency. It is also standard to ask what type of tobacco is used and history of past use. Most current users of tobacco are daily users, thus the standard screening question asks the person if they use tobacco products, if so, how much on average per day. The key is how the question is framed. The question should be "Have you ever used tobacco?" rather than "Do you smoke cigarettes?" Because tobacco use includes smokeless tobacco, cigars, pipes, and other forms of inhaling tobacco, it is important to identify those with a history of tobacco use. A good screening tool is to use the single-question approach recommended by the National Institute on Drug Abuse (NIDA), which can be combined with screening for alcohol, tobacco use, and other drug use by asking a single question related to at-risk use.[80] Because any current use of tobacco is considered at-risk, if the person is a current tobacco user, the next step in the screening process is to determine the person's readiness to quit. If they are, the next step is to assist the person. If they are not willing to quit, you can provide support to help motivate them to quit by offering information on smoking cessation. Finally, arrange for follow up. If the person is not a current tobacco user, it is important to determine if they are a former user of tobacco and if they are at risk for relapse. It is also important to determine if they are exposed to secondhand smoke.[73]

Smoking cessation can occur for some without any intervention. However, over the past 2 decades, strides have been made in the development of methods to assist those who wish to stop smoking. Most former smokers quit without using one of the treatments that scientific research has shown can work. According to the CDC, there are a number of evidence-based approaches to smoking cessation. They include: brief help by a health-care provider; counseling, including individual, group, or telephone; behavioral therapies; mobile phone-assisted treatment; and medications.[81] Medications used for smoking cessation include over-the-counter and prescription nicotine replacement products and prescription non-nicotine medications such as bupropion SR (Zyban®) and varenicline tartrate (Chantix®). A combination of some form of counseling and medication is more effective than using either one by itself.[81,82,83]

Policy Level Intervention to Reduce Tobacco-Related Harm: Local to Global

There are a number of events in U.S. history that coincided with changes in the smoking behavior of the American public, many of them associated with policy. Tobacco use in the U.S. rose steadily from the great depression, through World War II, and then peaked during the 1960s and 1970s. The period from 1934 to the end of World War II (1945) saw a consistent, almost 300% increase in number of cigarettes consumed.

Consumption dropped off again in the mid-1950s when the first evidence of the association of cancer and cigarette smoking was found. Both of those periods of reduced cigarette consumption were followed by a rebound to levels higher than they were before. In 1964, this phenomenon ceased.[84]

With the release of the first Surgeon General's report on Smoking and Health, a period began of reduced cigarette consumption that has continued over the past 3 decades. In addition, the Federal Communication Commission (FCC) applied the Fair-Trade Act of 1949 to tobacco advertising. The point of this was to offer a no-cost opportunity to present health information that was directed toward smoking cessation. The application of the Fair-Trade Act would have given the same amount of time to the anti-smoking initiatives (at no cost) as was purchased by the cigarette industry for advertising. Application of the Fair-Trade Act seemed to be associated with a marked decrease in number of cigarettes smoked. Shortly following the ban on television advertising, however, the resulting elimination of free anti-smoking advertising, and the smoker's rights movement in the 1970s, cigarette smoking increased again. The Great American Smoke Out of 1977 hosted by the American Cancer Society appears to be the beginning of a fairly consistent decline in cigarette consumption. This provided opportunities to encourage people to commit and quit smoking while increasing public awareness of harms associated with smoking. In the 1980s, nonsmokers' rights movements began with eventual changes in policies related to smoking in public places, advertising restrictions, and increased taxes.[84]

Currently, global public health efforts include both individual and population-level strategies with the objective of reducing tobacco related harm. The WHO's Report on the Global Health Epidemic 2017 uses the acronym MPOWER to lay out policy steps needed to reduce tobacco use and includes interventions at the individual and the population level (Table 11-3).[85] Since MPOWER was released, the number of countries that have implemented at least one of the recommended measures has risen from 42 to 121. Eight countries have implemented four or more of the measures. In tandem with adoption of these measures has been a global decline in current tobacco use globally from 24% in 2007 to 21% in 2015. One example of these types of population-level actions is smoke-free environments. Two cities in China, Shanghai and Shenzhen, instituted a smoking ban that included indoor public places, workplaces, and public transport as well as many outdoor public places. These measures require support at the

TABLE 11–3 ■ World Health Organization MPOWER: Effective Tobacco Control	
Monitor	Monitor tobacco use and prevention policies
Protect	Protect people from tobacco smoke
Offer	Offer help to quit tobacco use
Warn	Warn about the dangers of tobacco
Enforce	Enforce bans on tobacco advertising, promotion and sponsorship
Raise	Raise taxes on tobacco

Source: (84)

national level.[85] In the U.S., the CDC has published Best Practices for Comprehensive Tobacco Control Programs.[86] The five areas presented by the CDC include state and community interventions, mass-reach health communication interventions, cessation interventions, surveillance and evaluation, and infrastructure, administration, and management.

Drug Use

The opioid overdose epidemic brought the issue of drug use to the national forefront. In addition to opioid use, the use of stimulants such as methamphetamine and cocaine continues with subsequent adverse effects on individuals and communities, resulting in what has been called a public health crisis. Drug use affects individuals, families, and communities because it can cause serious health consequences, environmental pollution, increased crime, and, due to potential overdose, a significant increase in mortality.[87]

In 2017, it was estimated that a little more than 11% of Americans reported illicit drug use during the past 30 days, up from a little more than 8% in 2010.[2] The most prevalent illicit drug used was marijuana (9.6%) followed by nonmedical use of psychotherapeutics (sedatives, painkillers, stimulants) (2.2%), cocaine (0.8%), and hallucinogens (0.5%).[2] Males were more apt to report current illicit drug use. Illicit drug use varies across age groups with those 18 to 25 reporting the highest current use (24.2%).[2] There was an overall decline in current illicit drug use among 12 to 17-year-olds from a high of 11.6% in 2002 to 7.9% in 2017.[2] Those aged 65 years or older reported the lowest use at 3%.[2] However, current illicit drug use is higher among adults aged 50 to 59 with an increase from 2.7% in 2002 to 9.5% in 2009.[2] It is worth noting that rates of illicit use may be higher and likely to be underreported due to the illegality of these substances.

❱ SOLVING THE MYSTERY

The Case of the Morgue Pile Up: New Hampshire and the Opioid Epidemic

Public Health Science Topics Covered:
- Epidemiology
- Surveillance
- Program Planning

Up to this point, we have largely been talking about SUDs in relation to individuals or populations. The fact is, however, that substance abuse is a community-wide problem, affecting not just individuals but also the community and health-care providers confronted with the grim reality of the impact drug use has on a community.

In 2018, New Hampshire led the nation in per capita overdose deaths.[6,88] Reporter Katharine Seeley from the New York Times wondered why New Hampshire, one of the wealthier states in the country, was experiencing such a high prevalence of opioid use and subsequent high overdose mortality rate. She discovered a report that helped explain the multiple factors that contributed to the crisis.[88] The two main factors were access to opioids and lack of access to treatment. On the supply and demand side, New Hampshire borders Massachusetts, which has a large illicit drug distribution network, making access to opioids easier. In addition, the state has higher rates of prescribing opioids. On the treatment side, there are limited resources for those in need of treatment. Barriers to treatment include lengthy waitlists and trouble navigating the system. There is also little funding for treatment on the consumer and program side. There are also staffing shortages.[88]

Using the steps in program planning, the HotSpot report[89] demonstrates completion of the first step in the process, assessment. Based on their assessment, they found that overdoses increased in New Hampshire by almost 1,600% from 2010 to 2015. Based on these statistics, a number of groups partnered to do a Rapid "HotSpot" study in two phases. Phase one was with stakeholders and phase two was a survey conducted with opioid users (n = 76) and with first responders/emergency department personnel (n=36).

The collected data helped them identify the next steps in the process (Box 11-4).

The challenge in the program planning part is to decide what recommendations to act on and what barriers may further impede the ability to act on those recommendations. One barrier is the culture of New Hampshire, the state whose motto is "live free or die" with an emphasis on self-sufficiency. For example, the state does not have laws that require using seat belts and allows liquor stores to be next to major highways. Other issues include the lack of health-care providers in the field of substance use and the lack of needle exchange programs.

In alignment with the harm reduction recommendation from the report, in 2017, two Dartmouth medical students opened a needle exchange program in a soup kitchen.[90] The program uses a harm reduction model built on community partnerships including working with the fire chief, the police chief, the mayor, and community organizers such as Hope for Recovery within the county. The program is located in the Southwestern Shelter, across the street from a soup kitchen, and is open at the same time the kitchen is providing meals. The students distribute supplies such as clean needles and sharps containers for safe disposal. They also distribute naloxone and teach how to recognize signs of overdose and how to use naloxone.

BOX 11–4 ■ HotSpot Report: Understanding Opioid Overdoses in New Hampshire: Next Steps

Based on data from this study, preliminary considerations for New Hampshire's approach to tackling the opioid overdose crisis include:

- Increase public health funds targeting substance use
- Expand prevention programs in elementary and middle schools
- Strengthen treatment to include broader availability, non-prohibitive cost, and inclusion of medication-assisted options and holistic approaches
- Incentivize physicians to become buprenorphine-waivered providers
- Assist physicians with prudent prescribing of opioids, educating patients, and alternatives to pain management
- Support first responder and emergency department personnel with vicarious trauma associated with responding to overdoses
- Initiate needle exchange programs
- Collaborate with Massachusetts on addressing the manufacturing and trafficking of fentanyl and other opioids
- Launch programming to dispel stigma and fear:
  - Educate consumers (e.g., Narcan and Good Samaritan Law)
  - Educate physicians and pharmacists (e.g., chronic disease management and value of Narcan)
  - Educate law enforcement (e.g., alternative approaches to punitive measures)
  - Educate the public (e.g., opioid crisis is not isolated to one demographic/area and breaking the intergenerational cycle of addiction)

Source: (87)

One of the recommendations listed in the HotSpot Report was to increase the number of health-care providers able to deliver medication-assisted treatment. Placing those with an opioid use disorder on a similar acting medication has been controversial, yet evidence points to this approach as more effective in reducing relapse than an abstinence-based approach.

■ EVIDENCE-BASED PRACTICE
Medication Assisted Treatment (MAT)

The use of medications to treat an SUD has been in practice for many decades. With the opioid epidemic, there has been an increased focus on using MAT in conjunction with other treatments as an effective treatment for both opioid use disorders and AUDs. The use of MAT has also increased as a means to treat a nicotine use disorder. Some medications, especially buprenorphine and methadone, opioid agonists, result in long term maintenance while other medications, such as those used to treat a nicotine use disorder are used with the ultimate goal of abstinence.

Practice Statement: Increase availability of MAT to adults suffering from a SUD with FDA-approved effective medications.

Targeted Outcome: Reduction in health risks associated with substance use and to achieve abstinence from use.

Supporting Evidence: For an opioid use disorder in adults, MAT has been shown to be effective not only in reducing overdose deaths but also improving social functioning, reducing the risk of transmitting communicable disease, reducing criminal behavior, and for pregnant women improving neonatal outcomes.[1] The two medications approved for use by the FDA are buprenorphine and methadone. Both medications are opioid agonists and long-acting medications, thus reducing cravings and likelihood of subsequent relapse; both medications exemplify a harm reduction approach. In addition, both medications were associated with substantial reductions in mortality in people being treated for an opioid use disorder.[2] For an AUD, acamprosate calcium, disulfiram, oral naltrexone, and extended-release injectable naltrexone are approved for use in the treatment and have established effectiveness.[3] For nicotine use disorders, bupropion, nicotine replacement therapies (NRTs), and varenicline are approved for use and have established effectiveness.[4] For other substances such as cannabis, cocaine, or methamphetamine, there are no FDA-approved medications to treat an SUD. There is insufficient evidence on the effectiveness of MAT with adolescents or the possible negative impact on the developing adolescent brain.[5]

Recommended Approaches: The use of MAT is seen as part of a more comprehensive treatment plan that includes behavioral treatment. Access to MAT is an issue especially with the opioid epidemic.[4] Methadone clinics must comply with federal regulations. Physicians, nurse practitioners, and physician assistants who have completed the required training may now dispense Buprenorphine in primary care settings, yet few actually complete training. Social stigma related to SUDs can also impact the ability to open methadone clinics or for practitioners to complete the training and work with patients with a SUD.

References

1. Volkow, N.D., Frieden, T.R., Hyde, P.S., & Cha, S.S. (2014). Medication-assisted therapies — Tackling the opioid-overdose epidemic. *New England Journal of Medicine, 370*, 2063-2066. DOI: 10.1056/NEJMp1402780.
2. Substance Abuse and Mental Health Services Administration and National Institute on Alcohol Abuse and Alcoholism. (2015). *Medication for the treatment of alcohol use disorder: A brief guide.* HHS Publication No. (SMA) 15-4907. Rockville, MD: Substance Abuse and Mental Health Services Administration.
3. Sordo, L., Barrio, G., Bravo, M.J., Indave, B.I., Degenhardt, L., ... Pastor-Barriuso, R. (2017). Mortality risk during and after opioid substitution treatment: Systematic review and meta-analysis of cohort studies. *British Medical Journal, 26*, 357:j1550. doi: 10.1136/bmj.j1550.
4. National Institute on Drug Abuse. (2017). *Principles of adolescent substance use disorder treatment: A research-based guide.* Retrieved from https://www.drugabuse.gov/publications/principles-adolescent-substance-use-disorder-treatment-research-based-guide/evidence-based-approaches-to-treating-adolescent-substance-use-disorders/addiction-medications.
5. Vashishtha, D., Mittal, M.L., and Werb, D. (2017). The North American opioid epidemic: Current challenges and a call for treatment as prevention. *Harm Reduction Journal, 14*, 7. Retrieved from https://www.ncbi.nlm.nih.gov/pmc/articles/PMC5427522/ doi: 10.1186/s12954-017-0135-4.

In addition to opioids, methamphetamines (meth) have also negatively impacted communities. Persons who use meth present in a number of ways. They can appear euphoric, tremulous, anorexic, with dilated pupils, or with diaphoresis. Continued use results in weight loss, strong body odor, dry mouth, and tactile hallucinations that often take the form of imagined insects under the skin. These tactile hallucinations can result in infections and lesions on the skin where the user scratches or tries to remove the insects. In an attempt to relieve dry mouth, the user often drinks copious amounts of sugary beverages, which contributes to tooth decay in addition to other dental manifestations associated with methamphetamine use such as bruxism, gingival inflammation, decreased saliva production, and lower pH values.[91] Long-term use can result in cachexia, alopecia, corneal ulcerations, repetitive behavior patterns, and severe mental illness symptoms. Harm done to the family is predictably similar to the harm done by the use of other substances. Meth is less expensive than cocaine or heroin, so it appeals to those in the lower socioeconomic groups, that is, those who can least afford it financially.[92]

Meth is easily manufactured, particularly in states lacking laws regulating the sale of the key components for manufacture. Interestingly, the early centers of manufacture were the farming communities of the Midwest and Western U.S. The ease with which meth is manufactured and its increasing popularity facilitated the spread of meth "labs" throughout the U.S. and Mexico. These labs can be located in homes, apartments, trailers, campers, caves, or any place of shelter.[93]

Some of the chemical components of meth are quite caustic in their own right. They can include pool acid/muriatic acid, lye, acetone, brake fluid, brake cleaner, iodine crystals, lithium metal/lithium batteries, lighter fluid, drain cleaners, cold medicine containing pseudoephedrine or ephedrine, ethyl ether (in engine starting fluid), anhydrous ammonia (stored in propane tanks or coolers), sodium metal, and red phosphorous. Often, manufacturers of meth are either careless or lack knowledge regarding the proper handling of the components, which often leads to fires and explosions.[94]

Some "superlabs" can manufacture up to 100 pounds of meth per day. For every pound of meth produced, there are 5 to 6 pounds of toxic waste produced as well. This is an environmental disaster in the making. The manufacturers of meth dispose of the waste in a number of ways; flushing down the toilet, pouring into drains, burying, and pouring on the ground.[93]

Unlike other illicit drugs, pollution of the environment with a hazardous chemical is a major issue connected to the production of meth. The threat to the water supply, health of the soil, and people in the surrounding areas is clear. Toxic waste byproducts from meth production can be in suspension in the air and settle on furniture, carpeting, floors, tables, food, and toys, creating a serious threat to those who reside where the labs are located, especially children. Children in such environments not only suffer from neglect but also are exposed to hazardous materials.[95] When a meth lab is seized by law enforcement officials, assuming welfare of the children and treatment and/or incarceration for the users/manufacturers is only the beginning. For first responders, there are occupational health hazards that need to be addressed. Hazmat teams must be summoned to decontaminate and clean up the area where the lab was located. This process usually costs thousands of dollars or more, depending on the size of the lab.[93]

Consequences of Drug Use

The consequences of drug use for individuals vary based on the pharmacokinetics of the drug used. For example, cocaine is a stimulant; thus, while under the effect of the drug, the individual experiences a stimulation of the CNS. These effects include an increase in energy, a decreased need for sleep, and increased mental alertness. It also has a stimulant effect on the cardiovascular system including constriction of the blood vessels, dilated pupils, and increased heart rate and blood pressure. Once the drug has left the system, the person experiences a rebound effect, an understimulation of the CNS that can result in depression and decreased energy.[96] Persons who use drugs are at increased risk for comorbid mental disorders, sexually transmitted infections (STIs), and other adverse effects on health secondary to the use of the specific drug.[97]

Vulnerable Populations Across the Life Span

As with alcohol and tobacco, the portions of the population most vulnerable to the effects of drugs are the fetus, youth, and the young adult. Use of drugs has been associated with adverse maternal and infant outcomes. The variation of the adverse effects again relates to the pharmacokinetics of the drug used. Adverse effects include prematurity, small for gestational age, neonatal withdrawal, and birth defects. In addition, women who use illegal drugs during pregnancy are at higher risk for poor nutrition, are more apt to engage in prenatal care later during the gestational period or not at all, and are at greater risk for STIs.[98]

For youth and the young adult, the focus is on prevention of use. In 2015, 10.1% of youth age 12 to 17 reported current use of an illicit drug. In young adults, the rate increased to a little over one-fifth (22.3%) of those ages 18 to 25 reporting current illicit drug use. Three of the *HP 2020* objectives related to substance abuse focused on the adolescent, specifically increasing the proportion who report never using substances, who disapprove of substance use, and who perceive great risk associated with substance use.[6]

To address the issue of adolescent drug use, the NIDA published two guides, Principles of Substance Abuse Prevention in Early Childhood[99] and Principles of Adolescent Substance Use Disorder Treatment: A Research-Based Guide,[100] both aimed at preventing drug use and providing guidance for providers to help adolescents identified with a drug use disorder. Issues associated with drug use in adolescents include not only social consequences but cognitive development.[101] Researchers are beginning to identify possible adverse effects of marijuana on brain development.[101, 102, 103] These findings underscore the need for prevention of drug use and the importance of screening and offering age appropriate treatment when indicated.

Screening and Treatment for Drug Use

A number of screening instruments are available to screen for drug use. One widely used is the Drug Abuse Screening Test (DAST-10). It screens for drug use excluding alcoholic beverages. The DAST-10 has been shown to be reliable and valid with both English-speaking and Spanish-speaking populations, and with those individuals seeking treatment for Attention-Deficit/Hyperactivity

Disorder (ADHD).[104] Another tool is the NIDA ASSIST tool. It is available online and covers the different types of drugs of abuse.[105, 106]

As with alcohol and tobacco, there is a clinician's guide that incorporates both screening and interventions.[106] The guide gives the health-care provider an excellent overview of interventions that can be instituted at the individual level including pharmacological approaches, the use of self-help groups, and behavioral therapies. SAMHSA also recommends using the SBIRT framework to address drug use in the same way used for those with at-risk alcohol use.[107]

Policy Level Intervention to Reduce Drug Use–Related Harm

Policy related to drug use has been a hot topic for decades. Most policy has focused on controlling drug use through criminal means. In the U.S., drug policy has come under the title of a "war on drugs" complete with a federal level drug "czar." The Office of National Drug Control Policy (ONDCP) is the national level organization focused on drug policy. The purpose of the office is to "… reduce drug use and limit its consequences by leading and coordinating the development, implementation, and assessment of U.S. drug policy." This office also provides administrative and financial support to special commissions at the federal level such as the President's Commission on Combating Drug Addiction and the Opioid Crisis, established by Executive Order on March 29, 2017.[108] Under President Obama, the focus of the ONDCP shifted from prosecution to increasing access to treatment. Under President Trump, the focus has shifted back to a focus on criminalization of drug use and a "just say no" approach to prevention.

Substance Use and Communicable Diseases

A prime example of how substance use contributes to the burden of disease is the association between substance use and communicable diseases. This occurs across multiple levels starting with the increased the risk of transmission of a communicable disease down to the cellular level.

Many communicable diseases such as hepatitis, HIV/AIDS, sexually transmitted infections, and tuberculosis are associated with substance use. Since the beginning of the HIV epidemic, substance use and increased risk of transmission of HIV have been strongly correlated. In a landmark study, McKusick, Horstman, and Coates (1985) examined the relationship between sexual behavior and HIV.[109] Subsequent research over the past 30 years has established that substance use often leads to impulsive behaviors, as a result of altered judgment, and engagement in high-risk sexual behavior (i.e., sexual intercourse without a condom, transactional sex, or sex-work) thus placing persons at risk for sexually transmitted infections.

Other issues also contribute to an increased risk of poorer outcomes. People living with HIV and who have been diagnosed with an SUD are also less likely to be engaged in care, to be adherent to antiretroviral treatment, and to achieve viral suppression, and are thus more likely to spread HIV to others.[110] Additionally, particular substances such as methamphetamine have also been linked to increased HIV viral load in the brain as well as neuronal damage, which leads to the development of HIV-associated neurocognitive disorders (HAND).[110,111]

Substance Use and Stigma

Substance use has a long history of being viewed from a moral standpoint. Moral views of substance use vary based on ethnic culture, social practices, the specific substance in question, and the gender of the substance user. Often the person who engages in risky substance use suffers stigma. **Stigma** is defined as a mark of disgrace or reproach. The person who is suffering from stigma often experiences shame, which in turn impacts their engagement in treatment.

Stigma has not always been experienced with substance use if the use is seen as a social norm. For example, tobacco use was a culturally acceptable practice for men in the United States, especially during the early to mid-20th century. However, women who smoked before World War II were perceived negatively. Many of the early tobacco ads aimed at getting women to smoke suggested that women should defy this moral stand and smoke. By the 1960s and early 1970s, some tobacco companies took this one step further and created a specific brand for women, such as Virginia Slims, and created ads that linked cigarette use to the feminist movement. By the 1990s, cigarette smoking shifted from acceptable social practice to a culturally reprehensible practice. The scientific evidence that ETS resulted in adverse effects for the nonsmoker, coupled with a growing intolerance of the odor of tobacco smoke in public places, resulted in bans against public smoking with a subsequent benefit to the population as a whole. But has this shift also resulted in a moral shunning of the tobacco user?

The stigma related to alcohol use has, for the most part, focused on risky use or those with an AUD. One exception is the temperance movement in the late 1800s and early 1900s that resulted in the passing of the 18th amendment in 1919. This amendment, also known as Prohibition, effectively turned alcohol into an illicit drug. It was repealed in 1933, and alcohol use once again became a socially acceptable and normative practice. However, the judgment that a person who had an AUD was morally reprehensible did not change. The stigma associated with being an "alcoholic" resulted in the creation of confidentiality as a core principle in 12 step programs.

An example of a cultural shift related to alcohol use is the banning of drinking and driving. In the 1950s, the phrase "one for the road" was socially acceptable. Although law enforcement attempted to deal with drunk driving, it was hard to determine what constituted drunkenness. A number of events contributed to a cultural shift in our view of driving under the influence (DUI).[112] These include the advent of the Mothers Against Drunk Driving movement, technological advances in measuring BAC, and evidence related to what constituted impaired driving. A cultural shift began in relation to public tolerance of the drunk driver. Today, all states have laws that restrict impaired driving in some capacity. Most states have laws that stipulate a precise BAC that, when present, constitutes proof that the individual is too impaired to drive. In addition, the law has evolved to the point that most states allow for proof of impairment through other means, such as specific field sobriety tests. All of these laws represent an attempt to discourage individuals from driving when they have been drinking or using drugs because it is often difficult for an individual to determine when they have had too much to drink.

Stigma is a continuing concern for persons who engage in risky drug use, especially when it becomes a barrier to treatment.[113-115] Stigma is pervasive in the general and medical community. Examples of stigma in the nursing literature can be found, including articles about pregnant women engaged in illicit drug use or nurses who may be impaired.[115-119] Stigma arises from the perception that risky substance use is a personal choice and the consequences are self-inflicted. The ONDCP support of midstream interventions reflects a growing emphasis on educating the national population on the benefits of treatment and the potential cost of continuing to treat substance use from a legal "war on drugs" approach. In addition, people with a SUD often experience discrimination and health inequities that further impede access to quality health-care services.[118,119]

Improving care delivery to this population by implementing a patient-centered approach and harm reduction interventions will address the issue of stigma and advance health outcomes.[120]

Summary Points

- At-risk substance use affects the overall health of the individual, family, and the community.
- Substance use results in adverse consequences from the cellular to the global level.
- Substance use varies across the life span with increased vulnerability for youth, young adults, and pregnant women.
- Evidence-based practices exist in relation to prevention programs, screening, brief intervention, and treatment.
- Substance use, especially use of tobacco and alcohol, are serious public health issues, and policy initiatives exist at the global, national, state, and local levels aimed at reducing the harm associated with at-risk substance use.
- Cultural context for substance use has shifted over time, but stigma continues to be a barrier for entrance into treatment for the person with at-risk use or an SUD.

▼ CASE STUDY

Implementing an Opioid Overdose Prevention Program

Learning Outcomes

- Apply program planning to the development and implementation of a health program.
- Examine current standards of care related to opioid overdose treatment
- Identify strategies for training the public in recognizing opioid overdose and steps need to prevent overdose death.

You have been asked to work with a community group to address the opioid epidemic. You suggest implementing a program in your county based on the program implemented by the medical students at Dartmouth College that combined a clean needle exchange program with a program for distribution of Naloxone.

- Outline the basic steps for building this program (see Chapters 4 and 5) and who you would involve in each step.

- Identify:
  - The main partners you would bring on board for the program.
  - At least one barrier to implementing the program and steps you would take to overcome the barrier.
  - Key data you will need to collect to evaluate the program.
- What strategies would you use achieve sustainability?

REFERENCES

1. America's Opioid Epidemic. (2017). *CBS News*. Retrieved from https://www.cbsnews.com/opioid-epidemic/.
2. Center for Behavioral Health Statistics and Quality. (2018). *2017 National Survey on Drug Use and Health: Detailed Tables*. Rockville, MD: Substance Abuse and Mental Health Services Administration. Retrieved from https://www.samhsa.gov/data/sites/default/files/cbhsq-reports/NSDUHDetailedTabs2017/NSDUHDetailedTabs2017.pdf.
3. Azofeifa, A., Mattson, M.E., Schauer, G., McAfee, T., Grant, A., Lyerla, R. (2016). National estimates of marijuana use and related indicators — National Survey on Drug Use and Health, United States, 2002–2014. *MMWR Surveillance Summary, 65*(No. SS-11), 1–25. DOI: http://dx.doi.org/10.15585/mmwr.ss6511a1.
4. National Institute on Alcohol Abuse and Alcoholism. (2017). *Alcohol facts and statistics*. Retrieved from https://www.niaaa.nih.gov/alcohol-health/overview-alcohol-consumption/alcohol-facts-and-statistics.
5. Centers for Disease Control and Prevention. (2017). *Fast facts: Smoking and tobacco use*. Retrieved from https://www.cdc.gov/tobacco/data_statistics/fact_sheets/fast_facts/index.htm.
6. World Health Organization. (2017). *Management of substance abuse*. Retrieved from http://www.who.int/substance_abuse/en/.
7. United Nations Office on Drug Control. (2017). *World drug report*. Retrieved from https://www.unodc.org/wdr2017/index.html.
8. World Health Organization. (2018). *Fact sheet: Alcohol*. Retrieved from http://www.who.int/news-room/fact-sheets/detail/alcohol.
9. World Health Organization. (2018). *Global status report on alcohol and health 2018*. Geneva, Switzerland: WHO Press.
10. United Nations. (2017). *Report of the International Narcotics Control Board for 2016*. Retrieved from https://www.incb.org/documents/Publications/AnnualReports/AR2016/English/AR2016_E_ebook.pdf.
11. The International Association of Chiefs of Police (2019). *7 Drug Categories*. Retrieved from https://www.theiacp.org/7-drug-categories
12. Mahmud, K.F.M., Mitchell, A., Finnell, D.S., Savage, C.L., Puskar, K.R. (2017). A concept analysis of substance misuse to inform contemporary terminology. *Archives of Psychiatric Nursing*. DOI: 10.1016/j.apnu.2017.06.004.
13. Centers for Disease Control and Prevention. (2017). *FACTS about FASD*. Retrieved from https://www.cdc.gov/ncbddd/fasd/facts.html.
14. Tapert, S.F., Caldwell, L., & Burke, C. (2004). *Alcohol and the adolescent brain—Human studies*. Alcohol Research & Health, National Institute on Alcohol Abuse and Alcoholism. Retrieved from https://pubs.niaaa.nih.gov/publications/arh284/205-212.htm.
15. Feldstein, S.W., Ewing, F., Sakhardandeb, A., Blakemoreb, S.J., (2014). The effect of alcohol consumption on the adolescent brain: A systematic review of MRI and fMRI studies of alcohol-using youth. *NeuroImage: Clinical, 5*, 420-437. Retrieved from https://doi.org/10.1016/j.nicl.2014.06.011.
16. Vetreno, R.P., & Crews, F.T. (2018). Adolescent binge ethanol-induced loss of basal forebrain cholinergic neurons and neuroimmune activation are prevented by exercise and indomethacin. *PLoS One, 13*(10), e0204500.
17. Han, B.H., & Moore, A.A. (2018). Prevention and screening of unhealthy substance use by older adults. *Clinical Geriatric Medicine, 34*, 117–129. doi:org/10.1016/j.cger.2017.08.005.
18. World Health Organization. (2015). *Alcohol fact sheet*. Retrieved from http://www.who.int/mediacentre/factsheets/fs349/en/.
19. Degenhardt, L., Hall, W.D., Farrell, M., & Whiteford, H.A., (2014). Illicit drug dependence across the globe: Results from the Global Burden of Disease 2010 Study. *Psychiatric Times, 31*(2).
20. Degenhardt, L. & Hall, W. (2016). Extent of illicit drug use and dependence, and their contribution to the global burden of disease. *Lancet, 379*(9810), 55-70. DOI:10.1016/S0140-6736(11)61138-0.
21. Britton, J. (2017). Death, disease, and tobacco. *Lancet, 389*. Published Online. April 5, 2017. http://dx.doi.org/10.1016/S0140-6736(17)30867-X.
22. Global Commission on Drug Policy. (2011). *War on drugs: Report of the Global Commission on Drug Policy*. Retrieved from http://online.wsj.com/public/resources/documents/GlobalCommissionReport0601.pdf.
23. American Psychiatric Association. (2013). *Diagnostic and statistical manual of mental disorder: DSM-5* (5th ed.). Arlington, VA: American Psychiatric Association.
24. Centers for Disease Control and Prevention. (2017). *Fact sheets - Binge drinking*. Retrieved from https://www.cdc.gov/alcohol/fact-sheets/binge-drinking.htm.
25. National Institute on Alcohol Abuse and Alcoholism. (2017). *What is a standard drink?* Retrieved from https://www.niaaa.nih.gov/alcohol-health/overview-alcohol-consumption/what-standard-drink.
26. National Institute on Drug Addiction. (2012). *Principles of drug addiction treatment: A research-based guide* (3rd ed.). Retrieved from https://www.drugabuse.gov/publications/principles-drug-addiction-treatment-research-based-guide-third-edition.
27. Institute of Medicine (IOM) Prevention Model. (1997). *Drug abuse prevention: What works*. Rockville, MD: National Institute of Drug Abuse, pp 10-15.
28. International Harm Reduction Association. (n.d.). *What is harm reduction?* Retrieved from https://www.hri.global/files/2010/05/31/IHRA_HRStatement.pdf.
29. Beirness, D.J., Jesseman, R., Notaradrea, R., & Perron, M. (2008). *Harm reduction, what's in a name*. Canadian Center

on Substance Abuse. Retrieved from http://www.ccsa.ca/ Resource%20Library/ccsa0115302008e.pdf#search=harm %20reduction.

30. U.S. Department of Health and Human Services. (2017). *Healthy People 2020 topics and objectives: Substance abuse.* Retrieved from http://www.healthypeople.gov/2020/ topicsobjectives2020/overview.aspx?topicid=40.

31. National Center for Health Statistics. (2016). *Chapter 40, Substance Abuse in Healthy People 2020 Midcourse Review.* Hyattsville, MD: National Center for Health Statistics.

32. Wolf, L., et al. (2017). Factors associated with pediatric mortality from motor vehicle crashes in the United States: A state-based analysis. *Journal of Pediatrics.* DOI: 10.1016/ j.jpeds.2017.04.044.

33. Centers for Disease Control and Prevention. (2017). *Impaired driving, get the facts.* Retrieved from https://www. cdc.gov/motorvehiclesafety/impaired_driving/impaired-drv_factsheet.html.

34. Substance Abuse and Mental Health Services Administration (US); Office of the Surgeon General (US) (2016). *Chapter Two; The neurobiology of substance use, misuse and addiction, in facing addiction in America: The Surgeon General's Report on alcohol, drugs, and health.* Washington, DC: U.S. Department of Health and Human Services.

35. Centers for Disease Control and Prevention. (2017). *Fact sheets: Alcohol and your health.* Retrieved from https://www.cdc.gov/alcohol/fact-sheets/alcohol-use.htm.

36. U.S. Department of Health and Human Services. (2018). *Healthy People 2020 topics and objectives: substance abuse.* Retrieved from https://www.healthypeople.gov/2020/ topics-objectives/topic/substance-abuse/objectives.

37. National Institute on Alcohol Abuse and Alcoholism. (n.d.). *Alcohol's effects on the body.* Retrieved December 2, 2018, from https:www.niaaa.nih.gov/alcohol-health/alcohols-effects-body.

38. U.S. Department of Health and Human Services. (2018). *Healthy People 2020 Leading Health Indicators; Substance abuse.* Retrieved from https://www.healthypeople.gov/ sites/default/files/HP2020_LHI_Subs_Abuse.pdf.

39. LoConte, N.K., Brewster, A.M., Kaur, J.S., Merrill, J.K., & Alberg, A.J. (2018). Alcohol and cancer: A statement of the American Society of Clinical Oncology. *Journal of Clinical Oncology, 36*(1), 83-93.

40. Seitz, H.K., & Mueller, S. (2015). Alcohol and cancer: An overview with special emphasis on the role of acetaldehyde and cytochrome P450 2E1. In: Vasiliou, V., Zakhari, S., Seitz, H., Hoek, J.B. (eds). *Biological basis of alcohol-induced cancer.* New York: Springer International Publishing.

41. Rogers, R.G., Boardman, J.D., Pendergast, P.M., & Lawrence, E.M. (2015). Drinking problems and mortality risk in the United States. *Drug and Alcohol Dependence, 151*, 38–46. DOI: http://dx.doi.org/10.1016/j.drugalcdep.2015.02.039.

42. Tembo, C., Burns, S., & Kalembo, F. (2017). The association between levels of alcohol consumption and mental health problems and academic performance among young university students. *PLoS One, 12*(6), e0178142. https:// doi.org/10.1371/journal.pone.0178142.

43. Martinez, P., Neupane, S.P., Perlestenbakken, B., Toutoungi, C., & Bramness, J.G. (2015). The association between alcohol use and depressive symptoms across

socioeconomic status among 40- and 45-year-old Norwegian adults. *BMC Public Health, 15,* 1146. http://doi.org/ 10.1186/s12889-015-2479-6.

44. Centers for Disease Control and Prevention. (2017). *Fetal alcohol spectrum disorders: Diagnosis.* Retrieved from https://www.cdc.gov/ncbddd/fasd/diagnosis.html.

45. Lange, S., Probst, C., Gmel, G., Rehm, J., Burd, L., & Popova, S. (2017). Global prevalence of fetal alcohol spectrum disorder among children and youth: A systematic review and meta-analysis. *JAMA Pediatrics, 171*(10), 948–956. doi:10.1001/jamapediatrics.2017.1919.

46. Patrick, M.E., & Schulenberg, J.E. (2014). Prevalence and predictors of adolescent alcohol use and binge drinking in the United States. *Alcohol Research: Current Reviews, 35*(2), 193.

47. National Institute on Alcohol Abuse and Alcoholism. (2011). Alcohol screening and brief intervention for youth. Retrieved from https://pubs.niaaa.nih.gov/publications/Practitioner/ YouthGuide/YouthGuide.pdf.

48. Centers for Disease Control and Prevention. (2018). *Fact sheets – Underage drinking.* Retrieved from https://www.cdc.gov/alcohol/fact-sheets/underage-drinking.htm.

49. Maimaris, W., & McCambridge, J. (2014). Age of first drinking and adult alcohol problems: Systematic review of prospective cohort studies. *Journal of Epidemiology Community Health, 68*, 268-274.

50. Goldstein, N.S., Hodgson, N., Savage, C.L., & Walton-Moss, B. (2015). Alcohol use and the older adult woman. *The Journal for Nurse Practitioners, 11*(4), 436-442.

51. National Institute on Alcohol Abuse and Alcoholism. (2017). *Facts about aging and alcohol.* https://www.nia.nih.gov/ health/facts-about-aging-and-alcohol.

52. World Health Organization. (2017). *Management of substance use: Screening and brief intervention for alcohol problems in primary health care.* Retrieved from http://www. who.int/substance_abuse/activities/sbi/en/.

53. Savage C.L., & Finnell, D. (2015). A comparative review of guides for implementing alcohol screening and brief interventions in trauma and primary care settings. *Journal of Addictions Nursing, 26*(1), 47-50.

54. National Institute on Alcohol Abuse and Alcoholism. (2005). *Helping patients who drink too much: A clinician's guide.* Rockville MD: National Institute on Alcohol Abuse and Alcoholism.

55. American College of Surgeons Committee on Trauma. (n.d.). *Alcohol screening and brief intervention for trauma patients.* Retrieved from http://www.facs.org/trauma/ publications/sbirtguide.pdf.

56. Oncology Nursing Society. (2014). *Cancer pain management.* Retrieved November 26, 2014 from https://www.ons.org/ advocacy-policy/positions/practice/pain-management.

57. National Cancer Institute. (2017). *Cancer trends progress report 2017.* Retrieved November 24, 2018, from https:// progressreport.cancer.gov/sites/default/files/archive/ report2017.pdf.

58. Substance Abuse and Mental Health Services Administration. (2011). *Screening, brief intervention and referral to treatment (SBIRT) in behavioral healthcare.* Retrieved November 26, 2014, from http://www.samhsa.gov/sites/ default/files/sbirtwhitepaper_0.pdf.

59. López-Pelayo, H., Miquel, L., Altamirano, J., Blanch, J.L., Gual, A., & Lligoña, A. (2016). Alcohol consumption in upper aerodigestive tract cancer: Role of head and neck surgeons' recommendations. *Alcohol, 51,* 51-56.

60. World Health Organization. (2010). *The ASSIST-linked brief intervention for hazardous and harmful substance use: Manual for use in primary care.* France: WHO.

61. Centers for Disease Control and Prevention. (2014). *Planning and implementing screening and brief intervention for risky alcohol use: A step-by-step guide for primary care practices.* Atlanta, Georgia: Centers for Disease Control and Prevention, National Center on Birth Defects and Developmental Disabilities.

62. Jeong, H.S., Park, S., Lim, S.M., Ma, J., Kang, I., Kim, J., ... Kim, J.E. (2017). Psychometric properties of the alcohol use disorders identification test-consumption (AUDIT-C) in public first responders. *Substance Use & Misuse, 52* (8), 1069-1075. doi: 10.1080/10826084. 2016.1271986.

63. Osaki, Y., Ino, A., Matsushita, S., Higuchi, S., Kondo, Y., Kinjo, A. (2014). Reliability and validity of the alcohol use disorders identification test - consumption in screening for adults with alcohol use disorders and risky drinking in Japan. *Asian Pac Journal on Cancer Prevention, 15*(16), 6571-4.

64. Higgins-Biddle, J.C., & Babor, T.F. (2018). A review of the alcohol use disorders identification test (AUDIT), AUDIT-C, and USAUDIT for screening in the United States: Past issues and future directions. *The American Journal of Drug and Alcohol Abuse, 44*(6), 578-586.

65. Smith, P., Schmidt, S., Allensworth-Davies, D., & Saitz, R. (2010). A single-question screening test for drug use in primary care. *Archives of Internal Medicine, 170*(13), 1155–1160.

66. Barbor, T.F., McRee, B.G., Kassebaum, P.A., Grimaldi, P.L., Ahmed, K., & Bray, J. (2007). Screening. Brief intervention, and referral to treatment (SBIRT): Toward a public health approach to the management of substance abuse. *Substance Abuse, 28*(3), 7-30.

67. Higgins-Biddle, J., Hungerford, D., & Cates-Wessel, K. (2009). Screening and brief interventions (SBI) for unhealthy alcohol use: A step-by-step implementation guide for trauma centers. Atlanta, GA: Centers for Disease Control and Prevention, National Center for Injury Prevention and Control.

68. World Health Organization. (2018). *Management of substance abuse: Global strategy to reduce harmful use of alcohol.* Retrieved from http://www.who.int/substance_abuse/activities/gsrhua/en/.

69. World Health Organization. (2017). *Tobacco.* Retrieved from http://www.who.int/mediacentre/factsheets/fs339/en/.

70. Centers for Disease Control and Prevention. (2017). *Smoking and tobacco use: Fact sheet.* Retrieved from https://www.cdc.gov/tobacco/data_statistics/fact_sheets/fast_facts/index.htm.

71. U.S. Department of Health and Human Services, Centers for Disease Control and Prevention, National Center for Chronic Disease Prevention and Health Promotion, Office on Smoking and Health. (2014). *The health consequences of smoking – 50 years of progress: A report of the Surgeon General.* Retrieved from https://www.surgeongeneral.gov/library/reports/50-years-of-progress/full-report.pdf.

72. MacLean, R.R., Sofuoglu, M., & Rosenheck, R. (2017). Tobacco and alcohol use disorders: Evaluating multimorbidity. *Addictive Behavior, 78,* 59-66. doi: 10.1016/j.addbeh. 2017.11.006.

73. American Cancer Society. (2015). *Secondhand smoke.* Retrieved from https://www.cancer.org/cancer/cancer-causes/tobacco-and-cancer/secondhand-smoke.html.

74. Centers for Disease Control and Prevention. (2017). *Smoking and tobacco use: Data and statistics.* Retrieved from https://www.cdc.gov/tobacco/data_statistics/index.htm.

75. Centers for Disease Control and Prevention. (2017). Tobacco use among adults with mental illness and substance use disorders. Retrieved from https://www.cdc.gov/tobacco/disparities/mental-illness-substance-use/index.htm.

76. Nguyen, K.H., Marshall, L., Brown, S., & Neff, L. (2016). State-specific prevalence of current cigarette smoking and smokeless tobacco use among adults — United States. *Morbidity and Mortality Weekly Report,* 1045–1051. DOI: http://dx.doi.org/10.15585/mmwr.mm6539a1.

77. National Center for Health Statistics. (2016). *Chapter 41, Tobacco use in Healthy People 2020 Midcourse Review.* Hyattsville, MD: National Center for Health Statistics.

78. US Department of Health and Human Services. (2019). Healthy People 2020 Topics: Tobacco. Retrieved from https://www.healthypeople.gov/2020/topics-objectives/topic/tobacco-use

79. National Cancer Institute. (2019). Cancer Trends Progress Report: Tobacco Use Initiation. Retrieved from https://www.progressreport.cancer.gov/prevention/smoking_initiation.

80. National Institute on Drug Abuse. (n.d.). *NIDA quick screen V1.0.* Retrieved from https://www.drugabuse.gov/sites/default/files/files/QuickScreen_Updated_2013%281%29.pdf.

81. Dept. of Health and Human Services, Centers for Disease Control and Prevention, National Center for Chronic Disease Prevention and Health Promotion, Office on Smoking and Health. (2012). *Preventing tobacco use among youth and young adults: A report of the Surgeon General.* Washington, D.C.: Dept. of Health and Human Services.

82. Agency for Healthcare Research Quality. (2014). *Helping smokers quit, a guide for clinicians helping smokers quit.* Rockville, MD: Agency for Healthcare Research and Quality. Retrieved from http://www.ahrq.gov/professionals/clinicians-providers/guidelines-recommendations/tobacco/clinicians/references/clinhlpsmkqt/index.html.

83. Centers for Disease Control and Prevention. (2017). *Smoking and tobacco use: Quitting smoking.* Retrieved from https://www.cdc.gov/tobacco/data_statistics/fact_sheets/cessation/quitting/index.htm.

84. Centers for Disease Control and Prevention. (1999). Achievements in public health, 1900-1999: Tobacco use-United States, 1900-1999. *Morbidity and Mortality Weekly Report,* 48(43), 986-993.

85. World Health Organization. (2017). *Report on the Global Tobacco Health Epidemic 2017.* Geneva, Switzerland: World Health Organization. Retrieved from http://apps.who.int/iris/bitstream/10665/255874/1/9789241512824-eng.pdf?ua=1&ua=1.

86. Centers for Disease Control and Prevention. (2014). *Best practices for comprehensive tobacco control programs—2014.* Atlanta, GA: U.S. Department of Health and Human Services, Centers for Disease Control and Prevention, National Center for Chronic Disease Prevention and Health Promotion, Office on Smoking and Health.

87. U.S. Department of Health and Human Services. (2017). *About the epidemic.* Retrieved from https://www.hhs.gov/opioids/about-the-epidemic/.

88. Seeley, K. (January 21, 2018). How a 'perfect storm' in New Hampshire has fueled an opioid crisis. *New York Times.* Retrieved from https://www.nytimes.com/2018/01/21/us/new-hampshire-opioids-epidemic.html

89. Meier, A., Moore, S.K., Saunders, E.C., Metcalf, S.A., McLeman, B., Auty, S., & Marsch, L.A. (2017). *HotSpot report: Understanding opioid overdoses in New Hampshire.* Retrieved from https://ndews.umd.edu/publications/hotspot-report-understanding-opioid-overdoses-new-hampshire.

90. Green, S. (August 16, 2017). Geisel students confront granite state's opioid epidemic. *Geisel School of Medicine News.* Retrieved from http://geiselmed.dartmouth.edu/news/2017/geisel-students-confront-granite-states-opioid-epidemic/.

91. Rommel, N., Rohleder, N.H., Wagenpfeil, S., Haertel-Petri, R., & Kesting, M.R. (2015). Evaluation of methamphetamine-associated socioeconomic status and addictive behaviors, and their impact on oral health. *Addictive Behaviors, 50,* 182-187.

92. WA Methamphetamine Campaign. (2016). *WA methamphetamine campaign community toolkit.* Retrieved from http://drugaware.com.au/media/1193/161128_da_meth_communitykit_final.pdf.

93. Indiana State Public Health Department. (n.d.). *Methamphetamine lab response: Potential hazards and health concerns.* Retrieved from https://www.in.gov/isdh/26410.htm.

94. NIDA. (n.d). Methamphetamine abuse and addiction. How is methamphetamine abused? *NIDA News – Research Report Series.* Retrieved from http://www.nida.nih.gov/researchreports/methamph/methamph3.html.

95. Castaneto, M.S., Barnes, A.J., Scheidweiler, K.B., Schaffer, M., Rogers, K.K., Stewart, D., & Huestis, M.A. (2013). Identifying methamphetamine exposure in children. *Therapeutic Drug Monitoring, 35*(6), 10.1097/FTD.0b013e31829685b2. http://doi.org/10.1097/FTD.0b013e31829685b2.

96. National Institute on Drug Abuse. (2016). *Info facts: Cocaine.* Retrieved from https://www.drugabuse.gov/publications/drugfacts/cocaine.

97. National Institute on Drug Abuse. (2017). *Info facts.* Retrieved from http://www.drugabuse.gov/publications/term/160/InfoFacts.

98. March of Dimes. (2017). *Street drugs and pregnancy.* Retrieved from https://www.marchofdimes.org/pregnancy/street-drugs-and-pregnancy.aspx.

99. National Institute on Drug Abuse. (2016). *Principles of substance abuse prevention in early childhood.* Retrieved from https://www.drugabuse.gov/publications/principles-substance-abuse-prevention-early-childhood/index.

100. National Institute on Drug Abuse. (2014). *Principles of adolescent substance use disorder treatment: A research-based guide.* Retrieved from https://www.drugabuse.gov/publications/principles-adolescent-substance-use-disorder-treatment-research-based-guide/acknowledgements.

101. Price, J.S., McQueeny, T., Shollenbarger, S., Browning, E.L., Wieser, J., & Lisdahl, K. M. (2015). Effects of marijuana use on prefrontal and parietal volumes and cognition in emerging adults. *Psychopharmacology, 232*(16), 2939-2950.

102. Jacobus, J., & Tapert, S.F. (2014). Effects of cannabis on the adolescent brain. *Current Pharmaceutical Design, 20*(13), 2186–2193.

103. Meruelo, A.D., Castro, N., Cota, C., & Tapert, S.F. (2017). Cannabis and alcohol use, and the developing brain. *Behavioral Brain Research, 325*(Pt A), 44-50. doi: 10.1016/j.bbr.2017.02.025. Epub 2017 Feb 20.

104. McCann, B.S., Simpson, T.L., & Ries, P.R. (2000). Reliability and validity of screening instruments for drug and alcohol abuse in adults seeking evaluation for attention-deficit/hyperactivity disorder. *American Journal on Addictions, 9*(1), 1-9. doi:10.1080/10550490050172173.

105. National Institute on Drug Abuse. (n.d.). *NIDA quick screen.* Retrieved from http://www.drugabuse.gov/nmassist/.

106. National Institute on Drug Abuse. (2010). *Screening for drug use in medical settings.* Retrieved from http://www.drugabuse.gov/publications/resource-guide.

107. Substance Abuse and Mental Health Administration. (2017). *About screening, brief intervention, and referral to treatment (SBIRT).* Retrieved from https://www.samhsa.gov/sbirt/about.

108. Office of National Drug Control Policy. (2018). *National drug control strategy.* Retrieved from https://obamawhitehouse.archives.gov/ondcp/policy-and-research/ndcs.

109. McKusick, L., Horstman, W., & Coates, T.J. (1985). AIDS and sexual behavior reported by gay men in San Francisco. *American Journal of Public Health, 75*(5), 493-496.

110. Paolillo, E.W., Gongvatana, A., Umlauf, A., Letendre, S.L., & Moore, D.J. (2017). At-risk alcohol use is associated with antiretroviral treatment nonadherence among adults living with HIV/AIDS. *Alcoholism: Clinical and Experimental Research, 41*(8), 1518-1525.

111. Marcondes, M.C., et al., (2010). Methamphetamine increases brain viral load and activates natural killer cells in simian immunodeficiency virus-infected monkeys. *American Journal of Pathology, 177*(1), 355-61.

112. Mann, H., Garcia-Rada, X., Hornuf, L., & Tafurt, J. (2016). What deters crime? Comparing the effectiveness of legal, social, and internal sanctions across countries. *Frontiers in Psychology, 7,* 85.

113. Fortney, J., Mukherjee, S., Curran, G., Fortney, S., Han, X. & Both, B.M. (2004). Factors associated with perceived stigma for alcohol use and treatment among at-risk drinkers. *Journal of Behavioral Health Services Research, 31*(4), 418-429.

114. Weine, E.R., Kim, N.S., & Lincoln, A.K. (2015). Understanding lay assessments of alcohol use disorder: Need for treatment and associated stigma. *Alcohol and Alcoholism, 51*(1), 98-105.

115. Van Boekel, L.C., Brouwers, E.P., Van Weeghel, J., & Garretsen, H.F. (2013). Stigma among health professionals towards patients with substance use disorders and its consequences for healthcare delivery: Systematic review. *Drug & Alcohol Dependence, 131*(1), 23-35.

116. Savage, C.L. (2009). Clinical reviews: A proposed framework related to the care of addicted mothers. *Journal of Addictions Nursing, 19*(3), 158-160.

117. Savage, C.L. (2016). Substance use and substance abuse – What's in a name? *Journal of Addictions Nursing, 27*(1).

118. Neville, K., & Roan, N. (2014). Challenges in nursing practice: Nurses' perceptions in caring for hospitalized medical-surgical patients with substance abuse/dependence. *Journal of Nursing Administration, 44*(6), 339-346.

119. Pauly, B.B., McCall, J., Browne, A.J., Parker, J., & Mollison, A. (2015). Toward cultural safety: Nurse and patient perceptions of illicit substance use in a hospitalized setting. *Advances in Nursing Science, 38*(2), 121-135.

120. McNeil, R., Kerr, T., Pauly, B., Wood, E., & Small, W. (2016). Advancing patient-centered care for structurally vulnerable drug-using populations: A qualitative study of the perspectives of people who use drugs regarding the potential integration of harm reduction interventions into hospitals. *Addiction, 111*(4), 685-694.

Chapter 12

Injury and Violence

Christine Savage

LEARNING OUTCOMES

After reading the chapter, the student will be able to:

1. Describe the impact of injury and violence on the health of a population.
2. Define the burden of disease related to injury and violence using current epidemiological frameworks.
3. Use appropriate frameworks in the assessment of injury and violence.
4. Understand the role of policy in injury and violence prevention.
5. Apply current evidence-based population interventions to the prevention of injury and violence.

KEY TERMS

Acquaintance violence
Alcohol-impaired driving
Child maltreatment
Collective violence
Community violence
Emotional abuse
Emotional neglect
Family violence
Fire-related injury
Haddon Matrix

Injury
Intentional injury
Interpersonal violence
Intimate partner violence
Motor vehicle crashes
   (road traffic injuries)
Physical abuse
Physical neglect
Physical violence
Poison

Post-traumatic stress
  disorder (PTSD)
Psychological/emotional
  violence
Road traffic injury (RTI)
Self-directed violence
Sexual abuse
Sexual violence
Stalking
Stranger violence

Suicide
Threat of physical/sexual
  violence
Unintentional injury
Unintentional poisoning
Violence
War
Youth violence

Introduction

School shootings. Motor vehicle crashes. Suicide bombings. War. It seems almost daily these events end up in the headlines creating a stir on social media. Every one of them contributes to increased mortality and morbidity. How do we address injury and violence from a public health perspective? What are the implications for nursing? Injury, both intentional and unintentional, results in both long-term health consequences and increased risk for death, and is a major reason for an emergency department (ED) visit. Of the 136.9 million ED visits annually, 39 million (28%) are injury related.[1]

Overview of Injury

Injury is a serious public health issue that kills more than 5 million people globally and causes harm to many more. Injury occurs as the result of a wide variety of events, including motor vehicle crashes (MVC), drowning,

poisoning, falls, burns, assault, self-inflicted violence, or acts of war. According to the World Health Organization (WHO), 9% of global mortality is attributable to injury, which is 1.7 times the deaths attributable to AIDS/HIV, tuberculosis, and malaria combined.[2]

Globally, road injury was the 10th leading cause of death in lower-income countries and lower-middle-income countries, and the eighth leading cause of death in upper-middle-income countries.[3] In the U.S., in 2016, unintentional injury (accidents) was the fourth leading cause of death, and intentional injury (suicide) was the 10th leading cause of death. In contrast to the U.S., injury is not one of the top 10 leading causes of death in other high-income countries.[3,4]

Unintentional injury disproportionately affects the young and the impoverished, and in the United States is the number one cause of death for those aged 1 to 44.[5] In addition, intentional injury (suicide and homicide) were in the top five causes of death for those ages 10 to 44, and homicide was the third leading cause of death for those aged 1 to 9.[5] Injury not only affects the person who is injured but also can have an effect on family members, friends, coworkers, employers, and communities.[6] Injury is a serious public health issue due to mortality, disability, health-care costs, and the need for emergency care.

Types of Injuries

An **injury** is damage or harm done to or suffered by a person or thing. There are two types of injury, unintentional and intentional.[7] An **unintentional injury** is an injury to a person that occurs in a short period of time for which there is no predetermined intent to injure another or oneself.[8] Unintentional injuries include motor vehicle traffic injuries, drowning, falls, poisoning, burns, and other injuries. Although the media use the term *accident* when referring to unintentional injuries, these injuries are often predictable and preventable, and not the result of random unavoidable accidental events.

In the United States, unintentional injuries account for more than 146,000 deaths and more than 30 million ED visits annually. Among unintentional injuries, the highest number of deaths are related to poisonings followed by motor vehicle traffic deaths and falls (Box 12-1).[9] The population most at risk is males under the age of 45. More than a third (37%) of all deaths for children aged 1 to 19 are related to injury, making it the leading cause of death in this age group. For infants under the age of 1 year and newborns, it is the fifth leading cause of death.[10] Unintentional injuries not only contribute to premature death, but nonfatal injuries also have consequences that range from temporary pain to long-term disability, chronic pain, and a diminished health-related quality of life. Following a serious injury, a person often requires hospitalization and/or rehabilitation services.

Intentional injuries are injuries that occur because of a deliberate act that causes harm either to the self or to others.[11] **Violence** refers to physical force used to violate, damage, or abuse others or oneself. It is a broader term and is used in conjunction with intentional injury in the public health literature. According to the WHO, violence is among the leading causes of death for those aged 15 to 44 years.[12] Violence constitutes a serious threat to a community and often occurs along with mental illness and/or substance use (Chapters 10 and 11). In 2016 in the United States, more than 19,000 people were victims of homicide and nearly 45,000 people died by suicide.[13] Of the $671 billion price tag for injuries in the United States, suicide accounted for $50.8 billion and homicide for $26.4 billion.[14]

Types of Violence

The WHO presented a topology that separates violence into two contexts, family violence and community violence, and three categories, self-inflicted violence, interpersonal violence, and collective violence. **Self-inflicted violence** is violence in which the perpetrator and victim are one and the same and includes suicide and self-inflicted injury. **Interpersonal violence** occurs between individuals and includes two different contexts in which the violence occurs. The first is **family violence**, which includes intimate partner violence (IPV), child abuse/maltreatment, and elder abuse. The second is **community violence**, which occurs in the context of the community and includes **acquaintance violence**, violence between individuals who know each other, and **stranger violence**, violence that occurs between individuals who do not know each other. **Collective violence** occurs when a large group of people engage in violent behavior and covers various types of violent acts such as conflicts between nations and groups, terrorism instigated by groups or states, rape as a weapon of war, and gang warfare.[12]

Violent acts are broken out into four types of violence: (1) neglect, (2) psychological violence, (3) physical violence, and (4) sexual assault. The topology proposed by the WHO helps demonstrate the context in which violence occurs and the four types of violence that can occur (Fig. 12-1).[12]

Injury and violence are of major concern worldwide, and in the United States *Healthy People 2020 (HP 2020)* health topics included prevention of unintentional injury and violence. This topic area was included because of the mortality and disability associated with injury. Under

---

BOX 12–1 ■ Top Three Causes of Unintentional Mortality and Intentional Mortality, All Ages, 2015

Unintentional injury deaths:

1. Poisoning 14.8 deaths per 100,000 population
2. Motor vehicle injury 11.7 deaths per 100,000 population
3. Falls 10.4 deaths per 100,000 population

Intentional injury deaths:

1. Suicide 13.7 deaths per 100,000 population
2. Homicide 5.5 deaths per 100,000 population

Note: Crude death rate for the U.S. in 2015 was 844 per 100,000 population

Source: (9)

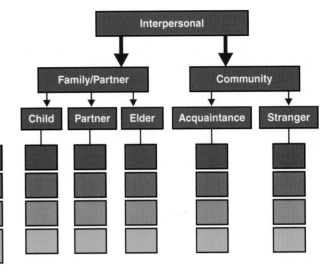

Figure 12-1 The topology of violence. *(From the World Health Organization, Violence Prevention Alliance. [2018]. Definition and typology of violence. Retrieved from* http://www.who.int/violenceprevention/approach/definition/en/)

this topic, there were a total of 43 objectives: 28 related to unintentional injury and 15 related to violence.[15]

■ **HEALTHY PEOPLE**
Injury and Violence Prevention

Goal: Prevent unintentional injuries and violence and reduce their consequences

Overview: Injuries and violence are widespread in society. Both unintentional injuries and those caused by acts of violence are among the top 15 killers for Americans of all ages.[1] Many people accept them as accidents, acts of fate, or as part of life. However, most events resulting in injury, disability, or death are predictable and preventable. The Injury and Violence Prevention Objectives for 2020 represent a broad range of issues that, if adequately addressed, will improve the health of the nation.[15]

Midcourse Review: Of the 65 objectives, 1 was archived, 9 were developmental, and 55 were measurable. Of those that were measurable, 9 met or exceeded the goal, 11 were improving, 26 had little or no change from baseline, and 9 were getting worse (Fig. 12-2).[16]

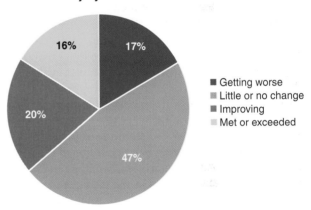

Healthy People 2020 Midcourse Review: Injury and Violence Prevention

- Getting worse
- Little or no change
- Improving
- Met or exceeded

Figure 12-2 HP 2020 Injury and Violence Prevention Midcourse Review.

Surveillance of Injury and Violence

Injury surveillance is conducted via various reporting mechanisms at the local, state, and national levels. In relation to unintentional injury, various tracking methods exist. For example, motor vehicle traffic incidents are tracked through the department of motor vehicles, department of transportation, and, for fatal motor vehicle incidents, through vital statistics. Some categories of injury, such as poisoning, are tracked through the department of public health. Some injuries are not routinely tracked at the governmental level, such as injury due to falls, but are tracked by institutions for patient-related falls and through public health departments and child protective services for child-related falls.

Tracking of intentional injury became more centralized in 2002 when the Centers for Disease Control and Prevention (CDC) received funding to establish the National Violent Death Reporting System. This system collects data on violent deaths from various state-level databases to create an anonymous database that could help states develop programs and monitor outcomes. Sources of data include death certificates, police reports, medical examiner reports, and other available data.[17] Thus, multiple sources of data can be used to examine the impact of injury at the population level.

Determining Risk for Injury or Violence

Tracking the incidence of injury is only one part of the puzzle. A key step in prevention of injury is to determine who is at greater risk for incurring an injury. The risk factors for injury vary based on the type of injury but come under the same main categories as chronic disease, behavioral, environmental, and socioeconomic risk factors. For example, in an MVC, several factors come into play. The behavioral level assessment includes evaluation of such issues as wearing seat belts, texting while driving, or driving under the influence of alcohol. In addition, environmental factors such as weather conditions and traffic control may play a role. Socioeconomic factors also play a role; for example, those with fewer economic resources may have older cars that may not be adequately maintained, and poorer countries, states, or municipalities may not be able to maintain safe roads. Analysis of risk for a particular injury requires a complex evaluation of a number of factors.

The Haddon Matrix

A common method used to determine injury risk is the **Haddon Matrix**. This matrix was developed based on the epidemiological triangle (see Chapter 3) and incorporates the three constructs in the triangle: (1) agent, (2) host, and (3) environment. It was designed by William Haddon, Jr., the first head of what is now the National Highway Traffic Safety Administration (NHTSA). The original purpose was to examine the problem of traffic safety.[18]

The Haddon Matrix has a minimum of 12 empty boxes to be filled in. The rows reflect the time around the event—"pre-event," "event," and "post-event"—and the columns are related to the host, agent, and environment (Fig. 12-3). Filling in the boxes provides a method of viewing the factors that contributed to the event and helps in the planning of injury interventions and prevention strategies. The matrix can also help set up the process for data collection. The process helps identify interventions that could occur at multiple points by preventing the injury (pre-event) or by mitigating the impact of the event (event or post-event).

Although this matrix was originally developed for the evaluation of MVCs, it can be used for any category of injury. Because it uses a classic epidemiological framework, it has applicability across settings. For example, it could be useful in an acute care setting to evaluate patient falls. It also provides needed information to develop primary prevention strategies (prevention of the event) and mitigation of the impact of the event, both during the event and following the event (secondary and tertiary prevention).

Figure 12-3 includes a blank Haddon Matrix and a partially filled-out matrix related to motor vehicle crashes (MVCs) that can be used with your own county or city data. If you continue filling out the partially completed form, you can begin to identify areas where interventions could be developed at all three levels: pre-crash, crash, and following the crash. The first part of the matrix provides vital information on what contributes to the injury and the consequences of the injury, and the second dimension provides vital information to help planners compare possible interventions on a variety of dimensions. The matrix becomes three dimensional by adding decision criteria for each level and includes consideration of the effectiveness, cost, feasibility, and other identified criteria used to decide what would be the best intervention.[18] This can help planners choose from a variety of possible interventions.

Prevention of Injury and Violence

Prevention of injury and violence is a major public health initiative. The CDC has a national center dedicated to injury prevention. The homepage for this center illustrates the current main areas for prevention including suicide, opioid overdose prevention, traumatic brain injury, home and recreation safety, motor vehicle safety, and violence prevention. The injury center not only collects surveillance data on injury, it also provides leadership and funds research aimed at reducing injury.[19]

Nursing Role in Prevention

Nurses play a key role in addressing the issue of injury and violence through the care they provide, the interventions they develop, and their active role in policy making. There is constant national attention from the media on injury issues that help raise awareness and, in many cases, result in policy-level interventions. For example, the issue of violence against women has received international attention, especially with the #metoo movement. Nurses directly helped shape policy here in the United Sates to help prevent violence against women. For example, public health nurse researchers, such

Phases	Host/Human	Agent Vehicle/Equipment	Physical Environment	Social Environment
Pre-Event				
Event				
Post-Event				

Partially Filled-In Haddon Matrix: Analysis of a Motor Vehicle Crash

Complete the matrix by filling in possible factors for agent and environment based on the time phases.

Assess the contributing factors or characteristics from the perspective of:

1. *Host/Human:* What were the Host or Human Factors that contributed to the event?

2. *Agent Vehicle/Equipment:* What was the crash worthiness of the vehicle?

3. *Physical Environment:* What was the status of the roadway design or safety features?

4. *Social Environment:* For example, passage and enforcement of seat belt laws.

Combine with time phases:

1. *Pre-Event:* What factors affect the host before the event occurs?

2. *Event:* What are factors related to the crash phase?

3. *Post-Event:* What are the factors related to the post-event crash phase?

Phases	Host/Human	Agent Vehicle/Equipment	Physical Environment	Social Environment
Pre-Event	Poor vision Texting/Cell phone Reaction time Alcohol Risk taking Driving experience	Failed brakes Missing lights	Narrow shoulders Rain storm	
Event	Failure to wear seat belt	Malfunctioning seat belts		
Post-Event	High susceptibility Alcohol			

Figure 12-3 Twelve boxes of the Haddon Matrix.

Dr. Jacquelyn Campbell, and nursing organizations, especially the American Nurses Association (ANA), were actively involved in the passing of the 2013 Violence Against Women Act. Nurses also play a role on the front lines every day providing care for persons following injury, especially in trauma centers. Dr. Nancy Glass used results from her research to develop an evidence-based app, myPlan, that women can use to help prevent relationship abuse.[20] Nurses like Dr. Glass and Dr. Campbell have championed the cause of preventing violence against women not only here in the U.S. but globally.

Other nursing organizations also focus on injury prevention. The Society of Trauma Nurses (STN) includes injury prevention and education in its mission statement. It has an active committee dedicated to injury prevention.[21] In line with the STN priorities, trauma nurses at Cincinnati Children's Hospital Medical Center (CCHMC) initiated an injury prevention program. The nurses developed and implemented a child passenger safety program. The program was offered to low-income families and was conducted at 46 "fitting" stations located in the community, including fire stations and health departments, so that parents could receive help on car seat installation, which is "fitting" the seats into their cars. These nurses also initiated a bike safety program, conducted community health fairs, and participated in leadership of the Safe Kids Coalition.

Because injury prevention is an essential component of what nurses provide to their communities, how would you begin? A good place to start is to examine the injury data related to the setting in which you work and the population for whom you care. If you work in the ED, you are most likely confronted with injury on a daily basis. As almost all injury is preventable, it is important to take an upstream approach while tending to the victims downstream, as did the nurses at CCHMC. To review from Chapter 2, the upstream metaphor in public health refers to the following: people are drowning in a river and rescue workers are pulling them out to save them from drowning. Pretty soon, the rescuers realize that, no matter how hard they work at pulling people out, more keep floating downstream. They decide to walk upstream to find out why people are falling into the river in the first place. Effort is then put into fixing the problem upstream that is causing people to fall into the river.

The problem for the individual nurse is that it feels as though there is no time to walk upstream. There are just too many patients coming for nursing care who have already fallen into the water. Luckily, the upstream approach is done as a collaborative effort across disciplines and entities. Take, for example, the child safety initiative at CCHMC.[22] The programs were offered in community settings and included nurses at the hospital, the public health department, the fire department, and the police department. The key is to have someone ask the question, "What is happening upstream?" and then have a team not only ready to find out but also committed to fixing the issues upstream.

Policy Aimed at Prevention of Injury and Violence

Many examples of policies aimed at preventing injury exist at the state and local levels. For example, most local municipalities require that a fence be placed around a swimming pool to prevent accidental drowning. Pedestrian laws and signs at crosswalks are in place to prevent injury to pedestrians. The list is long and demonstrates that policy efforts are effective in reducing injury. Seat belt laws alone have resulted in a reduction in fatal motor vehicle injuries and death. Policies aimed at reducing violence often come through the judicial system. However, other approaches are also effective, such as creating neighborhood watch groups, increasing lighting on streets at night, and reducing density of alcohol outlets. Policy initiatives often arise from the grassroots, and effectiveness is often contingent on neighborhood buy-in (Chapter 4).

Epidemiology of Unintentional Injury: Motor Vehicle Crashes

Motor vehicle crashes (MVCs) are a major public health concern worldwide, particularly for the young. An MVC is the collision of a motor vehicle with another vehicle, a stationary object, or a person that results in injury or death. The term *crash* has been substituted for the term *accident* because most MVCs are not random accidental events but are related to preventable causes. To help encompass the broader issue of road-related injury, the WHO uses the term **road traffic injury** (RTI). The WHO's definition of an RTI is similar to the definition of an MVC, but it includes the term *public road*. Thus, its definition is an injury that occurs as the result of a collision on a public road with involvement of at least one vehicle.[23,24]

In the United States, for persons aged 15 to 24, MVCs are the leading cause of unintentional injury deaths.[25] The annual number of MVC deaths in the U.S. is 32,000 and there are more than 2 million MVC-related nonfatal injuries.[26] There has been a decline over time in MVC-related injury, which may reflect an increase in the use of seatbelts, car seats, and booster seats.[26] Policy can help reduce MVC-related injury and death. For example, variation in alcohol-related MVC deaths are associated with alcohol policies.[27]

Risk Factors for Motor Vehicle Crashes

As noted earlier, when considering motor vehicle traffic, a number of factors come into play. The behavioral level includes such issues as wearing seat belts, texting while driving, or driving under the influence of alcohol. In addition, environmental factors may play a role, for example, weather conditions and traffic control. Socioeconomic factors also play a role; for example, those with fewer economic resources may have older cars that may not be adequately maintained, and poorer countries, states, or municipalities may not be able to maintain safe roads.

The CDC uses data from the National Vital Statistics System (NVSS) to estimate the economic burden of both fatal and nonfatal injuries.[28] The annual cost of medical care and productivity losses associated with injuries and deaths from MVCs exceeds $63 billion.[29,30] Other sources of data that can help determine which risk factors are associated with MVC injuries are the Fatality Analysis Reporting System (FARS) and the Behavioral Risk Factor Surveillance System (BRFSS).[31] In one study, Beck, Downs, Stevens, and Sauber-Schatz explored the underlying risk factors related to the higher MVC rate in rural areas versus urban areas. In 2015, although an estimated 19% of the U.S. population lived in rural areas, 57% of passenger-vehicle–occupant deaths occurred on rural roads, with a higher proportion of rural MVCs resulting in death. Based on their review of the data, they concluded that, because there was a lower rate of seat belt use in rural areas, efforts to reduce MVC mortality should focus on improving seat belt use in rural areas.[31]

Two major risk factors for MVCs are alcohol use and distracted driving. **Alcohol-impaired driving** is driving with a blood alcohol level at 0.08 or above, and laws have been enacted that make it illegal to drive impaired. **Distracted driving** is defined as diversion of attention from activities critical for safe driving. There are three main types of diversions: visual (taking your eyes off the road), manual (taking your hands off the wheel), or cognitive (taking your mind off of driving).[32,33] Distraction can include use of handheld devices, eating, driver drowsiness, and adjusting the radio, and in 2015, these accounted for 10% of fatal crashes and 15% of injury crashes.[33,34]

Speed is another major contributing factor to the severity of the injury associated with MVCs. Speed contributes more than any other factor because of its impact on reaction time, the amount of kinetic energy created, and ability to control the vehicle.[35] Other contributing factors include weather, road conditions, and vehicle safety features.[35] Once again, behavioral and environmental factors and socioeconomic status play roles. Other injury issues exist when the broader context of all RTIs is considered. Passengers and operators of other vehicles such as all-terrain vehicles, motorcycles, and bicycles are at risk for injury in the case of an RTI. Pedestrians are also at risk. Potential injuries in these circumstances are major public health issues, especially because of the high mortality rates associated with these types of injuries. The same risk factors apply across all RTIs.

Prevention of Motor Vehicle Crashes

Reduction in MVC-associated injury has, in part, occurred due to changes at the policy level. Laws related to the use of seat belts, car seats, booster seats, and handheld phones have helped reduce injury and mortality. A case in point is the issue of texting while driving. Under the Haddon Matrix, this risk factor would come under the Host/Human column as a pre-crash factor (see Fig. 12-3). This risk factor came to the forefront of media attention in 2009 based on data indicating that an increasing number of motorists were texting while driving prior to an MVC. The CDC now includes texting as one of the examples of distracted driving often equated with driving while intoxicated. Response to this risk factor has been reflected in laws making texting while driving illegal.

Much of the prevention efforts at the primary level in the United States have focused on reducing risky behaviors such as alcohol-impaired driving and on increasing public education about the importance of using proper safety measures. Back in the late 1970s, hospitals enacted policies that all parents must have a car seat in place prior to taking their newborns home from the hospital. Another approach has been to put in place a graduated driver licensing system aimed at reducing MVCs where teenagers are the drivers.

Other prevention efforts are aimed at the environment: improving roads, installing traffic lights, and installing pedestrian walkway signs. These types of prevention approaches are more difficult to put in place in low- and middle-income countries (LMICs) that lack the resources and that have not placed a strong emphasis on injury prevention.[24] The WHO adopted a global plan for road safety for the decade 2011–2020. The plan has five pillars, or categories, of prevention efforts. These include: "1) building road safety management capacity; 2) improving the safety of road infrastructure and broader transport networks; 3) further developing the safety of vehicles; 4) enhancing the behavior of road users; and 5) improving post-crash care."[24]

In the United States, there have been dramatic improvements in post-crash care, resulting in a reduction in MVC-associated mortality and morbidity. Much of this is due to the development of Level I trauma units, use of flight teams to bring helicopters to the crash site and transport victims directly to a trauma center, and the development of interventions aimed at decreasing the time from initial trauma to initiation of treatment. Such efforts to improve post-crash care help reduce long-term disability and survival rate of injury associated with MVCs.

Epidemiology of Unintentional Injury: Burn-Related Injuries

Burn-related injuries include "… an injury to the skin or other organic tissue primarily caused by heat or due to radiation, radioactivity, electricity, friction, or contact with chemicals. Skin injuries due to ultraviolet radiation, radioactivity, electricity, or chemicals, as well as respiratory damage resulting from smoke inhalation, are also considered to be burns."[36] Globally, the annual estimate of burn-related deaths from fires is 265,000. This figure does not include deaths that occur from burns that occurred due to scalding, electrical burns, and other non-fire-related forms of burns.[36] More than 96% of the fatal burns occur in LMICs, with more than half occurring in Southeast Asia.[36] Burns are among the most devastating of all injuries and are almost always preventable. They are difficult to treat even in high-income countries and, with limited resources, even more difficult to treat in LMICs.[37, 38]

In the United States, an estimated 486,000 people received medical treatment for burns in 2016. Fires and smoke inhalation accounted for 3,275 deaths. Of those burned, 40,000 required hospitalization. Seventy-three percent of burn injuries occurred in the home. The majority (68%) of those burned were male. According to the American Burn Association, one civilian death due to burns occurs every 2 hours and 41 minutes.[39] More than 300 children and adolescents are treated in emergency rooms for burn-related injuries each day, and two of those die.[40]

Younger children are more likely to sustain injuries from scald burns caused by hot liquids or steam, whereas older children are more likely to sustain injuries from flame burns caused by direct contact with fire.[40] However, in LMICs, the epidemiology of pediatric burn injury is different from what it is in high-income countries in that burn mortality is often higher. Burn mortality among children is closely associated with maternal deprivation and varies by region and income level, with the highest mortality burden in Sub-Saharan Africa.[41, 42]

Risk Factors for Burn Injuries

Using the epidemiological data, the associated risk factors for burn injuries are influenced by behavioral, social, cultural, and economic factors. Women and children in LMICs are at greatest risk because they spend more time at home using open fires to cook food and heat water. In LMICs in colder climates, there is exposure to heaters and stoves to keep homes warm.[42] Behavioral risk factors include alcohol use, tobacco use, history of seizures, and history of a psychiatric disorder. Environmental risk factors include the safety of the built environment, population density, the work environment, and the natural environment. To address these risk factors, in 2008, the WHO published a burn prevention plan (see Box 12-2) that addresses the main risk factors for burns, and it is still relevant today.[42,43]

Prevention of Burn Injuries

Prevention is an essential component in any burn management program, especially with the high incidence in LMICs.[41,42] As in all injuries, the main focus is on reduction of risk. For burns, primary prevention focuses on environmental measures in the home and behavioral changes. In the United States, many of the public health interventions focus on children and on measures that can be taken to reduce risk. In LMICs, the challenge for prevention is greater, where there is less governmental emphasis on prevention of injury as well as limited resources.[37,38,42]

In the United States, policy has played a large role in reducing fire-related morbidity and mortality. In 1911, a devastating fire in the Triangle Shirtwaist factory in New York City took the lives of 146 garment workers, most of them women. Based on that event, laws were put in place

BOX 12–2 ■ A WHO Plan for Burn Prevention and Care

Specific recommendations for individuals, communities, and public health officials to reduce burn risk:

- Enclose fires and limit the height of open flames in domestic environments.
- Promote safer cookstoves, fewer hazardous fuels, and educate regarding loose clothing.
- Apply safety regulations to housing designs and materials and encourage home inspections.
- Improve the design of cookstoves, particularly with regard to stability and prevention of access by children.
- Lower the temperature in hot water taps.
- Promote fire safety education and the use of smoke detectors, fire sprinklers, and fire-escape systems in homes.
- Promote the introduction of and compliance with industrial safety regulations, and the use of fire-retardant fabrics for children's sleepwear.
- Avoid smoking in bed and encourage the use of child-resistant lighters.
- Promote legislation mandating the production of fire-safe cigarettes.
- Improve treatment of epilepsy, particularly in developing countries.
- Encourage further development of burn-care systems, including the training of health-care providers in the appropriate triage and management of people with burns.
- Support the development and distribution of fire-retardant aprons to be used while cooking around an open flame or kerosene stove.

Sources: (42, 43)

to improve safety of the workplace. Another fire, the Coconut Grove fire that occurred in Boston in 1942, resulted in the deaths of 462 people, the deadliest nightclub fire in U.S. history. The club was decorated in a South Pacific motif using decorations made of flammable materials that covered exit signs. The fire spread rapidly, engulfing the club within 5 minutes of the first flame. The main entrance was a single revolving door that quickly became jammed as panicked customers tried to escape. This fire resulted in the institution of fire code regulations that are in place today, such as restriction on the use of flammable materials as decorations and requirements for clearly marked exit signs. It also resulted in the mandate that two regular doors equipped with panic bars flank all revolving doors. The next time you go through a revolving door, you will notice that this safety measure is always in place.

Secondary prevention focuses on what to do in the event of a fire. Stop, Drop, and Roll is an example of a successful campaign to teach children, workers, and others what to do if their clothes or hair are on fire (Fig. 12-4). The purpose is to mitigate the extent of the burns by using a technique that is effective in extinguishing the flames. Strides have also been made in the management of burns, resulting in a worldwide decline in fire-related mortality.[42] Care of a fire-related injury must also consider the issues of disability, disfigurement, emotional impact, and pain.

▶ SOLVING THE MYSTERY
The Case of the Exploding Barrel
Public Health Science Topics Covered:

- Assessment
- Epidemiology
- Health planning

In May 2020, Ben Smith, RN, moved from a large metropolitan area to a rural region of the country. He took a job working in the ED in a regional medical center serving six counties. After working there for 2 months, he became concerned about the number of injuries from firecrackers that he saw, especially injuries to teenagers. His concern grew when two teenagers were admitted to the ED. They had sustained eventually fatal injuries after placing a 50-gallon metal barrel over a sparkler bomb. After this event, Ben approached his supervisor about his concerns, and the supervisor commented that this was something they saw every summer, especially in July. Ben wanted to know whether the number of injuries was up this year and whether their ED had been involved in any prevention efforts. His supervisor thought that was a good question and suggested that Ben look into the issue.

Ben applied basic public health principles that he had learned in his undergraduate community health courses to begin investigating the problem. He began

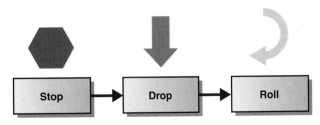

Figure 12-4 Stop, Drop, and Roll.

by reviewing their records for the number of fireworks-related injuries treated in the ED during the past 5 years, including age of the patient, month the injury occurred, and the severity of the injury based on triage level. This first phase of his investigation required a basic understanding of epidemiology (see Chapter 3), specifically how to calculate incidence rates, track the rates over time, and compare them with national rates. It also required basic community assessment skills. In this case, he did a focused assessment (see Chapter 4), that is, he started with a specific focus of fireworks-related injury. He found that the Consumer Product Safety Commission (CPSC) had a fireworks safety page and a three-step guide to fireworks safety.[44] This helped guide his investigation because the site provided information on the most common risk factors, current laws and regulations, and possible solutions. Through a link to firework injury data available on the CPSC site, Ben found that in 2016 there were an estimated total of 11,100 injuries in the U.S that required medical treatment at an ED.[45]

Using 5 years of data from their own hospital, Ben found that the two deaths he had encountered in the ED were the only deaths in the past 5 years, but various fireworks-related injuries had been treated during that time period that were similar to national data; most of the injuries had occurred to the fingers, hands, and eyes, and the majority were burns. He calculated incidence rates for the entire population living in the region served by the medical center, using population estimates for each of the 5 years (Box 12-3). He then looked at the frequency of injuries based on separate age groups including children under the age of 5, children aged 6 to 12, youths aged 13 to 18, and adults over the age of 18, and for each county. Based on that information, he determined that the overall incidence rate for the five-county region was higher than the national rate. He also found that the injury rate had decreased in children under the age of 6 but had increased in those aged 6 to 18. Starting in 2014, the majority of cases were between the ages of 13 and 18.

Ben then looked into community information that might help explain the decreased incidence rate in one age group and the increased rate in the other age group. After talking with his colleagues in the pediatric units, he discovered that the community had introduced a fireworks safety initiative with new parents in 2014. The health departments in all five counties had developed a brochure that was handed out at all the well-baby clinics and was provided to the pediatricians as well. For

BOX 12–3 ■ Estimating Injury Rates

The populations of the following five counties are considered here when estimating injury rates:

County Q	44,516
County R	42,316
County X	40,383
County Y	17,934
County Z	28,093

- The total population for the preceding counties in 2012 = 173,242.
- The total number of ED visits for fireworks injuries = 25.
- Rate of fireworks-related injury for the region = 12.9 per 100,000.
- The 2012 population for the United States as a whole = 313,780,968.
- The estimated number of ED visits in the United States for fireworks-related injury in 2012 = 9,300.
- Rate of fireworks-related injury in the United States = 2.9 per 100,000.

children less than 5 years of age, the prevention program from the public health departments appeared to have been effective. But why was the rate going up in the older children, especially among teenagers?

Ben did some further research on the laws surrounding the sale of fireworks. He found that there was a wide variance in the state laws. The state in which he was working had strict laws that went beyond the Federal Hazardous Substances Act, which prohibits the sale of highly dangerous fireworks and the components used to make them. However, the region his hospital served was close to the border of another state that had more lax laws and allowed the sale of fireworks that were just under the legal limit of no more than 50 milligrams of explosive powder and no more than 130 milligrams of flash powder. In 2015, two new fireworks stores had opened right across the state border. This increased availability was a possible factor in the increased incidence.

He then applied the Haddon Matrix to the problem. He started with the incident that had resulted in the death of the two teenagers and filled out the Haddon Matrix using factors related to the two boys, pre-event, event, and post-event. He accessed local news reports, police reports, and fire department reports on fireworks-related injuries and filled in the matrix. He found that the social environment pre-event played a big role, with a growing peer-related interest in using more dramatic fireworks. He also found that most of the injuries were clustered in the counties closest to the state border.

The Haddon Matrix assisted Ben in his assessment in another way. It helped him examine whether there were factors during the event or post-event that also influenced the outcome of the injury. The two counties that were closest to the state border were also farthest from the regional medical center and were quite rural. For some of the events, the time for emergency personnel to arrive on the scene was 20 minutes or more. Transportation to the regional medical center averaged 25 minutes from the time the emergency personnel arrived on the scene to the time the victim arrived at the medical center.

Following his assessment, Ben identified possible action that could be taken by the hospital in conjunction with the public health departments, the schools, the emergency providers, and other stakeholders to reduce the number of these incidents. The actions he recommended included prevention at the three levels of pre-event (e.g., public service announcements on firework safety), event (e.g., increasing safety measures at the county firework displays, emergency personnel preparedness), and post-event (e.g., a formal process for the evaluation of each event to identify contributing factors at the individual and community level). In some cases, his information opened the door for a discussion on injury prevention in the region at a higher level. Ben felt that the post-event issue related to emergency response time was bigger than just the fireworks injury issue. Ben's approach to a problem led to the development of a comprehensive fireworks prevention program spearheaded by the regional hospital that built on the work done with the preschool children. Ben now had baseline data to track the effectiveness of the intervention. Based on his work, the community put an injury prevention committee in place.

Epidemiology of Unintentional Injury: Drowning

Drowning is defined by the WHO as "… the process of experiencing respiratory impairment from submersion/immersion in liquid." The end result of drowning includes death, morbidity, or no morbidity.[46] The WHO estimates that there are 3,536 deaths from drowning annually, or 10 per day. Drowning is among the top 10 leading causes of death in children and young adults globally. This holds true in the U.S., with 10 deaths associated with unintentional drowning per day. Children ages 1 to 4 have the highest drowning rates. Those who receive emergency care for nonfatal submersion frequently require a high level of hospitalization, and if they suffer brain damage, they can become a heavy burden to society.[47]

Risk Factors for Drowning

We know that age is a risk factor for drowning. This is true in the U.S. and globally. Age plays a role for the older adult as their swimming ability declines. For young children, risk is tied to multiple issues. Their inquisitiveness and their lack of coordination make them susceptible to falls into bodies of water such as swimming pools, lakes, ponds, ditches of water, bathtubs, and buckets. Children aged 1 to 4 have the highest drowning rate. In the United States, young males are 10 times more likely to drown than young females, with 80% of all drowning victims being male.[47] In the United States, the most common sites for drowning are home swimming pools. Drowning rates for all rural residents are three times higher than for urban residents with drowning usually occurring in open water such as ponds, rivers, irrigation canals, and lakes. Children usually die of drowning in sites where they are without adequate supervision.[47] Another risk factor is hair or body entrapment in drains of pools or spas. There are multiple risk factors associated with drowning (Box 12-4) that help guide development of prevention programs including swimming lessons, use of barriers around swimming pools, increased supervision especially of children, and use of life jackets. Alcohol also increases the risk of drowning among adolescents and adults due to impairment of balance, coordination, and judgment. These effects of alcohol increase with sun exposure and heat.[47]

BOX 12–4 ■ Risk Factors for Drowning in the U.S.

What factors influence drowning risk?

- Lack of swimming ability
- Lack of barriers, such as pool fencing
- Lack of close supervision
- Location: people of different ages drown in different locations
- Failure to wear life jacket
- Alcohol use
- Seizure disorders

Source: (47)

Not having the ability to swim is a significant risk factor and is more common in females than males, and more common in African Americans than whites.[47] The tragic event that occurred on the Red River near Shreveport highlights this issue when six teens from two African-American families drowned. One unknowingly stepped off the shallow edge and slipped into the deep river, and six more teens went in to rescue him. Only one made it back. None of them knew how to swim and neither did their parents, watching from the shore.[48] In the United States, African-American children aged 5 to 19 are five times more likely to drown in swimming pools than white children.[47] Thus, the fact that no one in a family knows how to swim increases the risk, because family members often are the only ones supervising children when they swim.

Prevention of Drowning

Prevention requires a concerted effort on the part of health-care providers, public health officials, and family members. The American Academy of Pediatrics (APA) policy statement issued in 2010 remains the standard for prevention. The policy is aimed at increasing the role that pediatricians can play in preventing drowning in children and serves as a guide to nurses. The policy statement focuses on prevention interventions aimed at both primary and secondary levels of prevention. The scope is broad and includes supervising, learning to swim (both caretakers and children), and making changes to the environment such as installing fences and drain covers.[49] The CDC breaks down primary prevention into the following categories: barriers, supervision, learning to swim, life jacket use, and alcohol use.[47] From a secondary prevention viewpoint, both the APA and CDC recommend learning cardiopulmonary resuscitation (CPR). The CDC also includes recommendations to help prevent drowning in natural bodies of water. There is a clear consensus on the actions that can be taken to prevent drowning and, in the event of a drowning, to provide early and effective treatment to prevent mortality (Box 12-5).

Epidemiology of Unintentional Injury: Falls in Children

The WHO defines a fall as "… an event which results in a person coming to rest inadvertently on the ground or floor or other lower level".[50] The two populations at greatest risk for fall-related injuries are children and older adults (see Chapter 19). Globally each year there are 646,000 fall-related deaths and 37.3 million falls that

---

BOX 12–5 ■ Primary Prevention for Drowning in the United States

Tips to help you stay safe in the water:

- Pool fencing on all four sides at a 4-foot height would reduce drowning by 83%.
- Supervise when in or around water.
- Use the buddy system.
- Seizure disorder safety.
- Learn to swim.
- Learn cardiopulmonary resuscitation (CPR).
- Air-filled or foam toys are not safety devices.
- Avoid alcohol.
- Don't let swimmers hyperventilate before swimming underwater or try to hold their breath for long periods of time.
- Know how to prevent recreational water illnesses.
- Know the local weather conditions and forecast before swimming or boating.
- Do not use personal flotation devices, as they are not designed to keep people safe.

Sources: See reference (47).

---

require medical attention.[50] In the U.S., falls are the leading cause of nonfatal injury in children under 19 years of age.[51]

Risk Factors for Falls in Children

In the U.S., the majority of falls in children occur on the playground, from windows, from beds or other furniture, from baby carriers or with baby walkers/riders that allow an infant to independently move from place to place, including ride-on toys and circular walkers.[51,52,53] Age, socioeconomic status, and gender play roles as well. The type of fall changes based on the age and stage of development of the child. When examining the contributing factors that increase the risk for falls in children, it is important to consider the evolving developmental stages of children and adolescents. These include the innate curiosity of children in relation to their surroundings and increasing levels of independence. In addition, other factors include inadequate adult supervision, poverty, being a single parent, and hazardous environments.[50] Fall risk increases once an infant becomes mobile. In mobile infants and toddlers, falls are usually from furniture or on the stairs. Preschool and school-age children are at risk for playground-related falls.[51,52] As children enter middle school and engage in athletics, sports-related falls predominate. Window-related falls are perhaps the most dramatic, as underscored by Eric Clapton's song "Tears in Heaven." In 1991, his 4-year-old son Conor fell from a 53rd floor apartment window in New York City. Window falls occur most often in urban, low-income, and multidwelling settings.

Prevention of Falls in Children

Prevention efforts begin with home safety interventions. Parents are encouraged to put stair and window guards in place to prevent falls and, as with drowning prevention, maintain supervision of children in the home and on the playground.[54] Product regulation has also played a role in increasing the safety of baby walkers and playground equipment. The U.S. Consumer Product Safety Commission has a playground equipment safety guideline publication that clearly outlines how to prevent playground-related injury.[55] Window guards, baby walkers, and other nursery products must meet product safety requirements.

■ EVIDENCE-BASED PRACTICE
Use of Window Guards

Practice Statement: Window guards should be placed on all windows in multidwelling buildings.
Targeted Outcome: Reduction in incidence of window-related falls in children
Evidence to Support: The majority of the evidence is linked to surveillance data tracking the incidence of window-related falls in children before and after the enactment of window guard laws. In New York City, the incidence dropped 35% in the 2 years following the enactment of the requirement for window guards.
Recommended Approaches: Legislative approaches that require landlords and owners of multidwelling buildings to install window guards, provide access to window guards for those who may not be able to purchase them, and distribute public information on preventing window-related falls in children (Box 12-6).

Source: (56)

Epidemiology of Unintentional Injury: Poisonings

According to the CDC, "A **poison** is any substance, including medications, that is harmful to your body if too much is eaten, inhaled, injected, or absorbed through the skin. An **unintentional poisoning** occurs when a person taking or giving too much of a substance did not mean to cause harm."[57] Globally, more than 80% of all unintentional poisonings occur in LMICs with a resulting loss

BOX 12–6 ■ New York City Window Guard Program

In 1976, the New York City Board of Health enacted legislation known as *Health Code Section 131.15,* the window guard law. It requires owners of multiple dwellings (buildings of three or more apartments) to provide and properly install approved window guards on all windows, including first floor bathroom and windows leading onto a balcony or terrace in an apartment where a child (or children) 10 years of age or younger reside and in each hallway window, if any, in such buildings.

The exceptions to this law are:

- Windows that open onto fire escapes
- A window on the first floor that is a required secondary exit in a building in which there are fire escapes on the second floor and up

If tenants or occupants want window guards for any reason, even if there are no resident children in the covered age category, they should request them in writing, and they may not be refused. Examples:

- Grandparents who have visiting children
- Parents who share intermittent custody
- Occupants who provide childcare

If required or requested and window guards have not been installed, if they appear to be insecure or improperly installed, or if there is more than 4.5 inches of open, unguarded space in the window opening, a complaint should be made immediately to **311**.

For more information on Window Guards, call **311**.

Source: (56)

of more than 10.7 million years of healthy life (disability-adjusted life years [DALYs]).[57]

In 2015, in the U.S., 47,478 persons died from unintentional poisoning, a mortality rate of 14.8 per 100,000.[58] Most concerning has been the rise in drug poisoning mortality, attributable to the rise in opioid drug overdoses (see Chapter 11). From 1999 to 2016, for all ages, the mortality rate for drug poisoning rose from 6.1 to 19.8 per 100,000 (Fig. 12-5).[59] However, for non-Hispanic whites, the rate for all ages went from 8.7 in 1999 to 48.7 per 100,000. For non-Hispanic white males aged 25-34 the rate rose from 12.2 to 68.4 per 100,000. By comparison, for non-Hispanic black males during the same time period, the rate rose from 12.2 to 27.2 per 100,000 (Fig. 12-6).[59]

The National Poison Data System, an electronic surveillance system documenting all calls made to poison centers across the United States, is a source for data to monitor poisonings. In 2016, analgesics (11.2%), household

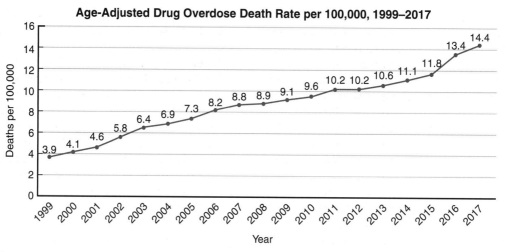

Figure 12-5 Age-Adjusted Drug Poisoning Rate U.S. 1999–2016. (*Data from* https://www.cdc.gov/nchs/data-visualization/drug-poisoning-mortality/)

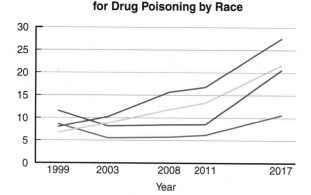

Figure 12-6 Age-adjusted drug poisoning by race. (*Data from* https://www.cdc.gov/nchs/data-visualization/drug-poisoning-mortality/)

cleaning substances (7.54%), cosmetics/personal care products (7.20%), sedatives/hypnotics/antipsychotics (5.84%), and antidepressants (4.74%) were the top five poison exposures in the U.S.[60] For children 5 years of age and under, the top five poison exposures were cosmetics/personal care products (13.3%), household cleaning substances (11.1%), analgesics (9.21%), foreign bodies/toys/miscellaneous (6.48%), and topical preparations (5.07%).[61] From a global perspective, lead poisoning, especially in children, is a leading cause of poisoning.

According to the WHO, 494,550 deaths annually are due to lead exposure. Furthermore, there is a loss of 9.3 million DALYs due to the long-term effects that exposure to lead has on health, with the highest burden occurring in LMICs.[61] In the U.S., the Flint, Michigan, water crisis demonstrated the real threat of lead poisoning due to the built environment (see Chapter 6).

Risk Factors for Unintentional Poisonings

As noted earlier, there are differences in unintentional poisoning mortality rates based on demographic characteristics such as age, gender, and ethnicity. Children younger than 6 years of age account for most poisoning events (46%), followed by adults (39%) and teens (7%).[62] The most common poisoning in adults age 20 or older was related to pain medication and, in children, the most common poisonings were related to cosmetics and personal care products.[62]

A major issue related to children and poisoning is the home environment. Most childhood poisonings occur in the home.[63,64] Children who live in older homes are at greater risk for lead poisoning as a result of the presence of lead-based paint or carbon monoxide poisoning from older heating systems. The other issue is ingestion of poisonous substances found in the home such as chemicals and medications.

Prevention of Unintentional Poisoning

With the predominant problem of overdose related to prescription medications, the most obvious approach to prevention is a focus on proper use and labeling of medications, not sharing medications, proper storage of medications, and proper disposal of medications.[63,64] Due to the opioid overdose epidemic, much of the focus has been on reducing prescription of opioids for the treatment of pain (see Chapter 11). With children at greatest risk, prevention efforts related to poisoning reduction in children are also important. The American Association of Poison Control Centers provides valuable guides to prevention that cover a wide range of potential poisons as well as environmental issues related to exposure.[65] The United States Consumer Product Safety Commission also has a Web site that provides guidance for prevention and highlights current hazards such as single load liquid laundry packets and tiny button batteries. They also provide a link to recent recalls.[66] Another major mechanism for prevention of morbidity and mortality is the network of poison control centers throughout the U.S. [65]

Prevention efforts globally include efforts to reduce lead poisoning and poisoning from pesticides. The WHO has an International Program on Chemical Safety (IPCS). Their work includes promoting and establishing poison centers, providing information on poisoning, and developing peer-reviewed guidelines on the prevention and management of poisoning.[67]

Epidemiology of Self-Directed Violence: Suicide

Self-directed violence (SDV), both fatal and nonfatal, is a serious public health issue and is defined as "... anything a person does intentionally that can cause injury to self, including death".[68] It includes **suicide**, defined as "death caused by self-directed injurious behavior with an intent to die as a result of the behavior."[69] Other suicidal acts include suicide attempt, defined as "a nonfatal, self-directed, potentially injurious behavior with an intent to die as a result of the behavior; might not result in injury", and suicidal ideation, defined as "thinking about, considering, or planning suicide."[69] SDV also includes non-suicidal acts such as cutting, head banging, self-biting, and self-scratching with some non-suicidal acts being unintentional and occurring in response to something environmental.[68]

Currently, due to a rise in the suicide rate, prevention of suicide has become a primary public health focus. In the U.S., there has been an alarming statistically significant rise in the suicide rate from 1999 to 2016 from 10.5 to 13.4 per 100,000. By 2016, suicide was the 10th leading cause of death in the U.S. Breaking it down by age group,

suicide was the second leading cause of death for persons aged 10 to 34, and the fourth leading cause of death among persons aged 35 to 54.[70]

There were more than twice as many suicides (44,965) in the United States as there were homicides (19,362).[70,71] The media helped focus national attention on the problem, especially with the high-profile celebrity deaths in 2018 of Anthony Bourdain and Kate Spade. One of the frequently referenced risk factors for suicide has been a history of mental health problems, but in a recent study of state surveillance data, 54% of those who committed suicide in 27 states had no known mental health condition.[71]

Globally, suicide is the 17th leading cause of death accounting for 1.4% of all deaths with an annual suicide rate of 10.7 per 100,000. It is also the second leading cause of death worldwide for persons aged 15-29. Almost a third (30%) are due to ingestion of pesticides. The other two most common methods globally are death by use of a firearm and hanging.[72] There is no clear pattern globally with socioeconomically diverse countries in the top five: Guyana, Lithuania, South Korea, Kazakhstan, and Sri Lanka.[73]

Overall, in 2016, 4% of the U.S. population reported suicidal ideation (Fig. 12-7), and 0.5% reported a suicide attempt. Women and young people are more likely to attempt suicide than men and older adults. For that same year, 1.3 million adults attempted suicide, and 1 million reported making suicide plans.[70]

Risk Factors for Suicide

Although in the United States suicide has been viewed as a moral problem or a sign of personal weakness by some (see Chapter 10), the underlying risk factors are complex and often multifactoral.[71] Based on an analysis of suicide surveillance data, half of all persons who die by suicide had not been diagnosed with mental health disorder at the time of death. This brings into question limiting prevention to persons with a known mental health disorder. Those with mental health disorders often have other risk factors as well such as job or relationship problems or physical health issues.[71] According to the WHO, some suicides are an impulsive action in a time of crisis with the person losing the ability to cope with life stressors. Other triggers "... experiencing conflict, disaster, violence, abuse, loss, or a sense of isolation are strongly associated with suicidal behavior."[72] In addition, specific groups that experience discrimination are at increased risk including refugees; migrants; indigenous peoples; prisoners; Lesbian, Gay, Bisexual, Transgender, Queer (LGBTQ+) persons; and prisoners.[72] There are a

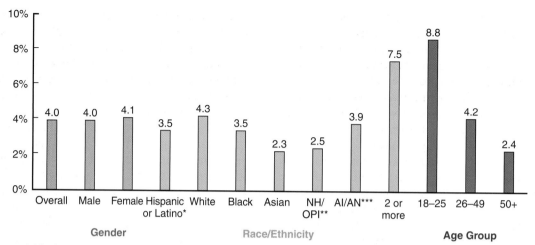

Figure 12-7 Past Year Prevalence of Suicidal Thoughts Among U.S. Adults. (2016) *(Data courtesy of SAMHSA; figure source* https://www.nimh.nih.gov/health/statistics/suicide.shtml*)*

number of protective factors as well including both family and community support (Box 12-7).

■ CULTURAL AWARENESS AND COMPETENCY AROUND SUICIDE PREVENTION

Taking into account the cultural context of different communities is central to the building of effective suicide prevention programs as evidenced by the Substance Abuse and Mental Health Services Administration's publication *To Live to See the Great Day that Dawns: Preventing Suicide by American Indian and Alaska Native Youth and Young Adults – 2010*. The publication utilizes culturally appropriate guidance to American Indian and Alaska Native communities drawing on cultural strengths and narratives to address suicide risk.[75]

According to the Indian Health Service, "Factors that protect AI/AN youth and young adults against suicidal behavior are a sense of belonging to one's culture, a strong tribal/spiritual bond, the opportunity to discuss problems with family or friends, feeling connected to family, and positive emotional health."[76] Building a prevention program should not only address risk factors but build on cultural strengths within a community.

Veterans are another vulnerable group at higher risk for suicide in the U.S., especially those experiencing

---

BOX 12–7 ■ World Health Organization: Prevention of Suicide

Suicides are preventable. There are a number of measures that can be taken at population, subpopulation, and individual levels to prevent suicide and suicide attempts. These include:

- Reducing access to the means of suicide (e.g., pesticides, firearms, certain medications)
- Reporting by media in a responsible way
- Introducing alcohol policies to reduce the harmful use of alcohol
- Early identification, treatment, and care of people with mental and substance use disorders, chronic pain, and acute emotional distress
- Training of non-specialized health workers in the assessment and management of suicidal behavior
- Follow-up care for people who attempted suicide and provision of community support

Source: (72)

---

homelessness. The attempted suicide rate among veterans who are housed is 1.2% compared to 6.9% of those experiencing homelessness.[77] The rate of suicidal ideation in the past 2 weeks is also higher among those experiencing homelessness (19.8% versus 7.4%). In Montana, between 2013 and 2016, veterans accounted for 20% of all suicides.[78] Comparing suicide rates among veterans versus civilian populations is complicated, and recent statistics can be misleading because it is important to be clear about who is counted as a veteran. In addition, suicide rates for the general population includes adolescents to older adults. Thus, when comparing the suicide rate in veterans to the adult population, it is important to use an age-adjusted rate as well as a clear definition of who is classified as a veteran.

Place of residence also plays a role. Both veterans and non-veterans living in rural areas in Montana and in the U.S. are at increased risk for suicide.[73,79] Also, states with stricter gun laws have lower suicide rates as well as states with gun seizure laws.[80] Nevada, a state that put in place suicide prevention programs, has seen a drop in the suicide rate, although the rate remains high.

Prevention of Suicide

Prevention occurs from the individual to the policy level. As evidenced by the reduction of suicide rate in states with stricter gun control laws, upstream polices that address a risk factor, in this case easy access to guns, can help reduce the suicide rate. One set of authors recommended the use of the socioecological model (Chapter 2) in the development of suicide prevention programs using access to guns as the targeted risk factor. Using this approach, prevention occurs across the continuum of societal, community, relationship, and individual interventions.[81] Examples of societal approaches include policy and system level strategies. Novel approaches such as social networking for youth are emerging to address specific populations within the context of their daily lives. This is an example of a relationship approach.[82]

The Zero Suicide (ZS) model is an example of a health systems-level approach. ZS uses a multilevel approach to help implement evidence-based practices for suicide prevention in the behavioral health setting. The components of the program include four aspects of clinical care (Identify, Engage, Treat, and Transition) and three components on the administrative level (Lead, Train, and Improve).[83] The CDC published a guide to suicide prevention programs that illustrates that multiple evidenced-based prevention programs exist.[84] From a global perspective, prevention requires attention to the multiple factors that contribute to suicide (Table 12-1). Suicide was listed in *HP 2020* under mental health rather than injury and violence.[85] Given that approximately 50% of persons who commit suicide in the U.S. had not been diagnosed with a mental health disorder,[71] suicide is relevant to both the mental health topic and to the violence and injury topic in *Healthy People 2030*.

TABLE 12–1 ■ Suicide: Risk Factors and Protective Factors

Risk Factors	Protective Factors
• Family history of suicide • Family history of child maltreatment • Previous suicide attempt(s) • History of mental disorders, particularly clinical depression • History of alcohol and substance abuse • Feelings of hopelessness • Impulsive or aggressive tendencies • Cultural and religious beliefs (e.g., belief that suicide is noble resolution of a personal dilemma) • Local epidemics of suicide • Isolation, a feeling of being cut off from other people • Barriers to accessing mental health treatment • Loss (relational, social, work, or financial) • Physical illness • Easy access to lethal methods • Unwillingness to seek help because of the stigma attached to mental health and substance abuse disorders or to suicidal thoughts	• Effective clinical care for mental, physical, and substance abuse disorders • Easy access to a variety of clinical interventions and support for help seeking • Family and community support (connectedness) • Support from ongoing medical and mental health care relationships • Skills in problem solving, conflict resolution, and nonviolent ways of handling disputes • Cultural and religious beliefs that discourage suicide and support instincts for self-preservation • Substance abuse disorders or suicidal thoughts

Source: (74)

Epidemiology of Violence Against Children and Women

Violence against women and children occurs both within and outside of the family context. **Family violence** includes violence between intimate partners (IPV), maltreatment of children, and elder abuse. The context of the violence is the family and occurs between individuals. The victims and the perpetrators have an established family-based relationship and can include violence against children and women. Violence against children that occurs outside the family includes community-based violence (see later), bullying, and school-based violence (see Chapter 18). Violence against women other than IPV includes stalking and sexual assault by persons other than intimate partners.

Child Maltreatment

Child maltreatment is defined by the federal Keeping Children and Families Safe Act of 2003 (P.L. 108-36) as "any recent act or failure to act on the part of a parent or caretaker which results in death, serious physical or emotional harm, sexual abuse or exploitation" or "an act or failure to act which presents imminent risk or serious harm."[87] The WHO points out that maltreatment of a child can lead to serious adverse consequences both immediately and long term. Violence against children not only leads to death, serious injury, and potential disability but also causes stress that negatively impacts brain development with damage to the nervous and immune systems. Thus, victims of child maltreatment may have "… delayed cognitive development, poor school performance and dropout, mental health problems, suicide attempts, increased health-risk behaviors, revictimization, and the perpetration of violence."[88]

Child neglect is the most prevalent form of child maltreatment and includes both physical neglect and emotional neglect. **Physical neglect** includes the withholding of food, shelter, clothing, and/or medical or dental care, whereas **emotional neglect** involves the omission of caring, nurturing, and acceptance. **Emotional abuse** is defined as extreme debasement of feelings, whereas **physical abuse** is nonaccidental physical harm such as bruising, bites, thermal burns or cigarette burns, severe fractures, and even death. **Sexual abuse** defined by the federal Child Abuse Prevention and Treatment Act[87] and as amended by the Keeping Children and Families Safe Act of 2003 is "the employment, use, persuasion, inducement, enticement, or coercion of any child to engage in, or assist any other person to engage in, any sexually explicit conduct or simulation of such conduct for the purpose of producing a visual depiction of such conduct; or the rape, and in cases of caretaker or inter-familial relationships, statutory rape, molestation, prostitution, or other form of sexual exploitation of children, or incest with children."[87]

At both the global level and in the U.S., one in four adults have a history of physical abuse as a child.[89,90] The National Child Abuse and Neglect Data System is the surveillance system that monitors trends of child maltreatment by collecting child protective service reports from 50 states, Puerto Rico, and the District of Columbia.[91] In 2016, in the U.S., child protective services received reports of 676,000 victims of child maltreatment of whom an estimated 1,750 died.[91] Also in 2016, children younger than a year old had the highest rate of child maltreatment at 24.8 per 1,000. American Indian or Alaska Native children had the highest rate (14.2 per 1,000) followed by African-American children (13.9 per 1,000). The fatality rate was highest in African-American children at 4.65 per 100,000, which is twice as high as the rate for white children (2.10 per 100,000) and three times as high as Hispanic children (1.58 per 100,000).[91] Because these data represent only those cases reported to child protective services, the actual incidence may be higher. The estimated cost of child maltreatment in the U.S. is $124 billion each year.[90]

Risk Factors for Child Maltreatment

Risk factors for childhood maltreatment include three levels of risk: individual, family, and community (Table 12-2).[92] Parental socioeconomic factors play a role. For example, the level of mother's education and poverty, and parental behavioral issues such as mental health disorders or substance use place a child at higher risk.[90, 92,93] For some, a parent's history of child

TABLE 12–2 ■ Child Maltreatment: Risk Factors and Protective Factors

Risk Factors for Victimization

Individual Risk Factors

- Children younger than 4 years of age
- Special needs that may increase caregiver burden (e.g., disabilities, mental health issues, and chronic physical illnesses)

Risk Factors for Perpetration

Individual Risk Factors

- Parents' lack of understanding of children's needs, child development, and parenting skills
- Parental history of child abuse and or neglect
- Substance abuse and/or mental health issues including depression in the family
- Parental characteristics such as young age, low education, single parenthood, large number of dependent children, and low income
- Nonbiological, transient caregivers in the home (e.g., mother's male partner)
- Parental thoughts and emotions that tend to support or justify maltreatment behaviors

Family Risk Factors

- Social isolation
- Family disorganization, dissolution, and violence, including intimate partner violence
- Parenting stress, poor parent-child relationships, and negative interactions

Community Risk Factors

- Community violence
- Concentrated neighborhood disadvantage (e.g., high poverty and residential instability, high unemployment rates, and high density of alcohol outlets), and poor social connections.

Protective Factors

Family Protective Factors

- Supportive family environment and social networks
- Concrete support for basic needs
- Nurturing parenting skills
- Stable family relationships
- Household rules and child monitoring
- Parental employment
- Parental education
- Adequate housing
- Access to health care and social services
- Caring adults outside the family who can serve as role models or mentors

Community Protective Factors

- Communities that support parents and take responsibility for preventing abuse

Source: (90)

abuse in the family of origin is significant,[93] whereas for other families current substance abuse and/or mental health issues including depression in the family are predictors of child maltreatment.[90,92] Other risk factors include parents' lack of understanding of children's needs, child development, and parenting skills, or parental thoughts and emotions that tend to support or justify maltreatment behaviors.[90] Maternal IPV (see later) is another strong risk factor for child maltreatment.[94] The presence of a nonbiological, transient caregiver in the home is another risk factor for sexual abuse in particular (e.g., mother's male partner).[90] Community-level risk factors include low socioeconomic status and living in an impoverished community.[90,92]

A history of childhood maltreatment can lead to lifelong health issues in adults.[90]

Prevention of Child Maltreatment

The focus of childhood maltreatment prevention programs is often on parental education, support, and/or public awareness campaigns in an effort to strengthen the protective factors within the home and community (Table 12-3).[92,95] Tertiary prevention is also important to prevent recurrence of abuse or to decrease impairment. Home visitation (see Chapter 17) in particular has been implemented for the prevention of child maltreatment. Focusing on selective protective factors is the focus of many of these programs. Protective factors for child maltreatment include nurturing parenting skills, promoting stable family relationships, promoting household rules and child monitoring, and assisting with parental employment, adequate housing, or access to health care and social services.[95] Home visitation programs include the Nurse Family Partnership Model, which has undergone rigorous evaluations and shows promise for the prevention of child maltreatment.[96] Examples of other programs aimed at reinforcing protective factors in families and communities include the Triple P program and Family Connections.[97,98]

Violence Against Women and Intimate Partner Violence

Intimate partner violence is violence that occurs between two people in an intimate relationship. It includes physical violence, sexual violence, and/or psychological/emotional violence as well as threats of physical and/or sexual violence. It can occur between both heterosexual and same sex partners.[99] Globally, more than one-third of women (38%) have experienced either physical and/or sexual violence with 30% of them experiencing IPV. In addition, 38% of all homicides of women are perpetrated by an intimate partner.[100]

Physical violence is the intentional use of physical force with the potential for causing death, disability, injury, or harm. Physical violence includes, but is not limited to, scratching, pushing, shoving, throwing, grabbing, biting, choking, shaking, slapping, punching, burning, use of a weapon, and use of restraints or one's body, size, or strength against another person. **Sexual violence** is divided into three categories: (1) use of physical force to

---

TABLE 12–3 ■ Childhood Maltreatment Prevention Programs

Strategy	Approach
Teach safe and healthy relationship skills	• Social-emotional learning programs for youth • Healthy relationship programs for couples
Engage influential adults and peers	• Men and boys as allies in prevention • Bystander empowerment and education • Family-based programs
Disrupt the developmental pathways toward partner violence	• Early childhood home visitation • Preschool enrichment with family engagement • Parenting skill and family relationship programs • Treatment for at-risk children, youth and families
Create protective environments	• Improve school climate and safety • Improve organizational policies and workplace climate • Modify the physical and social environments of neighborhoods
Strengthen economic supports for families	• Strengthen household financial security • Strengthen work family supports
Support survivors to increase safety and lessen harms	• Victim-centered services • Housing programs • First responder and civil legal protections • Patient-centered approaches • Treatment and support for survivors of IPV

Source: (112)

compel a person to engage in a sexual act against his or her will, whether or not the act is completed; (2) attempted or completed sexual act involving a person who is unable to understand the nature or condition of the act, to decline participation, or to communicate unwillingness to engage in the sexual act (e.g., because of illness, disability, the influence of alcohol or other drugs, or because of intimidation or pressure); and (3) abusive sexual contact. **Threat of physical or sexual violence** is the use of words, gestures, or weapons to communicate the intent to cause death, disability, injury, or physical harm. **Psychological/ emotional violence** involves trauma to the victim caused by acts, threats of acts, or coercive tactics. Psychological/ emotional abuse can include, but is not limited to, humiliating the victim, controlling what the victim can and cannot do, withholding information from the victim, deliberately doing something to make the victim feel diminished or embarrassed, isolating the victim from friends and family, and denying the victim access to money or other basic resources. **Stalking** is defined as "… a pattern of harassing or threatening tactics used by a perpetrator that is both unwanted and causes fear or safety concerns in the victim."[101,102]

About 1 in 4 American women and about 1 in 10 males reported a lifetime impact of contact sexual violence, physical violence, and/or stalking.[102] Surveillance of IPV occurs through various databases. This abuse can start early in dating relationships.[102] LGBTQ+ persons also experience IPV at levels equal to or higher than the heterosexual population.[103]

IPV has significant negative effects on health. These effects are both short- and long-term and include physical, mental, sexual, and reproductive adverse health consequences for women and their children.[100,104] There are also serious negative social and economic consequences for women, their families, and their communities.[100,104] Abused women are also more likely to use medical services including outpatient primary care, EDs, and mental and substance abuse services.[105] Femicide (Box 12-8) is the most extreme negative outcome.[106]

■ CULTURAL CONTEXT

As part of a series on violence prevention, the WHO examined how cultural and social norms can encourage violence, including IPV. Some examples of cultural norms from different countries provided by the WHO include the following: "a man has a right to assert power over a woman and is socially superior (India, Nigeria, Ghana); a man has a right to 'correct' or discipline female behavior (India, Nigeria, China); a woman's freedom should be restricted (Pakistan); and physical violence is an acceptable way to resolve conflicts within a relationship (South Africa, China)."[107] Deviation from norms results in disgracing the entire family, which can then lead to honor killings such as the honor killing of a couple who married for love in Pakistan in 2018. The role culture plays in violence against women has been in the spotlight with calls to stand up against a cultural acceptance of men perpetuating violence against women, especially sexual violence. Thus, at the global level, a cultural shift is occurring to not only accept women who speak out and report perpetrators but also to make violence against women unacceptable. *Time* magazine choosing the founders of the #metoo movement as their Person of the Year in 2017 is evidence of the cultural shift.

Risk Factors for Intimate Partner Violence

Risk for IPV occurs at many levels. At the individual level, risk factors include female gender, young age, being unmarried, being uninsured or on medical assistance, low income, and having a history of child maltreatment.[100,108] In addition, at-risk alcohol use by either partner or both is associated with IPV perpetration.[100,108] Other risk factors include low self-esteem, mental health problems, unemployment, or desire for power and control in relationships.[100,108] At the family level, exposure as an adolescent to severe IPV between caregivers increases the risk for relationship violence in early adulthood.[100,108] At the community level, residence in an area characterized by poverty and social disadvantage as well as by an increased density of alcohol outlets are factors associated with IPV–related ED visits.[100,108,109]

BOX 12–8 ■ World Health Organization Definition of Femicide

Femicide is the intentional murder of women.

- Femicide is usually perpetrated by men, but sometimes female family members may be involved.
- Femicide differs from male homicide in specific ways. For example, most cases of femicide are committed by partners or ex-partners, and involve ongoing abuse in the home, threats or intimidation, sexual violence, or situations where women have less power or fewer resources than their partner.

Source: (106)

The majority of studies have focused on risk factors in relation to the female victim. Globally, there is a lack of research related to the perpetrator. In addition, outside of the U.S., there is little research on the community level related to IPV.[110] In a ground-breaking study by Campbell et al., risk factors for femicide included a history of prior abuse, a history of perpetrator unemployment, availability of guns, and presence of the victim's child from another relationship in the home.[111]

Prevention of Intimate Partner Violence

In 2017, the CDC published *Preventing Intimate Partner Violence Across the Lifespan: A Technical Package of Programs, Policies, and Practices,* an evidence-based review of prevention strategies across the continuum aimed at reducing IPV and reducing negative consequences in persons who have experienced IPV.[112] The main categories of prevention include: (1) Teach safe and healthy relationship skills, (2) Engage influential adults and peers, (3) Disrupt the developmental pathways toward partner violence, (4) Create protective environments, (5) Strengthen economic supports for families, and (6) Support survivors to increase safety and lessen harms. This broad overview of prevention requires promoting change at all levels of the socioecological model (Chapter 2): individual, relationship, community, and society. Examples of evidence-based prevention strategies presented in the CDC technical program package include early childhood visitation programs, organizational and workplace policies, and family-based programs.[112]

At the secondary prevention level, screening and referral for treatment are two key steps for prevention of further IPV in women who have a history of prior IPV or are at risk for IPV.[110] Nurses have advocated for universal screening for IPV.[110,111,113] A number of screening tools are available, such as the DOVE tool developed by a nurse and tailored for screening during a home visit. DOVE is an evidence-based screening tool developed to help identify women who may be at risk for perinatal IPV and includes steps for implementing interventions during a perinatal home visit aimed at reducing violence.[114] Disclosure of IPV requires action by the provider, further assessment, appropriate referrals, and discussion of a safety plan. To help practitioners, the Agency for Healthcare Research and Quality reviewed the evidence to support screening for IPV in women who did not have signs of abuse. Their fact sheet provides the evidence to support screening as well as for resources for implementing screening in healthcare settings.[115]

Epidemiology of Community Violence

Community violence is an event that includes crime, weapons use, and violence or potential violence, and is perpetrated in a public place by individuals who do not have a relationship with the vicitms.[116] Examples of community violence include violent acts or victimization by strangers perpetrated by one or more individuals, sniper attacks, gang wars, and drive-by shootings.[117]

The impact of violence on a community is widespread. Exposure to the constant stress of living within an unsafe community takes its toll on all of its citizens. It can lead to a sense of isolation for older adults who limit their activity outside their home because of violence. It can lead to a lack of physical activity in children and families because parents are concerned about the safety of their children. It can lead to psychiatric sequelae because of the feelings of fear and stress.[116,117]

Community violence can also occur in towns and neighborhoods where violence is not the norm, such as the killing of 20 children and 6 adults at Sandy Hook Elementary School in Newtown, Connecticut; the killing of church members in South Carolina; or the school shootings in Parkland, Florida. These events sent shock waves through the nation and brought calls for stricter gun control laws. Understanding the causative factors behind community-level violence is complex and can include individual level factors such as a history of mental illness or terrorism, as was the case in the Boston Marathon bombing and the events on September 11, 2001.

In 2016, in the U.S., 5.7 million people aged 12 or older experienced violent victimization at a rate of 21.2 per 1,000. The rate of violent victimization by a stranger was higher than the rate for IPV (8.2 per 1,000 versus 2.2 per 1,000).[118,119] These statistics reflect actual reported events of violent crime. At the community level, violence not only affects the victim(s), it also affects those who witness the violence and can create a community-level reaction of concern for safety. For some communities, it is an unexpected event that takes a community unaware, and in others, the violence is part of everyday life. In the case of war, one expects to be exposed to death, trauma, and stress. Unfortunately, certain neighborhoods in our cities have often been compared to war zones where it is not uncommon to be exposed to severe violence on a regular basis.

Exposure to community violence (i.e., seeing someone shot; someone being stabbed, molested, raped, mugged, threatened with a knife, gun or weapon; or someone being beaten up or hurt) is often associated with psychiatric sequelae including post-traumatic stress disorder (PTSD).[115,116] **Post-traumatic stress disorder** is a type of anxiety disorder in children and adults who witness horrific events. PTSD can develop in response to a variety of traumatic events such as witnessing a violent act or crime, experiencing a natural or unnatural disaster, and experiencing physical or sexual abuse.[116] Other comorbid psychiatric symptoms include anxiety and major depressive episodes. Substance use and behavior problems are also seen in children exposed to violence.[116]

Risk and Protective Factors for Community Violence

For the most part, economically depressed and disorganized communities with fewer resources and an increased access to guns are at greater risk for community-level violence.[120] Truly understanding risk and protective factors for community violence continues to be a challenge. Risk factors often not addressed include racism, discrimination, prisoner reentry, and other conditions of vulnerability and invisibility.[121] Protective factors at the community level include norms supporting gender equity and robust economic/job opportunities in communities.

A particular concern with violence in the community is **youth violence**, which occurs when youths hurt peers unrelated to them that they may or may not know well.[122] Young people perpetrate violent acts at a higher rate than any other age group. The risk factors for youth violence occur at the individual, family, peer, and community level. They include low socioeconomic status, poor parental supervision, delinquent peers, and harsh parenting. At the community level, risk factors for violence are similar and include living in disorganized communities with fewer resources, lower socioeconomic status, and a higher rate of transiency.[122]

Promoting youth development is one strategy used to decrease youth violence within the community. This is based on the fact that social connectedness is a protective factor inversely associated with rates of crime at the community level.[122] Resilience is the ability to successfully adapt and function despite exposure to chronic stress and adversity. Resilience is achieved through support from a family, school, or peer group. The CDC has published a guide to evidence-based programs aimed at reducing youth violence. The recommendations include six areas: (1) promote family environments that support healthy development, (2) provide quality education early in life, (3) strengthen youth skills, (4) connect youth to caring adults and activities, (5) create protective community environments, and (6) intervene to lessen harms and prevent future risk. This technical prevention package provides links to evidence-based programs, many of which can be implemented at the community level.[123]

Epidemiology of War: An Example of Collective Violence

War as defined by the online Merriam Webster dictionary is "a state of usually open and declared armed hostile conflict between states or nations."[124] This excludes individuals or families fighting, gangs fighting, and other smaller community entities. Traditional war is thought of as the fighting between two political states or countries, but just as common is the fighting between two groups within a state (civil war) that are aspiring to become the political entity for the state. War is a violent way of determining who will govern. War and its violence create serious social consequences that affect all the political communities involved. These consequences can be a result of a prolonged conflict, extreme aggression, excessive mortality and morbidity, and/or high financial cost, all of which reduce resources for social needs.

In their book *On War and Public Health*, Levy and Sidel write:

> *War accounts for more death and disability than many major diseases combined. It destroys families, communities, and sometimes whole cultures. It directs scarce resources away from protection and promotion of health, medical care, and other human services. It destroys the infrastructure that supports health. It limits human rights and contributes to social injustice. It leads many people to think that violence is the only way to resolve conflicts—a mindset that contributes to domestic violence, street crime, and other kinds of violence. And it contributes to the destruction of the environment and overuse of nonrenewable resources. In sum, war threatens much of the fabric of our civilization (p. 3, 138).[125]*

War affects more than the combatants. In the 20th century, it was estimated that 136.5 to 148.5 million people died in war and conflict.[126] However, the largest death toll comes not from the direct conflict but from both the short- and long-term residual effects of the war such as disease and malnutrition.[127,128]

Worldwide, in 2018, examples of ongoing wars included those in Afghanistan, Syria, Yemen, Somalia, and Myanmar. More than 40 wars (both between nations and civil wars) began in the 1990s compared with fewer than

10 in the first decade of this century. There also were fewer deaths caused directly by war-related violence. For example, the number of all battle-related deaths in conflicts in 2016 was 87,432.[129] One contributing factor to lower mortality is that the nature of war has changed. There are no longer huge armies in battle with massive human destruction. However, more countries have access to weapons of mass destruction, and the number of countries with active nuclear warheads has grown from two in the 1940s to nine by 2013.

With the use of social media, there has also been more reporting of wars and their atrocities. The reporting occurs almost at the moment they occur. It makes the violence seem greater, because of the immediacy with which it is being reported. When traditional reporting by journalists is impeded, as occurred in the Syrian conflict, social media has provided an alternative source of news for those inside and outside the country.

Even with fewer wars and numbers of deaths, the war-related effects of current conflicts are enormous. There is an obvious breakdown in public health systems with the displacement of resources to war and away from health services including prevention services, increases in disease transmission, and other changes in the social systems that had previously kept the population healthy. There are many other examples of the destructiveness of war: the use of child soldiers resulting in severe physical and emotional abuse of the children, making it very difficult for them to reintegrate into civil society; the forced movements of refugees and displaced persons from their own homes to areas with decreased health and safety; and the increased acceptability of violence as a solution to problems.

■ CELLULAR TO GLOBAL
The Impact of War

Advances in health care have reduced the immediate impact of combat injuries, reducing mortality and long-term morbidity substantially in the time between the American Civil War and today. So, on the surface, it appears we have vastly improved our ability to address the impact of war on combatants at the cellular level. Taking the wider view of the impact of war on the communities where the conflict occurs demonstrates the more complex relationship between armed conflict and health not only due to injury but malnutrition, destruction of community infrastructure, housing, and access to clean water. On the psychological level, both combatants and non-combatants suffer from short- and long-term PTSD. On the global level, war in one section of the world flows over into other countries, especially with the current crisis related to war refugees coming into western countries and ensuing resistance from citizens of western countries to accept refugees (see Chapter 7). Hogopian argued that war should be reframed as a public health issue due to the serious consequences to the health of populations that result during war and its aftermath.[130] White took a global view and proposed that collaboration among nations was essential in the prevention of war.[131] Advances in treating injury resulting from war at the cellular level has improved survival rate for combatants, yet a global international approach may be needed to reduce the short- and long-term impacts on non-combatants including those who stay and those who are forced to seek refuge from a war zone.

Role of the Nurse in War

Starting with primary prevention, the nurse can support actions to prevent war. If war ensues, the nurse may try to minimize the effects of the war as part of secondary prevention. After the war is over, the nurse, at the tertiary level, may help treat the victims of the war and minimize the political, economic, social, and environmental destruction. Nurses can help in surveillance and documentation of what happens during the war and report it to the appropriate agencies, advocate for the use of nonviolence, advocate to minimize the results of war, and work with the refugees and displaced persons from the war, either in the United States or in other countries, to improve their health and social reintegration into society. With additional training, nurses can provide the emergency relief frequently needed during and immediately at the end of the war. Nurses can also help document and understand the most appropriate interventions for refugees and displaced persons, which are frequently specific to the affected population. Using this additional information, the reintegration of individuals into post-war social systems can be facilitated.

■ Summary Points

- Injury is a major public issue that includes both intentional and unintentional injury, most of which is preventable.
- Risk factors associated with injury and violence are complex and include a combination of individual behaviors, environment, socioeconomic status, and culture.

- Violence can occur at the family or community level, with the most vulnerable being children, women, and older adults.

▼ SUICIDE AND VULNERABLE POPULATIONS
Learning Outcomes

At the end of this case study, students will be able to:

- Compare dependent rates (Chapter 3).
- Compare the effectiveness of different approaches to prevention based on the target population.
- Explain the role of health-care providers and key stakeholders in prevention program planning.
- Discuss the benefits of incorporating cultural components into a health program.
- Compare and contrast different levels of prevention as well as the applicability of the socioecological model when developing a health program.

Suicide rates are rising in the U.S. with a rate of 15.6 per 100,000 in 2016, up from 11.3 per 100,000 in 2007. Split into teams and have each team choose a different specific subpopulation (e.g., adolescents, older adults, veterans). Subpopulations can be further divided based on demographic variables such as race and gender. Examine the most recent statistics on suicide rates in this population as well as the most recent statistics at the national and global level. Then examine the current evidence-based approaches to prevention and decide on a specific prevention approach. As part of your assessment and program planning:

1. Compare the suicide rate in your chosen population with the suicide rate in the general population and decide if there is a significant difference.
2. Examine possible evidence-based approaches to suicide prevention within the context of a particular health-care setting (e.g., ED, primary care, public health department) and the chosen population. Choose one to implement.
3. Determine the level of intervention based on whether it is primary, secondary, or tertiary as well as whether it is universal, selective, or indicated.
4. Develop a draft plan of the program. Be sure to address possible cultural concerns, key stakeholders, and access to care.
5. Compare plans between teams. If you could only implement one program, which would you chose? Support your choice using a public health perspective.

REFERENCES

1. Centers for Disease Control and Prevention. (2017). *Emergency department visits.* Retrieved from https://www.cdc.gov/nchs/fastats/emergency-department.htm.
2. World Health Organization. (2014). *Injury and violence: The facts.* Geneva, Switzerland: Author.
3. World Health Organization. (2018). *Top ten causes of death.* Retrieved from http://www.who.int/mediacentre/factsheets/fs310/en/index1.html.
4. Centers for Disease Control and Prevention. (2017). *Leading causes of death.* Retrieved from https://www.cdc.gov/nchs/fastats/leading-causes-of-death.htm.
5. Centers for Disease Control and Prevention. (2018). *Leading causes of death by age group, United States 2016.* Retrieved from https://www.cdc.gov/injury/images/lc-charts/leading_causes_of_death_age_group_2016_1056w814h.gif.
6. Centers for Disease Control and Prevention, Healthy People 2020. (2018). *Injury and violence prevention.* Retrieved from https://www.healthypeople.gov/2020/topics-objectives/topic/injury-and-violence-prevention and https://www.cdc.gov/nchs/data/hpdata2020/HP2020MCR-C24-IVP.pdf.
7. World Health Organization. (2018). *Injuries.* Retrieved from http://www.who.int/topics/injuries/en/.
8. Maine Center for Disease Control and Prevention. (2018). *Maine injury prevention program: Unintentional injury.* Retrieved from http://www.maine.gov/dhhs/mecdc/population-health/inj/unintentional.html.
9. Centers for Disease Control and Prevention. (2017). *Fast stats: Accidents or unintentional injuries.* Retrieved from https://www.cdc.gov/nchs/fastats/accidental-injury.htm.
10. Murphy, S.L., Xu, J., Kochanek, K.D., Curtin, S.C., Arias, E. (2017). Deaths: Final data for 2015. *National Vital Statistics Reports, 66*(6).
11. Maine Center for Disease Control and Prevention. (2018). *Maine injury prevention program: Intentional injury.* Retrieved from http://www.maine.gov/dhhs/mecdc/population-health/inj/intentional.html.
12. World Health Organization, the United Nations Development Programme, and the United Nations Office on Drugs and Crime. (2014). *World report on violence and health.* Geneva, Switzerland: Author.
13. Centers for Disease Control and Prevention. (2019). *NVDRS Frequently Asked Questions.* Retrieved from https://www.cdc.gov/violenceprevention/datasources/nvdrs/faqs.html.
14. Centers for Disease Control and Prevention. (2016). *Cost of injury and violence in the United States.* Retrieved from https://www.cdc.gov/injury/wisqars/overview/cost_of_injury.html.
15. Centers for Disease Control and Prevention. (2018). *Healthy People 2020: Injury and violence prevention.* Retrieved from https://www.healthypeople.gov/2020/topics-objectives/topic/injury-and-violence-prevention.
16. Centers for Disease Control and Prevention. (2017). *Healthy People 2020 Midcourse Review: Chapter 24, injury and violence prevention.* Retrieved from https://www.cdc.gov/nchs/data/hpdata2020/HP2020MCR-C24-IVP.pdf.
17. Centers for Disease Control and Prevention. (2017). *National violent death reporting system.* Retrieved from http://www.cdc.gov/ViolencePrevention/NVDRS/.

18. Haddon, W., Jr. (1999). The changing approach to the epidemiology, prevention, and amelioration of trauma: The transition to approaches etiologically rather than descriptively based. *Injury Prevention, 5*(3), 161-162.

19. Centers for Disease Control and Prevention. (2018). *Injury prevention and control*. Retrieved from https://www.cdc.gov/injury/index.html.

20. myPlan. (2018). *Our story: The science of safety*. Retrieved from https://www.myplanapp.org/about.

21. Society of Trauma Nurses. (2018). *Vision and mission*. Retrieved from http://www.traumanurses.org/about/mission-vision.

22. Cincinnati Children's Medical Center. (2018). *Comprehensive children's injury center*. Retrieved from https://www.cincinnatichildrens.org/service/c/ccic/child-passenger-safety.

23. World Health Organization. (2018). *Violence and injury prevention: Road traffic injuries*. Retrieved from http://www.who.int/violence_injury_prevention/road_traffic/en/.

24. World Health Organization. (2018). *Global plan for the decade of action for road safety 2011–2020*. Retrieved from http://www.who.int/roadsafety/decade_of_action/plan/en/index.html.

25. World Life Expectancy. (2017). *U.S. life expectancy*. Retrieved from http://www.worldlifeexpectancy.com/usa-cause-of-death-by-age-and-gender.

26. Sauber-Schatz, E.K., Ederer, D.J., Dellinger, A.M., & Baldwin, G.T. (2016). Vital signs: Motor vehicle injury prevention - United States and 19 comparison countries. *MMWR: Morbidity & Mortality Weekly Report, 65*(26), 672-677. doi:10.15585/mmwr.mm6526e1.

27. Naimi, T.S., Ziming Xuan, Z., Sarda, V., Hadland, S.E., Lira, M.C, Swahn, M.H., Heeren, ... T.C. (2018). Association of state alcohol policies with alcohol-related motor vehicle crash fatalities among U.S. adults. *JAMA Internal Medicine*. Published online May 29, 2018. doi:10.1001/jamainternmed.2018.1406.

28. Centers for Disease Control and Prevention. (2018). *WISQARS*. Retrieved from https://wisqars-viz.cdc.gov/.

29. Centers for Disease Control and Prevention. (2018). *Motor vehicle safety: Cost data and prevention strategies*. Retrieved from https://www.cdc.gov/motorvehiclesafety/costs/index.html.

30. Centers for Disease Control and Prevention. (2018). *Injury prevention and control: Cost of injuries and violence in the United States*. Retrieved from https://www.cdc.gov/injury/wisqars/overview/cost_of_injury.html.

31. Beck, L.F., Downs, J., Stevens, M.R., Sauber-Schatz, E.K. (2017). Rural and urban differences in passenger-vehicle–occupant deaths and seat belt use among adults — United States, 2014. *MMWR Surveillance Summary, 66*(No. SS-17), 1–13. DOI: doi.org/10.15585/mmwr.ss6617a1.

32. U.S. Department of Transportation, Federal Motor Carrier Safety Administration. (2015). *CMV driving tips - Driver distraction*. Retrieved from https://www.fmcsa.dot.gov/safety/driver-safety/cmv-driving-tips-driver-distraction.

33. Centers for Disease Control and Prevention. (2017). *Distracted driving*. Retrieved from https://www.cdc.gov/motorvehiclesafety/distracted_driving/index.html.

34. National Center for Statistics and Analysis. (2017). *Distracted driving: 2015, in traffic safety research notes. DOT HS 812 381*. Washington, D.C.: National Highway Traffic Safety Administration.

35. U.S. Department of Transportation, National Highway Traffic Safety Administration. (2018). *Speeding*. Retrieved from https://www.nhtsa.gov/risky-driving/speeding.

36. World Health Organization. (2018). *Violence and injury prevention: Burns*. Retrieved from http://www.who.int/violence_injury_prevention/other_injury/burns/en/.

37. World Health Organization. (2018). *Fact sheet: Burns*. Retrieved from http://www.who.int/en/news-room/fact-sheets/detail/burns.

38. Smolle, C., Cambiaso-Daniel, J., Forbes, A.A., Wurzer, P., Hundeshagen, G., Branski, L.K., & Kamolz, L. (2017). Recent trends in burn epidemiology worldwide: A systematic review. *Burns (03054179), 43*(2), 249-257. doi:10.1016/j.burns.2016.08.013.

39. American Burn Association. (2018). *Burn incidence fact sheet: Burn incidence and treatment in the United States: 2016*. Retrieved from http://ameriburn.org/who-we-are/media/burn-incidence-fact-sheet/.

40. Centers for Disease Control and Prevention. (2016). *Protect the ones you love: Child injuries are preventable. Burn prevention*. Retrieved from https://www.cdc.gov/safechild/burns/index.html.

41. Sengoelge, M., El-Khatib, Z., & Laflamme, L. (2017). The global burden of child burn injuries in light of country level economic development and income inequality. *Preventive Medicine Reports, 6*, 115–120. http://doi.org.ezp.welch.jhmi.edu/10.1016/j.pmedr.2017.02.024.

42. World Health Organization. (2018). *Burns fact sheet*. Retrieved from http://www.who.int/en/news-room/fact-sheets/detail/burns.

43. World Health Organization. (2008). *A WHO plan for burn prevention and care*. World Health Organization. http://www.who.int/iris/handle/10665/97852.

44. United States Consumer Product Safety Commission. (2017). *Fireworks safety: 3-step guide to a safer celebration*. Retrieved from https://onsafety.cpsc.gov/blog/2017/06/27/fireworks-safety-3-step-guide-to-a-safer-celebration/.

45. United States Consumer Product Safety Commission. (2017). *2016 fireworks annual report: Fireworks-related deaths and emergency department treated injuries*. Retrieved from https://www.cpsc.gov/s3fs-public/Fireworks_Report_2016.pdf?t.YHKjE9bFiabmirA.4NJJST.5SUWIQJ.

46. World Health Organization. (2018). *Violence and injury prevention: Drowning*. Retrieved from http://www.who.int/violence_injury_prevention/other_injury/drowning/en/.

47. Centers for Disease Control and Prevention. (2016). *Home and recreational safety. Unintentional drowning: Get the Facts*. Retrieved from https://www.cdc.gov/homeandrecreationalsafety/water-safety/waterinjuries-factsheet.html.

48. Claiborne, R., Francis, E. (Aug 3, 2010). 6 teens drown while wading in Louisiana's Red River. *ABC News*. Retrieved from https://abcnews.go.com/WN/teens-drown-wading-louisianas-red-river/story?id=11312631.

49. Committee on Injury, Violence and Poison Prevention, & America Academy of Pediatrics. (2010). Policy statement: Prevention of drowning. *Pediatrics, 126*. Retrieved from http://pediatrics.aappublications.org/content/early/2010/05/24/peds.2010-1264.full.pdf+html. doi:10.1542/peds.2010-1264.

50. World Health Organization. (2018). *Falls: Key facts.* Retrieved from http://www.who.int/en/news-room/fact-sheets/detail/falls.

51. Centers for Disease Control and Prevention. (2016). *Child safety and injury prevention: Fall prevention.* Retrieved from https://www.cdc.gov/safechild/falls/index.html.

52. Tuckel, P., Milczarski, W., & Silverman, D.G. (2018). Injuries caused by falls from playground equipment in the United States. *Clinical Pediatrics, 57*(5), 563-573. doi:10.1177/0009922817732618.

53. Gaw, C.E., Chounthirath, T., & Smith, G.A. (2017). Nursery product-related injuries treated in United States emergency departments. *Pediatrics, 139*(4), 1-11. doi:10.1542/peds.2016-2503.

54. Centers for Disease Control and Prevention. (2017). *Falls: Children.* Retrieved from https://www.cdc.gov/HomeandRecreationalSafety/Falls/children.html.

55. The U.S. Consumer Product Safety Commission. (2017). *Public playground safety handbook.* Washington D.C.: Author.

56. New York City Department of Health and Mental Hygiene. (n.d.). *Window guards: Preventing falls.* Retrieved from https://www1.nyc.gov/site/doh/health/health-topics/window-guards-preventing-falls.page.

57. Centers for Disease Control and Prevention. (2015). *Home and recreational safety poisoning.* Retrieved from https://www.cdc.gov/homeandrecreationalsafety/poisoning/index.html.

58. Centers for Disease Control and Prevention, National Center for Health Statistics. (2017). *Accidents and unintentional injuries.* Retrieved from https://www.cdc.gov/nchs/fastats/accidental-injury.htm.

59. Rossen, L.M., Bastian, B., Warner, M., Khan, D., Chong, Y. (2017). *Drug poisoning mortality: United States, 1999–2016.* National Center for Health Statistics. Retrieved from https://www.cdc.gov/nchs/data-visualization/drug-poisoning-mortality/.

60. Gummin, D.D., Mowry, J.B., Spyker, D.A., Brook, D.E., Fraser, M.O., & Banner, W. (2017). 2016 annual report of the American Association of Poison Control Centers' national poison data system (NPDS): 34th annual report. *Clinical Toxicology, 55*, 1072-1254. doi: 10.1080/15563650.2017.1388087.

61. World Health Organization. (2018). *Lead poisoning and health.* Retrieved from http://www.who.int/en/news-room/fact-sheets/detail/lead-poisoning-and-health.

62. National Capital Poison Center. (2018). *Poison statistics: National data 2016.* Retrieved from https://www.poison.org/poison-statistics-national.

63. Safe Kids Worldwide. (2015). *Poisoning safety fact sheet.* Retrieved from https://www.safekids.org/sites/default/files/documents/skw_poisoning_fact_sheet_feb_2015.pdf.

64. Centers for Disease Control and Prevention. (2017). *Poisoning prevention.* Retrieved from https://www.cdc.gov/safechild/Poisoning/index.html.

65. American Association of Poison Control Centers. (n.d.). *Prevention.* Retrieved from http://www.aapcc.org/prevention/.

66. United States Consumer Product Safety Commission. (n.d.). *Poison prevention information center.* Retrieved from http://www.aapcc.org/prevention/.

67. World Health Organization. (2018). *International programme on chemical safety: Poisoning prevention and management.* Retrieved from http://www.who.int/ipcs/poisons/en/.

68. Centers for Disease Control and Prevention. (2017). *Self-directed violence and other forms of self-injury.* Retrieved from https://www.cdc.gov/ncbddd/disabilityandsafety/self-injury.html.

69. Centers for Disease Control and Prevention. (2017). *Definitions: Self-directed violence.* Retrieved from https://www.cdc.gov/violenceprevention/suicide/definitions.html.

70. National Institute of Mental Health. (2018). *Suicide.* Retrieved from https://www.nimh.nih.gov/health/statistics/suicide.shtml.

71. Stone, D.M., Simon, T.R., Fowler, K.A., Kegler, S.R., Yuan, K., Holland, K.M., & Crosby, A.E. (2018). Vital signs: Trends in state suicide rates — United States, 1999–2016 and circumstances contributing to suicide — 27 states, 2015. *Morbidity and Mortality Weekly Report, 67*(22), 617–624. doi:10.15585/mmwr.mm6722a1

72. World Health Organization. (2018). *Mental health: Suicide data.* Retrieved from http://www.who.int/mental_health/prevention/suicide/suicideprevent/en/.

73. Dyer, O. (2018, 12 June). U.S. suicide rate is climbing steadily with highest prevalence in sparsely populated western states. *British Medical Journal, 361*, k2586. doi:10.1136/bmj.k2586.

74. Centers for Disease Control and Prevention. (2017). *Suicide: Risk and protective factors.* Retrieved from https://www.cdc.gov/violenceprevention/suicide/riskprotectivefactors.html.

75. U.S. Department of Health and Human Services. (2010). To live to see the great day that dawns: Preventing suicide by American Indian and Alaska Native youth and young adults. DHHS Publication SMA (10)-4480, CMHS-NSPL-0196, Printed 2010. Rockville, MD: Center for Mental Health Services, Substance Abuse and Mental Health Services Administration, 2010.

76. Indian Health Service. (n.d.). *Suicide prevention and care program.* Retrieved from https://www.ihs.gov/suicideprevention/.

77. Tsai, J., Trevisan, L., Huang, M., & Pietrzak, R.H. (2018). Addressing veteran homelessness to prevent veteran suicides. *Psychiatric Service.* doi: 10.1176/appi.ps.201700482. [Epub ahead of print].

78. Montana Department of Health and Human Services: Office of Epidemiology and Scientific Support. (2018). *Veteran suicide in Montana, 2013-2016.* Retrieved from https://dphhs.mt.gov/Portals/85/publichealth/documents/Epidemiology/VSU/VSU_Veteran_Suicide_2013-2016.pdf.

79. U.S. Department of Health and Human Services, Administration for Children and Families. (n.d.). *Keeping Children Safe Act.* Retrieved from https://www.childwelfare.gov/systemwide/laws_policies/federal/index.cfm?event=federalLegislation.viewLegis&id=45.

80. Smith, M. (2018, June 8). 5 takeaways on America's increasing suicide rate. *New York Times.* Retrieved from https://www.nytimes.com/2018/06/09/us/suicide-rates-increasing-bourdain.html.

81. Allchin, A., Chaplin, V., Horwitz, J. (2018). *Injury Prevention, 0,* 1–5. doi:10.1136/injuryprev-2018-042809.

82. Bailey, E., Rice S., Robinson J., Nedeljkovicc, M., & Alvarez-Jimenezab M. (2018). Theoretical and empirical foundations of a novel online social networking intervention for youth suicide prevention: A conceptual review. *Journal of Affective Disorders, 238*, 499-505. https://doi.org/10.1016/j.jad.2018.06.028.

83. Brodsky, B.S., Spruch-Feiner, A., & Stanley, B. (2018). The zero suicide model: Applying evidence-based suicide prevention practices to clinical care. *Frontiers in Psychiatry, 9*, 33. http://doi.org.ezp.welch.jhmi.edu/10.3389/fpsyt.2018.00033.

84. Stone, D.M., Holland, K.M., Bartholow, B., Crosby, A.E., Davis, S., & Wilkins, N. (2017). *Preventing suicide: A technical package of policies, programs, and practices.* Atlanta, GA: National Center for Injury Prevention and Control, Centers for Disease Control and Prevention.

85. U.S. Health and Human Services: Healthy People 2020. (2017). *Topics and objectives: Mental health and mental disorders.* Retrieved from https://www.healthypeople.gov/2020/topics-objectives/topic/mental-health-and-mental-disorders.

86. U.S. Health and Human Services: Healthy People 2020. (2017). *Healthy People 2020 Midcourse Review: Chapter 28, mental health and mental disorders (MHMD).* Retrieved from https://www.cdc.gov/nchs/data/hpdata2020/HP2020MCR-C28-MHMD.pdf.

87. Keeping Children and Families Safe Act of 2003. (2003). *P.L. 108-36.* Retrieved from https://www.acf.hhs.gov/sites/default/files/cb/capta2003.pdf.

88. World Health Organization. (2018). *Violence and injury prevention: Child maltreatment (abuse).* Retrieved from http://www.who.int/violence_injury_prevention/violence/child/en/.

89. World Health Organization. (2017). *World health statistics 2017: Monitoring health for the SDGs.* Geneva, Switzerland: Author.

90. Centers for Disease Control and Prevention. (2018). *Child abuse and neglect prevention.* Retrieved from https://www.cdc.gov/violenceprevention/childabuseandneglect/index.html.

91. U.S. Department of Health & Human Services, Administration for Children and Families, Administration on Children, Youth and Families, Children's Bureau. (2018). *Child maltreatment 2016.* Available from https://www.acf.hhs.gov/cb/research-data-technology/statistics-research/child-maltreatment.

92. Centers for Disease Control and Prevention. (2018). *Child abuse and neglect: Risk and protective factors.* Retrieved from https://www.cdc.gov/violenceprevention/childabuseandneglect/riskprotectivefactors.htmL

93. Dittrich, K., Boedeker, K., Kluczniok, D., Jaite, C., Attar, C.H., Fuehrer, D., ... Bermpohl, F. (2018). Child abuse potential in mothers with early life maltreatment, borderline personality disorder, and depression. *The British Journal of Psychiatry, 213*,412-418. https://doi-org.ezp.welch.jhmi.edu/10.1192/bjp.2018.74.

94. Ahmadabadi, Z., Najman, J.M., Williams, G.M., Clavarino, A.M., d'Abbs, P., Abajobira, A.A. (2018). Maternal intimate partner violence victimization and child maltreatment. *Child Abuse and Neglect, 82*(August 2018), 23-33. https://doi.org/10.1016/j.chiabu.2018.05.017.

95. Centers for Disease Control and Prevention. (2018). *Child abuse and neglect: Prevention strategies.* Retrieved from https://www.cdc.gov/violenceprevention/childabuseandneglect/prevention.html.

96. Nurse Family Partnership Program. (2018). *About us.* Retrieved from https://www.nursefamilypartnership.org/About/.

97. Triple P Program. (2018). *Find out about Triple P.* Retrieved from https://www.triplep.net/glo-en/find-out-about-triple-p/.

98. Family Connections. (2018). *Home.* Retrieved from http://familyconnections.org/.

99. Centers for Disease Control and Prevention. (2018). *Intimate partner violence.* Retrieved from https://www.cdc.gov/violenceprevention/intimatepartnerviolence/index.html.

100. World Health Organization. (2018). *Violence against women.* Retrieved from http://www.who.int/news-room/fact-sheets/detail/violence-against-women.

101. Breiding, M.J., Basile, K.C., Smith, S.G., Black, M.C., & Mahendra, R.R. (2015). *Intimate partner violence surveillance: Uniform definitions and recommended data elements, version 2.0 [PDF 283KB].* Atlanta, GA: National Center for Injury Prevention and Control, Centers for Disease Control and Prevention.

102. Centers for Disease Control and Prevention. (2018). *National intimate partner and sexual violence survey: 2015 data brief.* Retrieved from https://www.cdc.gov/violenceprevention/nisvs/2015NISVSdatabrief.html.

103. Walters, M.L., Chen J., & Breiding, M.J. (2013). *The national intimate partner and sexual violence survey (NISVS): 2010 findings on victimization by sexual orientation.* Atlanta, GA: National Center for Injury Prevention and Control, Centers for Disease Control and Prevention.

104. Centers for Disease Control and Prevention. (2017). *Intimate partner violence: Consequences.* Retrieved from https://www.cdc.gov/violenceprevention/intimatepartnerviolence/consequences.html.

105. Hoelle, R.M., Elie, M., Weeks, E., Hardt, N., Wei, H., Hui, Y., & Carden, D. (2015). Evaluation of healthcare use trends of high-risk female intimate partner violence victims. *Western Journal Of Emergency Medicine: Integrating Emergency Care With Population Health, 16*(1), 107-113. doi:10.5811/westjem.2014.12.22866.

106. World Health Organization. (2012). *Femicide.* Retrieved from http://apps.who.int/iris/bitstream/handle/10665/77421/WHO_RHR_12.38_eng.pdf;sequence=1.

107. World Health Organization. (2009). *Changing cultural and social norms supportive of violent behavior.* Retrieved from http://www.who.int/violence_injury_prevention/violence/norms.pdf.

108. Wathen, C.N., MacGregor, J.D., & MacQuarrie, B.J. (2018). Relationships among intimate partner violence, work, and health. *Journal Of Interpersonal Violence, 33*(14), 2268-2290. doi:10.1177/0886260515624236.

109. Yakubovich, A.R., Stöckl, H., Murray, J., Melendez-Torres, G.J., Steinert, J.I., Glavin, C.Y., & Humphreys, D.K. (2018). Risk and protective factors for intimate partner violence against women: Systematic review and meta-analyses of prospective-longitudinal studies. *American Journal Of Public Health, 108*(7), e1-e11. doi:10.2105/AJPH.2018.304428.

110. Alvarez, C., Fedock, G., Grace, K.T., & Campbell, J. (2017). Provider screening and counseling for intimate partner violence: A systematic review of practices and influencing factors. *Trauma, Violence & Abuse, 18*(5), 479-495. doi:10.1177/1524838016637080.

111. Campbell, J., Webster, D., Koziol-McLain, J., Block, C., Campbell, D., Curry, M., ... Laughon, K. (2003). Risk factors for femicide in abusive relationships: Results from a multi-site case control study. *American Journal of Public Health, 93*(7), 1089-1097. doi:10.2105/AJPH.93.7.1089.

112. Niolon, P.H., Kearns, M., Dills, J., Rambo, K., Irving, S., Armstead, T., & Gilbert, L. (2017). *Preventing intimate partner violence across the lifespan: A technical package of programs, policies, and practices.* Atlanta, GA: National Center for Injury Prevention and Control, Centers for Disease Control and Prevention.

113. Ghandour, R.M., Campbell, J.C., & Lloyd, J. (2015). Screening and counseling for intimate partner violence: A vision for the future. *Journal of Women's Health (15409996), 24*(1), 57-61. doi:10.1089/jwh.2014.4885.

114. Sharps, P.W., Bullock, L.F., Campbell, J.C., Alhusen, J.L., Ghazarian, S.R., Bhandari, S.S., & Schminkey, D.L. (2016). Domestic violence enhanced perinatal home visits: The DOVE randomized clinical trial. *Journal of Women's Health (15409996), 25*(11), 1129-1138. doi:10.1089/jwh.2015.5547.

115. Agency for Healthcare Research and Quality. (2015). *Intimate partner violence screening.* Retrieved from http://www.ahrq.gov/professionals/prevention-chronic-care/healthier-pregnancy/preventive/partnerviolence.html.

116. Hamblen, J. & Goguen, C. (2016). *U.S. Department of Veterans Affairs: Community violence.* Retrieved from https://www.ptsd.va.gov/professional/trauma/other/community-violence.asp.

117. The National Child Traumatic Stress Network. (n.d.). *Community violence.* Retrieved from https://www.nctsn.org/what-is-child-trauma/trauma-types/community-violence.

118. Office of Justice Programs, Bureau of Justice Statistics. (n.d.). *Crime in the United States.* Retrieved from https://www.bjs.gov/index.cfm?ty=tp&tid=31.

119. Office of Justice Programs, Bureau of Justice Statistics. (2017). *Criminal victimization, 2016.* Retrieved from https://www.bjs.gov/index.cfm?ty=pbdetail&iid=6166.

120. New York State Office of Mental Health. (n.d.). *Violence prevention: Risk factors.* Retrieved from https://www.omh.ny.gov/omhweb/sv/risk.htm.

121. Armstead, T.L., Wilkins, N., Doreson, A. (2018). Indicators for evaluating community- and societal-level risk and protective factors for violence prevention: Findings from a review of the literature. *Journal of Public Health Management and Practice, 24S,* S42- S50. DOI: 10.1097/PHH.0000000000000681.

122. Centers for Disease Control and Prevention. (2018). *Youth violence.* Retrieved from https://www.cdc.gov/violenceprevention/youthviolence/index.html.

123. David-Ferdon, C., Vivolo-Kantor, A.M., Dahlberg, L.L., Marshall, K.J., Rainford, N. & Hall, J.E. (2016). *A comprehensive technical package for the prevention of youth violence and associated risk behaviors.* Atlanta, GA: National Center for Injury Prevention and Control, Centers for Disease Control and Prevention.

124. Merriam Webster Dictionary. (2018). *Definition of war.* Retrieved from https://www.merriam-webster.com/dictionary/war.

125. Levy, B., & Sidel, V. (Eds.). (2007). *War and public health* (2nd ed.). Oxford, England: Oxford University Press.

126. Leitenberg, M. (2006). *Deaths in wars and conflicts in the 20th century.* Retrieved from http://www.cissm.umd.edu/papers/files/deathswarsconflictsjune52006.pdf.

127. Johnson, S.A. (2017, Jan 12). The cost of war on public health: An exploratory method for understanding the impact of conflict on public health in Sri Lanka. *PLoS One, 12*(1), e0166674. doi: 10.1371/journal.pone.0166674. eCollection.

128. Elsafti, A.M., van Berlaer, G.A., Safadi, M., Debacker, M., Buyl, R., Redwan, A., & Hubloue, I. (2016). Children in the Syrian Civil War: The familial, educational, and public health impact of ongoing violence. *Disaster Medicine and Public Health Preparedness, 10*(6), 874-882. doi: 10.1017/dmp.2016.

129. Roser, M. (2018). *War and peace.* Retrieved from https://ourworldindata.org/war-and-peace.

130. Hogopian, A. (2017). Why isn't war properly framed and funded as a public health problem? *Medicine Conflict Survival, 33*(2), 92-100. doi: 10.1080/13623699.2017.1347848. Epub 2017 Jul 10.

131. White, S.K. (2017). Public health and prevention of war: The power of transdisciplinary, transnational collaboration. *Medicine and Conflict Survival, 33*(2), 101-109. doi: 10.1080/13623699.2017.1327155. Epub 2017 May 25.

Public Health Planning

Chapter 13

Health Planning for Local Public Health Departments

Susan Bulecza, Laurie Abbott, and Barbara Little

LEARNING OUTCOMES

After reading the chapter, the student will be able to:

1. Describe the historical development of public health departments (abbreviated in this chapter as PHDs).
2. Describe the structure and services of PHDs.
3. Describe the interdisciplinary workforce in PHDs.
4. Analyze key roles and responsibilities of public health nurses (PHNs) in PHDs.
5. Discuss current issues related to delivery of essential public health services by PHDs.

6. Investigate the role of PHDs in community assessment and planning for health needs of the community.
7. Identify the most frequent activities and services provided by PHDs.
8. Discuss financial and information technology resources needed to support PHDs.
9. Describe the challenges facing PHDs.
10. Discuss accreditation and evaluation of services provided by PHDs.

KEY TERMS

Behavioral Risk Factor Surveillance System (BRFSS)
Categorical funding
Centralized system
Community health assessment

Decentralized system
Directly observed therapy
Geographic information system (GIS)
Federally qualified health centers (FQHCs)
Fetal death

Healthy Start
Medication electronic monitoring system
Public health department (PHD)
Public health informatics
Public health system

Public health systems and services research
Shared or mixed system
Vital statistics
Women, Infants, and Children (WIC)

▓ Introduction

An official governmental body responsible for assuring the health of citizens residing within a county, municipality, township, or territory is called a **public health department (PHD)**. PHDs are considered trusted conveners that facilitate partnerships and coalitions to assess and address local public health issues.

The basic mandate of the PHD is to protect and improve health in partnership with the community (see Chapter 1). Citizens generally think that the PHD is responsible for providing services related to communicable diseases or immunization services. However, they may not be aware of the overarching mission of the PHD to promote and protect the health, defined more broadly than communicable diseases, of all people in the community. This mission can only be accomplished through a host of health-care providers and community partners who pool together resources and coordinate services. These partners and their services make up the **public health system**.[1] Although the PHD is not responsible for providing all health services for a population, governmental agencies are responsible for assuring essential community health services.[2]

The purpose of this chapter is threefold. It is important for all nurses to be aware of the role of local health departments to (1) facilitate linkages between clients and services, (2) describe the role of the public health nurse in a PHD, and (3) discuss current challenges affecting PHDs.

History of Public Health Departments

Local official agencies in the United States developed out of local boards of health in the late 18th century.[3] The first city to form a board of health was Philadelphia (1794), followed by Baltimore (1797), Boston (1799), Washington, DC (1802), New Orleans (1804), and New York City (1805).[4] The concerns at that time were focused on communicable diseases within densely populated cities. In part because of a growing understanding of the connection between proper sanitation and disease, there was an expansion of municipal health departments in the 1880s and early 1900s.[5] Another major growth period occurred with the passage of the Social Security Act in 1935, which provided millions of dollars for maternal and child health services for public health.[4]

The delivery of public health services in rural community settings presented unique challenges. Prior to the establishment of formalized governmental units in rural areas, district nurses provided much of the work of public health.[5] The progression of time and population growth within rural communities influenced the formation of county health departments, which provided public and environmental health services including sanitation. In 1908, the first PHD to provide public health services was established in Jefferson County, Kentucky, and in 1911, two others were formed. Guilford County, North Carolina, expanded school health programs, and Yakima County, Washington, responded to a typhoid epidemic.[5] The first exclusively rural county health department was in Robeson County, North Carolina.[5] By 1921, the county movement had spread to 186 counties in 23 states, often with the help of private foundations.[6,7] The Rockefeller Foundation developed rural programs between 1910 and 1913 to:[5]

- Educate medical professionals and the public about hookworm disease;
- Provide funds to sanitize communities for protection against hookworm and typhoid diseases;
- Fund the employment of personnel to continue work in the counties.

The financial support from the Rockefeller Foundation and other private foundations including the

Commonwealth Fund, W.K. Kellogg Foundation, and, eventually, the Public Health Service (PHS) contributed to the rapid increase in county health departments during the early 20th century, from 1 in 1908 to 610 in 1932.[5]

Mission of Public Health

The mission of public health had its beginnings in the mid-19th century when physicians, housing reformers, advocates for the poor, and scientists trained in housing and civil engineering came together to target health problems associated with urbanization, industrialization, and immigration.[8] The focus was largely on housing conditions and communicable diseases. The work of social reformers at Hull House in Chicago or the Henry Street Settlement with Lillian Wald (Chapter 1) are examples of this work.

Beginning in the 1920s, the Committee on Administrative Practice of the American Public Health Association (APHA) sought to define the mission of public health agencies.[3,9] In 1933, the Committee on Administrative Practice of APHA listed two primary goals for local public health agencies:[3]

- Control of communicable diseases
- Promotion of child health

These goals reflected the basic public health needs of the time, recognizing that children suffered the most from communicable diseases. By 1940, another APHA statement produced a clearer listing of the six minimum functions of local health departments:[10]

- Vital statistics
- Environmental sanitation
- Communicable disease control
- Public health laboratories
- Maternal and child health
- Public health education

The mission of public health was revisited with the Institute of Medicine (IOM) report in 1988. At that time, public health was redefined (see Chapter 1), and the mission was defined as fulfilling society's interest in assuring conditions in which people can be healthy.[11] The three core functions of assurance, assessment, and policy formation evolved from this work.

Structure of Public Health Departments

As hospitals have different corporate and organizational structures, so does the infrastructure for public health agencies vary on the state and local levels. Thus, the adage, "When you have seen one health department, you have seen one health department,"[1] means that no two health departments are alike. Knowing how the PHD is organized is of key importance for nurses to understand how public health services are delivered in their state and community. Generally, PHDs are organized by one of three major delivery modes:

- **Centralized (state) system:** PHDs are operated by a state health agency or board of health, and the PHD functions under the state agency (five states).
- **Decentralized (local) system:** PHDs are operated by local government with or without a board of health (27 states).
- **Shared or mixed system:** PHDs are operated under shared or combined authority of the state health agency, board of health, and local government (16 states).[12,13]
- Hawaii and Rhode Island have state, not local, PHDs.[12]

Similar to the size of the hospital (number of beds) and nurse-to-patient ratio, the size of the population the PHD serves is a critical factor in local public health service delivery. Figure 13-1 illustrates the percentage of small, medium, and large PHDs and the percentage of the U.S. population served by these PHDs. It is interesting to note that 51% of the population is served by only 6% of large PHDs, whereas 62% of small PHDs cover 10% of the population.[12]

The type of jurisdiction or territory served by the PHD is another organizational factor. The majority of PHDs

(69%) are county-based with smaller percentages serving a city or town (20%) as well as city/county (3%) areas such as Miami-Dade in Florida[12] (Fig. 13-2). Proposed as a method for strengthening public health services in rural areas, multicounty or regional jurisdictions encompass 8% of all PHDs.[12,13]

PHDs located in rural areas are challenged by infrastructural issues related to limited resources and isolation.[14] And yet, they are often called upon to address widening health disparities and worsening health outcomes than those in urban areas.[15] For example, morbidity and mortality rates reported for rural areas are often higher, and the environmental health challenges related to agricultural pollution and unsafe mining and logging practices contribute to the problem. People living in rural areas are typically older, poorer, and more likely to have been diagnosed with chronic diseases.[15] In fact, the more remote the rural area is, the lower the life expectancy.[15]

Public Health Workforce

The PHD workforce is interdisciplinary, and the majority of PHDs have fewer than 100 employees. The types of occupations typically found in PHDs include physicians, environmental health specialists, dietitians, social workers, pharmacists, epidemiologists, information technology (IT) specialists, health educators, public information specialists, and nurses. The 2016 National Association of City and County Health Officials (NACCHO) survey reported that registered nurses comprised 18% of the public health workforce composition, a notable decrease from 24% in 2005 (Fig. 13-3).[12] Depending on the jurisdiction, some PHDs employ mental health service providers (2%), physicians (1%), and licensed practical nurses (2%).[12] Staffing patterns vary depending on the size and services provided by the PHD.

Historically, the sociodemographic characteristics of the public health workforce have not adequately represented the diversity of the communities served. The reported findings of a study by NACCHO were that the local health department workforce is predominately Caucasian (72.2%).[16] The PHD employees belonging to specific racial and ethnic minority groups (overall, 27.8%) were African American (15.8%), American Indian/Alaska Native (0.5%), Asian (3.8%), Native Hawaiian/Other Pacific Islander (1.9%), and Some Other Race/Two or more Races (5.8%).[16] Regarding ethnicity, a small percentage of all PHD employees are Hispanic (10.5%), but most are Not Hispanic or Latino (89.5%).[16] The larger the size of the population served, the greater the percentage of diverse workers employed by the PHD.[16]

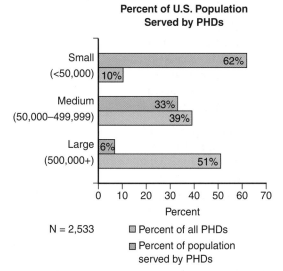

Percent of U.S. Population Served by PHDs

N = 2,533

■ Percent of all PHDs
■ Percent of population served by PHDs

Figure 13-1 Percentage of PHDs and percentage of U.S. population served, by size of population served. (© 2017. *National Association of County and City Health Officials. The 2016 national profile of local health departments. Retrieved from* http://nacchoprofilestudy.org/wp-content/uploads/2017/10/ProfileReport_Aug2017_final.pdf)

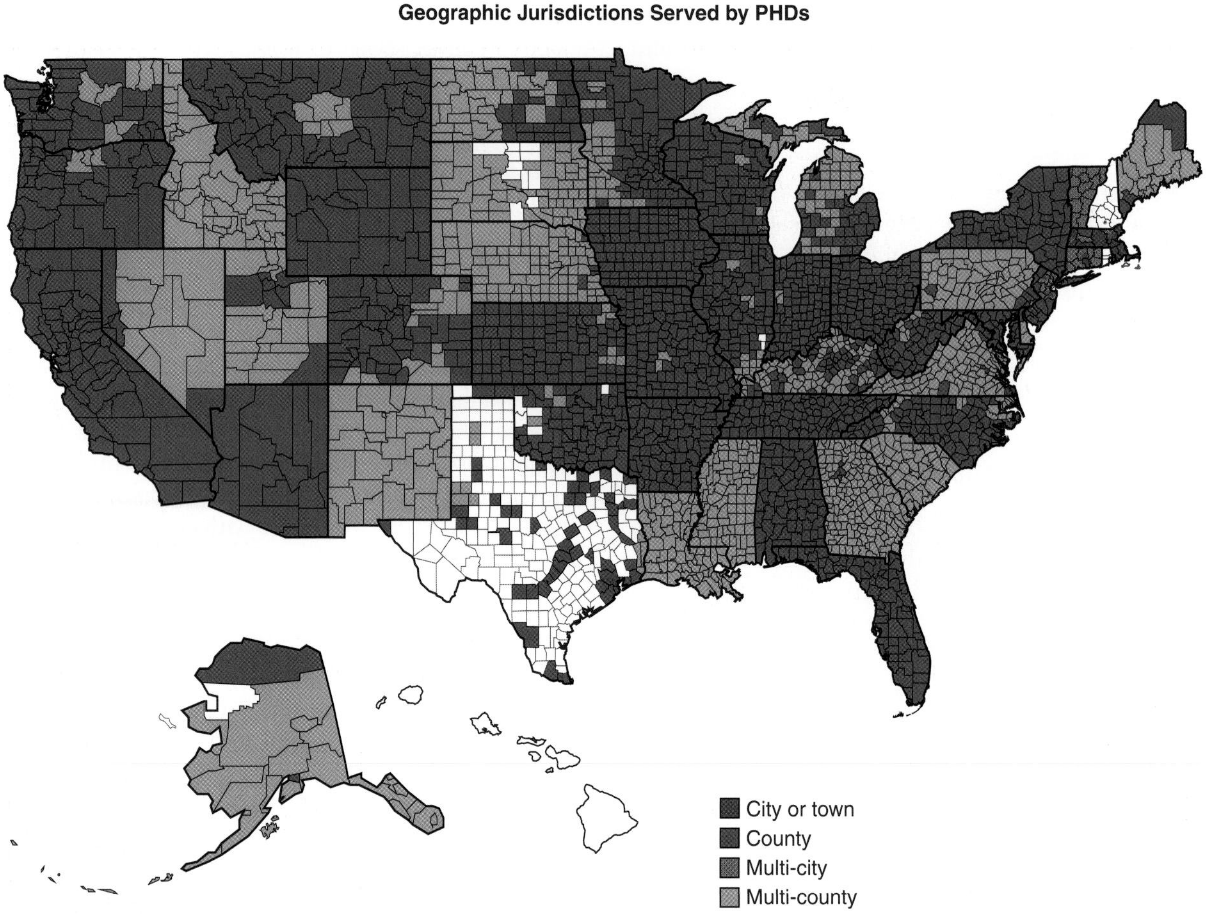

Geographic Jurisdictions Served by PHDs

City or town
County
Multi-city
Multi-county

Figure 13-2 Percentage distribution of PHDs by type of geographical jurisdiction. (*© 2017. National Association of County and City Health Officials. The 2016 national profile of local health departments. Retrieved from* http://nacchoprofilestudy.org/wp-content/uploads/2017/10/ProfileReport_Aug2017_final.pdf)

Role of Public Health Nurses in Public Health Departments

Nurses who work within a PHD are usually considered public health nurses (PHNs). PHNs make up one of the largest professional groups within the health department. Not all PHNs work within an official agency.

The relevance of nursing to public health was recognized in the early 1920s when C.E. Winslow's definition of public health highlighted the role of nursing services:[17]

Public health is the science and art of preventing disease, prolonging life, and promoting physical and mental health well-being through organized community effort for the sanitation of the environment, the control of communicable infections, the organization of medical and nursing services for the early diagnosis and prevention of disease, the education of the individual in personal health, and the development of social machinery to assure everyone a standard of living adequate for the maintenance or improvement of health.

In addition, APHA's 1933 and 1940 statements of the mission of public health emphasized the role of public health nursing in several functions of the health department, especially communicable disease and maternal-child health.[3]

Core Functions

Today, PHNs who work in PHDs promote and protect the health of the entire population in a community through the three core public health functions:[11]

- Population assessment
- Assurance of a well-coordinated system of health promotion and health-care services
- Policy development to support the health of the community

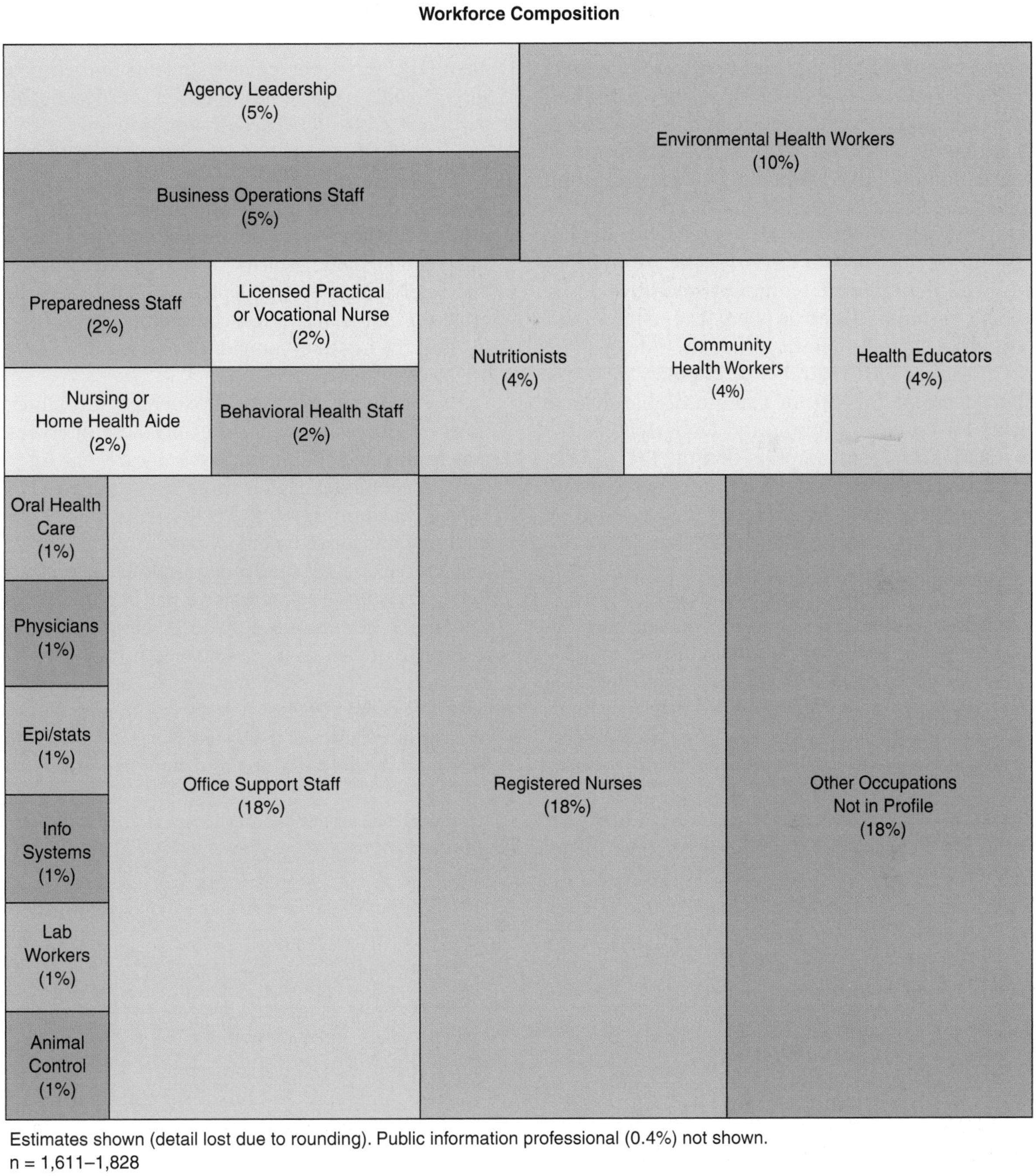

Workforce Composition

Estimates shown (detail lost due to rounding). Public information professional (0.4%) not shown.
n = 1,611–1,828

Figure 13-3 Percentage distribution of occupations in the PHD workforce. (© 2017. National Association of County and City Health Officials. The 2016 national profile of local health departments. Retrieved from http://nacchoprofilestudy.org/wp-content/uploads/2017/10/ProfileReport_Aug2017_final.pdf)

These functions and their related essential services[18] were introduced in Chapter 1 (see Box 1-1), and their relevance for guiding local health departments is further explored in this chapter.

We can apply the core functions to public health nursing within a PHD setting using immunization as

an example of an intervention to promote the health of a population/community. Assessment is illustrated when PHNs working in PHDs gather epidemiological data to determine the rate of children fully immunized against specific communicable diseases (e.g., measles, H1N1 influenza). A high immunization rate (>70%) is needed to provide a community level of immunity (herd immunity) to protect the population (see Chapter 8).[19] Another example of the application of core functions by PHNs in PHDs is their involvement in writing and implementing policies that require immunizations for entry into day care, schools, and colleges to help ensure that herd immunity level is obtained for the protection of students, staff, and families. If the rate is lower, PHNs assure immunization services are provided by mobilizing community partners to target specific groups that have low immunization rates and by providing easily accessible immunizations in pediatric clinics and schools. This example demonstrates the role of PHD PHNs in assessment, assurance, and policy development to decrease the risk of communicable disease transmission in their community. Underlying these three functions is the assumption that the PHN working in the PHD will provide ethical and moral leadership in providing public health services as outlined by the Public Health Leadership Society[20] (Box 13-1).

Essential Services

The core functions of a PHD are further delineated in the 10 essential public health services that illustrate to legislators and the general public what public health does (see Chapter 1) (Fig. 13-4). For example, the assurance function is further defined in the essential public health service of linking people to needed personal health services and assuring the provision of health care when otherwise unavailable.[18] Continuing with the immunization example, PHD PHNs refer college students to their primary care provider, college health center, or local health department to obtain needed immunizations.

Public Health Interventions

A useful conceptual framework for understanding how a health department provides population-based care is the Intervention Wheel, which was introduced in Chapter 2.[21] The Intervention Wheel depicts 17 PHN interventions provided on the individual, community, or systems level to affect the health of individuals and families that make up the community.

PHD PHNs usually provide several types of interventions to address a single issue and these interventions may be directed at different levels of care. The Intervention Wheel model depicts three levels of care: (1) individual, (2) community, and (3) systems.[21] For example, interventions for reducing tobacco use can be provided for all three levels of care. On the individual level, a PHD PHN may counsel a pregnant woman about ways to stop smoking. A community-level intervention may be used to have an impact on more smokers through group education. The PHD PHN may teach tobacco cessation classes that target teens. Nurses working in PHDs also direct interventions at the systems level, which affects the health of the populations and may have the greatest

---

BOX 13–1 ■ Principles of the Ethical Practice of Public Health

- Public health should principally address the fundamental causes of disease and requirements for health, aiming to prevent adverse health outcomes.
- Public health should achieve community health in a way that respects the rights of individuals in the community.
- Public health policies, programs, and priorities should be developed and evaluated through processes that ensure an opportunity for input from community members.
- Public health should advocate and work for the empowerment of disenfranchised community members, aiming to ensure that the basic resources and conditions necessary for health are accessible to all.
- Public health should seek the information needed to implement effective policies and programs that protect and promote health.
- Public health institutions should provide communities with the information they have that is needed for decisions on policies or programs and should obtain the community's consent for their implementation.

- Public health institutions should act in a timely manner on the information they have within the resources and the mandate given to them by the public.
- Public health programs and policies should incorporate a variety of approaches that anticipate and respect diverse values, beliefs, and cultures in the community.
- Public health programs and policies should be implemented in a manner that most enhances the physical and social environment.
- Public health institutions should protect the confidentiality of information that can bring harm to an individual or community if made public. Exceptions must be justified on the basis of the high likelihood of significant harm to the individual or others.
- Public health institutions should ensure the professional competence of their employees.
- Public health institutions and their employees should engage in collaborations and affiliations in ways that build the public's trust and the institution's effectiveness.

Source: (18)

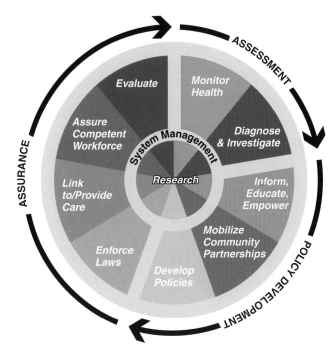

Figure 13-4 Essential services and core functions of public health. *(From the Public Health Functions Steering Committee, 1995. Retrieved from http://www.health.gov/phfunctions/public.htm)*

potential for improving health-care outcomes. For example, in considering a population, intervening on the systems and policy levels to levy tobacco taxes is likely more effective for tobacco cessation at a community level than individually counseling people to quit smoking[22] (see Chapter 11).

What does intervening at a systems level mean? For at least 10 years, the Tobacco Control Research Branch of the National Cancer Institute studied a transdisciplinary initiative to explore systems thinking approaches and methods in tobacco prevention and control, resulting in a 2007 monograph titled *Greater Than the Sum: Systems Thinking in Tobacco Control.*[23] The complexity involved in systems thinking was discussed, for example, by presenting a framework for investigating the social ecology of tobacco use. The multiple factors at play included actions of the tobacco industry, regulatory systems (smoke-free laws, taxation levels), and the tobacco use control subsystem (quit lines, social marketing, multilevel networks).[24,25] One can address any of these factors from a systems perspective.

Ideally, PHD PHNs and community partners work together to implement the core functions, essential services, and public health nursing interventions to ultimately meet the *Healthy People 2030 (HP 2030)*-proposed vision of a "society in which all people achieve their full potential for health and well-being across the life span."[26] To help illustrate how this is done, the next section describes how a PHD implements core functions, essentials services, and interventions to address high infant mortality rates in their community (Fig. 13-5).

▌ **SOLVING THE MYSTERY**
The Case of the Dying Babies
Public Health Science Topics Covered:

- Assessment
- Epidemiology
- Surveillance
- Rates

Health problems are identified in a variety of ways, often simultaneously. In hypothetical Beach County, the death of a 5-month-old infant of a 14-year-old mother was highly publicized in the local media, and community members were outraged that this occurred in their "backyard." A nurse leader at the PHD was asked to convene a community work group to assess the issues, especially because this was not viewed as an isolated case, and to make recommendations for addressing infant mortality in her community.

The nurse leader decided to begin by conducting an assessment on the population level. **Community health assessments** (see Chapter 4) are ongoing activities by PHDs, and formal community health assessments are usually conducted every 3 to 5 years.[25] There are several frameworks for conducting a community health assessment, including the Community Health Assessment and Group Evaluation tool (CHANGE) (see Chapters 4 and 5). Beach Health Department selected the Mobilizing for Action Through Planning and Partnerships (MAPP) because of its emphasis on a community-driven process facilitated by the PHD.[25] This framework, which consists of four different types of assessments, allows communities to apply strategic thinking to prioritize public health issues and identify resources to address them (see Chapters 4 and 5). In this case, the PHD was very concerned about the infant mortality issue and decided to focus its assessment on a specific population: mothers and babies. Because a comprehensive assessment was due in approximately 2 years, this phase was viewed as a narrower perspective for identifying the issues surrounding the infant mortality problem.

Vision: A healthy and safe community where individuals can thrive and prosper
Mission: Collaborate with community partners to promote and assure high quality, accessible health and human services for local residents

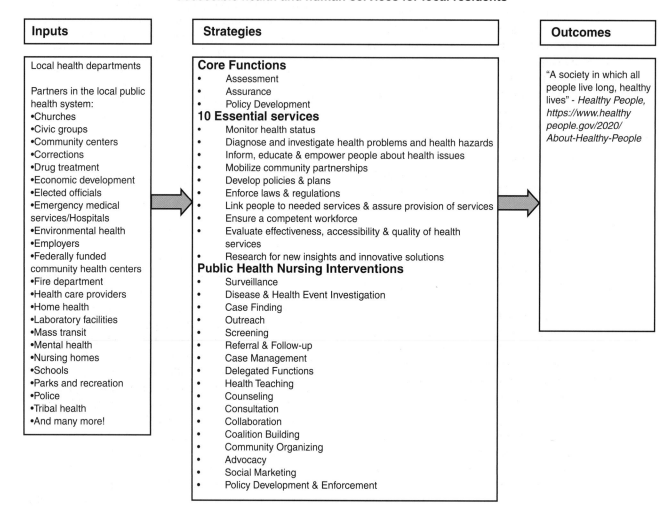

Inputs	Strategies	Outcomes
Local health departments Partners in the local public health system: •Churches •Civic groups •Community centers •Corrections •Drug treatment •Economic development •Elected officials •Emergency medical services/Hospitals •Environmental health •Employers •Federally funded community health centers •Fire department •Health care providers •Home health •Laboratory facilities •Mass transit •Mental health •Nursing homes •Schools •Parks and recreation •Police •Tribal health •And many more!	**Core Functions** • Assessment • Assurance • Policy Development **10 Essential services** • Monitor health status • Diagnose and investigate health problems and health hazards • Inform, educate & empower people about health issues • Mobilize community partnerships • Develop policies & plans • Enforce laws & regulations • Link people to needed services & assure provision of services • Ensure a competent workforce • Evaluate effectiveness, accessibility & quality of health services • Research for new insights and innovative solutions **Public Health Nursing Interventions** • Surveillance • Disease & Health Event Investigation • Case Finding • Outreach • Screening • Referral & Follow-up • Case Management • Delegated Functions • Health Teaching • Counseling • Consultation • Collaboration • Coalition Building • Community Organizing • Advocacy • Social Marketing • Policy Development & Enforcement	"A society in which all people live long, healthy lives" - *Healthy People, https://www.healthy people.gov/2020/ About-Healthy-People*

Figure 13-5 Framework for the delivery of population-focused health services on the local level. *(Created by B. Little and S. Bulecza, 2013.)*

There were several steps involved in the assessment, all exhibiting evidence of the essential services. The nurse leader contacted the state department of health and arranged for training on MAPP, thus assuring a competent workforce, the eighth essential public health service. A MAPP committee was formed to guide the health planning process, with broad representation of the community and local public health system including community members, nurses, and health-care providers from the local hospital, schools, and private practices. Elected officials were asked to join as well as a pregnant woman and teen mothers.

This committee is an example of the fourth essential public health service: mobilizing community partnerships to identify and solve health problems. The assessment was initiated by the PHD in this case, bringing not only a public health perspective to the issue but also a governmental legitimacy and sense of urgency.

The committee began with a brainstorming activity to formulate a shared community vision and values statements to guide the community-driven planning process. A timeline was established, and a preliminary plan was written that identified the work to be done.

As explained in Chapter 4, MAPP is divided into four assessments:[25]

1. The **Community Themes and Strengths Assessment** provides a deep understanding of the issues that residents feel are important by answering the open-ended questions about what is important to the community. In this case, it might involve some key informant interviews or focus groups assessing the strengths and problems surrounding the care of mothers in the community.
2. The **Local Public Health System Assessment** focuses on the organizations and entities that contribute to the public's health. In this case, it would be important to assess the organizations providing services to mothers and babies.
3. The **Community Health Status Assessment** identifies priority community health and quality of life issues. It includes identifying the indicators focused on maternal-child health and gathering secondary and primary data related to these indicators.
4. The **Forces of Change Assessment** focuses on identifying forces such as legislation, technology, and other impending changes that affect the context in which the community and its public health system operate. In this case, a key question was focused on the impending changes regarding funding for maternal-child services in the county.

The members of the core steering committee divided themselves according to interest or expertise into one of four groups. The nurse and the PHD epidemiologist provided support to each of the subcommittees. This assessment illustrates how the PHD implements the essential services of monitoring health status to identify, diagnose, and investigate health problems and health hazards in the community.

During the next several months, subcommittees met on a regular basis and periodically reported on progress and findings to each other. For example, the Forces of Change subcommittee reported on a newly funded grant for the development of a federally funded health center in a neighborhood where there was a high infant mortality rate. The Community Health Status subcommittee asked the PHD epidemiologist for additional vital statistics and geographic information systems (GIS) data, described later in this chapter, and assistance with analyzing the rate of infant mortality and teen births by ZIP code, race, and age. The committee also gathered secondary data from the state and county **Behavioral Risk Factor Surveillance System (BRFSS)**

survey data about high-risk behaviors as well as county data about neonatal mortality, infant mortality, percentage low birth weight, percentage very low birth weight, percentage of prenatal care initiated in the first trimester, percentage of mothers who smoke, and the prevalence of sudden infant death syndrome (SIDS). BRFSS is a behavioral and noncommunicable disease surveillance system sponsored by the Centers for Disease Control and Prevention (CDC).[26] The surveys are conducted via land line telephones and recently expanded to include cell phones. The Community Themes and Strengths Assessment group decided to focus on a series of listening or focus groups with minority residents and youth, whereas the Local Public Health System Assessment group focused on identifying resources within the community addressing health concerns. They conducted an Inventory of Resources (see Chapter 4).

After the subcommittees completed their assessments, the nurse leader compiled the results and prepared a presentation and agenda for the next MAPP committee meeting. The report consisted of county-specific data, health status compared with state objectives, trends, disparities, assets, and summary conclusions. The results showed that the infant mortality rate was 9.6 deaths per 1,000 live births compared with 7.1 for the state. There were racial differences, also: a rate of 12.7 deaths per 1,000 live births for African Americans and a rate of 6.2 for the white population. Only 68.4% of the African American population received prenatal care in the first trimester compared with 80% for the total population. Fifteen percent of pregnant women smoked in Beach County compared with 12% statewide. The percentage of low birth weight was much higher for the minority population (12%) compared with that of the white population (7.8%). Low birth weight was similar to the state findings. The teen birth rate was 71 per 1,000 live births compared with 67 per 1,000 live births only 2 years earlier.

The core committee met to review the data. Community issues were discussed and a list of four issues were identified and arranged by priority. In Beach County, some of the issues directly related to infant mortality were delayed prenatal care, increased low birth weight, high birth rates among teens, and tobacco use during pregnancy. Each issue was further researched for best practices, and goals and strategies were developed. In addition, the committee established a community goal for reducing infant mortality to 6 per 1,000 live births within 3 years.

This MAPP example illustrates the PHD role in conducting community assessments, facilitating health planning, and collaborating with partners to target high-priority issues. During the next year, the MAPP committee entered the action cycle and sought funding from public and private donors to establish a Nurse-Family Partnership[27,28] community health program with nurse home visits for low-income, first-time mothers. Through administration of the home visitation program, the PHD addressed the essential service of linking people to needed personal health services and assuring the provision of health care when otherwise unavailable.

Sources:
1. Nurse-Family Partnership.[27] (2018a). *Overview.* Retrieved from https://www.nursefamilypartnership.org/wp-content/uploads/2017/07/NFP_Overview.pdf
2. Nurse-Family Partnership.[28] (2018b). *Research trials and outcomes.* Retrieved from https://www.nursefamily partnership.org/wpcontent/uploads/2017/07/NFP_Research_Outcomes_2014.pdf
3. Nurse-Family Partnership.[29] (2018c). *Nurses and mothers.* Retrieved from https://www.nursefamily partnership.org/wpcontent/uploads/2017/07/NFP_Nurses_Mothers.pdf

■ EVIDENCE-BASED PRACTICE

The Nurse-Family Partnership Model for Providing Home-Visiting for Low-Income, First-Time Mothers and Their Children

Practice Statement: Nurses provide prenatal and child health education, care coordination, and life coaching during home visits that begin during pregnancy and continue through the child's second birthday.

Targeted Outcome: Improved prenatal health, fewer childhood injuries, fewer subsequent pregnancies, increased intervals between births, increased maternal employment, improved school readiness

Evidence to Support: Randomized controlled trials and economic analysis suggest improved long-term outcomes for mothers and children in the nurse-family partnership home visitation program. Nurse-family partnership programs are available in 43 states and participate in a web-based data collection and evaluation system that allows programs to measure progress toward meeting nurse-family partnership benchmarks for maternal and child health outcomes.

Recommended Approaches: The nurse-family relationship is the cornerstone of the home-visiting program that is based on a client-centered, strengths-based approach to support personal and family functioning. Nurses are equipped with tools, education, and resources to improve family outcomes. The nurse-family partnership agency provides the infrastructure to ensure high quality implementation and ongoing program evaluation in local communities.

Local Health Department Activities

In 2016, PHDs were surveyed by NACCHO to identify not only structure but also function and capacity of local PHDs. The role of PHDs has changed during the past century and has been shaped by historical events. The events of September 11, 2001, brought to the forefront an awareness of the role of PHDs in disasters. The recent natural disasters in the United States including hurricanes, wildfires, and floods as well as manmade tragedies such as mass shootings have emphasized the necessity of public health services to an even greater degree.

The following section describes a contemporary view of the activities of PHDs and recognizes that separating out activities solely performed by local health departments is indeed difficult. The 2016 NACCHO survey asked PHDs to report those activities performed only by the PHD, those done in concert with the state, and those done by contracting out to other members of the public health system. The 10 most frequent activities and services provided by PHDs directly are found in Table 13-1.[12] It is clear that more than three-fourths of PHDs provide these services. Other services are provided through contractual relationships with other organizations such as lab services, by other governmental agencies (animal control), or through nongovernmental organizations (NGOs). The contractual agreements are one way for PHDs to assure that needed health services are available to its citizens.[29]

There are five categories used to summarize the major activities of PHDs:[30]

1. Environmental health services
2. Data collection and analysis: health and vital statistics
3. Individual and community health
4. Disease control, epidemiology, and surveillance
5. Regulation, licensing, and inspection

TABLE 13–1 ■ Percentage of Public Health Department Jurisdictions With 10 Most Frequent Activities and Services

Available Through PHDs Directly

Activity or Service	Percentage of Jurisdictions
Adult Immunization Provision	90%
Communicable/Infectious Disease Surveillance	93%
Child Immunizations Provision	88%
Tuberculosis Screening	84%
Food Service Establishment Inspection	79%
Environmental Health Surveillance	85%
Food Safety Education	77%
Tuberculosis Treatment	79%
Schools/Day Care Center Inspection	74%
Population-Based Primary Prevention: Nutrition	74%

Source: (12)

Environmental Health Services

Environmental health services are focused on ensuring that communities have safe water, safe food, and sanitary environments. For example, local health departments located near beaches are responsible for conducting periodic water sampling to ensure that the water does not contain high levels of contaminants or bacteria. If bacteria or contaminants are found at levels out of the normal range that pose a risk to persons swimming at the beach, then local health departments have the authority to close the beach until levels return to an acceptable range.

Environmental services are the backbone of public health infrastructure in developed countries and have eliminated such problems as cholera and diarrheal disease. In fact, in 1940, environmental sanitation was viewed as a minimum function of local health departments to address proper public and private water supply systems and sewage disposal, restaurant inspections, insect and rodent control, housing inspections, and environmental complaints.[3] The development of solid waste management is interesting. At the time of the infectious epidemics in the 1800s, funding was not available for a regional approach to solid waste management, which resulted in municipal approaches to dealing with the problems.[30] Today, solid waste management is largely handled by municipalities and operated by private companies.

Environmental concerns today are often seen as the responsibilities of both local and state agencies as well as other local governmental agencies or NGOs. In the most recent NACCHO 2016 survey, food safety education and vector control activities were most often connected with the PHD as the resource. State health departments were most often listed as resources for indoor air quality, groundwater protection, noise pollution, hazardous waste disposal, air pollution, and radiation control.[12] With any of these activities, there is a great deal of variability, with many agencies often assuming some level of responsibility. In another study examining the combined roles of state and local health departments, the PHD was typically found to oversee private water supplies and septic systems.[31] A list of typical environmental concerns is found in Box 13-2 (see also Chapter 6).

BOX 13–2 ■ Environmental Health Services Potentially Provided by Public Health Departments

- Inspect and investigate food service and outlets, from wholesale to retail.
- Inspect and investigate wastewater management systems, either community or individual homes (septic tanks).
- Inspect and investigate solid and hazardous waste site investigations.
- Conduct sanitary surveys of potential or existing water systems and watersheds.
- Conduct investigations of facilities, institutions, and licensed establishments.
- Inspect swimming pools and recreational facilities.
- Investigate hazardous materials and radiation hazards or spills.
- Manage occupational health and safety programs.
- Investigate and analyze potential toxic exposures.
- Conduct community education and provide expertise on environmental conditions.
- Assure animal and vector control including rabies surveillance.
- Address sanitary nuisances.

Source: Centers for Disease Control and Prevention. (2014). *Environmental public health performance standards*. Retrieved from http://www.cdc.gov/nceh/ehs/envphps/Docs/EnvPHPSv2.pdf

Data Collection and Analysis: Health and Vital Statistics

Most data collection and analysis activities are state-level functions, although the process of collecting statistics begins at the local level. **Vital statistics** are data collected regarding births, deaths, marriages, and divorces. Data are forwarded to the state, where they are compiled and sent to the CDC National Vital Statistics System.[32] This is the oldest process for sharing public health data across governmental agencies. It requires that these agencies share standards and procedures so that the National Center for Health Statistics can monitor, store, and disseminate the nation's official vital statistics.

When a baby is born, the hospital completes a birth form that is submitted to the PHD. The PHD then issues the official birth certificate to the child's parents. The birth record includes data that can be found on the official birth certificate such as the birth date, place of birth, and parents' names. It also includes a wealth of other information not listed on the official birth certificate. These data include neonatal outcomes, risk factors related to adverse outcomes, and protective factors related to positive outcomes.[33] Information is included on parental demographic and behavioral variables such as age, level of education, race, and maternal use of alcohol, tobacco, and other drugs during pregnancy. Information is also collected related to the pregnancy and delivery, such as the number of prenatal visits, when the trimester prenatal care began, and the type of delivery. Finally, data are collected on the newborn. In addition to weight, head circumference, and length, data are collected on information related to the neonate's weeks of gestation and congenital defects. Data are obtained from the medical record, the health provider of record, and from family members. These data provide important information needed to understand population-level trends related to birth and facilitates evaluation of how well *Healthy People* objectives are being met.

Likewise, PHDs collect mortality data based on the information obtained from death records. The first part of the document includes basic demographic information about the deceased that is completed by the funeral director or other person in charge of internment. This same person is also responsible for filing the certificate with the registrar in the location where the death occurred. The medical examiner or coroner certifying the death completes the second section of the document that specifies the cause of death. The certificate contains essential demographic data as well as date and time of death, where the death occurred, and the primary cause of death. Like the birth record, the death record includes more data than what is contained in the death certificate. The death record includes information about the conditions that contributed to the death, history of tobacco use, race, and other variables.[33] These data are used to evaluate mortality trends at the population level. If the death was due to an injury, information related to the injury is also collected. Data regarding causes of death are compiled from death certificates and used to determine specific disease, injury, or mode of death rates within communities and the state. For example, death data are used to determine the number of cancer deaths in a community and to help during community assessments and health system planning. For infants aged less than 1 year, linked birth and death certificate files provide information to determine significant risk factors that influenced fetal mortality.

Another required vital record is fetal death. **Fetal death** is a spontaneous intrauterine death of a fetus at any time during pregnancy. Again, the record includes a section to complete the basic information related to parental demographic data, time and date of delivery, and gender of the fetus. The second section relates to the cause of death and conditions contributing to the fetal death. The data not only provide an official record of the death, the additional information also facilitates population-level assessments and program planning. Most states report fetal deaths of at least 20 weeks of gestation and/or birth weight of 350 grams or more.

Although states are responsible for the analysis of most data, the PHD is typically responsible for the collection and analysis of data regarding the Reportable Diseases category.[12] In addition, in some states with local boards of health, morbidity data are sometimes collected at the local level.

There are many uses for vital statistics. Birth and death certificates are used to legally establish citizenship and obtain drivers licenses and Social Security cards, and are required in the probating of a will. Vital statistics help genealogists conduct family research and establish ties between individuals. Most importantly, vital statistics from a global perspective are vital to understanding the health of populations, determining life expectancy, and helping to guide interventions aimed at improving health.

■ CULTURAL CONTEXT

The Future of the Public's Health in the 21st Century[35]

"A healthy community is a place where people provide leadership in assessing their own resources and needs, where public health and social infrastructure and policies support health, and where essential public health services, including quality health care, are available. In a healthy community, communication and collaboration among various sectors of the community and the contributions of ethnically, socially, and economically diverse community members are valued. In addition, the broad array of determinants of health is considered and addressed, and individuals make informed, positive choices in the context of health-protective and supportive environments, policies, and systems."

Individual and Community Health

The role of some PHDs in assuring the health of populations sometimes involves providing direct individual care as well as providing care at the community level. Direct individual care provided by PHDs can include a variety of services such as prenatal and well-baby clinics, clinics for communicable diseases (e.g., tuberculosis [TB], sexually transmitted infections [STIs]), primary care clinics, school health services, and vaccination clinics. Comparing PHDs, there is probably no area within the local public health system with as much diversity in programs for the provision of direct individual care. Some health departments provide no direct care at all, whereas others provide a wide variety of care. The City of Cincinnati Health Department, for example, includes home-care services, pharmacy, school nursing, and multiple clinics.[34] Other PHDs contract out services or the services are available only through NGOs.

At one time, the provision of primary care services (see Chapter 15), particularly to underserved and economically disadvantaged citizens (and areas), was part of the mainstream of public health activities. There has been a national effort to have governmental public health services return their attention to more population-based public health services.[35] Consequently, a transfer of services has taken place, and this has been done in many different formats. PHDs have contracted or networked with their local hospital system to fund primary care services as a more cost-effective alternative to emergency room visits for the same service. In some cases, the most recent 2016 NACCHO survey found that certain activities were exclusively provided through contracts:[12]

- Laboratory services, 14%
- HIV/AIDS treatment, 9%
- HIV/AIDS screening 8%
- STI screening, 8%
- STI treatment 7%
- Population-based tobacco prevention services, 7%
- TB treatment, 7%

- Cancer screening, 6%
- Oral health, 6%

Another process for PHDs to obtain funding for providing care is through federally qualified health centers. **Federally qualified health centers (FQHC)** are funded through the Health Resources and Service Administration (HRSA) under section 330 of the Public Health Service Act. There are multiple benefits for having a FQHC, including enhanced reimbursement from Medicare and Medicaid. FQHC must serve an underserved area or population, offer a sliding fee scale, and provide comprehensive services.[36] They must also have an ongoing quality assurance program with a governing board of directors.

Maternal and Child Health

Maternal-child services have traditionally been a key component of any PHD (see Chapter 17). This goes back to the early 20th century as evidenced in the APHA mission statements.[9,10] The overall goal of maternal-child services has been to improve the health of mothers and children through the delivery of preventive interventions. Although these efforts have changed over time, they are still an important aspect of PHD services. PHDs either provide these services directly or help to link their constituents with available services. For maternal-child health services overall, the 2016 NACCHO survey shows that the current services provided most often in PHDs are **Women, Infants, and Children (WIC)** services (66%), MCH home visits (60%), and family planning (53%).[12] The importance of these programs was underscored by HRSA in 2017 when they provided $342 million in funding to 55 states, territories, and nonprofit organizations through the Maternal, Infant, and Childhood Home Visiting Program.[37] The money is awarded to provide evidence-based home visiting services to pregnant women and families with young children from birth until entry into kindergarten.[37]

One example of a comprehensive maternal-child health program is **Healthy Start**, which focuses on reducing infant mortality and low birth weight. The Healthy Start initiative was signed into law in 1991 and is funded through HRSA.[38] In this program, nurses working at PHDs engage in multiple services from group-level activities, such as health education for expectant and new mothers to individual care in prenatal and well-baby clinics or home visiting. Healthy Start addresses multiple issues such as providing adequate prenatal care, meeting basic health needs, reducing barriers to access, and empowering clients. There is growing evidence that these programs have been successful in reducing infant mortality rates, increasing access to early prenatal care, and providing community services to lower preterm delivery and incidence of low birth weight.[39]

In addition to maternity care programs, PHDs provide nutritional support for pregnant women and children through the federally funded WIC programs.[12] WIC was established as a pilot program in 1972, made permanent in 1974, and is administered at the federal level by the Food and Nutrition Service of the U.S. Department of Agriculture. In April 2014, there were 9.3 million women, infants, and children enrolled in the WIC program, and almost three-quarters of them (74.2%) were at or below the poverty line.[40] Nurses and dietitians work collaboratively to provide nutrition counseling and breastfeeding support.

Family planning programs are a third example of maternal-child health care in PHDs. Family planning programs in the United States were implemented in the 1960s and 1970s in response to the reproductive needs of populations at some level. Family planning grew out of federal legislation, originally the Office of Economic Opportunity in 1965 and then the enactment of Family Planning Services and Population Research Act of 1970, or Title X.[41] Family planning programs did not share a universal acceptance upon their inception. These programs coincided with the approval of oral contraceptives and were associated with the changing societal attitudes regarding sexual activity. Many communities initially resisted the provision of these services. Over the years, levels of acceptance of these programs have risen and fallen, with most of the controversy focusing on whether there should be public financing of family planning. This demonstrates the role that public opinion plays in public health policy. Core family planning services have centered on individual counseling regarding contraceptive method selection, annual physicals, and follow-up services.

An example of comprehensive family planning services can be found at the New York State Department of Health website: http://www.health.state.ny.us/health_care/medicaid/program/longterm/familyplanbenprog.htm. The purpose of the program is to "…increase access to confidential family planning services and to enable teens, women, and men of childbearing age to prevent and/or reduce the incidence of unintentional pregnancies."[42]

School Health

School health is concerned with assuring the health of the entire school population, students, and staff (Chapter 18). As the health-care expert in the school setting, school nurses take a leadership role in developing policies and providing clinical care activities that promote health and assure safe health-care practices in a nonmedical setting. School nursing services include medication administration, immunizations, and response to emergencies during medical crises and disasters. School-based screening programs identify children with potential health problems associated with vision, hearing, and obesity that may be barriers of academic achievement. When underlying medical conditions are detected, the school nurse will make referrals to specialists and other health-care providers and conduct follow-up activities to assure access to care and adherence to treatment (see Chapter 18).[43] By delivering case management services, school nurses coordinate care and help families locate resources for medical, social, and mental health services. School-based wellness programs are designed to address common childhood issues such as obesity; dental caries; asthma; and health education needs related to growth and development, communicable diseases, and sexuality. Funding and staffing patterns for school nurses employed by PHDs and school districts vary between states and counties. Not every school has a school nurse, and for the 5% of children without health insurance, the school nurse may be their only access to health screening and care.[44]

Immunization and Health Protection Programs

Providing immunizations to protect a population from communicable diseases is an essential component of public health. Vaccinations are mandated by school districts and in some cases employers, especially in health-care settings. If an outbreak of disease occurs, the PHD is often the entity responsible for mass immunization, as occurred in the H1N1 influenza outbreak in 2009.

Immunization practices have been in place for centuries. For example, variolation (the exposure of well persons to material from an infected person such as pus or scabs) was used to prevent smallpox. Although variolation resulted in death for some, the overall death rate related to smallpox fell. In the late 1700s, Edward Jenner, a physician, discovered that milkmaids exposed to cowpox, a less deadly disease, developed immunity to smallpox. The term *vaccine* comes from the word *vaca*, which means "cow" in Latin. He exposed a small boy to pus from a milkmaid with cowpox and then exposed him to smallpox. The boy did not contract the disease. Although it took a while for vaccinations to enter into mainstream practice, by 1800, the use of vaccines spread across Europe and to other parts of the globe.[45] Today, through the successful efforts of a global campaign, smallpox has been eradicated worldwide.

Immunizations are a major responsibility of PHDs. PHDs manage the program requirements associated with administration and utilization of vaccines for preventable diseases. Immunization administration may be integrated into the PHD clinical service program. Immunization program components include ordering and tracking vaccines, ensuring that individual immunizations are recorded into registries if used in that jurisdiction, and coordinating special immunization clinics. In addition, immunization programs coordinate the Vaccine for Children program. This program facilitates the delivery of adequate supplies of vaccines to health-care providers who provide services and vaccines to children. This ensures that all children, regardless of ability to pay, have access to immunizations for vaccine-preventable diseases.

In addition to childhood vaccination programs, PHD immunization programs provide services to other populations at risk. This includes international travel vaccinations and the rabies postexposure prophylaxis vaccine. PHDs often work with community partners to provide clinics where anyone can come for immunizations for diseases such as influenza. These types of clinics help increase a community's level of immunity from these diseases. PHNs often coordinate the planning and implementation of these open clinics. Schools have often been a place where immunizations and other child-focused services are provided. Through these activities, not only does the PHD protect individuals who receive the vaccine, but it also reduces the overall prevalence of communicable diseases, thus reducing the opportunity for the spread of disease and providing herd immunity (see Chapter 8).

Role of Nurses in Providing Individual Care

Nurses are often employed by PHDs to provide the direct individual care at the clinics. The nursing care provided often includes one-on-one clinical interventions such as vaccinations, prenatal care, and dispensing of medications for STIs or TB. In addition, PHNs often provide home visiting and a focus on high-risk families as part of these services.[46] Establishing working relationships with these families has been a strength of public health nursing, and home visitations by registered nurses has been associated with improved outcomes.[47,48] A recent qualitative study illustrates that PHNs are flexible and especially adept at recognizing the sociohistorical factors that influence families while simultaneously focusing on strengths and chaotic life situations.[46]

Community Health Primary Prevention Efforts

As described in Chapter 2, primary prevention is a strategy used to avert occurrences of illness or injury. In addition to services focused on individuals, PHDs provide a wide array of primary prevention services aimed at health promotion and protection at the community level. Health promotion includes activities that focus on improving the ability of individuals and populations to practice healthy living. Health protection interventions involve protecting individuals and populations from disease by improving the immune system through vaccination for individuals or providing protective barriers such as the use of personal protective equipment by health-care providers.

Health promotion efforts at the community level include educating about healthy lifestyles. Examples of health education include HIV prevention education for teens or Back to Sleep campaigns for reducing SIDS. The Back to Sleep campaigns began in 1994 and focused on educating parents, caregivers, and health-care providers about ways to reduce the risk of SIDS. Since the campaign started, there has been a 50% reduction in SIDS deaths, and the percentage of babies being placed on their backs to sleep has increased significantly.[49] Unfortunately, health promotion interventions and the latest advances in primary prevention and screening activities are less likely to be delivered among vulnerable populations having lower socioeconomic status, racial and ethnic minorities, and people living in rural and remote areas of the United States.[50,51] Culturally relevant, evidence-based health promotion interventions can be especially useful for improving health and reducing disease risk among at-risk populations.

Communication is a key component to the provision of primary prevention programs for PHDs. In today's world, there are multiple methods for communicating important health data and health promotion information. For example, during the H1N1 influenza outbreak in 2009, PHDs used multiple methods to communicate with communities regarding the locations where immunizations were available as well as potential public health priorities associated with vaccinating certain groups, such as pregnant women and children, before the general population. Technological strategies traditionally used to communicate public health messages include television, radio, newspapers, and sending printed information home with school-aged children. During this century, PHDs are increasingly using computer-mediated technologies, including social media such as YouTube, Twitter, and Facebook, as effective avenues for providing health information.

A Healthy Community: Sarasota, Florida: An example of a community-wide health promotion initiative is the Community Health Improvement Partnership in Sarasota, Florida.[52] The Sarasota PHD led this partnership and brought together many stakeholders from the community. Partners included community organizations, individual citizens, and health-care professionals. Together, they identified evidence-based strategies and chose those that had the most applicability to their community. These strategies were multipronged; that is, they used different venues and methods to engage the community in a healthier lifestyle. They developed Healthy Living kiosks throughout the community. These kiosks provided information about health insurance options, health-care resources, and consumer tips. Users were able to access a county health scorecard that provided data on health status and linkage to a community pharmacy where those who were uninsured or underinsured could have access to needed medications. The development of this required that PHD nurses understand the basics of public health science so that they could develop an intervention based on the community priority health needs and service gaps within the community. It also required understanding implementation and evaluation strategies to determine whether the kiosk was an effective intervention. PHDs provide essential leadership and skills in the promotion of the health of the community they serve.

Disease Control, Epidemiology, and Surveillance

Disease Control

Because communicable disease is a primary concern of PHDs, their ability to provide necessary training and services surrounding communicable diseases is important. This will vary depending on the size of the public health system. Many small health departments gather private physician case reports and provide the information to a regional or central office for analysis and compilation. Larger PHDs may have internal units devoted to the communicable disease program, including core epidemiological services and biostatistical analysis of the determinants of diseases in animals and man.

Tuberculosis Management: TB management is one of public health's oldest communicable disease programs for one of the oldest diseases noted in history. With the advent of effective therapies, elimination of TB was

considered a possibility. However, this remarkable organism continues to be a major threat to public health both globally and in the United States. A resurgence of the disease is sometimes now accompanied by a rise in multidrug-resistant TB (MDR-TB), which is defined as TB resistant to the two most effective first-line therapeutic drugs, isoniazid and rifampin. The CDC established a task force to develop a plan of action to address the issue of drug-resistant TB.[53] TB is a complex interaction of medical, societal, behavioral, and economic factors.

Because of the communicability of TB, PHDs and PHNs take a leading role in both the prevention and treatment of TB. One approach by state and PHDs is to provide TB clinics that include screening assessment, diagnosis, and treatment components. Efforts at the local, state, and national levels have resulted overall in a reduced incidence of TB.[54] It is possible that TB could be eliminated in the United States. It will take continued efforts on the part of PHDs to continue to screen those at risk, assess persons with positive screens, and treat those with active disease.

● APPLYING PUBLIC HEALTH SCIENCE

The Case of the Tuberculosis Neighborhood Investigation

Public Health Science Topics Covered:

- Surveillance
- Disease investigation
- Prevention

Sara Johnson, communicable disease nurse at Creek County Health Department, received a call from the infection control nurse at Providence Hospital reporting a newly diagnosed case of TB in a hospitalized patient. The patient was a 40-year-old male (Mr. H.) who worked for the grounds maintenance unit of the local college. Sara advised the infection control nurse that she would come to the hospital that day to review the chart and interview the patient. She remembered that there had been another university employee from the same unit diagnosed a year ago and that all of the employees had received appropriate TB testing. No other cases had been identified during that case follow-up, so she was somewhat concerned about the appearance of this case.

Sara learned the following from her chart review and patient interview:

- The patient had only been employed with the university for 4 months.

- He lived with his girlfriend and her two daughters.
- He presented with classic TB symptoms—night sweats, weight loss, no appetite, and persistent cough. His sputum was acid-fact bacillus (AFB) positive and his chest x-ray was indicative of pulmonary TB. Pharmacological therapy was consistent with the CDC's TB treatment protocols. He would be hospitalized in isolation until three consecutive AFB sputum smears were negative.
- Names of coworkers, family, and friends were obtained.
- He wasn't sure whether he had been around anybody with TB. One of his neighbors had been sick a few months ago with similar symptoms, but the patient didn't know what the neighbor had.

Based on this information, Sara ruled out that he had been exposed from the previous case and began to prioritize the contact list for follow-up. What criteria should Sara use to prioritize the contacts? To answer this question and the rest of the questions related to this case, see Box 13-3.[53–55]

Sara contacted the patient's girlfriend and arranged for her and her daughters to come to the health department for evaluation and tuberculin skin testing because they had closest contact with the patient. Then, she contacted the patient's supervisor to advise him of the situation and the need to interview coworkers. To minimize disruption to the workers, Sara agreed to bring a small interview team to the site to conduct evaluations and provide tuberculin skin testing. She agreed to go back to the site to read the tests 72 hours later so the workers would not have to miss work.

After about a week, Sara received notification from the hospital that the patient was ready for discharge and he would need to be on **directly observed therapy** for several months to ensure adherence to the medication regimen. It was decided that Sara would meet the patient at his home the next day after he was discharged. During this meeting, Sara reviewed activity restrictions and the medication plan, explained the process of directly observed therapy, and told him that she would be coming to his home each day to watch him take the medications.

Two key issues in the treatment of TB are the length of treatment and the emergence of MDR-TB. For the most part, MDR-TB occurred because of nonadherence to recommended treatment. That is, those with an active infection did not complete the

---

1. How is the infectious period for TB defined?
2. What is the difference between active and latent TB infection?
3. What factors had an impact on the decision to initiate a contact investigation? What are the goals of a contact investigation?
4. What groups are most at risk for TB infection? How should the nurse prioritize contact for follow-up?
5. What factors would require a contact be placed on chemoprophylaxis?
6. Directly observed treatment is a resource-intensive intervention. How should the nurse prioritize contacts for it?
7. If the neighborhood had been different, what other interventions could have been used to reach the neighbors?
8. Discuss challenges with and solutions for providing directly observed therapy with someone who is homeless.
9. This investigation may attract the attention of the media. What strategies should the nurse use for communicating with the media?

The following are recommended sources for answering the preceding questions:

Centers for Disease Control and Prevention. (2005). Guidelines for the investigation of contacts of persons with infectious tuberculosis. *Morbidity and Mortality Weekly Report, 54*(RR15), 1-37. Retrieved from http://www.cdc.gov/mmwr/preview/mmwrhtml/rr5415a1.htm
CDC TB Web site: http://www.cdc.gov/tb/

---

required drug regimen, and the bacterium became resistant to the drug. Today, the World Health Organization (WHO) recommends treatment to continue for 6 months or longer.[56] In the United States, the populations most at risk for active TB are often those hardest to reach (e.g., foreign-born persons from countries with a high TB prevalence, those exposed to persons with active TB, those who are immune-compromised, persons with alcohol or substance abuse, and persons with latent TB infections [they are infected but do not have active disease]).[55] To assist with this, nurses working in PHDs often function as case managers to help ensure that patients with TB follow through with the required treatment. Nurses apply their holistic approach to care and are able to appreciate and mitigate factors that exist in the patient's life.

A key function of TB case management is ensuring adherence to the medication regimen. As noted earlier, one of the oldest ways of ensuring adherence is through the use of directly observed therapy, in which the patient takes the required daily medication in the presence of a public health-care provider, often a nurse. Either the patient goes directly to the PHD, or the public health-care provider comes to the patient's home. As with other areas of health care, technology has been developed that enhances the ability to monitor medication adherence. One example is a **medication electronic monitoring system**, which tracks adherence to a medication regimen through a chip placed in the medication bottle cap that uploads the date and time the cap is opened.[57] Other examples include use of text messaging, phone call reminders, and e-mail reminders.

With case management under way in the case of Mr. H., it was critical to continue to investigate for additional exposures. In trying to determine how he may have been exposed, Sara began reviewing previous cases. She found that the case from the prior year lived on the same street as the patient, and there had been several contacts who could not be found. She also determined that there had been another earlier case on the same street. Based on this information, should Sara expand the contact investigation? Sara determined that there needed to be outreach to all the neighbors to ensure there were not any additional undiagnosed cases. She decided to learn more about the neighborhood by conducting a windshield survey of the street. Her findings were the following: (1) The street was isolated and not connected to a larger neighborhood; (2) there were about 15 houses; (3) there appeared to be children of all ages living on the street; and (4) there were several open, grassy areas on the street.

Sara decided that a community information fair and testing clinic would be the best way to provide outreach services to the neighbors without compromising the patient's privacy. She developed the plan and presented it to the health department administrator for approval. After the plan was approved, she identified a Saturday for the event, recruited health department staff to assist, and solicited other health department programs to participate or provide information or give-away items. The event was very successful, with many of the neighbors receiving testing and information. Fortunately, no new cases were identified, but several people with latent TB infection were placed on prophylaxis therapy.

Sexually Transmitted Infections: Communities also rely on PHDs to provide surveillance, prevention, and treatment of STIs. Most STIs are reportable diseases and the PHD reports each case to the state department of health, which then reports to the CDC. PHDs also combine clinical care for the diagnosis and treatment of the disease with a strong field investigative component needed to identify and notify contacts. Many PHDs conduct primary prevention programs, especially with teens, aimed at preventing STIs with outreach to schools, correctional facilities, bathhouses, and other community settings.

There is an enormous burden of STIs in the United States with more than 1.5 million cases of chlamydia infections, 468,514 cases of gonorrhea, 27,814 cases of syphilis, and 39,782 new cases of HIV infection in 2016.[58] With a disease burden of this magnitude in addition to the costs for society, the investigative role of PHDs is critical. The investigation of STIs includes three steps:

1. Screening for possible infection. Persons with suspected STIs are screened using appropriate tests. Depending on the STI, a positive screen may require further laboratory confirmation.
2. Treatment.
3. Screening all known sexual contacts of the person with the confirmed STI and treat if necessary.

PHNs often conduct the follow-up investigations for persons diagnosed with an STI such as syphilis. The PHN follows up with the patient to ensure he has adhered to the prescribed medications and obtain contact information for any sexual contacts before he was treated.

In 2012, NACCHO published a policy statement about the prevention and control of STIs.[59] PHDs have traditionally fulfilled a critical role in this arena but there is a current threat to this coverage because of dwindling funds. In 2011, 57% of PHDs had to make cuts in their core programs, which in some cases resulted in an elimination of programs and services.[60]

● APPLYING PUBLIC HEALTH SCIENCE

The Case of the Unintended Death

Public Health Science Topics Covered:

- Surveillance
- Community Organizing
- Advocacy
- Policy Development and Enforcement

Community members seek assistance from PHDs for a variety of health issues. In hypothetical Beach County, Mrs. McIntire requested a meeting with the director of the PHD to discuss her concern about misuse of prescription drugs by young adults in the county. She shared that her son accidently died from an overdose of prescription pain drugs and alcohol. She explained her concern that this was a growing problem in the county and that she wasn't the only person in the community that lost their son or daughter. The PHD director listened to her and agreed to take a look at the data on prescription drug misuse and overdose.

Data analysis by the PHD epidemiologist revealed the county had the highest rates in the state. The director called a meeting with Mrs. McIntire and the PHD leadership team to discuss what to do next. They decided to bring up the issue at the next meeting of the Behavioral Health Consortium to see if they were aware of this disturbing trend and if this was something that the Consortium could address as a community concern. The Consortium consisted of a variety of community agencies including social services, law enforcement, health care, mental health, substance use, as well as advocacy groups. During the meeting, Mrs. McIntire told the story of her son's accidental overdose. PHNs from the Healthy Start program also shared stories of young families with at-risk substance use issues and children who were orphaned as a result of their parent's unintentional deaths. The epidemiologist presented data on mortality rates related to substance abuse.

The Numbers

Deaths caused by drugs, medications, and biological substances are categorized as unintentional poisoning. Mortality data showed the county experienced a 22% increase in unintentional poisonings, which was twice that of the state rate. The crude death rate for ages 15-29 due to unintentional poisoning steadily increased over the previous 4 years from a rate of 7.3 (N=3) to 52.9 (N=24). In comparison to the state rate, the county rate was statistically higher (52.9 county, 15.7 state). In addition, there was a 90% increase in patients admitted to local Addictions Receiving Facilities for prescription drug misuse over the previous 4 years. The epidemiologist explained these rates reflect the health and well-being of this age group as well as the quality of the health care available, particularly mental health and substance abuse counseling.

Collaboration

The Consortium members agreed to work together to address this urgent public health problem by collaborating with local governments and organizations to identify existing services and designate available resources. The next steps involved making a similar presentation to local hospital administrators. The medical examiner in attendance reported that approximately 40% of the deaths were related to the combined use of prescription opioids and alcohol. The hospital agreed to join in the effort to educate the public, police, and local governmental officials and to develop solutions.

Meetings with the Sheriff's Office revealed that several new pain management clinics had recently opened in the county and were thought to be contributing to increased access to prescription pain medications. The Sheriff reported a pattern of illegal drug use and distribution associated with clinics that dispense narcotics on-site and were trafficked by users from other states. Increased arrests for drug trafficking near some of these clinics were also reported. Addressing the source of prescription drugs through regulation of pain management clinics was proposed as a solution and presented to the Board of County Commissioners.

Implementation of Strategies

The PHD Consortium and community partners implemented an array of strategies to address the epidemic including the following.

The PHD and Sheriff's Office worked with the county government to develop legislation that regulated pain clinics and placed a moratorium on new occupational licenses for pain management clinics. The PHD Community Health Improvement Project (CHIP) worked with local hospitals and medical providers to present educational programs for clinicians regarding the epidemic. This included the need to inform patients of the risks of opioids and to monitor them closely. A public awareness campaign was implemented by CHIP to inform the public of the problem and available community resources. A local database was established to track narcotic prescriptions by patients and providers. This was later implemented on the state level.

Conclusion

The rates of unintended poisonings declined over the next few years. This case illustrates the role of the PHD in:

- Being open to early identification of problems facing the community
- Using data to validate the depth and breadth of the problem
- Bringing key community leaders to work together to create a comprehensive array of solutions
- Utilizing public health practices related to surveillance, community organizing, policy development, and advocacy (see Box 13-4 for discussion questions)

BOX 13–4 ■ Questions Related to The Case of the Unintended Death

1. What are the rates for deaths caused by unintentional poisoning in your community?
2. How is your local and state PHD involved in addressing the issue? What other community agencies are addressing the issue?
3. What types of substance abuse services are provided in your community? Is there a waiting list for inpatient services?
4. How is the community informed about the problem and community resources?
5. What types of prevention programs are offered in the schools?
6. What are the challenges to addressing substance abuse in your community?
7. Would the strategies in Beach County work in your community? Review the literature on best practices for addressing the opioid crisis. What additional strategies would you recommend for your community?

The following are recommended sources:

1. National Institute on Drug Abuse. *Opioid crisis.* https://www.drugabuse.gov/drugs-abuse/opioids/opioid-overdose-crisis
2. National Institute on Drug Abuse. *Opioid summaries by state.* https://www.drugabuse.gov/drugs-abuse/opioids/opioid-summaries-by-state
3. Department of Health & Human Services. *National opioids crisis-help, resources & information.* https://www.hhs.gov/opioids/

Epidemiology and Surveillance

Emerging or Re-emerging Infections: As we move ahead into the 21st century, PHDs will face two significant challenges: increased mobility due to globalization and emergence of new human pathogens. Joshua Lederberg coined the term *emerging infections* for the IOM in 2000.[61] Morens and Fauci (2013) define emerging infections as "diseases that are recognized in the human host for the first time "and re-emerging diseases as "diseases that historically have infected humans, but continue to appear in new locations or in drug-resistant forms, or that reappear after apparent control or elimination (p. 1)."[62]

Our global society and rapid transit around the globe can result in the rapid dissemination of pathogens throughout the world. Examples of emerging infectious diseases include the 2009 H1N1 pandemic influenza, severe acute respiratory syndrome (SARS), and Middle East Respiratory Syndrome (MERS). SARS originated in China and was rapidly spread across the globe as infected persons traveled by airplane from China to other countries. As noted in Chapter 8, SARS infected 8,437 people with a case fatality rate of 9.6% (813 people).[63] Other recent examples of rapid global dissemination of a communicable disease are that of H1N1 and H7N9 (see Chapter 8). For H1N1, the Mexican government disseminated a wide array of pamphlets and posters to alert their population about mitigating the impact of H1N1 by slowing the transmission and lowering mortality.[64]

Besides globalization, there are a number of factors that influence emergence and re-emergence of disease. These factors include climate/natural disasters, economic development/urbanization, poverty, limited or lack of public health services, war/social disruption, and famine. Population movement has been associated with the re-emergence of Dengue virus and West Nile virus in the United States and Caribbean countries. Likewise, the global emergence of antibiotic resistant organisms is linked to antibiotic overuse and inadequate antibiotic stewardship, medical tourism, and economic globalization. This has resulted in multidrug-resistant TB and malaria, and bacterial diseases like vancomycin-resistant enterococci.[62]

Zoonotic Diseases: Another challenge in the modern world is the growth of cities and suburbia, which encroaches on the natural habitats of wild animals. Across the United States, deer, fox, and other wild animals are now living in suburbia and even in urban settings, increasing the likelihood of the transmission of zoonotic disease. Zoonotic diseases are diseases transmitted from animals to humans in the community through direct contact, as with rabies, or indirect contact through a vector, such as Lyme disease[65] (see Chapter 8). PHDs are called on to conduct surveillance of zoonotic disease and institute prevention programs.

Rabies is a preventable viral disease of mammals usually transmitted through the bite of a rabid animal such as a dog or a raccoon. Efforts from PHDs, both at the local and state levels, have reduced the incidence of rabies in the United States dramatically during the past 100 years.[66] Through public health campaigns to vaccinate domestic animals, 90% of all cases reported to the CDC are now in bats and wild carnivores. Human deaths due to rabies rarely occur because of effective and early intervention with post-bite exposure prophylaxis. The PHD provides education to health-care providers; tracks and reports all known cases to the state department of health, both animal and human; and works in partnership with animal control programs and veterinarians

Disaster Preparedness: An increasingly prominent role of PHDs, especially PHNs, is public health preparedness for responding to emergencies and disasters. Prior to the events of 2001, the preparedness functions were dictated by the regularity of events that affected the population and the health-care systems. Southeastern coastal states regularly face hurricanes. Midwestern states continually experience tornados. West Coast states are constantly threatened by earthquakes and fires. All have created robust emergency response systems. However, the realities of the 21st century have placed an additional responsibility on these systems because of threats caused by humans. Disaster planning programs evolved into "all hazards" planning. For example, a biological event, whether it is an anthrax attack or a widely distributed *Escherichia coli* contamination, calls for a concerted response action. Preparedness has five major requirements PHDs need to address (see Chapter 22):

- Preparedness
- Mitigation
- Response
- Recovery
- Evaluation

In 2002, the *Bioterrorism and Emergency Readiness Competencies for All Public Health Workers* was developed and became the standard for ensuring the public health workforce was prepared and ready to respond to emergencies and disasters.[67] As more experience has been gained through public health response and more discipline-specific competencies have been developed, these initial competencies have evolved into the *Public Health Preparedness & Response Core Competency Model*.[67b] The Association of Public Health Nurses integrated this model into its 2013 *The Role of Public Health Nurses in Emergency and Disaster Preparedness, Response, and Recovery* position paper, which provides guidance to PHNs on how to work in a disaster or emergency.[67]

Preparedness functions and planning rely heavily on the use of partners and data sets to achieve success. Each community is different in the resources it can bring to bear in dealing with an emergency or disaster. Consistently, the PHD is looked to as the community lead, in collaboration with local emergency management, for health and medical response activities in an emergency or disaster. PHNs have key roles to play in disaster planning and preparedness efforts. A key preparedness function uses a basic public health nursing skill, community assessment. By knowing the aspects of the community, plans can be written to meet the unique needs of that community during an emergency or disaster. During the disaster, the PHN's role may center on staffing emergency shelters for persons with special health and medical needs or providing tetanus immunizations in the community for persons engaged in clean-up activities. During the recovery phase of a disaster, the PHN may be assigned to go into the community to assess the current and long-term needs of the area. Identification of these needs is essential to ensure the delivery of services to the community so that normal functioning may return.

Regulation, Licensing, and Inspection

Regulatory, licensing, and inspection activities are common roles for a PHD. The 2016 NACCHO survey of PHDs revealed that the areas of particular focus in PHD were food service, schools/daycare centers, swimming pools, septic systems, and smoke-free ordinances.[12] Other areas included private drinking water, body art (tattoos/piercings), camps, campgrounds, and, in some cases, housing.

Public Health Department Challenges for the Future

Healthy People

As one thinks about the future, the objectives for *HP* provide some insight into the issues of importance to the functioning of local health departments. *HP*'s goal is to increase public health infrastructure. It is this infrastructure that provides the foundational capacity for national, state, and local actions to prevent disease and promote health. An example of an objective is "to increase the proportion of tribal and state public health agencies that provide or assure comprehensive laboratory services to support essential public health services."[68]

Other objectives relate to assuring the workers' competencies, monitoring performance, and assuring practice is guided by standards. In an effort to highlight the need to strengthen the public health workforce, increased workforce diversity and reducing the shortage are critical and are reflected in the objectives added to *HP 2020* that targeted public health education and competencies.

Other challenges of PHDs include issues of relevance to the public health workforce, IT, quality improvement and PHD accreditation, and PHD financing, especially as it relates to the economic recession.

■ HEALTHY PEOPLE

Healthy People 2020 Objectives Relevant to Public Health Department Infrastructure

Selected Objectives:

PHI-1: Increase the proportion of federal, tribal, state, and local public health agencies that incorporate core competencies for public health professionals into job descriptions and performance evaluations.

PHI-2: Increase the proportion of Tribal, State, and local public health personnel who receive continuing education consistent with the Core Competencies for Public Health Professionals.

PHI-3: Increase the proportion of Council on Education for Public Health (CEPH) accredited schools of public health, CEPH accredited academic programs, and schools of nursing (with a public health or community health component) that integrate Core Competencies for Public Health Professionals into curricula.

PHI-4: Increase the number of public health or related graduate degrees, post-baccalaureate certificates, and bachelor's degrees awarded.

PHI- 5: (Developmental) Increase the proportion of 4-year colleges and universities that offer public health or related majors and/or minors consistent with the core competencies of undergraduate public health education.

PHI-6: Increase the proportion of 2-year colleges that offer public health or related associate degrees and/or certificate programs.

PHI-11: Increase the proportion of tribal and state public health agencies that provide or assure comprehensive laboratory services to support the essential public health services.

PHI-12: Increase the proportion of public health laboratory systems (including state, tribal, and local)

which perform at a high level of quality in support of the 10 Essential Public Health Services.

PHI-13: Increase the proportion of tribal, state, and local public health agencies that provide or assure comprehensive epidemiology services to support essential public health services.

PHI-14: Increase the proportion of state and local public health jurisdictions that conduct a public health system assessment using national performance standards.

PHI-15: Increase the proportion of tribal, state, and local public health agencies that have developed a health improvement plan and increase the proportion of local health jurisdictions that have a health improvement plan linked with their state plan.

PHI-16: Increase the proportion of tribal, state, and local public health agencies that have implemented an agency-wide quality improvement process.

PHI-17: Increase the number or proportion of tribal, state and local public health agencies that are accredited.

Midcourse Review: Of the 61 objectives for this topic, 2 were archived, 6 were developmental, and 53 were measurable. Of the measurable objectives, 12 met or exceeded their 2020 targets, 9 improved, 4 demonstrated little or no change, 7 were getting worse, 17 only had baseline data, and 4 were informational (Fig. 13-6).[68b]

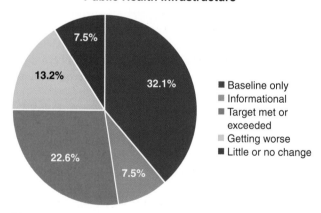

Healthy People 2020 Midcourse Review: Public Health Infrastructure

- Baseline only
- Informational
- Target met or exceeded
- Getting worse
- Little or no change

Figure 13-6 HP 2020 Midcourse Status of the Public Health Infrastructure Objectives.

Public Health Workforce

Currently, there is a shortage of public health workers, and this shortage is projected to increase in the coming years. In 2016, the Association of State and Territorial Health Officials conducted a survey of state agencies. It found an average of 14% of state health agency positions were vacant, an average of 365 positions per state health agency. There are a number of factors contributing to this shortage, including budget reductions and hiring freezes, a rapidly aging workforce whose average age was 47, and 25% of the workforce eligible to retire by 2020.[69] All of these issues raise concern for PHDs as well.

The U.S. public health workforce has been of sufficient interest to policy makers during the past 4 decades to lead to regular efforts to enumerate it. In 1980, there was a ratio of public health workers to the general population of 220/100,000, and in 2000 that had dropped to 158/100,000.[70] Although there is an overall shortage, the critical shortage of PHNs is a threat to the public's health and of great concern because they make up a large sector of the public health workforce.[71,72] Executive leadership for PHDs is also a major concern, especially in light of the aging public health workforce and projected shortages.[73]

Core competencies for various public health workers or in specific functions have been developed to enhance the public health workforce capacity. These include the *Public Health Nursing: Scope and Standards of Practice,*[74] *Public Health Preparedness and Response Core Competencies,*[75] *Council on Linkages: Core Competencies for Public Health Professionals,*[76] and *Competencies for Public Health Informaticians.*[77]

Because the public health workforce comprises a broad range of educational backgrounds and training, these competencies provide a common framework for measuring and improving public health workforce skills and abilities (Box 13-5). To further support public health workforce competency, public health workers have the ability to become certified in public health through the National Board of Public Health Examiners.[78]

Sustainment of the public health workforce is a major concern and is influenced by several factors. First, many of the health-care professions have experienced shortages in available workers, thus many health-care facilities are competing for the same candidates. Second, many PHD jurisdictions are located in rural or remote areas, making recruitment of qualified personnel difficult. Third, limited financial resources may make it difficult for PHDs to provide compensation that is competitive with private-sector entities. Finally, there are faculty shortages within the academic setting that limit the ability of colleges and universities to graduate large numbers of qualified individuals.[79] Currently, there are critical PHN nursing faculty shortages that have significantly limited the exposure to and specialization in public health nursing.[80]

Information Technology

IT is a key infrastructure component within a PHD, from clinical records management to supporting a PHD Web site. IT is used in every aspect of operations. All persons working in a PHD use IT at varying degrees. The level of use and knowledge required is position-dependent. For example, an administrative assistant would require just basic knowledge and skills to use IT for general office functions, whereas an epidemiologist will need more advanced knowledge and skills for data collection and analysis. IT is much more than just using computer equipment and programs. The field of **public health informatics** focuses on the use of IT by public health professionals. There are several definitions for public health informatics, all of which essentially define it as public health information systems and infrastructure that are population-based and used for surveillance, program outcome evaluation, quality assurance, systems analysis, and evidence-based disease management.[81]

In 2002, the CDC created a work group of subject matter experts to define overarching public health informatics competencies for all persons working in public health. These competencies focused on three areas: (1) information for public health practice, (2) use of IT by the public health professional to enhance personal performance, and (3) utilization of IT projects to improve PHD effectiveness.[77] These competencies provide the framework to ensure that PHDs have the capacity to adequately perform in today's technologically demanding environment.

Although PHDs use IT to support general business operations, new regulations and technology create new demands on PHDs to enhance IT use. Two key examples

---

BOX 13–5 ■ Public Health Core Competencies

- Core Competencies for Public Health Workers.
  http://www.phf.org/resourcestools/Documents/Core_Competencies_for_Public_Health_Professionals_2014June.pdf
- Public Health Preparedness and Response Core Competencies
  https://www.cdc.gov/phpr/documents/perlcpdfs/preparednesscompetencymodelworkforce-version1_0.pdf
- PHN Scope and Standards of Practice
  http://www.nursesbooks.org/Main-Menu/Standards/O—Z/Public-Health-Nursing.aspx
- Public Health Informatics Competencies
  https://www.cdc.gov/informaticscompetencies/

of this are **geographic information system (GIS)** application and electronic health records. Both of these activities have required PHDs to expand staff knowledge and hardware capacity to effectively integrate these applications into daily operations.[82] The use of GIS has transformed a number of functions within PHDs. It can be used to visualize data geographically within a designated area. For example, in a disease outbreak, the case data can be entered into a GIS program and maps can then be created to show various characteristics of the cases. An epidemiology nurse can easily identify where cases may be clustering geographically or identify density of cases through a color-coding system. Likewise, the PHN can use GIS to identify potential exposure risk from environmental hazards by applying layers of demographic data to environmental data layers. GIS technology is a very effective tool for understanding the dynamics between health status, health system access, and physical environment.

Regulations and requirements to move health records from paper-based systems to electronic systems have resulted in a paradigm shift for medical record management. PHDs have faced unique challenges in implementing these systems because public health practitioners' health focus is much broader than that in clinical care. Public health electronic systems need to (1) integrate clinical data from all providers for public health use, such as disease surveillance and investigation, and (2) include expanded capacity for psychosocial, behavioral, and environmental client data collected by PHDs. The impact of electronic health record implementation affects public health systems in two ways: (1) There is a need to implement an electronic system for individual patient care, and (2) PHDs need to maintain the ability to conduct population-based core functions such as assessment, policy development, and assurance through interfaced integration of electronic data from providers. This will require public and private providers to come together to ensure electronic health record systems include a public health orientation. By effectively integrating this focus, reporting duplication can be reduced and community decision making can be enhanced through more comprehensive data availability.[83]

Quality Improvement and Public Health Department Accreditation

The emerging areas of PHD accreditation and **public health systems and services research** expand our knowledge about the relationship between characteristics of PHDs, local public health system performance, and public health outcomes. Continuous quality improvement initiatives are led by multidisciplinary teams to systematically apply evidence-based practice, improve service delivery, and achieve the best outcomes. In the NACCHO 2016 survey of PHDs, 89% of PHDs reported conducting some type of quality improvement activities.[12] The Public Health Accreditation Board has developed a national voluntary accreditation program for state and PHDs to formalize and advance quality and performance of PHDs and improve population health outcomes. In early 2018, more than 200 state and local PHDs had received national accreditation.[84] Accredited PHDs have reported many benefits from the accreditation process. These benefits include increased transparency, stronger management processes, and increased ability to identify organizational weaknesses. However, the most significant benefit identified was the increased use of quality improvement information in decision making and a more robust quality improvement culture.[85,85b]

Studies show that the strongest predictor of PHD performance is the size of the jurisdiction population.[73,85] In general, PHDs serving larger populations with greater numbers of staff and higher funding per capita perform better than PHDs serving populations of less than 50,000.[2] PHD leadership structure also influences the staffing model and service focus. Bekemeier and Jones[86] found there were distinct differences between programmatic service delivery and the core functions of assessment and planning in PHDs led by nurse executives and non-nurse executives. PHDs under nurse executive leadership had stronger prevention programs to address unintended pregnancy, obesity, injury prevention, immunization, and maternal-child health than non-nurse-led PHDs. However, assessment and planning functions were performed less by nurse executives than by medical or nonclinical senior executives, indicating the need for additional training in these areas.[86]

Public Health Department Financing

Public health systems have historically been designed as a function of local (county or city) government operations. The structure of PHDs previously described has an impact on PHD financing. The vast majority of states have county-operated systems, usually governed by local boards of health, but large metropolitan areas, such as Los Angeles or New York City, may have city structures as well. Some states (e.g., Florida) have a state-centered program with contractual agreements with counties for provision of public health services. The financing of PHD operations can become very complex, related to disparities in county size, needs, and local community capabilities to provide services. There is an inverse relationship between per person expenditures and revenues and size of population served. Small PHDs have higher per person expenditures ($49) and revenues ($51) compared to large PHDs ($31 expenditures and $33 revenues). Due to decreasing funding, PHD per person expenditures have declined from an average of $63 in 2008 to $48 in 2016. This translates into fewer services available to populations the PHD serves.[12] However, the 2016 NACCHO survey noted that more PHDs reported higher budget amounts than in any previous survey. Hopefully, this increasing revenue trend will continue.

The three primary funding streams for PHDs are federal (24%), state (21%), and local (55%)[12]. There is not an overriding formula for any of these financing layers. However, there are guidelines developed to assure that allocations are used appropriately and may be designated for specific programs or services. These funds, often called **categorical funds**, are usually federal funds either directly disbursed to PHDs from the federal government through grants or received by the states and reallocated to the PHDs. Either way, budgets must show the expenditures by category (personnel, expenses, fixed capital) and require annual reporting back to the federal government.[87] An example of this might be a PHN position that performs family planning, STI, and school-based health services. The PHN will then need to record her time spent in each service area to ensure her time is allocated to the appropriate funding source. This is a common occurrence in PHDs; therefore, tracking systems and reporting procedures have been developed to manage the funding reporting requirements.

A significant part of PHDs clinical service funding is through insurance billing such as Medicaid or Medicare. The amounts generated through billing will vary greatly among PHDs depending on the types of services provided and the robustness of their billing process to fully leverage the revenue return. For example, Alabama PHDs have been able to generate 29.5% of their total revenue through Medicare and Medicaid billing. Whereas, Georgia only generated 1.3% of revenue from Medicaid or Medicare billing.[91] Maximizing billing opportunities allows PHDs to utilize other public funds to provide more clinical services to uninsured or underinsured populations.

The 2016 NACCHO survey of PHDs found a loss of 43,000 employees since 2008. The economic recession had a significant impact on jobs, budgets, and programs. Many of the PHDs reported that the cuts are most often in local and state funding, and that the dramatic cuts threaten the general use funds that enable PHDs to respond to urgent community needs not covered by specific disease grants.[10]

One way the PHDs have survived these changes has been through one-time funding for diseases, such as the H1N1 influenza outbreak and Ebola virus preparedness. What is needed, however, is stable, long-term funding. The key to funding the PHD in the future will be the ability to clearly articulate its mission. Policy makers will need to support PHDs by ensuring an adequate investment in public health by assuring that prevention dollars do go to PHDs to help build their capacities. This is critical, considering the important role that PHDs play in keeping communities safe. "[PHDs] have been described as the country's 'best kept secret.' As one PHD official states, 'Unless there is an outbreak, no one even knows that we exist. We operate diligently and quietly in the background, keeping our community healthy and safe.'"[88]

Additional Challenges

Keeping the community healthy and safe is key. Although there is a growing emphasis on emerging or re-emerging communicable diseases or on disaster preparedness, a major threat to the health of populations is noncommunicable disease. PHDs often lack structure as well as money to address noncommunicable disease and contributing factors like obesity. This challenge raises issues of what strategies to use in addressing multiple health issues as well as how to finance new initiatives. Some health departments provide an exemplar of what can be done. In a local collaboration between the PHD, the school board, and city of Anchorage, a multiyear project was initiated to reduce childhood obesity using a broad set of policies. These policies included increased weekly physical education in public schools and day care centers, no sodas sold during school hours, healthier school lunches, and increased healthier food options in campus vending machines as well as a public awareness campaign on the consequences of childhood obesity. Because of these efforts, elementary and middle school obesity rates declined by 2.2%.[89]

In an effort to engage communities more effectively within a limited funding environment, 12 Utah PHDs collaborated to initiate a month long social media campaign to promote healthy family meals and family dinner together. They used a variety of social media platforms with videos, competitions, and a designated interactive Web site. Some of the results were an average of 121 individuals visited the Web site daily, Facebook likes had reached 1,454, and Twitter followers were 255 by the month's end. The authors estimate between 10% and 12% of the target population was reached. Additionally, the campaign was cost effective at an overall cost of

27 cents per engagement.[90] The PHDs built their capacity by relying on categorical funding supplemented by flexible funding and sometimes the use of state revenue as well as creative community collaborations.

■ CELLULAR TO GLOBAL

Multidimensional interventions, such as those previously discussed, are frequently implemented by PHDs in communities across this country. However, middle- to low-income countries are challenged to implement even the most basic interventions, such as directly observed therapy for TB control or bed net distribution for malaria prevention, due to the lack of resources and public health infrastructure. Lack of a robust public health workforce with high quality training and strong leadership at local and national levels significantly affects a nation's ability to provide basic services or response to expanding disease threats.[92]

■ Summary Points

- The basic mandate of the PHD is to protect and improve health in partnership with the community.
- PHDs are organized by three major delivery modes: centralized system, decentralized system, and shared or mixed system.
- The PHD workforce is interdisciplinary, with nurses making up 17% of it.
- The 10 most frequent activities and services available through the direct services of the PHD are: adult immunization provision, communicable disease surveillance, child immunization provision, TB screening, food service establishment inspection, environmental surveillance, food safety education, TB treatment, schools/day-care center inspections, and population-based nutrition services.
- PHDs also work in collaboration with the state or contract with other partners to fulfill the core functions of public health.
- The major responsibilities of PHDs lie with environmental health services, data collection and analysis (which includes the collection of vital statistics), assurance of individual and community health, communicable diseases, epidemiology and surveillance, and licensing.
- Nurses' roles within health departments include providing primary prevention efforts, making health policy, designing health programs, and providing care at the individual and community levels. The role of the nurse in a PHD varies depending on

the services being provided and the level of expertise needed.
- Challenges for PHDs include the shortage of public health workers, using IT to enhance care, quality improvement, and financing efforts in the future.
- PHD accreditation is a voluntary program to advance quality and performance of PHDs.
- The mission of public health is to assure conditions in which people can be healthy. Although there are emerging and re-emerging infections from a global concern that affects population health, noncommunicable diseases, which are additional challenge for PHDs, are the major threats to the health of populations.

▼ CASE STUDY
Collaborating with Community Partners

Learning Outcomes

At the end of this case study, the student will be able to:

- Investigate the role of PHDs in community assessment and planning for health needs of the community.
- Describe the structure and services of your PHD.
- Identify the major partners involved in community health planning.

You have been asked by your hospital to be the representative on a community needs assessment. This will involve measuring and evaluating health status and developing collaborative programs that will address the health needs of your community. You realize that you need to learn more about your local health department and the population that it serves. Research your local health department and answer the following questions:

1. What type of public health system is used in your state (centralized, decentralized, mixed, shared)?
2. What type of jurisdiction does your PHD serve (city, town, county, multiple county, district, region)?
3. Is there a local board of health and, if so, what is its role and function?
4. What types of assessment and planning are under way? Who are the main community partners?
5. Where is the PHD located? Are there branch offices?
6. What types of services are provided? What services exist that (a) ensure a safe environment; (b) provide

preventive and/or primary health care; (c) monitor, detect, and investigate disease outbreaks; (d) track and record health data about the community; (e) promote healthy behaviors; and (f) prepare the health department to support communities during times of disasters or emergency?

7. What roles and services do nurses perform? How many nurses are employed? What are the educational and certification requirements?

REFERENCES

1. Scutchfield, F.D., Knight, E.A., Kelly, A.V., Bhandarie, M.W., & Vasilescu, I.P. (2004). Local public health agency capacity and its relationship to public health system performance. *Journal of Public Health Management Practice, 10*(3), 204-215.

2. Erwin, P.C. (2008). The performance of local health departments: A review of the literature. *Journal of Public Health Management and Practice, 14*(2), E9-E18.

3. Jekel, J.F. (1991). Health departments in the U.S. 1920–1988: Statements of mission with special reference to the role of C.E.A Winslow. *The Yale Journal of Biology and Medicine, 64,* 467-479.

4. Fee, E., & Brown, T. (2007). The unidentified promise of public health: Déjà vu all over again. *Health Affairs, 26*(6), 31.

5. Meit, M., & Knudson, A. (2009). Why is rural public health important? A look to the future. *Journal of Public Health Management and Practice, 15*(3), 185-190.

6. U.S. Public Health Service. (1936). *Health of county health organizations in the United States: 1908–1933.* Washington, DC: US Government Printing Office.

7. Hiscock I. V. (1937). *History of County Health Organizations in the United States, 1908-33—Bulletin 222, U. S. Public Health Service. American Journal of Public Health and the Nations Health, 27*(1), 90.

8. Fairchild, A.L., Rosner, D., Colgrave, J., Bayer, R., & Fried, L.P. (2010). The exodus of public health. *American Journal of Public Health, 100*(1), 54-63.

9. Vaughan, H.F. (1972). Local health services in the United States: The story of the CAP. *American Public Health Association, 62,* 95-111.

10. APHA. (1940, September). An official declaration of attitude of the American Public Health Association on desirable standard minimum functions and suitable organization of health activities. *American Journal of Public Health,* (9) 1099-1106.

11. Institute of Medicine. (1988). *The future of public health.* Washington, DC: National Academies Press.

12. National Association of County and City Health Officials. (2017). *2016 national profile of local health departments.* Washington, DC: Author. Retrieved from http://nacchoprofilestudy.org/wp-content/uploads/2017/10/ProfileReport_Aug2017_final.pdf.

13. Association of State and Territorial Health Officers (ASTHO). (2017). *ASTHO profile of state and territorial public health.* Retrieved from http://www.astho.org/Profile/Volume-Four/2016-ASTHO-Profile-of-State-and-Territorial-Public-Health/.

14. Kansas Health Institute. (2006). *Local public health at the crossroads: The structure of health departments in rural areas.* Topeka, KS: Author. Retrieved from http://media.khi.org/news/documents/2009/09/02/40-0601HealthDeptStructureHRSABrief.pdf.

15. Meit, M., Knudson, A., Gilbert, T., Yu, A., Tanenbaum, E., Ormson, E., ... Popat, S. (2014). The 2014 update of the rural-urban chartbook. *Rural Health Research and Policy Centers.* Retrieved from https://ruralhealth.und.edu/projects/health-reform-policy-research-center/pdf/2014-rural-urban-chartbook-update.pdf.

16. National Association of County & City Health Officials. (2010). *The local health department workforce.* Retrieved from http://archived.naccho.org/topics/infrastructure/profile/upload/NACCHO_WorkforceReport_FINAL.pdf.

17. Winslow, C.E.A. (1920). The untilled fields of public health. *Science, 51,* 23-33.

18. Centers for Disease Control and Prevention. (n.d.). *Ten essential public health services.* Retrieved from http://www.cdc.gov/od/ocphp/nphpsp/essentialphservices.htm.

19. Lahariya, C. (2016). Vaccine epidemiology: A review. *Journal of Family Medicine and Primary Care, 5(1),* 7-15.

20. Public Health Leadership Society. (2002). *Principles of the ethical practice of public health, version 2.2.* Retrieved from http://www.phls.org/home/section/3-26/.

21. Keller, L., Strohschein, S., Lia-Hoagberg, C., & Schaffer, M. (2004). Population-based interventions: Innovations in practice, teaching and management. Part II. *Public Health Nursing, 21*(5), 469-487.

22. Golechha, M. (2016). Health promotion methods for smoking prevention and cessation: A comprehensive review of effectiveness and the way forward. *International Journal of Preventive Medicine, 7,* 7. http://doi.org/10.4103/2008-7802.173797.

23. National Cancer Institute. (2007). *Greater than the sum: Systems thinking in tobacco control.* Retrieved from http://cancercontrol.cancer.gov/Brp/tcrb/monographs/18/monograph18.html.

24. Marcus, S.E., Leischow, S.J., Mabry, P.L., & Clark, P.J. (2010). Lessons learned from the application of systems science to tobacco control at the National Cancer Institute. *American Journal of Public Health, 100*(7), 1163-1165.

25. Borland, R., Young, D., Coghill, K., & Zhang, J.Y. (2010). The tobacco use management system: Analyzing tobacco control from a systems perspective. *American Journal of Public Health, 100*(7), 1229-1236.

26. U.S. Department of Health and Human Services. (n.d.). *Healthy People 2020.* Retrieved from http://www.healthypeople.gov/hp2020/objectives/framework.aspx.

27. Nurse-Family Partnership. (2018a). *Overview.* Retrieved from https://www.nursefamilypartnership.org/wp-content/uploads/2017/07/NFP_Overview.pdf.

28. Nurse-Family Partnership. (2018b). *Research trials and outcomes.* Retrieved from https://www.nursefamilypartnership.org/wpcontent/uploads/2017/07/NFP_Research_Outcomes_2014.pdf.

29. Nurse-Family Partnership. (2018c). *Nurses and mothers.* Retrieved from https://www.nursefamilypartnership.org/wpcontent/uploads/2017/07/NFP_Nurses_Mothers.pdf.

30. Bazzoli, G.J., Stein, R., Alexander, J.A., Conrad, D.A., Sofaer, S., & Shortell, S.M. (1997). Public-private collaboration in

health and human service delivery: Evidence from community partnerships. *The Milbank Quarterly, 75*(4), 533-561.

31. Shah, G., Luo, H., & Sotnikov, S. (2014) Public health services most commonly provided by local health departments in the United States. *Front Public Health Serv Syst Res, 3*(1), DOI: 10.13023/FPHSSR.0301.02.

32. Centers for Disease Control and Prevention. (n.d.). *National vital statistics system.* Retrieved from http://www.cdc.gov/nchs/nvss.htm.

33. Centers for Disease Control and Prevention. (2017). *Revisions of the U.S. standard certificates and reports.* Retrieved from http://www.cdc.gov/nchs/nvss/vital_certificate_revisions.htm.

34. City of Cincinnati Health Department. (2018). *Health department: Celebrating 190 years of service to the people of Cincinnati, 1826—2016.* Retrieved from http://www.cincinnati-oh.gov/health/.

35. Institute of Medicine. (2003). *The future of the public's health in the 21st century.* Washington, DC: National Academies Press.

36. Rural Assistance Center. (2015). *What is a federally qualified health center and what are the benefits?* Retrieved from https://www.ruralhealthinfo.org/topics/federally-qualified-health-centers#faqs.

37. Maternal and Child Health Bureau. (2017). *HRSA awards $342 million to support families through the maternal, infant and early childhood home visiting program.* Retrieved from https://www.hrsa.gov/about/news/press-releases/hrsa-awards-342-million-miechv-program.html.

38. National Healthy Start Association. (2015). *Healthy start initiative.* Retrieved from http://www.healthystartassoc.org/hswpp6.html.

39. Health Resources & Services Administration Maternal & Child Health. (2018). *Healthy start.* Retrieved from https://mchb.hrsa.gov/maternal-child-health-initiatives/healthy-start.

40. U.S. Department of Agriculture, Food and Nutrition Service, Office of Research and Analysis. (2015). *WIC participant and program characteristics 2014.* Retrieved from https://www.fns.usda.gov/wic/wic-participant-and-program-characteristics-2014.

41. Office of Population Affairs. (2018). *Title X: Family planning.* Retrieved from http://www.hhs.gov/opa/familyplanning/index.html.

42. New York State Department of Health. (2017). *Family planning benefit program.* Retrieved from http://www.health.state.ny.us/health_care/medicaid/program/longterm/familyplanbenprog.htm.

43. National Association of School Nurses. (2018). *The role of the 21st century school nurse.* Retrieved from https://www.nasn.org/advocacy/professional-practice-documents/position-statements/ps-role.

44. Henry J. Kaiser Family Foundation. (2016). *Health insurance coverage of children 0—18.* Retrieved from https://www.kff.org/other/state-indicator/children-0-18/?currentTimeframe=0&sortModel=%7B%22colId%22:%22Location%22,%22sort%22:%22asc%22%7D.

45. Riedel, S. (2005). Edward Jenner and the history of smallpox and vaccination. *BUMC Proceedings, 18,* 21-25.

46. Browne, H., Reimer, J., MacLead, M., & McLellan, E. (2010). Public health nursing practice with "high priority" families: The significance of contextualizing "risk." *Nursing Inquiry, 17,* 27-38.

47. Sama-Miller, E., Akers, L., Mraz-Esposito, A., Zukiewicz, M., Avellar, S., Paulsell, D., & DelGrosso, P. (2016). *Home visiting evidence of effectiveness review: Executive summary.* Washington, D.C.: Office of Planning, Research and Evaluation, Administration for Children and Families, U.S. Department of Health and Human Services.

48. Olds, D., Robinson, J., O'Brien, R., Luckey, D., Pettitt, L., Henderson, C., ... Talmi, A. (2002). Home visiting by paraprofessionals and by nurses: A randomized, controlled trial. *Pediatrics, 110,* 486-496.

49. Safe to Sleep. (n.d.). *National Institutes of Health, Eunice Kennedy Shriver National Institute of Child Health and Human Development.* Retrieved from http://www.nichd.nih.gov/sids/.

50. Havranek, E.P., Barr, D.A., Cruz-Flores, S., Davey-Smith, G., Dennison-Himmelfarb, C.R., Lauer, M.S., ... Yancy, C.W. (2015). Social determinants of risk and outcomes for cardiovascular disease: A scientific statement from the American Heart Association. *Circulation, 132*(9), 873-898

51. Howard, G., Kleindorfer, D.O., Cushman, M., Long, D.L., Jasne, A., Judd, S.E., ... Howard, V.J. (2017). Contributors to the excess stroke mortality in rural areas in the United States. *Stroke 48*(7), 1773-1778.

52. Sarasota County Health Department. (n.d.). *Community health improvement partnership.* Retrieved from http://www.chip4health.org/whatwedo/index.htm.

53. LoBue, P., Sizemore, C., & Castro, K.G. (2009). Plan to combat extensively drug-resistant tuberculosis: Recommendations of the federal Tuberculosis Task Force. *Morbidity and Mortality Weekly Report, 5*(RR03), 1-43. Retrieved from http://www.cdc.gov/mmwr/preview/mmwrhtml/rr5803a1.htm?s_cid=rr5803a1_e.

54. Jeffries, C., LoBue, P., Chorba, T., Metchock, B., & Kashef, I. (2017). Role of the health department in tuberculosis prevention and control-Legal and public health considerations. *Microbiology Spectrum, 5*(2). doi:10.1128/microbiolspec.TNMI7-0034-2016.

55. Centers for Disease Control and Prevention. (2016). *Tuberculosis.* Retrieved from http://www.cdc.gov/tb/.

56. World Health Organization. (2009). *Treatment of tuberculosis guidelines.* Retrieved from http://whqlibdoc.who.int/publications/2010/9789241547833_eng.pdf.

57. van Heuckelum, M., van den Ende, C., Houterman, A., Heemskerk, C., van Dulmen, S., & van den Bemt, B. (2017). The effect of electronic monitoring feedback on medication adherence and clinical outcomes: A systematic review. *Plos ONE, 12*(10). https://doi.org/10.1371/journal.pone.0185453.

58. Centers for Disease Control and Prevention. (2017). *Sexually transmitted disease surveillance, 2016.* Atlanta, GA: U.S. Department of Health and Human Services.

59. National Association of County and City Health Officials. (2010). *Statement of policy prevention and control of sexually transmitted infections.* Retrieved from http://www.naccho.org/advocacy/positions/upload/09-10-Prevention-and-Control-of-STI.pdf.

60. National Association of County and City Health Officials. (2012). *Statement of policy-Sexually transmitted infections.* Washington, DC: Author.

61. Davis, J.R., & Lederberg, J. (Eds.). (2000). *Public health systems and emerging infections: Assessing the capabilities of the public and private sectors.* Washington, DC: National Academies Press.

62. Morens, D.M., & Fauci, A.S. (2013) Emerging infectious diseases: Threats to human health and global stability. *PLoS Pathog, 9*(7): e1003467. doi:10.1371/journal.ppat.1003467

63. World Health Organization. (2003). *Summary of probable SARS cases with onset of illness from 1 November 2002 to 31 July 2003.* Retrieved from http://www.who.int/csr/sars/country/table2004_04_21/en/index.html.

64. Stern, A.M., & Markel, H. (2009). What Mexico taught the world about pandemic influenza preparedness and community mitigation strategies. *JAMA, 302*(11), 1221-1222.

65. Centers for Disease Control and Prevention. (2018). *National center for emerging and zoonotic infectious diseases.* Retrieved from https://www.cdc.gov/ncezid/index.html.

66. Centers for Disease Control and Prevention. (2011). *Public health importance of rabies.* Retrieved from https://www.cdc.gov/rabies/location/usa/index.html.

67. Centers for Disease Control and Prevention. (2002). *Bioterrorism & emergency readiness: Competencies for all public helath workers.* Retrieved from http://training.fema.gov/emiweb/downloads/BioTerrorism%20and%20Emergency%20Readiness.pdf.

67b. Association of Schools of Public Health (ASPH). (2010). *Public health preparedness & response core competency model.* Retrieved from http://www.asph.org/userfiles/PreparednessCompetencyModelWorkforce—Version1.0.pdf

67c. Association of Public Health Nurses. (2013). *The role of public health nurses in emergency and disaster preparedness, response, and recovery.* Retrieved from http://www.achne.org/files/public/APHN_RoleOfPHNinDisasterPRR_FINALJan14.pdf.

68. Department of Health and Human Services. (2014). *Healthy People 2020 topics & objectives-public health infrastructure.* Retrieved from https://www.healthypeople.gov/2020/topics-objectives/topic/public-health-infrastructure.

68b. National Center for Health Statistics. (2016). *Chapter 35: Public health infrastructure. Healthy People 2020 midcourse review.* Hyattsville, MD: National Center for Health Statistics.

69. Association of State and Territorial Health Officials. (2017). *Profile of state public health* (Vol. 4). Retrieved from http://www.astho.org/Profile/Volume-Four/2016-ASTHO-Profile-of-State-and-Territorial-Public-Health/.

70. Merrill, J., Btoush, R., Gupta, M., & Gebbie, K. (2003). A history of public health workforce enumeration. *Journal of Public Health Management, 9*(6), 459-470.

71. Beck, A.J., Boulton, M.L., & Coronado, F. (2014). Enumeration of the governmental public health workforce, 2014. *American Journal of Preventive Medicine, 47*(5S3), S306-S313.

72. Beck, A. J., & Boulton, M. L. (2016). The public health nurse workforce in U.S. State and local health departments, 2012. *Public Health Reports, 131,* 145-152.

73. Little, R.G., Greer, A., Clay, M., & McFadden, C. (2016). Profile of public health leadership. *Journal of Public Health Management and Practice, 22*(5), 479-481.

74. American Nurses Association. (2013). *Public health nursing: Scope and standards of practice* (2nd ed.). Silver Spring, MD: Author.

75. Centers for Disease Control & Prevention. (2010). *Public health preparedness & response core competency model.* Retrieved from https://www.cdc.gov/phpr/documents/perlcpdfs/preparednesscompetencymodelworkforce-version1_0.pdf.

76. Public Health Foundation. (2014). *Council on linkages: Core competencies for public health professionals between academia and public health practice.* Retrieved from http://www.phf.org/resourcestools/Documents/Core_Competencies_for_Public_Health_Professionals_2014June.pdf.

77. U.S. Department of Health and Human Services. (2009). *Competencies for public health informaticians.* Retrieved from http://www.cphi.washington.edu/resources/PHICompetencies.pdf.

78. National Board of Public Health Examiners. (n.d.) *Credentialing public health leaders.* Retrieved from: https://www.nbphe.org/.

79. Council on Linkages Between Academia and Public Health Practice. (2016). *Recruitment and retention: What's influencing the decisions of public health workers?* Washington, DC: Public Health Foundation.

80. Collier, J., Davidson, G., Allen, C.B., Dieckmann, J., Hoke, M.M., & Sawaya, M.A. (2010). Academic faculty qualification for community/public health nursing: An association of community health nursing educators position paper. *Public Health Nursing, 27*(1), 89-93.

81. Baker, E.L., Fond, M., Hale, P., & Cook, J. (2016) What is "informatics"? *Journal of Public Health Management & Practice, 22*(4), 420-423.

82. Centers for Disease Control and Prevention. (2016). *GIS and public health at CDC.* Retrieved from https://www.cdc.gov/gis/index.htm.

83. Tomines, A., Readhead, H., Readhead, A., & Teutsch, S. (2013). Applications of electronic health information in public health: Uses, opportunities & barriers. *EGEMS, 1*(2). DOI: http://dx.doi.org/10.13063/2327-9214.1019.

84. Public Health Accreditation Board. (2018). *Public health department accreditation.* Retrieved from http://www.phaboard.org/

85. Laymon, B., Shah, G., Leep, C., Elligers, J. & Kumar, V. (2015). The proof's in the partnerships: Are affordable care act and local health department accreditation practices influencing collaborative partnerships in community health assessment and improvement planning? *Journal of Public Health Management and Practice, 21*(1), 12-17.

85b. Kronstadt, J., Meit, M., Siegfried, A., Nicolaus, T., Bender, K., & Corso, L. (2016). Evaluating the impact of national public health department accreditation-United States, 2016. *Morbidity and Mortality Weekly Report, 65,* 803-806.

86. Bekemeier, B., & Jones, M. (2010). Relationship between local public health agency functions and agency leadership and staffing: A look at nurses. *Journal of Public Health Management and Practice, 16*(2), E8-E16.

87. Leider, J., Resnick, B., Sellers, K., Kass, N., Bernet, P., Young, J., & Jarris, P. (2015). Setting budgets and priorities at state health agencies. *Journal of Public Health Management and Practice, 21*(4), 336-344.

88. National Association of County and City Health Officials. (2010). *Research brief: Local health department job losses and program cuts.* Retrieved from http://www.naccho.org/topics/infrastructure/lhdbudget/upload/Job-Losses-and-Program-Cuts-5-10.pdf.

89. National Collaborative on Childhood Obesity Research. (2015). *Signs of progress in childhood obesity declines-site*

summary report Anchorage, Alaska. Retrieved from https://www.nccor.org/downloads/CODP_Site%20Summary%20Report_Anchorage_public_clean1.pdf.

90. Lister, C., Royne, M., Payne, H., Cannon, B., Hanson, C. & Barnes, M. (2015). The laugh model: Reframing and rebranding public health through social media. *American Journal of Public Health,105*(11), 2245-2251.

91. Meit, M., Knudson, A., Dickman, I., Brown, A., Hernandez, N., & Kronstadt, J. (2013). *An examination of public health financing in the United States.* (Prepared by NORC at the University of Chicago) Washington, DC: The Office of the Assistant Secretary for Planning and Evaluation.

92. Yamey, G. (2012). What are the barriers to scaling up health interventions in low- and middle-income countries? A qualitative study of academic leaders in implementation science. *Globalization and Health, 8,* 11. https://doi.org/10.1186/1744-8603-8-11.

Chapter 14

Health Planning for Acute Care Settings

Kathleen Ballman, Christine Savage, and Mary Nicholson

LEARNING OUTCOMES

After reading the chapter, the student will be able to:

1. Describe the relationship between acute care and population health.
2. Identify the role of population-level data in the development of the discipline of critical care.
3. Discuss the relevance of cohort studies to the delivery of tertiary care.
4. Explain the application of health planning in an acute care setting.
5. Recognize the basic steps in the quality improvement process.
6. Identify key infection control issues related to the acute care setting.

KEY TERMS

Acute care
Acute coronary syndrome (ACS)
Acute myocardial ischemia
Cardiopulmonary resuscitation (CPR)
Critical care nursing
Critically ill/injured patients
Door-to-balloon time
Electronic medical record (EMR)

Epidemiology
Health care-associated infections (HAIs)
Hospital-associated pneumonia (HAP)
Hospital discharge rate
Hospital recidivism
Institutional review board
International Classification of Diseases, 9th Revision (ICD9)

International Classification of Diseases, 10th Revision (ICD10)
Major diagnostic category (MDC)
Multiple drug-resistant organisms
Plan-Do-Study-Act (PDSA) cycle
Patient populations
Polio

Performance improvement
Quality improvement
Sepsis
ST-elevation myocardial infarction (STEMI)
Surgical site infection (SSI)
Survival rate
Ventilator-associated pneumonia (VAP)

Introduction

Sixty-one percent of the nursing workforce works in an acute care setting.[1] **Acute care** is care provided during a severe episode of illness, following surgery, or following a traumatic injury. Acute care usually occurs in a hospital setting and requires skilled care provided by health-care providers. Acute care is provided for a short time during the severe episode and may be followed by chronic care in the home or a long-term care facility.[2]

Acute care occurs mostly at the tertiary prevention level (see Chapter 2), and the focus of the care is to prevent further morbidity and reduce disability related to the disease or injury. The majority of the care is clinical rather than environmental or even behavioral. Although an effort is made during the hospital stay to provide education on behavioral changes that will increase the chances of return to a healthier state and reduce the chances of death or disability, the primary focus of the hospital stay is direct clinical interventions.

Hospitals provide care to persons who are acutely ill, many of them critically ill. Adults who seek care in a hospital setting require highly skilled nurses competent to provide care to the individual addressing the acute episode of illness or aftermath of an injury. It would seem at first glance that the public health sciences have little to contribute to the acute care setting. However, the high level of care now available to patients experiencing an acute episode of illness or injury is based on a clear understanding of the natural history of disease that evolved out of cohort and case control studies (see Chapter 3). Our knowledge of the effectiveness of interventions is based on the findings from rigorous clinical trials (see Chapter 3). These research designs have their basis in epidemiology.

Nurses have a long history of applying population-level research and an understanding of determinants of health to their delivery of care at both the macro (population) level and the micro (individual) level. As hospitals strive to meet criteria for accreditation and recognition of excellence, the role of the staff nurse in improving patient outcomes includes actively applying public health science to the evaluation and improvement of the care they provide.

The Acute Care Setting and Population Health

Often, the distinction between the community/public health nurse (PHN) and the nurse working in a hospital is based on the concept of direct and indirect care as presented in the *Essentials of Doctoral Education for Advanced Nursing Practice*.[3] However, that distinction becomes blurred because many nurses who define themselves as PHNs provide direct care to individuals, for example, administering flu vaccines, whereas hospital-based nurses frequently tackle problems from a public health perspective, for example, reducing the rate of health care–associated infections (HAIs) (see following section on HAIs) or improving targeted patient outcomes for a particular population.

If, instead of a dichotomous concept of direct and indirect care, nursing practice is viewed across the continuum of care from micro/individual health to macro/population health, it is easier to demonstrate the application of public health science to nursing practice in acute care settings. Nurses in acute care settings are continuously involved in efforts to improve care for the populations they serve, not just for each individual. If nurses on a unit are working on a performance improvement project, they have moved along the continuum to look at an issue at the group level, the group they serve. Development of an understanding of the patient data they collect for the project requires the application of epidemiology such as computing discharge rates, establishing odds ratios (see Chapter 3), or looking at HAI rates. In most hospitals, the performance improvement committee provides frequent updates on care issues within the hospital and evidence to demonstrate whether efforts to address specific problems have resulted in improved patient outcomes.

The challenge is differentiating the term *population* used in public health and the term *population* used in a hospital setting. In Chapter 1, the term was defined as a mass of people that make up a definable unit to which measurements pertain. Chapter 1 explains that population health occurs within the context of the social, economic, cultural, and environmental influences on populations

and, thus, on individuals. This implies that, from a public health perspective, population includes persons who share a similar social setting, culture, and/or geographical community over a period of time. In a hospital setting, populations are instead grouped based on a particular health issue or a hospital unit with individuals rapidly entering and exiting the population. For example, within the hospital the concern may be the diabetic population being treated at the hospital, or it may be the **patient population** on a specific unit. Thus, the term *population* within a hospital context does not usually refer to a group of persons who share other attributes other than being admitted to the hospital on a certain unit and/or having a specific diagnosis.

> ## ❱ SOLVING THE MYSTERY
> ### The Case of the Nurse Who Wanted to Know "Who, Why, What, Where, and When?"
> Public Health Science Topics Covered:
> - Assessment
> - Epidemiology
>   - Computing rates
>   - Comparing rates with national rates
> - Health planning
>   - Conducting a setting-specific assessment
>   - Population-level conclusions: Identifying priorities
>
> A large midwestern teaching hospital contracted with a college of nursing to have a faculty member with research experience provide mentorship to the staff engaged in nursing practice research. A nurse researcher who was also a PHN, Cheryl, was assigned to the project. She found that the hospital had a history of nurses on the units initiating small nursing-practice studies; they also reviewed the literature to examine the evidence related to a particular nursing intervention. These projects were conducted by individual nurses and typically culminated in a brief report on their findings from the literature. The projects did not necessarily result in a change in practice. There was no information on the effect any of these activities had on patient outcomes. The newly appointed chief nursing officer (CNO), Janet, stated that she wanted to change the process to seek evidence that demonstrated whether these studies or projects resulted in a change in how nursing care was delivered and if there was a positive impact on patient outcomes. Janet asked Cheryl how to change the process so it was clear what

patient outcomes should be targeted, how to plan change, and how to evaluate the impact of the change.

Cheryl explained to Janet that a good starting point was to take a public health perspective. When Janet asked her to explain, Cheryl replied that a health-planning model that included an assessment phase and health program phase was the best approach (Chapters 4 and 5). Cheryl said the best place to begin was to answer the questions related to who, why, what, where, and when; that is, to find out who was being admitted to their hospital, why were they being admitted (diagnosis), what were their outcomes, where were they coming from, and whether there was a variation in these variables over the months and years.

As explained in Chapter 4, there are different types of community/population assessments. Cheryl proposed to Janet that the nursing department conduct a setting-focused assessment. In addition, Cheryl explained that this assessment would be conducted using an epidemiological model; that is, the assessment would focus on quantifying hospital-based data using existing data sources and would then compare these data with national data such as that available from the Healthcare Cost and Utilization Project (HCUP).[4] The purpose of the assessment would be to determine what patient issues were priorities for nursing practice research in the hospital. The choice of priorities would be based on the discharge diagnostic category with the highest volume, longest mean length of stay, and highest mean charges as well as trends over time.

The CNO liked this approach and, together with Cheryl, assembled a small team of graduate student nurses and nurses familiar with the nursing units. They were able to use a de-identified database (no patient names or other means of identification) that included all hospital discharges during a 5-year period. For each discharge, they had information on gender, diagnoses (including primary diagnosis and all other diagnoses applied during the hospital stay), procedures, length of stay, hospital charges, ZIP code, and payer source. They used the HCUP Web site[4] to access national-level data to compare these parameters with national statistics.

The team first calculated hospital discharge rates for each diagnostic category. A **hospital discharge rate** is the rate of a particular discharge diagnosis divided by the total number of discharges times a constant, and is computed in the same way other rates are computed (see Chapter 3). Thus, a hospital discharge rate represents the number of discharges for that diagnosis in

comparison with all other discharges for that time period. It is calculated using the number of discharges for the diagnostic category or group divided by all discharges times a constant, usually per 100 discharges (Box 14-1).

While doing the assessment, one of the students asked Cheryl to explain the difference between **International Classification of Diseases, 10th Revision (ICD-10)** codes and the Major Diagnostic Categories (MDC) used by HCUP. Cheryl explained that the **major diagnostic category (MDC)** is a taxonomy that groups the principal diagnosis of patients into similar diagnosis-related groups. There are 25 categories based on systems designed to be mutually exclusive.[4] Conversely, although *ICD-10* is also a taxonomy, it was developed to code very specific diagnoses related to the discharge rather than categories of diagnoses, although the codes can be collapsed into broader categories based on systems such the circulatory system or disease group such as neoplasms. A person with diabetes who has heart failure (HF) may be admitted primarily to treat an acute episode of HF. Therefore, the primary diagnosis coded using an *ICD-10* code would be specific to HF. They may have subsequent secondary and tertiary *ICD-10* codes entered related to the circulatory system and would have an *ICD-10* code for diabetes listed as the fourth or fifth diagnosis. *ICD-10* allows the hospital to code for billing a very specific diagnosis under the broader *ICD-10* category that indicates exactly what particular diagnoses were related to this admission. To help illustrate this for the student, Cheryl took the data for one admission from the database and demonstrated what *ICD-10* categories were entered for that patient including the primary diagnosis and all other diagnoses related to the admission

---

BOX 14–1 ■ Calculating a Discharge Rate

The total number of discharges assigned to the MDC Cardiovascular System was 4,179, and the total number of discharges was 29,585.

The discharge rate per 100 discharges is as follows:

$$4,179/25,585 \times 100$$

and is read as

$$14.1 \text{ per } 100 \text{ discharges in } 2009$$

Note: This reflects discharges, not patients.

(Table 14-1). She then pointed out that only one MDC category was applied to that specific admission. In this case, the MDC was used to identify the principal diagnosis for admission and was a broader category, whereas the *ICD-10* code identified for what specific diseases the patient was being treated during the admission (Table 14-1).

The team ran frequencies on the discharge data to determine the top five MDCs, which MDC had the highest mean length of stay, and which had the highest mean charges. They also calculated hospital discharge rates for each MDC. The MDC with the highest discharge rate was the circulatory system. They constructed a table that displayed the top 10 MDC discharge rate bases on gender and age (Table 14-2).

They then compared these data with the available national data related to hospital discharges. They found that although their discharge rate was higher, when compared with the national data, the hospital had a lower mean length of stay and mean charges for that MDC. Despite the evidence that they were better than the national norms on these two indicators, they concluded that, because of the high discharge rate, the patients admitted with an MDC related to the circulatory system would be a focus area for development of health programs aimed at improving outcomes.

The team had now answered the "why" question. They went on to answer the rest of the questions. They used gender, payer source, and place of residence to answer the "who" and "where" questions. They

TABLE 14-1 ■ Comparison of Major Diagnostic Category Listing and *ICD10* Codes for a Discharge

MDC	Major Diagnostic Category	*ICD10* Primary Diagnostic Category	*ICD10* Secondary Diagnostic Category	*ICD10* Tertiary Diagnostic Code
Discharge	6	D21.4	172	I11.2
Diagnoses	Diseases of the digestive system	Neoplasm of the abdomen	Diseases of arteries, arterioles, and capillaries	Hypertensive disease

TABLE 14-2 ■ Top 10 Major Diagnostic Categories for Nonmaternal Nonneonatal Hospitalizations

Major Diagnostic Category	Rank Males Aged 0–85+	Rank Females Aged 0–85+	Rank All Genders Aged 18–44	Rank All Genders Aged 45–64	Rank All Genders Aged 65+
Diseases of the circulatory system	1	1	4	1	1
Diseases of the respiratory system	2	2	6	4	2
Diseases of the digestive system	3	4	2	3	4
Diseases of the musculoskeletal system and connective tissue	4	3	3	2	3
Diseases of the nervous system	5	5	5	5	5
Diseases of the kidney and urinary tract	6	6	10	6	6
Mental disorders	7	7	1	8	12
Infectious and parasitic diseases	8	8	14	9	7
Diseases of the hepatobiliary system	9	11	7	7	9
Endocrine, nutritional, and metabolic systems	10	9	8	10	8
Diseases of the female reproductive system		10	9	12	15

completed the analysis for each of the 5 years of data and trending discharge rates during the 5 years and by month. They then used the discharge status variable to examine outcomes. This was an extensive project, but it provided answers to their questions and, most importantly, provided a clear picture of the patients they served and the subpopulations most at risk for poorer outcomes. They also identified other information that they wished to add to the assessment such as **hospital recidivism**, that is, readmission to the hospital within 30 days of discharge.

The assessment project not only helped the nursing department establish these priorities, but also provided baseline data from the past 5 years. In this way, the nursing department could track discharge rates and other quality indicators such as length of stay and charges over the next 5 years to help determine whether institution or revision of nursing interventions resulted in any changes in patient outcomes. At this hospital, the nursing department moved from focusing on the evaluation of effectiveness of nursing interventions on individual patient outcomes to an inclusion of the population-level perspective and the evaluation of the outcomes for both levels.

■ CULTURAL CONTEXT AND ACUTE CARE SETTINGS

Culture is an important aspect of nursing care within an acute care setting. Nurses understand the need for culturally relevant care for individuals and families, but it also helps if nurses working in an acute care setting are aware of the different cultures represented in their community. An excellent hypothetical example based on an actual story is the issue of the Burundian refugees who settled in a midwestern city. In this example, a total of 106 Burundian refugees came to the city with support from the Catholic Archdiocese of the city. They were able to find housing in one of the poorer sections of the city and faced multiple challenges, including obtaining health care. They had lived in refugee camps since the 1970s and were unable to speak English, with low literacy in their own language.

To address the challenges faced by these refugees, the parish nurse employed by a large urban hospital as part of their community outreach project began to work with the Burundians to help establish a means for them to access care and communicate with health-care providers. This required that she learn their culture and normative health-care practices. The parish nurse

located an interpreter and began meeting with the women in the community on a regular basis. Together they learned from one another: The Burundians learned the culture of their new country, and the parish nurse learned the culture of the Burundians. She was able to use this cultural knowledge to provide the hospital with key cultural insights into Burundian culture, especially in relation to health beliefs, so that the physicians and nurses providing care would understand health from a Burundian perspective. Without the work of the parish nurse, the hospital would have had difficulty not only in understanding the Burundians when they came for care but also in understanding their cultural perspective on the care received.

The Epidemiology of Populations Treated in Acute Care Settings in the United States

As defined in Chapter 3, **epidemiology** is the study and quantification of illness and disease within human and animal populations. From an acute care perspective, epidemiology provides the framework for the study of the frequency, distribution, cause, and control of diseases or injury in persons who receive care in an acute care setting. Thus, epidemiology revolves around several factors, including patients with noncommunicable diseases, communicable diseases, violence, abuse, and injury. Its purpose is to assist public health officials as well as the registered nurse (RN) to understand the causes of disease, the distribution and impact of disease, and the groups at risk so that prevention efforts along the continuum from primary to tertiary levels can be developed. Hospital morbidity and mortality rates are published each year by the Centers for Disease Control and Prevention (CDC) and the Agency for Healthcare Research and Quality (AHRQ). PHNs as well as nurses working in the acute care setting may access any of these databases to determine specific health risk factors based on age group, gender, and residence. This information may then be used to target interventions to improve the health of those they care for in acute care settings.

According to the CDC, in 2016 the top two leading causes of death in the United States were heart disease and cancer for both males and females. There were differences between genders; the third leading cause of death for males was unintentional injuries, and for females, it was chronic lower respiratory diseases (Table 14-3). Following cancer and chronic respiratory diseases were stroke, Alzheimer's disease, unintentional injury, diabetes,

TABLE 14–3 ■ 2015 Differences in Top 10 Leading Causes of Death by Gender

Leading Causes of Death Males	Percentage	Leading Causes of Death Females	Percentage
1. Heart disease	24.4	1. Heart disease	22.3
2. Cancer	22.8	2. Cancer	21.2
3. Unintentional injuries	6.8	3. Chronic lower respiratory diseases	6.2
4. Chronic lower respiratory diseases	5.3	4. Stroke	6.1
5. Stroke	4.2	5. Alzheimer's disease	5.7
6. Diabetes	3.1	6. Unintentional injuries	4.0
7. Suicide	2.5	7. Diabetes	2.7
8. Alzheimer's disease	2.0	8. Influenza and pneumonia	2.3
9. Influenza and pneumonia	2.0	9. Kidney disease	1.8
10. Chronic liver disease	1.9	10. Septicemia	1.6

influenza and pneumonia, kidney disease, and sepsis.[5] In 2016, 6.4% of the U.S. population aged 1 and older had at least one hospital stay, down from 7.8% in 1997. When broken down by age, 15.2% of those over the age of 64 had at least one hospital stay and for those over the age of 84, almost a quarter (22.5%) had at least one hospital stay.[6] The average length of stay was 6.1 days.[7] In 2015, The most common diagnosis for inpatient stays after live birth was septicemia (Table 14-4).[8]

TABLE 14–4 ■ 2015* U.S. National Inpatient Stays

Principal Diagnosis	Rate of Stays per 100,000
Liveborn	1,195
Septicemia (except in labor)	552
Osteoarthritis	339
Congestive heart failure; nonhypertensive	297
Pneumonia (except that caused by tuberculosis or sexually transmitted disease)	276
Mood disorders	267
Cardiac dysrhythmias	212
Complication of device; implant or graft	203
Acute myocardial infarction	196
Other complications of birth; puerperium affecting management of mother	195

*Maternal/Neonatal Stays Included
Source: (8)

Discharge Status of Hospitalized Patients

The goal on discharge is to return the patient to his optimal state of health and, if possible, to independent living. Return to independent living is attainable for the majority of all hospitalized adults in the U.S. Others are able to return to their home environment with home health-care services or are transferred to an extended care facility for both short-term and long-term stays. Finally, patients may have been discharged to another hospital, died, or left against medical advice.[8] Assessing patients at the time of admission and developing individual discharge plans will make the postdischarge transition easier for all of those involved. Tracking discharge status is another indicator of patient outcomes and could easily be added to an ongoing hospital population assessment such as the one conducted by Janet and Cheryl.

Inpatient Populations

Understanding public health science and its daily role in the hospital setting is an essential competency for all nurses working across various units including critical care, emergency departments (EDs), and medical-surgical units. They participate through their daily activities in the improvement of health for the patients for whom they care, the patients' families, and the communities to which those patients return. Understanding the patients they care for within the broader context of the community served by the hospital can be a challenge. As the nation takes its slow march toward health promotion and disease prevention, as evidenced in the Affordable Care Act of 2010,[9] the need for more health-care activities on the population end of the continuum continues to increase. Nurses working in acute care settings have an important role to play.

Within hospitals, there are numerous settings that are usually referred to as units. These units vary based on the type of services required (e.g., surgery, medical, emergency care) and the severity of the patients' condition (e.g., intensive care, trauma, step-down units). Hospitals also vary in relation to the level of care they provide, the communities they serve, and whether or not they are teaching hospitals. Some services, such as infection control, are provided across all units of the hospital. Community hospitals located in suburban or rural areas are less apt to provide care to high-level-of-acuity patients such as those requiring complex surgical procedures or trauma level-one care. By contrast, a large urban medical center, especially one affiliated with a large university, has a wide array of units, many of which provide complex or specialized services.

Critical Care

An excellent example of the relationship between public health science and acute care settings is the role that public health science has played in the development of critical care as a specialty in the acute care setting. **Critical care nursing** requires specialized skills related to human responses to life-threatening health problems,[9] and is usually provided within an area in the hospital designed to provide care to the most critically ill or injured patients. **Critically ill** or **injured patients** are patients who are at high risk for actual or potential life-threatening health-care problems.[10] Critical illness can result from a progressive disease such as chronic obstructive pulmonary disease or may occur in an acute situation such as myocardial infarction (MI). Acute illness can involve a rapid change in condition for the worse or a condition that arises quickly, such as an exacerbation of fluid overload in the patient with HF. Patients in the critical care arena have varied disease etiologies, background demographics, socioeconomic status, and complexities. Also, a patient may be in critical condition from blood loss due to an acute injury sustained in motor vehicle crash. The more critically ill the patient is, the more vulnerable they are for instability and threat to life, requiring intense and highly skilled nursing care.

The care of the critically ill patient takes place in several different arenas within the hospital setting. This patient population can be found in the intensive care units (ICUs), step-down or transitional care units, EDs, postanesthesia care units (PACU), cardiac catheter laboratories (cardiac cath lab), and cardiac care units. The focus of the critical care nurse is not only on the patient's responses to illness and optimal care but also on the family's response. Almost two-thirds of all working RNs work in the hospital setting (61%). Of those, more than a third work in the critical care area.[1,10,11] Critical care nurses rely on a vast body of knowledge, skill, and experience so that they can provide care to the patient and the patient's family while performing as a patient advocate and liaison. Included in the body of knowledge is public health science.

Although nurses working in critical care settings spend the majority of their time providing individual care to patients and families, hospital-based, population-level data are needed to evaluate the effectiveness of that care. Nurses use well-established epidemiological models to guide their health prevention activities, mostly at the tertiary prevention level. These activities include health education and careful discharge planning to promote recovery and reduce the risk of disability and mortality. In addition, over time critical care nurses actively engage in population-level care through performance improvement activities and participation in research studies aimed at gathering evidence to demonstrate the effectiveness of interventions for improving the outcomes of the patient populations they serve.

Evolution of Critical Care: Population Driven

Over the past few decades, critical care nursing has been recognized as a distinct and essential specialty, providing care to those who are the most severely ill or injured.[10] The origin and development of the critical care field occurred in response to several different factors, each of which was population driven. The initiating factors first occurred in response to wartime injury. The progression of critical care can be attributed to the advancement in technology and the utilization of an improvement process shaped by evidence-based practice (EBP).

War: Critical care, in part, was developed using knowledge and skill obtained during wartime efforts. The true origin has been difficult to establish, but Florence Nightingale[12] is considered to be the first to have used an ICU approach to help focus care on those who were in the need of the highest level of nursing care. She served with the British during the Crimean War from 1854 to 1856. In her book *Notes on Hospitals*, she wrote about the advantages of establishing a separate area of the hospital for the sickest or most severely injured soldiers. She maintained this area close to her nursing station where she could keep a close watch on their condition and provide quick help when needed. The next report of a similar effort was in 1929, when Dr. Walter Dandy of Johns Hopkins Hospital in Baltimore developed a specialized postoperative unit containing three beds for neurosurgical patients.[13]

Advancements in care for the critically ill also occurred as a consequence of wartime injuries. During World War I, the importance of recognizing shock and treating it with the intravascular volume replacement using saline and colloid solutions was demonstrated. Early in World War I, before the United States entered into the war, Bruce Robertson first introduced blood transfusion. He was a Canadian physician who, while training in the U.S., became convinced that whole blood was superior to saline infusions. The blood was collected from soldiers on the battlefield who were willing and ready to donate. It was not until World War II that the technique of blood transfusion was widely used. This war provided the stimulus for organized blood collection; as the war progressed, a national blood program was established, which provided massive quantities of blood for overseas use.[14]

Also, during World War II, advances in surgical techniques led to survival after injuries that were previously considered lethal. These injured soldiers subsequently needed prolonged supportive care for recovery. Shock wards were developed to resuscitate and care for soldiers injured in battle or undergoing surgery, and postoperative patients were admitted to recovery rooms to facilitate nursing care.[15]

With each subsequent war, advances have been made in the care of the critically ill and injured. In the Iraq and Afghanistan wars, significant advances were made in the treatment of traumatic brain injuries that resulted from roadside bomb explosions. These have translated into advances in caring for civilian injuries both unintentional, such as motor vehicle crashes (MVCs) and football injuries, and intentional, such as the mass shooting event that occurred at a high school in Parkland, Florida. These advances occurred because of the focus on the care of a population, in this case soldiers, and the particular type of injuries they were experiencing. This has resulted in a steady improvement in the mortality rate of soldiers in U.S. conflicts.[16,17] During the American Civil War, the chance of dying was about one in four (250 per 1,000). Only a fraction actually died during battle because much of the deaths were attributable to disease and infections of wounds sustained during battle.[17] By the time of the war in Vietnam, the death rate dropped to 21.8 per 1,000, which was five times higher than the death rate during the war in Iraq as measured between the beginning of the war under George Bush in 2003 and the functioning of the new Iraq government in 2006.[19] Some of these advancements were a result of innovations not that dissimilar to what Florence Nightingale did in the Crimean War. For example, in Iraq, medical teams were deployed closer to combat areas, and evacuation times were greatly improved.[19]

All of these innovations in care were driven by population-level data. In particular, these changes were made to improve the health outcomes of soldiers who had sustained life-threatening injuries or contracted diseases on the battlefield. The practices continued to be refined and used because population-level data demonstrated that survival rates improved. **Survival rate** is defined as the number of persons who survive an event divided by the total number of persons who experience an event. Thus, these innovative clinicians, including Florence Nightingale (see Chapter 1), effectively used public health science to improve the health of the critically ill.

Polio and Intensive Care: Critical care has evolved not only through the care of those injured during war but also through advances related to communicable diseases (see Chapter 8) and noncommunicable chronic diseases (see Chapter 9). Innovations in the delivery of care to those who are critically ill have developed in response to communicable disease outbreaks. In other cases, public health science findings have resulted in changes in how we care for chronic diseases.

A good example of how a communicable disease outbreak changed practices in critical care is the poliomyelitis (polio) epidemic that started in the late 1940s. **Polio**, one of the most dreaded diseases of childhood during the 20th century, is caused by the poliovirus, a human enterovirus member of the family Picornaviridae. It is transmitted from person to person via the fecal-oral route. Until the 20th century, the virus was readily transmitted via water, and most exposures to the virus occurred during infancy. At this young age, when most have at least partial protection via maternal antibodies, the resulting infection was subclinical. This asymptomatic infection in turn gave lifelong immunity. Only a few suffered from paralysis, which was labeled *infantile paralysis*. As advancements in water treatment took place, the early childhood exposure to the poliovirus decreased. As a consequence of better hygiene, the first exposure to the virus was more apt to occur during late childhood or young adulthood. In this older age group, the infection caused more severe sequelae: a paralysis syndrome. At the peak of the epidemic in 1952, there were more than 21,000 cases. With the introduction of the Salk vaccine, the incidence rapidly decreased. By 1965, there were only 61 cases, and the last known case caused by wild poliovirus was in 1993.[20]

Prior to the introduction of the vaccine, the epidemic in the late 1940s and early 1950s resulted in an increased demand on the health-care system. More than 90% of poliovirus infections are asymptomatic, however, in cases that do show symptoms, the most severe potential effect of the virus is paralysis. The paralytic syndromes range from paralysis of one or more limbs to respiratory muscle paralysis. The mortality rate from respiratory polio was greater than 90%. Boston Children's Hospital was the first to use a mechanical respiratory machine called the *iron lung* to prevent likely death (Fig. 14-1). Use of this respiratory therapy resulted in a significant reduction of mortality but was found to be cumbersome and expensive, which made it difficult to provide nursing care. As years passed, improvements were made to this mechanical respiratory unit, and it was broadly used throughout North America and Europe during severe polio outbreaks.

In 1952, during a large polio outbreak in Denmark, Bjorn Ibsen, an anesthesiologist in Blegdam Hospital, used the positive pressure ventilation concept used in the operating room for the respiratory support for the polio victims. Dr. Ibsen had his medical students hand-ventilate dozens of patients through tracheostomy tubes until the worst of the paralytic phase had passed. For efficiency and convenience, the patients who needed the respiratory support were placed in a single location within the hospital. This is often cited as the world's first ICU, "a ward where physicians and nurses observe and treat 'desperately ill' patients 24 hours a day."[13,21] It is considered the origin of today's ICU. Again, improved outcomes and decreased mortality for this particular hospital-based population drove the development of these interventions.

Despite the innovative use of an iron lung and an ICU concept, the polio pandemic spurred public health research aimed at primary prevention. Based on the epidemiological triangle reviewed in Chapters 3 and 8, clinicians had the choice to eradicate the virus, change the environment, or protect the host (humans). There was a major public health program using public service announcements that warned parents about the risk of polio with a focus on public swimming areas. Polio outbreaks often occurred during the summer months as a result of children swimming in contaminated water. Thus, initial efforts were to alter the chance of exposure. However, public health research concentrated on protecting the host through the development of a vaccine that would boost human resistance to the virus. It was the introduction of the Salk vaccine in 1952 and the Sabin vaccine in 1962 that dramatically reduced the incidence of polio to less than one per 100,000 persons annually in the early 1960s. Thus, public health science can often help bring solutions to health issues which result in the need for critical care. Since the initiation of the ICU concept during the polio pandemic, ICUs have come to provide care for many different kinds of patients, from the neonate to adults with specific intensive care needs (Box 14-2).

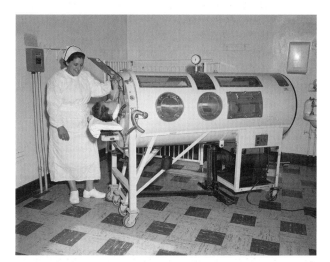

Figure 14-1 A 1960 historical photograph of a nurse caring for a victim of a Rhode Island polio epidemic, who is inside an Emerson respirator, also sometimes referred to as an "iron lung" machine. *(From Centers for Disease Control and Prevention, Public Health Image Library, No. 12009. Retrieved from* http://phil.cdc.gov/phil/details.asp)

BOX 14–2 ■ Specialized Types of Intensive Care Units

- Neonatal intensive care unit (NICU)
- Special care nursery (SCN)
- Pediatric intensive care unit (PICU)
- Psychiatric intensive care unit (PICU)
- Coronary care unit (CCU)
- Cardiac surgery intensive care unit (CSICU)
- Cardiovascular intensive care unit (CVICU)
- Medical intensive care unit (MICU)
- Medical surgical intensive care unit (MSICU)
- Surgical intensive care unit (SICU)
- Overnight intensive recovery (OIR)
- Neurotrauma intensive care unit (NICU)
- Neurointensive care unit (NICU)
- Burn wound intensive care unit (BWICU)
- Trauma intensive care unit (TICU)
- Surgical trauma intensive care unit (STICU)
- Trauma-neuro critical care (TNCC)
- Respiratory intensive care unit (RICU)
- Geriatric intensive care unit (GICU)
- Mobile intensive care unit (MICU)

Technology and Acute Care: Cardiopulmonary Resuscitation: Advances in technology have also resulted in changes in the delivery of critical care. The use of these technologies demonstrates a combination of population data, advances in the understanding of human physiology, and technological advances. As in the field of pharmacy, the randomized clinical trial (Chapter 3) is the gold standard for determining the effectiveness and efficacy of technological interventions in critical care. These advances often began with bench science; in the end, however, they translate into how care is provided because of positive changes in the outcomes of the patient populations involved. One of the most dramatic examples is the whole issue of **cardiopulmonary resuscitation (CPR)**, an emergency procedure that includes the use of external cardiac massage and artificial respiration for persons who experience sudden cardiac arrest. The technique was developed within the acute care setting and adopted for use by the general public. Overall, CPR has dramatically reduced mortality attributed to a variety of events that result in cessation of breathing, heartbeat, or both.

Peter J. Safar, the "father" of CPR, converted the method of CPR used in the hospital for use by the general public. He promoted the development of life-supporting first aid, which is known as basic life support. In 1957, he publicized the "A" (airway), "B" (breathing), and "C" (circulation system). Safar was a public health advocate who gave the first step to the general public to aid others in an emergency. He worked hard to popularize the procedure around the world and collaborated with a Norwegian company to create "Resusci Anne," the first CPR training mannequin. His contribution to life-saving medical technique has earned him a reputation as one of the pioneers of critical care medicine and has saved countless lives.[22]

In 1960, the American Heart Association (AHA) started a program to acquaint physicians with closed-chest cardiac resuscitation, and it became the forerunner of CPR training for the general public. Although only 40 communities in the United States regularly measure and report survival rates, these population-level data have proved invaluable in the evaluation of the success of CPR and the development of changes aimed at improvement of survival rates. Initially, it was recommended that laypersons administering CPR first clear the airway (A), then administer breaths (B), and then initiate chest compressions (C). In 2010, dramatic revisions were made to the CPR guidelines. The recommendations were for the three steps of CPR to be rearranged: the new first step is now chest compressions instead of first establishing the airway, and then administering breaths.

Newborns are an exception to the change. Thus, for the single rescuer, A-B-C has become C-A-B for compressions, airway, and breathing (Fig. 14-2). For laypersons, the AHA states that the most effective approach is to immediately deliver chest compressions at a rate of greater than 100 compressions per minute "the same rhythm as the beat of the Bee Gees' song, 'Stayin' Alive.'"[24] Although it is difficult to determine the exact outcomes associated with long-term survival, according to 2014 data, nearly 45% of out-of-hospital cardiac arrest victims survived when bystander CPR was started.[23] Using the AHA information to guide the administration of CPR, supportive programs such as public access defibrillation programs were implemented aimed at improving survival rates.[24,25]

Role of Cohort Studies in the Delivery of Acute Care

Population data have not only been gathered from within the hospital to help improve patient outcomes but have also been gathered from general populations. A longitudinal cohort study (see Chapter 3) provides valuable evidence on who will potentially develop disease based on different risk factors. At baseline, information is collected about the health of the individuals in the cohort and then these individuals are tracked over time to determine who develops disease and who does not. A cohort study can be focused on a particular disease, for example, the Framingham Health Study (FHS),[26] or a particular population, such as the Nurses' Health Study.[27]

The Framingham Heart Study and Cardiovascular Disease

As reported in Chapter 9, the leading cause of death in the United States is cardiovascular disease (CVD). Nearly 2,300 Americans die of CVD each day, an average of one death every 38 seconds. CVD claims more lives each year than all forms of cancer and chronic lower respiratory diseases combined. There are an estimated 92,100,000 American adults (more than one in three) with CVD.[28] The FHS is directly responsible for the remarkable advances made in the prevention of heart disease in the United States and throughout the world.

In 1948, the town of Framingham, Massachusetts, was selected as the study site by the U.S. Public Health Service, and 5,209 healthy residents between 30 and 60 years of age, both men and women, were enrolled as the first cohort of participants. It was the first major cardiovascular study to recruit women participants. At the time, little was known about the general causes of heart disease

CPR Guide
Hands-Only CPR vs. CPR with breaths

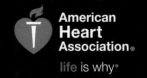
American Heart Association®
life is why®

HANDS-ONLY CPR

CALL 911

PUSH HARD AND FAST IN THE CENTER OF THE CHEST

Public awareness campaign to get more people to act when they encounter a cardiac arrest. Starting point to get more people to learn CPR.

Will not meet requirements if you need CPR for your job.

CPR Training

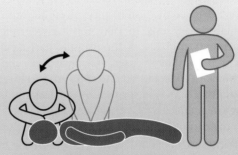

COMPRESSIONS + BREATHS

Offered through online or in-person classes. Provides more in-depth training with an instructor, including CPR with breaths and choking relief.

Often necessary for people who need CPR training for work.

How does it work?

Chest compressions are good for the *first few minutes* someone is in cardiac arrest pushing remaining oxygen through body to keep vital organs alive. Buys time until someone with more skills can provide help.

CPR with breaths combines chest compressions and breaths, providing additional oxygen to circulate throughout the body.

Who can I use it on?

Adults and teens.

Anyone who is in cardiac arrest, including: adults and teens, infants and children, and any victims of drowning, drug overdose, collapse due to breathing problems or prolonged cardiac arrest.

How do I learn?

Go to
heart.org/handsonlycpr
to learn the steps of Hands-Only CPR.

Go to
heart.org/cpr
and click on FIND A COURSE to find a class online or near you.

Figure 14-2 C-A-B for cardiopulmonary resuscitation. *(See [24]. Used with permission.)*

and stroke, but the death rates for CVD had been increasing steadily since the beginning of the 20th century and had become an American epidemic. The FHS became a joint project of the National Heart, Lung, and Blood Institute (NHLBI) and Boston University.[27]

The objective of the FHS was to identify the common risk factors that contribute to CVD by following its development over a long period of time in a large group of participants who had not yet developed overt symptoms of CVD or suffered a heart attack or stroke. Since 1948, the subjects have continued to return to the study every 2 years for a detailed medical history, physical examination, and laboratory tests. In 1971, the study enrolled a second generation, 5,124 of the original participants' adult children and their spouses, to participate in similar examinations. In 1994, the need to establish a new study including a more diverse community of Framingham was recognized, and the first Omni cohort (OMNI1) of the FHS was enrolled. Due to the predominantly white population in the first cohorts, the OMNI cohorts were enrolled as a way of representing the growing diversity of Framingham from a racial and ethnic perspective. In

April 2002, the study entered a new phase, the enrollment of a third generation of participants, who were the grandchildren of the original cohort. In 2003, a second group of Omni participants was enrolled.[26]

The FHS continues to make important scientific contributions by enhancing its research capabilities and capitalizing on its inherent resources. Some of the more recent data from the FHS, from the original and offspring cohorts (1980–2003), show that the average annual rate of first major cardiovascular events is on the rise. Events have gone from 3 per 1,000 in men at ages 35 to 44, to 74 per 1,000 at ages 85 to 94. For women, comparable rates occur 10 years later in life, and the gap narrows with advancing age. Before age 75, men suffer a higher proportion of CVD events due to coronary heart disease (CHD) than do women, and a higher proportion of events due to stroke occur in women. From 1996 to 2006, death rates from CVD declined 29.2%. Data from the FHS indicate that the lifetime risk for CVD is two in three for men and more than one in two for women at age 40.[26] Over time, the impact of the study on heart health is substantial (Box 14-3).[28,29]

BOX 14–3 ■ Framingham Heart Study Milestones

1960	Cigarette smoking found to increase the risk of heart disease.
1961	Cholesterol level, blood pressure, and electrocardiogram abnormalities found to increase the risk of heart disease.
1967	Physical activity found to reduce the risk of heart disease, and obesity found to increase the risk of heart disease.
1970	High blood pressure found to increase the risk of stroke.
1976	Menopause found to increase the risk of heart disease.
1978	Psychosocial factors found to affect heart disease.
1988	High levels of high-density lipoprotein cholesterol found to reduce risk of death.
1994	Enlarged left ventricle (one of two lower chambers of the heart) shown to increase the risk of stroke.
1996	Progression from hypertension to heart failure described.
1998	Development of simple coronary disease prediction algorithm involving risk factor categories to allow physicians to predict multivariate CHD risk in patients without overt CHD.
1999	Lifetime risk at age 40 years of developing CHD is one in two for men and one in three for women.
2001	High-normal blood pressure is associated with an increased risk of CVD, emphasizing the need to determine whether lowering high-normal blood pressure can reduce the risk.
2002	Lifetime risk of developing high blood pressure in middle-aged adults is 9 in 10.
2002	Obesity is a risk factor for heart failure.
2004	Serum aldosterone levels predict future risk of hypertension in non-hypertensive individuals.
2005	Lifetime risk of becoming overweight exceeds 70%; risk for obesity approximates one in two.
2006	The NHLBI of the National Institutes of Health announced a new genome-wide association study at the FHS in collaboration with Boston University School of Medicine to be known as the SHARe project (SNP Health Association Resource).
2007	Based on evaluation of a densely interconnected social network of 12,067 people assessed as part of the FHS, network phenomena appear to be relevant to the biological and behavioral trait of obesity, and obesity appears to spread through social ties.
2008	Based on analysis of a social network of 12,067 people participating in the FHS, researchers discover that social networks exert key influences on decision to quit smoking.

BOX 14-3 ■ Framingham Heart Study Milestones—cont'd

2008 Discovery by FHS and publication of four risk factors that raise probability of developing precursor of heart failure; new 30-year risk estimates developed for serious cardiac events.

2009 FHS cited by the AHA as being among the top 10 cardiovascular research achievements of 2009, "Genome-wide Association Study of Blood Pressure and Hypertension: Genome-wide Association Study Identifies Eight Loci Associated With Blood Pressure."

2009 A new genetic variant associated with increased susceptibility for atrial fibrillation, a prominent risk factor for stroke and heart failure, is reported in two studies based on data from the FHS.

2009 FHS researchers find parental dementia may lead to poor memory in middle-aged adults.

2010s Sleep apnea is tied to increased risk of stroke; Additional genes identified that may play a role in Alzheimer's disease; and hundreds of genes were discovered that are underlying major heart disease risk factors.

Source: (29)

Women and Cardiovascular Disease

CVD is the leading cause of death in women.[30] Initially CVD was perceived by many health-care providers as a predominately male disease linked to stress and lifestyle. It was thought that women had a low risk for developing CVD and were protected by female sex hormones. Since the 1990s, there has been an effort to increase the amount of research done to help understand heart disease in women. This research is leading to a better understanding of risk factors, early signs and symptoms, and treatment.[31,32]

As mentioned earlier, the FHS is one of the few long-term prospective studies of CVD that has included both men and women. Women participated from the very beginning, and investigators recognized that CVD occurs later in life and with lower frequency in females. With follow-up of 5,209 original study participants (2,873 women and 2,336 men), researchers have documented information about the incidence of CVD in the FHS women and risk factors unique to women.[29]

There are specific physiological, pathophysiological, clinical, and socioeconomic issues that differentiate women and men with CVD. Because of these differences, symptoms of an acute myocardial infarction (AMI) are different between genders. Women are more likely to experience atypical chest pain, abdominal pain, dyspnea, nausea, and fatigue during a cardiovascular event. Because these symptoms are different from the "elephant sitting on the chest" type of pain that males often experience, the atypical presentation may be missed or be attributed to another etiology. If the suspicion of CVD has not been raised by symptoms, underinvestigation and undertreatment may occur. Women typically wait longer to seek medical assistance; this may be due to the atypical presentation of symptoms.[32,33] Delay of treatment has a devastating effect on the outcome of a cardiovascular event, which certainly may be seen in the mortality rate for a woman following an AMI (Box 14-4). The risk of

BOX 14-4 ■ Facts About Women and Cardiovascular Disease

• CVD, particularly coronary heart disease (CHD) and stroke, remain the leading causes of death of women in America and most developed countries, with nearly 37% of all female deaths in the United States occurring from CVD.

• CVD is a particularly important problem among minority women. The death rate due to CVD is higher in black women than in white women.

• One in 2.7 females who die, die of heart disease, stroke, and other CVD compared with one in 30 who die of breast cancer.

• At age 40 and older, 23% of women compared with 18% of men will die within 1 year after a heart attack.

Source: (30)

CVD increases with age, and as the baby boomers age, the morbidity and mortality rate related to CVD in women will grow. Because of this increasing number, it is important to raise awareness of this major public health issue for older women.

● APPLYING PUBLIC HEALTH SCIENCE
The Case of the Waiting Women
Public Health Science Topics Covered:

• Health planning
  • Conducting a setting-specific assessment
  • Population-level conclusions: Identifying priorities

Two nurses, Susan and Maria, work together in a cardiac catheterization laboratory (cath lab) in a large urban tertiary center. The cath lab is a very busy area within this medical center. This specialized area holds diagnostic imaging equipment used to support diagnostic and interventional procedures. The cath lab is staffed by a multidisciplinary team including physicians (interventional cardiologists, vascular surgeons, or radiologists), nurses, and radiology technicians.

A diagnostic procedure called a cardiac catheterization is performed in the cath lab to determine the extent of disease present in the vascular system. Left heart catheterization (arterial) is performed to determine blockages in the coronary vascular system. Right heart catheterization (venous) is performed to determine how well the heart valves are functioning and how effectively the heart is pumping blood to the lungs. The method involves threading a catheter through a femoral artery or vein or the radial artery and then threading it into the heart. During cardiac cath, a radiopaque dye is injected through the catheter to highlight the coronary arteries. This test is called a *coronary angiogram* or *coronary arteriogram*.

Depending on what is found during the coronary angiogram, different interventions may be necessary during the cardiac cath. For example, an angioplasty that uses a balloon on the end of the catheter is able to open narrowed coronary arteries. Stents, which are small, mesh-like devices that act as supports, or scaffolds, inside of a vessel, may be placed at the time of angioplasty.

During one particularly busy shift in the cath lab, Susan relieved Maria for lunch and received a report on a patient who was coming from the ED with a diagnosis of a suspected AMI. The patient was a 60-year-old woman with no known history of CVD who arrived in the ED about an hour before with vague complaints of fatigue, shortness of breath, and chest pressure. After a detailed history and physical, this patient was found to have an **ST-elevation myocardial infarction (STEMI)**, a heart attack caused by a prolonged period of blocked blood supply.[33] While Susan was with this patient in the cath lab, the coronary angiogram showed a severely occluded left main coronary artery, a surprising discovery given her atypical complaints. Knowing that this type of obstructive disease holds an increased mortality risk, Susan wanted to know why this patient was in the ED for such a long time before the diagnosis was made. She was also concerned because the door-to-balloon time was just at the 90-minute mark.

Door-to-balloon time is defined as the amount of time between a patient's arrival at the hospital and the time he/she receives percutaneous coronary intervention, such as angioplasty.[33] Because "time is muscle," meaning that delays in treating an AMI increases the likelihood and amount of myocardial damage resulting from localized hypoxia, the American College of Cardiologists and the AHA guidelines recommend a door-to-balloon time of no more than 90 minutes. A national Door-to-Balloon Initiative was launched in November 2006 and has become a core quality measure for The Joint Commission.

When Maria returned from her lunch break, she and Susan discussed the circumstances of the patient with the STEMI. Susan voiced her concerns about the severity of the CVD in the presence of atypical complaints and the length of door-to-balloon time despite the success of the intervention. Maria was equally concerned in light of the fact that she had just cared for a postmenopausal patient with a STEMI who also presented with vague complaints earlier in the day that had gone beyond the 90-minute door-to-balloon time. After much discussion and a review of the recorded door-to-balloon times during the past several months, which showed other cases of women with prolonged times, both nurses felt strongly that they needed to take action so that they could make a difference in the care of women with CVD.

Unsure of what to do next, Susan and Maria decided to consult Karen, the director of nursing research at the hospital. They knew that their short-term goal was to discover the red flags that could be used to alert the ED personnel to the possibility of CVD in postmenopausal woman with atypical symptoms. After educating the ED staff, Susan and Maria then wanted to use this information to educate women at risk.

Karen encouraged the two nurses to learn more about the population at risk. Was the event that Susan witnessed unusual or more the norm in the ED? What was the evidence to support the door-to-balloon time frame? Were women at greater risk than men? Susan and Maria had hunches but no real data on the issue. Karen suggested that they conduct a retrospective chart review to answer these questions. She reminded them that they would have to follow the hospital policies related to chart reviews. The two nurses, with Karen's help, wrote up a proposal for doing the review.

Focused Assessment

The purpose of their review was not only to determine the length of time between arrival in the ED and treatment but also to determine the length of time between the point at which the women first had symptoms and their arrival at the ED. Thus, the team embarked on a focused assessment (Chapter 4) that allowed them to examine the population of women who arrived in the ED over a specified period of time. They collected data on all adult women who arrived with a non-trauma event and then compared the presenting symptoms for those who actually had STEMI with those who did not. They collected information on time from first symptoms to arrival at the ED and what those first symptoms were. All of these assessment data were needed not only to determine whether indeed the door-to-balloon time standard was or was not being met, but also to more accurately describe the presenting symptoms of the women with a STEMI compared with those without a STEMI. This vital information helped in the development of an intervention for health-care providers and for the educational program the nurses wanted to develop for women at risk for a STEMI. Both centered on how to recognize a possible STEMI, and both interventions used a population approach.

Ethics in an Acute Care Setting

One issue Susan and Maria faced was how to address the privacy of the patient information they obtained during their chart review. Karen showed them how to write a proposal, which they would then send to the institutional review board for approval. Karen explained to them that they could not access patient data without going through this process. In that way, they would design the review so that they would ensure the privacy of the patients and also allow them to disseminate their findings at an aggregate level with no personal identifiers.

Nurses interested in using population-level data to improve patient outcomes must be fully aware of the ethics of utilizing individual patient-level data for purposes other than what they were intended. There are two legal areas that nurses must remember at all times when conducting assessments or doing health program evaluations using patient data. The Health Insurance Portability and Accountability Act (HIPAA) of 1996 was designed to protect the use of electronic patient data. It set national standards for the security of electronic protected health information such as the **electronic medical record**. An EMR is a digital version of the patient chart that has replaced paper charts in most acute care settings. HIPAA also includes rules on the use of identifiable confidential patient information to analyze patient safety events and improve patient safety.[34]

Although patient information obtained during a hospital stay is protected under HIPAA, there are times when the information can be or must be shared. This represents the conflict between the individual's right to privacy and the public health perspective of protecting the health of the whole. The law includes regulations that recognize the need for public health authorities, and others mandated to protect the public safety, to have access to patient data. Thus, a physician may report information on dog bites or gunshot wounds to those with authority without violating HIPAA. Agencies with such authority include state and local health departments, the Food and Drug Administration (FDA), the CDC, and the Occupational Safety and Health Administration (OSHA). Situations in which individual information may be shared to help protect the public include child abuse or neglect, adverse events associated with an FDA-approved activity or product, and reportable communicable diseases. It is important to note that the information may only be released to agencies with recognized authority as stipulated in the law.[34]

HIPAA is an important factor for nurses who plan to collect patient data to conduct a study related to their care. For example, in some cases, nurses make changes to practice based on existing evidence and do this within the scope of their practice. They do not report the assessment data or the success of their program outside of their hospital because it is not a research study. Susan and Maria remembered covering human subjects' research in their research class but were not sure how to proceed. Their hospital had a policy that all projects that involved obtaining data from patient records and/or collecting patient data from patients must be reviewed by the institutional review board (IRB) prior to collecting any data. An **institutional review board** is a committee formally charged with reviewing biomedical and behavioral research conducted with human subjects to ensure the protection of research participants. These committees must comply with federal regulations related to conducting research with human subjects. The two nurses worked with the hospital nurse researcher to delineate exactly what their process was and then provided the information as required to their institution's IRB. They clarified that, when collecting the data from the medical records, they would include information on the residence of the patient and that they would need to link medical records from the two different areas. Although they were planning to use the information for an internal change in practice, they wished to also examine whether there was a difference between those patients who actually had a STEMI and those who did not, and then report those findings in a journal article or at a conference. Thus, they wished to generalize the findings of their assessment. They submitted their proposal with specific information on how they would protect the privacy of the patient's medical record. The IRB determined that it did constitute human subjects' research but met the requirements for an expedited review because it involved a review of medical records only, with minimal risk to the patients.

Thus, nurses working in acute care settings are faced with multiple ethical issues. From a public health perspective, the nurse must be aware of the need to protect the health of the public while protecting the right to individual privacy. In addition, as more hospitals encourage nurses working in acute care settings to engage in research, they must become aware of the ethical dilemmas posed in the collection of patient data. Improving patient outcomes requires a constant review of the evidence and health planning to improve practice. During this process, human subjects must always be protected from unnecessary risk.

The Nurses' Health Study

The Nurses' Health Study is similar to the FHS but focuses on the health of women rather than on incidence of a particular disease. It started in 1976 and has expanded to include two more cohorts, one in 1989 and one in 2008. Initially, the primary objective was to study the long-term consequences related to the use of oral contraceptives. However, the findings from the studies are providing insights into a broad array of health issues including breast cancer, diabetes, and CVD in women. Based on the results of the studies, researchers have concluded that diet, physical activity, and other lifestyle factors promote better health and reduce risk for disease to a significant degree.[35]

Health Planning and Acute Care

The first case study in this chapter, Solving the Mystery, is an example of a health planning approach to the delivery of nursing care in a hospital setting. The team completed the first step in heath planning, the assessment (see Chapter 4). The data from that step helped to identify populations at risk for poorer outcomes. Armed with these data, the nursing department could now move to the next steps, the development, implementation, and evaluation of a health program aimed at improving patient outcomes (see Chapter 5). For Cheryl, who wanted to know the who, what, why, when, and where, the final results of the assessment identified the areas in need of nursing activities related to searching for the evidence to support practice, as well as conducting research studies aimed at improving outcomes. For the CNO, the assessment provided her with the outcomes-focused approach and the baseline data she needed to evaluate change over time from an organizational perspective. The results were distributed to the nursing staff as a whole, and nursing units were encouraged to explore opportunities to develop population-level interventions that would improve outcomes for patients admitted with a diagnosis that matched those included in Table 15-2.

Noncommunicable Diseases and Acute Care Settings

Chapter 9 provided an overview of noncommunicable diseases and their contribution to the overall burden of disease. Acute care settings provide care to persons with noncommunicable diseases when they are experiencing an acute stage of the disease. They may come to the hospital when they have first been diagnosed, or the admission may be one of many related to the noncommunicable disease. Providing acute care for a disease process that will not result in a cure leaves the care provider focused on decreasing disease-related morbidity and disability, and reducing the risk of premature death. Thus, the nurse in the acute care setting who is caring for a person with a noncommunicable disease is providing tertiary prevention (see Chapter 2). This can be challenging for the nurse because of short hospital stays. The nurse must adapt the plan of care to fit the individual's needs. However, development of a program that addresses population-level barriers to care and improves the ability of patients to self-manage their disease upon discharge can make a big difference. This again requires using a population approach and often requires the identification of subpopulations within the patient population who may be experiencing significant barriers to self-management of their diseases.

The first step for the nurse working on a hospital unit who wishes to develop an intervention program is to identify the level of prevention involved in the intervention. For example, if a nurse wanted to develop a program focused on **acute coronary syndrome (ACS)**, she would have to begin with an understanding of the disease. ACS is defined by the AHA as any set of clinical symptoms associated with acute myocardial ischemia.

Acute myocardial ischemia presents as chest pain due to an insufficient blood supply to the heart muscle. The underlying cause is CAD. The majority of known risk factors for CAD are modifiable by specific preventive measures. Primary prevention focuses on prevention of disease in those who do not have the disease (see Chapter 2). The AHA goal for primary prevention is to educate all adults about the levels and significance of risk factors related to CAD. The AHA guide to primary prevention of CAD has a risk reduction focus. The major risk factors targeted include smoking, blood pressure control, dietary intake, blood lipid management, physical activity, and weight management. Comprehensive risk factor interventions can prevent disease from occurring. In addition, secondary prevention, early identification of those with subclinical disease, can extend overall survival, improve health-related quality of life, and decrease the need for interventional procedures, such as angioplasty and bypass grafting. Ultimately, the goal is to reduce the incidence of subsequent heart attack (MI). Examples of secondary prevention include identifying and treating people with established disease and those at very high risk of developing CAD. Examples of tertiary prevention include treating and rehabilitating patients who have had a heart attack or to prevent another cardiovascular event. *Healthy People (HP)* includes heart disease and stroke as one of its topics, and one objective is to reduce hospitalizations.[35] Meeting these objectives requires interventions across the prevention continuum and a population health perspective.

■ **HEALTHY PEOPLE**
HEART DISEASE AND STROKE

Goal: Improve cardiovascular health and quality of life through prevention, detection, and treatment of risk factors for heart attack and stroke; early identification and treatment of heart attacks and strokes; prevention of repeat cardiovascular events; and reduction in deaths from CVD.

Overview: Heart disease is the leading cause of death in the United States. Stroke is the fifth leading cause of death in the United States. Together, heart disease and stroke, along with other CVDs, are among the most widespread and costly health problems facing the nation today, accounting for approximately $320 billion in health care expenditures and related expenses annually. Fortunately, heart disease and stroke are also among the most preventable.[36.]

HP 2020 Midcourse Review: Of the 36 measurable objectives, 15 objectives had met or exceeded their 2020 targets, 8 objectives were improving, 7 objectives demonstrated little or no detectable change, and 2 objectives were getting worse. Three objectives had baseline data only, and 1 objective was informational (Fig. 14-3).[37] An example of an objective that exceeded its target was the age-adjusted rate of coronary heart disease deaths (HDS-2). By 2013, it had declined from 129.2 per 100,000 population in 2007 to 102.6 exceeding the 2020 target. Another example is that between 2009 and 2014, the percentage of heart attack patients receiving percutaneous intervention within 90 minutes of hospital arrival (HDS-19.2) increased from 90.4% to 95.9%. Despite moving toward the 2020 target, there is still a statistically significant difference based on gender, with women less likely to meet the 90-minute threshold.[37]

Performance Improvement and Acute Care Settings

One of the most important aspects in the progression of hospital-based health care has been the change in emphasis from the hospital as a location or a place that holds acutely ill patients to a focus on the provision of evidence-based care with documented improved patient outcomes. To achieve this goal, acute care settings use a specific process called quality improvement (QI) and/or performance improvement (PI) that works to provide safe and consistent care to the acutely ill and injured. This process is population-based and provides the appropriate framework for conducting studies that evaluate the effectiveness of actions taken. The type of studies conducted

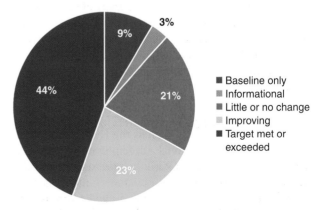

Healthy People 2020 Midcourse Review: Heart Disease and Stroke

- ■ Baseline only
- ■ Informational
- ■ Little or no change
- ■ Improving
- ■ Target met or exceeded

Figure 14-3 Midcourse Review Heart Disease and Stroke.

may involve the calculation of rates of infections, determining the impact of risks such as diabetes on MI, and developing interventions like a walking program to decrease risks of osteoporosis.

According to the Health Resources and Services Administration, **quality improvement** in health care "...consists of systematic and continuous actions that lead to measurable improvement in health care services and the health status of targeted patient groups.."[38] From a public health nursing perspective, **performance improvement** is a "process that considers the organizational context, describes desired performance, identifies gaps between desired and actual performance, identifies root causes, selects interventions to close the gaps, and measures changes in performances with the goal of achieving desired results or outcomes."[39]

The terms *quality improvement* and *performance improvement* are often used interchangeably; the difference is, PI takes a more bottom-up approach and acknowledges that improvement is an ongoing, rather than a static, process. For the purposes of this chapter, the term *PI* is used because it matches the term used in *Public Health Nursing: Scope and Standards of Practice*. Basically, the goal is to improve the care of hospitalized patients through the implementation of EBPs or system changes. No project is too small if it improves patient outcomes. For the majority of direct patient care staff, questioning a specific practice by asking, "Why do we do this task this way?" may initiate a PI project.

For programs to be successful, data collection must occur within the context of a continuous improvement strategy so that the caregivers in the acute care setting can implement changes that improve the quality of health care. Two examples of PI projects are (1) comparison of hospital antibiotic timing rates among patients who receive required preoperative antibiotics before the start of the operative procedure with data from the Centers for Medicare and Medicaid Services and (2) comparing the rates of postoperative infections against the national rates reported by the CDC.

Why Do We Need PI in Acute Care Settings?

A groundbreaking report published by the Institute of Medicine (IOM), now known as the Health and Medicine Division of the National Academies of Sciences, Engineering and Medicine (HMD), at the start of the 21st century entitled *To Err Is Human: Building a Safer Health Care System* created a stir in the health-care industry.[40] The findings from this report brought the lack of consistent quality programs in hospitals in the United

States to the forefront. The report identified the following deficiencies:

- In 1997, there were more than 33.6 million admissions to U.S. hospitals.
- Approximately 44,000 Americans die each year as a result of medical errors and other data suggest that the number may be as high as 98,000.
- More people die due to medical errors than MVAs, breast cancer, and AIDS each year.
- Total national costs (including loss of income, disability, and health-care costs) were estimated to be between $37 and $50 billion for all adverse events, and for preventable adverse events between $17 and $29 billion.
- In terms of lost lives, patient safety is as important as worker safety. More than 6,000 American workers die each year of workplace injuries as compared with the 7,000 lives lost to medication error deaths as reported in 1993.[40]

As a result of these findings, the group recommended a fundamental redesign of the entire health-care system. It recommended the following six aims for improving the system around the following core needs of health care:

1. Safe—Avoid injuries to patients.
2. Effective—Care should be evidence and scientifically based.
3. Patient centered—Care should be built upon patient preferences, needs, and values.
4. Timely—Reduce waits and delays.
5. Efficient—Avoid waste.
6. Equitable—Care should be equal to all persons regardless of age, gender, ethnicity, location, and socioeconomic status.[40]

Based on the IOM report and recommendations, the Institute for Healthcare Improvement (IHI) developed a patient safety initiative because it believes that patients deserve safe and effective health care. The IHI exists to close the gap between the health care we have and the health care we should have.[41] Thus, the IHI launched its 100,000 Lives Campaign and then its 5 Million Lives Campaign with positive results. According to IHI, the campaign resulted in "Hospitals ... demonstrating impressive results. At its formal close in December 2008, the Campaign celebrated the enrollment of 4,050 hospitals, with more than 2,000 facilities pursuing each of the Campaign's 12 interventions to reduce infection, surgical complication, medication errors, and other forms of unreliable care in facilities."[42] To assist hospitals in implementing these PI projects, the IHI supplies template tools to implement as well as tracks progress in achieving these goals. The IHI created steps for incorporating these QI initiatives (Box 14-5).

● APPLYING PUBLIC HEALTH SCIENCE

The Case of the Hospital Partners

Public Health Science Topics Covered:

- Epidemiology and biostatistics
- Determining rates
- Assessment

A group of 10 Cincinnati area hospitals collaborated to reduce HAIs as part of a patient safety initiative. One goal of the project was to reduce catheter-related bloodstream infections (CR-BSI) through the implementation of EBP. The hospitals

met monthly to discuss their progress and share information about their progress toward meeting their specific goal. A team was formed in Hospital A to work on their institutional-level efforts to meet the regional goals. The group not only used the IHI model described earlier but also applied the four-step Plan-Do-Study-Act (PDSA) cycle to their PI project. The **PDSA cycle** is an interactive process adopted from business, also known as the Deming Wheel, and has been around since the 1920s (Fig. 14-4). This cycle is based on action-oriented learning, provides shorthand for testing a change, and is accomplished through a cycle of planning the change, trying it, observing the results, and then acting on what is learned.[44]

The first step in the IHI process is to set an aim. For Hospital A, they decided their aim would be to reduce CR-BSIs. The second step is the measurement statement, in this case, a reduction in CR-BSI by 50% over the next 12 months. This was chosen based on the evidence that more than 200,000 CR-BSIs occur each year in the United States, with an associated mortality of 4% to 35%.[43] Hospital A determined that, to reduce the rates of CR-BSIs, they would first have to develop a tool to measure adherence to treatment with best practices outlined by the CDC (Box 14-6).[44] These best practices included performing hand hygiene before insertion of catheters, applying maximum sterile barriers (gowns, masks, head cover, and sterile gloves) prior to the insertion of central line catheters, covering the

---

BOX 14–5 ■ Institute for Healthcare Improvement Steps for Incorporating Quality Improvement Initiatives

- Set AIM—Defining the specific population to be studied and what the group wishes to accomplish.
- MEASURE results—Specific rate or number as a benchmark for comparison to determine whether the changes being made lead to improvement (e.g., reduction in bloodstream infections, or reduction in the wait time from ED visit to hospital room).
- TEST changes—This may be accomplished through the Plan (P) Do (D) Study (S) Act (A) cycle (PDSA) (Fig.14-4).
- Plan = Plan the change
  - Determine the key personnel
  - Where/when it will take place
  - How it will be tested
  - What data need to be collected
  - Who will collect the data and record the results
- Do = Test the change/intervention.
- Study = Determine the results—did it work?
- Act = Was the intervention/change successful?
  - If yes, can it be expanded to more patients?
  - If yes, then implement another PDSA cycle.
- If the intervention/change did not work:
  - Determine why it failed.
  - Reassess and develop a new plan and test it again.
- IMPLEMENT changes—Move the program on a broader scale. This may include other shifts on the nursing unit, similar nursing units, or hospital-wide.

Source: (41)

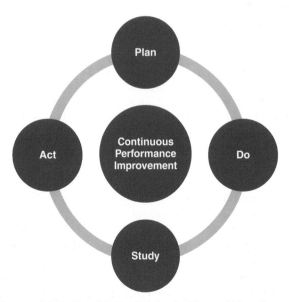

Figure 14-4 Plan (P) Do (D) Study (S) Act (A) cycle.

BOX 14–6 ■ Central Line Insertion Guidelines

With each central line insertion, the nursing staff collected data on each of the best practices and reported adherence back to all end-users on the following:

- Percentage adherence to hand hygiene
- Percentage adherence to maximum barriers (mask, head cover, surgeon gown, and sterile gloves)
- Percentage adherence to full body drapes
- Percentage adherence to chlorhexidine antiseptic for each central line insertion

Source: (84)

patient with a full body drape, and prepping the insertion site with a chlorhexidine-based product.

Once the nursing staff determined what they wanted to measure, they initiated the PDSA cycle (see Fig. 14-4). The **PLAN** identified the key personnel to be included in the central line insertion—the chief medical resident and patient's RN. The line insertion would take place in a patient's room on day shift in the medical intensive care unit (MICU). The data to be collected were outlined on a central line check sheet developed by Hospital A, and the person collecting the information would be the charge RN.

The next step is **DO**. Once it was determined there was a patient who needed a central line, the charge nurse gathered all the supplies including a central line insertion tray, surgical attire from the operating room, a large surgical thyroid drape with an opening (fenestration) near the top of the drape, and the chlorhexidine antiseptic swabs. The MICU RN and the chief resident donned the sterile garb. The MICU charge RN applied a mask and remained at the bedside to act as a circulating nurse to record the events and to complete the checklist. The medical resident and the MICU RN applied the drape and prepped the patient's insertion site with chlorhexidine. The resident inserted the central line per hospital protocol.

The next step is **STUDY**. During the covering with the sterile drape, several problems were encountered. First, neither the chief medical resident nor the MICU RN had much experience with applying a large surgical drape and had difficulty maintaining sterility. Thus, they went through several drapes during the application process. Using several drapes decreased the volume in the operating room. This resulted in placing an urgent order to the manufacturer. This had an impact on the cost of the procedure. Also, the current central line kit

was found to be missing some of the supplies needed to meet the CDC recommendations,[45] so the MICU charge RN had to leave the room several times to find the supplies not included in the current central line trays.

The final step is **ACT**. The group concluded that this first test was not successful, and they regrouped. They determined there were a number of processes that needed to be corrected before they proceeded with the next line insertion: requesting the OR staff provide the MICU nurses/residents with in-service teaching on the proper application of a full body drape, working with the purchasing department to have more drapes stocked in the MICU and the operating room, and reviewing the contents of the current central line kits to determine what supplies would be needed to meet the intent of the CDC recommendations to decrease the number of interruptions during the insertion process. The group asked the purchasing department to schedule meetings with the central line tray manufacturers to revise the trays to include the supplies needed.

The group concluded that employing the PDSA cycle allowed them to test the new protocols before instituting it in all the other ICUs and the hospital. This was a new approach, replacing the usual practice in which a policy was developed, and the users were then required to determine how they would adhere to it. They were able to determine what worked on a small scale and what needed to be corrected to provide their patients with the best care they deserved. Eventually, the group was able to work with the manufacturers of surgical drapes and central line insertion trays to develop efficient and EBP central line trays and surgical packs.

They collected data by using the check sheets, reported adherence to the best practices back to the end users, and published the rates in their respective units for staff, physicians, and families to review. The nurses were empowered to stop any procedure wherein any of the components on the checklist were not followed. Eventually, through repeated PDSA cycles, the MICU unit reduced their CR-BSI rates by more than 50%, and the process was instituted in the rest of the hospital. The checklist was followed throughout Hospital A for all central line insertions. Adherence rates continued to be reported to all users, and committees and infection rates were then posted in all ICUs, allowing for immediate action and the continuous use of the PDSA cycle.

Infection Control and Acute Care Settings

Health care-associated infections are infections caused by pathogens acquired as a consequence of a health-care intervention.[46] Prevention of HAIs requires an upstream population health approach.[2] HAIs may be localized or systemic responses to the presence of an infectious agent(s) or its toxin(s) that (1) occurs in a patient in a health-care setting (e.g., a hospital or outpatient clinic); (2) was not found to be present or incubating at the time of admission, unless the infection was related to a previous admission to the same setting; and (3) if the setting is a hospital, meets the criteria for a specific infection site as defined by the CDC.[46-48] The major issues include sepsis/bacteremias, pneumonia, and urinary tract infections (UTIs). Based on data collected by the CDC, it is estimated that approximately one in 25 U.S. patients contracts at least one infection in association with his or her hospital care.[49]

■ HEALTHY PEOPLE
Health Care-Associated Infections

Targeted Topic: Health care-Associated Infections
Goal: Prevent, reduce, and ultimately eliminate HAIs.
Overview: HAIs are infections that patients get while receiving treatment for medical or surgical conditions. They are among the leading causes of preventable deaths in the United States and are associated with a substantial increase in health-care costs each year.[50]
HP 2020 Midcourse Review: Both objectives for HAI in HP 2020 showed improvement. For central line infections, the rate fell from 1.0 standardized infection rate in 2006-2008 to 0.54 in 2013. Invasive health care-associated methicillin-resistant staphylococcus aureus (MRSA) infections dropped from 27.08 infections per 100,000 persons in 2007–08 to 18.23 infections per 100,000 persons in 2013.[51]

Sepsis

Globally, there are an estimated 30 million cases of sepsis annually with 6 million deaths.[52] In the U.S. at least 1.7 million people develop sepsis every year and 270,000 die. In addition, one in three patients who die in U.S. hospitals die of sepsis.[52] Infants, children, older adults, and pregnant and postpartum women are at higher risk for hospital-associated sepsis (HAS).[10] **Sepsis** is "…life-threatening organ dysfunction caused by a dysregulated host response to infection."[53,54] It is the body's response to the invasion of pathogenic microorganisms in which

severe sepsis and septic shock are the end results of the interaction between infecting organisms and the body's host responses. These responses cause inflammation, immunosuppression, abnormal coagulation, and blood flow and circulatory dysfunction, which lead to organ injury and cell death.[52,55]

When sepsis causes dysfunction in one organ, it is diagnosed as severe sepsis. Signs and symptoms of sepsis include (1) fever; (2) chills; (3) inflammatory responses such as increased WBC and increased serum concentrations of C-reactive protein; (4) hemodynamic symptoms of increased heart rate, increased cardiac output, low oxygen saturation rate; (5) metabolic responses such as increased insulin requirements; (6) tissue perfusion changes such as altered skin perfusion and decreases in urinary output; and, (7) organ dysfunction such as increases in urea and creatinine levels, decreases in platelets, and coagulation abnormalities.[55] If sepsis results in induced hypotension that does not respond to increased fluid challenges, then the diagnosis of septic shock is made.[53] There is a wide variety in patient presentation thus there is no "one-size-fits-all" approach to care of the patient with severe sepsis.[54]

Initial antibiotic therapies are based on the likely source of the infection and the most common pathogens. For instance, urosepsis treatment is based on the most likely source of UTIs such as *Escherichia coli* and enterococcal species. Antibiotic therapies should begin as soon as possible and always within the first hours of recognized sepsis and septic shock.[54,55] Blood, urine, and sputum cultures should be sent to the laboratory before antibiotics are given for proper identification of the incriminating organism. Once the organism is identified, antibiotic treatments should be reassessed to decrease the risk of antibiotic resistance.[54,59]

Ventilatory and volume support are also crucial for patient survival to combat hypotension and respiratory insufficiency. Hemodynamic support includes fluid replacement, crystalloids, or colloids. Vasopressor support includes dopamine and norepinephrine; inotropic therapy may include dobutamine. Steroids may be used when hypotension responds poorly to fluids and vasopressors. Other supportive measures may include blood products, glucose control, and renal replacement therapy (e.g., dialysis and continuous renal replacement therapy, deep venous thrombosis prophylaxis, and stress ulcer prophylaxis).[56-60]

Because of their increased age and variance of presenting symptoms, older adults frequently do not develop fever. Thus, initial treatment is geared toward antibiotic therapy, after urine, sputum, blood, or wound cultures have been analyzed. The initial antibiotics are geared toward a broader spectrum of suspected pathogens such as *E. coli* and MRSA. In addition to antibiotic therapy, fluid resuscitation as well as invasive monitoring for blood pressure, urinary catheters for renal output, and oxygen therapy must be considered and used as needed. Older adult patients do respond well to treatment protocols, but health-care providers need to have a high level of suspicion for sepsis in older adults so that treatment may begin in a timely manner.[56,60]

Cerebrospinal and Postoperative Central Nervous System Infections

Hospital-associated central nervous system (CNS) infections include meningitis, encephalitis, and intracranial abscesses. Meningitis is an inflammation of the meninges, the membrane that covers the brain and spinal cord.[61] There are four types of meningitis categorized based on the causative agent: bacterial, parasitic, fungal, and amoebic. Sometimes there are noninfectious causes of meningitis including cancer, lupus, and brain injury.[61] Globally, the World Health Organization (WHO) warned of a possible meningitis epidemic that could expand beyond sub-Saharan Africa to neighboring countries, with the main concern being the low stockpile of vaccines.[62,63] Universal vaccinations can help boost herd immunity and reduce the incidence of disease. In the U.S., the recommendation is to vaccinate all children aged 11 to 12 years old with a booster at age 16. In sub-Saharan Africa, national preventive campaigns were conducted.[64] Following the campaigns, routine vaccinations were recommended for children under the age of 1.[16] This illustrates the importance of understanding the incidence of community-acquired infections when examining the possibility of hospital-associated infections. In geographic areas with a high incidence of a communicable disease, the risk of a hospital-associated case of the disease increases.

High morbidity and mortality highlight the importance of preventing health care-associated meningitis and other CNS infections in the acute care setting.[65] Patients at greater risk are those who have had neurosurgery, those over the age of 65, children, and those who have a shunt, lumbar drain, or other foreign material placed in their CNS.[65] Steps can be taken from an institutional and population perspective using the CDC guidelines[21] to prevent hospital-acquired CNS infections.[65]

Early identification and treatment of a hospital-associated CNS infection is essential to prevent spread of the infection and reduce mortality.[66] If the infection is not diagnosed early and antibiotics are not initiated promptly, patients may develop sepsis (meningococcemia), which results in hypotension and bilateral adrenal hemorrhage. Thus, intravenous (IV) antibiotics must be initiated promptly.[67] With the rise in incidence of viral meningitis, there is an increasing need for further research on treatment.[68]

Surgical Site Infections

A **surgical site infection** (SSI) occurs after surgery or other invasive procedure in the area of the body where the surgery or procedure took place.[69,70] Up to one-fifth of all HAIs are SSIs; 5% of patients who had a surgical procedure later develop an SSI.[69] As many as 300,000 SSIs occur each year in the U.S. Most (55%) SSIs are preventable.[71,72] An SSI not only reduces the quality of life for patients but also increases the risk of morbidity and mortality as well as the cost of care.[70] Prevention includes actions taken preoperatively, intraoperatively and postoperatively.[70,72] Types of SSIs are separated into three categories: superficial incisional, deep incisional, and organ/space.[71]

Strategies to prevent SSIs begin with having a surveillance system within the acute care organization. Because the length of stay following a surgical procedure is short, it is important to incorporate a method for conducting surveillance post-discharge.[70] In the U.S., the CDC publishes guidelines on SSI prevention that provide the preventionists in the hospital, such as the infection control nurse, with an up-to-date evaluation of the evidence as to what works and what does not work over all three phases of prevention. For example, in 2017, the guidelines supported the administration of the appropriate antimicrobial agent prior to skin incision (versus at cord clamping) for patients having a caesarean section. The guidelines also included a list of strategies determined to be unnecessary to prevent an SSI such as antimicrobial prophylaxis after surgical closure (clean and clean-contaminated procedures).[72]

Based on programs in different states, taking a population-level approach to prevent SSIs has resulted in reduced rate of SSIs. For example, Georgia addressed the overuse of antibiotics by developing an Antibiotic Stewardship Committee of key stakeholders. These stakeholders established a strategic framework for statewide activities along with support for implementation. Some of their initiatives included implementing a method for determining baseline hospital prescribing practices and for tracking practices over time, and they instituted training programs for pharmacists and physicians on antibiotic use.[73]

Hospital-Associated Pneumonia and Ventilator-Associated Pneumonia

Pneumonia is the leading cause of HAI with an estimated rate of mortality associated with **hospital-associated pneumonia (HAP)** from 33% to 50%.[74] The majority of HAP infections are linked to gram-negative bacteria, whereas 20% to 30% of cases involve gram-positive cocci.[29] The mortality rate is high and is the leading cause of HAI deaths.[74]

The two main risk factors are intubation and mechanical ventilation. To help track these risk factors, experts have differentiated between cases of HAP, an episode of pneumonia that occurs after admission to the hospital that is not associated with mechanical ventilation, and **ventilator-associated pneumonia (VAP)**, pneumonia that presents more than 48 hours after endotracheal intubation.[75-77] Risk factors for developing HAP/VAP also differ based on geography, specific characteristics of the health care setting, length of stay before onset of the disease, and risk factors for multiple drug-resistant (MDR) pathogens (see Chapter 8).[76] Estimating the incidence of VAP is done by calculating the number of episodes per ventilator days within the health care setting. In the U.S., VAP incidence ranges from 2 to 16 episodes for 1,000 ventilator-days, with an attributable mortality of 3% to 17%.[75]

Prevention of HAP/VAP requires a systems-based population approach. The 2016 guidelines provide detailed information on steps to take both from a systems approach, to prevent HAP/VAP from occurring, as well as appropriate treatment to improve outcomes for those diagnosed with HAP/VAP. The main focus has been prevention of VAP with recommended bundling of treatments.[74] In addition, the 2016 guidelines provide guidance to hospitals on generating antibiograms aimed at reducing MDR organisms (MDROs).[75]

Catheter-Associated Urinary Tract Infections

Among UTIs acquired during a hospital stay, approximately 75% are associated with a urinary catheter. Because up to 25% of hospitalized patients receive urinary catheters while in the hospital, the risk for a catheter-associated urinary tract infection (CAUTI) is high. The main risk factor for a CAUTI is prolonged use of the urinary catheter. Thus, the main prevention step is to remove the urinary catheter as soon as possible.[79] Other risk factors include colonization of the drainage bag, diarrhea, diabetes, female gender, renal insufficiency, errors in catheter care, catheterization late in the hospital course, and immunocompromised or debilitated states.[80]

CAUTIs occur because the urethral catheter can actually inoculate pathogens into the bladder. They also help in the colonization of pathogens by providing a surface for bacterial adhesion and by causing mucosal irritation.[80] The CDC has set criteria for what qualifies as a CAUTI (Box 14-7).[81] Complications of an indwelling Foley catheter include: prostatitis, epididymitis, and orchitis in males; and cystitis, pyelonephritis, gram-negative bacteremia, endocarditis, vertebral osteomyelitis, septic arthritis, endophthalmitis, and meningitis in all patients.[81] Adverse consequences include: discomfort to the patient, prolonged hospital stay, and increased cost and mortality; an estimated 13,000 deaths annually are associated with UTIs.[82] Organisms most frequently associated with CAUTIs generally originate in the gastrointestinal tract such as enterococci (Fig.14-5).

Preventing CAUTIs includes the following key components:

- Practice hand hygiene before and after catheter insertion and when manipulating the catheter site or device.

BOX 14-7 ■ Catheter-Associated UTI (CAUTI)

- A UTI where an indwelling urinary catheter (IUC) was in place for >2 calendar days on the date of event, with day of device placement being Day 1,
- AND an indwelling urinary catheter was in place on the date of event or the day before.
  - If an indwelling urinary catheter was in place for >2 calendar days and then removed, the date of event for the UTI must be the day of discontinuation or the next day for the UTI to be catheter-associated.

Source: (81)

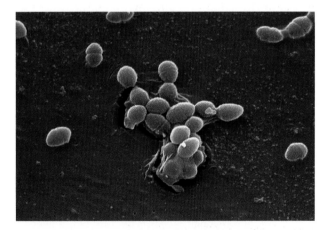

Figure 14-5 Enterococci, leading causes of nosocomial bacteremia, surgical wound infection, and urinary tract infection. *(From Centers for Disease Control and Prevention Public Health Image Library. Photograph by Pete Wardell.)*

- Use aseptic technique when inserting the catheter and obtaining urine samples, and always use sterile equipment.
- Properly secure the catheter to prevent movement and urethral traction.
- Consider using portable ultrasound devices to assess the volume of urine in the bladder and to reduce unnecessary catheterization.
- Maintain a closed drainage system and unobstructed flow of urine.[82]

QI programs have been implemented to promote proper usage of urinary catheters and to reduce the risk of CAUTIs. Key initiatives include appropriate use of catheters, removing catheters when no longer needed, monitoring adherence to hand hygiene practices and proper care of catheters, developing alert systems or reminders among patients with catheters for early removal, and developing protocols for placement of catheters, the use of ultrasound devices, and assessing the need for catheters.[82]

Central Line-Associated Bloodstream Infections

A central line-associated bloodstream infection (CLABSI) is defined by the CDC as an infection that occurs when pathogens enter the bloodstream through the central line.[83] The most common source of a health care-associated bloodstream infection is a central line. The estimated health care cost per case of a bloodstream infection is $25,000.[84] After the CDC instituted guidelines to prevent CLABSIs in 2009, incidence dropped, yet it is estimated that more than 30,000 health care-associated CLABSIs still occur.[84] Treatment of a CLABSI generally depends on the severity of the patient's clinical disease, risk factors for the infection, and the bacteria associated with the infection.[84,85] Complications may include septic thrombosis and infective endocarditis, which require long-term antibiotic treatment. A number of actions can be taken to prevent CLABSI. For example, in one study the use of antimicrobial-impregnated (AIP) peripherally inserted central catheters (PICCs) versus nonantimicrobial-impregnated (NAIP) catheters lowered the risk of CLABSIs.[86]

■ EVIDENCE-BASED PRACTICE
Prevention of CLABSI

Practice Statement: Patients in acute care settings are at risk of developing CLABSIs because of the need for invasive monitoring in critical care medicine. A patient safety goal for ICU patients is to reduce the risks of CLABSI through the adoption of best practices

including: hand hygiene, maximal sterile barriers, full body drapes, and chlorhexidine-based products for insertion site antisepsis.

Targeted Outcome: Reduction in CLABSI

Evidence to Support: The CDC has always supported the use of maximum sterile barriers and covering the patient with a full sheet during insertion of central lines as a means to reduce CLABSIs.[1] One hospital instituted a Comprehensive Unit-Based Safety Program (CUSP) that resulted in a reduction in CLABSIs from 1.95 to 1.04 per 1,000 central line days.[2] Another PI project in a Maryland hospital included interventions at the organizational and the unit level to reduce CLABSIs in a burn unit. Interventions included a "…development of new blood culture procurement criteria, implementation of chlorhexidine bathing and chlorhexidine dressings, use of alcohol-impregnated caps, routine performance of root-cause analysis with executive engagement, and routine central venous catheter changes". These interventions resulted in the reduction of CLABSI rates from 15.5 per 1,000 central-line days to zero with a sustained rate of zero CLABSIs over 3 years.[3]

Recommended Approaches and Resources:

- Insert central line catheters into the subclavian site when possible. Femoral sites have been associated with higher rates of infection.
- Perform hand hygiene before insertion of catheters as well as when manipulating or accessing central line catheters.
- Apply maximum sterile barriers (gowns, masks, head cover, and sterile gloves) prior to the insertion of central line catheters.
- Cover the patient with a full body drape.
- Prepare the insertion site using chlorhexidine-based products.
- Cover the insertion site with a sterile occlusive dressing.
- Use aseptic technique when accessing or changing central line dressing.
- Remove catheters when no longer needed.

Sources:

1. Marschall, J., Mermel, L., Fakih, M., Hadaway, L., Kallen, A., O'Grady, N., … Yokoe, D. (2014). Strategies to prevent central line–associated bloodstream infections in acute care hospitals: 2014 update. *Infection Control and Hospital Epidemiology, 35*(7), 753-771. doi:10.1086/676533.

2. Richter, J.P., & McAlearney, A. (2018). Targeted implementation of the Comprehensive Unit-Based Safety Program through an assessment of safety culture to minimize central line-associated bloodstream infections. *Health Care Management Review, 43*(1), 42–49. https://doi-org.ezp.welch.jhmi.edu/10.1097/HMR. 0000000000000119

3. Sood, G., Caffrey, J., Krout, K., Khouri-Stevens, Z., Gerold, K., Riedel, S., ... Pronovost, P. (2017). Use of implementation science for a sustained reduction of central-line–associated bloodstream infections in a high-volume, regional burn unit. *Infection Control & Hospital Epidemiology, 38*(11), 1306–1311. https://doi-org.ezp.welch.jhmi.edu/ 10.1017/ice.2017.191

Health Care-Associated Infections and Multiple Drug-Resistant Organisms

Multiple drug-resistant organisms pose a public health issue for hospitals. According to the CDC "…antibiotic resistance happens when germs like bacteria and fungi develop the ability to defeat the drugs designed to kill them."[87] According to the CDC, annually in the U.S., approximately 2 million people are infected with antibiotic-resistant bacteria; 23,000 deaths are associated with antibiotic-resistant bacteria.[87] According to the WHO, antibiotic resistance is increasing related to the treatment of malaria and HIV-related infections. In addition, 490 000 people developed multidrug-resistant TB globally.[88] Persons with resistant infections require more care resulting in increased cost.[88]

One example of an MDRO is the carbapenem-resistant enterobacteriaceae family of infectious agents. This family of pathogens presents a challenge to health-care workers in acute care settings because these infections are resistant to most front-line antibiotics. Some enterobacteriaceae are normally present in the human gut and can become carbapenem-resistant through enzymes that break down these antibiotics so that they are no longer effective.[89] Other MDROs include MRSA, *Clostridium difficile,* and vancomycin-resistant enterococci.

The most common mechanism for acquiring a MDRO in a hospital is patient-to-patient via the hands of a health-care worker. Prevention efforts include a wide range of interventions conducted at the organizational and individual levels. They require the application of public health principles and an understanding of how communicable diseases are transmitted. The CDC lists the following as components of an MDRO prevention program: education, judicious use of antimicrobials, MDRO surveillance, infection control precautions, and environmental controls aimed at reducing transmission.[90]

▮ Summary Points

- A public health perspective applies to the acute care setting.
- Focused assessments related to acute care population–level data provide the necessary information for setting priorities.
- The improvement of health-care delivery and patient outcomes in an acute care setting has occurred because of population-level interventions.
- Differences exist between males and females in relation to health care received in the acute care setting.
- The evolution of critical care has occurred at the population level.
- Health planning occurs in acute care settings using the same process used in community settings.
- PI within an acute care setting uses public health science and health planning principles throughout the process.
- The prevention of HAIs is a major public health issue and the responsibility of every nurse.

▼ CASE STUDY
Health Planning to Prevent Falls

Learning Outcomes

At the end of this case study, the student will be able to:

- Apply the techniques for a focused assessment.
- Identify risk factors associated with an identified patient safety issue.
- Apply program planning to the development, implementation, and evaluation of a hospital fall prevention program.

The recent safety reports for the medical units in a hospital caught the attention of the nursing department because there had been an increase in falls. The CNO asked the nurse managers of the medical units to determine what was behind the increased fall incidence rate. After examining the hospital incident report data, they found that three medical units had an increased fall rate and two did not. The nurse managers formed a committee of nurses across the five units to examine the issues related to falls and develop a fall prevention program.

To complete this case study, answer the following questions:

1. What further information do the nurse managers need for the assessment phase of their investigation (see Chapter 4)?
2. What are the risk factors associated with falls in an acute care setting from a national perspective?
3. How would you construct a hypothetical case control study for three of the major risk factors (see Chapter 3)?
   a. What sources of data would you use?
   b. Would this require IRB approval?
4. What evidence-based interventions are relevant to fall prevention in an acute care setting?
5. What recommendations would you make for implementing an intervention?
6. What outcome measures would be relevant to evaluating the effectiveness of the intervention?

REFERENCES

1. Bureau of Labor Statistics, U.S. Department of Labor (2018). *Occupational outlook handbook, registered nurses*. Retrieved from https://www.bls.gov/ooh/healthcare/registered-nurses.htm.
2. Acute care. (2018). *The free dictionary*. Retrieved from http://medical-dictionary.thefreedictionary.com/acute+care.
3. American Association of Colleges of Nursing. (2006). *The essentials of doctorate education for advanced nursing practice*. Washington, DC: Author.
4. U.S. Department of Health and Human Services, Agency for Health Research and Quality. (2018). *Healthcare cost and utilization project (HCUP)*. Retrieved from http://hcupnet.ahrq.gov/.
5. Centers for Disease Control and Prevention. (2018). *Leading causes of death*. Retrieved from http://www.cdc.gov/nchs/fastats/leading-causes-of-death.htm.
6. National Center for Health Statistics. (2017). *Health, United States, 2016; Trend Tables, Table 81. Persons with hospital stays in the past year, by selected characteristics: United States, selected years 1997–2016.* Retrieved from https://www.cdc.gov/nchs/data/hus/2017/081.pdf.
7. National Center for Health Statistics. (2017). *Health, United States, 2016; Trend Tables, Table 82. Hospital admission, average length of stay, outpatient visits, and outpatient surgery, by type of ownership and size of hospital: United States, selected years 1975–2015.* Retrieved from https://www.cdc.gov/nchs/data/hus/2017/082.pdf.
8. Agency for Healthcare Research and Quality. (2015). Healthcare cost and utilization project (HCUP), National Inpatient Sample (NIS). Retrieved from https://www.hcup-us.ahrq.gov/nisoverview.jsp.
9. U.S. Department of Health and Human Services. (2015). *Understanding the Health Care Reform Act*. Retrieved from http://www.healthcare.gov/law/introduction/index.html.
10. American Association of Critical Care Nurses. (n.d.). *About critical care nursing*. Retrieved from https://www.aacn.org/about-aacn.
11. U.S. Department of Labor, Bureau of Labor Statistics. (2018). *Occupational employment and wages, May 2018, 29-1141 registered nurses*. Retrieved from https://www.bls.gov/oes/current/oes291141.htm#ind.
12. Nightingale, F. (1863). *Notes on hospitals* (3rd ed.). London, England: Longmans, Green.
13. Hall, J.R. (1990). Critical-care medicine and the acute care laboratory. *Clinical Chemistry, 36*(8B), 1552-1556.
14. Hanson, C.W., III, Durbin C.G., Jr., Maccioli, G.A., Maccioli, G.A., Deutschman, C.S., ...Gattinoni, L. (2001). The anesthesiologist in critical care medicine: Past, present, and future. *Anesthesiology, 95*(3), 781-788.
15. Society of Critical Care Medicine. (n.d.). *History of critical care*. Retrieved from http://www.sccm.org/SCCM/History+of+Critical+Care/.
16. Okie, S. (2005). Retrospective TBI in the war zone. *New England Journal of Medicine, 352*, 2043-2047.
17. Warden, D. (2006). Military TBI during the Iraq and Afghanistan wars. *Journal of Head Trauma Rehabilitation, 21*(5), 398-410.
18. eHistory archive. (n.d.). *Statistics on the Civil War and medicine*. Retrieved from https://ehistory.osu.edu/exhibitions/cwsurgeon/cwsurgeon/statistics.
19. Preston, S.H., & Buzzell, E. (2006). *Mortality of American troops in Iraq*. Retrieved from http://repository.upenn.edu/cgi/viewcontent.cgi?article=1000&context=psc_working_papers.
20. Centers for Disease Control and Prevention. (2018). *Polio vaccination: What everyone should know*. Retrieved from http://www.cdc.gov/vaccines/vpd-vac/polio/dis-faqs.htm.
21. Berthelsen, P., & Cronqvist, M. (2003). The first intensive care unit in the world: Copenhagen 1953. *Acta Anaesthesiology Scandinavia, 47*(10), 1190-1195.
22. Milka, M. (2003). Father of CPR, innovator, teacher, humanist. *Journal of the American Medical Association, 289*(19), 2485-2486.
23. American Heart Association. (2015). *2015 AHA guidelines for CPR and ECC*. Retrieved from https://eccguidelines.heart.org/index.php/circulation/cpr-ecc-guidelines-2/part-5-adult-basic-life-support-and-cardiopulmonary-resuscitation-quality/.
24. American Heart Association. (2018). *CPR facts and stats*. Retrieved from https://cpr.heart.org/AHAECC/CPRAndECC/AboutCPRECC/CPRFactsAndStats/UCM_475748_CPR-Facts-and-Stats.jsp.
25. Kleinman, M., Goldberger, Z., Rea, T., Swor, R.A., Bowbrow, B., Brennan, E.E., ... Travers, A.H. (2017). *2017 American Heart Association focused update on adult basic life support and cardiopulmonary resuscitation quality: An update to the American Heart Association guidelines for cardiopulmonary resuscitation and emergency cardiovascular care*. Retrieved from: https://www.ahajournals.org/doi/pdf/10.1161/CIR.0000000000000539.
26. The Framingham Heart Study. (2018). *History of the Framingham Heart Study*. Retrieved from https://www.framinghamheartstudy.org/fhs-about/history/.
27. The Nurses' Health Study. (2016). Retrieved from http://www.channing.harvard.edu/nhs/.
28. American Heart Association. (2018). *Heart disease and stroke statistics 2018 at-a-glance*. Retrieved from:

https://www.heart.org/-/media/data-import/downloadables/heart-disease-and-stroke-statistics-2018—-at-a-glance-ucm_498848.pdf.

29. The Framingham Heart Study. (2018). *Key findings.* Retrieved from https://www.nhlbi.nih.gov/science/framingham-heart-study-fhs#key-findings.

30. Centers for Disease Control and Prevention. (2017). *Women and heart disease fact sheet.* Retrieved from https://www.cdc.gov/dhdsp/data_statistics/fact_sheets/fs_women_heart.htm.

31. Federal Drug Administration. (2018). *Research on heart disease in women.* Retrieved from https://www.fda.gov/ScienceResearch/SpecialTopics/WomensHealthResearch/ucm134670.htm.

32. Merz, C.N.B., Ramineni, T., Leong, D., & Bairey Merz, C.N. (2018). Sex-specific risk factors for cardiovascular disease in women-Making cardiovascular disease real. *Current Opinion in Cardiology, 33*(5), 500–505. https://doi-org.ezp.welch.jhmi.edu/10.1097/HCO.0000000000000543.

33. O'Gara, P., Kushner, F., Casey, D., Chung, M., de Lemos, J., Ettinger, S.M., ... Zhao, D.X. (2012). *2013 ACCF/AHA guidelines for the management of patients with ST-elevation myocardial infarction.* Retrieved from: https://www.ahajournals.org/doi/abs/10.1161/cir.0b013e3182742cf6

34. U.S. Department of Health and Human Services. (n.d.). *Health information privacy: Public health.* Retrieved from http://www.hhs.gov/ocr/privacy/hipaa/understanding/special/publichealth/index.html.

35. Nurse's Health Study. (2016). *About NHS.* Retrieved from nurseshealthstudy.org/about-nhs.

36. United States Department of Health and Human Services. (2018). *Healthy People 2020 topics: Heart disease and stroke.* Retrieved from http://www.healthypeople.gov/2020/topicsobjectives2020/objectiveslist.aspx?topicid=21.

37. United States Department of Health and Human Services. (2017). *Healthy People 2020 Midcourse Review: Chapter 21; Heart disease and stroke.* Retrieved from https://www.cdc.gov/nchs/data/hpdata2020/HP2020MCR-C21-HDS.pdf.

38. U.S. Health Resources & Services Administration. (n.d.). *Quality improvement.* Retrieved from https://hrsa.gov/quality/toolbox/methodology/qualityimprovement/.

39. American Nurses Association. (2013). *Public health nursing: Scope and standards of practice, second edition.* Silver Spring, MD: Nursesbook.org.

40. Kohn, L.T., Corrigan, J.M., & Donaldson, M.S. (1999). *To err is human: Building a safer health care system.* Washington, DC: Institute of Medicine, National Academies Press. Retrieved from http://www.nationalacademies.org/hmd/~/media/Files/Report%20Files/1999/To-Err-is-Human/To%20Err%20is%20Human%201999%20%20report%20brief.pdf.

41. Institute for Healthcare Improvement. (2018). *About.* Retrieved from http://www.ihi.org/engage/initiatives/completed/5MillionLivesCampaign/Pages/default.aspx http://www.ihi.org/about/Pages/default.aspx.

42. Institute for Healthcare Improvement. (2018). *Overview: 5 million lives campaign.* Retrieved from http://www.ihi.org/engage/initiatives/completed/5MillionLivesCampaign/Pages/default.aspx.

43. Agency for Healthcare Research and Quality. (2013). *Plan-Do-Study-Act (PDSA) Cycle* (2nd ed.). Retrieved from https://innovations.ahrq.gov/qualitytools/plan-do-study-act-pdsa-cycle.

44. Render, M., Brungs, S., Kotagal, U., Nicholson, M., Burns, P., Ellis, D., ... Hirschhorn, L. (2006). Evidence-based practices to reduce central line infections. *Joint Commission Journal on Quality and Patient Safety, 32*(5), 253-260.

45. Centers for Disease Control and Prevention. (2011). *Guidelines for the prevention of intravascular catheter related infections.* Retrieved from http://www.cdc.gov/hicpac/pdf/guidelines/bsi-guidelines-2011.pdf.

46. U.S. Department of Health and Human Services. (2017). *Health care-associated infections.* Retrieved from https://www.healthypeople.gov/2020/topics-objectives/topic/healthcare-associated-infections.

47. Cairns, S., Gibbons, C., Milne, A., King, H., Llano, M., MacDonald, L., ... Reilly, J. (2018). Results from the third Scottish National Prevalence Survey: Is a population health approach now needed to prevent healthcare-associated infections? *Journal of Hospital Infection, 99*(3), 312–317. https://doi-org.ezp.welch.jhmi.edu/10.1016/j.jhin.2018.03.038.

48. U.S. Department of Health and Human Services, Office of Disease Prevention and Health Promotion. (2018). *Health care-associated infections.* Retrieved from https://health.gov/hcq/prevent-hai.asp.

49. Centers for Disease Control and Prevention. (2017). *Current HAI progress report.* Retrieved from https://www.cdc.gov/hai/data/portal/progress-report.html.

50. U.S. Department of Health and Human Services, Healthy People 2020. (2018). *Hospital-acquired infections.* Retrieved from https://www.healthypeople.gov/2020/topics-objectives/topic/healthcare-associated-infections.

51. U.S. Department of Health and Human Services, Healthy People 2020. (2017). *HP 2020 midcourse review Chapter 19, Hospital-acquired infections.* Retrieved from https://www.cdc.gov/nchs/data/hpdata2020/HP2020MCR-C19-HAI.pdf.

52. World Health Organization. (2018). *Sepsis.* Retrieved from http://www.who.int/news-room/fact-sheets/detail/sepsis.

53. Centers for Disease Control and Prevention. (2018). *Sepsis: Data and reports.* Retrieved from https://www.cdc.gov/sepsis/datareports/index.html.

54. Rhodes, A., Evans, L., Alhazzani, W., Levy, M.M., Antonelli, M., Ferrer, R., ... Dellinger, R.P. (2017). Surviving sepsis campaign: International guidelines for management of sepsis and septic shock: 2016. *Critical Care Medicine, 45*(3), 486–552.

55. Ranzani, O.T., Prina, E., Menéndez, R., Ceccato, A., Cilloniz, C., Méndez, R., ...Torres, A. (2017). New sepsis definition (Sepsis-3) and community-acquired pneumonia mortality. A validation and clinical decision-making study. *American Journal of Respiratory & Critical Care Medicine, 196*(10), 1287–1297. https://doi-org. ezp.welch.jhmi.edu/10.1164/rccm.201611-2262OC.

56. Centers for Disease Control and Prevention. (2016, August). *CDC Vital signs: Making health care safer. Think sepsis. Time matters.* Retrieved from https://www.cdc.gov/vitalsigns/pdf/2016-08-vitalsigns.pdf.

57. Jaffee, W., Hodgins, S., & McGee, W.T. (2018). Tissue edema, fluid balance, and patient outcomes in severe sepsis: An organ systems review. *Journal of Intensive Care Medicine, 33*(9), 502–509. https://doi-org.ezp.welch.jhmi.edu/10.1177/0885066617742832.

58. Ladha, E., & House-Kokan, M. (2017). The ABCCs of Sepsis: A framework for understanding the pathophysiology of sepsis. *Canadian Journal of Critical Care Nursing, 28*(2), 38. Retrieved from http://search.ebscohost.com.ezp.welch.jhmi.edu/login.aspx?direct=true&db=rzh&AN=123094902&site=ehost-live&scope=site.

59. López-Mestanza, C., Andaluz-Ojeda, D., Gómez-López, J.R., & Bermejo-Martín, J.F. (2018). Clinical factors influencing mortality risk in hospital-acquired sepsis. *Journal of Hospital Infection, 98*(2), 194–201. https://doi-org.ezp.welch.jhmi.edu/10.1016/j.jhin.2017.08.022.

60. Ward, C. (2018). Overview of the incidence, early identification and management of sepsis. *Nursing Standard, 32*(25), 41–46. Retrieved from http://search.ebscohost.com.ezp.welch.jhmi.edu/login.aspx?direct=true&db=rzh&AN=128026946&site=ehost-live&scope=site.

61. Centers for Disease Control and Prevention. (2017). *Meningitis.* Available from https://www.cdc.gov/meningitis/index.html.

62. World Health Organization. (2018). *Risk of meningitis epidemics in Africa: High threat in 2018, 2019.* Retrieved from http://www.who.int/mediacentre/infographic/meningitis/meningitis-2018-2019.pdf?ua=1.

63. World Health Organization. (2018, April 6). Epidemic meningitis control in countries of the African meningitis belt, 2017. *Weekly Epidemiological Record, 93*(14), 173–184. http://www.who.int/wer.

64. Centers for Disease Control and Prevention. (2018). *Vaccines and preventable diseases: Meningococcal vaccine.* Retrieved from https://www.cdc.gov/vaccines/vpd/mening/index.html.

65. Lee, J.J., Lien, C.Y., Huang, C.R., Tsai, N.W., Chang, C.C., Lu, C.H., & Chang, W.N. (2017, Dec 15). Clinical characteristics and therapeutic outcomes of post neurological bacterial meningitis in elderly patients over 65: A hospital-based study. *Acta Neurol Taiwan, 26*(4), 144-153.

66. Anderson, D.J., Podgorny, K., Berríos-Torres, S.I., Bratzler, D.W., Dellinger, E.P., Greene, L., ... Kaye, K.S. (2014). Strategies to prevent surgical site infections in acute care hospitals: 2014 update. *Infection Control & Hospital Epidemiology, 35*(Suppl 2), S66–S88.

67. Mount, H.R., & Boyle, S.D. (2017). Aseptic and bacterial meningitis: Evaluation, treatment, and prevention. *American Family Physician, 96*(5), 314–322. Retrieved from http://search.ebscohost.com.ezp.welch.jhmi.edu/login.aspx?direct=true&db=rzh&AN=124575352&site=ehost-live&scope=site.

68. McGill, F., Griffiths, M.J., & Solomon, T. (2017). Viral meningitis: Current issues in diagnosis and treatment. *Current Opinion in Infectious Diseases, 30*(2), 248–256. https://doi-org.ezp.welch.jhmi.edu/10.1097/QCO.0000000000000355.

69. Centers for Disease Control and Prevention. (2012). *Surgical site infection (SSI).* Retrieved from https://www.cdc.gov/hai/ssi/ssi.html.

70. National Institute for Health and Care Excellence. (2017). *Surgical site infections: Prevention and treatment. Clinical guideline [CG74].* Retrieved from https://www.nice.org.uk/guidance/cg74/chapter/Introduction.

71. Anderson, D.J., Podgorny, K., Berríos-Torres, S.I., Bratzler, D.W., Dellinger, E.P., Greene, L., ... Kaye, K.S., et al. (2014). Strategies to prevent surgical site infections in acute care

hospitals: 2014 update. *Infection Control and Hospital Epidemiology, 35,* 605-627. DOI: 10.1086/676022.

72. Preas, M.A., O'Hara, L., & Thom, K. (2017). 2017 HICPAC-CDC guideline for prevention of surgical site infection: What the infection preventionist needs to know. *Prevention Strategist, Fall.* Retrieved from https://apic.org/resource_/tinymcefilemanager/periodical_images/api-q0414_l_ssi_guidelines_final.pdf.

73. Centers for Disease Control and Prevention. (n.d.). *HAI prevention stories from the states: Georgia.* Retrieved from https://www.cdc.gov/hai/state-based/pdfs/success_story-Georgia_stewardship.pdf.

74. Rodriguez, T. (2017). Challenges in managing hospital-acquired pneumonia. *Infectious Disease Advisor.* Retrieved from https://www.infectiousdiseaseadvisor.com/pneumonia/managing-hospital-acquired-pneumonia/article/681011/.

75. Kalil, A.C., Metersk, M.L., Klompas, M., Musceder, J., Sweeney, D.A., Palmer, L.B., ... Brozek, J.L. (2016). Management of adults with hospital-acquired and ventilator-associated pneumonia: 2016 clinical practice guidelines by the Infectious Diseases Society of America and the American Thoracic Society. *Clinical Infectious Diseases, 63*(5), e61-e111. doi: 10.1093/cid/ciw353.

76. Luyt, C.-E., Hékimian, G., Koulenti, D., & Chastre, J. (2018). Microbial cause of ICU-acquired pneumonia: Hospital-acquired pneumonia versus ventilator-associated pneumonia. *Current Opinion in Critical Care, 24*(5), 332–338. https://doi-org.ezp.welch.jhmi.edu/10.1097/MCC.0000000000000526.

77. Barbier, F., Andremont, A., Wolff, M., & Bouadma, L. (2013). Hospital-acquired pneumonia and ventilator-associated pneumonia: recent advances in epidemiology and management. *Current Opinion in Pulmonary Medicine, 19*(3), 216–228. https://doi-org.ezp.welch.jhmi.edu/10.1097/MCP.0b013e32835f27be.

78. Cunha, B.C., & Brusch, J.L. (2018). Hospital-acquired pneumonia (Nosocomial Pneumonia) and ventilator-associated pneumonia. *Medscape.* Retrieved from https://emedicine.medscape.com/article/234753-overview.

79. Centers for Disease Control and Prevention. (2017). *Catheter-associated urinary tract infections (CAUTI).* Retrieved from https://www.cdc.gov/hai/ca_uti/uti.html.

80. Brusch, J.L. (2017). Catheter-related urinary tract infection (UTI). *Medscape.* Retrieved from https://emedicine.medscape.com/article/2040035-overview.

81. Centers for Disease Control and Prevention. (2018). *Urinary tract infection (catheter-associated urinary tract infection [CAUTI] and non-catheter-associated urinary tract infection [UTI]) and other urinary system infection [USI]) events.* Retrieved from https://www.cdc.gov/nhsn/pdfs/pscmanual/7psccauticurrent.pdf.

82. Gould, C.V., Umscheid, C.A., Agarwal, R.K., Kuntz, G., & Pegues, D.A. (2010). Guideline for prevention of catheter-associated urinary tract infections. *Infection Control and Hospital Epidemiology, 31,* 319-26.

83. Centers for Disease Control and Prevention. (2011). *Central line-associated bloodstream infections: Resources for patients and healthcare providers.* Retrieved from https://www.cdc.gov/hai/bsi/clabsi-resources.html.

84. Pathak, R., Gangina, S., Jairam, F., & Hinton, K. (2018). A vascular access and midlines program can decrease hospital-acquired central line-associated bloodstream infections and

cost to a community-based hospital. *Therapeutics & Clinical Risk Management, 14,* 1453–1456. https://doi-org.ezp.welch.jhmi.edu/10.2147/TCRM.S171748.

85. Kagan, E., Salgado, C.D., Banks, A.L., Marculescu, C.E., & Cantey, J.R. (2018). Peripherally inserted central catheter-associated bloodstream infection: Risk factors and the role of antibiotic-impregnated catheters for prevention. *American Journal of Infection Control, pii,* S0196-6553(18)30749-1. doi: 10.1016/j.ajic.2018.07.006.

86. Tobar, S., Olmsted, R., & Kast, R. (2018). Intersection between sepsis not present on admission and central catheter–associated bloodstream infections: Connections aimed at patient safety...2018 National Teaching Institute Research Abstracts. Presented at the AACN National Teaching Institute in Boston, Massachusetts, May 21-24, 2018. *American Journal of Critical Care, 27*(3), e13. https://doi-org.ezp.welch.jhmi.edu/10.4037/ajcc2018805.

87. Centers for Disease Control and Prevention. (2018). *About antibiotic resistance.* Retrieved from https://www.cdc.gov/drugresistance/about.html.

88. World Health Organization. (2018). *Antimicrobial resistance.* Retrieved from http://www.who.int/en/news-room/fact-sheets/detail/antimicrobial-resistance.

89. Centers for Disease Control and Prevention. (2018). *Carbapenem-resistant Enterobacteriaceae in healthcare settings.* Retrieved from https://www.cdc.gov/hai/organisms/cre/index.html.

90. Centers for Disease Control and Prevention. (2018). *Antibiotic/antimicrobial resistance: Protecting patients and stopping outbreaks.* Retrieved from https://www.cdc.gov/drugresistance/protecting_patients.html.

Chapter 15

Health Planning for Primary Care Settings

Christine Colella

LEARNING OUTCOMES

After reading the chapter, the student will be able to:

1. Describe the evolution of primary care at the national and global levels.
2. Apply the principles of epidemiology to the primary care setting.
3. Discuss the integration of primary, secondary, and tertiary care interventions in the primary care setting.
4. Describe chronic disease management and case management.
5. Discuss current policy issues related to the delivery of primary care.
6. Describe the patient-centered medical home (PCMH) component of the Affordable Care Act.

KEY TERMS

Case management
Food desert
Health promotion

Health protection/risk reduction

Patient-centered medical home (PCMH)
Primary care

Primary health care
Vaccine

Introduction

"Primary health care now more than ever" was declared by the World Health Organization (WHO) in 2008.[1] More than a decade later, barriers remain from local obstacles to global challenges. Noncommunicable diseases (NCDs) such as cardiovascular disease, respiratory disease, diabetes, and cancer are the leading causes of death and disability across the world. Despite decades of research by Starfield and others, that demonstrated a positive association between access to primary care and better health outcomes, the supply of general primary care practitioners continues to be low.[2] The question then arises: "If the importance of primary care is known, why is it not realized?" The issue at the forefront in the United States, and the world, is that the demand for primary care providers continues to exceed the supply. Due to this trend, there is a projected shortfall of the primary care workforce by 2030.[3]

In response to the looming shortage, more states have sought to expand the role of advanced practice registered nurses (APRN). The APRN as nurse practitioner (NP) has increased access to primary care where it is needed. A report by the University of Michigan (2018)[4] demonstrated that more NPs worked in low-income areas. This effort has placed nursing in the center of the struggle to address the increasing demand for primary care services in the United States. What is behind the focus on primary care, and what does primary care have to do with public health? According to the WHO, the answer is found in the theme used for the 2018 World Health Day: "Universal Health coverage: Everyone, everywhere under the slogan: Health for All."[5]

Populations that have access to health care, especially preventive care on a primary and secondary level, are healthier.[1] Primary health care includes preventive care such as vaccines and immunizations, health education, health promotion, and monitoring of health status. **Primary care** provides individuals and families with vital secondary prevention such as screening and early treatment. These efforts can decrease the overall burden of disease experienced by a population through the prevention of disease and reduction of mortality and morbidity. Primary care is central to the health of the public, and primary health-care providers who apply public health science to their practice become active participants in the promotion of health in the populations they serve. Primary care is delivered across a continuum from the individual to the community (Fig. 15-1).

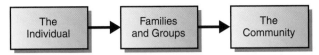

Figure 15-1 The continuum of primary care.

Evolution of Primary Care

According to the WHO, globalization is putting the social cohesion of countries under stress, and health-care systems are not performing at the level needed to adequately address the health-care needs of their citizens. The WHO reported that, in 2018, almost 100 million people were being pushed into extreme poverty by having to pay for health-care services out of their own pocket.[5] In their 2008 plea for increasing primary care, the WHO argued that primary health care would make a difference in the capability of health-care systems to respond better and faster to the need for services.[1] Despite overall improvement worldwide in health and life expectancy, the WHO explained that these improvements are not consistent across countries or populations. In addition, trends in the delivery of health-care services are problematic, especially the following:

- The focus by health-care systems is on curative care.
- The approach to disease control is short term and fragments service delivery.
- A laissez-fare approach to health systems has allowed unregulated commercialization of health care.[1]

United States

Primary care, as we think of it today in the United States, has evolved out of population demand and political changes. The definition of primary care is dependent on the services provided to the patient and the provider of that service, and for the most part focuses on the method for delivery of primary health-care services to individuals and families. In the past, the local general practitioner cared for a patient from birth to death. After World War II, that method of care delivery dwindled, and specialty care grew. Because of population demand, it was not until the late 1960s and early 1970s that family practice became a new specialty with the launch of family practice medical education programs in 1969.[6] According to the American Academy of Family Physicians (AAFP), to define primary care one must describe the nature of the services provided and identify the provider of these services.[6]

The patient is the core of primary care; patients must be partners in their care for it to be effective. Primary care is often referred to as the gatekeeper or control center for access to care. It is the entryway to the maze known as the health-care system. Although this is true, we should also see the opportunity that primary care brings to fully meet the needs of the patient. The services delivered encompass health promotion, disease prevention, health maintenance, counseling, patient education, diagnosis, and treatment of acute and chronic illness.[5] In addition to providing health care to patients, the primary care provider also acts as a patient advocate. The primary care environment promotes patient-centered care that is cost effective and focused on both accomplishing the goals of individual patients, and reducing morbidity and mortality in the population served through prevention, early detection of disease, and engagement in treatment. The importance of increasing access to care is part of the *Healthy People (HP)* objectives.[7]

■ HEALTHY PEOPLE

Topic: Access to Health-Care Services

Goal: Increase access to comprehensive quality health-care services

Overview: Access to comprehensive, quality health-care services, including oral care and prescription drugs, is important for promoting and maintaining health, preventing and managing disease, reducing unnecessary disability and premature death, and achieving health equity for all Americans.

There are three components of access to care:

- insurance coverage
- health services
- timeliness of care

Midcourse Review: Of the HP 2020 26 objectives, 6 were archived, 10 were developmental, and 10 were measurable. Of those that were measurable, 4 showed improvement, 5 showed little or no improvement, and 1 worsened (Fig. 15-2).[8]

Sources: (7, 8).

Global

In 1978, the International Conference on Primary Health Care in Alma-Ata, USSR, resulted in a declaration that urged action from all governments, health-care workers, and the global community to protect and promote the health of all peoples. The declaration defined primary health care as:

Primary health care is essential health care based on practical, scientifically sound, and socially acceptable methods and

**Healthy People 2020 Midcourse Review:
Access to Health Care Services**

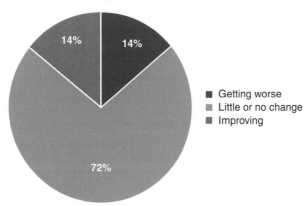

■ Getting worse
■ Little or no change
■ Improving

Figure 15-2 Healthy People 2020 midcourse review: Access to health services.

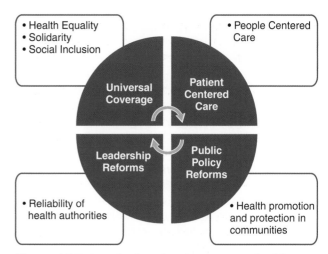

Figure 15-3 Social values that drive primary health care and the corresponding set of reforms. *(Adapted from the World Health Organization.)*

technology made universally accessible to individuals and families in the community through their full participation and at a cost that the community and country can afford to maintain at every stage of their development in the spirit of self-reliance and self-determination. It forms an integral part both of the country's health system, of which it is the central function and focus, and of the overall social and economic development of the community. It is the first level of contact of individuals, the family and community with the national health system, bringing health care as close as possible to where people live and work, and constitutes the first element of a continuing health-care process.[1]

The goal set at the end of the conference was to achieve an acceptable level of health care for all people of the world by 2000. Although this has not been achieved, a 2008 report by the WHO showed some progress in the building of primary health-care infrastructure. The report, however, also pointed to the existence of barriers. The WHO makes the argument that the core values of primary health care are equity, solidarity, and the active participation of people in the decisions that affect their health. These values then drive reforms that reflect concrete expectations of citizens within developing and developed societies (Fig. 15-3).[1]

■ CELLULAR TO GLOBAL

From a global perspective, the term **primary health care** has a broader meaning than it does in the United States. In the United States, the term primary health care is used to describe the level of delivery of care to individuals and families rather than to

populations. However, at the International Conference on Primary Health Care in Alma-Ata, USSR, in 1978, primary health care takes a broader approach that includes all aspects related to health, including access to health services, environment, and lifestyle. The difference in the definition of primary care from the global perspective is evident in the central values of the Alma-Ata Declaration related to the achievement of health for all. The declaration began a movement that tackled political, social, and economic inequalities in health care. The agenda for the 2008 WHO report was to renew the effort to reform health-care systems across the globe to achieve that equality.[1]

More than 10 years have passed since the 2008 agenda was set, yet equality is still not in place. The WHO 2018 Global Conference on Primary Care was focused on the goal of achieving universal health coverage (UHC) and meeting sustainable developmental goals (SDG).[9] On World Health Day, the WHO stated that, "we need to get 1 billion more people to benefit from universal health care by 2023 if we are to meet sustainable development goals by 2030".[5] Looking at the issue from a global perspective, 90% of a person's health needs in a lifetime can be covered by primary care.[9] The two perspectives of primary care come together in their central commitment to people-centered health care built on the development of a personal relationship between health-care providers and seekers of care. Both function under the belief that people are partners in the management of their health. Primary health care, as defined by the WHO, takes it one step further with the idea that primary care is responsible for the health of the community across the life span, and that primary care must tackle the determinants of ill health.[1]

This approach has brought criticisms. Some thought the Alma-Ata Declaration primarily supported the creation of one health-care delivery system with a narrow goal of providing adequate health care to the poor.[1] In reality, the declaration addressed much larger issues than just providing care to one group. Since 1978, large gaps have been exposed in the ability of current health systems to address the changing health needs of populations. Many systems are facing increased demands and changing expectations of what the health-care system should deliver. In addition, the issues raised by emerging chronic and communicable diseases are bringing to the forefront evidence that primary health care not only meets the needs of individuals, but also can improve the health of entire communities. The WHO General Director stated "Health is a human right. No one should get sick and die just because they are poor or because they cannot access the services they need."[9] This is very powerful language that speaks to the need and importance of primary care access for all. Primary care as defined in the Alma-Ata Declaration provides an overall model for the delivery of health care across the globe. Under this model, primary care should provide access to care from individuals to communities and address key health issues related to both communicable and noncommunicable disease, mental health, substance use, and injury from the cellular to global level.

UNICEF is another organization that looks at the health and well-being of children and their access to care and needs. Their Strategy for Health 2016-2030[10] speaks to some successes of countries improving health-care outcomes, but the need for continued achievement is paramount. For example, it discusses the tremendous achievement in improving the under-5 mortality rate as well as the maternal mortality rate, but is quick to note that, despite these achievements, unacceptable inequities remain within and among countries. UNICEF has also launched a global strategy for women's, children's, and adolescents' Health 2016-2030: Survive, Thrive, Transform initiative (Box 15-1).[11] The vision as presented by Ban Ki-moon, the UN Secretary-General, is explained as:

The three overarching objectives of the updated Global Strategy are Survive, Thrive, and Transform. With its full

---

BOX 15–1 ■ UNICEF Objectives and Targets

SURVIVE: End preventable deaths

- Reduce global maternal mortality to less than 70 per 100,000 live births
- Reduce newborn mortality to at least as low as 12 per 1,000 live births in every country
- Reduce under-5 mortality to at least as low as 25 per 1,000 live births in every country
- End epidemics of HIV, tuberculosis, malaria, neglected tropical diseases, and other communicable diseases
- Reduce by one-third premature mortality from noncommunicable diseases and promote mental health and well-being

THRIVE: Ensure health and well-being

- End all forms of malnutrition and address the nutritional needs of children, adolescent girls, and pregnant and lactating women
- Ensure universal access to sexual and reproductive health-care services (including for family planning) and rights
- Ensure that all girls and boys have access to good-quality early childhood development
- Substantially reduce pollution-related deaths and illnesses
- Achieve universal health coverage, including financial risk protection and access to quality essential services, medicines, and vaccines

TRANSFORM: Expand enabling environments

- Eradicate extreme poverty
- Ensure that all girls and boys complete free, equitable, and good-quality primary and secondary education
- Eliminate all harmful practices and all discrimination and violence against women and girls
- Achieve universal and equitable access to safe and affordable drinking water and to adequate and equitable sanitation and hygiene
- Enhance scientific research, upgrade technological capabilities, and encourage innovation
- Provide legal identity for all, including birth registration
- Enhance the global partnership for sustainable development

---

implementation—supporting country priorities and plans, and building the momentum of Every Woman and Every Child—no woman, child, or adolescent should face a greater risk of preventable death because of where they live or who they are. But ending preventable death is just the beginning. By helping to create an enabling environment for health, the Global Strategy aims to transform societies so that women, children, and adolescents everywhere can realize their rights to the highest attainable standards of health and well-being. This, in turn, will deliver enormous social, demographic, and economic benefit.[11]

According to the UNICEF State of the World's Children 2017 report,[12] changes have occurred, but there is significant room for improvement. Pneumonia and diarrhea, both treatable and preventable diseases, still claim 1.4 million young children every year. They report that one in four deaths among children under 5 is caused by either pneumonia or diarrhea. Low and lower middle-income countries are home to 62% of the world's under-5 population but account for 90% of global pneumonia and diarrhea deaths.[12] There has been a decline in the deaths however, because of the work being done. Between 2000 and 2015 the death rate fell from 2.9 million to the current 1.4 million. This is a significant decline, but as their publications state, even one death is too many.

The focus going forward is to continue to implement the interventions that have been successful. That includes a threefold strategy of protection, prevention, and treatment. Protection means that to decrease the number of deaths you must have healthier infants. The strategy is to encourage breastfeeding exclusively for the first 6 months with adequate complimentary feeding and vitamin A supplementation. Prevention places an emphasis on hand washing with soap, safe drinking water and sanitation, and vaccines for pertussis, measles, hepatitis B, PCV, and rotavirus. It also requires reducing household pollution and spread of HIV; approximately half of the deaths from pneumonia are associated with air pollution and HIV. Treatment means access to health care, which requires improved care seeking, case management, and availability of supplies such antibiotics.

What do these changes in the overall health of the population have to do with primary health care? The basic need is to have a health-care system that provides resources that can effect change. This requires a concerted effort of a government to put in place agencies and people dedicated to the health of their nation. To be successful at the population level, a primary health-care system must consider the social, economic, and political context in which it functions.

Epidemiology and Targeted Prevention Levels in Primary Care

Primary care encompasses all levels of prevention: primary, secondary, and tertiary. Interventions vary based on the level of prevention, gender, and age. Helping our country achieve optimal health requires a comprehensive understanding of the community. Health promotion and protection should be provided to all members of the community despite their disease status. Primary care nurses who apply public health science, including assessment and health-planning skills, will not only have a better chance of providing optimal care to individuals and families, but also are more apt to contribute to the building of a healthier community. Public health nurses (PHNs) who work in primary care settings develop health programs that help prevent disease and manage NCD. Examples of the programs implemented for populations include case management, health education programs, and community outreach.

A major challenge in the United States and globally is ensuring access to primary care services. The Patient Protection and Affordable Care Act (ACA) of 2010 (see Chapters 1 and 21) was built on the assumption that increasing access to care will improve the health of the U.S. population. Among other things, this legislation made funds available to create and support nurse-managed clinics that would focus on promoting and maintaining optimal health. Changes to the ACA later eroded away some of this support, but the primary care setting remains central to the reform bill. The interventions provided by nurses working in primary care are built on the application of public health science. This requires that nurses working in primary care settings have knowledge not only of the health of individuals seeking care but also an understanding of the context in which they live. Thus, nurses working in a primary care setting who are caring for individuals, families, and/or communities and populations must have current information on the prevalence of diseases within the community they serve, information on the current recommendations for primary and secondary prevention relevant to their community, and the ability to engage community partners in development of sustainable and effective interventions.

▶ **SOLVING THE MYSTERY**
The Case of the Sleeping Mom
Public Health Science Topics Covered:

- Assessment
- Advocacy

Nurses who know the community their clients live and work in have a great advantage in primary care. Sometimes they can intervene at a level that goes beyond assessment, diagnosis, and treatment. Consider Terry, a nurse working at a primary care clinic located in one of the poorer neighborhoods in New York City. Brenda, a single African American mother, came in with her 4-month-old baby for a routine well-baby checkup. The mother was seen initially by the primary care physician working in the clinic. He came out of the examining room and asked Terry to put together a social services referral. The physician told Terry, "This mother has real problems. When I was examining the baby, the mother fell asleep in the chair and I had to keep waking her up to answer questions. She obviously is not capable of caring for this child if she can't stay awake in the middle of the day!" Terry told the physician that she would go in and talk with the mother.

When Terry went into the room, she found the baby safely nestled in the car seat and Brenda asleep in the chair. Terry gently woke up Brenda up and identified herself. She asked Brenda to tell her about her baby. Brenda glowed and said that the baby was wonderful. Terry then told her that she noticed Brenda was asleep when she came in. Was there a reason for this? Brenda hesitated and said that it was nothing. Terry gently probed further, and Brenda explained that she has been staying up at night because the apartment in which she is living is infested with rats. If she doesn't stay awake, the rats will get into the baby's crib and hurt him. She was pleased that she has been able to keep her baby safe but worried that she was so tired that she may fall asleep during the night.

Terry asked her whether she had issued a complaint. Brenda said she had complained to the landlord, but nothing had happened. Terry assured her that there are steps that can be taken to address the issue and then began the process, not for a social service visit, but to work with the public health department and the housing authority to implement the process for getting the rodents eliminated from the building. In addition, Terry looked through the charts to find other families attending the clinic who lived in the same building and called each one to determine whether the rat problem was being experienced throughout the building. Many of the clients complained of a similar problem, and Terry helped the tenants begin to work together to address the issue as well. Within a short period of time, an effective program was put in place that included action from the public health department, the housing authority, and the newly formed tenants group. The result was landlord compliance with rodent eradication and elimination of rats from the building. Brenda was at last able to sleep at night.

Terry built on the knowledge she had obtained in her community health course. When she accepted the job, she took the time to learn about the community where the clinic was located, including identifying key contacts in the public health department. This knowledge had helped her in the past to address problems with immunization of children, distribution of flu vaccines, and now a problem with rodent infestation. Over time, she not only knew the patients who came to the clinic but also had a growing understanding of the environment in which they lived. This knowledge meant that she immediately understood the possibility that there was an alternative explanation for the sleeping mom. Her knowledge of key stakeholders helped her determine who had the power to act and effect change. In addition, her understanding of how a community works helped her to include the residents of the building in the problem-solving process.

An important component to all levels of prevention is education of patients about what they can do to minimize their own risk factors for disease (see Chapter 2). Understanding the relationship of diet, exercise, and maintaining a healthy weight can be key to disease prevention or minimizing complications of disease. The diabetic who controls his blood sugar will minimize micro- and macrovascular complications. The smoker who enters a smoking cessation program will reduce her risk of cardiovascular disease and chronic obstructive pulmonary disease. Other important items a nurse can address with a patient during a primary care visit include use of sunscreen, dental hygiene, and alcohol intake. When these risks occur across a group of patients, the nurse can develop population-level interventions such as education packets or working with the health department to implement the use of public safety announcements specific to their community.

Primary Prevention Within the Primary Care Setting

The first and desired level of intervention is primary prevention to keep a person free of disease (see Chapter 2). For individuals who are free of disease and seek primary care, the major focus for the nurse is to conduct a routine checkup, provide health education (see Chapter 2), support positive health practices, and provide information and support related to changing unhealthy behaviors. The challenge for the nurse working in a primary care setting is how to engage in primary prevention at the aggregate level as well as at the individual and family levels. This requires knowledge of the community, the resources available, leaders within the community, and the other stakeholders in the community who can support efforts to promote and protect the health of the community. Thus, it is important to know how to conduct a community assessment and make a plan (see Chapters 4 and 5).

Let's consider the example of the nurses working in a primary care setting in the Midwest, where a key behavioral issue that affects overall health is the high rate of tobacco use. According to the Centers for Disease Control and Prevention (CDC),[13] the Midwest has the highest regional prevalence of smoking; 19 out of every 100 adults smoke.[13] Furthermore, nearly 18 out of every 100 adult men and 14 out of every adult female smoke. A comprehensive smoking cessation program at a clinic in the Midwest should include not only efforts to help individuals quit, but also primary prevention programs at the community level. If nurses seek further information at the community level, they will identify the resources available to the community. They will also be able to identify cultural issues related to tobacco use that may influence the success of a smoking prevention campaign. Knowledge of the community will also help them engage other potential partners in the community in doing an anti-smoking campaign among the youth of the community.

Primary prevention is the first step in reducing the number of adults who smoke over the next decade. In the example of tobacco use in a Midwest community, the primary care nurse could collaborate with the school system to develop a culturally grounded anti-smoking campaign in the hope that, over time, they would see fewer patients in their clinic suffering from smoking-related adverse health consequences. Such a campaign could encompass the development of policies that not only reduce youth access to tobacco products but also reduce exposure to secondary smoke. Information would also be shared about vaping and electronic cigarettes as this activity is being seen in both adults and adolescents. As per the CDC,[14] electronic cigarettes are not safe for youth, young adults, pregnant women, nor adults who don't smoke. Vaping is also targeted by advertisers to young children and adults, and poses a threat to the smoking prevention process.

To be effective, primary prevention in a primary care setting requires both individual- and community-level interventions. It includes both health promotion and health protection activities. As defined in Chapter 2, **health promotion** at the individual and family levels helps people change their lifestyle to achieve optimal health.[15] Health promotion as defined by the WHO is "the process of enabling people to increase control over and to improve their health. It moves beyond a focus on individual behaviors toward a wide range of social and environmental interventions".[15] As stated in Chapter 2, **health protection/risk reduction** includes primary prevention interventions that protect the individual from disease by reducing risk and usually focuses on behavioral change with health education a main tool, whereas health protection involves a clinical intervention such as immunization (Table 15-1).

Health Promotion

Most health promotion in primary health-care settings is delivered at the individual and family levels. However, to be effective, these interventions should be developed, implemented, and evaluated from a population level (see Chapter 5). This requires an understanding of the community, including cultural, environmental, socioeconomic

---

TABLE 15–1 ■ Levels of Prevention in Primary Care and Recommended Interventions

Primary Prevention—Adult (to prevent illness from occurring)

Primary Prevention Focus	Examples
Health protection: Immunizations	• Flu shot • Pneumococcal vaccination • Tetanus booster (every 10 years) • Human papillomavirus (females aged 9–26) • Chicken pox (VZV) for those born after 1980
Health promotion: Education	• Healthy diet • Exercise • Weight loss • Smoking cessation • Low-risk alcohol use

TABLE 15–1 ■ Levels of Prevention in Primary Care and Recommended Interventions—cont'd

Secondary Prevention—Adult (to identify disease in a patient with asymptomatic illness)

Men	Age Range	Testing
	19–39	• Blood pressure (BP), body mass index (BMI), health risks • HIV discussion • Depression screening • Diabetes screening • Lipids for men at age 35
	40–49	• BP, BMI, health risks • HIV discussion • Depression screening • Diabetes screening • Lipids every 5 years
	50–70	• BP, BMI, health risks • HIV discussion • Depression screening • Diabetes screening • Colorectal screening (at age 50)
	70 and older	• BP, BMI, health risks • Depression screening • Diabetes screening • Colorectal screening until 75

Women	Age Range	Testing
	19–39	• BP, BMI, health risks • HIV discussion • Depression screening • Diabetes screening • Chlamydia/gonorrhea (sexually active women through age 24 and then as needed) • Cervical cancer (first should be done at age 21 or 3 years after first sexual contact, then every 3 years)
	40–49	• BP, BMI, health risks • HIV discussion • Depression screening • Diabetes screening • Cervical cancer (every 3 years) • Mammography (optional as a baseline every 2 years)
	50–70	• BP, BMI, health risks • Depression screening • Diabetes screening • Cervical cancer screening up to age 65 • Colorectal screening (at age 50) • Mammography (every 2 years) • Bone density (age 65 or women at a high risk for fractures per risk factors) • Lipids optional every 5 years until 70 as per risk factors

Continued

TABLE 15–1 ■ Levels of Prevention in Primary Care and Recommended Interventions—cont'd

Secondary Prevention—Adult (to identify disease in a patient with asymptomatic illness)

71 and over	• BP, BMI, health risks • Depression screening • Diabetes screening • Colorectal screening • Mammography every 1 to 2 years until 74, then optional

Tertiary Prevention—Adult (identifies the disease state the patient may have to minimize complications)

Diabetes	• Tight glycemic control • Lipid management • BP control • Healthy weight • Exercise • Foot care
Cardiovascular	• Lipid management • BP control • Healthy weight • Exercise

For further information on interventions in primary care refer to:

1. Agency for Healthcare Research and Quality (2014). Guide to Clinical Preventive Services, 2014. Rockville, MD, Author. Retrieved from http://www.ahrq.gov/professionals/clinicians-providers/guidelines-recommendations/guide/index.html
2. U.S. Preventative Services Task Force. (2018). Retrieved from http://www.uspreventiveservicesraskforce.org/BrowseRec/Index/browse-recommendations

aspects of the community, and the resources available in the community.

For example, if you worked in a primary care setting in Arizona with a high percentage of American Indians as clients, it would be important to know what diseases this population is most at risk for. Based on data from the CDC, a major concern would be prevention of type 2 diabetes in American Indian youth (Table 15-2).[16,17] This requires a review of population-level information related to risk factors. In the case of the American Indians, the risk factors include genetic predisposition and a shift in diet from traditional foods they grew themselves to processed foods.[14,15] Less than 100 years ago, diabetes was unknown in the American Indian population but

started be reported after World War II.[18] The Pima Indians of Arizona have the highest rates of diabetes in the world;[17] they have a higher incidence of long-term complications from diabetes, and their problems develop earlier in life. Based on these facts, primary prevention strategies would require buy-in from the community and need to begin as early as possible, even during the prenatal period instead of waiting until a problem develops. Partnering with the community would be a key first step prior to initiating evidence-based prevention strategies that have been used in other parts of the country. The Pima Indians have their own unique culture as well as a genetic predisposition that requires modification of any other programs to match the specific needs of the community. Fortunately, much work has been done in partnership with Pima Indians to understand how to improve their health.[18] Again, primary care requires a population perspective not only as the starting point but also for ongoing evaluation of the effectiveness of interventions delivered across the continuum in primary care (see Fig. 15-1).

Immunization and Health Protection

Immunization through the administration of a vaccine is one of the most frequently used health protection efforts conducted in primary care. As explained in Chapter 8, a

TABLE 15–2 ■ Prevalence of Type 2 Diabetes >18 yrs in the United States

Ethnic Group	Prevalence
American Indians	15.1%
Asian, non-Hispanic	8.0%
Black, non-Hispanic	12.7%
White, non-Hispanic	7.4%

Source: (16)

vaccine refers to the immunizing agent that is used to increase the host's resistance to viral, rickettsial, and bacterial diseases. They can be killed, modified, or become a variant form of the agent. In the United States, the CDC provides detailed guidance to the health-care provider related to the recommended vaccination schedule for all age groups. An example is the recommended adult immunization schedule compiled for the health-care provider (see https://www.cdc.gov/vaccines/schedules/hcp/imz/adult.html). The schedule includes immunizations recommended for all adults based on age group, including:

- Tetanus
- Human papillomavirus
- Varicella
- Measles, mumps, and rubella
- Influenza

Other vaccines are recommended if some risk factor is present, such as the occupational risk of exposure to hepatitis A and B for health-care providers.[19] The primary care nurse often administers the vaccine. Nurses providing the vaccines use population-level data related to risk, helping them identify persons who would most benefit from the vaccine. Recommendations for vaccination from the CDC are based on age, risk factors, and medical conditions.[20]

Immunizations are central to the patient's risk reduction and health promotion. Every interaction with the health-care team is an opportunity to assist the patient in making choices that will enhance his/her health. Patient education regarding how immunizations can affect health is often the role of the primary care nurse. With every interaction with each patient, the nurse has the opportunity to make the information relatable to that patient and his concerns or needs. The young mother who cannot miss work for illness needs to understand that getting the flu vaccine could decrease her risk for illness this year. The farmer working in the soil needs to understand how important his tetanus booster is to keep him working without a problem. The student starting a career in health care needs to see the relationship between getting his/her hepatitis B series and his/her new role. One of many things the primary care nurse does is show patients the relationship between their own needs and how preventive health care can help them meet those needs. The understanding and availability of immunizations such as the flu vaccine helps the patient adhere to this mandate. Thus, the primary care nurse actively participates in the achievement of the *HP* goal related to immunization.

The HP 2020 goals for immunization and communicable diseases were rooted in evidence-based clinical and community activities and services for the prevention and treatment of infectious diseases. Objectives new to HP 2020 focused on technological advancements ensuring that states, local public health departments, and nongovernmental organizations are strong partners in the federal attempt to control the spread of communicable diseases. Objectives for 2020 reflected a more mobile society and the fact that diseases do not stop at geopolitical borders.[7] Awareness of disease and completing prevention and treatment courses remain essential components for reducing transmission of communicable disease and meeting the proposed visions and mission of Healthy People 2030 (see Chapter 1).

■ HEALTHY PEOPLE
Immunization and Infectious Disease

Goal: Increase immunization rates and reduce preventable infectious diseases.

Targeted Topic: Immunizations and infectious diseases

Overview: The increase in life expectancy during the 20th century is largely due to improvements in child survival; this increase is associated with reductions in infectious disease mortality, due largely to immunization. However, infectious diseases remain a major cause of illness, disability, and death. Immunization recommendations in the United States currently target 17 vaccine-preventable diseases across the life span.

HP 2020 Midcourse Review: (See Chapter 8.)

Source: (7)

Secondary Prevention Within the Primary Care Setting

Secondary prevention is a major activity in primary care. Secondary prevention focuses on identifying individuals with subclinical disease and initiating early treatment. The activity usually associated with secondary prevention is screening. Most primary care settings follow the current recommendations for screening. Screening in primary care includes a wide range of tests, from taking weight and height done in the office to colonoscopies that require aesthesia. (For more detail on screening, see Chapter 2.) Primary care settings are where most screening occurs; thus, primary care providers are essential to the process of early detection and treatment. However, note again that aggregate-level approaches are also vital to the success of screening. Some screening procedures such as colonoscopy can be expensive and require access to health-care facilities that provide the service. Patients who are less likely to have a colonoscopy covered by their insurance, if they have insurance, can be offered a fecal for occult blood, which is less costly and a valid pretest for colon cancer. Knowledge about the community and the population served can help improve access to screening services, thus improving the health of the population served.

Screening

Here is an example of how nurses take an active role in screening and health promotion. Access to mammography screening in the rural communities of southeastern Indiana was limited. In response, nurses developed a screening program that has resulted in a regional drive to bring screening to the women living in these communities. This program, funded by the Susan G. Komen Foundation and others, uses the mammography van from a local hospital to go to the women who need the service. With advanced advertisement, women are registered for a screening, clinical breast exam, and education.

This example of a grassroots approach to breast cancer screening has been successful. Many women have been reached, screened, and referred for follow-up care. A parallel opportunity that came out of this project in southern Indiana was the development of a nurse-run clinic for the uninsured. This free clinic opens twice a month, staffed by nurses, a pharmacist, and an NP who offer education, episodic intervention, and referral to primary care providers in the community who will care for patients using an economic sliding scale. These interventions were implemented by nurses living in the area who identified a need and responded to it from a primary care perspective. Nurses in the community applied their understanding of the community to find a way to respond to that need. This included knowledge of the community demographics, the regional and ethnic cultural practices, and community resources such as treatment facilities available for those who screened positive for breast cancer. The focus was secondary prevention with the long-term goal of reducing morbidity and mortality in a population of women at risk.[21]

The CDC is an excellent source for recommendations related to screening in primary care settings. For example, it has a Web page dedicated to HIV screening in primary care with a recommendation that all patients aged 13 to 64 be screened.[22] The CDC also has recommendations on screening for cancer, including breast and colorectal cancers.[23]

Screening is basic to care because health-care providers are looking for illness that is asymptomatic. In the primary care population, we screen routinely for elevated blood pressure, cholesterol, and hyperglycemia. We screen for these because we know through evidence-based practice that people who have these underlying issues are at greatest risk for disease. Hypertension, hyperlipidemia, and diabetes are the root causes for diseases that have the highest incidence of mortality and morbidity. Taking a blood pressure is noninvasive and simple to do, uses minimal equipment, and can identify the patient who is at risk for coronary artery disease. To identify this patient and then offer the education and opportunities to improve their health is foundational to primary care. Screening must be followed up with education that includes information on lifestyle changes such as diet, exercise, weight loss, and medications. Screening without follow-up leaves the patient without the direction or knowledge to take charge of his health.

Ethics of Screening in Primary Care

Chapter 2 addressed the ethical issues related to screening in detail, but the importance of ethics in screening bears repeating here. A major issue in primary care is conducting screening when treatment is not available. Prior to screening, the primary care nurse must first know what to do if the patient screens positive. Is this something the patient wants to know? Does the family want to know? For example, you may have a woman with two sisters who wants to know whether she carries the gene for breast cancer, but the other sisters do not want to know. This can become an ethical issue for the family. Think about the family in which a member may have a disease for which there is no known cure, such as amyotrophic lateral sclerosis, also known as Lou Gehrig's disease. Do the children want to know whether they are carriers and how does this affect their lives going forward? Does the nurse know what facilities are available to the client to take the next steps—assessment, diagnosis, and treatment? Availability includes geographical availability, the patient's access to transportation to get the facility, and whether the patient can pay for the treatment. For example, if a surgical intervention is required and the patient is uninsured and has no savings, the only option may be Medicaid. The state Medicaid program may require that the patient sell any assets, such as a home, prior to qualifying for Medicaid. These ethical issues related to screening should be considered prior to conducting routine screening.

Tertiary Prevention Within the Primary Care Setting

Despite our best efforts with primary prevention, some people will become ill with either a communicable disease (Chapter 8) or an NCD (Chapter 9). Certainly, primary care plays a key role during the acute phase of the illness, but it also is crucial to successful tertiary care. The goal of tertiary prevention is to minimize the complications or sequelae to NCDs. All NCDs carry a risk of lifelong complications.

Nurses are familiar with the macro- and microvascular changes that occur if diabetes is not well controlled. A cerebral vascular accident or myocardial infarction can occur in the patient with uncontrolled hypertension or hyperlipidemia. It is the follow-up, management, and education of the patient with an NCD in primary care that reduce this risk. Reduction of risk of possible complications occurs through the careful evaluation of the patient done on a set schedule of appointments. However, care recommendations made to a patient are based not only on patient-specific data but also on population-level data. For example, the recommendations that the diabetic patient on insulin should be seen every 3 months and the diabetic patient on oral agents should be seen every 4 to 6 months are based on the epidemiological evidence that these time frames provide adequate coverage for the average patient. However, specific patients may need to be seen more often based on the management of their disease. This schedule of care minimizes complication by a careful evaluation on the success of the current plan of care or the opportunity to adjust the interventions.

Management of Noncommunicable Diseases

As reviewed in Chapter 9, management of NCDs is an essential component of care aimed at reducing the associated morbidity and premature death. For example, patients with diabetes require long-term management related to regulation of blood sugar, medications, foot care, diet, and exercise. Although management of diabetes is most frequently delivered to the individual, a population approach is also required. Primary care nurses rely on already developed health education materials to help teach their patients how to self-manage their disease. However, not all materials work across populations because of a lack of cultural relevance or health literacy levels (see Chapter 2). Based on one literature review, development of self-management interventions in populations with low income or low health literacy need careful review. Those that were most effective included three to four self-management skills especially when teaching patients to learn problem-solving skills.[24] The application of public health science in a primary care setting does not always require time-consuming, sophisticated studies. It can often be accomplished using simple assessment tools.

Case Management

Visits to primary care allow health-care workers to reinforce health education and answer questions. It is this follow-up that establishes the trust and provides the basis for outcomes that will improve the patient's overall health and well-being. To help guide this effort, nurses in primary care often use a case management approach. According to the Case Management Society of America, **case management** is "a collaborative process of assessment, planning, facilitation, and advocacy for options and services to meet an individual's health needs through communication and available resources to promote quality cost-effective outcomes."[25] Case management involves the monitoring and managing of a patient's health needs. The role can be designated in different ways. A case manager can be diagnosis-focused (diabetes, heart failure, multiple sclerosis), patient type-focused (homeless, older adult, obese, pediatric), or site-focused (hospital, clinic, shelter).

Nurse case managers actively participate with their clients to identify and facilitate options and services for meeting individuals' health needs to reduce fragmentation and duplication of care.[26] Contemporary case management began in the 1970s to assure both quality outcomes and cost containment.[27] The essence of case management is the incorporation of the client, the family, and the community in meeting the needs of the patient. Case management has a positive impact on cost containment and improves patient outcomes.[25-27] This focus on patient outcomes improves the quality of patient care and, therefore, the overall health of the community.

Public Primary Care

Primary care occurs in public settings such as health clinics run by public health departments, federally qualified health centers, and free clinics. Not all public health departments have primary care clinics, and most are located in urban areas. Federally qualified health centers provide health care to underserved populations on a sliding scale and have received grants under section 330 of the Public Health Service Act. These clinics qualify for enhanced reimbursement from Medicare and Medicaid. They must also provide comprehensive services.[28] These primary care settings are funded at the federal, state, or local level and aim to improve access to primary care for populations who have limited resources.

Another source of primary care for the underserved population is a free health clinic. The National Association of Free Health Clinics says the following about free health clinics:

> Free clinics are volunteer-based, safety-net health-care organizations that provide a range of medical, dental, pharmacy, and/or behavioral health services to economically disadvantaged individuals who are predominately uninsured. Free clinics are 501(c)(3) tax-exempt organizations or operate as a program component or affiliate of a 501(c)(3) organization. Entities that otherwise meet the previous definition, but charge a nominal fee to patients, may still be considered free clinics provided essential services are delivered regardless of the patient's ability to pay.[29]

These organizations are not directly supported by public funds and depend heavily on a volunteer workforce.

The ACA, enacted in 2010, brought an increased focus on primary care and the need to build the workforce. In 2010, the Department of Health and Human Services announced the availability of $250 million aimed at increasing the number of health-care providers working in primary care, especially in clinics that provide care to underserved populations. Congress has reduced this funding through changes to the ACA. One of the major aims of the ACA was to increase access to primary care with the goal of reducing the morbidity and mortality related to untreated disease and lack of preventive care.

Increasing the capacity of public primary care through public health clinics helps to provide care to those with limited access. One of the challenges for these clinics is matching care to the resources available to promote and protect health. Once again, nurses who restrict themselves to the individual level of care miss opportunities to maximize the ability of a community to support healthy living. In the case of one primary care nurse, the identification of the lack of nutritional resources led to a communitywide effort that far exceeded her initial one-on-one health education with her patients.

● APPLYING PUBLIC HEALTH SCIENCE

The Case of the Nurse Who Thought She Lived in the City—Not the Desert

Public Health Science Topics Covered:

- Assessment
- Collaboration
- Health planning

Katherine, a nurse, lived and worked in the inner city for many years. "I'm a city girl," she would often say, explaining that she could get whatever she needed in the city. However, she heard that there was a problem with hunger in the city. She noticed an article that discussed inner-city nutrition and the article used the term *food desert*. From a public health perspective, a **food desert** is a large, often isolated, geographical area where there is little or no access to the food needed to maintain an affordable and healthy diet.[30] In many major cities, large grocery stores are closing their doors in inner-city neighborhoods, especially poor neighborhoods, thus limiting access to fresh produce, food varieties, and nutritional choices. In the United States, food deserts tend to be in urban and rural low-income neighborhoods, where residents are less likely to have access to supermarkets or grocery stores that provide healthy food choices.

Through her review of the literature on food deserts, Katherine discovered that an increasing number of communities had few food retailers or supermarkets that regularly stocked fresh produce, low-fat dairy, whole grains, and other healthy foods.[31,32] This phenomenon has been slowly occurring over time with the movement of people out of the city, the economic downswing, and the loss of jobs. The 2008 Farm Bill directed the U.S. Department of Agriculture (USDA) to study food deserts in the United States, assess their incidence and prevalence, identify characteristics and factors causing and influencing food deserts, and determine the overall effect of food deserts on local populations.[33] Based on this, the USDA was asked to provide recommendations for addressing the causes and effects. There has been little improvement in accessibility to food, which results in poor nutrition that in turn affects the overall health of the individual. Seventy-five retailers opened 10,000 new locations between 2011 and 2015, and only 250 of those were in the country's food deserts.[30] A USDA report found that not only do low-income people have less access to healthy food, it costs more if they do have access. Nearly 10% of the U.S. population is low income and lives more than a mile from a grocery store with healthy options. There are some "convenient" markets in these locations, but they do not have fresh fruits and produce. Coupled with either the lack of transportation or the cost of transportation, you truly can be stranded on a desert island in the middle of the city when it comes to food.

Katherine realized that a major supermarket had left the community in which her clinic is located, and she wondered about the impact. With this on her mind, she began to ask the patients in the primary care clinic where she worked a simple question: "Where do you shop for food?" The responses of the patients began to identify this as a real concern. The convenience store or fast-food restaurants were the most common answers. The patients explained lack of transportation as the main reason for shopping at the convenience store even though the prices were higher. Ms. Reid, an older adult patient, related how hard it was for her to get on the bus and carry groceries home. James told Katherine that the convenience store was close by but so expensive that he could not purchase much food. The most disturbing comment came from Mary, the mother of four children, who said, "I know my children need fresh fruits and vegetables, but I cannot get that around here." All the patients, in one way or another, felt the impact of living in a "desert." Katherine did further reading and found that the economic and nutritional sequelae to this loss of access to supermarkets were far reaching. It is well documented that dietary choice may reverse or lessen the disease burden of many NCDs as well as prevent communicable diseases.[30-33]

When the choice is limited to red meats, fatty foods, added fats, desserts, and sweets, there is a substantially increased risk for obesity, type 2 diabetes, and heart disease.[34] The effect goes across the life span, affecting adults, older adults, and the younger population. The growth and development of the child and adolescent are compromised by the unavailability of quality foods. The long-term effect for the younger population is twofold; it affects their health, certainly, but it also provides a pattern of eating that will be detrimental for the rest of their lives. The goal of adequate nutrition in childhood is to prevent nutritional disorders such as malnutrition and obesity, as well as the increased morbidity and mortality that accompany them.[35] Nearly one in three children are overweight or obese, which puts them at risk for chronic long-term conditions that will negatively affect their health through their life span. Snack, convenience, and fast foods as well as sweets continue to dominate food advertisements viewed by children. The marketing of these items contributes to the fast-food consumption of U.S. children.[35,36] Children spend more time, an average of 44.5 hours per week, in front of a television, computer, and/or game screen; that's more than any other activity except sleeping.[36,37] They are repeatedly exposed to advertisements and often cannot distinguish between an advertisement and programming.[37] The other issue is the use of restaurants as opposed to cooking healthy food in the home. According to

the National Restaurant Association, in 2017,[38] 48% of the food dollar was spent in a restaurant with a total intake of $799 billion dollars spent at a restaurant.

Katherine and the other nurses at her clinic reviewed HP objectives related to nutrition and weight status and found a new objective. The goal was listed as "promote health and reduce chronic disease risk through the consumption of healthful diets, and achievement and maintenance of healthy body weights". To achieve this goal of a healthful diet and healthy weight, HP 2020 stated that it must encompass increasing household food security and eliminating hunger.[39]

Based on this, the nurses decided to attack this problem on two fronts. They realized that education must take place to inform and advise the patients on the importance of good nutrition. In addition, because the lack of availability of the food was a serious barrier to healthy eating, the food desert in their community needed to change first. Katherine decided to investigate ways to get a neighborhood farmer's market into the city. She learned that this concept helps bring fresh produce, eggs, and meats to the city as well as helps the small farm owner.[40] It can also be a method to develop local gardens, new business, employment, and camaraderie in a neighborhood. In a project in Florida, a town with issues such as elderly, no transportation, multiple chronic conditions, and no local store suffered from a severe food desert. They decided to make a change and developed a community garden. The results showed a true effect on the social determinates of health: increased access to fresh foods, increased physical activity, creation of social ties, and a greater feeling of community.[41] She realized that this was something doable and contacted a group in New York City, Greenmarket, to find out where to start. Greenmarket began in 1976 with 12 farmers and one farmers' market located in Manhattan. It grew to 54 markets and 230 family farms and fishermen.[42] The registered nurse group that Katherine worked with on this project used what they learned in their undergraduate public health nursing courses to tackle the problem. They knew they had to begin with an assessment but had little time in their busy clinic schedules to do this. One of the more recent graduates of a local school of nursing suggested that they enlist the help of the students and the nearby school of nursing. They added a member of the nursing faculty from the school to their planning group. The faculty member agreed to have students who were taking their public health nursing practicum help conduct the assessment and contribute to the planning and evaluation stages of the project. The nurses now had a team.

The team began with a geographical assessment of their community and the surrounding area, plotting the location of fast-food restaurants, convenience stores, and the closest supermarkets (see Chapter 4). They then plotted the public transportation routes. To help with the assessment, they asked members of the community to join their team. The community members described the realities of trying to shop for food. With the help of the community members, they conducted a more formal survey of the patients coming to their clinics, asking about their nutritional intake and for information on where they purchased their food. This provided them with baseline data.

Using the data from their community-specific assessment, the team constructed a viable plan to bring farmers' markets into the community, which included measurable objectives, impact, and outcomes (see Chapter 5). The plan included organizing local food cooperatives and farmers' markets to set up sites in the neighborhoods. Once availability of the food was in place, the group of nurses supplemented their nutritional education for patients with added knowledge of what was available in the community. They provided their patients with pamphlets and information about the new offerings. They put up posters in their office. After 6 months, they reissued their survey and found that the nutritional intake had improved, and patients reported easier access to healthy foods through the farmers' markets. Thus, Katherine's concern as well as application of basic public health assessments and program planning resulted in a change of the health of an entire neighborhood.

Private Primary Care

Primary care is also provided through private practices. Providers include physicians, NPs, nurses, and other health-care providers. Private practices do not receive direct federal support, but most accept payment through federal programs such as Medicaid and Medicare. The financial structure is based on a fee-for-service model. However, the delivery of care is the same. Again, the nurse must be attuned to the larger context of the community in which the patients of the clinic live. This understanding helps the nurse identify issues that require intervention at the community level.

▶ **SOLVING THE MYSTERY**
The Case of the Wobbly Men
Public Health Science Topics Covered:
- Surveillance and case finding
- Epidemiology
- Communication

Madelyn, a nurse who works as the intake nurse at the primary care office in Rivertown, Ohio, began her busy day reviewing the schedule. She noticed that James T., a 45-year-old male, was on the schedule again for a chief complaint of "feeling weak, a wobbly gait, and his wife says he is irritable." Madelyn recalled that James was at the clinic last month with a similar complaint, and he was not the only one. She wondered why the local men had been visiting the office so often recently. Usually, it is very difficult to get this age bracket of men into the office for risk prevention and routine checks. James was the fifth man this week with a similar complaint.

As she did the initial intake of James T's history, she noticed a listing of symptoms that she had heard recently from the other five middle-aged male patients. The complaints of weakness, unsteady gait, and feeling depressed and irritable were new for these patients. She decided to explore this change in the usual patient population. She realized that these symptoms can be attributed to many different diagnoses, but it was the similarity of the symptoms in a specific group of male patients in the same age group that got her attention.

Madelyn pulled the charts of all five of the men with similar chief complaints and started on a basic public health mission, looking for anything that might link these five men. They did not live on the same street, and they worked at different jobs. She then called each of the men and asked them other questions to try and find a link between them. She found one very quickly when she asked whether they knew each other. They reported that they had formed an informal fishing group and fished regularly for relaxation. Because most of their wives did not like to clean the fish or cook it, they ate most of the catch the same day on the boat. The rest they cleaned themselves and froze for eating during the week. They regularly caught Rock Bass, Smallmouth Bass, and Yellow Bullhead. They also threw back the smaller fish, even those that met regulations, and sought the bigger fish. When asked how many times a week they ate fish that they had caught, they replied that they ate between three and four meals per week. For Madelyn, the common denominator across this patient population was the ingestion of large quantities of river fish over the past few years. She found no other common denominator. She remembered hearing something about freshwater fish being contaminated with chemicals. She reviewed the men's symptoms again and noticed that the symptoms pointed to mercury poisoning. Madelyn's attention to detail and her understanding of basic epidemiology led her to a possible solution to the puzzle of the wobbly men. She explained her conclusions to the physician and the two NPs who worked in the clinic with her. She shared her information with the providers in the office, who then followed up on her recommendation to test the men for mercury poisoning. When the levels came back elevated in excess of 20 mcg/L (normal value is less than 5 mcg/L), the providers were able to initiate appropriate treatment. Madelyn also made a call to the county public health department to alert them to the cluster of cases.

Mercury poisoning has been around for centuries and noted as early as 1500 BC in Egyptian tombs. In the manufacture and processing of felt hats in the 18th and 19th centuries, chronic exposure of workers to the mercury used to process the felt led to the term "mad as a hatter." Mercury in any form is toxic. Exposure can be via ingestion, vapor inhalation, injection, and absorption through the skin.[43,44] The presentation of symptoms relates to the most commonly affected systems, which

are the neurological, gastrointestinal, and renal systems. The concentration of mercury is very low in most foodstuffs (below 0.02 mg Hg/kg). However, certain types of marine fish (such as shark, swordfish, and tuna) and certain fish taken from polluted freshwaters (such as pike, walleye, and bass) may contain high concentrations of mercury (Fig. 15-4).[44] In this setting, mercury is almost completely in the form of methylmercury. It is not uncommon that concentrations of methylmercury in these fish are 1 mg/kg or even higher.[44] Organic mercury can be found in three forms—aryl, short-chain, and long-chain alkyl compounds. Once absorbed, the aryl and long-chain alkyl compounds convert to their inorganic forms and possess similar toxic properties to inorganic mercury. The short-chain alkyl mercurials are readily absorbed in the gastrointestinal tract (90%–95%) and remain stable in their initial forms. Alkyl organic mercury has high lipid solubility and distributes uniformly throughout the body, accumulating in the brain, kidney, liver, hair, and skin. Organic mercurials also cross the blood-brain barrier and placenta and penetrate erythrocytes, attributing to neurological symptoms, teratogenic effects, and high blood to plasma ratio, respectively.[44]

The presentation of acute mercury poisoning includes burning of the throat, edema of oral mucous membranes, abdominal pain, vomiting, bloody diarrhea, and

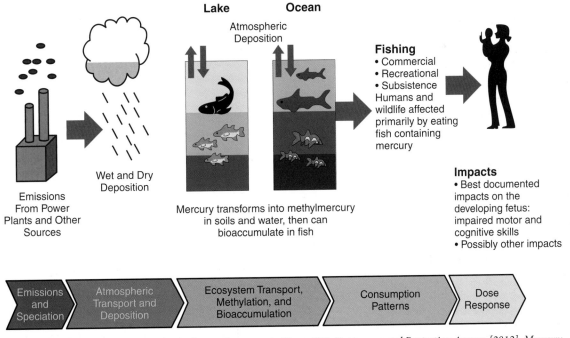

Figure 15-4 How mercury enters the environment. *(From U.S. Environmental Protection Agency [2012]. Mercury in your environment.)*

shock.[43] Chronic mercury poisoning, which these men were experiencing, causes weakness, ataxia, intentional tremors, irritability, and depression. Exposure to alkyl (organic) mercury derivatives from contaminated fish or fungicides used on seeds has caused ataxia, convulsions, and catastrophic birth defects.[43] Without a complete history, mercury toxicity, especially in older adults, can be misdiagnosed as Parkinson's disease, senile dementia, metabolic encephalopathy, depression, or Alzheimer's disease.[45] It is imperative to do a thorough history that includes occupation, hobbies, and level of seafood intake if clinical suspicion includes mercury exposure.

Based on her own research and her discussion with the public health department, Madelyn found that the Environmental Protection Agency (EPA) (see Chapter 6) released regular reports on the safety of freshwater fish with recommended levels of consumption (Table 15-3).[46] For the river flowing through Rivertown, the recommendation for consumption of Rock Bass, Smallmouth Bass, and Yellow Bullhead was one meal per month. These men were consuming 12 to 16 times more than the recommended amounts. Madelyn was concerned that, although this information was available on the Web site, the information was not getting out to the community.

Madelyn decided to contact the other two primary care groups in Rivertown and ask them whether they have seen anyone with similar complaints. The two other offices reported that they had, for a total of eight more patients, all male and all between aged 35 to 60. She joined forces with the nurses in these two clinics and proposed to the health department that a public campaign be launched to alert fishermen to the potential danger of eating a large quantity of fish caught in the local river. One of the men being treated told Madelyn that he belonged to a local fish and game club that had recently organized in the community. The nurses asked this club to help spread the word, thus reducing the risk of mercury poisoning in their community. Madelyn provided a valuable service to her community, not only because she solved the problem of the wobbly men, but also because she took it to the next step and worked at preventing more cases.

TABLE 15–3 ■ EPA Advisory Table: Small selection of Bodies of Water in Ohio

Body of Water	Area Under Advisory	Species	One Meal per Month or Two Months	Contaminant
Dicks Creek	Cincinnati – Dayton Road, Middletown to the Great Miami River (Butler County)	All species	Month	Mercury, Polychlorinated biphenyls (PCBs)
Great Miami River	Lowhead Dam at Monument Avenue (Dayton) to mouth (Ohio River) (Butler, Hamilton, Montgomery, Warren Counties)	All Suckers	Month	Mercury, PCBs
Little Scioto River	State Route 739, near Marion to Holland Road, near Marion (Marion County)	All species: Common Carp, Black Crappie, White Sucker 16" and over	Month	PCBs and PAHs
Lake Erie	All Waters (Ashtabula, Cuyahoga, Erie, Lake, Lorain, Lucas, Ottawa, Sandusky Counties)	Channel Catfish, Common Carp 27" and over, Lake Trout	2 Months	PCBs
		Chinook Salmon 19" and over, Coho Salmon, Common Carp under 27", Freshwater Drum, Smallmouth Bass, Steelhead Trout, White Bass, Whitefish, White Perch	Month	PCBs
		Brown Bullhead, Largemouth Bass	Month	Mercury

Source: (46)

Emerging Primary Care Public Health Issues

Public health issues that challenge primacy care continue to emerge. For example, issues with insufficient supply of flu vaccine or it not being affective against the flu are problematic. In a time when we want all people to be immunized, it shakes the faith of people in the effectiveness and can undermine usage of the flu vaccine. Widespread administration of the flu vaccine promotes herd immunity. Herd immunity means if a significant proportion of a population are vaccinated (the herd) it provides a measure of protection for individuals who are not able to receive the vaccine.[47] For example, if a person undergoing chemotherapy for cancer has a low white count and a compromised immune system, she is susceptible to the flu but not able to take the flu shot. If she is surrounded by people who are protected, she too will be protected because she has less of a chance being exposed to it. This requires that primary care nurses remain on top of the public health information.

Some public health issues reflect the emergence of health problem that can have a devastating effect on the community. A current problem is the opioid epidemic (see Chapter 11). This is an especially difficult problem for providers and health-care workers in primary care. Opioid comes from[48] the word opium, and these drugs were developed to replicate opium's pain-reducing properties. There are legal painkillers like morphine, oxycodone, or hydrocodone and illegal drugs like heroin or illicitly made fentanyl and carfentanil. Fentanyl is 100 times more powerful than morphine, and carfentanil is 10,000 times more potent than morphine; when these are added to heroin, the loss of life increases. How did this all start and why do people continue to use when they almost die from it? These are important questions that need to be understood so you can help your patient and their families try and understand.

Hydrocodone and oxycodone are semisynthetic opioids manufactured in labs with natural and synthetic ingredients. Between 2006 and 2014, the most widely prescribed opioid was hydrocodone (Vicodin). In 2014, 7.8 billion hydrocodone pills were distributed nationwide, and the second most prevalent opioid was oxycodone (Percocet). In 2014, 4.9 billion oxycodone tablets were distributed in the United States. The International Narcotics Control Board reported that, in 2015, Americans represented about 99.7% of the world's hydrocodone consumption.[49]

Those are staggering numbers, and they are where the problems begin. Looking at the management of pain historically gives us some insight. This is not the first opioid epidemic that has occurred with increased use; records show epidemics occurring as early as 1840.[50] The national supply of opium and morphine soared by 538% before the end of the 19th century, and those using were a diverse population. It included soldiers, persons with an alcohol use disorder, mothers and children, and Chinese immigrants. The model individual with an opioid use disorder was a native-born white woman with a chronic painful disorder; most were exposed to opium with child birth. In an interesting twist of history, heroin was first produced in 1898 by Bayer and was thought to be less addictive than morphine so it was used for people addicted to morphine. One reason that this first epidemic occurred was because cures for painful diseases were scarce. With the invention of the morphine injectable, it was easier to use and more effective. However, the institution of public health cleaned up some of the squalor that had caused the diarrhea and other diseases treated with opium; this helped to get the epidemic under control. In 1924, the Anti-Heroin Act banned the production and sale of heroin in the United States, and the prescribers of that time were educated against the practice. Later in the 20th century, transient nonmedical heroin use in urban areas affected disproportionately inner-city minority populations. In 1970, the Controlled Substance Act became law which created groupings (schedules) of drugs based on the potential for abuse.[50]

Heroin is a schedule 1 drug whereas morphine, fentanyl, oxycodone (Percocet, OxyContin), and methadone are schedule II. So how are we in the state today of such staggering loss of life related to opioid abuse? It starts with a drug company that did a small study in 1986. The study was of 38 patients with chronic pain who were treated with opioid pain relievers (OPR), and it was concluded that these were safe for long-term use. In 1995, this study was used as the advertising campaign to introduce the medication OxyContin, an extended release formulation of oxycodone. By 1996, the rate of opioid use was accelerating rapidly. Between 1996 and 2002, the manufacturer funded more than 20,000 pain-related educational programs through direct sponsorship or financial grants to encourage OPR use for non-cancer patients. This company provided financial support to the American Pain Society, American Academy of Pain Medicine, Federation of State Medical Boards, Joint Commission, and patient groups who then all advocated for more aggressive identification of and treatment of pain with OPRs.

In 1995, the American Pain Society introduced the campaign of "pain is the 5th Vital Sign" embraced by Veterans' Affairs health system and Joint Commission to increase identification and treatment with OPRs.

There was caution about imprudent prescribing, but it was overshadowed by assertions that the risk of tolerance and addiction were low, and abuse should not constrain prescribing.[50] Exaggerated benefits of long-term use of OPR was put forth without any high-quality long-tern clinical trials being conducted. Customer satisfaction was a Joint Commission survey criterion, and it may have influenced a study showing that physicians prescribed high-dose opioids in more than 50% of 1.14 million nonsurgical hospital admissions from 2009-2010. On May 10, 2007, the federal government brought criminal charges against the pharmaceutical company for misleadingly advertising OxyContin as safer and less addictive than other opioids.[50]

How does opioid misuse constitute a public health crisis? The National Institute on Drug Abuse estimates:[50]

- Half of all young people who inject heroin turned to it after abusing painkillers
- Three in four new heroin users start out using prescription drugs
- Overdose deaths related to heroin increased 533% between 2002 and 2016 from an estimated 2,089 in 2002 to 33,219 in 2016
- Every day, more than 90 Americans die after overdosing on opioids

The CDC estimates that the total "economic burden" of prescription opioid misuse alone in the United States is $78.5 billion a year, including the costs of health care, lost productivity, addiction treatment, and criminal justice involvement. Roughly 21% to 29% of patients prescribed opioids for chronic pain misuse them, and between 8% and 12% develop an opioid use disorder. It is crucial for primary care nurses and PHNs to understand the effect of this crisis. We need to think about who is at risk. It can be anyone: teens, college students, middle-aged adults, elderly adults, medical users of OPRs, or nonmedical users of OPRs.

We understand the physiology of pain, but what happens to cause addiction? The use of OPRs affects the reward circuit of the brain. The drug floods the brain with dopamine causing the person to feel pleasure, which is motivation to repeat the behaviors. Unfortunately, over time the brain adjusts to the excess dopamine resulting in tolerance, and the patient needs more and more to reach the desired high. This circuit is permanently changed, and other functions such as learning, judgment, decision making, stress, memory, and behaviors are affected.[51]

This change in circuitry leads to addiction, and overcoming that addiction is difficult for many. There is no one factor that means someone will develop an opioid use disorder; it is a combination of genetics, environment, and when they start. The issue is now what can be done. As with the first epidemic, we need to educate prescribers and the public. In primary care, it is imperative to screen appropriately, prescribe appropriately, and help patients recognize potential problems. Also, it is necessary to note any increases in "need or request" for more medications or unscheduled refills.[52] It is important for offices to use a state-wide automated reporting system, if available, to cut down on multiple medications and inappropriate refills. Having a contract with patients regarding opioid use is imperative as well as urine drug screens. Another important component is the overall reduction of the use of nonmedical OPR use and the issue of diversion concerns, that is, when persons who have been legally prescribed OPRs transfer this controlled substance to another person for illegal use.[52]

Many people think that they should never have pain and that there is a "pill" for everything; we need to educate our patients regarding appropriate use. The key recommendations for practice in primary care include:

- Identify cause of pain: History, assessment, testing, diagnosis
- Assess risk factors for medication use
- Appropriate for level of pain, physiologic risk to kidneys, liver, GI, history of abuse
- Use nonopioid analgesics when possible
- Scheduled as opposed to prn better control pain
- Use of adjunctives
- Avoid the use of extended release OPRs
- Limit supply to 3-5 days (some states have specified time)
- Reduce patient exposure and reduce the supply of OPRs in the home

Pain management guidelines,[53-57] patient education,[58] patient follow-up, and thoughtful care of the patient's needs are all factors that can help to manage the current crisis.

Ongoing Use of Public Health Science in the Primary Care Setting

Nurses working in primary care consistently apply public health science to their practice. This includes trending disease and risk factors in the community they serve. They do not have to collect the data themselves. They can use local, state, and national public health surveillance data to help identify significant trends in the population they serve. In addition, primary care nurses who actively employ public health communication skills will build a partnership with the community and key stakeholders.

Tracking Health Trends in the Community Served

Many issues, such as the opioid crisis, require a population perspective to effectively treat the individual. For example, recent trends might show a rise in emergency department admissions for exacerbations of asthma. Members of the community, such as parents, school teachers, or PHNs, raise the question—Why is there an increase? Upon investigation by these members of the community, it is discovered that a new factory has opened that manufactures aromatics released into the air. There is a direct correlation between this change in the environment and the rise in asthma exacerbations. A community seems to have a higher incidence of a certain cancer than another, and the cause must be addressed.

A rise in the population complaining of back and foot pain because they started a new job at a warehouse is evidence that education on proper body mechanics is needed. The community-focused approach to problems has patient/public education at its heart, and nurses as educators are foundational to the success of these programs. Knowing the community means understanding their needs, values, education level, and what is important to them. When this part of the community can be identified, the best approach can be developed, and success will occur. To develop a plan without the input and buy-in from a community will cause a weak foundation and result in failure.

Health-Care Policy and Primary Care

Due to funding available through the ACA, there has been an increased focus on the use of community health centers (CHCs). The ACA provided funding for existing and new CHCs and enabled them to serve an estimated 28 million new patients by 2018.[59] The CHCs were launched in 1965 by the Office of Economic Opportunity as part of Lyndon Johnson's War on Poverty. They were designed to reduce or remove the health-care disparities among the poor, racial and ethnic minorities, and the uninsured. The plan was that the governance of these facilities be centered in the host community. There are more than 8,000 urban and rural sites in every state and territory. They are federally funded but must meet budget requirements and offer services according to an economic sliding scale. CHCs are dedicated to the delivery of primary medical, dental, behavioral, and social services to the underserved populations, and they have

demonstrated their ability to provide care in a comprehensive fashion.[60] This may explain the influx of patients. The CHC core values coincide with the **patient-centered medical home (PCMH)** concept. The PCMH is built on the premise of a holistic approach that encompasses accessible, coordinated, and team-driven delivery of primary care that relies on outcome measurement and evidence-based practice.

Another issue is the inclusion of the medical home in the ACA. The PCMH is a model or philosophy of primary care that drives primary care excellence. The features of a Medical Home include: (1) patient-centered, (2) comprehensive, (3) coordinated, (4) accessible, and (5) committed to quality and safety. These five functions of a medical home are listed in more detail in Box 15-2.[61] The ACA includes the medical home as one of the required quality measures. Individuals with an NCD covered under Medicaid may choose a PCMH, which can be an individual provider (such as a CHC or comprehensive primary care clinic) or a health team. This PCMH would provide the care needed

---

BOX 15–2 ■ **Association for Health Care Research and Quality: The Medical Home Encompasses Five Functions and Attributes**

The five functions and attributes of the medical home are as follows:

1. **Patient-centered:** A partnership among practitioners, patients, and their families that ensures decisions respect patients' wants, needs, and preferences, and that patients have the education and support they need to make decisions and participate in their own care.
2. **Comprehensive care:** Team of care providers is wholly accountable for a patient's physical and mental health-care needs, including prevention and wellness, acute care, and chronic care.
3. **Coordinated care:** Care is organized across all elements of the broader health-care system, including specialty care, hospitals, home health care, community services and supports.
4. **Accessible:** Patients are able to access services with shorter waiting times, "after hours" care, 24/7 electronic or telephone access, and strong communication through health IT innovations.
5. **Committed to quality and safety:** Clinicians and staff enhance quality improvement to ensure that patients and families make informed decisions about their health.

Source: Patient-Centered Primary Care Collaborative. (2018). *Defining the medical home.* Retrieved from https://www.pcpcc.org/about/medical-home

to manage the NCD and could include care management, care coordination, health promotion, transitional care, family support, and referral to community and social support services when needed. The medical home should also use health information technology to link services.[62]

■ EVIDENCE-BASED PRACTICE
Patient-Centered Medical Home

Practice Statement: A PCMH is based on the integration of patients as active participants in their own health and well-being.

Targeted Outcome: Improved health outcomes, increased ability to self-manage NCDs, prevention of both NCDs and communicable diseases, improved quality of health care, and decreased health-care costs.

Evidence to Support: The move to a PCMH is a core concept in the ACA. Crabtree and colleagues[1] pointed out that, based on their own 15-year program of research, successful transformation of primary care settings to a PCMH model is unlikely to be successful unless a stronger theoretical foundation is established.[1] The evidence to support PCMH is growing.[2,3] Key aspects of PCMH included organizational access and increased knowledge as well as the interpersonal skills of the provider.[4,5] However, findings related to the effectiveness of PCMHs remains mixed.[6,7]

Sources

1. Crabtree, B.F., Nutting, P.A., Miller, W.L., McDaniel, R.R., Stange, K. C., Jaen, C.R., & Stewart, E. (2011). Primary care practice transformation is hard work: Insights from a 15-year developmental program of research. *Medical Care, 49,* S28-S35. doi:10.1097/MLR.obo13e318cad65c
2. Meo, N., Wong, E., Sun, H., Curtis, I., Batten, A., Fihn, S.D., & Nelson, K. (2018). Elements of the Veterans Health Administration patient-centered medical home are associated with greater adherence to oral hypoglycemic agents in patients with diabetes. *Population Health Management, 21*(2), 116-122. doi:10.1089/pop.2017.0039
3. Shippee, N.D., Finch, M., & Wholey, D. (2018). Using statewide data on health care quality to assess the effect of a patient-centered medical home initiative on quality of care. *Population Health Management, 21*(2), 148-154. doi:10.1089/pop.2017.0017
4. Bilello, L.A., Hall, A., Harman, J., Scuderi, C., Shah, N., Mills, J.C., & Samuels, S. (2018). Key attributes of patient-centered medical homes associated with patient activation of diabetes patients. *BMC Family Practice,* 191-8. doi:10.1186/s12875-017-0704-3
5. Platonova, E.R., Warren-Findlow, J., Saunders, W., Hutchison, J., & Coffman, M. (2016). Hispanics' satisfaction with free clinic providers: An analysis of patient-centered medical home characteristics. *Journal Of Community Health, 41*(6), 1290-1297. doi:10.1007/s10900-016-0218-2
6. Chou, S., Rothenberg, C., Agnoli, A., Wiechers, I., Lott, J., Voorhees, J., ... Venkatesh, A.K. (2018). Patient-centered medical homes did not improve access to timely follow-up after ED visit. *American Journal of Emergency Medicine, 36*(5), 854-858. doi:10.1016/j.ajem.2018.01.070
7. Marsteller, J.A., Hsu, Y.J., Gill, C., Kiptanui, Z., Fakeye, O.A., Engineer, L.D., ... Harris, I. (2018). Maryland multi-payor patient-centered medical home program: A 4-year quasiexperimental evaluation of quality, utilization, patient satisfaction, and provider perceptions. *Medical Care, 56*(4), 308-320. doi:10.1097/MLR.0000000000000881

Communication and Collaboration

One of the standards in public health nursing is collaboration. One of the characteristics of collaboration is that the nurse partners with key individuals, group, coalition, and organizations to effect change in public health policies, programs, and services to generate positive outcomes.[63] This standard holds true for the primary care nurse. Nurses working in primary care settings enhance their practice when they build collaborative relationships with these entities. In each of the case studies presented in this chapter, primary care nurses needed to communicate and collaborate with individual members of the community, with organizations, and with other stakeholders. The building of these relationships takes time and requires a conscious effort to do so that goes beyond creating a list of referrals for patients. It means building strong partnerships and requires specific skills. Although this is not unique to primary care nurses, there are partnerships that should be a part of every primary care nurse's practice.

Community Organizations

A good starting point is the local public health department (see Chapter 13). Primary care health providers are required to report certain diseases to the public health department (Table 15-4). This system is a good starting point and can be a two-way street. For example, some communicable diseases are rare enough that they may be missed during the first assessment, but if the primary care nurse knows that there has been an increase in a particular disease, the level of suspicion increases. Then, if a patient comes into the primary care clinic, the nurse is more apt to be on the alert for symptoms that match that disease.

Many initiatives begin with the local public health department and require buy-in by primary care providers.

TABLE 15–4 ■ Classification of Common Class A Notifiable Diseases Into Disease Type

Bloodborne (Excludes HIV/AIDS)	Enteric/Food-Borne	Vaccine Preventable	Sexually Transmitted	Other
Hepatitis B	Campylobacteriosis	Hepatitis A	AIDS	Aseptic meningitis
Hepatitis C	Cryptosporidiosis	Measles	Chlamydia	Meningococcal disease
	Giardiasis	Mumps	Gonorrhea	*Haemophilus influenzae*
	Escherichia coli 0157:H7	Pertussis	Syphilis (primary,	Tuberculosis
	Listeriosis		secondary, latent,	Legionellosis
	Salmonellosis		congenital)	Streptococcal group A,
	Shigellosis			invasive
	Yersiniosis			

Developing a relationship with the public health department brings a primary care clinic into the public health arena and increases the likelihood that the clinic's patients will benefit from these initiatives. Primary care nurses are in the "trenches" and often have a good grasp of the health issues faced by their patients. Collaborating with the public health department can result in the building of population-level initiatives that build on the experiences of the primary care nurses. This two-way communication can have a powerful effect on community-level public health that will work in the field.

There are a multitude of organizations with which primary care nurses can build a relationship to help better serve their patients. These include but are not limited to governmental organizations, other health-care providers, churches, community groups, and other primary care providers. Most student nurses learn how to conduct a community assessment (see Chapter 4), but once the course is completed, they fail to apply it when they move out into the real world of nursing care. In primary care, the community assessment component is essential. Consider the cases presented in this chapter. The nurses in these cases tapped into the resources available from various organizations such as the housing authority and the EPA.

Often, the collaboration can result in the building of coalitions. The role a primary care clinic can play in these coalitions is substantial. If a community wishes to address a specific health issue such as lead poisoning or secondary smoke exposure, the primary care setting is ideal for screening, distribution of health education materials, and other health protection and promotion activities.

Community Members

The primary care setting is not an island but exists within a community. Again, the lessons learned related to community assessment are essential to the primary care setting. The success of a primary care clinic depends on the trust built between the clinic and the population it serves. This requires reaching out to the community, not just persons in leadership positions such as a mayor or a school superintendent, but residents of the community. What is the nature of the community? Is it rich, poor, urban, suburban, or rural? How many people live in the community served by the clinic and what proportion uses the clinic? What are the age groups? What is the ethnic background of the community? These questions and more help to build a picture of the community and help primary care nurses tailor the services provided to the patients being served.

A case in point is a public primary care clinic located in a community of subsidized housing. This clinic operates on a first-come, first-served basis, using a sliding scale fee. The community is on the city bus line but is on the outskirts of the city and built next to the city landfill. It is also located close to a major interstate. The population is made up primarily of younger families, and there are no major grocery stores within walking distance. The nearest grocery store requires a transfer from one bus to another. The clinic is the only one in the community, and other clinics require at least one bus transfer to get to, but many residents opt to go to other clinics rather than to the clinic in their neighborhood.

The nurses working in the clinic struggle with a full waiting room, crying children, and clients who complain about the long waits. What can the nurses do? Where should they start? Contacting a few members in the community is a good place to start. This is the first step to looking outside the clinic, finding out what the residents think about the clinic, and beginning to work on ways to solve the problems. In this example, potential issues could include the long waiting times for mothers who do not have access to day care and must bring their children with them. The nurses providing the care might not fully understand the culture within the community. Another possibility is the perception of public assistance. If the nurses at the clinic begin to build a relationship with the community, they will include the community in solving these issues and truly form a partnership. These partnerships can result in multiple interventions that improve the health of all, not just those who come in for care on a given day. Without these partnerships, the primary care nurses may continue to create barriers to care without realizing it.

Public health science makes a strong contribution to the effectiveness of primary care nursing. It provides primary care nurses with the skills needed to be full members of the public health team, even if their focus is care of the individual and the family. Through active participation in disease surveillance and the building of partnerships with other organizations and the community itself, primary care nurses contribute to the health of the community in powerful ways.

Culture and Primary Care

As in any setting where nursing care is provided, culture is an important aspect of the provision of primary care. Cultural issues not only play a part in the assessment and development of a plan of care but also affect the availability of resources for the family and the community. Because primary care clinics are located in a community, it is important for the primary care providers to learn about the culture of their community. Patients seek health care within the context of their own culture, and that culture affects how they perceive illness, birth, and death. Learning about the culture of a community can be challenging, especially if the community is made up of culturally diverse populations. However, this process is essential to meet cultural competence requirements.

■ CULTURAL CONTEXT

Providing care to immigrant populations illustrates the complexity of integrating culture into the primary care setting. In Cincinnati, Ohio, a group of refugees from the small country of Burundi settled in a poor, largely African American community within the city. These refugees came from a different climate and did not share in the culture of the predominant group in the community. They experienced acculturation issues as they tried to fit in their new country. For the most part, they were young families and needed primary care services. However, they did not speak English and had low literacy in their own language. The primary care-givers located in the community had to not only locate an interpreter but also become knowledgeable about the health practices and beliefs of the Burundians. Aspects of the Burundian culture important to the delivery of care included understanding gender roles with women responsible for child care and housekeeping yet highly respected for their life-giving role. Kinship constitutes the core of Burundi social units with women becoming assimilated by their husband's family. Children are highly valued. Incorporating these cultural components into the care of Burundians seeking treatment, such as building on close kinship ties, will improve the success of interventions offered by primary care providers.

The patient does not need to be from another country to be from another culture. Often people in our own communities feel marginalized due to race, poverty, or other differences. Understanding the sensitive issues of the lesbian, gay, bisexual, and transgender populations (see Chapter 7), and providing opportunities for patients to provide information within a safe environment, is imperative to gaining trust. The trust needed to truly "hear" what the patient is saying begins at the first moment of the patient visit. Asking questions that are gender-neutral and done without judgment will allow the patient to completely have their needs met. If a patient feels that their health-care giver is judgmental, trust will not be formed. It is imperative to treat all with the respect and dignity that each human deserves. When we do that, we will be able to learn about all peoples and construct a safe environment.

Application of the community assessment approach described in Chapter 4 is essential if primary care–level interventions are going to be effective. The primary care provider, located in the community, is in an excellent position to gather this information and gain partners in developing culturally relevant interventions. Each day coming to work, the provider can observe the community by performing a brief windshield survey (see Chapter 4). Individuals and families can develop trusting relationships with the nurses who work in primary care settings, because this is often their only interaction with the health-care system. This is where they come for their physical checkups, where they bring their children for care, and where they go first when they do not feel well. An understanding of the cultural context of the persons seeking primary care enhances a nurse's ability not only to provide care to individuals and families but also to develop programs such as an immunization program. Failure to consider the culture of the persons served can result in poor follow-up care, miscommunication, and failure to build that essential trusting relationship.

▌ Summary Points

- Primary care in the United States is a delivery system, and primary health care from the WHO perspective is a movement to bring about health-care reform that will result in achieving equitable health care for all.
- Primary care encompasses all levels of prevention: primary, secondary, and tertiary.
- In the United States, primary care occurs in public settings such as health clinics run by public health departments as well as in private settings such as private practices and hospital-run clinics.
- Primary care is often the first line of action for emerging health issues such as the opioid epidemic.
- Primary care involves policy, advocacy, and collaboration in an effort to address public health issues and enhance the health of populations.
- The importance of primary care is growing along with the introduction of the PCMH.

▼ CASE STUDY
Measles Vaccination Program for Parents

Learning Outcomes

At the end of this case study, the student will be able to:

- Apply principles of descriptive epidemiology to trend a disease over time.
- Describe the steps taken to develop an intervention.
- Discuss national current recommendations for vaccination.

In 2018-2019, there was an increase in measles cases across the United States, particularly in New York City, with predictions that the incidence rate would be the highest it had been in that state for 50 years. Across the United States, efforts were made not just to immunize children but also to immunize adults. You have been assigned the task of developing a vaccination program for the parents and children who attend your public health well-baby clinic. Begin with the current incidence rates in the city or county nearest to you for measles in both children and adults. Then determine

the recommendations for immunizations on the CDC Web site located at https://www.cdc.gov/measles/vaccination.html

Based on your findings and building on what you learned about health assessment and planning in Chapters 4 and 5, develop a vaccination program for the clinic. Be sure you include the following:

- A summary of the incidence rates for your city or county compared with those for the state and the nation
- Have the incidence rates increased or declined in the past 5 years?
- Which population is at greatest risk?
- Current immunization recommendations from the CDC
- A plan to inform clinic patients and their families about vaccination that includes:
  - Communication methods (e.g., TV, flyers, school newsletters)
  - Cultural considerations
  - Other communication strategies
- A mechanism for handling potential increase in demand
- A plan to deal with a possible outbreak

REFERENCES

1. World Health Organization. (2008). *Primary health care: Now more than ever.* Geneva, Switzerland: Author.
2. Caley, M. (2013). Remember Barbara Starfield: Primary care is the health systems bedrock. *The BMJ, 347,* f4627.
3. Association of American Medical Colleges. (2018). *The complexities of physician supply and demand projections from 2016-2030.* Retrieved from: https://aamc-black.global.ssl.fastly.net/production/media/filer_public/85/d7/85d7b689-f417-4ef0-97fb-ecc129836829/aamc_2018_workforce_projections_update_april_11_2018.pdf.
4. Davis, M., Anthopolos, R., Tootoo, J., Titler, M., Bynum, J., & Shipman, S. (2018). Supply of healthcare providers in relation to county socioeconomic and health status. *Journal of General Internal Medicine, 33*(4), 412-414. doi: 10.1007/s11606-017-4287-4. Retrieved from https://www.sciencedaily.com/releases/2018/02/180227125629.htm.
5. World Health Organization. (2018). *World Health Day 2018: Universal health coverage: everyone, everywhere.* Retrieved from http://www.emro.who.int/media/news/world-health-day-2018-universal-health-coverage-everyone-everywhere.html.
6. American Academy of Family Physicians. (2018). *Primary care.* Retrieved from https://www.aafp.org/about/policies/all/primary-care.html.
7. U.S. Department of Health and Human Services. (2018). *Healthy People 2020 topics and objectives: Access to health services.* Retrieved from https://www.healthypeople.gov/2020/topics-objectives

8. U.S. Department of Health and Human Services, Healthy People 2020. (2017). *Healthy People 2020 midcourse review: Chapter 1: Access to health care services.* Retrieved from https://www.cdc.gov/nchs/data/hpdata2020/HP2020MCR-C01-AHS.pdf.

9. World Health Organization. (2018). *Global conference on primary health care: Achieving universal health coverage and the sustainable development goals.* Retrieved from http://www.who.int/primary-health/conference-phc/en/.

10. UNICEF. (2015). *UNICEF: Strategy for Health 2016-2030.* Retrieved from https://www.unicef.org/health/files/UNICEF_Health_Strategy_Final.pdf.

11. Every Woman Every Child. (2015). *Global strategy report for women's, children's, and adolescents' health 2016-2030.* Retrieved from http://globalstrategy.everywoma neverychild.org/pdf/EWEC_globalstrategyreport_200915_FINAL_WEB.pdf.

12. UNICEF. (2016). *One is too many: Ending child deaths from pneumonia and diarrhoea. Key findings.* Retrieved from: https://data.unicef.org/wp-content/uploads/2016/11/Pneumonia_Diarrhoea_brochure.pdf.

13. Centers for Disease Control and Prevention. (2018). *Smoking and tobacco use: Data and statistics.* Retrieved from: https://www.cdc.gov/tobacco/data_statistics/index.htm.

14. Centers for Disease Control and Prevention. (2018). *Smoking and tobacco use: Electronic cigarettes.* Retrieved from https://www.cdc.gov/tobacco/basic_information/e-cigarettes/.

15. World Health Organization. (2108). *Health promotion.* Retrieved from http://www.who.int/topics/health_promotion/en/.

16. Centers for Disease Control and Prevention. (2018). *National Diabetes Statistics Report, 2017.* Retrieved from https://www.cdc.gov/diabetes/pdfs/data/statistics/national-diabetes-statistics-report.pdf.

17. U.S. Department of Health and Human Services, Office of Minority Health. (2018). *Diabetes and American Indians/Alaska Natives.* Retrieved from https://minorityhealth.hhs.gov/omh/browse.aspx?lvl=4&lvlid=33.

18. Hsueh, W.C., Bennett, P.H., Esparza-Romero, J., Urquidez-Romero, R., Valencia, M.E., Ravussin, E., ... Hanson, R.L. (2018). Analysis of type 2 diabetes and obesity genetic variants in Mexican Pima Indians: Marked allelic differentiation among Amerindians at HLA. *Annals of Human Genetics, 82*(5), 287-299. doi: 10.1111/ahg.12252.

19. Centers for Disease Control and Prevention. (2018). *Vaccine recommendations: Health care workers.* Retrieved from https://www.cdc.gov/flu/faq/health-care-workers.htm.

20. Centers for Disease Control and Prevention. (2018). *Vaccines and immunizations schedules.* Retrieved from http://www.cdc.gov/vaccines/schedules/easy-to-read/adult.html.

21. Lane A., Martin, M., & Neuman, M.E. (2009). Breast cancer screening program targeting rural Hispanics in southeastern Indiana: Program evaluation. *Hispanic Health Care International, 7*(3), 153-159.

22. Centers for Disease Control and Prevention. (2018). *Act against AIDS.* Retrieved from https://www.cdc.gov/actagainstaids/campaigns/lsht/index.html.

23. Centers for Disease Control and Prevention. (2018). *HIV screening: Standard care.* Retrieved from https://www.cdc.gov/cancer/breast/.

24. Schaffler, J., Leung, K., Tremblay, S., Merdsoy, L., Lambert, S.D., Belzile, E., & Lambrou, A. (2018). The effectiveness of self-management interventions for individuals with low health literacy and/or low income: A descriptive systematic review. *Journal Of General Internal Medicine, 33*(4), 510-523. doi:10.1007/s11606-017-4265-x.

25. Case Management Society of America. (2018). *Glossary: Case management.* Retrieved from http://www.cmsa.org/about-cmsa/.

26. Nursing Explorer. (2018). *Case management nurse.* Retrieved from https://www.nursingexplorer.com/careers/case-management-nurse.

27. Cesta, T. (2017). *What's old is new again: The history of case management.* Retrieved from https://www.ahcmedia.com/articles/141367-whats-old-is-new-again-the-history-of-case-management.

28. U.S. Department of Health and Human Services. (2018). *Federally qualified health centers.* Retrieved from https://www.cms.gov/center/fqhc.asp.

29. National Association of Free & Charitable Clinics. (n.d.). *What is a free or charitable clinic.* Retrieved from http://www.nafcclinics.org/content/nafc-history.

30. Soergel, A. (2015, December 7). Millions of food desert dwellers struggle to get fresh groceries. *U.S. News & World Report.* Retrieved from https://www.usnews.com/news/articles/2015/12/07/millions-of-food-desert-dwellers-struggle-to-get-fresh-groceries.

31. Ver Ploeg, M. (2017). *Access to affordable, nutritious food is limited in food deserts.* Retrieved from https://www.ers.usda.gov/amber-waves/2010/march/access-to-affordable-nutritious-food-is-limited-in-food-deserts/.

32. Centers for Disease Control and Prevention. (2017). *A look inside food deserts.* Retrieved from https://www.cdc.gov/features/FoodDeserts/index.html..

33. U.S. Department of Agriculture. (2018). *Access to affordable and nutritious food-measuring and understanding food deserts and their consequences.* Retrieved from https://www.ers.usda.gov/data-products/food-access-research-atlas/documentation/.

34. Ohlhorst, S., Russell, R., Bier, D., Klurfeld, D., Zhaoping, L., Mein, J., ... Konopka, E. (2013). Nutrition research to affect food and a healthy life span. *The American Journal of Clinical Nutrition, 98*, 620-625.

35. American Heart Association. (2014). *Dietary recommendations for healthy children.* Retrieved from http://www.heart.org/HEARTORG/HealthyLiving/Dietary-Recommendations-for-Healthy-Children_UCM_303886_Article.jsp#.W3w3E_ZFw2w.

36. McManus, K. (2016). *The impact of food advertising on childhood obesity.* Retrieved from http://prowellness.vmhost.psu.edu/impact-food-advertising-childhood-obesity.

37. Campaign for Commercial Free Childhood. (n.d.) *Food marketing & childhood obesity.* Retrieved from http://www.commercialfreechildhood.org/issue/food-marketing-and-childhood-obesity.

38. National Restaurant Association. (2017). *Pocket fact book.* Retrieved from http://www.restaurant.org/Downloads/PDFs/News-Research/Pocket_Factbook_FEB_2017-FINAL.pdf.

39. U.S. Department of Health and Human Services. (2018). *Healthy People 2020: Nutrition and weight status.* Retrieved from https://www.healthypeople.gov/2020/topics-objectives/topic/nutrition-and-weight- status.

40. O'Connor, K. (2017). *Farmers market brings affordable produce to food deserts.* Retrieved from https://www.seattletimes.com/nation-world/farmers-market-brings-affordable-produce-to-food-deserts/.

41. Diaz de Villegas, C. & Rodriguez, K. (2015). *Medley food desert project.* Retrieved from https://www.epa.gov/sites/production/files/2016-05/documents/floridainternational universitymedleyfooddesertproject.pdf.

42. Greenmarket. (n.d.). *Greenmarket farmers.* Retrieved from http://www.grownyc.org/greenmarket.

43. Olsan, D.A. (2017). *Mercury toxicity.* Retrieved from http://emedicine.medscape.com/article/819872-overview.

44. U.S. Environmental Protection Agency. (2018). *Mercury in your environment.* Retrieved from http://www.epa.gov/hg/exposure.htm.

45. McPhee, S., & Papadakis, M. (2018). *Current medical diagnosis & treatment* (ed 57, pp 1611-1612). New York, NY: McGraw-Hill.

46. Ohio Environmental Protection Agency. (2018). *2018 Ohio sport fish health and consumption advisory.* Retrieved from http://www.epa.ohio.gov/dsw/fishadvisory/index.aspx.

47. Vaccines Today. (2018). *What is herd immunity?* Retrieved from https://www.vaccinestoday.eu/stories/what-is-herd-immunity/.

48. National Institute on Drug Abuse. (2016). *Understanding drug use and addiction.* Retrieved from https://www.drugabuse.gov/publications/drugfacts/understanding-drug-use-addiction.

49. Kolodny, A., Courtwright, D., Hwang, C., Kreiner, P., Eadie, J., Clark, T., & Alexander, G. (2015). The prescription opioid and heroin crisis: A public health approach to an epidemic of addiction. *Annual Review of Public Health, 36,* 559-74.

50. Mihm, S. (2017, July 17). This isn't the first opiate addiction crisis. *Bloomberg.* Retrieved from https://www.bloomberg.com/view/articles/2017-07-17/this-isn-t-the-first-u-s-opiate-addiction-crisis.

51. National Institute on Drug Abuse. (2018). *Drugs, brains, and behavior: The science of addiction.* Retrieved from https://www.drugabuse.gov/publications/drugs-brains-behavior-science-addiction/drugs-brain.

52. Politico Staff. (2016). *The opioid crisis: Changing the culture of prescribing.* Retrieved from https://www.politico.com/story/2016/03/opioid-crisis-prescriptions-working-group-221350.

53. American Academy of Family Physicians. (2013). *Acute pain guidelines.* Retrieved from http://www.aafp.org/afp/2013/0601/p766.html.

54. Centers for Disease Control and Prevention. (2016). *Chronic pain management.* Retrieved from https://www.cdc.gov/mmwr/volumes/65/rr/rr6501e1.htm

55. Chou, R., Gordon, D.B., de Leon-Casaola, O.A., Rosenberg, J.M., Bicker, S., Brennan, T., ... Wu, C.L. (2016). Management of postoperative pain: A clinical practice guideline from the American Pain Society, the American Society of Regional Anesthesia and Pain Medicine, and the American Society of Anesthesiologists' Committee on Regional Anesthesia, Executive Committee, and Administrative Council. *The Journal of Pain, 17*(2), 131–157. doi: 10.1016/j.jpain.2015.12.008

56. American Association of Colleges of Nursing. (2016). *Understanding the opioid epidemic: The Academic Nursing Perspective.* Retrieved from http://www.aacnnursing.org/Portals/42/Policy/Newsletters/Inside%20Academic%20Nursing/June-2016.pdf.

57. American Academy of Nurse Practitioners. (2018). *Education tools: Opioids.* Retrieved from https://www.aanp.org/education/education-toolkits/opioids-and-other-controlled-substances.

58. Junquist, C., Vallerand, A., Sicoutris, C., Kwon, K., & Polomano, R. (2017). Assessing and managing acute pain: A call to action. *American Journal of Nursing, 117*(3), Supplement 1-4.

59. National Association of Community Health Centers. (2018, August 12). *Community Health Centers August 2018.* Retrieved from http://www.nachc.org/wp-content/uploads/2018/08/AmericasHealthCenters_FINAL.pdf.

60. Vogt, H.B., Tinguely, J., Franken, J., Ten Napel, S. (2018). Community health centers in the Dakotas, 2018. *South Dakota Medicine, 8,* 355-360. doi:10.1056/NEJp1003729.

61. Patient-Centered Primary Care Collaborative. (2018). *Defining the medical home.* Retrieved from https://www.pcpcc.org/about/medical-home.

62. Patient-Centered Primary Care Collaborative. (2018). *PCMH success.* Retrieved from https://www.pcpcc.org/news-tags/pcmh-success.

63. American Nurses Association. (2013). *Public health nursing: Scope and standards of practice.* Silver Springs, MD: Author.

Chapter 16

Health Planning with Rural and Urban Communities

Paula V. Nersesian and Christine Savage

LEARNING OUTCOMES

After reading the chapter, the student will be able to:

1. Describe the unique characteristics of rural and urban environments.
2. Identify specific health needs of rural communities and of urban communities.
3. Discuss potential solutions to decrease disparities in rural areas.
4. Define and implement the concepts of community partnership, community linkage, and community collaboration.
5. Describe the steps in community organizing and coalition building; identify how these activities can be a tool for positive community change.
6. Discuss the potential role of the nurse and the impact on the health-care system in community-based participatory research, parish nursing, healthy communities/healthy cities, nurse-managed clinics, and community academic partnerships.

KEY TERMS

Community empowerment
Community organizing
Community partnerships
Coalition building
Collaboration
Community-based participatory research (CBPR)
Federally qualified health centers (FQHC)
Metropolitan statistical area (MSA)
Patient-centered medical homes
Rural
Telehealth
Urban
Urban agglomeration

Nursing In Partnership with Communities

Community members and leaders want to create a healthy and welcoming environment for their residents. To accomplish this, they form partnerships with collaborators and stakeholders. Consider the example of Chicago's Walking School Bus Program.[1] Through a partnership among community members, the school system, the City of Chicago, and the police department's Chicago Alternative Policing Strategy (CAPS), a strategy was developed to protect children from drugs, guns, strangers, and traffic on their way to and from school. Children need a safe, secure environment at school and in their community. Partnerships with key stakeholders can make this happen. The walking school bus program provides adult supervision for children as they walk to and from school. Parents rotate the responsibility of walking children to and from school through a carefully managed volunteer system. By walking the same route each day, parent volunteers pick up children at specified locations, like school bus stops. By reducing the number of children being dropped-off at school in a private vehicle, traffic congestion around schools and the increased risks that come with it, are reduced. Other positive outcomes include physically active and healthier children and adults, reduced noise and air pollution, increased interaction among community members, more "eyes on the street," exposure to positive adult role models, healthier relationships between adults and children, and decreased incidence of bullying.[2] The benefits of partnerships are greater than what an individual can create alone.

Definition of *Partnership*

Community partnerships are collaborative working relationships between local organizations, government entities, and sometimes private companies to achieve common goals. The groups may have a long-lasting relationship and guide their efforts with a formal agreement.

Or they may be in a temporary alliance to achieve a time-limited objective. A search of the term "community partnerships" reveals a large number of groups that seek to attain objectives through partnerships. They may be focused on a subpopulation, such as children with disabilities, improvements in a school setting, or elimination of a communicable disease. Community partnerships are often needed for health-promoting community services as those efforts are often fragmented. Communication among health services, the education system, job placement services, and affordable housing organizations can be challenging. This calls for effective collaboration among these entities, so that they can work together and reach outcomes that they cannot reach alone.

Collaboration is an essential component of successful nursing interventions. **Collaboration**, as defined in The Intervention Wheel from the Minnesota Department of Health (Minnesota Wheel)[3] (Chapter 2), is an activity that "commits two or more persons or organizations to achieve a common goal through enhancing the capacity of one or more of the members to promote and protect health."[4] From a family perspective, a collaborative relationship exists when clients and nurses view each other as partners, with both providing expertise and knowledge that will help the family reach its goals. Interpersonal and communication skills are essential for successful collaboration. Partnerships are based on respect and equity, whether the partnership is between a nurse and a family or among multiple organizations. A successful partnership has synergy; it is larger than the sum of its parts. The participating agencies and their clients realize benefits that could not be achieved by a single organization. Successful partnerships are built on clear roles and responsibilities, a shared vision of desired outcomes, processes that are transparent, frequent open communication among members, and strategic use of resources.

The Center on Education and Training for Employment at The Ohio State University created a six-step guide that facilitates development of community collaboration by creating linkages among agencies.[5] By linking them together, client needs are served better because the emphasis is on community needs, not the needs of the individual agency.

Step 1: Assess the need to work in partnership with other agencies. The first step involves assessing whether an interagency partnership is needed and whether the local climate favors a partnership. Sometimes it's best to have a single agency solve local problems. Sometimes problems are best addressed or needs are best filled by the involvement of multiple agencies. Questions to help identify whether a partnership makes sense include: How might relationships with other agencies improve client outcomes? What challenges could be addressed more effectively through interagency linkages?

Step 2: State the key challenges; articulate why they are better addressed by multiple agencies; and name potential key players. Also, during this step, existing linkages are identified.

Step 3: Identify the key players. Narrow the potential key player agencies down to a priority list and name the people who will represent each agency. Agency representatives should either be decision makers or have access to their agency's decision makers to maximize efficiency and effectiveness of the group.

Step 4: Establish effective collaboration among the agencies. Cooperation is important, but not sufficient. Funders want to see evidence of collaborative efforts among the agencies. Coalitions that collaborate have a better chance of using resources effectively and producing better results.

Step 5: Create a harmonious planning environment among agencies and then establish mutual goals, objectives, and a plan that includes administrative support from all the partners.

Step 6: Implement the plan.[5]

Importance of Partnerships

Partnerships among collaborative agencies can improve client access to programs, referrals between agencies, coordination of limited resources, working relationships, and an understanding of the aims of each partner agency and how to work together.[5] Linkages between local health departments and community members often focus on a specific purpose or subpopulation. A collaboration between local health departments and communities can range from low levels of collaboration to high levels. To improve health-care coordination and utilization of resources, partnerships between health department officials and community leaders should be promoted so that community health priorities, objectives, and strategies can be set jointly.[6]

Formulating joint priorities, objectives, and strategies requires a robust partnership among the organizations. To build strategic partnerships, a range of skills is required. First, the lead organization must have a keen understanding of the type of partnership they desire. Then, they need to identify possible partners, develop a relationship, and negotiate the partnership. Finally, the partnership must be maintained in such a way that all parties enjoy benefits.[7]

● APPLYING PUBLIC HEALTH SCIENCE

The Case of the Polluting Incinerator

Public Health Science Topics Covered:

• Organized community effort
• Environmental science
• Public Health Nursing Skills
• Assessment
• Program planning
• Intervention: Advocacy

Federally qualified health centers (FQHC) are a critical component of the health-care safety net, and health centers that receive this designation receive funding support under Section 330 of the Public Health Service Act. There are more than 1,400 FQHC in the United States serving more than 26 million clients. The clinics are community-based and provide comprehensive primary care and behavioral and mental health services to patients regardless of their ability to pay.[8]

A public health nurse (PHN) who worked at an urban FQHC wanted to obtain additional resources to augment the services provided to the lower-income community members who attended the clinic. The PHN discussed her ideas with the professional staff at the clinic—primarily family nurse practitioners (FNPs) and primary care physicians. They were very supportive, discussed potential challenges, and encouraged the PHN to identify potential linkages with other agencies. They identified multiple agencies serving the community including a Head Start program, social service agencies, schools, and local community organizers. The PHN explored opportunities to link the efforts of the FQHC with these agencies to provide more comprehensive services to the clients at the FQHC.

The agencies all agreed that building a partnership with the FQHC would be advantageous, and several mentioned a newly formed group that included the identified agencies, community representatives, business owners, and religious leaders. The agency representatives said the group was quite diverse and that new members were welcome if they agreed to attend the meetings and make a commitment to the process. The PHN met with the social worker who started the group, and thereafter the PHN began participating.

The PHN was involved with the group for more than 4 years and learned a great deal about linkages and partnerships. When all the participants were sitting around a table, communication was clearer, and decisions were made. It became abundantly clear that forming partnerships took considerable time, trust had to be earned, and larger organizations had less flexibility. Making the process work was time-consuming and frequently frustrating, thus it required significant commitment.

Soon after the PHN joined the group, a community organizer and members of a small neighborhood in the larger community discussed their concerns about a municipal incinerator that deposited pollutants in their neighborhood. The participants representing the neighborhood affected by the incinerator expressed concern that representatives of the larger community had not challenged the placement of the incinerator. They felt that they were not invited to participate because the residents of their neighborhood were poor, had low education levels, and had no influence on city officials. The residents of the neighborhood said they tried to discuss the dangers associated with the incinerator with city representatives, but they felt ignored. Likewise, health department staff did not respond when information was presented to them. Everyone around the larger community table agreed that the incinerator was a public health menace. They also agreed that as a group they might be able to have an impact. The diversity of the partnership resulted in a wide range of actions. The community organizers considered how public demonstrations could show the city leadership how they felt. Other group members contacted faculty at the local university to request assistance in measuring air quality and identifying other health risks stemming from the incinerator. Other members of the group developed a social media campaign and explored other communication channels to get their message out. They were successful in accumulating many followers on social media, getting coverage in print newspapers, radio interviews, and television coverage. An issue that had been hidden was now quite public, and city officials ultimately shut down the incinerator. The outcome wasn't achieved quickly, but it was achieved, and the group was energized. They took on a specific issue and made a difference in their community.

Some members of the group who thought the effort was a waste of time recommitted to it after seeing that linking agencies and communities can result in meaningful change. By working together on a community issue, people got to know each other, developed trust, and communicated. Now they could see the possibility of organizing around other issues. While the PHN worked with the group, they convinced the police department to resume foot patrols in designated high-crime areas that had large numbers of robberies, aggravated assaults, and homicides. The police patrolled in pairs starting at 10 a.m. and stopping at 2 a.m. They engaged community members while on patrol and stopped suspicious cars and individuals. After initiation of the foot patrols, the crime rate dropped by 24% in the patrolled area, and there was little displacement of crime to nearby areas. All of the partners declared the foot patrol initiative a success.

The partnership set up other linkages, such as one with the high schools in their catchment area with the goal to decrease violence. After the first meeting, they determined that students needed tutoring. The group mobilized volunteers to support an after-school tutoring program at the school. It was clear that community concerns about student performance needed to be met before the school-based violence prevention program could be implemented.

This community group, flush with agency linkages, is intact and active. It became a respected model in the community and is enmeshed in working toward a healthier community that includes all the immediate and distal causes of poor health. No one agency could achieve this alone; it took partnerships, linkages, dedicated work, and authentic community participation.

This case demonstrates that the process of building a collaborative partnership is multidimensional and requires a long-term vision for change. Trust among collaborators is fostered over time. The appropriate group structure is not always immediately apparent; time and experience working together helps to clarify participant roles and ways to organize the group. Recognizing and mobilizing people to create change requires commitment over time and a focus on outcomes. Ensuring diversity by including people from a wide variety of backgrounds will help the group form a complete view of the community strengths and needs. It is essential to have participants invested in the goals and activities of the partnership.[7]

Rural Communities

People living in rural communities have strengths and needs that differ from people living in an urban environment. Statistical data show increased health disparities among residents of rural communities. These disparities reflect the economic opportunities, educational systems, social and cultural factors, and geographic isolation in rural areas. Demographic differences between rural and urban Americans are complex. For example, children living in rural areas have lower rates of poverty than their urban counterparts. However, more children are uninsured in rural areas compared to urban areas. Rural Americans are older and less likely to have a bachelor's degree.[9] The Health Resources and Services Administration (2018) Federal Office of Rural Health Policy points to several striking observations about the health of people who live in rural areas:

- About one-third of rural dwellers lose all of their teeth by age 65 for lack of dental services and fluoridation.
- Some 2,000 rural communities have only one pharmacist, who often is the only local health-care provider.
- Rural residents experience greater rates of chronic disease than any other segment of the U.S. population.
- Racial and ethnic minorities comprise 15% of the total rural population and 30% of the rural poor population.[10]

The National Rural Health Association represents more than 21,000 individual and organizational members in providing leadership on rural health issues. They track statistics and trends about the health of people living in rural areas to fulfill their mission of advocacy, communication, education, and research about rural health. The Association cites that, for individuals who live in rural areas of the United States:

- The patient-to-primary care physician ratio in rural areas is only 39.8 physicians per 100,000 people, compared to 53.3 physicians per 100,000 in urban areas.
- There are 22 generalist dentists per 100,000 residents in rural areas versus 30 per 100,000 in rural areas.
- On average, per capita income in rural areas is $9,242 lower than the average per capita income in the United States, and rural Americans are more likely to live below the poverty level than Americans in general.
- People who live in rural America rely more heavily on the Supplemental Nutrition Assistance Program (SNAP) …as 14.6% of rural households receive SNAP benefits, while 10.9% of metropolitan households receive assistance.
- Rural youths over the age of 12 are more likely to smoke cigarettes (26.6% versus 19% in large metro areas). They are also far more likely to use smokeless

tobacco, with usage rates of 6.7% in rural areas and 2.1% in metropolitan areas.

- Fifty-three percent of rural Americans lack access to 25 Mbps/3 Mbps of bandwidth, the benchmark for Internet speed according to the Federal Communications Commission.
- In rural areas, there is an additional 22% risk of injury-related death.
- Rural youth are twice as likely to commit suicide.[11]

Since 2004, stakeholders in rural areas have been informing priorities through the Rural Healthy People initiative. *Rural Healthy People 2010 (RHP 2010)* was a companion document to *Healthy People 2010 (HP 2010)* that identified unique needs of the rural population in the United States. The top concerns selected by respondents in the first round of *RHP 2010* was access to quality health care.[12] The document proved to be a valuable resource for policy makers, rural health providers, and rural communities for planning and policy making, so new survey data were collected between 2010 and 2012 following the release of *Healthy People 2020*. The rural health priorities for the *RHP 2020* changed from the earlier survey. The top five concerns, with access to quality health care still the number one priority, are shown in Table 16-1.[13,14]

TABLE 16–1 ■ Top 10 Priorities from *Rural Healthy People 2020 National Survey* by rank

Rank	Priority
1	Access to quality health services
2	Nutrition and weight status
3	Diabetes
4	Mental health and mental disorders
5	Substance abuse
6	Heart disease and stroke
7	Physical activity and health
8	Older adults
9	Maternal, infant, and child health
10	Tobacco use

Source: (13) and (14)

Bolin, J.N., Bellamy, G.R., Ferdinand, A.O., Vuong, A.M., Kash, B.A., Schulze, A., & Helduser, J.W. (2015). Rural Healthy People 2020: New decade, same challenges. *Journal of Rural Health, 31*(3), 326–333. https://doi.org/10.1111/jrh.12116.

Bolin, J.N., Bellamy, G., Ferdinand, A.O., Kash, B.A., Helduser, J.W. (Eds.). (2015). *Rural Healthy People 2020*. Vol. 1. College Station, Texas: Texas A&M Health Science Center School of Public Health, Southwest Rural Health Research Center.

■ RURAL HEALTHY PEOPLE (RHP)

The Promotion of the Health of Americans Living in Rural Communities

Goal: To identify rural health priorities and strategies

Overview: The purpose of *Rural Healthy People 2020 (RHP 2020)* is to advance the promotion of the health of Americans living in rural communities by identifying rural health priorities, supporting rural health leaders and researchers, and promoting effective rural health programs. Through the coordinated *RHP 2020* initiative, rural communities will benefit by increased ability to identify and implement right-sized, effective health programs for rural residents. Like *RHP 2010* a decade ago, *RHP 2020* provides policy makers, rural providers, and rural communities with a valuable resource to inform planning while also documenting successes and challenges. Specifically, *RHP 2020* identifies and promotes rural-specific health priorities; documents what is known about health in rural areas; identifies rural evidence-based best practice programs, community practices, and interventions; and promotes rural healthy communities.[13]

Midcourse Review of Healthy People 2020: Health disparities persist between urban and rural areas. The Midcourse Review of Healthy People 2020 analyzed data according to whether people lived in metropolitan areas (i.e., urban areas) or nonmetropolitan areas (i.e., rural areas). Disparities by geographic location were found for 339 of the 625 population-based trackable objectives. Populations in urban areas had more favorable rates than populations in rural areas for 65.8% of the 339 objectives that showed disparities.[15] This demonstrates the need for public health nurses to be vigilant in addressing the health needs of rural populations.

Health-care providers have additional challenges working in rural communities given their small numbers in relation to number of people served. In the United States, as in most countries, there is unequal distribution of health-care providers. Most often health-care providers stay in the metropolitan areas after they complete their education or purposefully select to settle in urban areas, attracted by well-resourced health-care centers, cultural and recreational opportunities, better housing, better work options for their family members, and a perceived higher quality of life for the family. In

2014, the Health Resource and Service Administration reported that there was a higher proportion of health providers living in rural areas that were from occupations requiring less education and training (e.g., emergency medical technicians) than those in occupations requiring more education (e.g., physicians). For example, in rural areas, there are 13.1 physicians per 10,000 population compared to 31.2 per 10,000 population in urban areas.[16]

Definition of *Rural*

Rural is defined based on population size, population density, or by proximity to larger metropolitan areas. Federal agencies, in defining a rural community, frequently first define an urban area and then, by exclusion, the remaining area is considered rural. The most commonly used definitions of *rural* come from the U.S. Census Bureau and the U.S. Department of Agriculture (USDA).

An urbanized area (UA) has a central city or core and a surrounding area that contains at least 50,000 people. According to the U.S. Census Bureau, areas that are not urban are considered rural. They can be in areas designated as metropolitan or nonmetropolitan. The term metropolitan is commonly used and is defined as an area and the population in a metropolitan statistical area (MSA). An MSA comprises an area that includes one or more counties with an urbanized core of at least 50,000 (Fig. 16-1).[17] People living in adjacent counties connected to the urban area as commuters are included in the MSA.[18]

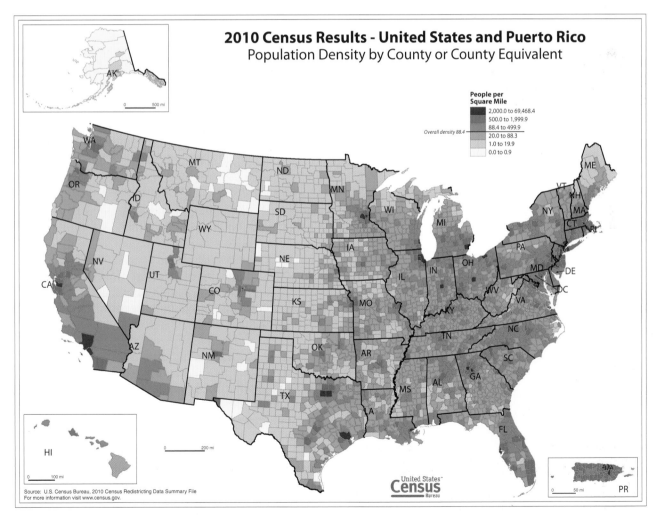

Figure 16-1 2010 Population Density by County or County Equivalent—United States and Puerto Rico. (*Retrieved from https://www2.census.gov/geo/maps/dc10_thematic/2010_Profile/2010_Profile_Map_United_States.pdf.*)

The USDA uses a code of 0 to 9 to differentiate urban and rural. Metropolitan counties are distinguished by size with a ranking of 0 to 3 and nonmetropolitan counties with 4 to 9. A code of 9 is equal to completely rural, or a population of fewer than 2,500 and not adjacent to a metropolitan area. In 2011, only 16% of the population was considered rural (51 million living in rural areas and 258 million in urban areas), the lowest ever; in 2000, 20% was rural, compared with 72% back in 1910.[19,20] Rural areas include open spaces and longer distances between neighbors (Fig. 16-2).

Specific Health Needs of Rural Communities

A major barrier to obtaining health care in rural settings is access. Residents of rural communities commonly travel long distances to access care, and tertiary care facilities are often even farther away. It is not uncommon for rural health facilities to have funding shortfalls and staffing challenges.[21] Local governments in rural areas often lack the resources and capability to establish safety net programs. Primary prevention resources such as gyms and hiker/biker trails are not commonly available, or they are located an inconveniently long distance away.

Potential Solutions to Decrease Health Disparities in Rural Areas

Addressing scope-of-practice barriers may increase the number of nurse practitioners in the rural areas and partially address the disparities faced by people living in rural areas. A recent study found that states with full scope-of-practice regulations had a higher supply of nurse

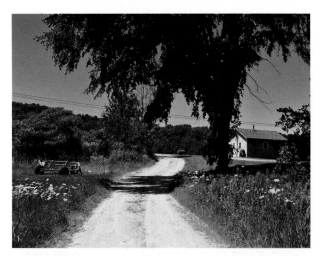

Figure 16-2 Rural landscape: Maine, U.S. *(Photo by Paula V. Nersesian, 2018.)*

practitioners in rural areas than states with more restrictive scope-of-practice.[22] The Affordable Care Act (ACA) (2010) provides incentives for educating and training health-care providers, including nurses and primary care nurse practitioners, to work in rural areas.[23] However, a survey of rural health clinics 4 years after passage of the ACA demonstrated challenges recruiting physicians, physician assistants, and nurse practitioners. The respondents anticipated an increase in their patient population accompanied by a feeling of being ill-prepared to work in an environment of value-based care.[24] This suggests that, despite the original intentions of the ACA, attempts to increase the number of health-care providers in rural areas may not have been successful.

Another strategy employed to meet the challenge of providing care in rural areas, especially for people with chronic illness, is the use of the **patient-centered medical home (PCMH)** model. The PCMH is an approach to primary care that aims to make care accessible, continuous, coordinated, family-centered, comprehensive, compassionate, and culturally competent. The main components of the model, as defined in the Bolin article,[25] include:

- Patient- and family-centered full scope of care
- Access in time and location
- Coordinated, team-based (integrated) care
- Medication coordination and management
- Community linkages with transition
- Electronic records and other information systems support

Bolin and colleagues suggest that using this model in rural communities would help address issues such as access, efficiency, quality, and sustainability. At the same time, it would increase linkages, improve integration of services, and achieve interdisciplinary practice. The ACA of 2010 was designed to contribute resources to facilitating the PCMH model in rural settings.[23,25] This is an innovative example of partnerships and linkages that can decrease rural health disparities. There is emerging evidence that it is successful in rural settings. In one rural Mississippi example, researchers found patients with chronic illness enrolled in a PCMH attend follow-up appointments more consistently than patients not enrolled in a PCMH.[26] PCMHs in rural areas face barriers to implementation linked to administration of electronic medical records and reimbursement, for example. Centralized health care systems, such as the Veterans Health Administration, do not face these obstacles and have a greater PCMH implementation in rural than urban areas.[27]

Telehealth, first developed in the 1970s, has also been shown to be useful in increasing access to health services, decreasing some of the costs of health care, and increasing the efficiency of providing the care. **Telehealth** is a broad term that includes using a telecommunication device to transfer information that enables a health-care professional to provide health-related services when there is a distance between client and health-care provider. Telehealth has been shown to decrease frequency of hospital visits and emergency department-initiated hospital admissions and to improve management of chronic illnesses. Nurses use telehealth services while providing home care, conducting health clinics, and delivering care in schools and prisons. Telehealth can also be used in hospitals to augment existing clinical services by obtaining expert opinion, for example.

Telehealth nursing is defined and explained in a fact sheet created by the members of the Telehealth Nursing Special Interest Group of the American Telemedicine Association.[28] The association describes how nurses use telehealth technology in a variety of practice settings. For example, nurses working in rural areas can tele-present a patient to a health-care provider at a higher-level facility when further assessment or treatment is needed. This can be done for conditions that are nonemergent and emergent. Home health nurses use monitoring systems that transmit physiological data (e.g., blood pressure, pulse, respiratory peak flow) and images through telephone lines or the Internet. Telehealth also includes routine communications such as when patients call their nurse to review how to give insulin or change a dressing. Nurses also play key roles in conceptualizing, designing, developing, and implementing telehealth innovations that benefit communities and their members. Nurse scientists are exploring communication technologies and their influence on health care and quality.

Urban Communities

Migration of people from rural to urban areas occurs worldwide. Sub-Saharan Africa and Asia have the highest rates of urbanization, which is the proportion of a national population living in urban areas, and urban population growth rates, which are the number of people living in urban areas. Rural-to-urban migration contributes to urbanization, but it has a limited contribution to urban growth, which is primarily attributable to natural population growth.[29] In 2014, the United Nations Department of Economic and Social Affairs estimated urbanization at 54% worldwide.[30] Migration occurs between countries, especially regionally, and within countries, sometimes to an extreme extent, such as in China where hundreds of millions of people living in rural areas have moved to urban areas for more favorable work opportunities. People also move to seek security and asylum, and others move to seek a better life for themselves and their families. A better life does not always result for people who end up living in urban areas, particularly those who reside in slums.[31]

■ CELLULAR TO GLOBAL

Much of who we are is embedded in our DNA, but our families, social settings, and physical environment also influence us. When faced with difficult experiences, changes can occur in our epigenome through epigenetic modification[32], our physiology, our relationships, and our communities. Difficult experiences, such as food scarcity, neglect, and war can have lasting effects on a person's epigenome and their community. Here, we examine the civil war in Syria, which began in 2011, and how it has affected communities. We do not know if the people who have been forced to move have epigenetic modifications, but their experience of community has most certainly changed. Millions of Syrians have been affected by the war. The United Nations estimates that at least 400,000 Syrians have died as a result of the war, and the number is likely much higher.[33] Six million people have been internally displaced, five million people have fled to neighboring countries in the Middle East and North Africa, about one million people are in Europe as refugees or asylees, and about 100,000 have sought refuge in North America.[34] Syria has a complex ancient and modern history, periodic droughts, limited arable land, and high population density. Their economic growth was around 2%, and income was about U.S. $5,000 gross domestic product per capita just before the war. This allowed Syrian families to enjoy relatively comfortable middle-class lives in urban and rural areas. They are well-educated and enjoyed high literacy levels.[35] The war changed all that for the millions of families that were forced to move. Now, Syrians are seeking to find safety, stability, and a means of survival. The extreme experiences faced by millions of Syrians will have lasting repercussions for individuals, families, and communities. Changes at the community level will be felt in the places that they left and the places where they ultimately reside. The biological aftermath of this tragedy may persist for a lifetime and possibly through generations via epigenetic modification.[36] For those who move to countries with cultures very different from their own, the impact on their lives will be pervasive. They will have to acculturate, build new social supports, integrate into schools, find new places of worship, learn new skills, obtain employment, and mourn great loss. And the existing members of their new communities—in rural and urban settings within the Middle East, Europe, and North America —will also face challenges as they welcome their new community members and seek to find a way for everyone to live in harmony.

The largest metropolitan areas are called **urban agglomerations**. They form when cities integrate. These urban clusters, which include all the built continuous UA within a specified location, may include several municipalities. This poses a challenge to elected officials and administrators tasked with addressing needs across jurisdictions, such as transportation. As agglomerations expand, they can cross international borders [37] such as the San Diego–Tijuana agglomeration spanning the United States and Mexico, and the one in Lille–Kortrijk spanning France and Belgium. Table 16-2 lists the 10 largest agglomerations in 1975 and 2000, and projecting to 2035. It is interesting to note the changes in location of the largest agglomerations and the significant increase in population for each of them.[38]

Definition of *Urban*

The U.S. Census Bureau defines **urban** according to the density of a population (Box 16-1).[39] A **metropolitan statistical area**, colloquially called a metro area, is a term used by the U.S. Office of Management and Budget to describe an UA and adjacent counties or county equivalents that link the population to the urbanized core through commuting ties. MSAs or metro areas have at least one urban core area of at least 50,000 residents. A central UA

TABLE 16–2 ■ Top 10 Largest Urban Agglomerations 1975, 2000, and Projected for 2035

Cities 1975	Millions of Inhabitants	Cities 2000	Millions of Inhabitants	Cities 2035	Projected Millions of Inhabitants
1. Tokyo, Japan	34	1. Tokyo, Japan	37	1. Delhi, India	43
2. Kinki M.M.A. (Osaka), Japan	19	2. Delhi, India	26	2. Tokyo, Japan	36
3. Ciudad de México (Mexico City), Mexico	17	3. Shanghai, China	23	3. Shanghai, China	34
4. New York-Newark, USA	17	4. Ciudad de México (Mexico City), Mexico	21	4. Dhaka, Bangladesh	31
5. São Paulo, Brazil	16	5. São Paulo, Brazil	21	5. Al-Qahirah (Cairo), Egypt	29
6. Mumbai (Bombay), India	14	6. Mumbai (Bombay), India	19	6. Mumbai (Bombay), India	27
7. Delhi, India	12	7. Kinki M.M.A. (Osaka), Japan	19	7. Kinshasa, Democratic Republic of the Congo	27
8. Kolkata (Calcutta), India	12	8. Al-Qahirah (Cairo), Egypt	19	8. Ciudad de México (Mexico City), Mexico	25
9. Al-Qahirah (Cairo), Egypt	12	9. New York-Newark, USA	19	9. Beijing, China	25
10. Buenos Aires, Argentina	12	10. Beijing, China	18	10. São Paulo, Brazil	24

Source: (38)
United Nations Population Division Department of Economic and Social Affairs. (2018). *World urbanization prospects*. Retrieved from
https://esa.un.org/unpd/wup/

is a contiguous area of relatively high population density. The counties containing the urbanized core are called central counties of the MSA. When the surrounding counties, called outlying counties, are strongly connected socially and economically to the central counties, they are included in the MSA.[40] Some outlying counties are actually rural in nature and are often called bedroom communities because people live in those areas and commute to the urban area. According to the 2010 Census, 84% of the U.S. population lived in metro areas. The five most populous metro areas were New York, Los Angeles, Chicago, Dallas-Fort Worth, and Philadelphia. The three least populous metro areas were all located in the Mountain Division of the U.S.: Carson City, NV; Lewiston, ID-WA; and Casper, WY.[41] And within metro areas, most people reside in cities—also called incorporated places.[40]

Health problems are present in both rural and urban areas. Although there are more documented health issues with higher morbidity and mortality in rural areas of the United States, the specific health problems of city-dwellers reflect the conditions of our cities. Medical historian David Rosner wrote, "One lesson from history is that we create our own environment and hence we create the conditions within which we live and die."[42] Health problems can arise and perpetuate from migration, crowded living conditions, poverty, homelessness, racism, and other social determinants of health. Creating a healthful environment can improve people's health in both rural and urban settings.

■ CULTURAL CONTEXT

UNESCO Global Report on Culture for Sustainable Urban Development [43]

The United Nations Educational, Scientific, and Cultural Organization (UNESCO) draws on the 2030 Agenda for Sustainable Development and its associated goals—the Sustainable Development Goals or SDGs—to identify entry points to address culture. They include SDG 2 (Zero Hunger), SDG 3 (Good Health and Well-being), SDG 4 (Gender Equality), and many others. Three policy areas categorize approaches to addressing culture in urban areas: people, environment, and policies. These drive the specific recommendation described in the *Global Report*. Health and well-being are subsumed in most if not all the recommendations, and standouts include enhancing the livability of cites, ensuring social inclusion, promoting a livable built and natural environment, improving resilience, regenerating linkages with rural areas, and promotion of a participatory process. These recommendations directly and indirectly affect health by improving access to green space for physical activity, to clean water, and to health services. They also foster opportunities for employment and social connections by promoting local culture and integrating people from diverse cultures.

BOX 16-1 ■ Definitions of Urban and Rural

U.S. Census Bureau Definitions

Urban: Areas of densely developed territory, specifically all territory, population, and housing units in urbanized areas and urban clusters. "Urban" classification cuts across other hierarchies except for census block and can be in metropolitan or non-metropolitan areas.

Urban area (UA): Collective term referring to urbanized areas and urban clusters.

Urban Cluster (UC): A densely developed territory that contains a minimum residential population 2,500 people but fewer than 50,000.

Urban Growth Area: Legally defined entity defined around incorporated places and used to regulate urban growth. They are delineated cooperatively by state and local officials and then confirmed by state law. UGAs are a pilot project, first defined for Census 2000 in Oregon, and added in Washington for the 2010 Census.

Urbanizacion: An area, sector, or residential development, such as a neighborhood, within a geographic area in Puerto Rico.

Urbanized Area: An area consisting of a densely developed territory that contains a minimum residential population of at least 50,000 people.

Rural: Territory, population, and housing units not classified as urban. "Rural" classification cuts across other hierarchies and can be in metropolitan or non-metropolitan areas.

Metropolitan: Refers to the area and population located in metropolitan statistical areas.

Metropolitan statistical area (MSA): A geographic entity delineated by the Office of Management and Budget for use by federal statistical agencies. Metropolitan statistical areas consist of the county or counties (or equivalent entities) associated with at least one urbanized area of at least 50,000 population, plus adjacent counties having a high degree of social and economic integration with the core as measured through commuting ties.

Source: (39)
U.S. Department of Commerce. (2018). *Glossary: United States Census Bureau.* Retrieved June 8, 2018, from https://www.census.gov/glossary/

Characteristics of the Urban Population

With our concern about how the public's health is related to urbanization, it is important to consider not only the number of people in an urban environment, but also the size, density, and economic status of the cities in which individuals live (Fig. 16-3). From a public health perspective, we look at the influence of upstream and downstream factors on urban living conditions and health disparities that result from environmental exposures. Too often, the interactions between culture, social factors, and the physical environment are not examined together to deconstruct the health disparities in urban settings.[44] Urban environments also have marked disparities in socioeconomic status (see Chapter 7), crime rates, violence (see Chapter 12), and psychosocial distress.[45] Mental health stressors and exposure to violence and trauma can cause or exacerbate mental health disorders (see Chapter 10). In densely populated areas, exercise resources may be limited, and air quality may be poor, which puts people with chronic respiratory disease at risk (Chapter 6). The American Lung Association's *State of the Air 2018* reports that 133.9 million people in the U.S. are exposed to unhealthy levels of ozone and particulate pollution, which increase the risk of lung cancer and decrease the life span.[46] A key feature of the ACA was to improve health insurance coverage for Americans, and it has largely achieved that outcome.[47] One study found that previously uninsured low-income adults who were eligible for subsidies under the ACA health insurance marketplaces had a significant decline in insurance rates.[48] Medicaid expansion also played a key role in increasing coverage. In states where Medicaid was expanded, the uninsured rate declined 56.7% between 2013 and 2017; in states where Medicaid expansion was not adopted, the uninsured rate dropped 25% in the same period.[47] In addition, the 2018 dissolution of the individual health insurance mandate may result in some self-employed people and families with low income dropping their coverage or switching to catastrophic plans that don't include the preventive services outlined in the ACA. Undocumented immigrants remain a hard-to-insure group because they are not included in any of the safety net programs and therefore they must either pay directly for services or obtain individual health insurance coverage, and both tend to be expensive.

Despite the barriers to insurance coverage, people living in urban areas have access to emergency department services, whether they are insured or not, given the substantial number of hospitals located in cities and their mandate to not turn people away. Urban areas also have more safety net services. These include FQHCs, health department clinics, community health centers, and specialty clinics. Living in cities also offers opportunities for social well-being and improved health of its residents. Urban areas also usually include more economic and educational options, access to diverse social networks, and more and better-quality health and social resources closer to the population. To reach diverse populations, decision makers and community partnerships should consider the cultures, values, and languages represented by members of the community. Listening to and understanding the needs of diverse populations in urban areas may improve efforts to provide critical resources because communities are influenced by the cultures they represent and the history of the residents.

Role of the Public Health Nurse

Community assessment, diagnosis, program planning, interventions, and evaluation are essential public health nursing skills for both rural and urban environments (see Chapters 4 and 5). The PHN either in an urban or in a rural setting seeks to build collective efficacy among community members. A community with strong neighborhood cohesion usually has residents willing to contribute to the common good, which can promote health. A cohesive group can access resources not available to individuals and can respond to threats from inside and outside the community. The community can form partnerships and linkages with local government, organizations, and other communities, increasing the possibility for positive change. This exemplifies social capital of a social group, which might be people in a workplace, within a voluntary organization, or in a residential community.

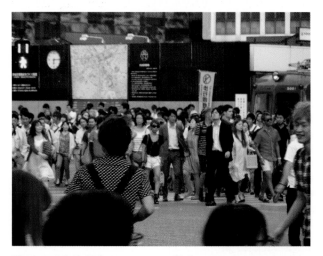

Figure 16-3 Urban cityscape: Tokyo, Japan. *(Photo by Paula V. Nersesian, 2012.)*

Within the social group, resources might include an ability to exchange favors, maintain group norms, and trust among members. These are attributes that can be enjoyed by individual group members or by the entire group. Research on social capital has demonstrated improved health outcomes in communities with higher levels of social capital.[49]

Community upheaval can occur in poor urban areas where the perception is that injustices have run unchecked or an injustice has occurred. An example of this upheaval is the riots in Baltimore following the death of Freddie Grey. This is an example of community violence (see Chapter 12). As is the case with community violence, businesses are often affected, disrupting the microeconomy, and buildings are often damaged beyond repair, requiring demolition. In some settings, communities remain damaged for decades before urban renewal occurs.

Sometimes gentrification occurs in these distressed neighborhoods often displacing residents with few resources to relocate. If not conducted in partnership with the local community, gentrification can force residents out of their lifelong neighborhoods as taxes rise with increasing property values. When people lose their homes and social network, they can experience significant stress and grief. Demolition of buildings can also expose community members to environmental threats such as lead, asbestos, and airborne particulates. Abandoned buildings that remain standing foster proliferation of rodents. When communities are disorganized, environmental and social problems flourish. The social milieu changes and resources become more difficult to obtain, which creates challenges in the conduct of daily life. Informal ties within a community are important to its functioning.

These factors are important to consider given the health inequities linked to whether you reside in a distressed or prosperous community. Several online interfaces allow exploration of these factors. The County Health Rankings and Roadmaps derives from a well-established framework developed by the University of Wisconsin Population Health Institute; it links physical environment, social and economic factors, clinical care, and health behaviors to health outcomes. The County Health Rankings and Roadmaps online interface contains comprehensive statistics for each county in the U.S.[50] Information about policies and programs, and the level of evidence to support them is also included.[51] The City Health Dashboard focuses exclusively on cities and includes 36 measures of social and economic factors, physical environment, health behavior, health outcomes, and clinical care. The project team has data for the 500 largest cities in the United States, which is designed for policy makers and community leaders.[52] The Distressed Communities Index measures seven metrics to describe communities in relation to education, income, employment, housing, and businesses. According to these metrics, in 2016 the number of Americans living in prosperous zip codes rose from 10.2 million in 2007 to 86.5 million. During that same time period the number of Americans living in distressed zip codes decreased by 3.4 million to a total of 50 million.[53]

Community Organizing and Public Health Nursing

Effective partnerships and community linkages may be the difference between sustained success in addressing public health needs—whether in urban or rural settings—and brief programs that fail to produce long-lasting favorable outcomes.

Community Organizing

Community organizing is a public health nursing activity in both rural and urban communities. It is a useful tool for creating positive change domestically and internationally.

Definition of Community Organizing

Using the knowledge and the definition of **community organizing** by experts in the field, the Minnesota Wheel[3] (Chapter 2) defines this activity as helping "community groups to identify common problems or goals, mobilize resources, and develop and implement strategies for reaching the goals they collectively have set."[3]

Minkler and colleagues pointed out the importance of including the concept of community empowerment as a logical component of community organizing. Without empowering the community, the organizing has not been successful.[54] The World Bank defines **empowerment** of communities as the social action "process of increasing the capacity of individuals or groups to make choices and to transform those choices into desired actions and outcomes."[55] A focus area of the World Bank's social development efforts is community-driven development (CDD). Essential elements of CDD include transparency, participation, local empowerment, demand-responsiveness, greater downward accountability, and enhanced local capacity.[56] It expands the concept of community empowerment and its elements of access to information by the community, inclusion and participation of community members in decision-making forums, power to hold the decision makers accountable, having the capacity and resources to organize, take on roles as partners with government and private agencies, and make decisions about things that affect their interests.[56]

Nurses and health-care providers utilize empowerment and community-driven development to help improve the health of communities. The actions taken include partnering with local groups such as religious congregations, local community centers, neighborhood associations, educational institutions, and civil rights and social justice organizations to help improve the health of communities. Amendola's (2011)[57] metasynthesis of empowerment of Hispanic and Latinx populations revealed that shared power with health providers and agencies and a sense of empowerment was possible to attain. Attaining these results required health-care professionals to incorporate strategies for empowerment into their practice. Davis' (2016)[58] work with people experiencing homelessness who have diabetes found that people who served as a peer educator for 4 weeks were empowered, and people who participated in the education sessions were found to be more knowledgeable about diabetes and how to manage it. Importantly, the sense of empowerment felt by peer educators decreased over time, albeit not significantly. Benoit's (2017)[59] work in Canada with sex workers had similar findings where empowerment and knowledge gains were reported after serving as a peer educator.

Usefulness as a Tool for Change

Community organizing is an important facet of public health nursing. When providing health education or introducing a new program or intervention, addressing community priorities and addressing their perceived needs is respectful and has a higher likelihood of success. In fact, the process of organizing a community and soliciting participation of community members in social action can contribute to improved health outcomes.[60]

Successful examples of community organizing go back to the 1900s in the U.S. when women successfully organized and obtained the right to vote, and when labor organizers established a 40-hour workweek. More recently, in the 1960s and 1970s, organizing took on the fight for civil rights and protested against the war in Vietnam. Current organizing campaigns have focused on LGBTQ+ rights, protection of natural resources, abortion rights, and efforts targeting racial discrimination such as the Black Lives Matter movement. Social media has transformed modern community organizing.

An inspiring example of community organization driving change occurred in Kwara State, Nigeria, where the local Community Social Development Agency advocated for and succeeded in bringing electricity to this rural area. Now, the residents can not only charge their phones easily, but they can also store food safely and study after the sun sets.[61] In the U.S., a community group in Maine uses resources from a tool box called *Resources for Organizing and Social Change*. The resources adhere to seven principles for creating social change through community organizing:

1. Use nonviolence in creating change.
2. Identify the root causes of the problems, look upstream, and create solutions that will improve the situation for everyone.
3. Provide communities an opportunity to work with each other and the support they need to solve their problems.
4. Address equity and basic needs of community members.
5. Facilitate the ability of people to gain power over their lives and the access they need to be involved in the decision-making processes that affect them.
6. Promote social equality by enabling participation and leadership roles for those who experience discrimination.
7. Build momentum in the movement for social change.[62]

Other suggestions on how to organize a community include doing something interesting or unique to attract the attention of community members so they engage in the process. Be sure your colleagues understand the issues and can communicate them to community members, so they can effectively engage them. Recruit people face-to-face, follow-up, and encourage diverse leadership. Identify existing assets and make fundraising a regular part of the program. Involve as many people in the group as possible, seek multiple assets and sources of income, and keep good records.[7] With the necessary resources, communities have the capability to make their own decisions. The people who assist, organize, and provide resources should not lead the organization and dictate policy decisions and action. Rather, they should amplify the voices of the community members.

Although community organizing is often a tool for change regarding a contentious topic, such as the removal of an incinerator or the use of a street patrol to decrease crime, it can also be used to mobilize the community to initiate public health programs, such as adolescent pregnancy prevention and reducing smoking.[7,63] In a college town, community organizing was used to form coalitions between the university and the surrounding community with the goal of decreasing high-risk drinking behavior by college students. Equity in the partnership was given special attention because universities typically appear to be more powerful than the communities in which they exist; they tend to drive partnerships. Because of this, a study was conducted that examined community organizing and the interventions. Schools that used community organizing were compared with control schools that did not. At the end of 3 years, in the schools that used community organizing, there was a decrease in severe consequences resulting from student drinking and alcohol-related injuries experienced by others. The community organizing approach resulted in new programs, changed institutional policies, and increased law enforcement efforts to prevent underage drinking on campus and in the community.[64]

Process of Community Organizing

There are several steps in the process of community organizing. PHNs can immerse themselves in the community, participate in activities, talk with residents, make home visits, and meet with formal and informal leaders. Development of mutual respect, trust, and familiarity takes time. Through community assessment, the nurse will develop an understanding of the structure of the community, issues of concern, and strengths. But it is more than community assessment because the nurse is seeking to assimilate into the community. It is only after doing so that the nurse can start to understand the strengths and problems the community has identified and begin to understand what role they might play in helping the community to organize, become empowered, and create social change.

Once an understanding begins to develop, the nurse must integrate local leaders into a core group that can identify and organize the community around public health needs. Then, the group can motivate others to respond to the same issues, encouraging collective action. After the problems have been identified and an interested group with essential leadership skills forms, the group is ready to act and mobilize the community. Clear goals must be formed before mobilization. They must also know what resources are available and identify who will hinder and who will support the action. Group reflection after action is taken will help the group evaluate outcomes and determine next steps. A more permanent organization may be formed with shared leadership under a simple structure. Then, the PHN can step back and let the community own the organization independently.[3]

Coalition Building

Coalition building is another tool that PHNs can use to enhance community capacity.

Definition of Coalition Building

According to the Minnesota Wheel (Chapter 2), **coalition building** "promotes and develops alliances among organizations or constituencies for a common purpose. It builds linkages, solves problems, and/or enhances local leadership to address health concerns."[3] Since 1991, The Prevention Institute's eight-step guide to developing effective coalitions has been a key resource on the topic. The groups that form a coalition must be clear about their objectives and the coalition's needs. The right people must be recruited. Objectives and activities must be detailed and address diversity among the membership. The coalition must be convened after careful preparation that includes drafting a mission statement and structure, which will be finalized at a later date. Assets must be mapped, and a budget developed. And the vitality of the coalition must be maintained and evaluated.[65]

> ▶ **SOLVING THE MYSTERY**
> ## The Case of the Mysterious Rise in Sexually Transmitted Infections
> ### Public Health Science Topics Covered
>
> - Epidemiology
>   - Surveillance
>   - Comparison of rates
> - Health planning
>   - Community organizing
>   - coalition building
> - PHN Skills
>   - Assessment
>   - Health planning
>   - Community diagnosis
>   - Organization and management
>   - Community partnerships
>
> Health-care providers from two FQHCs, three private clinics, and one university-sponsored clinic in an underserved urban community formed a partnership with the goal to better serve the community's health needs. They met monthly to discuss innovative strategies and share information about innovative programs, especially in the area of primary prevention. The agenda for the current meeting was how to best serve the clients who fall through the cracks of the ACA and are left without health insurance coverage. Each clinic was approaching the problem from a different perspective and all parties agreed that a unified plan made more sense. While discussing options, a nurse from the university clinic mentioned the marked increase in

clients without health insurance who tested positive for at least one sexually transmitted infection (STI). An FNP from the FQHC said she was also seeing more STIs in the family planning clinic. By the end of the meeting, the group had devised a plan to better serve the uninsured and establish STI surveillance for each clinic. The surveillance data would allow them to gather data on current levels of STIs and compare it with STI rates from 1 year ago.

At the next meeting, representatives of all six clinics reported a 6%-15% increase in STIs, especially gonorrhea and chlamydia. The increase was almost exclusively among young adults ages 18-28 years. The PHN at the clinic suggested that they contact other agencies in the community to see whether they would be interested in forming a linkage to help address the problem. Health-care providers from other agencies agreed. All of the providers agreed that they would begin asking their patients what they thought contributed to the increase in STIs. One of the members of the partnership suggested they involve the health department and other official agencies.

The following week, while speaking with a local police officer, the PHN was told that there had been a raid on a gambling operation in the community, and several residents had been arrested. As part of the arrest processing, the young men received several health screenings. The police officer told the PHN that they were shocked at the number who tested positive for STIs as they had never seen such numbers.

The PHN worked with a group of community organizers who were helping empower the community to achieve better health outcomes. When she met with them later in the week, she mentioned the increase in the number of young men and women with STIs in the community. They said they would put this on the agenda for their next meeting. This group had been meeting over the past 2 years, had developed a shared vision and mission, and had achieved a number of successes. The PHN, providers from the university clinic, and representatives of two of the FQHCs attended the next community meeting. The problem of the increased STIs was presented. The health-care providers reported that their patients were surprised that there was an increase in numbers but said they were glad that they could be seen without insurance because the free health department STI clinic closed 9 months ago. Some community leaders said the health department downsized and closed the clinic even though community members had wanted it to remain open. They stated that the closest free STI clinic was now more than 10 miles away in a different ethnic and racial community, and required two bus transfers to reach it. The group decided to focus on solving this problem.

Using their organizational linkages and collaborative relationships, the community members collected and analyzed the STI data, figured out the cost-benefit of reopening the health department clinic, and talked to key informants in the community including people who previously used the clinic. The informants said it had been a well-attended walk-in clinic. Prior users of the clinic said it was difficult to pay for treatment now because they wanted to avoid going to the other community for care. And because the alternatives for care required an appointment, they no longer had the convenience of being able to walk in when they sensed symptoms. Without involvement of the local health department clinic, there was no active case-finding of sexual contacts, and the patients found to have an STI were reluctant to notify their sexual contacts. Without reopening the health department walk-in clinic, it looked like the surge in STIs had no end in sight. Two community residents were chosen to represent the community at the next health department meeting. The health department officials listened respectfully to the community presentation and were both receptive and surprised by all the information the group had collected. Within 8 weeks, the health department formally agreed that it was appropriate to reopen the clinic and concurred that a member of the community organization could be on the board of directors of the new STI clinic to enhance communication, service, and evaluation.

Community-Based Participatory Research

Community-based participatory research (CBPR) involves community members in research projects that include and affect them. Partnerships and coalition building are tools employed in CBPR. These tools enable shared power, respect, and equity between the researchers and the community. Public health nurses that are already active in communities serve as excellent resources for CBPR. They can introduce community members to researchers, participate in developing research protocols, and help interpret the collected data. Actively engaging the community equitably in all aspects of the research process, ideally starting with a topic of importance to the community, promotes shared knowledge, expertise, and responsibility. Active engagement improves the validity of research outcomes and facilitates translation of the findings into practice.[66] Effectively engaging the community can also promote community development and address health disparities as was demonstrated in studies that decreased environmental hazards through policy-making initiatives.[67]

The Secretary's Advisory Committee on National Health Promotion and Disease Prevention provides recommendations to the Secretary of Health and Human Services about Healthy People 2030 (HP2030). The Committee considered community capacity and other issues, such as behavior and health outcomes, interventions, and socioenvironmental conditions as they developed the list of objectives for HP2030. Community capacity is a community's ability to plan, implement, and evaluate health strategies.[68] Because communities are in the best position to identify their needs and create change to address public health problems using their collective knowledge, skills, and resources, community capacity is inherent in CBPR. In one study, collaboration between members of a low-income community and researchers on the presence of chemicals that trigger asthma in their community increased community members' understanding and facilitated action among the community to improve health.[69]

Public health nurses practicing in the community can introduce researchers to the community. A challenge facing nurses who engage in CBPR is addressing ethical issues that arise. Typically, ethical considerations in the conduct of human-subject research focus on protecting the individual, but also CBPR requires addressing ethical issues related to protecting the community.[69] These issues include ensuring that the community will benefit from the research, sharing leadership roles, and establishing protocols for data-sharing. Bastida, Tseng, Mckeever, and Jack (2010) provide six principles that address these ethical issues and can help guide the nurse participating in this type of research (Box 16-2).[70]

BOX 16–2 ■ Six Principles for the Ethical Conduct of Community-Based Participatory Research

Principle 1. Respect
Principle 2. Fiduciary transparency
Principle 3. Fairness
Principle 4. Informed consent: Always voluntary
Principle 5. Reciprocity
Principle 6. Equal voice and disclosure

Source: (70)
Bastida, E., Tseng, T., McKeever, C., & Jack, L., Jr. (2010). Ethics and community-based participatory research: Perspective from the field. *Health Promotion Practice*, *11*(1), 16-20. doi:10.1177/1524839909352841

Population Nursing Roles in the Community

In public health nursing, there are many types of employment where the community is the primary client. Examples of specific areas where PHNs provide care within the community include parish nursing and nurse-managed health centers (NMHCs) that occur in urban and rural environments.

Parish Nursing/Faith Community Nursing

Faith community nursing is a specialty practice with its own scope and standards. Although parish nursing began in Christian congregations, it has grown to encompass an inclusive approach to nursing within the context of a spiritual community and is practiced around the world. It is defined as follows:

Faith community nurses are licensed, registered nurses who practice holistic health for self, individuals, and the community using nursing knowledge combined with spiritual care. They function in paid and unpaid positions as members of the pastoral team in a variety of religious faiths, cultures, and countries. The focus of their work is on the intentional care of the spirit, assisting the members of the faith community to maintain and/or regain wholeness in body, mind, and spirit.[71]

Parish nursing was first envisioned by Reverend Dr. Granger Westburg and first practiced in 1985 as a pilot project in Park Ridge, Illinois, a suburb of Chicago. The specialty has grown rapidly, and networks of faith community nursing exist in 30 countries.[71] The activities of parish nurses include:

- Health promotion, health education, and personal health counseling for the congregation
- Monitoring and screening for health problems
- Advocacy for individuals and groups
- Collaboration within the church and with organizations outside the church. Frequently, it involves establishing linkages with government and health-care agencies and local nongovernmental organizations to establish services for the congregation.
- Congregational health assessment of the faith community followed by analysis and program implementation
- Spiritual care through shared faith beliefs individually and in groups, such as grief counseling, and at-risk substance use.[72]

Nurse-Managed Health Centers

NMHCs are increasingly important and common in the U.S. They are staffed and often owned by advanced practice nurses and provide primary care for U.S. residents.[73] Currently, NMHCs serve as a significant safety net for the medically underserved. Given the preventive care services included in the ACA, there is an increase need for primary care providers to deliver those preventive care services. The National Nursing Centers Consortium currently includes more than 200 NMHCs and serves 2.5 million patients in urban and rural setting across the U.S.[74] NMHCs provide high-quality, affordable care and serve as training sites for future advance practice nurses.

Healthy Communities

In recent decades, there has been a groundswell of interest in healthy communities. In 1986, the World Health Organization (WHO) launched The Healthy Cities movement in several industrialized countries and then expanded it to developing countries in 1994. Currently, more than 1,000 cities around the world are part of the Health Cities Network.[75] The approach emphasizes collaboration between government health authorities, such as ministries or departments of health, and local organizations to address priority health issues in a climate of social justice and equity.[76] For example, in Europe, where at least 90 cities have participated, the goal has been to emphasize equity and health in all government sectors, especially at the local level, using community participatory governance and emphasis on the determinants of health.[75] This local involvement can promote public health leadership and create environments that allow for healthier living. There is an authentic opportunity for PHNs working with communities that are ready to embrace the healthy cities and communities' initiatives. These strategies offer the chance to decrease disparities, especially health disparities.

● APPLYING PUBLIC HEALTH SCIENCE

The Case of a Family Struggling to Find Health Care

Public Health Science Topics Covered:

- Health service systems
- Intervention: advocacy

Mary and James Wilson and their two young children lived in a small rural community and had received primary care from a health maintenance organization (HMO) through James's health insurance plan at work.

The family lost their health insurance when James lost his job. The manufacturing company closed after moving its operations overseas. Mary and James eventually found part-time work, but neither received benefits. They met most of their expenses with very careful financial management. They checked the health insurance rates on their state exchange, but even the bronze plan seemed out of their reach. Because the ACA no longer required them to carry health insurance, they decided to go without coverage. But without health insurance, they had to pay for all their health-care costs. The closest clinic was 20 miles from their home. It was a private facility and, without any health insurance coverage, the fees were very expensive. On top of the cost of the care, a visit to the health-care facility would mean they would have to miss a day of work. Mary was able to take the children to the local health department for one well-child visit and to obtain their immunizations. But the health department was in the process of closing the clinic as the state finally opted for Medicaid Expansion. Mary and James perceived themselves as young and healthy, so they thought they could get by without medical care.

Things were fine for about 9 months, but then one of the children got sick and then the other became ill too. The private clinic was too expensive, and the children did not improve with over-the-counter medications. Mary turned to the PHN at the health department and was told that a rural nurse-managed primary care clinic had just opened in a nearby town. They saw uninsured patients and used a sliding scale based on actual income to determine the fees.

They were able to get an appointment right away and were relieved that the cost would be manageable. Mary was pleased with the pediatric nurse practitioner (PNP) who appeared competent in their examination and treatment, was friendly, and talked directly with the children, which put them at ease. The PNP spoke with Mary about what she could do to help manage the children's illness and prevent it. Mary felt the PNP authentically listened to the issues and family concerns and understood their economic challenges. The nurse practitioner suggested they apply for the State Children's Health Insurance Program, often called CHIP, because it was likely that they qualified, and the plan would cover the medical care cost for the children (see Chapter 18). Mary was reassured and made an appointment for herself to receive preventive exams for cervical and breast cancer. That night, she told her spouse that she felt that they once again had a medical home and a practitioner upon whom they could rely.

Community-Academic Partnerships

Universities and community organizations often form partnerships to enable service learning. As students work with agency staff, they learn about the challenges faced by community members and the resources to address them. Learning in the community about community outreach and community health enables the development of skills in program planning, implementation, and evaluation.[77]

Sometimes community groups or employers form a partnership with a university on a focused topic, such as raising awareness of the complexity and pervasiveness of chronic illness and seeking how to address or prevent them.[78] A focused topic unites the partners to work together for change. Multiple entity partnerships are strengthened when organizations with different foci are included, such as those focusing on health, social services, business development, and various religions. Inclusiveness emphasizes community engagement in social action and positive change.

■ EVIDENCE-BASED PRACTICE
Multipronged Home-Based Care Intervention Promotes Aging in Place for Older Adult

As the proportion of older adults in rural and urban areas increases, there is increased attention on how to enable older adults to safely reside in their homes. For some, this is an economic necessity. For others, it is a preference.

Practice Statement: The Community Aging in Place, Advancing Better Living for Elders (CAPABLE) Program is an interprofessional approach that aims to enable older adults to remain in their homes as they age while enjoying a reduction in the impact of their disabilities.

Targeted Outcomes: The targeted outcomes include: (1) reduced difficulty with activities of daily living (ADL), (2) improvement in ability to perform instrumental activities of daily living (IADL), (3) improvement in symptoms of depression, and (4) reduced costs.

Supporting Evidence: Many older adults experience pain, depression, and functional limitations. This impacts well-being and the ability to live safely and comfortably at home. The CAPABLE program was a randomized controlled trial funded by the Center for Medicare and Medicaid Innovation.[1] It was first piloted in 2009, and the evidence supporting this intervention has grown in subsequent applications. CAPABLE demonstrated a 75% reduction in difficulty performing ADLs, a 65% decrease in difficulty performing IADLs, and a 53% improvement in symptoms of depression.[2,3] A substantial cost-saving was found for CAPABLE participants who were dually eligible for Medicare and Medicaid; over an average of 17 months, Medicaid spending on CAPABLE participants was $867 less per month than matched comparisons who did not participate in CAPABLE.[4]

Recommended Approaches: An interprofessional team includes a public health nurse, occupational therapist, and handyman. Over a 5-month period, the nurse made four home visits to the participant, the occupational therapist visited six times, and the handyman provided up to one full day's work. The structured program includes application of a semistructured interview and goal-setting by the participant on three priorities under each discipline (nursing and occupational therapy). A home improvement workplan is developed jointly by the therapist and the participant, and a work order is developed for the handyman.

References

1. Johns Hopkins Medicine. (2018). *CAPABLE: Aging in place.* Retrieved from https://www.johnshopkinssolutions.com/solution/capable/
2. Smith, P.D., Becker, K., Roberts, L., Walker, J., & Szanton, S.L. (2016). Associations among pain, depression, and functional limitation in low-income, home-dwelling older adults: An analysis of baseline data from CAPABLE. *Geriatric Nursing, 37*(5), 348–352. https://doi.org/10.1016/j.gerinurse.2016.04.016
3. Szanton, S.L., Leff, B., Wolff, J.L., Roberts, L., & Gitlin, L.N. (2016). Home-based care program reduces disability and promotes aging in place. *Health Affairs, 35*(9), 1558–1563. https://doi.org/10.1377/hlthaff.2016.0140
4. Szanton, S.L., Alfonso, Y.N., Leff, B., Guralnik, J., Wolff, J.L., Stockwell, I., ... Bishai, D. (2018). Medicaid cost savings of a preventive home visit program for disabled older adults. *Journal of the American Geriatrics Society, 66*(3), 614–620. https://doi.org/10.1111/jgs.15143

■ Summary Points

- Partnerships among community agencies, healthcare providers, and community residents create mutual benefits that are greater than an individual agency or a group of community residents can accomplish alone.
- Rural and urban dwellers experience health disparities.
- Rural Americans (nearly 20% of the U.S. population), compared to Americans in urban areas, have more problems accessing health and dental care, paying for

health care, and covering the costs associated with education, transportation, food, and other necessities.

- Innovations designed to address health disparities in rural communities include providing incentives for health-care providers, establishing PCMHs, and developing telehealth services.
- When impoverished urban communities experience social upheaval, the disruption can lead to poorer health in the community.
- Community organizing and coalition building can result in community empowerment—useful tools for positive change. Community-based participatory research can build a community's capacity to understand their assets and challenges and is an important approach that can lead to positive change.
- PHNs can play many roles in population-based care at the community level in both urban and rural environments: parish nursing, care provision in nurse-managed clinics, and membership in community-academic partnerships.

▼ CASE STUDY

Forming a Partnership to Improve Access to Primary Care a Rural Community

In a small town in rural Colorado, there was no primary health-care provider or facility. The closest provider was 35 miles away, and the nearest hospital was 45 miles away. The health department provided immunizations and well-child care once a month at the local library. All other health department services were provided in the county seat 26 miles away. The residents of the community of 4,000 people started talking about the limited health services in their town, and they got organized. Through the efforts of a small group of people identified to represent the town's interests, a partnership was formed with a health system that had facilities in the region. They explored opening a primary care center in the town, and after several meetings with the health system executives, a primary care center was opened. The community had to present a compelling argument for the center that demonstrated the facility would be used. The health system also had to demonstrate that they would accept the health insurance policies that the town residents carried.

1. Explore health care issues encountered in rural areas. https://www.ruralhealthinfo.org/ and https://www.ruralhealthinfo.org/topics

2. Describe approaches used by rural communities and their partners to solve this problem.
   Community-driven solutions to improve health: https://www.rwjf.org/en/blog/2017/11/rural-america-healthier-with-community-driven-solutions.html
   A solution that includes service-learning in another industrialized country: http://www.health.gov.au/internet/budget/publishing.nsf/Content/budget2018-factsheet21.htm
   A solution in a middle-income country that incorporates telehealth: https://www.huffingtonpost.com/entry/improving-rural-healthcare-in-india_us_5928a67fe4b08861ed0cc96f

3. Who can provide the primary care?
   Reimagining Rural Health Care: https://www.commonwealthfund.org/publications/newsletter-article/2017/mar/focus-reimagining-rural-health-care
   The expansion of nurse practitioners in rural areas: https://www.forbes.com/sites/brucejapsen/2018/06/05/nurse-practitioners-boost-presence-by-43-in-rural-america/#5452017a648b

REFERENCES

1. Prevention Institute. (n.d.) *Walking school busses: Chicago, Illinois.* Retrieved from https://www.preventioninstitute.org/location/walking-school-buses-chicago-illinois.
2. National Center for Safe Routes to School. (n.d.) *Start a walking school bus.* Retrieved from http://www.walkingschoolbus.org/.
3. Minnesota Department of Health, Public Health Nursing Section. (2001). *Public health interventions applications for public health nursing practice. Public health nursing practice for the 21st century.* St. Paul, Minnesota. Retrieved from http://www.health.state.mn.us/divs/opi/cd/phn/docs/0301wheel_manual.pdf.
4. Heinemann, E.A., Lee, J.L., & Cohen, J.I. (1995). Collaboration: A concept analysis. *Journal of Advanced Nursing, 21,* 103-109.
5. Imel, S. (1995). A *guide for developing local interagency linkage teams.* Retrieved from http://literacy.kent.edu/CommonGood/Guide/.
6. Luo, H., Winterbauer, N.L., Shah, G., Tucker, A., & Xu, L. (2016). Factors driving local health departments' partnerships with other organizations in maternal and child health, communicable disease prevention, and chronic disease control. *Journal of Public Health Management and Practice*, 22(4), E21–E28. https://doi.org/10.1097/PHH.0000000000000353.
7. John Snow, Inc. (2012). *Engaging your community: A toolkit for partnership, collaboration, and action.* Boston. Retrieved from https://www.jsi.com/JSIInternet/Inc/Common/_download_pub.cfm?id=14333&lid=3.

8. Health Resources and Services Administration. (2017). *Health center program.* Retrieved from https://bphc.hrsa.gov/about/healthcenterfactsheet.pdf%0Ahttps://bphc.hrsa.gov/about/healthcenterfactsheet.pdf%0Ahttps://bphc.hrsa.gov/about/healthcenterfactsheet.pdf.

9. U.S. Census Bureau. (2016). *American community survey: 2015: New census data show differences between urban and rural populations.* Retrieved from https://www.census.gov/newsroom/press-releases/2016/cb16-210.html.

10. Health Resource and Service Administration, U.S. Department of Health and Human Services. (2018). *Federal office of rural health policy.* Retrieved from https://www.hrsa.gov/about/organization/bureaus/orhp/index.html.

11. National Rural Health Association. (2018). *About rural health care.* Retrieved from: https://www.ruralhealthweb.org/about-nrha/about-rural-health-care#_ftn1.

12. Gamm, L. (2007). Keynote address: Rural *Healthy People 2010* and sustaining rural population. In L. Morgan & Fahs, P. (Eds.). *Conversations in the disciplines: Sustaining rural populations* (pp 1-12). Binghamton University: Global Academic Publishing.

13. Bolin, J.N., Bellamy, G.R., Ferdinand, A.O., Vuong, A.M., Kash, B.A., Schulze, A., & Helduser, J.W. (2015). Rural Healthy People 2020: New Decade, Same Challenges. *Journal of Rural Health*, 31(3), 326–333. https://doi.org/10.1111/jrh.12116.

14. Bolin, J.N., Bellamy, G., Ferdinand, A.O., Kash, B.A., Helduser, J.W. (Eds.). (2015). *Rural Healthy People 2020.* Vol. 1. College Station, Texas: Texas A&M Health Science Center School of Public Health, Southwest Rural Health Research Center.

15. U.S. Centers for Disease Control and Prevention. (2017). *Overview of midcourse progress and health disparities.* Atlanta. Retrieved from https://www.cdc.gov/nchs/data/hpdata2020/HP2020MCR-B03-Overview.pdf.

16. Health Resources and Services Administration. (2014). *Distribution of U.S. health care providers residing in rural and urban areas.* Retrieved from: https://bhw.hrsa.gov/sites/default/files/bhw/nchwa/nchwafactsheet.pdf.

17. U.S. Census Bureau. (2010). *2010 Census: United States profile population density by county.* Retrieved from http://www2.census.gov/geo/maps/dc10_thematic/2010_Profile/2010_Profile_Map_United_States.pdf.

18. Ratcliffe, M. (2016). *Defining rural at the U.S. census bureau.* Retrieved from https://www2.census.gov/geo/pdfs/reference/ua/Defining_Rural.pdf.

19. U.S. Department of Agriculture. (2016). *What is rural?* Retrieved from https://www.nal.usda.gov/ric/what-is-rural.

20. Ingram, D. & Franco, S. (2013). *2013 NCHS Urban – Rural classification scheme for counties.* Retrieved from https://www.cdc.gov/nchs/data/series/sr_02/sr02_166.pdf.

21. Kaufman, B.G., Thomas, S.R., Randolph, R.K., Perry, J.R., Thompson, K.W., Holmes, G.M., & Pink, G.H. (2016). The rising rate of rural hospital closures. *Journal of Rural Health*, 32(1), 35–43. https://doi.org/10.1111/jrh.12128.

22. Xue, Y., Kannan, V., Greener, E., Smith, J.A., Brasch, J., Johnson, B.A., & Spetz, J. (2018). Full scope-of-practice regulation is associated with higher supply of nurse practitioners in rural and primary care health professional shortage counties. *Journal of Nursing Regulation*, 8(4), 5–13. https://doi.org/10.1016/S2155-8256(17)30176-X.

23. Patient Protection and Affordable Care Act. (2010). *124 Stat. 119 thru 124 Stat. 1025 H.R. 3590.* Retrieved from http://www.gpo.gov/fdsys/pkg/PLAW-111publ148/content-detail.html.

24. Wright, B., Damiano, P.C., & Bentler, S.E. (2015). Implementation of the Affordable Care Act and rural health clinic capacity in Iowa. *Journal of Primary Care and Community Health*, 6(1), 61–65. https://doi.org/10.1177/2150131914542613.

25. Bolin, J., Gamm, L., Vest, J., Edwardson, N., & Miller, T. (2011). Medical homes. Will health care reform provide new options for rural communities and providers? *Family Community Health*, 34(2), 93-101.

26. James, W., Matthews, K., Albrecht, P., & Church, A. (2018). Improving the health of rural America's chronically ill: A case study of a patient-centered medical home clinic in Mississippi. *Population Health Management*, 21(1), 83–83. https://doi.org/10.1089/pop.2017.0054.

27. Johnson, V., Wong, E., Lampman, M., Curtis, I., Fortney, J., Kaboli, P., ... Nelson, K. (2018). Comparing patient-centered medical home implementation in urban and rural VHA clinics: Results from the Patient Aligned Care Team Initiative. *Journal of Ambulatory Care Management*, 41(1), 47–57. https://doi.org/10.1097/JAC.0000000000000212.

28. American Telemedicine Association. (2018). *Telehealth nursing fact sheet.* Retrieved from https://higherlogicdownload.s3.amazonaws.com/AMERICANTELEMED/3c09839a-fffd-46f7-916c-692c11d78933/UploadedImages/SIGs/Telehealth_Nursing_Fact_Sheet_04_25_2018.pdf.

29. Tacoli, C., McGranahan, G., & Satterthwaite, D. (2014). *Urbanization, rural–urban migration and urban poverty: World Migration Report 2015 background paper.* Geneva. Retrieved from https://www.iom.int/sites/default/files/our_work/ICP/MPR/WMR-2015-Background-Paper-CTacoli-GMcGranahan-DSatterthwaite.pdf.

30. International Organization for Migration. (2015). *World migration report: Migrants and cities: New partnerships to manage mobility.* Geneva: International Organization for Migration.

31. International Organization for Migration. (2018). *World Migration Report.* Geneva: International Organization for Migration. Retrieved from https://www.iom.int/wmr/world-migration-report-2018 https://doi.org/10.1017/CBO9781107415324.004.

32. Feinberg, A.P. (2018). The key role of epigenetics in human disease prevention and mitigation. *New England Journal of Medicine*, 378(14), 1323–1334. https://doi.org/10.1056/NEJMra1402513.

33. Specia, M. (2018). How Syria's death toll is lost in the fog of war. *The New York Times*, pp. 2016–2018. Retrieved from https://www.nytimes.com/2018/04/13/world/middleeast/syria-death-toll.html.

34. Connor, P. (2018). *Where Syrian refugees have resettled worldwide.* Retrieved from http://www.pewresearch.org/fact-tank/2018/01/29/where-displaced-syrians-have-resettled/.

35. Polk, W.R. (2013). Understanding Syria: From Pre-Civil War to Post-Assad. *The Atlantic*, 1–20. Retrieved from https://www.theatlantic.com/international/archive/2013/12/understanding-syria-from-pre-civil-war-to-post-assad/281989/.

36. Brockie, T.N., Heinzelmann, M., & Gill, J. (2013). A framework to examine the role of epigenetics in health disparities

among Native Americans. *Nursing Research and Practice*, 2013, 1–9. https://doi.org/10.1155/2013/410395.

37. Fang, C., & Yu, D. (2017). Urban agglomeration: An evolving concept of an emerging phenomenon. *Landscape and Urban Planning*, 162, 126–136. https://doi.org/10.1016/j.landurbplan.2017.02.014.

38. United Nations Population Division Department of Economic and Social Affairs. (2018). *World urbanization prospects.* Retrieved from https://esa.un.org/unpd/wup/.

39. U.S. Department of Commerce. (2018). *Glossary: United States Census Bureau.* Retrieved from https://www.census.gov/glossary/.

40. Cohen, D.T., Hatchard, G.W., & Wilson, S.G. (2015). Population trends in incorporated places: 2000 to 2013. *Current Population Reports*, (March 2015), 1–19.

41. Wilson, S.G., Plane, D.A., Mackun, P.J., Fischetti, T.R., Goworowska, J., Cohen, D.T., ... Hatchard, G.W. (2012). Patterns of metropolitan and micropolitan population change: 2000 to 2010. *Census Special Reports*, (September), 1–102. https://doi.org/C2010SR-01.

42. Rosner, D. (2006). Public health in U.S. cities, a historical perspective. In N. Freudenberg, S. Galea, & D. Vlahov. (Eds.), *Cities and the health of the public* (p. 140). Nashville, TN: Vanderbilt University Press.

43 UNESCO. (2016). *Global report on culture for sustainable urban development heritage and creativity culture.* Paris: United Nations Educational, Scientific, and Cultural Organization. Retrieved from http://unesdoc.unesco.org/images/0024/002459/245999e.pdf.

44. Corburn, J. (2017). Urban place and health equity: Critical issues and practices. *International Journal of Environmental Research and Public Health*, 14(2), 1–10. https://doi.org/10.3390/ijerph14020117.

45. Gong, Y., Palmer, S., Gallacher, J., Marsden, T., & Fone, D. (2016). A systematic review of the relationship between objective measurements of the urban environment and psychological distress. *Environment International*, 96, 48–57. https://doi.org/10.1016/j.envint.2016.08.019.

46. American Lung Association. (2018). *State of the air.* Retrieved from https://www.lung.org/our-initiatives/healthy-air/sota/.

47. Long, S.K., Bart, L., Karpman, M., Shartzer, A., & Zuckerman, S. (2017). Sustained gains in coverage, access, and affordability under the ACA: A 2017 update. *Health Affairs*, 36(9), 1656–1662. https://doi.org/10.1377/hlthaff.2017.0798.

48. Goldman, A.L., McCormick, D., Haas, J.S., & Sommers, B.D. (2018). Effects of the ACA's health insurance marketplaces on the previously uninsured: A quasi-experimental analysis. *Health Affairs*, 37(4), 591–599. https://doi.org/10.1377/hlthaff.2017.1390.

49. Villalonga-Olives, E., Wind, T.R., & Kawachi, I. (2018). Social capital interventions in public health: A systematic review. *Social Science and Medicine*, 212(July), 203–218. https://doi.org/10.1016/j.socscimed.2018.07.022.

50. Remington, P.L., Catlin, B.B., & Gennuso, K.P. (2015). The County Health Rankings: Rationale and methods. *Population Health Metrics*, 13(1), 1–12. https://doi.org/10.1186/s12963-015-0044-2.

51. University of Wisconsin Population Health Institute. (2018). *County health rankings and roadmaps.* Retrieved from http://www.countyhealthrankings.org/.

52. NYU Langone Health. (2018). *City health dashboard.* Retrieved from https://www.cityhealthdashboard.com/dc/washington/city-view.

53. Economic Innovation Group. (2018). From the Great Recession to Great Reshuffling: Charting a decade of change across American Communities. Retrieved from https://eig.org/wp-content/uploads/2018/10/2018-DCI.pdf.

54. Minkler, M. (Ed.). (2012). *Community organizing and community building for health and welfare* (3rd ed.). New Brunswick, NJ: Rutgers University Press.

55. The World Bank. (2016). *Empowerment.* Retrieved from http://web.worldbank.org/WBSITE/EXTERNAL/TOPICS/EXTPOVERTY/EXTEMPOWERMENT/0,,contentMDK:20245753~pagePK:210058~piPK:210062~theSitePK:486411,00.html.

56. The World Bank. (2018). *Community-driven development.* Retrieved from http://www.worldbank.org/en/topic/communitydrivendevelopment.

57. Amendola, M.G. (2011). Empowerment: Healthcare professionals' and community members' contributions. *Journal of Cultural Diversity*, 18(3), 82–89. Retrieved from http://web.b.ebscohost.com.hal.weber.edu:2200/ehost/pdfviewer/pdfviewer?vid=2&sid=c3f4d181-f68b-41f3-ab4e-012a683249fc%40sessionmgr120.

58. Davis, S., Keep, S., Edie, A., Couzens, S., & Pereira, K. (2016). A peer-led diabetes education program in a homeless community to improve diabetes knowledge and empowerment. *Journal of Community Health Nursing*, 33(2), 71–80. https://doi.org/10.1080/07370016.2016.1159435.

59. Benoit, C., Belle-Isle, L., Smith, M., Phillips, R., Shumka, L., Atchison, C., ... Flagg, J. (2017). Sex workers as peer health advocates: Community empowerment and transformative learning through a Canadian pilot program. *International Journal for Equity in Health*, 16(1), 1–17. https://doi.org/10.1186/s12939-017-0655-2.

60. Rifkin, S.B. (2014). Examining the links between community participation and health outcomes: A review of the literature. *Health Policy and Planning*, 29(July), ii98-ii106. https://doi.org/10.1093/heapol/czu076.

61. The World Bank. (2018). *Nigeria's poor communities in the driver's seat of their development journey.* Retrieved from http://www.worldbank.org/en/news/feature/2018/02/16/nigerias-poor-communities-in-the-drivers-seat-of-their-development-journey.

62. Marysdaughter, K., & Dansinger, L. (2000). *Community organizer's guide.* Monroe, ME: Resources for Organizing and Social Change. Retrieved from http://resourcesforsocialchange.org/index.php/publications.

63. American Lung Association. (2014). *Community organizing.* Retrieved from http://center4tobaccopolicy.org/community-organizing/.

64. Wagoner, K., Rhodes, S., Lentz, A., & Wolfson, M. (2010). Community organizing goes to college: A practice-based model to implement environmental strategies to reduce high-risk drinking on college campuses. *Health Promotion Practice*, 11, 817. doi:10.1177/1524839909353726.

65. Cohen, L., Baer, N., & Satterwhite, P. (2002). *Developing effective coalitions: An eight step guide.* Oakland, CA. Retrieved from https://www.preventioninstitute.org/publications/developing-effective-coalitions-eight-step-guide.

66. Center for Community Health and Development. (2018). *Chapter 36, Section 2: Community-based participatory research.* Retrieved from https://ctb.ku.edu/en/table-of-contents/evaluate/evaluation/intervention-research/main.

67. Cacari-Stone, L., Wallerstein, N., Garcia, A.P., & Minkler, M. (2014). The promise of community-based participatory research for health equity: A conceptual model for bridging evidence with policy. *American Journal of Public Health, 104*(9), 1615–1623. https://doi.org/10.2105/AJPH.2014.301961.

68. Secretary's Advisory Committee on National Health Promotion and Disease Prevention: Objectives for 2030. (2017). Report #2: *Recommendations for developing objectives, setting priorities, identifying data needs, and involving stakeholders for Healthy People 2030.* Rockville, MD. Retrieved from https://www.healthypeople.gov/sites/default/files/Advisory_Committee_Objectives_for_HP2030_Report.pdf.

69. Perovich, L.J., Ohayon, J.L., Cousins, E.M., Morello-Frosch, R., Brown, P., Adamkiewicz, G., & Brody, J.G. (2018). Reporting to parents on children's exposures to asthma triggers in low-income and public housing, an interview-based case study of ethics, environmental literacy, individual action, and public health benefits. *Environmental Health, 17,* 48. https://doi.org/10.1186/s12940-018-0395-9.

70. Bastida, E., Tseng, T., McKeever, C., & Jack, L., Jr. (2010). Ethics and community-based participatory research: Perspective from the field. *Health Promotion Practice, 11*(1), 16-20. doi:10.1177/1524839909352841.

71. Westberg Institute. (2018). *Foundations of faith community nursing.* Retrieved from http://www.parishnurses.org/.

72. Swinney, J., Anson-Wonkka, C., Maki, E., & Corneau, J. (2001). Community assessment: A church community and the parish nurse. *Public Health Nursing, 18*(1), 40-44.

73. Family Practice and Counseling Network. (2018). *How we help.* Retrieved from https://www.fpcn.com/how-we-help.

74. Raise the Voice Edge Runner. (2015). *Nurse managed health centers: National nursing centers consortium & institute for nursing centers* Retrieved from http://www.aannet.org/initiatives/edge-runners/profiles/edge-runners—nurse-managed-health-centers.

75. World Health Organization. (2018). *Healthy cities.* Retrieved from http://www.who.int/healthy_settings/types/cities/en/.

76. Goldstein, G. (2000). Healthy cities: Overview of a WHO international program. *Reviews on Environmental Health. 15,* 1-2.

77. Voss, H., Mathews, L., Cohn, S., Fossen, T., Scott, G., & Schaefer, M. (2015). Community-academic partnerships: Developing a service-learning framework. *Journal of Professional Nursing, 31*(5), 395–401. https://doi.org/10.1016/j.profnurs.2015.03.008.

78. Schouw, D., Mash, R., & Kolbe-Alexander T.L. (2018). Transforming the workplace environment to prevent non-communicable chronic diseases: Participatory action research in a South African power plant. *Global Health Action,* under review(1). https://doi.org/10.1080/16549716.2018.1544336.

Chapter 17

Health Planning for Maternal-Infant and Child Health Settings

Erin M. Wright, Phyllis Sharps, Joanne Flagg, and Deborah Busch

LEARNING OUTCOMES

After reading the chapter, the student will be able to:

1. Describe maternal, infant, and child health from a global and national perspective.
2. Identify key concerns for public health planning for maternal, infant, and child health.
3. Apply health promotion planning to maternal, infant, and child health.
4. Integrate cultural perspectives into planning for maternal, infant, and child health interventions.
5. Discuss strategies for community engagement and consensus building for maternal, infant, and child health planning.

KEY TERMS

Fishboning
Infant mortality rateLow
  birth weight
Mainstream smoke
Maternal health
Maternal mortality

Maternal mortality rate
Maternal mortality ratio
Preterm birth
Preterm labor
Secondhand smoke
Side stream smoke

Sudden infant death
  syndrome (SIDS)
Sudden unexplained infant
  death
Teen pregnancy
Teen pregnancy birth rate

Under-5 mortality rate
Upstream approach
Very low birth weight

▮ Introduction

Maternal, infant, and child health is a global health priority. According to the World Health Organization (WHO), the number of children under the age of 5 who die each year is 5.6 million, or approximately 625 per hour.[1] More than 46% of these deaths occur in the first 28 days of life.[1] The top five leading causes of death are preterm birth complications, pneumonia, birth asphyxia, diarrhea, and malaria.[1] Most deaths of children under 5 are related to malnutrition and are preventable simply by providing affordable interventions.[1] Nurses working in settings that provide care to mothers and their children play a key role in the interventions aimed at improving the health of mothers and their children.

Maternal Mortality

Maternal mortality is defined as the death of a woman while pregnant or within 42 days of the end of a pregnancy.[2] Approximately 850 pregnant women and women giving birth die of preventable causes per day.[2] Most common causes are bleeding, pregnancy-related hypertension (pre-eclampsia and eclampsia), infections and sepsis, complications from delivery, and unsafe abortion.[2] Nearly all these deaths are preventable. Although almost 99% of maternal mortality takes place in developing countries, more resource advantaged counties are not immune.[2] Since 1987, rates of maternal mortality in the United States have skyrocketed from 7.2 to a high of 17.8 maternal deaths per 100,000 births in 2016.[3] Causes of pregnancy related deaths in the U.S. differ slightly from global sources. These include cardiovascular disease, cardiomyopathy, noncardiovascular disease, hemorrhage, pulmonary embolism, cerebrovascular accidents, hypertensive disorders, and infection.[3] There are considerable racial disparities in the U.S. concerning the **maternal mortality rate (MMR)**, which represents the number of pregnancy-associated deaths per 100,000 births.[3] White women experience the lowest rates at 12.7 deaths per 100,000 live births, whereas black women have 3 to 4 times that rate at 43.5 deaths per 100,000 live births.[3] The inequities in outcomes exist in part due to inequities in social determinants of health.[4] These include pregnancy intention, access to an obstetric care provider, level of education among household members, employment and economic opportunities, social support, and health insurance coverage.[4]

Maternal health specifically refers to the woman's health during pregnancy, childbirth, and the postpartum period. Infant health includes the health of newborns, that is, infants up to 28 days of age, and children younger than 1 year. In this chapter, child health focuses on the health of children under the age of 5. This age group is the recipient of much of the focus on child health because of the high risk of morbidity and mortality during this age span.[1] The issue of maternal, infant, and child health spans the globe, with major public health initiatives aimed at improving the health of this vulnerable population.

Historical Perspectives

Lillian Wald was one of the earliest pioneers in population approaches to health and is considered the founder of public health nursing (see Chapter 1).[5] Her work at the Henry Street Settlement addressed health disparities among expectant mothers and children. The interventions she planned and implemented focused on the health priorities of the population living in the Lower East Side of New York City during the last decades of the 19th century and the first decades of the 20th century. Through this work, she developed maternity services at Henry Street, including health classes for mothers and home visits for maternal-infant health assessment and teaching. She addressed health reform for sanitation and public health, and developed prevention programs for mothers, infants, and children. Considered the founder of school health services and visiting nursing, she also developed what became known as the Children's Bureau.[5]

Unfortunately, more than a century later, health disparities and high rates of morbidity and mortality persist for pregnant women and their infants worldwide. Although the leading causes of mortality and morbidity have changed somewhat during the past 100 years, there is a continued need for nurses to use public health science to address maternal-child health issues. Nurses use the science of epidemiology to examine morbidity and mortality data and identify priorities for maternal and infant health.

Cultural Contexts for Pregnancy and Childbirth in the United States

Family and children are highly valued in U.S. culture with specific practices in place at birth and during the postpartum period. However, due to advances in obstetric and neonatal care, pregnancy, birth, and early childhood are, for the most part, safe for families and children. In the United States, 99% of births take place in hospitals rather than in the home. Additionally, safe and available contraceptive methods and choices are available to most women, resulting in improved family planning. This in turn has increased opportunities for women related to education, employment, and building a career. These have long-term effects on population growth with a predicted decrease in U.S. birth rates through 2060.[6] The majority of the population growth is increasingly associated with people immigrating to the U.S., leading to increasing diversity in the population.[6]

With this diversity comes a broad range of cultural practices surrounding birth. Culture shapes expectations at birth. Expectations include personal control during the birthing process, support from the partner, and health of the baby and pain management during childbirth provided by health-care providers.[7,8] These expectations vary across cultures.[7] From a nursing perspective, understanding a mother's expectations of the birthing process based on her cultural background during the birthing process is an important component of the nursing care provided.

Although major shifts occur in birth rates and how the U.S. population grows, healthy pregnancy, childbirth, and parenting requires an emphasis on family-centered care. This includes access to medical care from preconception through the prenatal and postpartum period. In addition to medical care providing parents with paid time off from work to allow for attachment and bonding and to initiate breastfeeding further promotes health and wellbeing for both the mother and the newborn. Finally, based on the increasing diversity in the U.S. population efforts to promote healthy mothers and babies requires the incorporation of evidence-based practices that integrate diverse cultural norms and reflect the diversity of the maternal population served.

■ CULTURAL CONTEXT FOR PREGNANCY AND CHILDBIRTH IN THE 21ST CENTURY IN THE UNITED STATES

The biological process of childbirth has not changed over time. Advances in care over the past century, however, have greatly reduced infant and maternal mortality. In addition to these medical advances, cultural perceptions of childbirth have changed including women's expectations of childbirth, methods of pain management, the economics of childbirth, health-care systems, and delivery options. Other advances include being able to plan pregnancies and increased ability to care for newborns. Cultural norms surrounding these changes are still in flux with polarizing political views of planning pregnancies and abortion.

In the U.S., the delivery of care during labor and childbirth has changed with the rate of cesarean sections approaching 30% of all deliveries in the United States. In addition, the development of the vacuum extractor has decreased the use of forceps, although both are still used frequently. Inductions of labor are becoming increasingly more common; currently, an estimated 40% of all women are induced, despite estimates that only 10% of women need to be induced for a medical reason.[8] These changes reflect a cultural shift in the U.S. that has occurred over the last 100 years, from most births occurring in the home to most deliveries occurring in the hospital. In the latter half of the last century birthing centers began to incorporate the family setting back into births by including family members and utilizing birthing rooms that reflected a setting closer to the home versus a hospital operating room.

Despite these changes in the U.S., cultural practices in other countries that put both the mother and the newborn at risk continue. For example, in Ethiopia, food taboos can result in poor maternal nutrition.[9] When providing care to pregnant women from cultures different from their own, midwives and nurses encounter complex factors that influence the health care expectations of pregnant women. These cultural differences include family relationships, religion, authoritative knowledge, and how information is communicated.[10] Thus, it is essential to assess cultural preferences and practices of women during the pregnancy and incorporate that into the plan of care throughout the pregnancy, labor and delivery, and the postpartum period.

Trends in Maternal, Infant, and Child Health

In the United States, maternal, infant, and child health remains central to the improvement of the health of the country's population. It was a key topic area in *Healthy*

People 2020 (HP 2020) with 33 main topics and a total of 73 objectives.

■ HEALTHY PEOPLE

Targeted Topic: Maternal, infant, and child health
Goal: Improve the health and well-being of women, infants, children, and families.
Overview: Improving the well-being of mothers, infants, and children is an important public health goal for the United States. Their well-being determines the health of the next generation and can help predict future public health challenges for families, communities, and the health-care system. The objectives of the Maternal, Infant, and Child Health topic area address a wide range of conditions, health behaviors, and health system indicators that affect the health, wellness, and quality of life of women, children, and families.[11]

HP 2020 Midcourse Review: Maternal, Infant, and Child Health Objectives: Of the 73 HP 2020 objectives related to maternal, infant, and child health (MCH), 64 objectives were measurable with 26.6% of objectives (n=17) having met or exceeded their 2020 targets; another 26.6% of the objectives (n=17) are improving; 18.8% of the objectives (n=5) have shown little or no detectable change, and 7.8% of the objectives (n=5) are getting worse (see Fig. 17-1). Twelve objectives were baseline only, and one objective was informational. Among the leading MCH indicators that have exceeded the 2020 targets are: infant deaths under 1 year, preterm births less than 37 weeks, adolescents using illicit drugs, adolescent cigarette smoking, and children exposed to secondhand smoke. Important MCH indicators that are improving are children receiving recommended vaccinations by ages 19-35 months. Little or detectable change was noted among these MCH indicators: family planning services among sexually active women ages 15-44 years, obesity among adults 20+ years, and obesity among children and adolescents 2-19 years. MCH objectives getting worse were oral health/annual dental visits among children, adolescents, and adults aged 2+ years.[12]

To understand trends in maternal, infant, and child health, it helps to begin with three indicators often used to evaluate this population: infant mortality rate (IMR), MMR, and under-5 mortality rate. Infant mortality is the death of a child before his or her first birthday. **Infant mortality rate** is the number of infant deaths for every 1,000 live births.[13] It does not include fetal demise or

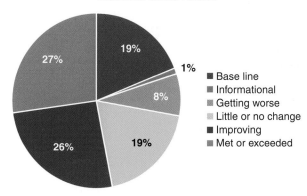

Healthy People 2020 Midcourse Review: Maternal Child Health

- Base line
- Informational
- Getting worse
- Little or no change
- Improving
- Met or exceeded

Figure 17-1 Healthy People 2020 Midcourse Review Maternal Child Health.

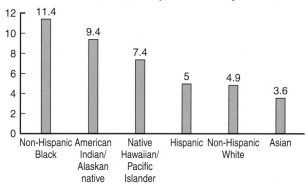

U.S. Infant Mortality Rate 2016 by Race

Figure 17-2 Infant mortality rate by race and ethnicity, 2016. Rate per 1,000 live births.

miscarriage. The MMR is the number of maternal deaths per 100,000 births. To be classified as a maternal death, the woman must be pregnant or within 42 days of the termination of a pregnancy, and the death must be directly related to pregnancy, not including accidental or incidental causes.[2] The **under-5 mortality rate** of children is technically not an actual rate but rather represents the probability of a child born in a specific year dying before the age of 5. It is calculated per 1,000 births.[14]

Infant Mortality Rate

Across the world, IMR is used as an indicator of population health. It reflects the quality of pre- and postnatal care in that population and is an indicator of access to medical care, socioeconomic conditions, and public health practices.[1] Although some have challenged the legitimacy of IMR as an indicator of the health of an entire population, it has withstood the test of time. In addition, in countries with few resources to monitor other health indictors, IMR is an easily calculated indicator.[13] As of 2017, and based on estimated infant mortality data, the United States ranked 53rd worldwide for infant mortality with a rate of 5.8 per 1,000 live births.[15]

Vulnerable Populations and IMR in the U.S.

Within the United States, there are differences among ethnic/racial groups concerning IMR. For example, in 2016 the IMR for babies whose mothers were non-Hispanic black women was double the IMR for babies whose mothers were white non-Hispanic women (11.4 per 1,000 live births vs. 4.9 per 1,000 live births) (see Fig. 17-2).[13] The top five leading causes of infant

death in the United States in 2016 were birth defects, preterm birth and low birth weight (LBW), sudden infant death syndrome (SIDS), maternal pregnancy complications, and injuries.[13]

Preterm Birth

Globally, two of the top leading causes of all childhood deaths under the age of 5 nearly are preterm birth and birth asphyxia, with almost 50% of deaths in this age group occurring in infants.[12] **Preterm birth** is defined as a birth occurring less than 37 weeks of gestation. **Low birth weight** is defined as a birth weight less than 2,500 grams (5 lbs. 8 oz.). The number of preterm babies born annually worldwide is 15 million, with 1 million infants dying annually because of preterm births.[14,16] Countries in Asia and Africa are most significantly affected, with almost 60% of all preterm births occurring in those areas.[15]

Maternal Mortality Rate

Globally, the MMR is on the decline and has shown a 37% reduction since 2000.[17] Despite this success, the **maternal mortality ratio**, defined as the proportion of mothers who do not survive childbirth compared to those who do survive, is still 14 times higher than in developing regions compared to developed regions.[17] The United States is the only industrialized nation to show an increase in the rates of maternal mortality (Fig. 17-3). Between 1987 and 2014, the U.S. MMR rose from 7.8 per 100,000 live births to 18 per 100,000 live births.[18] Globally, under Sustainable Development Goal number 3 (SDG 3) the objective is to reduce the global rates of maternal mortality to less than 70 per 100,000 live births by 2030.[17] Promising progress has been made at meeting the SDG 3 objectives related to maternal health with an

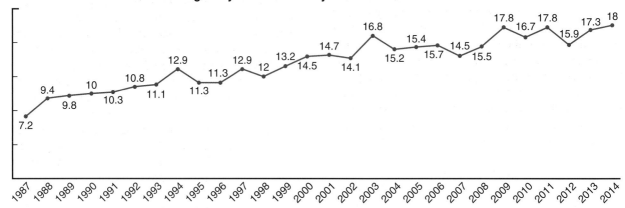

Figure 17-3 Trends in pregnancy-related mortality in the United States: 1987-2014. (Note: This represents the pregnancy-related mortality ratio.)

increase in prenatal care, a decrease in the number of teens giving birth, and an increase in meeting family planning needs.[17]

■ EVIDENCE-BASED PRACTICE

Practice Statement: Prevent postpartum hemorrhage
Targeted Outcome: Reduce the incidence of postpartum hemorrhage, a leading risk factor for maternal mortality.
Supporting Evidence: Based on a promising new study from the WHO, a new drug used to reduce maternal hemorrhaging following delivery may help reduce the MMR. In June of 2018, the WHO stated in a press release:

Currently, WHO recommends oxytocin as the first-choice drug for preventing excessive bleeding after childbirth. Oxytocin, however, must be stored and transported at 2–8 degrees Celsius, which is hard to do, in many countries, depriving many women of access to this life-saving drug. When they can obtain it, the drug may be less effective because of heat exposure.

The study, published today in the New England Journal of Medicine, has shown an alternative drug – heat-stable carbetocin – to be as safe and effective as oxytocin in preventing postpartum hemorrhage. This new formulation of carbetocin does not require refrigeration and retains its efficacy for at least 3 years stored at 30 degrees Celsius and 75% relative humidity.

Recommended Approaches: Based on these findings, the WHO stated that the next step was to submit the findings for regulatory review and approval by countries. The WHO Guideline Development Group will then "… consider whether heat-stable carbetocin should be a recommended drug for the prevention of postpartum hemorrhage."

References:

1. World Health Organization. (2018, June 27). WHO study shows drug could save thousands of women's lives. *WHO News Release*, Geneva. Retrieved from http://www.who.int/news-room/detail/27-06-2018-who-study-shows-drug-could-save-thousands-of-women's-lives
2. Widmer, M., Piaggio, G., Nguyen, T.M.H., Osoti, A., Mistra, S., ... WHO Champion Trial Group. (2018). Heat-stable carbetocin versus oxytocin to prevent hemorrhage after vaginal birth. *New England Journal of Medicine, 379*(8), 743-752. doi: 10.1056/NEJMoa1805489

Vulnerable Populations and MMR in the U.S.

There are racial disparities in the U.S. with regard to the MMR.[3] During 2011-2014, the maternal mortality ratios were 12.4 for white women, 40.0 or African American women, and 17.8 for other racial/ethnic groups.[3] The inequities in outcomes exist in part due to inequities in social determinants of health.[4] These include pregnancy intention, access to obstetric care providers, level of education among household members, employment and economic opportunities, social support, and health insurance coverage.[4] However the higher rates that African American women experience goes beyond social determinants of health and includes systemic racism that can occur in health care. An example is the case of new mother and tennis phenomenon Serena Williams. Although she does not experience poverty or lack of access to care, she had a life-threatening complication after childbirth. Despite her known history of a clotting disorder and previous pulmonary embolisms, she was told that she was just having pain from her delivery and was initially offered a test that would not properly diagnose her condition. She had to forcefully advocate for the appropriate testing and treatment to diagnose the pulmonary embolism she knew she was experiencing after childbirth.

Geographic differences also exist in relation to the U.S. MMR rates. Rural and more impoverished counties in the United States lack appropriate obstetric care resources, especially in the Southeastern region of the country.[19,20] Vulnerable populations such as the homeless, those who are incarcerated, and the LGBTQ+ community experience greater disparities in access to health care.[20] Although the rate of maternal mortality among the LGBTQ+ community has not yet been examined in a systematic fashion, there appear to be greater disparities in this population related to health care access.[21] There are also differences in relation to sources of social support within and outside of the LGBTQ+ community.[22] In 2012, The American College of Obstetricians and Gynecologists (ACOG) released a white paper advocating for equitable care for LGBTQ+ persons who are pregnant. They stated that "The American College of Obstetricians and Gynecologists endorses equitable treatment for lesbians and bisexual women and their families, not only for direct health-care needs, but also for indirect health-care issues."[23] Since the release of that statement, new issues that have emerged for the LGBTQ+ community include pregnancy and transgender persons who may become pregnant.

■ CELLULAR TO GLOBAL: MATERNAL HEALTH

The SDG 3.1 target is aimed at reducing the global maternal mortality ratio to less than 70 per 100,000 births by 2030[2]; under the HP 2020 topic of Maternal Child Health, the MICH 5 objective is to reduce the maternal mortality to 11.4 per 100,000 births by 2020.[11] Not only did the U.S. fail to meet the target of 11.4, but the MMR rose to 18 by 2014 (Fig. 17-3).[24] To help reduce the MMR requires a population approach as outlined by the United Nations in SDG 3. According to the WHO, 75% of maternal deaths globally are caused by preventable causes including severe bleeding (mostly bleeding after childbirth), infections (usually after childbirth),

high blood pressure during pregnancy (pre-eclampsia and eclampsia), complications from delivery, and unsafe abortion. The other 25% of maternal deaths are caused by or associated with diseases such as malaria and AIDS during pregnancy. Every day around the world, 830 women die from these preventable causes related to pregnancy and childbirth.[2] Worldwide, since 2000, the MMR dropped by 37%.[18] However, even though 99% of all maternal deaths occur in developing countries, maternal mortality remains a challenge in the United States, where about 700 women die each year from complications during pregnancy or childbirth.[24] In addition, in the U.S., **severe maternal morbidity** (SMM), defined as the most severe complications of pregnancy, annually affects more than 50,000 women every year.[25]

Based on recent trends, the global burden of maternal mortality continues to be recognized as a public health problem. The Years of Life Lost (see Chapters 3 and 9) is an issue because mothers are relatively young.[26,27] These maternal deaths impact the community not only as a loss to the workforce but as providers of child care. Addressing the primary causes of maternal mortality at the individual level across the continuum of prevention requires improving access to care from preconception through the postpartum period.[26] This often requires changes at the policy level. Nurses and midwives have continued to be an important part of the strategy to promote maternal health and optimal pregnancy outcomes. Nurses and midwives not only provide direct services to pregnant women, they also serve as advocates for universal access to prenatal care, for training to increase the number of skilled birth attendants at every birth, and for an increase in policies that support safe motherhood and baby-friendly hospitals.[2,17]

Mortality Rate for Children Under the Age of 5

Great strides have been made over the past 3 decades to reduce the rates of mortality for children under the age of 5. Since 1990, there has been a drop in the child mortality rate from 12 million to 5.6 million in 2016.[1] One of the objectives under the SDG 3 is to reduce the rate of child mortality under the age of 5 to at least as low as 25 per 1,000 live births by 2030.[17] As mentioned earlier, the leading causes of death for children under the age of 5 that are not birth-related are pneumonia, diarrheal diseases, and malaria.[1] By contrast, in the

United States, the leading causes of death in children between the ages of 1 and 4 are unintentional injury, developmental/genetic conditions present at birth, and assault (homicide) (Table 17-1).[8]

Population Focus on Maternal, Infant, and Child Health

A population focus to improve the health of mothers, infants, and children under the age of 5 is essential. The following examples are reminders of the importance of this perspective for maternal, infant, and child health. Using principles of epidemiology, changes in clinical practice and policies greatly reduced the leading causes of death for pregnant women and infants. In the first example, during the 1840s, Dr. Ignaz Semmelweis, a Hungarian working in Austria, discovered that hand washing reduced the incidence of puerperal fever (also called childbed fever) or septicemia that follows delivery. This serious condition caused deaths among 30% of those women who delivered their newborns in the hospital. He observed that women who delivered their babies at home where a midwife assisted with the birth had better outcomes than those who delivered in the hospital. Noting that the medical students came to the delivery ward directly from the autopsy room at the hospital without washing their hands, Semmelweis ordered a change in hand washing policy. Once the policy change took place, the maternal death rate decreased from 12% to 1% within 2 years.[29] His work is an early record of the importance of epidemiology for improving health outcomes.

Sudden unexpected infant death (SUID) is defined as a sudden unexpected death in a child less than 1 year of age in which the cause is not evident without further investigation. It usually occurs in or around the infant's sleep area. The four main causes of SUID are (1) **Sudden Infant Death Syndrome (SIDS)**, (2) accidental deaths (such as suffocation and strangulation), (3) sudden natural deaths (such as those caused by infections, cardiac or metabolic disorders, and neurological conditions), and (4) homicides.[30] SIDS is defined as an infant death that cannot be explained after an extensive examination that includes a review of the clinical history, a complete autopsy, and complete assessment of the site where the death occurred. SIDS is the third leading cause of death for all infants in the United States and the leading cause of death for infants from 1 to 12 months of age.[13] In the U.S. in 2016, there were approximately 3,600 SUIDs with SIDS the most common type of a SUID.[30]

The results of initial population-based studies conducted in the late 1980s and 1990s established that babies placed on their backs were at a lower risk of SIDS than those placed on their stomachs.[30-33] In response to these findings, in the United States, a national Back to Sleep campaign was instituted in 1992 that encouraged parents to place infants in the supine position. The campaign, now referred to as the Safe to Sleep Campaign, is an excellent example of a universal prevention program (see Chapter 2) using a public service approach. The campaign also demonstrates the power of collaboration between agencies. Safe to Sleep is a public education campaign supported by the Eunice Kennedy Shriver National Institute of Child Health, and Human Development, the Maternal and Child Health Bureau, the American Academy of Pediatrics, the SIDS Alliance, and the Association of SIDS and Infant Mortality Programs (see Box 17-1).[34] It is also an example of how these type of primary prevention programs can be effective. The SUID rate fell from 154.6 deaths per 100,000 live births

TABLE 17-1 ■ Leading Causes of Death in Children Aged 1 to 4

United States	Worldwide
Unintentional Injury	Pneumonia
Congenital malformations, deformations, and chromosomal abnormalities	Diarrhea
Assault (Homicide)	Malaria

Sources: (1) and (25)

BOX 17-1 ■ Safe to Sleep Campaign Parental Guide

There are ways parents and caregivers can reduce the risk of Sudden Infant Death Syndrome (SIDS) and other sleep-related causes of infant death. Learn how to create a safe sleep environment for the baby.

- Select the crib.
- Always place the baby on his or her back to sleep, for naps and at night, to reduce the risk of SIDS.
- Use a firm sleep surface, such as a mattress in a safety-approved crib, covered by a fitted sheet, to reduce the risk of SIDS and other sleep-related causes of infant death.
- Give the baby a dry pacifier—not attached to a string—for naps and at night to reduce the risk of SIDS.
- Do not let the baby get too hot during sleep.
- Have the baby share your room, but not your bed.
- Keep soft objects, toys, crib bumpers, and loose bedding out of the baby's sleep area to reduce the risk of SIDS and other sleep-related causes of infant death.

Source: (34)

in 1990 to 91.4 deaths per 100,000 live births in 2016 with the majority of the decline occurring from the start of the Back to Sleep campaign and 2000. Since then, the rate has leveled off.[35] During the same time period, SIDS rates declined from 130.3 deaths per 100,000 live births to 38.0 deaths per 100,000 live births in 2016.[35] Unfortunately, accidental suffocation and strangulation in bed (ASSB) mortality rates increased with a rate of 21.8 per 100,000 births in 2016.[35]

In the U.S., disparities have persisted along racial lines with regard to SUID over the past 3 decades. American Indian/Alaskan Native and non-Hispanic black infants were more than twice as likely to die of SUID than Hispanic and Pacific Islanders, who hold the lowest rates of SUID.[36] Underlying reasons for this disparity are not clearly understood. Parks, Lambert, and Shapiro-Mendoza (2017) suggested that public health campaigns aimed at reducing SUID may not be "… reaching certain races/ethnicities, not addressing the most important risk factors for these groups, or not being framed in the most effective way to ensure uptake among diverse populations."[36] For example, one of the main risk factors of SUID is preterm birth. With the preterm birth rate highest in both American Indian/Alaskan Native and non-Hispanic black infants than other racial/ethnic groups,[37] a Safe to Sleep campaign may not adequately

address underlying risks across all populations. Preventing preterm births in at-risk populations may be needed as well.

Upstream to Prevention Across the Maternal-Child Health Continuum

An important aspect of a population focus is the **upstream approach**, a metaphor for looking at factors that contribute to illness and disease (see Chapter 2). It is based on the idea that if one only focuses on pulling drowning people out of the river, one may miss the fact that they are falling off the bridge upstream. If they are prevented from falling off the bridge in the first place, no one will have to save them from drowning further down stream. Nurses and other health providers are urged to focus upstream on the social, political, economic, and behavioral causes of disease and unhealthy health events to prevent disease in the first place and potentially poor health outcomes for mother and child.

The health and safety of the mother, the health of the developing fetus, safe birth for the newborn, and continued healthy development of the child are the top priorities for nurses who work in maternal-child health. If the mother is healthy throughout the pregnancy and delivers a healthy child, the nurse working in the hospital only interacts with the mother/child dyad (group of two) for a brief time along this continuum. Therefore, it is essential for nurses to think upstream about the root causes of health problems and to prepare new mothers and families for their future health back in the community. The maternal-child health continuum spans the time from preconception and continues as the child develops. The health and well-being of the woman throughout her pregnancy and perinatal period, and the healthy growth and development of the fetus and child continue for decades. The potential impact of upstream approaches to health and safety for the maternal-child health continuum is significant in health, social, and economic terms, particularly for children. For this reason, nurses use public health approaches to ensure adequate nutrition, appropriate prenatal care, safe delivery for the newborn, and care of mother and child during the postpartum period.

Review of Assessment and Planning in Maternal, Infant, and Child Health Settings

Nursing approaches to improve health for maternal-child populations often involve interdisciplinary teams that bring the breadth of expertise necessary for strong programs. As a key member of that team, the nurse is vital for creating successful and effective programs. Assessment at the population level involves analysis of data from national, state, and local data sources (see Chapters 4 and 5). Such data allow the nurse planner to identify risks and protective factors related to maternal-child health. International, national, state, and local data that track risks and adverse outcomes are available through numerous governmental and nongovernmental agencies such as the CDC, the National Center for Health Statistics, and the Office of Minority Health. Another excellent source of data at the state level is the Pregnancy Risk Assessment Monitoring System.[38] These data help nurses identify risks related to the population for which they are caring. Another useful example is the PeriStats data supported by the March of Dimes Foundation.[39] Once risks are identified, other assessment strategies such as interviews, community forums, and identification of local resources can follow to aid in the planning process.

Models for community assessment, discussed in Chapter 4, illustrate the need to include social, political, economic, and cultural contextual perspectives in epidemiological investigations. In addition, the strengths or assets are always identified in any population-level assessment. Data collected for the assessment can include archival data, health indicator data, interviews, observational surveys, formal surveys, focus groups, and community forums. Other sources of local data include hospital records, local health surveys, and agency records.

Health problems, as well as community or organizational assets, can be identified from the analysis of the data collected in the community assessment. A variety of methods for prioritization exist. Most are based on the perceived severity of the health problem and the importance placed on the problem by the community or organization. In the case of maternal-child health, serious immediate risks for maternal or infant mortality often rank higher than long-term morbidity risks. Although obesity is a significant risk factor related to maternal, neonatal, and child health,[40] other immediate risks can take priority. For example, in the fall and winter of 2009–2010, the H1N1 pandemic became the immediate priority because of the high risk to the health of pregnant women and their fetuses, resulting in a nationwide effort to immunize pregnant women.[41] Despite continued suboptimal vaccination rates, research demonstrates the safety of the influenza vaccine in pregnancy.[42] Another example is the pertussis outbreak that began in 2012 that was responsible for 18 deaths as of January 2013.[43] This has resulted in pertussis immunization becoming a priority for infant and child health and in a reduction of pertussis cases from 48,277 in 2012 to 17,972 in 2016.[43]

In addition, the feasibility and likelihood of positive change as a result of the planned interventions is important for prioritization. Short-term programs with a greater likelihood of success often receive a higher prioritization ranking for funding.

Once the priority needs for the maternal-child population of interest are identified, planning can begin (Chapter 5). As explained in Chapter 5, program goals and objectives are created. The goals must be both long- and short-term and must address positive health outcomes; the objectives must be measurable. The identified goals guide the evaluation process. Planning must include the exploration of resources as well as constraints to the planned interventions, which include political, economic, and time constraints. Before any interventions can begin, a budget must be developed; staffing needs must be met; supplies, equipment, and space need to be obtained; required protocols must be followed; and permissions must be granted. Interventions that are well planned can be completed successfully. Clear evaluation plans that include both process and outcome measures document the success of the program.

In maternal-child health, the challenge is to identify significant health risks in maternal-infant populations across different health settings, set priorities for planning, suggest strategies for interventions to address the risks, and discuss evaluation plans for the selected interventions. For the nurse working in maternal-child health acute care and primary care settings, this requires building alliances with other disciplines, agencies, and members of the community. There are a variety of risks for the mother and child across the continuum from preconception to childhood.

Health promotion with this population begins with prevention of high-risk pregnancy and reduction of shared exposures to risk for both the pregnant mother and the developing fetus. These efforts to promote the health and safety of mother and developing fetus can reduce the incidence of preterm birth, LBW, birth defects, and IMR. Nurses who seek to address health risks for maternal-infant settings must apply assessment and planning strategies of public health science.

● APPLYING PUBLIC HEALTH SCIENCE

The Case of the Teenage Pregnancy Epidemic

Public Health Science Topics Covered:

- Assessment
- Program development
- Program evaluation

Nurses in the local hospital in City A, a moderate-sized city in an economically depressed area, responded to a state health department call for funding for teen pregnancy prevention and the initiation of a community program to address the growing teen pregnancy rate. **Teen pregnancy** is defined as a pregnancy in which the mother is between 15 and 19 years of age, and the **teen pregnancy birth rate** is calculated as the number of births per 1,000 women in this age group.[44] The nurses felt they could contribute to the development of a teen pregnancy program because of their expertise in working with pregnant teens who came to their hospital for care across the perinatal period and through their infants' first year of life. These nurses included those working in the labor and delivery room, the hospital-run prenatal clinic for teens, the neonatal unit, and the pediatric unit. They felt that addressing teen pregnancy would also address the larger issue of the high IMR in the community as recommended by authorities in the field.[44]

The nurses began by reviewing the literature related to teen pregnancy. They found that commonly reported teen pregnancy adverse outcomes increased the risk for both the mother and infant. These adverse outcomes included maternal death, risk for sexually transmitted infections, and greater risk for cephalopelvic disproportion, wherein the infant's head is too large to fit through the mother's pelvis. In addition, they found that teen mothers are less likely to seek prenatal care early and more likely to deliver low birth weight infants.[44] Based on these national statistics, the team became curious about the teens who were served by their hospital and decided further assessment was needed.

The team also recognized the importance of the various legal and ethical concerns when working with adolescents who are minors in the eyes of the law. Nurses who work with programs to prevent teen pregnancy face several ethical concerns. Because teens are often under the age of 18 and must have parental consent for most of their interactions with health-care providers, the nurse must consider whether a planned intervention will require parental consent. In addition, many school settings where teens spend most of their days also control the content of the information made available to students. Various issues should be addressed up front from an ethical perspective to best protect this vulnerable population (Box 17-2).[45,46]

To begin the work, these nurses created an interdisciplinary team of key stakeholders to help identify

---

BOX 17–2 ■ Legal and Ethical Issues Related to Preventing Teen Pregnancy

Individuals under the age of 21 come under the definition of a vulnerable population. In addition, women who are pregnant are also considered vulnerable. Caution must be taken to protect their privacy and the confidentiality of their information. There are differing laws concerning the emancipation of minors and the dispensing of information related to pregnancy. Pediatric obstetrical ethics represents the intersection between pediatric/adolescent ethics and obstetrical ethics and includes ethical decisions made by, with, and for pregnant adolescents. Community buy-in presents another important issue because various community groups, including parents, political bodies, and religious groups, have differing opinions on:

- Sexual behaviors
- Abstinence
- Safer sexual practices
- Use of illegal substances
- Use of tobacco and alcohol products
- Contraception options
- Abortion counseling
- Birth options

Sources: (45) and (46)

---

critical issues related to teen mothers in the community they served and to develop a program based on those findings. These stakeholders included key personnel from the hospital's maternal-child health services and community-based health service providers such as the federally qualified community health center, the director of the teen clinic at the health center, the director of the Planned Parenthood center, and the nursing director from the local department of public health. They also felt it was essential to invite representatives from the public and private schools in the community, the director of immigrant services, leaders of the four ethnic/cultural groups in the community, and the director of the U.S. Department of Agriculture's Women, Infants, and Children nutrition program. In addition, the nurses reached out to the community and invited women living in the community to join the nurse team to help complete the assessment and create a program based on their findings.

The team believed that they needed to begin with a focused assessment to identify the risk factors associated with the problem of teen pregnancy specific to their community (see Chapter 4). Their approach included a mapping of community assets related to maternal, infant, and child health, and identification of adolescent programs that included females.

They began their assessment using a technique referred to as **fishboning**, also known as the Ishikawa cause-and-effect diagram, which provides an easy and fast method of identifying root causes of a complex issue or problem. This technique begins with the forming of a root cause diagram (Fig. 17-4).[47] The planning team assembled their diagram with a facilitator leading the process. In this case, the team identified social causes such as poverty, minority status, and access to adequate prenatal care. They also identified maternal behavioral risk factors, including substance use and maternal stress. Finally, they identified issues related to teen maternal health and pregnancy outcomes, including nutrition and prior birth history.[48] The outcome they wished to address was preterm birth and LBW, with teen pregnancy as one of the root causes.

Using the results of the fishbone diagram process based on national data, the team then searched the epidemiological data from their community to identify whether the issues they found were significant in their community. First, they reviewed the overall demographics of the city. They found that, in City A,

50.1% of the residents had less than a high school education compared with 20% of the state residents. The city reported that 25.7% of the households were below the poverty line, whereas in the state in general, only 13.2% of households were below the poverty line. Thirty percent of high school female teens reported using tobacco in City A, compared with 17.5% at the national level, and 28% met the definition for obesity, compared with 20.9% nationally. Next, they looked at the publicly available birth data and discovered that the teen birth rate was 35.5 per 1,000 births, compared with 20.3 at the national level and 25.2 at the state level. Also, teen mothers in City A had a preterm birth rate of 17.8%, which was significantly higher than the 11.6% rate for all pregnancies at the national level. Another critical issue was access to prenatal care, with teen mothers 20% less likely to receive adequate prenatal care or breastfeed their babies than women in the state overall.

They then requested information from the city health department on the rates of LBW, IMR, prenatal care, maternal obesity, prematurity, and tobacco use among teen moms based on the birth certificate data. The city agreed to provide this information and reported back that the IMR for teen mothers overall

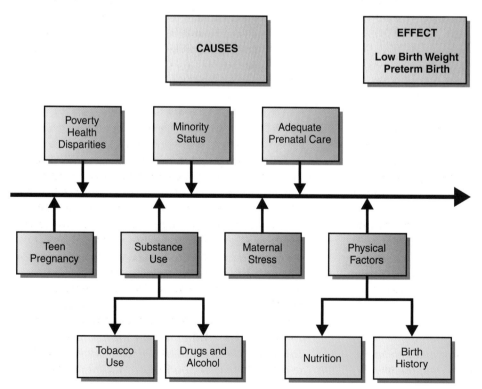

Figure 17-4 Ishakawa fishbone template for low birth weight and prematurity outcomes.

was 8.7 per 1,000 births, and for African American teen mothers it was 16.8 per 1,000 births. The health department reported similar disparities in relation to preterm birth and LBW. Tobacco use in white teen mothers (25%) was higher than in African American teen mothers (10%), compared with 23.8% and 8.4%, respectively, of female teens at the national level. There was a slight difference in the initiation of prenatal care between the two groups, with 71% of white teen mothers and 68% of African American teen mothers initiating prenatal care in the first trimester. The percentage of obese teen moms was similar in both groups, with a 27.5% prevalence of obesity in white teen mothers and 29.3% in African American teen mothers.

Based on the data they gathered, the team concluded that, for their community, City A, the teen pregnancy rate was the highest in the state and represented a significant health problem. In addition, tobacco use and obesity among adolescent females during pregnancy was a problem. The team decided that obesity and tobacco use would be the target of their program.

Obesity and Pregnancy

Based on these facts, the team next took a closer look at the link between maternal obesity and neonatal outcomes. Based on the studies they read, they found that obesity has been linked to multiple adverse outcomes for both the mother and the baby. Researchers have demonstrated that babies born to obese mothers are at greater risk for mortality during their first month and during their first year of life.[49] Infants born to obese mothers were more likely to have macrosomia, that is, they have an excessive birth weight.[50] This often resulted in higher rates of maternal birth canal trauma, shoulder dystocia, and perinatal asphyxia.[50,51] Mothers who were obese during pregnancy were also found to be at greater risk of developing gestational diabetes, hypertension, and preeclampsia.[50] Children born to mothers with gestational diabetes were found to have an elevated body mass index (BMI) during their lifetime. Additionally, women who were obese during pregnancy were also more likely to use medical services, have longer hospital stays, and were twice as likely to have a cesarean section delivery with an increase in health-care costs.[50,51]

Tobacco Use and Pregnancy

They next examined the issue of tobacco use among pregnant teens. Smoking poses risks for both the mother and the infant. Women who smoke during pregnancy, when compared to women who do not smoke, are at increased risk for premature rupture of membranes, placenta previa, or placental abruption.[52] Further, among pregnant nonsmokers, those who are exposed to secondhand tobacco smoke are more likely to give birth to a low birth weight baby than are those pregnant mothers who are not exposed to secondhand tobacco smoke during pregnancy.[52] **Secondhand smoke** includes **side-stream smoke**, which is defined as smoke from the lighted end of a tobacco product, and **mainstream-smoke**, which is defined as smoke exhaled by the smoker.

Tobacco use poses a significant health risk for the baby.[52] E-cigarettes pose a threat as well because they contain nicotine, and nicotine is a known reproductive toxicant that has adverse effects on fetal brain development.[53] Babies born to women who use tobacco are more likely to be born prematurely and are more likely to be born with LBW (less than 2,500 grams or 5.5 pounds).[53] Overall, babies born to mothers who use tobacco weigh 200 grams less on average than babies born to nonsmoking mothers.[52] In addition, babies born to mothers who smoke are likely to die of SIDS.[53]

Infants and children exposed to secondhand smoke related to tobacco use are more likely to experience adverse health issues.[55,56] Exposure to secondhand smoke causes premature death and disease in children exposed in their home or daycare environment. These children experience higher rates of ear infections and respiratory problems that include bronchitis, asthma, and pneumonia.

Based on their findings, the team decided on a multifaceted approach. Programs that address issues such as teen pregnancy, healthy weight preconception, appropriate weight gain during pregnancy, and tobacco use generally focus on outcomes such as a reduction in number of pregnant teens, reduction in the rate of obesity among childbearing women, recommended weight gain during pregnancy, and reduction in tobacco use by pregnant mothers. Achieving the target measures for these outcomes should improve the health of teenage mothers and infants in City A. A more significant outcome would be the actual decline in the maternal mortality or IMRs.

In the case of City A, the team considered a variety of approaches that had been successful in other locations, such as community programs that strengthened parent-child communication and school-based programs.[57] From their assessment, they elected to work with the hospital outreach program and the local neighborhood health center. The nurses at the hospital would serve as the hospital's representatives on the team. The nurses' role included two aspects. First, they provided nutrition education to pregnant teens attending the teen pregnancy clinic based in their hospital, with a focus on healthy eating and achieving a healthy weight gain over the course of the pregnancy. They also put together a smoking cessation program that included the development of a smoking cessation peer-led support group. The hospital provided space for the teens to meet, and the nurses filled the role of facilitator. Once again, the support program was put in place in conjunction with the teen pregnancy clinic. The hospital agreed to give the nurses time within their workweek to provide this service. In addition, the nurses worked with community members and stakeholders on the team to look for opportunities to extend the nutritional education program out into community settings and link it back to the care given in the prenatal clinics. Finally, the nurses agreed to take the responsibility for collecting the needed evaluation data to establish whether the program was successful. They collected baseline and outcome data using specific outcome measures. For the teens who participated in the program, the nurses collected data on overall weight gain during the pregnancy, the percentage of participants who smoked and were able to quit, as well as recording maternal birth outcomes such as pregnancy complications, birth weight, gestational age, and other physical outcome measures related to maternal and neonatal outcomes chosen by the team.

Based on the statistics for City A, the team decided that they should also seek funding to expand the program to address other key areas they had identified during their assessment. They hoped by demonstrating success with their teen pregnancy clinic program, they would be able to secure funding to expand the program and thus have a more significant impact on the problem of teen pregnancy in City A.

Before submitting a grant, the nurses reconvened the larger team and discussed the need for community buy-in and consensus to expand the program. After demonstrating the success of their original program, they received funding from the hospital and some of the stakeholders to support a communitywide forum to be held at the city high school. The team held five

work meetings prior to the community meeting, in which logistics and format were planned, donated refreshments were solicited, and meeting details and advertising were arranged. Representatives of all community service agencies were invited to the planning meeting.

During the community forum planning, the team scheduled the mayor to speak to the assembly of 110 attendees, followed by local politicians at the state and national levels. This confirmed the importance of the work. Then, the audience broke into five small workgroups. Members of the planning team who were skilled in consensus building used the *nominal group process*.[56] Nominal group process or technique refers to the process wherein a larger group can come to a consensus for prioritizing needs in a brief meeting time. To be successful, all participants must agree that they will accept the results of the group process to represent their position for program planning. The first step is often called brainstorming, in which each participant is given a pad of paper and instructed to write down every important issue he or she can think of related to the broad topic of the forum. After about 5 to 8 minutes for this brainstorming, the participants post their written papers in clusters on a whiteboard. With input from the group, the facilitator arranges the clusters into smaller categories. In this community forum, the smaller groups contained about 22 participants. Next, the 90 ideas that were generated were consolidated into 12 categories. Through a process of voting to rank the order of the topics/categories, the group was able to identify their top three concerns or problems:

1. Teen pregnancy prevention
2. High rates of smoking by pregnant adolescents
3. Obesity among adolescent females

They also concluded that LBW was an issue, but it was being addressed in another program. Based on the initial success of the nurses' tobacco cessation and healthy nutrition program with pregnant teens, the community felt the team had the experience to take on a more comprehensive primary prevention program that focused on preventing pregnancy, tobacco use, and obesity in females under the age of 20.

The nurses were now working with a larger community team. They were able to secure support from the chief nursing officer at their hospital by demonstrating the value of the potential program to the hospital and its community outreach initiative. Together with the community team, the nurses developed the following goals for females aged 12 to 19 in City A:

1. Reduce the number of pregnancies.
2. Reduce the rate of obesity.
3. Reduce the initiation of tobacco use.

For both goals 1 and 2, the team developed a healthy living program that used the school-based health clinic system. They based the program on evidence from other programs.[58,59] The nurses on the team brought the school nurses into the planning process. The program extended over the academic year and included support groups for female students aimed at building self-esteem and healthy lifestyles with a focus on healthy sexual practices and healthy eating. There was some resistance from individual members of the community related to the information that might be provided in the support groups, so materials used in the program were developed in conjunction with parent groups. The program was expanded to include faith-based settings for alternative support groups that would provide the same intervention but with an emphasis on abstinence from sexual relations for parents and teens who were only willing to consider abstinence-based approach.

The nurses established three measurable outcome objectives:

- 75% of the teens who participate in the healthy lifestyles program will demonstrate an increase in self-esteem.
- 75% of participants who report they are not sexually active at the beginning of the program will report they are still abstinent at the end of the program, and 75% of those who report that they are sexually active will report that they are practicing safe sex.
- 75% of the participants will demonstrate healthy eating habits and daily exercising; 50% of participants with a BMI above normal will have a BMI within the normal range within 5 months of starting the program.

When developing the nutrition intervention, they considered the fact that there may be cultural issues that should be addressed in the program. Food is fundamental to a person's social and racial identity. In many parts of the world, health is determined by traditional dietary rules and practices. Recommendations given by a nurse or health-care provider are often in direct conflict with cultural rules. As a result,

women make food choices before conception, during pregnancy, when planning feedings for their newborn, and during their postpartum period based on their cultural and social history. To address this, they included an assessment of the cultural context related to the nutritional aspect of their program prior to implementing the program.

For goal 2, the community team chose to take a universal approach and target enforcement of existing laws in City A. The nurses helped the team develop a campaign to stop sales of tobacco products to underage customers, targeting stores selling tobacco located close to schools and playgrounds. The team's objectives were that 100% of all these stores in City A would comply with laws that prohibit sales of tobacco products to minors. The community team also decided to initiate a media campaign aimed at female middle school children, using social networking sites at the beginning of the school year. Their objective was that there would be no change in the percentage of students who reported they did not use tobacco from the beginning of the school year to the end.

During the entire process, the nurses who had initiated the project had the opportunity to work with an interdisciplinary team that included key stakeholders and members of the community. They personally implemented the team's first intervention because of their expertise and their ability to evaluate the success of the program. They were then able to work with a larger community team to develop a more ambitious primary prevention program titled the Healthy Teens and Healthy Families program. They were able to partner with nurses in a school setting to deliver part of the program. They had actively advocated for their patients and helped fill a gap in their community while building on available community resources, such as the hospital-affiliated prenatal clinic for teens and the school-based health clinics.

■ EVIDENCE-BASED PRACTICE
Culture and Nutrition During Pregnancy

Practice Statement: Food is fundamental to a person's social and racial identity. In many parts of the world, health is determined by traditional dietary rules and practices. Recommendations given by a nurse or health-care provider are often in direct conflict with cultural practices. As a result, women make food choices during the preconception period, during pregnancy, for feeding for their newborn, and during their postpartum period based on their cultural and social backgrounds.

Targeted Outcome: Healthy nutrition throughout pregnancy that is congruent with cultural practices.

Evidence to Support: Development of a nutritious diet plan for pregnant women requires that nurses learn about and respect the food practices of the diverse clients with whom they work. Strong evidence exists that early nutrition has a positive effect on the growth and development of the fetus and the child. However, limited nursing research has been conducted on the cultural aspect of nutrition during pregnancy. Nurses who plan health promotion programs for maternal-infant settings must consider race, ethnicity, and sociocultural influences to plan culturally appropriate interventions. Differences exist from a cultural perspective in relation to weight gain and nutrition. Cultural issues were seen as both support for and barriers to healthy nutrition. Other issues that emerged were economic disadvantage and lack of food security. Studies have shown the impact of cultural practices on food consumption during pregnancy. A study performed by Santiago and his associates of 200 predominately Hispanic women in California revealed that the majority of the women's diets included fresh fruits, meat, milk and juice, and prenatal vitamin supplements. However, large percentages of the women reported eating high-sugar sweet desserts, and high fat and salty fast foods more than once a week. They also found a high proportion of the women unknowingly consumed foods with BPA, methylmercury, caffeine, alcohol, and certain over-the-counter medications, all of which have been shown to have adverse effects on the developing fetus. In another study, Coronios-Vargas et al. showed the effects of cultural choices on food cravings and aversion of 160 women from four ethnic groups: Black, Cambodian, Hispanic, and White. Women were all enrolled in WIC programs and completed questionnaires about their food preferences during pregnancy. The Cambodian women craved more meat and spicy/salty foods than the other three groups. Additionally, educational level and number of years spent in the U.S. were positively correlated with significantly more cravings for traditional western American foods such as

chicken, peanut butter, and hotdogs. Aversions for less typical American food such as fermented fish and pigs' feet also increased with higher educational level and more years of residence in the U.S. Further evidence is needed that evaluates the effectiveness of cultural tailoring of pregnancy nutritional protocols and guidance for diverse populations.

Recommended Approaches: Conducting a cultural assessment prior to implementing a nutritional program for pregnant women is a critical first step. Understanding the cultural norms for nutrition can help in the development of a pregnancy nutrition curriculum that incorporates cultural supports and addresses possible cultural barriers.

A comprehensive cultural assessment is essential to developing a culturally appropriate plan and guidance for pregnant women of diverse backgrounds. The assessment should include collecting information about all aspects of the woman's background all of which may influence access to food, patterns of consumption, and preference. Items to assess include home/geographical setting (e.g., urban, rural, tribal), race and ethnicity, language, gender, age, spiritual/religiosity/faith beliefs, disability status, immigrant or refugee status, educational and literacy levels, health literacy level, sexual orientation, socioeconomic status, and military status. Understanding how each of these may influence nutrition during pregnancy, as well as developing a plan that incorporates these influences, is critical to adequate nutrition during pregnancy. Linguistic considerations should also be accommodated both in verbal and written communications. Providers should also avoid bias, prejudice, and stereotypes in working with diverse populations and their cultural and food practices. The goal is to help women develop a nutritional plan that recognizes their cultural practices as well as supports a healthy outcome for the pregnancy and the developing fetus.

Sources:

1. Koletzko, B., Brands, B., Grote, V., Kirschberg, F., Prell, C., Rezehak, P., ... Weber, M. (2017). Long-term health impact of early nutrition: The power of programming. *Annals of Nutrition and Metabolism, 70,* 161-169. doi.org/10.1159/000477781
2. Ramakrishnan, U., Grant, F., Goldenberg, T., Zongrone, A., & Martorell, R. (2012). Effect of women's nutrition before and during early pregnancy on maternal and infant outcomes: A systematic review. *Paediatric and Perinatal*

Epidemiology, 26(Suppl. 1), 285–301. doi:10.1111/ j.1365-3016.2012.01281.x

3. Bravo, I., & Noya, M. (2014). Culture in prenatal development: Parental attitudes, availability of care, expectations, values and nutrition. *Child and Youth Care Forum, 43*(4), 521-538.

4. Whitaker, K., Wilcox, S., Liu, J., Blair, S., & Pate, R. (2016). Patient and provider perceptions of weight gain, physical activity and nutritional counseling during pregnancy: A qualitative study. *Women's Health Issues, 26*(1), 116-122.

5. Coast, E., Jones, E., Lattof, S., & Portela, A. (2016). Effectiveness of interventions to provide culturally appropriate maternity care in increasing uptake of skilled maternity care: A systematic review. *Health Policy and Planning, 31*(10), 1479-1491.

6. Iwelunmor, J., Newsome, V., Airhihenbuwa, C. (2013). Framing the impact of culture on health: A systematic review of the PEN-3 cultural model and its application in public health research and interventions. *Ethnicity & Health, 1*(19), 20. DOI: 10.1080/13557858.2013.857768

7. Coronios-Vargas, C., Toma, R.V., Tuveson, R.V., Schultz, I.M., & Schutz, M. (2010). Cultural influences on food cravings and aversions during pregnancy. *Ecology of Food and Nutrition, 27*(1), 43-49. DOI:10.1080/03670244.1992.9991224

8. Santiago, S.E., Park, G.H., & Huffman, K.J. (2013). Consumption habits of pregnant women and implications for developmental biology: A survey of predominantly Hispanic women in California. *Nutrition Journal, 12*(91), 1-14.

9. Bronheim, S., & Goode, T. (2013). *Documenting the implementation of cultural and linguistic competence: Guide for maternal and child health bureau funded training programs.* Washington, D.C.: National Center for Cultural Competence, Georgetown University Center for Child and Human Development.

Prematurity and Low Birth Weight

As discovered by the nurses in City A, preterm birth and LBW are associated with increased morbidity and mortality during the first year of life as well as with developmental delays that can extend across childhood. LBW is defined as a birth weight less than 5.5 pounds, or 2,500 grams, whereas **very low birth weight (VLBW)** is defined as a birth weight less than 3.3 pounds, or 1,500 grams. Babies born with a LBW have a variety of morbidities that correspond to the severity of their LBW.[59]

Strongly associated with LBW is preterm birth. **Preterm birth** is defined as the birth of a live infant before 37 weeks of gestation, whereas a very preterm infant is born at less than 32 weeks gestation (Fig. 17-5). Frequently, babies born prematurely face health problems such as respiratory distress due to immature lungs and respiratory system, problems with feeding, difficulty with thermoregulation, jaundice, neurological problems with brain development, cerebral palsy, and risk for learning disabilities, blindness, and hearing loss. They are also at a greater risk for death.[59] In addition, there are significant costs. In the United States, those costs amount to approximately $26 billion per year.[60]

Most infants born prematurely meet the definition of LBW, but not all infants with a LBW are premature. A way to help separate the two terms is to evaluate the infant's weight, head circumference, and length against standardized growth charts based on gestational age. An infant born at 30 weeks who weighs 1,490 grams may meet the definition of VLBW but is actually close to the 50th percentile for his gestational age. But an infant born at 38 weeks who weighs 2,400 grams not only meets the definition of LBW but also is in the 5th percentile for his gestational age. Therefore, there are differences between preterm birth and LBW. From an epidemiological perspective, both prematurity and LBW are used as measures of the overall neonatal health of a population despite the overlap between the two terms.

The difficulty is determining the risk factors associated with each of these health indicators. In almost one-half of all preterm births, the cause is unknown. Risks associated with preterm labor include bacterial infection in the mother. It is thought that the infectious process sets

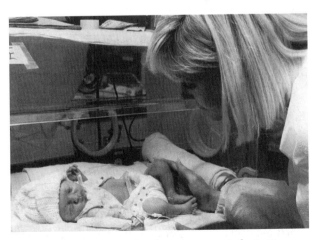

Figure 17-5 Nurse caring for premature infant. *(From the CDC public health awareness campaign to promote prenatal care; Centers for Disease Control and Prevention Public Health Images Library #8291.)*

off an immune response in the body of the pregnant mother that contributes to preterm labor and delivery. Another risk is psychological stress in the mother that results in fetal stress which triggers early uterine contractions. Corticotrophin-releasing hormone (CRH), a stress-related hormone, can be triggered by chronic psychosocial stress in the mother or physical stress to the fetus. The release of CRH is thought to precipitate uterine contractions that lead to premature labor and delivery. Maternal complications, such as placental abruption, are also linked to prematurity. In response to the bleeding, blood clotting stimulates uterine contractions. When there are multiple fetuses or abnormalities of the uterus or placenta, the uterus can become overstretched, and premature contractions may occur. Infants born as multiple births are about nine times more likely to be premature and have an LBW than singleton (one baby) births. Other medical risks include diabetes, hypertension, mother being underweight before pregnancy, obesity, and a short time between pregnancies. Finally, interventions such as inductions and cesarean sections can also lead to preterm births.[61]

Vulnerable Populations and Low Birth Weight Disparity

Differences exist in the risk of having an LBW infant based on race and socioeconomic status. Globally tracking LBW has been hampered as the LBW database has not been updated since October 2014. According to UNICEF, one of the problems is that "… nearly half of all babies are not weighed at birth. Moreover, the babies that are weighed are more likely to be born in health facilities, urban areas and of better-educated mothers, which can lead to an underestimation of LBW incidence."[62] UNICEF, in collaboration with other organizations, is working on updating the data base and hopes to have LBW data in their 2019 report.[62] Based on data from 2014, approximately 22 million, or 16%, of all babies fell into the LBW category.[63] In 2016, the U.S. LBW rate was 8.17% percent, the VLBW rate was 1.4%, and the percent of preterm births was 9.85%.[64]

In the U.S., racial disparities exist with regard to the incidence of LBW. The African American rate of LBW is almost two times higher than that of non-Hispanic white infants (13.7% vs. 7%).[65] The temptation in the U.S. is to ascribe this disparity solely to assumed genetic differences. Yet the role of environment, access to prenatal care, and systematic issues of inequality all conspire to create social determinants of health resulting in poor outcomes for persons of color.

Global and National Initiatives to Reduce LBW

■ HEALTHY PEOPLE
HP 2020 Maternal Infant Child Health (MICH) Objectives Related to Low Birth Weight

MICH objective 8.1: Reduce low birth weight (LBW)

Baseline: 8.2% of live births were low birth weight in 2007
Target: 7.8%
Target-Setting Method: Projection/trend analysis
Source: National Vital Statistics System–Natality (NVSS–N), CDC, NCHS

MICH objective 8.2: Reduce very low birth weight (VLBW)

Baseline: 1.5% of live births were VLBW in 2007
Target: 1.4%
Target-Setting Method: Projection/trend analysis
Source: National Vital Statistics System–Natality (NVSS–N), CDC, NCHS
Midcourse Review: In 2013, these objectives met or exceeded the 2020 targets. LBW was 8.0% in 2013, and VLBW 1.4% in 2013.[12] In 2016, there was no change in these rates.[64]

March of Dimes Prematurity Campaign

Building on their earlier Prematurity Campaign, "… In 2017, the March of Dimes began the Prematurity Campaign Collaborative to address the persistent health inequities and the rising rate of preterm birth in the United States".[66] This campaign provides information and services for families of newborns in neonatal intensive care units, creates community intervention programs to increase awareness of the problem, and includes funding for basic research to improve practice both in the United States and globally. In addition, the campaign helps health-care providers identify risks for premature birth and increases their ability to detect these risks in pregnant women. Since the initiation of the campaign, the March of Dimes has funded research and advocated for the PREEMIE Act (Prematurity Research Expansion and Education for Mothers Who Deliver Infants Early) that became law in 2006. The Prematurity Campaign supports activities in five main areas: research and discovery; care innovation and community engagement; advocacy; education; and family-centered newborn intensive care units (NICUs).[66]

Knowledge of strategies to effect change in the modifiable risk factors for infant mortality, specifically preterm birth and LBW, include education of women about preconception health, and the risks of smoking, alcohol use, and illegal drug use. In addition, all health-care providers involved with pregnant women as well as pregnant women themselves must be aware of the signs of **preterm labor**, defined as the presence of uterine contractions between 20 and 37 weeks that result in progressive dilation and effacement of the cervix. Nurses must reach out to diverse population groups and integrate culturally-sensitive messages into their educational materials and programs. Additionally, nurses must advocate for legislation, support federal and state legislation to increase research on prematurity, and work to expand maternity care services.

● APPLYING PUBLIC HEALTH SCIENCE

The Case of the Small Babies
Public Health Science Topics Covered:

- Epidemiology
- Focused assessment
- Health planning
- Coalition building

To determine additional priority areas for nursing interventions, epidemiological and demographic data should be used for assessment. In response to the work begun with the Healthy Teens and Healthy Families program, the nurse team from City A also worked to obtain funding to address the preterm birth rate in the city. They were aware that their city had not met the *HP 2020* objective to reduce LBW and VLBW. To further evaluate the data, the nurse team compared the local rates with the state's, using the national morbidity data set. Their findings confirmed that the rate of preterm births exceeded the state and national rates as well as the *HP 2020* goals and had increased over the past decade from 15.5% to 22.2%; this was a little more than double the national rate. The team decided to conduct a more in-depth epidemiological investigation to identify determinants of this health issue as well as strategies for addressing the problem in City A. To plan an intervention that would address preterm birth and LBW, the team partnered with the state department of maternal-child health and the local chapter of the March of Dimes. Both entities had a long-standing commitment to the improvement of maternal and infant outcomes, and were able to

provide some funding. They adopted a model of partnership proposed by two public health nurses (PHNs), Leffers and Mitchell, that included the following components:[66]

- *Participation* by multiple constituencies to strengthen the community support for the interventions
- *Collaboration* because it is necessary to address health problems and is fundamental to partnerships
- *Issues of diversity* that are addressed respectfully and appropriately, with representation of the various diverse groups in the community
- *Expertise and resources* that grow stronger with broad partners working together
- *Partnership relationships* as they are essential for the sustainability of interventions.

Another issue that the team addressed was disparities in preterm births and LBW related to ethnicity. At the national level, both the LBW rate and the preterm birth rate were higher for African American mothers than they were for any other ethnic group, with the LBW rate almost double in these mothers compared with non-Hispanic white mothers (13.68 vs. 6.97 in 2016). When they examined the literature to look for the underlying causes of the disparity, two of the possible causes were limited or lack of access to care and lower income. In a classic study, researchers dispelled the notion of the likelihood of genetic differences. The study's findings indicate that the rates of LBW and VLBW for first-generation African American women were similar to the rates for U.S.-born, non-Hispanic white women and were significantly less than the rate for U.S.-born, African American women.[67] Since then, much of the evidence supports a strong link between LBW and VLBW infants and social determinants, poverty, racial discrimination, and chronic stress.[13] In addition, African American mothers are at higher risk for having LBW infants.[13]

Based on their analysis of the data that confirmed significant disparities among racial and ethnic groups in City A, the team developed a citywide Healthy Babies, Healthy Families program that used the *HP* objectives as goals:

- **Goal 1.** Reduce preterm births.
- **Goal 2.** Reduce the number of LBW and VLBW infants.

The program included multiple interventions, including a media campaign and an outreach to underserved neighborhoods within the community using trained lay health workers, aimed at increasing prenatal care and promoting healthy living. The risk factors targeted by their program included the issues addressed in their first program with pregnant teens, tobacco use, and obesity, because these are associated with preterm births and LBW, while adding an intervention aimed at improving access to and utilization of prenatal care. They planned to expand their intervention to all women of childbearing age. In addition, to reach their goals to reduce preterm births and LBW, they needed to assess outcomes over an extended period to identify changes that could be attributed to the program in City A. The goals and objectives for the prematurity and LBW initiatives would be measured by both immediate outcomes and long-term impact evaluation (see Chapter 5).

In addition to the impact evaluation, the nurses were involved with a process evaluation (see Chapter 5). For the citywide Healthy Babies, Healthy Families program, the team created an advisory committee to strengthen the collaboration with the community and provide feedback. In the process evaluation, issues of implementation such as efficiency and effectiveness for the components of the program were addressed. In this case, the team evaluated the performance by team personnel, the lay health workers, educational resources and process, program participation and compliance with program elements, degree of fidelity to program interventions, timeliness, and budget expenditures. They located resources for protocols and tools for evaluation.[69] The primary long-term outcome of the Healthy Babies, Healthy Families program was a reduction in the number of preterm births, LBW infants, and VLBW infants in City A, with a subsequent reduction in IMR as well.

Applying Public Health Science to Acute Maternal, Infant, and Child Health Settings

The use of a population-level approach is helpful in acute maternal-infant health settings as well. Often, the nurses are the first to become aware of a trend in the health of infants and small children, and reach out to the community to implement a prevention program. For example, as mentioned in Chapter 12, the trauma nurses at the Cincinnati Children's Hospital Medical Center developed and implemented a child passenger safety program based on their exposure to severe trauma in children who were not properly restrained in a car. The program was offered to low-income families at 46 fitting stations located in the community, including fire stations and health departments, so that parents could receive help on car seat installation. In other cases, nurses implemented changes in procedures within the hospital setting to help provide better care, as illustrated in the use of an intensive care approach to care for children with polio in the 1950s (see Chapter 14). This requires applying public health science to the problem and determining whether the intervention was effective.

● APPLYING PUBLIC HEALTH SCIENCE
The Case of One State's Approach to Decrease Infant Mortality Rates
Public Health Science Topics Covered:
- Epidemiology
- Surveillance
- Infant Mortality Rates
- Health planning

The State of South Carolina, for many years, has had an IMR higher than the U.S. rate of 5.8 deaths per 1,000 live births.[70] South Carolina's IMR in 2005 was 9.5 – placing it among the highest rates in the U.S. In 2009, the IMR had decreased to 7.1, and in 2017 South Carolina's IMR was 6.7.[71] The drops in the IMR are impressive even though South Carolina's rate is still higher than the overall U.S. IMR of 5.8.[15] South Carolina adopted a new model of care that has had a positive effect on the IMR both in terms of health-care outcomes and the cost of health care.

South Carolina's IMR, similar to other locations in the U.S., was highest among African American women and poor women. Across the state, health-care providers, including nurse midwives, were concerned about the persistently high IMR. This IMR placed the state among the last out of all the states, and these health-care providers wanted to determine what could be done to address this health disparity and improve birth outcomes for mothers and infants. Nurses, nurse midwives, other health-care providers, and public health MCH providers were aware of many of the risk factors and barriers for many women that make it difficult for them to engage in and remain in prenatal care. Their needs assessment identified late entry into prenatal care and inconsistent use of prenatal care.

To complete their assessment of barriers and risks, state-level data from 2008 and 2009 were reviewed. The leading causes of infant deaths (42.6%) were congenital malformation and deformation disorders related to short gestation (premature birth), LBW, and SIDS.[71] Although the number of deaths due to maternal complications decreased by 47.2% between 2008 and 2009, and deaths due to dental causes such as unintentional suffocations and strangulations decreased, there was almost no change in infant deaths due to disorders related to short gestation and LBW.[71]

The state's health-care providers, especially the nurses and nurse midwives, believed a new model of delivery of prenatal care was needed to address the continued high rate of IMR. Some nurses and nurse midwives had heard about group prenatal care and the positive impact it was having on maternal and infant pregnancy and birth outcomes. The group model for prenatal care was known as CenteringPregnancy. The model was initially developed and implemented in the 1990s by Yale-trained nurse midwife Sharon Rising, CNM, MSN, FACM. MCH care providers were interested in exploring the model for potential implementation in the state to address the perinatal health disparities.[72]

The CenteringPregnancy model is an evidence-based model built on findings from research that prenatal education and social support have significant positive effects on birth outcomes, such as reduced risk for LBW babies and less substance use among at-risk mothers. The findings from other studies provided additional strong evidence about the benefits of the CenteringPregnancy model, including a reduction in the likelihood of preterm delivery, a reduction in the risk of NICU admissions, and a reduction in fetal demise.[73,74] Additional benefits included improved mental health for some participants and an increased likelihood that they would engage in breastfeeding.[73] The CenteringPregnancy model is implemented with groups of 8 to 12 women; groups are formed around gestational age and due dates. The groups meet around routine scheduled prenatal care visits and involve 10 visits of 90 minutes to 2 hours duration. Each session includes a physical assessment completed by the providers and some self-assessments such as weight, blood pressure, and recording their own health data. The groups have informal discussions among the participants and the facilitator. These discussions include educational content and provide an opportunity to discuss a variety of topics and concerns that women

have about their pregnancy, their health, their infant, and their family's health. The model and published research about positive impact on birth outcomes, especially LBW, and women's satisfaction with the model of care convinced providers in South Carolina to implement a CenteringPregnancy model of prenatal care groups. During 2009, with a $1.7 million grant, the South Carolina Department of Health and Environmental Control (SCDHEC) implemented the CenteringPregnancy model of care. The objectives included:

- Reducing IMR disparities
- Reducing C-Section rates
- Reducing preterm births
- Increasing adequate prenatal care utilization
- Decreasing gestational diabetes

The CenteringPregnancy groups were implemented across South Carolina at 24 sites, primarily for women who were Medicaid recipients. Along with implementing the CenteringPregnancy model, South Carolina health-care providers implemented increased access to long-acting reversible contraception (LARC) and targeted breastfeeding by encouraging hospitals to achieve the Baby Friendly Hospital designation.

There have been several state reports and presentations of the South Carolina CenteringPregnancy program outcomes.[74-76] Five years after the project was implemented, an analysis of the data provided evidence that there was increased prenatal care, decreased preterm births, decreased gestational diabetes, decreased C-section rates, and increased breastfeeding rates among the mothers who participated. Overall, there was a 34% reduction in the odds of having a preterm birth, and among African American women there was a 60% reduction in the odds of having a preterm birth. In terms of reducing the disparities in the IMR, there was also a significant reduction in IMR. In 2011 the overall state IMR was 7.4/1,000 live births, and for African American mothers it was 12.6/1,000 births. By 2014, the state rate was 6.5/1,000 live births, and for African American mothers it was 9.3/1,000 live births.[76]

A retrospective 5-year cohort study of women who were recipients of Medicaid and who had participated in the CenteringPregnancy programs showed significantly improved outcomes.[73] Findings revealed a 36% reduced risk for preterm birth and a 44% decreased incidence of delivering a LBW infant. Also, the infants of mothers who had participated in CenteringPregnancy programs had a 28% reduced risk of a NICU stay. Gareau concluded that the South Carolina's $1.7 million investment yielded an estimated $2.3 million return on their investment. It was concluded that CenteringPregnancy, a nurse-led model of care, was effective in reducing perinatal health disparities, improving health outcomes, and achieving cost savings.[73]

Maternal-Infant and Early Childhood Home Visiting

Home visiting has been a key component of public nursing since the turn of the last century, as exemplified in work done by Lillian Wald in New York City in the early 1900s (see Chapter 1). Nursing home health visits have traditionally included the delivery of health care in the home. It is not a specific, single intervention but rather represents a systematic approach to the delivery of services within the home setting that combines resources and supports available in the community. Common elements across home visiting programs for mothers and children include provision of social support to parents, connecting families to community services, and providing education to parents on childhood development.[77] The majority of home visiting programs target at-risk pregnant women or parents, or both, to assist them to engage in prenatal care, which is associated with improved pregnancy and birth outcomes, and to assist them to provide a home environment that supports optimal infant growth and development.[77] Published research has provided evidence that high-quality home visiting programs are associated with better maternal and infant outcomes, increased school readiness for children, reduced rates of child neglect and abuse, and higher levels of parent education and income.[78] A rigorous study by the RAND Corporation showed that high-quality home visiting programs are a good investment.[79] There is $5.70 return for every tax dollar spent on a home visit due to reduced expenditures for health care and welfare services.

The Affordable Care Act and Maternal, Infant, and Early Child Home Visiting

Prior to the implementation of the Affordable Care Act (ACA), approximately 450,000, or about 2% of U.S. children and their families, received home visiting services. To help increase that number, the 2010 ACA authorized federal funding for Maternal Infant and Early Child Home Visiting (MIECHV) programs. These were defined as programs that included home visiting as a primary service delivery strategy.[80] These programs were set up to be offered voluntarily to pregnant women with children age 5 or under. The goal was to improve maternal-child health outcomes.[81] In 2012, $71,900,246 was awarded to 10 state-level organizations. The purpose was to implement home visiting programs to provide links to services as well as early childhood education.[82] As part of the grant application process, organizations had to conduct a needs assessment (Chapter 4) using a public health approach to identify the needs of the population, and then tailor the program to the specific needs of that population.

Data from a FY2017 review of home visiting models provides ample evidence of the effectiveness of the MIECHV programs. Each year approximately 156,000 parents and children received services through 942,000 home visits. Services were provided in 27% of U.S. counties, (22% rural counties and 36% urban counties), and 72% of participating families had household incomes at or below 100% of the federal poverty guidelines ($24,600 for a family of 4). More than 80% of all funded programs showed significant improvements in the benchmarks, which include improved maternal and child health outcomes; improved school readiness and achievement; improved family economics and sufficiency; reduced child injuries, abuse, and neglect; reduced domestic violence; and improved coordination for referrals for community resources.[81]

Home Visiting Program Models: What Works?

Astero and Allen pointed out that evidence is divided over what works, but across studies there is evidence that home visiting programs have resulted in positive outcomes.[80] Central to the effectiveness of programs is the inclusion of a systematic approach to the delivery of services. Kahn and Moore completed a systematic review of 66 studies that included a home visiting component. They found that high-intensity early childhood programs were effective for one or more childhood outcomes.[81] The Health Resources and Services Administration has compiled a list of home visiting programs and encourages the collection of further evidence to support the use of a home visiting approach.[82]

Many of these interventions are delivered by PHNs. For example, in Washington County, Oregon, the Web site related to maternal-child home visits states that "the Field Team consists of experienced PHNs who make home visits to pregnant or postpartum women and families with newborn infants or young children with special health-care needs."[83] These nurses meet with families in their homes, provide education, and help link the families with needed resources. The focus is to help decrease the disparity in childhood outcomes related to socioeconomic status.[83]

The Health Resources Services Administration (HRSA) published a list of evidence-based programs that meet their criteria (Box 17-3). The benchmarks chosen for the MIECHV programs are consistent with the goal of the program to reduce disparity in health outcomes in children. They include six areas (Box 17-4). The evidence-based programs listed by the HRSA are, for the most part, based on a developmental theoretical framework. For example, the Child First program is based on research related to early brain development. The program focuses on building a nurturing environment for at-risk children based on the hypothesis that nurturing is protective in relation to brain development.

PHNs providing maternal, infant, and child home visits are actively engaged in prevention using a selective approach (Chapter 2) providing interventions to mothers and children at greater risk for more impoverished childhood outcomes. Recently HRSA has contracted with Mathematica Policy Research to conduct a systematic review of home visiting research. The HRSA HomVee review included only program models that used home visiting as the primary mode of service across eight domains and aimed to improve outcomes in at least one of the eight domains. The eight domains were: (1) maternal health, (2) child health, (3) positive parenting practices, (4) child development and school readiness, (5) reductions in child maltreatment, (6) family economic self-sufficiency, (7) linkages and referrals to community resources and supports, and (8) reductions in juvenile delinquency.[84] The study included 45 program models, and among those programs, 20 met the DHHS criteria for evidence-based early childhood home visiting

---

BOX 17–3 ■ Evidence-Based Home Visiting Service Delivery Models

Home Visiting Evidence of Effectiveness (HomVEE), a program within the U.S. Department of Health and Human Services, has reviewed 45 home visiting models that meet the DHHS criteria for evidence-based models, including at least one high- or moderate-quality impact study with favorable, statistically significant impacts in two or more of the eight outcome domains; at least one of the impacts is from a randomized controlled trial and has been published in a peer-reviewed journal; and at least one of the impacts was sustained for at least 1 year after program enrollment. Of the programs reviewed, 20 met the DHHS criteria for an evidence-based early childhood home visiting program model.

- Attachment and Biobehavioral Catch-Up (ABC) intervention
- Child First
- Early Head Start—Home Visiting
- Early Intervention Program for Adolescent Mothers
- Early Start (New Zealand)
- Family Check-Up
- Family Connects
- Family Spirit
- Healthy Access Nurturing Development Services
- Healthy Beginnings
- Healthy Families America (HFA)
- Healthy Steps (National Evaluation 1996 Protocol)
- Home Instruction for Parents of Preschool Youngsters (HIPPY)
- Maternal Early Childhood Sustained Home Visiting Program
- Minding Baby
- Nurse Family Partnership (NFP)
- Oklahoma Community-Based Family Resource and Support Program
- Parents as Teachers (PAT)
- Play and Learning Strategies (PALS) Infant
- Safe Care Augmented

Source: (84)

BOX 17–4 ■ Benchmark Areas to Demonstrate Improvement to Reduce Health Disparities in Children

The eight domains (benchmark areas) in which to demonstrate improvement among eligible families participating in the Maternal, Infant, and Early Childhood Home Visiting Program (MIECHV) are:

1. Maternal health
2. Child health
3. Positive parenting practices
4. Child development and school readiness
5. Reductions in child maltreatment
6. Family economic sufficiency
7. Linkages and referrals to community resources and support
8. Reductions in juvenile delinquency, family violence and crime

Source: (84)

programs. In terms of program impacts, one program model, Healthy Families, had one or more effects on each of the eight domains. Healthy Families America had the widest range of favorable impacts in all eight domains using primary or secondary measures. Nurse Family Partnership was next with favorable outcomes in seven domains. Interestingly, none of the 20 evidence-based programs showed favorable impacts on juvenile delinquency or family violence using a primary measure.[84]

Programs receiving MIECHV funds have mandated content that must be included in the home visit curriculum. All home visits must include: (1) preventive health and prenatal care practices, (2) assisting mothers with infant care and to maintain breastfeeding, (3) increasing parents knowledge and understanding of infant and child development milestones and behaviors, (4) providing parents with techniques that promote their use of praise and other positive parenting techniques, and (5) helping mothers to set goals for the future, including continuing their education, finding employment, and securing appropriate, affordable child care solutions. The home visitor provides knowledge and informational resources, and demonstrates and models strategies for maternal health practices, infant care, and parenting techniques.

Summary Points

- Maternal, infant, and child health is a major indicator of the health of populations.
- Globally, the IMRs and MMRs continue to be major health issues.
- Preterm birth is a leading cause of infant mortality worldwide.
- Nurses working in maternal-child health settings can actively engage in efforts to improve the health of mothers and children through the implementation of programs at the community level and within an acute care nursing unit.

▼ CASE STUDY
Planning a Breastfeeding Promotion Program

Learning Outcomes

At the end of this case study, the student will be able to:

1. Apply assessment strategies for accessing secondary data.

2. Describe assessment strategies for obtaining primary data.
3. Identify evidence-based practice relevant to perinatal health promotion.
   a. Describe the Ten Steps of the Baby Friendly Hospital Initiative.
4. Describe strategies for the development of a community support program.

The nurses in an urban hospital in Baltimore attended a professional development in-service regarding the newly updated WHO/UNICEF Baby Friendly Hospital Initiative Ten-Steps (BFHI) (2018), CDC Guide (2013), Surgeon General's Call to Action (2011), and the Healthy People 2020 Breastfeeding goals (CDC, 2018). The in-service emphasized the role of nurses working in perinatal, mother-baby unit, and newborn nursery settings to promote breastfeeding by applying the BFHI Ten-Steps to improve exclusivity rates and durations.

On return to work, they decided to review their current breastfeeding support program and identify: opportunities for aligning with the updated BFHI Ten Steps program, and ways to connect with resources in the community. They invited lactation consultant nurses from the Maryland Breastfeeding Coalition to help them review the existing data about breastfeeding and to discuss developing a community support program or clinic and partnership.

The lactation consultants directed them to available Web sites including:

- BFHI: http://www.who.int/nutrition/bfhi/ten-steps/en/
- Healthy People 2020 Breastfeeding Goals: http://www.usbreastfeeding.org/p/cm/ld/fid=221
- CDC Breastfeeding Report Card: https://www.cdc.gov/breastfeeding/data/reportcard.htm
- CDC's Guide to Strategies to Support Breastfeeding Mothers and Babies: https://www.cdc.gov/breastfeeding/pdf/BF-Guide-508.PDF
- U.S. Breastfeeding Committee and Coalition: http://www.usbreastfeeding.org/coalitions-support
- U.S. Surgeon General's Call to Action to Support of Breastfeeding: https://www.surgeongeneral.gov/library/calls/breastfeeding/index.html

Using their approach, answer the following questions that apply to assessment and planning.

1. Review the CDC BF Report Card. How does Maryland and your own state's current breastfeeding data compare with other states and national data?

2. Reflect on the BFHI Ten Steps and how these steps can increase breastfeeding rates.

3. Which of the Ten Steps reflects community support?

4. Review Healthy People Breastfeeding goals and Maryland State BF rates (or choose your own state). Does the data indicate a need for a breastfeeding support program or clinic?

5. Reflect on national initiatives to improve community breastfeeding support, such as the USBC, CDC, and the U.S Surgeon General. What are specific initiatives noted that aim to improve community breastfeeding support?

6. What information is essential to develop a needs assessment?

7. Consult nursing research to determine evidence-based strategies for nurses working in maternal-infant settings to improve breastfeeding support in the community setting. Review the Kaiser Permanente tool-kit (2013).

8. How will the problems, objectives, and goals be prioritized?

9. Describe the process of partnership. Who will be likely partners for the nurse team? Any other additional community stakeholders or agencies?

10. Develop a plan for one intervention, including the objectives and outcome goal for a community program or clinic in a chosen state or region.

Resources

1. Centers for Disease Control and Prevention. (2013). *Strategies to prevent obesity and other chronic diseases: The CDC guide to strategies to support breastfeeding mothers and babies.* Atlanta: U.S. Department of Health and Human Services. Retrieved from http://www.cdc.gov/breastfeeding

2. Centers for Disease Control and Prevention. (2018). *Breastfeeding report card: United States 2018.* Retrieved from: https://www.cdc.gov/breastfeeding/data/reportcard.htm

3. Kaiser Permanente. (2013). *Improving hospital breastfeeding support: Implementation toolkit.* Retrieved from http://kpcmi.org/wp-content/uploads/2013/03/kaiser-permanente-breastfeeding-toolkit.pdf

REFERENCES

1. World Health Organization. (2018). *Children: Reducing mortality.* Retrieved from http://www.who.int/news-room/fact-sheets/detail/children-reducing-mortality.

2. World Health Organization. (2018). *Maternal mortality.* Retrieved from http://www.who.int/news-room/fact-sheets/detail/maternal-mortality.

3. Centers for Disease Control and Prevention. (2017). *Pregnancy mortality surveillance system.* Retrieved from https://www.cdc.gov/reproductivehealth/maternalinfanthealth/pregnancy-mortality-surveillance-system.htm.

4. American Congress of Obstetrics and Gynecology. (2015). Racial and ethnic disparities in obstetrics and gynecology - Committee Opinion No. 649. *Obstetrics and Gynecology, 126e,* 130-134.

5. Buhler-Wilkerson, K. (1993). Bringing care to the People: Lillian Wald's legacy to public health nursing. *American Journal of Public Health, 83*(12), 1778-1786.

6. Colby, S.L., & Ortman, J.M. (2015). *Projections of the size and composition of the U.S. Population: 2014-2060, U.S. Census Bureau Report Number P25-1143.* Retrieved from https://www.census.gov/library/publications/2015/demo/p25-1143.html.

7. Moore, M.F. (2016). Multicultural differences in women's expectations of birth. *ABNF Journal, 27*(2), 39–43. Retrieved from http://search.ebscohost.com.ezp.welch.jhmi.edu/login.aspx?direct=true&db=rzh&AN=114898947&site=ehost-live&scope=site.

8. Liggett, K., & Ringdahl, D. (2016). *How has childbirth changed in this century? Taking charge of your health and wellbeing.* Regents of University of Minnesota. Retrieved from https://www.takingcharge.csh.umn.edu/explore-healing-practices/holistic-pregnancy-childbirth/how-has-childbirth-changed-century.

9. Vasilevski, V., & Carolan, O.M. (2016). Food taboos and nutrition-related pregnancy concerns among Ethiopian women. *Journal of Clinical Nursing, 25*(19/20), 3069–3075. https://doi-org.ezp.welch.jhmi.edu/10.1111/jocn.13319.

10. Goodwin, L., Hunter, B., & Jones, A. (2018). The midwife-woman relationship in a South Wales community: Experiences of midwives and migrant Pakistani women in early pregnancy. *Health Expectations, 21*(1), 347–357. https://doi-org.ezp.welch.jhmi.edu/10.1111/hex.12629.

11. Centers for Disease Control and Prevention, Health Resources and Services Administration. (2018). *Healthy People 2020 Topics: Maternal-child health.* Retrieved from https://www.healthypeople.gov/2020/topics-objectives/topic/maternal-infant-and-child-health.

12. Centers for Disease Control and Prevention, Health Resources and Services Administration. (2017). *Healthy-People 2020 - Midcourse Review Chapter 26: Maternal, infant, and child health.* Retrieved from https://www.cdc.gov/nchs/data/hpdata2020/HP2020MCR-C26-MICH.pdf.

13. Centers for Disease Control and Prevention. (2018). *Infant mortality.* Retrieved from: https://www.cdc.gov/reproductivehealth/MaternalInfantHealth/InfantMortality.htm.

14. World Health Organization. (2018). *Under-five mortality.* Retrieved from http://www.who.int/gho/child_health/mortality/mortality_under_five_text/en/.

15. Central Intelligence Agency. (2018). *The World Factbook: Infant mortality rate.* Retrieved from: https://www.cia.gov/library/publications/the-world-factbook/rankorder/2091rank.html. Accessed June 27, 2018.

16. World Health Organization. (2018). *Preterm birth*. Retrieved from: http://www.who.int/news-room/fact-sheets/detail/preterm-birth.

17. United Nations. (2018). *Sustainable development goals: Goal 3: Ensure healthy lives and promote well-being for all at all ages*. Retrieved from https://www.un.org/sustainabledevelopment/health/.

18. Centers for Disease Control and Prevention. (2018). *Pregnancy mortality surveillance system*. Retrieved from https://www.cdc.gov/reproductivehealth/maternalinfanthealth/pregnancy-mortality-surveillance-system.htm.

19. ACOG Committee. (2014). Opinion No. 586: Health disparities in rural women. *Obstetrics and Gynecology, 123*(2 Pt 1), 384-388.

20. Schroeder, S.A. (2016). American health improvement depends upon addressing class disparities. *Preventive Medicine, 92*, 6–15. https://doi-org.ezp.welch.jhmi.edu/10.1016/j.ypmed.2016.02.024.

21. Alencar Albuquerque, G., de Lima Garcia, C., da Silva Quirino, G., Alves, M.J., Belém, J.M., dos Santos Figueiredo, F.W., ... Adami, F. (2016). Access to health services by lesbian, gay, bisexual, and transgender persons: Systematic literature review. *BMC International Health and Human Rights, 16*, 2. https://doi-org.ezp.welch.jhmi.edu/10.1186/s12914-015-0072-9.

22. Manley, M.H., Goldberg, A.E., & Ross, L.E. (2018). Invisibility and involvement: LGBTQ Community connections among plurisexual women during pregnancy and postpartum. *Psychology Sexual Orientation and Gender Diversity, 5*(2), 169-181. doi: 10.1037/sgd0000285.

23. The American College of Obstetricians and Gynecologists, Committee on Health Care for Underserved Women. (2012). *Health care for lesbians and bisexual women*. Retrieved from https://www.acog.org/Clinical-Guidance-and-Publications/Committee-Opinions/Committee-on-Health-Care-for-Underserved-Women/Health-Care-for-Lesbians-and-Bisexual-Women.

24. Centers for Disease Control and Prevention. (2018). *Pregnancy related deaths*. Retrieved from https://www.cdc.gov/reproductivehealth/maternalinfanthealth/pregnancy-relatedmortality.htm.

25. Centers for Disease Control and Prevention. (2018). *Pregnancy complications*. Retrieved from: https://www.cdc.gov/reproductivehealth/maternalinfanthealth/pregnancy-complications.html.

26. GBD 2015 Eastern Mediterranean Region Maternal Mortality Collaborators. (2018). Maternal mortality and morbidity burden in the Eastern Mediterranean Region: Findings from the Global Burden of Disease 2015 study. *International Journal of Public Health, 63*, 47–61. https://doi-org.ezp.welch.jhmi.edu/10.1007/s00038-017-1004-3.

27. GBD 2015 Maternal Mortality Collaborators. (2016). Global, regional, and national levels of maternal mortality, 1990-2015: A systematic analysis for the Global Burden of Disease Study 2015. *Lancet, 388 North American Edition*(10053), 1775–1812. https://doi-org.ezp.welch.jhmi.edu/10.1016/S0140-6736(16)31470-2.

28. Centers for Disease Control and Prevention. (2018). *Preterm birth*. Retrieved from https://www.cdc.gov/reproductivehealth/maternalinfanthealth/pretermbirth.htm.

29. Potter, P. (2001). About the cover: Ignaz Philipp Semmelweis (1818–65). *Emerging Infectious Diseases, 7*(2). doi:10.3201/eid0702.AC0702.

30. Centers for Disease Control and Prevention. (2017). *Sudden unexplained infant death*. Retrieved from https://www.cdc.gov/sids/aboutsuidandsids.htm.

31. Dwyer, T., & Ponsonby, A.L. (1995). SIDS epidemiology and incidence. *Pediatric Annals, 24*(7), 350-352, 354-356.

32. Fleming, P.J., Blair, P.S., Bacon, C., Bensley, D., Smith, I., Taylor, E., ... Tripp, J. (1996). Environment of infants during sleep and risk of the sudden infant death syndrome: Results of 1993-5 case-control study for confidential inquiry into stillbirths and deaths in infancy. Confidential enquiry into stillbirths and deaths regional coordinators and researchers. *BMJ, 313*(7051), 191-195.

33. Mitchell, E.A., Tuohy, P.G., Brunt, J.M., Thompson, J.M.D., Clements, M.S., Stewart, A.W., ... Taylor, B.J. (1997). Risk factors for sudden infant death syndrome following the prevention campaign in New Zealand: A prospective study. *Pediatrics, 100*(5), 835-840.

34. U.S. Department of Health and Human Services, National Institutes of Health. (2018). *Safe to Sleep*. Retrieved from https://safetosleep.nichd.nih.gov/.

35. Centers for Disease Control and Prevention. (2018). *Sudden unexpected infant death and sudden infant death syndrome*. Retrieved from https://www.cdc.gov/sids/data.htm.

36. Parks, S.E., Erck Lambert, A.B., Shapiro-Mendoza, C.K. (2017). Racial and ethnic trends in sudden unexpected infant deaths: United States, 1995-2013. *Pediatrics, 139*(6), pii: e20163844. doi: 10.1542/peds.2016-3844.

37. Raglan, G.B., Lannon, S.M., Jones, K.M., & Schulkin, J. (2016). Racial and ethnic disparities in preterm birth among American Indian and Alaska Native women. *Maternal Child Health Journal, 20*, 16–24. doi: 10.1007/s10995-015-1803-1.

38. Centers for Disease Control and Prevention. (2018). *What is PRAMS?* Retrieved from https://www.cdc.gov/prams/index.htm.

39. March of Dimes Foundation. (2018). *Peristats*. Retrieved from https://www.marchofdimes.org/peristats/Peristats.aspx.

40. Meehan, S., Beck, C., Mair-Jenkins, J., Leonard-Bee, J., & Puleston, R. (2014). Maternal obesity and infant mortality: A meta-analysis. *Pediatrics, 133*(5), 863-71.

41. Lieberman, R.W., Bagdasarian, N., Thomas, D., & Van De Ven, C. (2011). Seasonal Influenza A (H1N1) infection in early pregnancy and second trimester fetal demise. *Emerging Infectious Disease, 17*(1). Retrieved from http://wwwnc.cdc.gov/eid/article/17/1/09-1895_article.htm.

42. Hvid, A. (2017). Association between pandemic influenza A (H1N1) vaccination in pregnancy and early childhood morbidity in offspring. *Journal of American Medical Association, Pediatrics, 171*(3), 239-248.

43. Centers for Disease Control and Prevention. (2018). *Pertussis outbreak trends*. Retrieved from http://www.cdc.gov/pertussis/outbreaks/trends.html.

44. Centers for Disease Control and Prevention. (2017). *Teen pregnancy*. Retrieved from https://www.cdc.gov/teenpregnancy/about/index.htm.

45. Mercurio, M.R. (2016). Pediatric obstetrical ethics: Medical decision-making by, with, and for pregnant early adolescents. *Seminars in Perinatology, 40* (4), 237-246.

46. Fischer, M., Shlomo, I.B., Solt, I., & Burke, Y.Z. (2015). Pregnancy prevention and termination of pregnancy in adolescence: Facts, ethics, law, and politics. *Israel Medical Association Journal, 17*(11), 665-8.

47. American Society for Quality. (2018). *Fishbone (Ishikawa) diagram*. Retrieved from http://asq.org/learn-about-quality/cause-analysis-tools/overview/fishbone.html.

48. Center for Disease Control and Prevention. (2018). *Pregnancy complications*. Retrieved from: https://www.cdc.gov/reproductivehealth/maternalinfanthealth/pregcomplications.htm#Research.

49. American College of Obstetricians and Gynecologists (ACOG). (2016). *Obesity and pregnancy*. Retrieved from https://www.acog.org/Patients/FAQs/Obesity-and-Pregnancy.

50. Vernini, J.M., Brogin Moreli, J., Garcia Magalhães, C., Araújo Costa, R.A., Cunha Rudge, M.V., & Paranhos Calderon, I.M. (2016). Maternal and fetal outcomes in pregnancies complicated by overweight and obesity. *Reproductive Health, 13*, 1–8. https://doi-org.ezp.welch.jhmi.edu/10.1186/s12978-016-0206-0.

51. Araujo Júnior, E., Peixoto, A.B., Zamarian, A.C.P., Elito Júnior, J., & Tonni, G. (2017). Macrosomia: Best practice & research. *Clinical Obstetrics & Gynaecology, 38*, 83–96. https://doi-org.ezp.welch.jhmi.edu/10.1016/j.bpobgyn.2016.08.003.

52. Centers for Disease Control and Prevention. (2018). *Smoking during pregnancy*. Retrieved from https://www.cdc.gov/tobacco/basic_information/health_effects/pregnancy/index.htm.

53. Centers for Disease Control and Prevention. (2016). *Information for health care providers: Preventing tobacco use and pregnancy*. Retrieved from https://www.cdc.gov/reproductivehealth/maternalinfanthealth/tobaccousepregnancy/providers.html

54. Mohlman, M., & Levy, D. (2016). Disparities in maternal child and health outcomes attributable to prenatal tobacco use. *Maternal & Child Health Journal, 20*(3), 701–709. https://doi-org.ezp.welch.jhmi.edu/10.1007/s10995-015-1870-3.

55. Centers for Disease Control and Prevention. (2017). *Health effects of second-hand smoke*. Retrieved from https://www.cdc.gov/tobacco/data_statistics/fact_sheets/secondhand_smoke/health_effects/index.htm.

56. Hoyt, A.T., Canfield, M.A., Romitti, P.A., Botto, L.D., Anderka, M.T., Krikov, S.V., & Feldkamp, M.L. (2018). Does maternal exposure to secondhand tobacco smoke during pregnancy increase the risk for preterm or small-for-gestational age birth? *Maternal & Child Health Journal, 22*(10), 1418–1429. https://doi-org.ezp.welch.jhmi.edu/10.1007/s10995-018-2522-1.

57. Center for Disease Control and Prevention. (2016). *Communitywide initiatives*. Retrieved from https://www.cdc.gov/teenpregnancy/projects-initiatives/communitywide.html.

58. Van de Ven, A.H., & Delbecq, A.L. (1972). The nominal group as a research instrument for exploratory health studies. *American Journal of Public Health, 62*(3), 336-342.

59. Center for Disease Control and Prevention. (2017). *Preterm birth*. Retrieved from https://www.cdc.gov/reproductivehealth/maternalinfanthealth/pretermbirth.htm

60. March of Dimes. (2015). *March of Dimes prematurity campaign: Activities and milestones*. Retrieved from https://www.marchofdimes.org/mission/march-of-dimes-prematurity-campaign.aspx.

61. Wood, S., Tang, S., & Crawford, S. (2017). Caesarean delivery in the second stage of labor and the risk of subsequent premature birth. *American Journal of Obstetrics and Gynecology, 217*(1), 63.e1–63.e10.

62. UNICEF. (2017). *Low birth weight*. Retrieved from https://data.unicef.org/topic/nutrition/low-birthweight/.

63. UNICEF. (2014). *Low birth weight, current status and progress*. Retrieved from: https://data.unicef.org/topic/nutrition/low-birthweight/.

64. Centers for Disease Control and Prevention, National Center for Health Statistics. (2018). *Birthweight and gestation*. Retrieved from https://www.cdc.gov/nchs/fastats/birthweight.htm.

65. Martin, J., Hamilton, B., Osterman, M., Driscoll, A., & Drake, P. (2018). *National Vital Statistics Report Vol 67, No. 1*. Hyattsville, MD: National Center for Health Statistics.

66. March of Dimes. (2018). *Fighting premature birth: The Prematurity Campaign*. Retrieved from https://www.marchofdimes.org/mission/prematurity-campaign.aspx.

67. Leffers, J., & Mitchell, E.M. (2011). Conceptual model for partnership and sustainability in global health. *Public Health Nursing, 28*(1), 91-102.

68. David, R.J., & Collins, J.W. (1997). Differing birth weight among infants of U.S. born blacks, African born blacks and U.S. born whites. *New England Journal of Medicine, 337*, 1209-1214.

69. McKenzie, J.F., Neiger, B.L., & Thackeray, R. (2017). *Planning, implementing & evaluating: Health promotion programs: a primer* (7th ed.). San Francisco, CA: Pearson/Benjamin Cummings.

70. Mathews, T.J., & Driscoll, A.K. (2017). *Trends in infant mortality data in the United States, 2005-2014*. NCHS Data Brief, No. 279. CDC.

71. SDHEC. (2011). *At a Glance: 2009 Infant Mortality Statistics. Division of Biostatistics, Pregnancy Risk Assessment System, South Carolina of Health and Environmental Control*. Retrieved from: http://www.scdhec.gov.

72. South Carolina Healthy Connections. (2015). *Centering pregnancy: A successful model for group prenatal care*. Retrieved from: https://www.scdhhs.gov/boi.

73. Gareau, S. (2016). Group prenatal care results in Medicaid savings with better outcomes: A propensity score analysis of centering programs in South Carolina. *Maternal and Child Health Journal, 20*(7). DOI: 10.1007/s10995-016-1935.

74. Trotman, G., Chhatre, G., Darolia, R., Tefera, E., Damle, L., & Gomez-Lobo, V. (2015). The effect of centering pregnancy versus traditional prenatal care models on improved adolescent health behaviors in the perinatal period. *Journal of Pediatric and Adolescent Gynecology, 28*, 396-401. https://doi.org/10.1016/j.jpag.2014.12.003.

75. Picklesimer, A.H. (2015). *Centering Pregnancy: Healthy communities- One group at a time*. https://prezi.com/f0qev54qopdj/the-south-carolina-centeringpregnancy-story/

76. Van De Griend, K., Billings, D., Marsh, C., & Kelley, S. (2015). *Centering pregnancy: Expansion in South Carolina process evaluation: Final Report 2015*. University of South Carolina.

77. Kahn, J., & Moore, K.A. (2010). *What works for home visiting programs: Lessons from experimental evaluations of programs and interventions. Child trend fact sheets (Publication*

No. 2010). Retrieved from http://www.childtrends.org/wp-content/uploads/2005/07/2010-17WWHomeVisit.pdf.

78. Child and Family Research Partnership. (2017). *Retaining families in home visiting programs by promoting father participation.* The University of Texas at Austin. Retrieved from www.childandfamilyresearch.org.

79. Dodge, K.A., Goodman, W.B., Murphy, R.A., O'Donnell, K., Sato, J., & Guptill, S. (2014). Implementation and randomized controlled trial evaluation of universal postnatal nurse home visiting. *American Journal of Public Health, 104*(51), 5136-2143. http://www.ncbi.nlm.nih.gov/pmc/articles/PMC4011097/.

80. Astero, J., & Allen, L. (2009). Home visiting and young children: An approach worth investing in? *Social Policy Report, 23*(5), 3-21.

81. Health Resources and Services Administration. (n.d.). *Maternal infant and early childhood home visiting program.* Retrieved from http://mchb.hrsa.gov/programs/homevisiting/.

82. Health Resources and Services Administration, Maternal Child Health. (n.d). *Home visiting.* Retrieved from https://mchb.hrsa.gov/maternal-child-health-initiatives/home-visiting-overview.

83. Washington County, Oregon. (n.d.). *Maternal and child health field team.* Retrieved from https://www.co.washington.or.us/HHS/PublicHealth/MCHFT/index.cfm.

84. U.S. Department of Health and Human Services. (n.d.). *Home visiting evidence of effectiveness.* Retrieved from: https://homvee.acf.hhs.gov/

Chapter 18

Health Planning for School Settings

Donna Mazyck and Joan Kub

LEARNING OUTCOMES

After reading the chapter, the student will be able to:

1. Define school nursing.
2. Present the contribution of school health to the achievement of Healthy People objectives.
3. Describe the components and tenets of the student-centered Whole School, Whole Community, Whole Child model.
4. Summarize the key principles of the 21st Century Framework for School Nursing Practice.
5. Discuss the role of school nurses in addressing health disparities and social determinants of health among vulnerable students.
6. Describe the role of policy in understanding school nursing practice.
7. Discuss challenges to school health nursing for the future.

KEY TERMS

Asthma action plan
Body mass index (BMI)
Cyberbullying
Delegation
Disabilities
Framework for 21st Century School Nursing Practice
Individualized education program (IEP)
Individualized family service plan (IFSP)
Individualized Healthcare Plan
Least restrictive environment
National Health Education Standards
School-based health center
School nursing
Title I
Whole School, Whole Community, Whole Child (WSCC)

▮ Introduction

Did you have a school nurse while going through K-12 education? School nurses provide health promotion and disease prevention for student populations, which in 2017 numbered 55.9 million students enrolled in public and private U.S. schools.[1] The opportunities and rewards in school nursing include helping students reach education goals while learning positive health behaviors; seeing students with chronic health conditions learn to manage their health; creating a culture of health in the school community so that students are healthy, safe, and ready to learn; and collaborating with school staff and community members to reduce social determinants that create barriers to student health and learning. Challenges in school nursing include inconsistent fiscal investment in school nursing positions and misconceptions about the role of school nurses as health professionals in education settings.

For children and adolescents throughout the world, attending school represents a foundational way in which to enter adulthood; however, gender and disparities in wealth keep about 263 million children and adolescents between ages 6-17 years out of school.[2] Students who are in school benefit from school nurses providing disease prevention and health promotion that facilitate student access to learning.

The National Association of School Nurses (NASN) defines **school nursing** as:

A specialized practice of nursing that protects and promotes student health, facilitates optimal development, and advances academic success. School nurses, grounded in ethical and evidence-based practice, are the leaders who bridge health care and education, provide care coordination, advocate for quality student-centered care, and collaborate to design systems that allow individuals and communities to develop their full potential.[3]

School nurses use the nursing process to provide individual and population-based care in schools to facilitate the school nurse's goal of supporting the health and academic achievement of students:

- Assessment
- Diagnosis
- Outcome identification
- Planning
- Implementation
- Evaluation

School nurses may be employed by local school districts, health departments, hospitals, or other entities. Health priorities and educational goals converge in school nursing, requires the school nurse to understand and function in two cultures: the worlds of health and education. Translation of these two cultures is a vital role for school nurses as they advocate for students. The school nurse knows both education and health priorities, goals, policies, and legal requirements in the implementation of school health services. This knowledge places school nurses in a central role as coordinators and connectors in the school setting. NASN published the Code of Ethics to set forth "a commonality of moral and ethical conduct" for school nurses. The code of ethics for school nurses focuses on three aspects: NASN core values, *NASN Code of Ethics,* and professional standards of practice.[4]

● APPLYING PUBLIC HEALTH SCIENCE
The Case of the Weeping Student
Public Health Science:

- Screening
- Referral and Follow-up
- Collaboration

After the second full week of the new school year, Mark, the freshman high school English teacher, visited the school nurse after the students left the building. Mark described a student who barely spoke in class and often wiped tears from her eyes. He knew that the student, Mary, and her family had settled in the U.S. after her family arrived as refugees in early June. Pat, the school nurse, agreed to meet with the student on Monday during her English class time. Mary came to the health room door and hesitated before entering. Pat stood up to meet Mary at the door, inviting her to come into the room. Pat and Mary sat in the private room at the back of the office. Pat told Mary that her English teacher was concerned because he saw her crying during each class. Pat asked Mary what had happened to her, and Mary talked about adjusting to a new country after living for 2 years in a refugee camp overseas. Pat understood that addressing "primary areas of concern for refugee children, such as mental health, nutrition, communicable and vaccine-preventable diseases, and oral health, is paramount to improving health care and learning outcomes" for children and youth who came to the country as refugees.[5] Pat did a nursing assessment that included Mary's health history, refugee status, and journey. Mary shared with Pat that, after she completed screening at the refugee center, the center staff connected her with a mental health therapist. Pat and Mary developed a rapport where they connected weekly. While reviewing literature on needs of students who are refugees, Pat learned that access to education is lower for children and youth who are refugees as compared to children who are not refugees.[6] In the Student Services Team meeting, Pat shared her concern about Mary's lack of confidence in certain school subjects with colleagues on the team (school counselor, school psychologist, school social worker, and school administrator) and her recommendation that Mary may need educational assessments to appropriately develop her schedule. The team agreed to work with Mary to develop a plan for her high school year.

Historical Foundations of School Nursing

School nursing has emerged as a specialty within the broader field of public health nursing. In the beginning of the 20th century, the convergence of compulsory education laws in the United States and medical exclusion of students with contagious diseases paved the way for Lillian Wald to collaborate with the New York City Board of Education and Board of Health to hire a school nurse to work with students and families in four schools where there were high numbers of student absenteeism and medical exclusions.[7] On October 1, 1902, Lina Rogers Struthers's work began as a month-long experiment when she took the role of a school nurse in those four New York City schools. By December, Struthers's use of school nurse assessments, planning, interventions, evaluations, and documentation yielded increased school time for children and an expansion of the school nurse staff from one nurse to 12 nurses.

Struthers, who became the superintendent of school nurses for New York City schools, and those who worked with her were the first school nurses hired by a municipality. The advent of school nursing resulted in students being able to remain in schools if possible and only excluded children with communicable diseases.[7] The presence of school nurses proved effective. From October 1902 to October 1903, student health-related exclusions from New York City public schools decreased by more than 90%, from 10,567 students to 1,101 students.[8] Based on this groundbreaking work by the New York City school nurse demonstration project, school nursing spread throughout the United States and Canada. From the inception of school nursing, school nurses focused on whole school populations and individual student case coordination. School nurses are an integral part of school-based health programs in the 21st century.

Healthy People and School Nursing

Two new topics were identified in *Healthy People 2020 (HP 2020)* that have particular relevance to school nursing—those of early and middle childhood and adolescent health. Both of these topics emphasize the link between behavioral patterns established in either early childhood or adolescence to adult health and the role of the school setting in promoting health. Thus, school nurses have a very important role to play in influencing health outcomes in children and adolescents as well as the long-term health of these children in the future.

■ HEALTHY PEOPLE
School Health

HP 2020 Topic relevant to School Health: Early and Middle Childhood

Goal: Document and track population-based measures of health and well-being for early and middle childhood populations over time in the United States.

Overview: There is increasing recognition in policy, research, and clinical practice communities that early and middle childhood provide the physical, cognitive, and social-emotional foundation for lifelong health, learning, and well-being. Early childhood, middle childhood, and adolescence represent the three stages of child development. Each stage is organized around the primary tasks of development for that period.

Selected *HP 2020* Objectives: Early and Middle Childhood

EMC–1: (Developmental) Increase the segment of children who are ready for school in all five domains of healthy development: physical development, social-emotional development, approaches to learning, language, and cognitive development.
Midcourse Review: There is no data for this developmental objective that had no national baseline value (see Fig. 18-1).
Source: (9)
EMC–4: Increase the segment of elementary, middle, and senior high schools that require school health education.
Midcourse Review: Ten objectives check school health education standards related to EMC-4. Three out of the 10 objectives worsened as noted in the following:
EMC-4.3.1: Between 2006 and 2014, the segment of elementary schools requiring that cumulative health education instruction meet the U.S. National Health Education Standards decreased from 7.5% to 1.7%.
EMC-4.3.2: Between 2006 and 2014, the segment of middle schools requiring that cumulative health

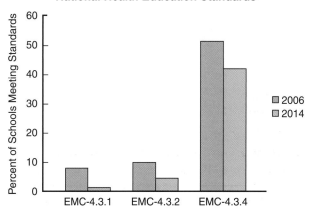

Healthy People 2020 Midcourse Review: National Health Education Standards

EMC-4.3.1: Elementary schools requiring cumulative health education instruction

EMC-4.3.2: Middle schools requiring cumulative health education instruction

EMC-4.3.4: Health education classes taught by an instructor who had received professional development within the past 2 years related to teaching skills or behavioral development

Figure 18-1 Healthy People 2020 Midcourse Review.

education instruction meet the U.S. National Health Education Standards decreased from 10.3% to 4.2%.

EMC-4.4: Between 2006 and 2014, the segment of health education classes taught by an instructor who had received professional development within the past 2 years related to teaching skills for behavioral development declined from 52.5% to 41.2%.

Source: (9)

HP 2020 Topic relevant to School Health: Adolescent Health

Goal: Improve the healthy development, health, safety, and well-being of adolescents and young adults.

Overview: Adolescents (aged 10 to 19) and young adults (aged 20 to 24) make up 21% of the population of the United States. The behavioral patterns established during these developmental periods help determine young people's current health status and their risk for developing noncommunicable diseases in adulthood.

Selected HP 2020 Adolescent Health Objectives

AH–2: Increase the segment of adolescents who participate in extracurricular and out-of-school activities.

Midcourse Review: From 2007 to 2011–2012, the segment of adolescents aged 12–17 participating in extracurricular and/or out-of-school activities demonstrated little or no detectable change (82.5% in 2007 and 82.7% in 2011-2012).

Source: (10)

AH–5: Increase educational achievement of adolescents and young adults.

Midcourse Review:

AH-5.1: The segment of students who graduated from high school 4 years after starting the ninth grade increased from 79% in 2010–2011 to 81% in 2012–2013. In 2012–2013, nine states met the national 2020 target.

AH-5.2: From 2007–2008 to 2012–2013, the segment of students aged 14–21 served under the Individuals with Disabilities Education Act (IDEA) who graduated from high school with a diploma increased from 59.1% to 65.1%.

AH-5.5: The segment of adolescents aged 12–17 who considered schoolwork meaningful and important increased from 26.4% in 2008 to 27.7% in 2013. In 2013, there were statistically significant disparities by race and ethnicity and family income in the segment of adolescents aged 12–17 who considered schoolwork meaningful and important.

AH-5.6: There was little or no detectable change in the segment of adolescents aged 12–17 who missed 11 or more days of school due to illness or injury from 2008 (5.0%) to 2014 (4.4%).

AH-5.3.1: The segment of fourth graders with reading skills at or above grade level increased from 33.0% in 2009 to 35.2% in 2013.

AH-5.3.2: The segment of eighth graders with reading skills at or above grade level increased from 32.4% in 2009 to 36.1% in 2013.

Source: (10)

Midcourse Review:

AH–6: Increase the segment of schools with a school breakfast program.

The segment of public and private elementary, middle, and high schools with a school breakfast program increased from 68.6% in 2006 to 77.1% in 2014.

Source: (10)

Midcourse Review:

AH–7: Reduce the segment of adolescents who have been offered, sold, or given an illegal drug on school property.

There was little or no detectable change in the segment of adolescents in grades 9–12 who have been offered, sold, or given an illegal drug on school property from 2009 (22.7%) to 2013 (22.1%).

Source: (10)

Midcourse Review:

AH–8: Increase the segment of adolescents whose parents consider them to be safe at school.

The segment of adolescents aged 12–17 whose parents considered them to be safe at school increased from 86.4% in 2007 to 90.9% in 2011–2012.[10]

Source: (10)

HP 2020 also includes a topic on educational and community-based programs. This topic includes schools as one of the targeted settings for delivery of these programs aimed at improving health.[11] An important objective under this topic is objective number 5: "Increase the segment of elementary, middle, and senior high schools that have a full-time registered school nurse-to-student ratio of at least 1:750 per student."[11] The midcourse status reveals that, between 2006 and 2014, the segment of schools with a registered nurse to student ratio of at least 1:750 increased for all schools (elementary, middle, and senior high schools—ECBP-5.1: 40.6% and 51.1%); senior high schools (ECBP-5.2: 33.5% and 37.9%); and elementary schools

(ECBP-5.4: 41.4% and 58.1%), exceeding their respective 2020 targets.[12] Instead of ratios, NASN deems that staffing for school nursing services must consider the range of health care required to meet the students' needs, including social determinants of health and student health care needs.[13] The educational and community *HP 2020* topic also includes objectives related to the provision of health-related educational programs including such topics as unintentional injury, violence, suicide, tobacco use and addiction, alcohol or other drug use, unintended pregnancy, HIV/AIDS and sexually transmitted infections (STIs), unhealthy dietary patterns, and inadequate physical activity.[11]

Whole School, Whole Community, Whole Child

With more than 55 million students spending a significant portion of their lives in school, schools are one of the most powerful social institutions shaping the next generation. The primary mission of schools is education, but health is also important because educational outcomes are inextricably linked to health. However, health and education sectors developed their individual approaches to meeting the needs of students. The Centers for Disease Control and Prevention (CDC) promotes a systems approach for **coordinated school health**. **The coordinated school health model** is an integral set of planned, sequential, school-affiliated strategies, activities, and services designed to promote the optimal physical, emotional, social, and educational development of students.[14,15] The concept of a comprehensive school health program is not new. The model is built on the inclusion of four main supportive structures:

- School health advisory council
- School health coordinator
- School-based health teams
- School board policy[16]

In the education sector, ASCD (formerly the Association of Supervision and Curriculum) developed five tenets for the development of the Whole Child: every student will be healthy, safe, engaged, supported, and challenged. In 2014, ASCD and CDC released the Whole School, Whole Community, Whole Child (WSCC) model, which expanded on the original eight components of the coordinated school health model and incorporated the five tenets of the Whole Child initiative.[17] ASCD and CDC collaborated with leaders across education, health, public health, and school health sectors to develop the WSCC model (see Fig. 18-2).[17]

In the WSCC model, positioned in the center are five tenets. That each student:

1. Enters school **healthy** and learns about and practices a healthy lifestyle.
2. Learns in an environment that is physically and emotionally **safe** for students and adults.
3. Is actively **engaged** in learning and is connected to the school and broader community.
4. Has access to personalized learning and is **supported** by qualified, caring adults.
5. Is **challenged** academically and prepared for success in college or further study and for employment and participation in a global environment.[19]

Between the Whole Child tenets and the components of coordinated school health, the WSCC model calls out the need to coordinate policies, processes, and practices with collaborations in learning and health. Surrounding the student, the WSSC model places the 10 components of coordinated school health, which expanded from the original eight.[18]

WSCC Components

Health Education

The health education component provides structured learning for students with information and skills.[19] The goal is to motivate and assist students in maintaining and improving their health, preventing disease, and reducing health-related risk behaviors. The comprehensive health education curriculum includes a variety of topics such as personal health, family health, community health, consumer health, environmental health, sexuality education, mental and emotional health, injury prevention and safety, nutrition, prevention and control of disease, and substance use and abuse. According to the CDC, National Health Education Standards "were developed to establish, promote and support health-enhancing behaviors for students in all grade levels—from pre-kindergarten through grade 12."[20] These standards provide the framework for the curricula and the methods used to deliver the curricula. They also provide guidelines for assessing student progress as well as expectations for school-based health education programs.[20]

Physical Education and Physical Activity

Physical education and physical activity comprise part of a national framework: comprehensive school physical activity program (CSPAP) with physical education being

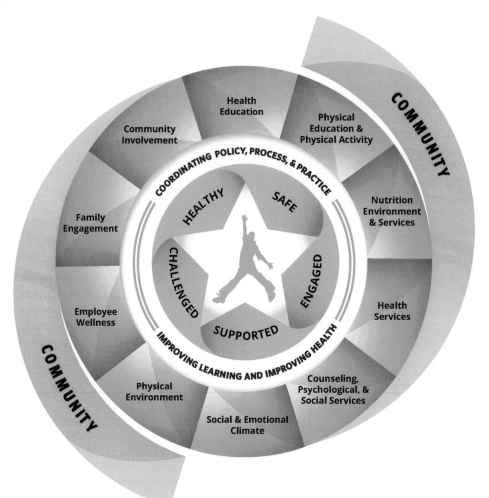

Figure 18-2 Whole School, Whole Community, Whole Child Model: A Collaborative Approach to Learning and Health. Retrieved from https://www.cdc.gov/healthy-schools/wscc/index.htm.

the foundation (see Fig. 18-3).[19] CSPAP includes five components: physical education, physical activity during school, physical activity before and after school, staff involvement, and family and community engagement.[19,21] Physical education curricula should be based on national physical education standards.[21]

Nutrition Environment and Services

School nutrition services promote access to a variety of nutritious and appealing meals that accommodate the health and nutrition needs of all students. School nutrition programs reflect the U.S. Dietary Guidelines for Americans and other criteria to achieve nutrition integrity. The school nutrition services offer students a learning laboratory for classroom nutrition and health education and serve as a resource for linkages with nutrition-related community services. It is recommended that qualified child nutrition professionals provide these services.[16]

School-based programs can influence the extent to which youth eat breakfast. In 2016—2017, the nationwide School Breakfast Program provided breakfast for approximately 12.2 million low-income children, representing a 0.6% increase over the previous school year [22] One of the factors thought to influence the growing problem of obesity in children and youth is the availability of junk food in vending machines and the lack of nutritious foods in school lunches. The school nutrition environment gives students "opportunities to learn about and practice healthy eating through nutrition education, messages about food in the cafeteria and throughout the school campus, and available food and beverages, including in vending machines, 'grab and go' kiosks, school stores, concession stands, food carts, classroom rewards and parties, school celebrations, and fundraisers."[19]

In 2010, the Healthy Hunger-Free Kids Act was signed into law. The bill allows the U.S. Department of

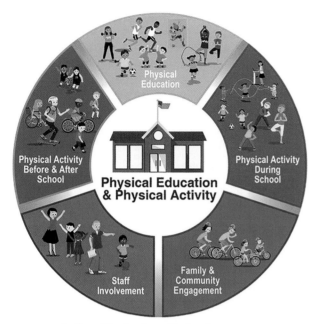

Active Students = Better Learners
www.cdc.gov/healthyschools/PEandPA

Figure 18-3 Comprehensive School Physical Activity Program (CSPAP). Retrieved from https://www.cdc.gov/healthyschools/physicalactivity/index.htm.

Agriculture (USDA) to update nutritional standards for all food sold in schools, including vending machines. It also provided an increase in funding for school lunch programs. The three broad initiatives of the bill are to (1) improve nutrition with a focus on reducing childhood obesity, (2) increase access to healthy school meals, and (3) increase program monitoring and integrity.[23] School nurses played a significant role in advocating for this law.

Health Services

The health services component is a service provided to students that assesses, protects, and promotes health. These services are designed to ensure access or referral to primary care services, foster appropriate use of primary care services, prevent and control communicable disease, provide emergency care for illness or injury, promote and provide optimal sanitary conditions for a safe school facility and school environment, and provide educational and counseling opportunities for promoting and maintaining individual, family, and community health.[16] School nurses are leaders of school health services, providing population-focused nursing care to all students in schools.[24] These health services include emergency services, acute care evaluations, noncommunicable

disease management, health education, and preventive services.

School nurses are primarily employed by education entities and funded with general or special education dollars. Other sources for school nurse funding include health departments, and local and state organizations (see Box 18-1).[25] School nurses facilitate access to providers (some providers may be in the building through school-based health center [SBHC] services), collaborate with community services, and work with families to support a healthy and safe school environment.[19] Details about school nursing in the 21st century are discussed later in this chapter.

Counseling, Psychological, and Social Services

Counseling, psychological, and social services prevention and intervention services seek to improve students' mental, emotional, and social health, as well as supporting their learning process.[19] Mental health disorders in children include attention deficit-hyperactivity disorder (ADHD), which is the most prevalent (11% among U.S. children 4-17 years old) as well as mood disorders, anxiety disorders, behavioral disorders, major depression, and eating disorders.[26] Over a lifetime, approximately 22.2% of 13- to 18-year-olds will experience a severe disorder.[27] Services to address severe disorders include individual and group assessments, interventions, and referrals. Organizational assessment and consultation skills of counselors, psychologists, and social workers contribute not only to the health of students but also to the health of the school environment. Professionals such as certified school counselors, psychologists, and social workers provide these services.[14]

Counseling, psychological, and social services programs provide education, prevention, and intervention services, which are integrated into all aspects of the students' lives. Early identification and intervention with academic and personal/social needs are essential in removing barriers to learning and promoting academic

---

BOX 18–1 ■ School Nurse Employed by Schools in the United States

35.3% of schools employ part-time school nurses (< 35 hours)
    39.3% of schools employ full-time school nurses (> 35 hours)
    Across the country, 25.2% of schools did not employ a school nurse.

Source: (25)

achievement. School-based mental health programs may include collaborations with school-employed mental health professionals and community-based mental health professionals. In seeking optimum outcomes for students, schools must focus on challenges to collaboration in school-based mental health programs, which include integrating education and mental health systems, coordinating staffing, and working with resources from both systems.[28]

Social and Emotional Climate

The psychosocial environment in schools influences the social and emotional development of students.[19] Violence within schools is one factor that can undermine academic learning within a school (see Chapter 12). In some cases, children are exposed to extreme acts of violence or trauma in homes, communities, or within schools, as in Newtown, Connecticut, at Sandy Hook Elementary School[29] (see Chapter 12) and at Marjory Stoneman Douglas High School in Parkland, Florida. School shootings are an example of the trauma and violence that can adversely impact student educational outcomes.[30] Violence can take the form of bullying behavior in schools but also includes other forms of peer victimization. These include physical assault, physical intimidation, emotional victimization, sexual victimization, property crime, and internet harassment.[31] This victimization can also occur within the context of a dating relationship. Overt signs of violence within schools can also include carrying weapons, an act that can intimidate students from attending school. Based on the data collected from the Youth Risk Behavior Surveillance System survey in 2017, 6.0% of high school students were threatened or injured with a weapon, such as a gun, knife, or club, on school property during the past year, and 6.7% reported not going to school in the past 30 days because of concern for safety.[32] Some states and school districts implement periodic climate surveys to assess and examine school social and emotional climate. The U.S. Department of Education (USDE) set forth three factors of school climate: engagement, safety, and environment; one study's findings support the USDE's three-factor model of school climate.[33] Increasingly, schools provide for safe emotional environments by establishing trauma-informed schools that consider any trauma that children experience in and out of schools.[34]

Physical Environment

The healthy school environment is focused on providing the physical and aesthetic surroundings of the school to promote an environment conducive to learning. Factors that influence the physical environment include the school building and the area surrounding it, such as any biological or chemical agents detrimental to health of students and staff as well as factors such as temperature, noise, and lighting.[16] To address a school's physical condition requires attention to everyday operations as well as during renovation with the goal of protecting staff and students in schools from physical threats, biological, and chemical agents in the air, water, or soil.[19]

Indoor air quality is one example of a physical condition that has gained significant attention. The Environmental Protection Agency (EPA) developed a tool kit, the Indoor Air Quality Tools for Schools Action Kit, which guides schools in developing a practical plan to remediate air problems.[35] Some of the sources of problems are classroom pets and plants, water/moisture accumulation, eating facilities attracting vermin, secondhand smoke, combustion problems from furnace rooms and kitchens, and ventilation systems.[32] Select interventions have been outlined by the EPA.[35] In addition to the EPA toolkit, the Healthy Schools Campaign, a national nonprofit organization advocating for green cleaning in schools, publishes a guide focused on the practical steps in implementing a green program.[36]

Another intervention aimed at providing a safe environment for students is the Safe Walk to School national program, a federal safe route to school program started in 2005. Then, in 2012, new transportation bill MAP-21 combined this program with safe transportation programs related to walking and bicycle use, giving more discretion to states for funding these programs.[37] Thus, safety concerns for schoolchildren exist both inside the school and in the community surrounding the school.

Employee Wellness

The school community consists of employees as well as students. Generally, employee policies and benefits originate on the school district level, but employee wellness initiatives may also occur at individual schools. In a coordinated school health initiative, the school nurse provides opportunities, often through an interdisciplinary team, for school employees to improve their health status through health assessments, health education, and health-related fitness activities through interdisciplinary teams. A variety of tools and activities to engage school employees can be used in health promotion activities. Employee wellness programs and initiatives have the potential to reduce staff health risks and improve quality of life.[38]

The value of encouraging school staff, especially teachers, to pursue a healthy lifestyle that can contribute to their improved health status and improved morale has meaning in schools focused on climate. Teachers experience stress and burnout, which can have implications in student outcomes.[39]

Family Engagement

A healthy school environment benefits from meaningful engagement with parents (i.e., biological parents, relatives, or non-biological parents or guardians). The influence of parents on their children and adolescents makes them ideal partners with schools in supporting healthy school environments, especially in nutrition services and environment, physical activity, and school health services.[40] The CDC sets forth three aspects for school staff to consider with parent engagement: connecting with parents, engaging parents in school health activities, and sustaining parent engagement in school health.[40]

Building capacity for school staff and families to act as partners requires more than programs. The Dual Capacity-Building Framework for Family and School Partnerships provides a compass for building family and school partnerships that include relational, developmental, interactive, and collective/collaborative learning networks.[41]

Community Involvement

The 10th component focuses on involving and integrating the community with school efforts for the purpose of enhancing the well-being of the students. Partnerships to promote school health and student learning exist with community organizations, local businesses, social service agencies, faith-based organizations, health clinics, and colleges and universities.[19] Schools and university schools of nursing/colleges partner in ways that enhance school health services policies, school nurse education, school nurse practice, and research that ultimately benefits students.[42]

Framework for 21st Century School Nursing Practice™

Looking more deeply into the school health services of the WSCC model led the National Association of School Nurses to develop the Framework for 21st Century School Nursing Practice™ (Framework), which depicts student-centered school nursing practice (see Figs. 18-4 and 18-5).[43] The five key principles of the Framework exist in a nonhierarchical and overlapping structure that surrounds the student, family, and school community; the key principles are standards of practice, care coordination, leadership, quality improvement, and community/public health. School nurses provide student-centered care within these key principles while also connecting with other WSCC components and community connections. The Framework helps guide individual school nurse practice as well as school district-level school health services.

Population-Based School Nursing Practice

School nurses care for individual students with acute and chronic health concerns, and also provide population-based interventions.[47] These school nurse population-based interventions can be clearly seen in the Framework components and are also depicted in the interventions outlined in the Minnesota model for public health nursing practice known as the *Intervention Wheel* or the *Minnesota Wheel* (see Chapter 2).[44] The Intervention Wheel describes 17 public health interventions that are population-based. A population-based approach considers intervening at three possible levels of practice. Interventions may be directed at one of the following, or all three: the entire population within the school's community, the systems that affect the health of those populations, or the individuals and families within those populations known to be at risk.

Primary Prevention

School nurses have an important role to play in selecting, implementing, and evaluating comprehensive educational efforts at the school level. At least four of the *HP 2020* Healthy Educational and Community-Based Programs objectives addressed the provision of comprehensive health education in schools to prevent health problems.[11] Areas of importance to school health include sexuality, mental health promotion, substance abuse/violence prevention, and health education including life skills.

Immunizations

Providing well-child services has been an important role of school nurses since the development of the specialty. Monitoring vaccinations among children and adolescents

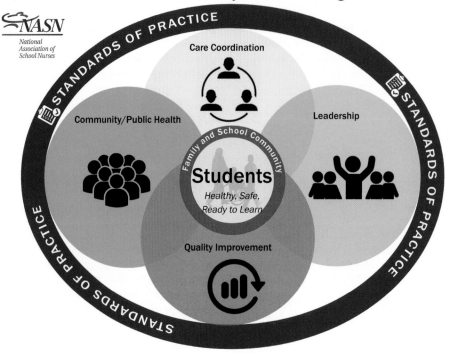

© National Association of School Nurses, 2015   *BETTER HEALTH. BETTER LEARNING.™*   Rev. 10/6/16

Figure 18-4 Framework for 21st Century School Nursing Practice™ [*Venn Diagram*]. NASN's Framework for 21st Century School Nursing Practice (Framework) provides structure and focus for the key principles and components of current day, evidence-based school nursing practice. It is aligned with the Whole School, Whole Community, Whole Child model that calls for a collaborative approach to learning and health (ASCD & CDC, 2014). Central to the Framework is student-centered nursing care that occurs within the context of the students' family and school community. Surrounding the students, family, and school community are the nonhierarchical, overlapping key principles of Care Coordination, Leadership, Quality Improvement, and Community/Public Health. These principles are surrounded by the fifth principle, Standards of Practice, which is foundational for evidence-based, clinically competent, quality care. School nurses daily use the skills outlined in the practice components of each principle to help students be healthy, safe, and ready to learn.

to assure compliance with state mandates is an important school nurse role related to surveillance. School nurses support the use of state immunization information systems to identify fully immunized children as well as those who are not fully immunized and consequently at risk. This also helps to prevent duplication of vaccinations. The school nurse also increases student and family awareness of other recommended vaccinations.

The CDC keeps an updated list on its Web site of many resources related to vaccinations for both health professionals and families.[45,46] Other sources of current vaccine recommendations include the National Network for Immunization Information and the American Academy of Pediatrics immunization schedules, also available online. These recommendations are updated annually because of changes in risk, changes in pathogens such as the flu virus, and changes in the evidence related to best practices for different vaccines. School nurses play a crucial role in counseling families and staff about immunizations across the life span. The CDC urges school nurses to specifically promote preteen vaccines.[47]

The seasonal influenza vaccine is of particular interest in school nursing practice. The primary resource for nurses

Framework for 21st Century School Nursing Practice™

NASN's *Framework for 21st Century School Nursing Practice* (the *Framework*) provides structure and focus for the key principles and components of current day, evidence-based school nursing practice. It is aligned with the Whole School, Whole Community, Whole Child model that calls for a collaborative approach to learning and health (ASCD & CDC, 2014). Central to the *Framework* is student-centered nursing care that occurs within the context of the students' family and school community. Surrounding the students, family, and school community are the non-hierarchical, overlapping key principles of *Care Coordination, Leadership, Quality Improvement,* and *Community/Public Health*. These principles are surrounded by the fifth principle, *Standards of Practice*, which is foundational for evidence-based, clinically competent, quality care. School nurses daily use the skills outlined in the practice components of each principle to help students be healthy, safe, and ready to learn.

 Standards of Practice	 **Care Coordination**	**Leadership** 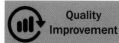	**Quality Improvement**	**Community/ Public Health** 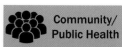
• Clinical Competence • Clinical Guidelines • Code of Ethics • Critical Thinking • Evidence-based Practice • NASN Position Statements • Nurse Practice Acts • Scope and Standards of Practice	• Case Management • Chronic Disease Management • Collaborative Communication • Direct Care • Education • Interdisciplinary Teams • Motivational Interviewing/ Counseling • Nursing Delegation • Student Care Plans • Student-centered Care • Student Self-empowerment • Transition Planning	• Advocacy • Change Agents • Education Reform • Funding and Reimbursement • Healthcare Reform • Lifelong Learner • Models of Practice • Technology • Policy Development and Implementation • Professionalism • Systems-level Leadership	• Continuous Quality Improvement • Documentation/Data Collection • Evaluation • Meaningful Health/ Academic Outcomes • Performance Appraisal • Research • Uniform Data Set	• Access to Care • Cultural Competency • Disease Prevention • Environmental Health • Health Education • Health Equity • Healthy People 2020 • Health Promotion • Outreach • Population-based Care • Risk Reduction • Screenings/Referral/ Follow-up • Social Determinants of Health • Surveillance

ASCD & CDC. (2014). *Whole school whole community whole child: A collaborative approach to learning and health.* Retrieved from http://www.ascd.org/ASCD/pdf/siteASCD/publications/wholechild/wscc-a-collaborative-approach.pdf

BETTER HEALTH. BETTER LEARNING.™   Rev. 10/6/16

Figure 18-5 Framework for 21st Century School Nursing Practice™ [*Text & Categories*]. NASN's Framework for 21st Century School Nursing Practice (Framework) provides structure and focus for the key principles and components of current day, evidence-based school nursing practice. It is aligned with the Whole School, Whole Community, Whole Child model that calls for a collaborative approach to learning and health (ASCD & CDC, 2014). Central to the Framework is student-centered nursing care that occurs within the context of the students' family and school community. Surrounding the students, family, and school community are the nonhierarchical, overlapping key principles of Care Coordination, Leadership, Quality Improvement, and Community/Public Health. These principles are surrounded by the fifth principle, Standards of Practice, which is foundational for evidence-based, clinically competent, quality care. School nurses daily use the skills outlined in the practice components of each principle to help students be healthy, safe, and ready to learn.

is the Advisory Committee on Immunization Practices, a division of the CDC. The committee periodically updates the influenza vaccine recommendations, including recommendations for school-age children.[48] In 2017, the committee recommended annual influenza vaccination for everyone aged 6 months or older.[48] School-located vaccination programs have become a viable option for reaching the target populations and are likely to continue. The models for providing this care vary; in some locales, school nurses lead school district vaccination programs and administer the vaccines, and in other cases, public health department staff members administer the vaccine in the schools.[49] The roles of school nurses in school-located vaccination range from providing direct care to working at a community and systems levels to assure coverage from a population perspective.

Sexuality and Sex Education

Nearly half of the most common STI, chlamydia, occurs in young women aged 15 to 24.[50] Primary prevention of high-risk behaviors related to sexuality is a priority for school populations. It is estimated that 39.5% of high school students have had sexual intercourse, and most adolescents who have ever had sexual intercourse remain sexually active.[51] About 9.7% have had multiple partners. The prevalence of being currently sexually active (past 90 days) was 28.7%. Of the 28.7% of students who are presently sexually active, 3.8% reported that neither they nor their partner had used any method of contraception to prevent pregnancy during their last sexual intercourse.[51]

One approach to prevention within a school setting is sex education. The topic of sex education is controversial. At the local, state, and national levels, educational experts have discussed who should decide what would be taught in schools. Factors that play into those decisions are parental concerns, public health prevention concerns, and the role the educational system plays in public health prevention versus parental rights. School nurses can help inform the discussion by presenting empirical data related to the magnitude and consequences of teen births and sexual activity among adolescents in their own school district and by suggesting evidence-based practices related to prevention. In addition, the school nurse must take into consideration cultural and environmental issues specific to their school and the children who attend their school. Standard 5 of the National Health Education Standards from the CDC provides a sound basis for curriculum development in this area. Standard 5 states: "Students will demonstrate the ability to use decision-making skills to enhance health."[52] Once general content is outlined, there are many resources available to assist local educators in selecting appropriate curricula to promote healthy sexuality.[53-54]

Violence Prevention

Cyberbullying: Student-to-student violence takes various forms within the school setting. Bullying, defined as unwanted aggressive behavior by one or more youth toward another youth who is not a sibling or dating partner, occurs in various contexts.[55] Cyberbullying represents a context in which bullying occurs via electronic methods using technology.[55] Researchers note that bullying in schools and cyberbullying combine to adversely impact the student's mental health.[56] The school nurse has the potential to play a role in the prevention and early identification of cyberbullying and in the provision of treatment to victims of violence.

● APPLYING PUBLIC HEALTH SCIENCE

The Case of the Frequent Flyer

Public Health Science Topics Covered:

- Assessment
- Program planning
- Program evaluation

Carly, an eighth-grader, recently entered a new middle school when her family moved midyear from a rural area to a large urban center after her father obtained a job transfer. Carly had spent her entire life in the rural area and was apprehensive about the move. For the first few weeks, things seemed to go well. She was welcomed by a group of girls who were the "popular" girls in the class. They offered to include her in activities outside of class, including football games and parties. To Carly's surprise, within a month she had received an upsetting e-mail from someone she did not know accusing her of sexual behavior. She learned that several derogatory remarks about her had been posted on a social media site that left her feeling alone and depressed. As these postings continued, her enthusiasm about school decreased, and she became more withdrawn. She was afraid to log on to her computer for fear that she would be bullied or picked on online.

Bob, the school nurse, began to suspect something was going on when Carly kept showing up in the health suite with nondescript, vague symptoms. Because he had heard through the student grapevine that a new girl was being bullied online, he wondered whether it might be Carly. After some initial probing about her adjustment to her new school, he learned about Carly's situation. Bob began to provide direct care to Carly to help her address the bullying, and with Carly's permission included her parents. He also included the school administration. Bob took this case very seriously given the recent cases in the news in which cyberbullying had resulted in the victim committing suicide. Counseling was sought for Carly, and she began to show improvement,

Helping Carly was only half of the problem; preventing further bullying was the other half. The school administration asked Bob to spearhead a school team charged with the task of finding an educational program for the school. Bob found evidence-based programs and decided to include students, teachers, and parents on his team to help choose the program most appropriate for his school. The team agreed that, in addition to putting an educational program in place, they should also assess the extent of the problem. Bob located a resource with tools to measure bullying, published by the CDC.[55] The team conducted a survey of the students and discovered that it was more widespread than they had initially thought.

To help the team, Bob found a definition of *bullying* that helped them understand the broad scope of the problem. According to the CDC, bullying involves a youth being bullied or victimized when he or she is exposed, repeatedly and over time, to negative actions on the part of one or more students.[55] Bob explored the issue further and found that the phenomenon of bullying includes three groups: the bully, the victim, and persons who are both bully and victim. He found that in 2015, 21% of students ages 1–18 reported being bullied at school, and in high schools alone, the prevalence was 19%. Additionally, girls were bullied at a greater percentage than boys.[57,58]

Because the school was specifically concerned with cyberbullying, Bob looked for a clear definition. Based on what he read, he reported to the team that **cyberbullying** is the purposeful and repeated harm inflicted through the use of computers, cell phones, and other electronic devices.[55,56] To help the team understand the seriousness of the problem, Bob explained to them that bullying can result in severe consequences for the victim, including elevated levels of depression, anxiety, poor self-esteem, psychosomatic problems, suicide ideation, suicide attempts, and suicide.[56] Using an ecological understanding of the bullying behavior and with Bob's help, the team concluded that whatever program they implemented should be based on the components of the Olweus Bullying Prevention Program. This program consists of school-level, classroom-level, individual-level, and community-level components.[59,60] The principles guiding this evidence-based program are that adults should:[59,60]

- Show warmth and positive interest in their students
- Set firm limits for unacceptable behavior
- Use consistent nonphysical, nonhostile negative consequences when rules are broken
- Function as positive roles models

The team completed their assessment and, based on their findings, put together an antibullying campaign for the school. The campaign included educational sessions for students, teachers, and parents; public service announcements posted throughout the school; an anonymous hotline for reporting suspected bullying; and the institution of a bullying intervention program to help with early identification of, and intervention with, victims. Because the team had collected initial assessment data, they were able to demonstrate significant improvement over time after the implementation of the campaign.

Dating Violence: Dating violence is another form of violence that is not unfamiliar to adolescents. Results from the 2017 Youth Risk Behavior Surveillance System (YRBSS) indicated that, of the 68.3% U.S. high school students who date, 6.9% described being forced to perform sexual acts, which included touching, kissing, or being forced to have sexual intercourse.[61] Also in the 2017 YRBSS, of the 69% of U.S. high school students who reported experiencing physical violence while on a date, 8% were hurt on purpose; the hurt was described as being hit, slammed into something, or injured with an object or weapon.[61] In the above violent situations, the prevalence of experiencing sexual dating violence at least once in the past 12 months was higher in females: 9.1% versus 6.8% in males.[61] There is a need to screen adolescents for teen dating violence, especially those with certain high-risk behaviors, including alcohol use and drug use.[62] Social-emotional skills are particularly important in addressing healthy relationships, and school-based interventions are increasingly being designed and tested.[62] Different strategies and approaches to engage adolescents in interventions are being explored, including treatment to lessen harms of youth exposed to violence and treatment to prevent problem behavior and further exposure to violence.[62]

Outreach to Immigrant Populations

Student populations are becoming increasingly diverse in the United States, given the growing number of immigrant parents. The percentage of all children living in the United States with at least one foreign-born parent rose from 15% in 1994 to 25% in 2016.[63] Children of immigrants often face many challenges, including cultural differences, poverty, lack of health insurance, lack of access to public assistance, limited English proficiency, and high levels of psychological distress in those who have experienced war and other adverse events. Outreach to these populations is one intervention in which school nurses can play an integral part. The multiple roles connected with outreach might include: developing a welcoming orientation for the students, developing student support teams, facilitating the integration of the students into after-school activities, and serving as an overall advocate for the families.

■ CULTURAL CONTEXT

School nurses work with a growing number of students and families from varied cultures in the context of school health services. NASN published survey results that pointed to school nurses knowing the demographics, languages spoken, health disparities, social determinants, and environment of the population they served.[64] Survey respondents expressed their need for additional knowledge and skills to provide culturally competent care. Specifically, school nurses saw gaps in (1) their ability to communicate health information in families' language of origin, (2) the availability the of school nurse-specific resources on the topic, and (3) their ability to navigate work barriers, such as time constraints and lack of administrative support.[64] Actions that addressed the expressed needs included providing school nurse education and a compilation of Web-based resources on cultural competence. With increased knowledge and skills, school nurses can provide culturally competent care for all students. A study demonstrated that a health promotion intervention used by school nurses and health teachers enabled secondary school-age students in a migrant education program to enhance their learning by developing student-made videos.[65] The study used a transcultural nursing framework and tailored the curriculum to the ethnicity of the student population.[65] School nurses grow in their influence on positive outcomes for students when engaging in understanding their identities and cultural differences, being culturally responsive, identifying social injustices, and committing to lifelong learning.[66]

Secondary Prevention

Health Screening of Children and Adolescents

Screening is another vital role of school nurses in addressing the actual and potential health problems of children. School nurses conduct vision and hearing screenings as well as BMI screenings, depending on the regulations within the jurisdictions. Other screenings can include postural or scoliosis screening, blood pressure reading, drug use screening, and screening for mental health problems, type 2 diabetes, cholesterol level, asthma, tuberculosis, and head lice. In all of these cases,

it is essential to assess the value of the screening program, to estimate the costs versus the benefits, and to assure that there is not any inadvertent harm that evolves from the program. The sensitivity and specificity of the screening tools are also critical to evaluate (see Chapter 2).

Some screening procedures, such as screening for scoliosis, have fallen out of favor over the past decade in some areas. In 2018, the U.S. Preventive Services Task Force concluded "the current evidence is insufficient to assess the balance of benefits and harms of screening for adolescent idiopathic scoliosis in children and adolescents aged 10 to 18 years."[67] Screening guidelines can vary by state, and it is important for school nurses to access information on requirements at both the national and state levels.

Vision Screening: Vision screening in schools has a history dating back to 1899, when the Snellen eye chart was first used. Although the Snellen chart continues to be prominent in the toolbox of school nurses, there is a need to evaluate the vision screening tools used based on national and international eye chart design guidelines and to apply best practices based on research.[68] It is equally important to use an eye chart that matches the cognitive level of the child. States generally require only distance acuity screening; when students do not meet the criteria to pass the screening, school nurses refer for eye exams and follow-up as directed by policy.[69]

Audiometric Screening: Screening for hearing problems is another vital school nursing activity. The American Academy of Audiology has specific childhood hearing screening guidelines. Minimum grades for screening include preschool, kindergarten, and grades 1, 3, 5, and either 7 or 9. It is also important to screen any student who enters a new school system without evidence of having had a previous hearing screening (Box 18-2).[70] Although these criteria are specific to hearing screening, the principles of proper communication, referral, follow-up, and effective treatment are equally important.

Screening for Obesity: It is evident from the National Health and Nutrition Examination Survey (NHANES) that obesity is a significant problem among U.S. adolescents and children. In 2015-2016, the prevalence of obesity among U.S. youth was 18.5%. Overall, the prevalence of obesity among adolescents (12–19 years) (20.6%) and school-aged children (6–11 years) (18.4%) was higher than among preschool-aged children (2–5 years) (13.9%). School-aged boys (20.4%) had a higher prevalence of obesity than preschool-aged boys (14.3%). Adolescent

BOX 18–2 ■ Position Statement: American Academy of Audiology

The position statement on early childhood and school-age population screening is as follows:

"The American Academy of Audiology endorses detection of hearing loss in early childhood and school-aged populations using evidence-based hearing screening methods. Hearing loss is the most common developmental disorder identifiable at birth, and its prevalence increases throughout school age due to the additions of late-onset, late-identified, and acquired hearing loss. Under-identification and lack of appropriate management of hearing loss in children has broad economic effects as well as a potential impact on individual child educational, cognitive, and social development. The goal of early detection of new hearing loss is to maximize perception of speech and the resulting attainment of linguistic-based skills. Identification of new or emerging hearing loss in one or both ears followed by appropriate referral for diagnosis and treatment are first steps to minimizing these effects. Informing educational staff, monitoring chronic or fluctuating hearing loss, and providing education toward the prevention of hearing loss are important steps that are needed to follow mass screening if the impact of hearing loss is to be minimized."

Source: (70)

---

girls (20.9%) had a higher prevalence of obesity than preschool-aged girls (13.5%).[71,72] In 2013-2014, the prevalence of obesity reported for all U.S. children aged 2 to 19 years was 17.2%.[72]

For non-Hispanic black (22.0%) and Hispanic (25.8%) youth, the rate was higher than among both non-Hispanic white (14.1%) and non-Hispanic Asian (11.0%) youth. There were no significant differences in the prevalence of obesity between non-Hispanic white and non-Hispanic Asian youth or between non-Hispanic black and Hispanic youth.[72,73] This disparity in obesity rates is the result of a complex set of risk factors including genetics, cultural nutritional practices, environments, and socioeconomic differences. Obesity adversely affects children and adolescents by increasing the risk for type 2 diabetes, hypertension, and depression, as well as increasing the possibility of arthritis, cancer, and cardiovascular disease later in life. Prevention and intervention efforts rely on multiple partnerships using multiple angles.

The primary screening method for obesity in children is the calculation of BMI. BMI is a number calculated from a child's weight and height, and is a reliable indicator of body fatness. To screen for obesity in children, the BMI by itself is not sufficient. The BMI number is plotted on a growth chart specific to girls or boys, and a percentile ranking is obtained. This percentile indicates where the child is in relation to other children of the same age and sex.[73] The categories are further broken down into underweight, healthy weight, overweight, and obese (Box 18-3).[73] School nurses can use the CDC Body Mass Index Child and Teen Calculator to calculate the BMI as well as the percentile ranking in children. In addition to height and weight, the calculator uses information on sex, date of birth, and date of measurement to calculate the percentile.[74] Communication of the results of the BMI to the family as well as the child's health-care provider is important. It is a challenge to design effective prevention and intervention programs, because cultural norms and perceptions must be taken into consideration.[75] Examining obesity trends within a particular school allows the school nurse to be an advocate at a community and systems level through his or her involvement in school wellness policies.

BOX 18–3 ■ BMI-for-Age Weight Status Categories and the Corresponding Percentiles

After BMI is calculated for children and teens, the BMI number is plotted on the CDC BMI-for-age growth charts (for either girls or boys) to obtain a percentile ranking. Percentiles are the most commonly used indicator to assess the size and growth patterns of individual children in the United States. The percentile indicates the relative position of the child's BMI number among children of the same sex and age. The growth charts show the weight status categories used with children and teens (underweight, healthy weight, overweight, and obese). BMI-for-age weight status categories and the corresponding percentiles are shown in the following table:

Weight Status Category	Percentile Range
Underweight	Less than the 5th percentile
Healthy weight	5th percentile to less than the 85th percentile
Overweight	85th to less than the 95th percentile
Obese	Equal to or greater than the 95th percentile

Source: (71)

Screening Vulnerable Populations and Social Determinants of Health

School nurses work with a vulnerable population – children and youth. The environment where students live, play, and learn (social determinants) has an impact on their health.[76] Racial and ethnic diversity among students is increasing, with the greatest growth in Hispanic children, 24.7% (2015) and 24.9% (2016).[63] Students who are or who have family members in immigrant or refugee status represent a vulnerable population; 25% of U.S. children ages 0–17 years have one foreign-born parent. An increasing number of children ages 5–17 speak a language other than English at home: 21.9% (2014) and 22.2% (2015).[63] Access to health care and safe housing are social issues impacting student health and learning. Children ages 0–17 with no usual source of health care has increased 3.6% (2014) and 4.4% (2015).[63] In addition to social determinants, vulnerable students have needs that require support in school settings. Students might have complex chronic health conditions, such as type 1 diabetes, asthma, and undiagnosed mental health illness; these complex health issues, along with social concerns, can lead to chronic absenteeism, which in turn limits school success.[77] School nurses collaborate with other school staff and community-based partners to provide students with the support they need to attend and complete school.

● APPLYING PUBLIC HEALTH SCIENCE

The Case of the Student with a Mysterious Growth

Public Health Science Topics Covered:

- Secondary prevention
- Referral and follow-up

Dana worked as a school nurse in a suburban high school. In her role, she connected with students by standing in the doorway of the health room during change of classes. Some students walking down the halls never came into the health room for services. Dana and those students greeted one another simply verbally or with a nod. Sue was one of the students who did not come to see Dana but enjoyed sharing brief verbal exchanges of greetings. After a semester of observing Sue from the health room door, Dana noticed Sue's abdomen growing larger. One day, Dana motioned to Sue to come near the health room door as she walked down the hallway. The school nurse

asked Sue if she would stop by for a visit during her study period, which Sue did the next day. When Sue arrived in the health room, Dana asked her to come to a quiet office area. After exchanging pleasantries, Dana asked Sue how she was feeling. Sue mentioned that she was fine. Dana shared her observations of Sue's growing abdomen over the past 4 months. Sue quickly stated, "I'm not pregnant!" Dana assured Sue she was not making any assumptions. Dana asked Sue if she would mind answering health-related questions. Sue replied no, so Dana asked, specifically "Do you have abdominal pain?" and "Do you have constipation or urinary frequency?" Dana explained that, after checking Sue's vital signs, she would call Sue's mother to share her recommendation for a medical referral.

On exam, Dana recorded the following: *Vital Signs:* BP 130/70, P 80, R 20, Temp 97.8°F, BMI 33. Dana also documented her observations and Sue's self-report. When Dana contacted Sue's mother, she heard the mother's concern that Sue might be pregnant. Dana referred Sue's mother to Sue's health-care provider. The school nurse documented her call. On the next school day, Sue popped her head into the office to say, "I have a medical appointment in 3 weeks." A month went by, and Dana had not heard back from Sue after her appointment. She also did not see Sue in the hallway. Dana called the home and spoke with Sue's mother. The abdominal growth occurred because of a large simple ovarian cyst that had gone undetected. The cyst was 20×10×25 cm in size and benign. Sue had surgery, which included removal of her right ovary and was at home recovering. Sue's mother thanked Dana for not ignoring her observations of Sue's growing abdomen. Dana inquired if Sue was in contact with the school counselor to arrange for resuming her studies.

Tertiary Prevention

Life-Threatening Emergencies in the School Setting

School nurses are a primary connection to medical and public health entities when schools experience emergencies.[78] Following the Sandy Hook shooting in 2012, there has been increased awareness of the potential for school-based violence (see Chapter 12). The CDC reports that less than 2.6% of child homicides occur at school.[79] Despite the low incidence rate, the school nurse must be prepared for the potential of a life-threatening violent act occurring at a school. These life-threatening emergencies require well-equipped schools, staff trained in first aid and cardiopulmonary resuscitation, and lay-rescuer automated external defibrillators (AEDs) [79] One approach for emergency preparedness in schools is to have a designated medical emergency response plan on record. A recommendation is that schools practice the plan a number of times each year. The other recommendation is to identify who within the system is authorized to make emergency medical decisions and make sure AEDs are available to the staff.[80]

Food Allergies: Exposure to a food allergen is another example of a potentially life-threatening event. Between 2009 and 2011 the reported prevalence of food allergies was 5.1% among children under age 18 years.[81] In a recent national survey of U.S. households with children under age 18 years, food allergy prevalence was 8.0%. The food allergen most prevalent in this survey was peanuts (2.5% of children) followed by milk, shellfish, and tree nuts.[82]

Prevention is crucial and demands adequate management plans, successful food allergy avoidance, recognition of food allergy reactions, preparation for appropriate treatment of acute allergic reactions, knowledge of treatments, and access to autoinjectable epinephrine.[83]

Episodic Care in the School Setting: An important role of the school nurse is to provide episodic care and to conduct disease and health investigations. School nurses provide care and care coordination for students with chronic health conditions and students with acute health concerns. Where SBHCs are located or linked with schools, school nurses determine if a student's acute health condition will benefit from a primary care referral to the SBHC. The School-Based Health Alliance recognizes the critical and foundational role of school nurses for the entire student population. SBHCs enhance foundational school health services:

> The **school nurse** is the building's health ambassador, on the frontline for day-to-day oversight and management of the school population's health. **School-based health care** complements the work of school nurses by providing a readily accessible referral site for students who are without a medical home or in need of more comprehensive services such as primary, mental, oral, or vision health care.[84]

School nurses spend a significant portion of their day caring for acute injuries and illnesses as well as administering medication and providing episodic care for minor ailments, such as headaches, stomachaches, pain, and hay fever. School nurses know the value of quality improvement, especially the collection, analysis, and use of data to improve outcomes for students. The interprofessional work of school nurses is noted when they participate in school team meetings as well as when they collaborate with community partners.

Although 83% of U.S. children under 18 years of age have very good or excellent health, noncommunicable disease affects their well-being and has the potential to have a great impact on school outcomes.[85] Noncommunicable diseases (see Chapter 9) include asthma, diabetes, allergies, cancer, and other medical disorders. Fourteen percent of children have asthma; 10% of children ages 3–17 years have attention deficit hyperactivity disorder (ADHD); and 6% of children have unmet dental needs due to lack of family funds.[85] Often, the health-care needs of a child with a noncommunicable disease are complex and require careful planning, appropriate referrals, safe management, and delegation of nursing tasks to licensed and unlicensed assistive personnel (UAP).[86] Mental disorders (see chapter 10) are also common among children. The global prevalence of mental disorders among children and adolescents is 13.4%.[87]

Noncommunicable diseases and mental health disorders in children and adolescents require coordination between family members, school personnel, and health-care providers. Care coordination of noncommunicable diseases and mental health disorders contributes to positive academic and health outcomes. One systems-level approach to care coordination sets forth a model with a focus on access to care that is student- and family-centered and is led by a school nurse whose initial priority is to set up a channel of communication across systems.[88] A system of care coordination includes five components:

1. School health-care teams that support and share processes and forms for care planning, partner agreements, tracking care, monitoring, evaluating, and reporting.
2. Interagency partnerships that enable services and solutions to assist students and families in care. Partner agreements support ease of communication.
3. Documentation with electronic health records to help with monitoring quality and efficiency of school health services through surveillance and tracking systems.
4. Clinical expertise and evidence-based guidelines that provide tools to help the school nurse give high-quality care.
5. Performance improvements and outcome evaluations that call for systems-level analysis of the care coordination implementation, and outcome reports that are shared with the care team, including families.[88]

Care coordination is based on a thorough assessment by the school nurse and involves activities that not only help the child deal with problems but also prevent and reduce their reoccurrence. Care coordination includes nursing care directed toward the child and coordination and communication with parents, teachers, and other care providers. The interventions are goal-oriented, based on the specific needs of the child, and evaluated based on their impact.[88]

Case management begins when the primary care provider (PCP) confirms a diagnosis, for example, of ADHD. Symptoms of ADHD in school-age children can be marked by academic difficulties, inattention, impulsiveness, oppositional behavior, poor self-esteem, excessive motor activity, low frustration tolerance, increased risky behavior, aggressive and antisocial behavior, and less adaptive behaviors.[98] The overall prevalence in school-age children is about 10%.[85] The school nurse is often the designated professional that helps bridge the gap between teachers, who often first see the behaviors suggestive of a diagnosis of ADHD, and the PCP, who can make an appropriate diagnosis. The school nurse also oversees the delivery of medications.[89]

In addition to providing individual care, the application of a population perspective allows the school nurse to develop programs at the school level to help identify students with ADHD and provide evidence-based options for care. The school nurse performs behavioral classroom observations that focus on early diagnosis and treatment of ADHD for purposes of decreasing academic failure, social isolation, high-risk behaviors, family conflict, and adversity later in life for these children.[90]

Asthma: In 2011, 14% of children under 18 had been diagnosed with asthma.[85] Asthma is a significant noncommunicable disease among adolescents. Over the past 20 years, asthma in children has increased when measured by prevalence, ambulatory visits, morbidity, and mortality.[91] The presence of a full-time registered school nurse is important to provide care and care coordination for students with asthma. In addition, the school nurse provides instruction to school staff concerning the recognition of and action steps for severe respiratory symptoms. School nurses often take the lead in providing school-based education to improve asthma management. School nurse leaders in one school-based asthma program recognized the crucial role of school district readiness to implement evidence-based asthma care.[92]

Diabetes: Diabetes is another noncommunicable disease that requires self-management and coordination of care within the school setting. There are two types of diabetes. Type 1 is an autoimmune disease in which the body forms antibodies to insulin, thus affecting the body's ability to produce insulin; previously type 1 was known as insulin-dependent disease. Diabetes is one of the most common noncommunicable diseases in children younger than 20 years in the U.S.; approximately 30.3 million people or 9.6% of the U.S. population over 18 years have diabetes.[93] Type 2 occurs when cells do not respond correctly to insulin, resulting in insulin resistance. Type 2 diabetes is a complex metabolic disorder with social, behavioral, and environmental risk factors including being overweight, a family history of type 2 diabetes, or other conditions such as high blood pressure, polycystic ovary syndrome, or abnormal cholesterol. The increasing frequency of diabetes types 1 and 2 in children is concerning. About 17,900 children under the age of 20 are diagnosed with type 1 every year, and 5,300 children ages 10–19 years old already have type 2 diabetes.[94]

One of the roles of the school nurse is to identify children with diabetes, or who are at risk of developing type 2 diabetes, and refer them to care. Once a diagnosis has occurred, the school nurse has an important role in encouraging self-care, which includes increasing knowledge and skills such as blood glucose testing, insulin injection, preparation of the insulin, diet management, and hypoglycemic treatment.[95,96] Additionally, assessing for signs of stress and providing needed support are important. The school nurse works closely with the student, family, and community-based health-care providers to develop a plan for managing children with diabetes.[96]

Disabilities: Students with disabilities represent another population that requires case management from the school nurse.[97] The IDEA of 2004 provides a comprehensive definition of a child with disabilities (Box 18-4).[98]

School health services enable students with disabilities to attend school. Student needs may include medication administration, treatments, emergency care plans, individualized health-care plans, health teaching, and health counseling.[99] School nurses maintain referral sources so that students and families may be appropriately referred for care and services. In addition, the school nurse is responsible for providing a safe and healthy environment. In the case of children with disabilities, this may mean wheelchair access, special furniture, elevators, restroom accommodations, or dedicated space in the health room for diaper changes, tube feedings, medication administration, or rest.

National policy has resulted in the integration of children with disabilities into the school setting. These laws help define the rights of children with disabilities as well as define the role of the school nurse. One law that had a significant impact on school nursing is the Education for

---

BOX 18–4 ■ Individuals with Disabilities Education Act—Definitions of a Child With a Disability

Child with a disability.—

"(A) In general.—The term 'child with a disability' means a child—

"(i) with mental retardation, hearing impairments (including deafness), speech or language impairments, visual impairments (including blindness), serious emotional disturbance (referred to in this title as 'emotional disturbance'), orthopedic impairments, autism, traumatic brain injury, other health impairments, or specific learning disabilities; and

"(ii) who, by reason thereof, needs special education and related services.

"(B) Child aged 3 through 9.—The term 'child with a disability' for a child aged 3 through 9 (or any subset of that age range, including ages 3 through 5), may, at the discretion of the State and the local educational agency, include a child—

"(i) experiencing developmental delays, as defined by the State and as measured by appropriate diagnostic

Child Ages 3 Through 9 (or any subset of that age range): May, at the discretion of the State and the local educational agency, include a child (i) experiencing developmental delays, as defined by the State and as measured by appropriate diagnostic instruments and procedures, in 1 or more of the following areas: physical development; cognitive development; communication development; social or emotional development; or adaptive development; and (ii) who, by reason thereof, needs special education and related services."

Source: (98)

All Handicapped Children Act (EAHCA) of 1975.[100] The ages covered under this law include birth to 2-year-olds in infant and toddler programs, as well as 3- to 21-year-old students. EAHCA appropriated federal funding to states for the provision of free appropriate public education in the **least restrictive environment**. The purpose of a least restrictive environment is to provide disabled students with the opportunity to be educated with their nondisabled peers.[100] This was followed by the IDEA, passed in 2004.[101] This law builds on the original 1974 legislation and provides a mechanism for continual updating of available resources. It addresses the same issues for children as the EAHCA does but encompasses the issues for all individuals with disabilities. Thus, the needs of people with disabilities are now covered across the life span. IDEA has undergone several amendments, with the most current in 2004. The current iteration of IDEA

specifies school nursing as one of the related services that will meet the needs of the student.[101]

A central component of these laws is the **individualized education program (IEP)**. An individualized education program is an individualized plan for a child with a disability; the goal of the plan is to help the child meet their educational objectives. School nurses are integral members of the team. If the student's disability requires the services of a nurse, the school nurse contributes to the individualized education program, which is both a process and a plan. School nurses, as part of the team, provide resources and information when transition planning begins for students with special educational services. An **individualized family service plan (IFSP)** is indicated for qualified birth to 3-year-old children. It is similar to an IEP and is provided to children with developmental delays to help address their issues. Once a child turns 3, an individualized education plan replaces the IFSP.

Other laws that affect children with disabilities, such as Section 504 of the Americans With Disabilities Act, are seen in Table 18-1.[102,103] Although school administrators are required to accommodate children with disabilities, school administrators, faculty, and staff are not required to accommodate limitations due to other characteristics such as poor literacy skills (that are not due to learning disabilities), low educational levels, inability to meet the minimum entrance requirements of the learning environment, or lack of credentials. Parents and students can ask for reasonable accommodations based on functional limitations secondary to a medical condition. These accommodations are made by teachers and other staff via adjustments to their standard practices to meet specific needs of the student.

Mental Health Disorders: The prevalence of mental health disorders in children and adolescents is, on average, about 13%, with ADHD being the most common at around 10%.[85,87] A comprehensive school-based health program must incorporate mental health care. One approach is to provide a minimum elementary school counselor-student ratio to help improve the overall school climate; this helps to reduce disruptions within classrooms that result from fighting, cutting class, stealing, or using drugs.[104]

Integrating learning and behavioral health with an overall focus on improving functioning and not just symptom reduction is a topic receiving increased emphasis.[104,105] Integrating social-emotional learning into school health education is needed. This can be accomplished on an individual basis or by developing and implementing school-wide programs to address positive behavioral support.[104,105]

TABLE 18–1 ■ Description of Federal Laws for Children With Special Needs

Law	Description	Special Considerations
Pub. L. No. 94-14. Education for All Handicapped Children Act (EAHCA) of 1975. Renamed the Individuals with Disabilities Education Act (IDEA) in 1990. Source: http://www.scn.org/~bk269/94-142.html	This law appropriates federal funding to states for the provision of a free and appropriate public education in the least restrictive environment to those students with disabilities who qualify.	An individualized education program (IEP) is mandated for each student in special education. An individualized family service plan (ISFP) is indicated for qualified birth to 3-year-old children.
Section 504 of the Rehabilitation Act of 1973 and current amendments (2008). 29 U.S.C. § 794. Source: http://www2.ed.gov/about/offices/list/ocr/504faq.html	This is a civil rights law that prohibits discrimination based on disabilities by entities receiving federal funds, including local education agencies; several amendments to the law expanded provisions in 2008.	Public elementary and secondary schools must provide Free Appropriate Public Education for qualified students with a disability.[30] A 504 plan is written by the child's treatment team. Section 504 expands disabilities beyond learning to a mental or physical impairment that substantially limits one or more life activities.
Americans With Disabilities Act (ADA) 1990 Americans With Disabilities Act (ADA) Amendment 2008. P.L. 110-325. Source: http://www.ada.gov/pubs/adastatute08.pdf	The ADA is another civil rights law that prohibits discrimination based on disability.	The provisions of this law apply to agencies with or without the receipt of federal funds.

School nurses also have a significant role in the early identification of mental health needs. Some children frequently visit the school nurse's office with unexplained physical symptoms. These frequent visitors ("frequent flyers," or what some have called "somatizers") account for a disproportionate use of resources in the school.[106] Once a physical etiology has been ruled out, somatization should be recognized as an early identifier of potential mental health needs and stress in school-age children. The school nurse can (1) monitor school-based mental health care; (2) act as a care coordinator; (3) advocate for the student; and (4) act as a liaison between the family, school, clinic, and primary provider for these children.[107] In addition, the nurse develops the health portion of the individualized education program and the **Individualized Healthcare Plan** for children with identified mental health needs. The nurse may be the first person to recognize the need for counseling. Consider the following examples of student visits to the school nurse:

Example 1: This first example illustrates how the school nurse can identify a problem that can be addressed with a simple solution. Jason came to the health room on a regular basis with complaints of coughing and shortness of breath due to asthma. His physical examination often did not correlate with his complaints. After recognition of a pattern of these complaints, it was found that these visits to the health room occurred only during math class. During consultations with the counselor, family, and his math teacher, it was learned that Jason was not getting good grades and was anxious about not doing well in class. Referral to tutoring services recommended by the counselor was an acceptable solution to this problem for all concerned, including Jason. After a few weeks, Jason was better prepared for class and did not complain of any more asthma symptoms during class.

Example 2: The second example is more complex. The PE teacher referred Annie, a 14-year-old middle school student, to the school nurse. Annie was at the point of failing PE; she could not participate in the activities because she forgot to bring her PE clothes to school. The PE teacher asked whether the nurse could talk to Annie. Annie and the nurse talked in private to discuss PE. Annie felt uncomfortable undressing and changing her clothes in front of other girls. There were no private dressing areas. She was self-conscious about her weight. When the nurse talked to Annie's mother, she discovered that Annie had not asked her mother for money for the PE clothes. Her mother did not have a lot of money, and Annie did not want to be an additional financial burden. The final plan was to allow Annie to change her clothes in the privacy of the health room and then go to PE. There were extra used but clean PE clothes available that were given to Annie. When Annie got dressed, the nurse noted healed and new linear wounds on both her upper forearms. They sat and talked. The nurse shared her assessment of the old scars and new wounds as being self-inflicted. Annie agreed. She had not wanted her classmates or teachers to know. The school counselor, the nurse, the mother, and Annie met to discuss the implications of the self-inflicted wounds. Annie and her mother agreed that Annie would see a psychologist, and she would attend PE with a long-sleeved PE shirt. The nurse met with Annie weekly to discuss healthy eating habits and daily physical activity. Along with counseling by a trained psychologist, increased daily exercise, and a change in dietary habits, Annie began to lose weight, passed PE, and had a group of friends by the end of the year.

These two examples differ in the severity of the issues. Jason did not have a mental health disorder, but Annie's symptoms were indicative of possible mental health issues. The right decision was to refer her for further assessment and possible treatment. Both examples exemplify a very important point. Although the mental health field has traditionally focused on psychopathology, the absence of mental illness does not necessarily equate with positive mental health.[108] Children who have low psychopathology and low subjective well-being are also at risk for academic and behavior problems, and can benefit from counseling.

The links between mental health and academic achievement have been well established.[108] In addition, the CDC has stated that, if mental health disorders are left untreated, adolescents are more likely to experience higher rates of suicide, violence, school dropout, family dysfunction, juvenile incarceration, alcohol use, drug use, and unintentional injuries.[108] These examples support the role of the school nurse in providing counseling and in conducting programs focused on prevention.

Delegation: Delegation is an intervention that has particular relevance to the school nurse in addressing noncommunicable diseases and mental health disorders in schools. According to the National Council of State Boards of Nursing (1995), delegation is defined as transferring the authority to perform a selected nursing task in a selected situation to a competent individual.[109] Because of budgetary constraints resulting in the lack of school nurses, delegation is given to UAPs to meet the health needs of student populations. One of the challenges of delegation is the fact that laws, regulations, scopes of practice, and standards vary by state, and there is a potential conflict between state laws and nurse practice acts. Another challenge is that of assuring safe and effective delegation in school settings. The school nurse must consider "the needs of the student, the stability of the student, the complexity of the task, the competence of the UAP, the expected outcomes, and the needs of other students in determining the appropriateness of delegating a specific task to a UAP."[110]

■ EVIDENCE-BASED PRACTICE
School Screening for Adolescent Idiopathic Scoliosis

Practice Statement: Routine school screening for adolescent idiopathic scoliosis is not recommended.
Targeted Outcome: School nurses advocate for review of state law and regulations requiring school scoliosis screening programs.
Evidence to Support: The most common form of scoliosis is adolescent idiopathic scoliosis, which affects 2%-4% of youth ages 10-18 years old. The U.S. Preventive Services Task Force (USPSTF) finds insufficient evidence to recommend screening adolescents for idiopathic scoliosis. From the current evidence, the USPSTF cannot assess benefits or harms of screening. School scoliosis screening programs are thought to over-refer for follow-up care, which incurs costs in dollars and anxiety. In addition, school screening may be duplicative because pediatric primary care clinicians screen for scoliosis in well-child visits. The majority of states do not require school scoliosis screening programs; 15 states have mandates for such school screening. The question to answer is: Are school scoliosis screening programs functioning out of tradition or evidence?

Recommended Approaches: School nurses lead in advocacy that results in optimum health for students. School nurses, especially through state school nurse organizations, can convene other groups of child and adolescent health and education professionals, student advocates, and families to:

- review current school scoliosis screening law and regulations
- review current evidence-based guidance on the topic
- discuss what is best for students
- advocate with one voice for the evidence-based course to take

Sources

1. American Academy of Orthopedic Surgeons and Scoliosis Research Society. (2015). *Position statement: Screening for idiopathic scoliosis in adolescents.* Rosemont, IL: American Academy of Orthopedic Surgeons. Retrieved from https://www.srs.org/about-srs/news-and-announcements/position-statement—-screening-for-the-early-detection-for-idiopathic-scoliosis-in-adolescents
2. Dunn, J., Henrikson, N.B., Morrison, C.C., Blasi, P.R., Nguyen, M., & Lin, J.S. (2018). Screening for adolescent idiopathic scoliosis evidence report and systematic review for the U.S. Preventive Services Task Force. *JAMA, 319*(2),173-187. doi:10.1001/jama.2017.11669
3. Horne, J.P., Flannery, R., & Usman, S. (2014). Adolescent idiopathic scoliosis: Diagnosis and management. *American Family Physician, 89*(3),193-198. Retrieved from https://www.ncbi.nlm.nih.gov/pubmed/24506121
4. Jakubowski, T.L. & Alexy, E.M. (2014). Does school scoliosis screening make the grade? *NASN SN, 29*(5), 258-265. https://doi.org/10.1177/1942602X14542131
5. Mabry-Hernandez, I., & Tannis, C. (2018). Screening for adolescent idiopathic scoliosis. *American Family Physician, 97*(10), 666-667.

Consultation

Because of health expertise, the school nurse is likely to provide consultation within schools to address health issues. This can be in the role of the school nurse for individualized education program evaluations, in which nurses have a critical role in determining student eligibility for 504 plans. A 504 plan for a student with a disability provides for reasonable accommodations that help a student to attend, participate in, and be successful at school.[103] ADA amendments went into effect in January 2009, making more health-related functions fit the criterion of major life activities. The list now includes reading, concentrating, thinking, sleeping, eating, performing manual tasks, and other major bodily functions.[111]

In addition to local school nurses, there is a state school nurse consultant in 39 states. This person provides consultation to nurses practicing in schools and is in a position to advocate for state-level policies and local school nursing practices.[112] The National Association of State School Nurse Consultants (NASSNC) has a position paper that provides the rationale for having a state school nurse consultant in every state. The NASSNC rationale for having a state school nurse consultant (SSNC) is as follows: The SSNC "is responsible for promoting statewide quality standards for school health policies, nursing scope of practice and clinical procedures, documentation, and for initiating and coordinating a quality assurance program for accountability. S/he works in collaboration with the state board of nursing, provides guidance in health program development and planning, establishes a continuum of staff development, and serves as a liaison and resource expert in school nursing practice and school health program(s)."[112] The position paper goes on to outline the responsibilities of the SSNC (Box 18-5).

Advocacy

Advocacy by the school nurse occurs on multiple levels. The school nurse can advocate for the student population and their families through efforts to influence policy at the local, state, and/or national levels.[113] The school nurse also serves as a direct advocate for healthcare consumers, in this case, students, families, and school communities. The role of advocate can include advocating for culturally competent and developmentally appropriate care, optimal utilization of resources, and promotion of a healthy environment.[114]

▶ **SOLVING THE MYSTERY**

The Case of the Missing Student Assessment

Public Health Science Topics Covered:

- Interdisciplinary collaboration
- Program planning

Tameka, the school nurse in a large inner-city charter high school, served on the attendance review

BOX 18–5 ■ Responsibilities of State School Nurse Consultants

The responsibilities of the state school nurse consultant include:

- Serving as liaison and resource expert in school nursing and school health program areas for local, regional, state, and national school health-care providers, and policy setting groups;
- Providing consultation and technical assistance to local school districts, parents, and community members;
- Coordinating school health program activities with public health, social services, environmental, and educational agencies as well as other public and private entities;
- Monitoring, interpreting, synthesizing, and disseminating relevant information associated with changes in health and medical care, school nursing practice, legislation, and legal issues that have an impact on schools;
- Facilitating the development of policies, standards, and/or guidelines. Interprets updates and disseminates policies, standards, guidelines, and/or procedures to enhance coordinated school health programs;
- Fostering and promoting staff development for school nurses. This may include planning and providing orientation, coordinating, and/or providing educational offerings and networking with universities and other providers of continuing education to meet identified needs;
- Promoting quality assurance in school health services by initiating and coordinating a quality assurance program that includes a needs assessment, data collection and analysis, and evidence-based practice;
- Participating in state-level public interagency/private partnerships with statewide stakeholders to foster a coordinated school health program, representing school nurses in multidisciplinary collaborations;
- Initiating, participating in, and utilizing research studies related to a coordinated school health program, the health needs of children and youth, school nursing practice, and related issues; and
- Serving as legislative liaison regarding school health issues with the state department of health.

Source: (112)

committee. Because attendance in school is critical to learning, the school administration had convened the committee to include those who could provide the most insight into underlying factors that might contribute to attendance problems. The current emphasis on educating the whole child by the Every Student Succeeds Act (ESSA) furnished the initial rationale for convening the committee. The school administration understood that academic achievement is linked to students being present in class,[115] and reduction of absenteeism was a major strategic goal for the school. The committee was composed of the vice principal, two teachers, the school social worker, and Tameka. During one meeting, the committee discussed one student, Aisha, who was in danger of losing credits for courses she was passing because of excessive absenteeism. Aisha had recently moved into the school district and had no record of a health problem. The committee decided that Tameka would contact the student and parent or guardian for additional information.

As a first step, Tameka asked Aisha to come to the health suite. Aisha told Tameka that she was an only child and her mother, Monique, was a single parent who had a night-shift job that paid the minimum wage. To make up for the low wages, Monique worked as much overtime as she could get. They had moved to the city to be closer to extended family. Aisha had made a few friends in school and in her neighborhood. She worked hard at staying current with her schoolwork, despite school absences.

After some probing, Aisha explained that she had juvenile rheumatoid arthritis (JRA), specifically, polyarticular disease, but had not reported it because she was sure she could cope with it on her own. She was diagnosed with JRA 4 years ago. She described a typical morning on school days; it took her about 2 to 3 hours to get dressed and ready for school because of extreme discomfort in her joints. Her mother usually did not return from her shift until after the time Aisha needed to leave for school. Aisha sometimes gave up trying to get ready in time to make the walk to school. Although it was only four blocks, some mornings the pain made it very difficult to walk.

When Tameka spoke with Aisha's mother, Tameka discovered that they did not have a car and traveling on the city bus to see her PCP was difficult for Aisha as it required two bus changes. The mother then admitted that Aisha had not actually seen a PCP since they had moved to the city. The prescribed medication regimen was abandoned by the family because of a lack of finances. Aisha primarily relied on over-the-counter NSAIDs for pain relief, which she described as "okay, sometimes."

Tameka concluded that her priority regarding Aisha was to help connect her with health care, including support for medication costs. Tameka referred

Monique to the local health department for assistance with completing the state Children's Health Insurance Plan (CHIP) application. With approval of the application, Aisha began visits to health-care providers.

The attendance review committee helped set up a class schedule to allow Aisha a first period study hall so that she could get to school in time for classes. The social worker also worked with Aisha and Monique to get documentation approved for the possibility of Aisha receiving home instruction in the event of an exacerbation of JRA. Tameka also arranged for Aisha to receive transportation to school if needed. It was hoped that, with proper management as well as accommodations within the school setting, Aisha would not miss school.

Intervening on Aisha's behalf was only the beginning of Tameka's job as an advocate. Through a collaborative approach, the school team had helped address an issue for Aisha and also identified a gap in how they collected health information on new students. Tameka proposed that they develop a new student process that would help to identify students at risk for adverse educational outcomes due to health issues such as Aisha's. The team identified other team members who needed to be on their committee, including the staff who did the initial intake. In Aisha's case, she had not reported the problem, but when the team reviewed her transcript form from the other school, they found a notation on Aisha's condition that had been missed. Changing the intake process was a crucial step for the school in the process of advocating for their students who needed additional support services.

Tameka modeled the nurse's role by illustrating the importance of health services that support learning, health, and student achievement. She began by focusing on individual student advocacy and then helped lead the team in advocating for the student body as a whole.

Policy Development and Enforcement

Policy plays a significant role in influencing school health and the health services provided to students. This role can be seen in the Focus on School Health section of *HP*, federal and state laws, and local regulations governing services. The advocacy role of school nurses includes advancing school health policy, whether it is local school policy, state policy, or national policy affecting children and adolescents.[113]

Local Laws and Regulations

From a local school perspective, implementing wellness policies and practices reflecting the goals of *HP* is one example of how nurses intervene at this level. In Wisconsin, a guide has been published titled *What Works in Schools: Healthy Eating, Physical Activity, and Healthy Weight*; the guide provides approaches that nurses can perform for prevention of obesity.[116] School nurses play an important role on school health advisory councils (wellness committees, school wellness advisory councils) where they can advocate for comprehensive health programs and recommend, review, and facilitate the implementation of district policies.[117] These policies relate to key components that support school health including the built environment, school wellness policies, or changing longstanding policies that are no longer supported by evidence. Changing practice involves changing beliefs, which requires collaborative community relationships, identification of hierarchy structures in school policy development, and system education.[113]

State Laws and Regulations

Variations in legislative mandates for school nurses occur within and among states in the United States. School nurses practice under state nurse practice acts and codes. That means nurses must not only understand the scope and standards of school nursing practice but also the specific state-level regulations related to their scope of practice, the required level of education, and other relevant laws. For example, school nurses need to know if state nurse practice acts provide for delegation of certain nursing tasks to UAPs, or the minimum level of education required to practice as a school nurse.

State immunization regulations govern the criteria for required vaccines for enrollment in schools. School nurses must be alert to changes in immunization regulations and requirements to inform parents and guardians of changes and to review compliance.

States mandates vary with respect to student screening for certain health conditions. More than 70% of states require hearing and vision screening to detect potential hearing or vision problems.[118] School nurses conduct these screenings in schools. In some school districts, technicians, not school nurses, are responsible for conducting hearing and vision screenings, and school nurses focus on following up with those students referred for exams.

Federal Laws

School nurses also play a significant role in adhering to federal laws and promoting the development of federal policies. The laws with particular relevance to children with disabilities were reviewed in preceding sections. Other laws also important to the role of the school nurse are discussed here.

Elementary and Secondary Education Act

School health services are influenced by a number of federal laws, beginning with the Elementary and Secondary Education Act (ESEA), also referred to as ESSA (Public Law 115).[119] This legislation provides federal funding for improved academic achievement for students, including students with disabilities. ESSA sets the stage for education policy and reform from the federal, state, and local levels, and sets the atmosphere in which schools work, including school health services. The act has come under some criticism because it includes a requirement for standardized testing. Under President Obama, the Act was modified to allow states to apply for a waiver from the requirements of the Act. States need to apply and demonstrate how they will improve academic achievement.[119] Title I of the ESSA is aimed at improving the academic outcomes of the disadvantaged. It provides a mechanism for state education agencies to provide funding to local education agencies that apply for grants to resource programs aimed at improving the academic achievement of students.

Child Abuse Prevention and Treatment Act

The Child Abuse Prevention and Treatment Act (CAPTA) was first passed into law in 1974 as Public Law 93-247 and has undergone numerous amendments over the years. CAPTA includes provisions for funding state child welfare agencies, among other provisions.[120] School nurses, along with other school staff, are required to report suspected child abuse and neglect according to their state laws and regulations.

Family Educational Rights and Privacy Act

The **Family Educational Rights and Privacy Act (FERPA)** provides for the protection of privacy for parents and eligible students as related to education records maintained by educational agencies and institutions that receive funds from the U.S. Department of Education. Because private and religious schools do not generally receive funds from the U.S. Department of Education, they would not be subject to FERPA. With FERPA, parents and students have certain rights to review, inspect, and request amendments to a student's education record. FERPA sets forth the parameters for educational agencies and institutions for disclosure of personally identifiable information from education records.[121] For example, student health records are often considered part of the education record, and the school nurse must maintain the privacy of the records under FERPA. According to FERPA, "At the elementary or secondary level, a student's health records, including immunization records, maintained by an educational agency or institution subject to FERPA, as well as records maintained by a school nurse, are 'education records' subject to FERPA."[143] From this perspective, school health records are considered education records. HIPAA sets out requirements for electronic health-care transactions to protect the privacy and security of individually identifiable health information.[121] Thus, it is important for school nurses to know which act applies in their school district.

Children's Health Insurance Program

In 1997, the U.S. Congress passed legislation titled the **Children's Health Insurance Program (CHIP)**, which was reauthorized as the Children's Health Insurance Reauthorization Act of 2018 (Pub. L. 115-123).[122] CHIP provides health insurance to approximately 9.4 million children whose family incomes are too high to qualify for Medicaid and too low to afford health insurance. The federal government provides matching funds to states. The states can implement the program as an extension of Medicaid, a separate program from Medicaid, or a combined CHIP-Medicaid program.[123] The reauthorized Act extends the requirement that states maintain coverage for children from 2019 through 2023; after October 1, 2019, the requirement is limited to children in families with incomes at or below 300% federal poverty level (FPL).[122] The reauthorization continues the 23 percentage point CHIP-enhanced federal match rate established by the Affordable Care Act for FY2018 and FY2019, decreases it to 11.5 percentage points in FY2020, and returns to the regular CHIP match rate for FY2021 through FY2023. [122]

School nurses serve a vital role in facilitating student enrollment in CHIP. School nurses are often the only health-care providers who see students on a regular basis. They collaborate with local health departments to provide information and outreach to parents and families of children about enrolling in CHIP. School nurses work one-on-one with families with ill children who need to seek primary health care but are hesitant to do so because of a lack of or inadequate health-care insurance.

Healthy Hunger-Free Kids Act

Another example of a federal law that impacts schools is the Healthy Hunger-Free Kids Act of 2010 (Pub. L. 111-296), which was signed into law on December 13, 2010. This law allows the USDA to update the school nutrition standards and provides funding to increase the national school lunch program.[124] School nurses have taken leadership in testifying for and supporting this new law.

Challenges for the Future

Time spent in childhood poverty has been linked with poor child health status, with African American children disproportionately affected.[125] Poor health status plays a role in limiting educational achievement of adolescents.[126] Addressing health disparities that have an impact on education, such as vision, asthma, teen pregnancy, aggression and violence, physical activity, lack of breakfast, and inattention and hyperactivity, has a role in promoting educational attainment among low-income and minority adolescents.[127] School nurses are in a position to lead health-promoting efforts and reform to help address health disparities in school-age children, and to transform educational and health systems to achieve health and educational equity.

Health-Care Reform

With the passage of the federal ACA as Public Law 111-148, school nursing has a role in certain provisions. Highlights of those provisions of Public Law 111-148 include:[128]

- Access to health insurance for people with preexisting conditions
- Streamlined enrollment procedures for Medicaid and CHIP
- Development of standards and protocols for health information technology
- Teen pregnancy prevention strategies and services
- Increased access to clinical preventive services through school-based health centers
- Oral health-care prevention activities
- Funding for a childhood obesity demonstration project

School nurses must remain aware of activities related to health-care reform. Partnerships with local health departments enable school nurses to know what resources exist for children and families.

School Health Services Funding

With few funded mandates for school nursing, financing school health services generally happens with local government dollars: either education or public health. What would it take for both health and education to support funding for school health services? The health needs of schoolchildren must be met. The answer may require

building creative and collaborative linkages between schools and community health services.[91]

Data on the cost-effectiveness of school nursing will allow critical and strategic decision making related to funding school health services. A study of the economic value of hospital nurses indicates the need to look at the broader values that nurses deliver in care and compassion as well as economics.[129] Demonstrating the economic value of professional nursing in the school setting may facilitate the provision of appropriate school nurse staffing to meet the health needs of students.

■ CELLULAR TO GLOBAL: WORLD HEALTH ORGANIZATION SCHOOL HEALTH INITIATIVE

According to the WHO:

WHO's Global School Health Initiative, launched in 1995, seeks to mobilize and strengthen health promotion and education activities at the local, national, regional, and global levels. The Initiative is designed to improve the health of students, school personnel, families, and other members of the community through schools.

The goal of WHO's Global School Health Initiative is to increase the number of schools that can truly be called "Health-Promoting Schools". Although definitions will vary, depending on need and circumstance, a Health-Promoting School can be characterized as a school constantly strengthening its capacity as a healthy setting for living, learning, and working.

The general direction of WHO's Global School Health Initiative is guided by the Ottawa Charter for Health Promotion (1986); the Jakarta Declaration of the Fourth International Conference on Health Promotion (1997); and the WHO's Expert Committee Recommendation on Comprehensive School Health Education and Promotion (1995).

The main strategies of this initiative are:

- Research to improve school health programs
- Building capacity to advocate for improved school health programs
- Strengthening national capacities
- Creating networks and alliances for the development of health-promoting schools[130]

According to the WHO, efforts to improve health in school-aged children and adolescents will improve health globally through the reduction of adverse health behaviors. These include:

- tobacco use
- behavior that results in injury and violence

- alcohol and substance use
- dietary and hygienic practices that cause disease
- sedentary lifestyle
- sexual behavior that causes unintended pregnancy and disease[131]

■ Summary Points

- School nursing provides care to individuals, families, and communities within the educational system.
- *HP* sets specific goals related to promotion of optimal health in school-age children and adolescents.
- The Whole School, Whole Community, Whole Child model informs a collaborative way to address learning and health needs for children and adolescents within a school setting. The Framework for 21st Century School Nursing Practice™ represents a student-centered structure for school nursing practice based on five key principles and is aligned with the WSCC model.
- Public health science informs school nursing practice, especially in relation to levels of prevention.
- Specific federal, state, and local laws apply to school nursing practice. School nurses serve as advocates for students, their families, and their communities in obtaining resources, protecting rights, and promoting reform.

▼ CASE STUDY
The Case of the New Nurse

Learning Outcomes

At the end of this case study, the student will be able to:

- Discuss how to prioritize steps for building a school health program.
- Identify opportunities for collaboration.
- Apply evidence-based school health programs to a specific population.
- Identify applicable education-related regulations.
- Apply components of health planning, assessment, and program development to the school setting.

Nesrin started her new job as a school nurse in a K–5 charter school in New York City that had just been established and was due to open its doors in 3 months. The school was located in a district where the population was 40% non-black Hispanic, 30% African American, 10% non-Hispanic white, and had a growing Arabic population. She took the job because the charter schools in New York have more freedom to create their own programs. She was included as part of the leadership team charged with creating a healthy learning environment. Based on her recommendation, the team decided to construct their program using the elements of the Whole School, Whole Community, Whole Child (WSCC) model created in collaboration with CDC.[18]

1. What would her first steps be from a public health perspective?
2. Compare your answers with your classmates' answers, make a master list, and prioritize the steps.
3. Once you have completed these first steps, put together a comprehensive health program for the school.
   a. Who would you put on your planning team?
   b. What essential elements are needed for the program?
   c. What resources are needed?
4. Put together a draft program based on available evidence of best practices.
5. Be sure to address the different developmental needs of the students.
6. How will you address special health needs, including accommodations for students with disabilities?
7. How will health education play a part in your plan?
8. What federal, state, and local regulations must you include in the plan?

REFERENCES

1. National Center for Education Statistics. (n.d.). *Fast facts: Back to school statistics.* Retrieved from https://nces.ed.gov/fastfacts/display.asp?id=372.
2. UNESCO Institute for Statistics (UIS) and Global Education Monitoring Report (GEMR). (2016). *"Leaving no one behind: How far on the way to universal primary and secondary education?"* GEMR policy paper 27/UIS fact sheet No.37. Montreal and Paris: UIS and GEMR. Accessed at http://unesdoc.unesco.org/images/0024/002452/245238E.pdf.
3. National Association of School Nurses. (2017). *Definition of school nursing.* Retrieved from https://www.nasn.org/nasn/about-nasn/about.
4. National Association of School Nurses. (2016). *Code of ethics.* Retrieved from https://www.nasn.org/nasn-resources/professional-topics/codeofethics.
5. Johnson, J., Beard, J., & Evans, D. (2016). Caring for refugee youth in the school setting. *NASN School Nurse, 32*(2), 122-128. doi.org/10.1177/1942602X16672310.
6. Mendenjall, M., Russell, S.G., & Buckner, E. (2017). *Urban refugee education: Strengthening policies and practices for*

access, quality, and inclusion. New York, NY: Columbia University, Teacher's College.

7. Zaiger, D. (2013). Historical perspectives of school nursing. In J. Selekman (Ed.), *School nursing: A comprehensive text,* *2e.* Philadelphia, PA: F.A. Davis.

8. Struthers, L.R. (1917). *The school nurse.* New York, NY: Putnam.

9. National Center for Health Statistics. (2016). *Chapter 10: Early and Middle Childhood.* Healthy People 2020 Midcourse Review. Hyattsville, MD.

10. National Center for Health Statistics. (2016). *Chapter 2: Adolescent Health.* Healthy People 2020 Midcourse Review. Hyattsville, MD.

11. U.S. Department of Health and Human Services. (2015). *Healthy People 2020: Educational and community-based programs.* Retrieved from http://www.healthypeople.gov/2020/topicsobjectives2020/overview.aspx?topicId=11.

12. National Center for Health Statistics. (2016). *Chapter 11: Educational and Community-Based Programs.* Healthy People 2020 Midcourse Review. Hyattsville, MD.

13. National Association of School Nurses. (2015). *School nurse workload: Staffing for safe care* (Position Statement). Silver Spring, MD: Author.

14. Centers for Disease Control and Prevention. (2015a). *The case for coordinated school health.* Retrieved from http://www.cdc.gov/healthyyouth/cshp/case.htm.

15. Centers for Disease Control and Prevention. (2015b). *Components of a coordinated school health program.* Retrieved from http://www.cdc.gov/healthyyouth/cshp/components.htm.

16. Allensworth, D.D., & Kolbe, L.J. (1987). The comprehensive school health program: Exploring an expanded concept. *Journal of School Health, 57,* 409-412.

17. Association for Supervision and Curriculum Development (ASCD). (2007). *The learning compact redefined: A call to action.* Alexandria, VA: ASCD. Retrieved from http://www.ascd.org/ASCD/pdf/Whole%20Child/WCC%20Learning%20Compact.pdf.

18. Lewallen, T.C., Hunt, H., Potts-Datema, W., Zaza, S., & Giles, W. (2015). The Whole School, Whole Community, Whole Child Model: A new approach for improving educational attainment and healthy development for students. *The Journal of School Health, 85*(11), 729-739. https://doi.org/10.1111/josh.12310.

19. Chiang, R.J., Peck, L., Hurley, J., & Labbo, B. (2017). *The Whole School, Whole Community, Whole Child Model: A guide to implementation.* Atlanta, GA: National Association of Chronic Diseases. Retrieved from http://www.ashaweb.org/wp-content/uploads/2017/10/NACDD_WSCC_Guide_Final.pdf.

20. Centers for Disease Control and Prevention. (2016). *National health education standards.* Retrieved from https://www.cdc.gov/healthyschools/sher/standards/index.htm.

21. Centers for Disease Control and Prevention. (2017). *Increasing physical education and physical activity: A framework for schools.* Atlanta, GA: Centers for Disease Control and Prevention, U.S. Dept of Health and Human Services. Retrieved from https://www.cdc.gov/healthyschools/physicalactivity/pdf/17_278143-A_PE-PA-Framework_508.pdf.

22. Food Research and Action Center. (2018). *School breakfast scorecard school year 2016–2017.* Washington, DC: Author. Retrieved from http://frac.org/wp-content/uploads/school-breakfast-scorecard-sy-2016-2017.pdf.

23. U.S. Department of Agriculture, Food and Nutrition Service. (2017). *Healthy Hunger-Free Kids Act.* Retrieved from https://www.fns.usda.gov/school-meals/healthy-hunger-free-kids-act.

24. Anderson, L.J.W., Shaffer, M.A., Hiltz, C., O'Leary, S.A., Luehr, R.E., & Yoney, E.L. (2017). Public health interventions: School nurse practice stories. *Journal of School Nursing, 34*(3), 192-202. doi.org/10.1177/1059840517721951.

25. Willgerodt, M.A., Brock, D. M., & Maughan, E.M. (2018). Public school nursing practice in the United States. *Journal of School Nursing, 34*(3), 232-244. doi.org/10.1177/1059840517752456.

26. National Institute of Mental Health. (n.d.). *Health statistics: Attention deficit hyperactivity disorder.* Retrieved from https://www.nimh.nih.gov/health/statistics/attention-deficit-hyperactivity-disorder-adhd.shtml#part_154906.

27. Merikangas, K.R., Jian-ping, H., Burstein, M., Swanson, S.A., Avenevoli, S., Cui, L., ... Swendsen, J. (2010). Lifetime prevalence of mental disorders in U.S. adolescents: Results from the National Comorbidity Study-Adolescent supplement (NCS-A). *Journal of American Academy Child Adolescent Psychiatry, 49*(10), 980-989. doi.org/10.1016/j.jaac.2010.05.017.

28. Stephen, S.H., Sugai, G., Lever, N., & Connor, E. (2015). Strategies for integrating mental health in schools via a multi-tiered system of support. *Child and Adolescent Psychiatric Clinics, 24*(2), 211-231. doi.org/10.1016/j.chc.2014.12.002.

29. Bethell, C.B., Newacheck, P., Hawes, E., & Halfon, N. (2014). Adverse childhood experiences: Assessing the impact on health and school engagement and the mitigating role of resiliency. *Health Affairs, 33*(12), 2106-2115.

30. Fry, D., Fang, X., Elliott, S., Casey, T., Zheng, X., Li, J., Florian, L., & McCluskey, G. (2017). The relationships between violence in childhood and educational outcomes: A global systematic review and meta-analysis. *Child Abuse and Neglect, 75,* 6-18.

31. Turner, H.A., Finkelhor, D., Shattuck, A., Hamby, S.L, & Mitchell, K. (2014). Beyond bullying: Aggravating elements of peer victimization episodes. *School Psychology Quarterly, 30*(3), 1-19. doi.org/10.1037/spq0000058.

32. Centers for Disease Control and Prevention. (2018). *Youth Risk Behavior Survey Data summary & trends report 2007-2017.* Retrieved from https://www.cdc.gov/healthyyouth/data/yrbs/pdf/trendsreport.pdf.

33. Bradshaw, C.P., Waasdorp, T.E., Debnam, K.J., & Johnson, S. (2014). Measuring school climate in high schools: A focus on safety, engagement, and the environment. *Journal School Health, 84,* 593-604. doi.org/10.1111/josh.12186.

34. Wiest-Stevenson, C., & Lee, C. (2016). Trauma-informed schools. *Journal of Evidence-Informed Social Work, 13*(5), 498-503. doi: 10.1080/23761407.2016.1166855.

35. Environmental Protection Agency. (2015). *Creating healthy indoor environments in schools.* Retrieved from http://www.epa.gov/iaq/schools/.

36. Healthy Schools Campaign. (n.d.). *Specialized green cleaning guides.* Retrieved from https://greencleanschools.org/resources/specialized-guides/.

37. Safe Routes to School National Partnership. (2018.). *Keep calm and carry on to school: Improving arrival and dismissal.* Retrieved from https://www.saferoutespartnership.org/sites/default/files/resource_files/improving_arrival_and_dismissal_for_walking_and_biking_1.pdf.

38. Centers for Disease Control and Prevention. (2018). *Workplace health promotion.* Retrieved from https://www.cdc.gov/workplacehealthpromotion/index.html.

39. Herman, K.C., Hickman-Rosa, J., & Reinke, W.M. (2018). Empirically derived profiles of teacher stress, burnout, self-efficacy, and coping and associated student outcomes. *Journal of Positive Behavior Interventions, 20*(2), 90-100.

40. Centers for Disease Control and Prevention. (2015). *Parents for healthy schools: A guide for getting parents involved from K–12.* Atlanta: U.S. Dept. of Health and Human Services.

41. Mapp, K.L., & Kuttner, P.L. (2013). *Partners in education: A dual capacity-building framework for family-school partnerships.* Austin: SEDL.

42. King, B.M., Gordon, S.C., Barry, C.D., Goodman, R., Jannone, L.T., Foley, M., Resha, C., & Hendershot, C. (2017). Town and gown: Building successful university-school partnerships. *NASN School Nurse, 32*(1),14-18. doi: 10.1177/1942602X16681819.

43. National Association of School Nurses. (2016). Framework for 21st century school nursing practice. *NASN School Nurse, 31*(1), 45-53. doi:10.1177/1942602X15618644.

44. Shaffer, M.A., Anderson, L.J.W., & Rising, S. (2016). Public health interventions for school nursing practice. *The Journal of School Nursing, 32*(3), 195-208. doi: 0.1177/1059840515605361.

45. Seither, R., Calhoun, K., Street. E.J., Mellerson, J., Knighton, C.L., Tippins, A., & Underwood, M. (2017, October 13). Vaccination coverage for selected vaccines, exemption rates, and provisional enrollment among children in kindergarten — United States, 2016–17 School Year. *MMWR Morbidity Mortality Weekly Report, 66*(40), 1073–1080. doi.org/10.15585/mmwr.mm6640a3.

46. Centers for Disease Control and Prevention. (2017). *State school and childcare vaccination laws.* Retrieved from https://www.cdc.gov/phlp/publications/topic/vaccinations.html.

47. Centers for Disease Control and Prevention. (2017). *National Association of School Nurses: Partners and programs in the spotlight.* Retrieved from https://www.cdc.gov/hpv/partners/spotlights/nasn.html.

48. Centers for Disease Control and Prevention, Advisory Committee for Immunization Practices. (2018). *Prevention and control of seasonal influenza vaccines: Recommendations of the ACIP—United States, 2017–2018.* Retrieved from https://www.cdc.gov/flu/professionals/acip/2017-18summary.htm.

49. Wilson, D., Sanchez, K.M., Blackwell, S.H., Weinstein, E., & El Amin, A.N. (2013). Implementing and sustaining school-located vaccination clinics: Perspectives from five diverse school districts. *The Journal of School Nursing, 29*(4), 303-314. doi.org/10.1177/1059840513486011.

50. Centers for Disease Control and Prevention. (2016). *CDC fact sheet: Reported in the United States: High burden of STDs threaten millions of Americans.* Retrieved from https://www.cdc.gov/nchhstp/newsroom/docs/factsheets/STD-Trends-508.pdf.

51. Centers for Disease Control and Prevention. (2017). Youth risk behavior surveillance—United States 2016. *Morbidity and Mortality Weekly Report, 67*(8).

52. Centers for Disease Control and Prevention. (2016). *National health education standards.* Retrieved from http://www.cdc.gov/healthyyouth/sher/standards/5.htm.

53. Arons, A., Decker, M., Yarger, J., Malvin, J., & Brindis, C. (2016). Implementation in practice: Adaptations to sexuality education curricula in California. *Journal of School Health 86*(9), 669-676. doi.org/10.1111/josh.12423.

54. U.S. Department of Health & Human Services, Office of Population Affairs, Office of Adolescent health. (2017). *Adolescent health: Think, Act, Grow (TAG).* Retrieved from https://www.hhs.gov/ash/oah/tag/index.html.

55. Gladden, R.M., Vivolo-Kantor, A.M., Hamburger, M.E., & Lumpkin, C.D. (2014). *Bullying surveillance among youths: Uniform definitions for public health and recommended data elements, Version 1.0.* Atlanta, GA; National Center for Injury Prevention and Control, Centers for Disease Control and Prevention and U.S. Department of Education. Retrieved from https://www.cdc.gov/violenceprevention/pdf/Bullying-Definitions-FINAL-a.pdf.

56. Hinduja, S., & Patchin, J.W. (2018, August). Connecting adolescent suicide to the severity of bullying and cyberbullying. *Journal of School Violence.* doi:10.1080/15388220.2018.1492417.

57. Musu-Gillette, L., Zhang, A., Wang, K., Zhang, J., & Oudekerk, B.A. (2017). *Indicators of school crime and safety: 2016 (NCES 2017-064/NCJ 250650), May. 74-80.* National Center for Education Statistics, U.S. Department of Education, and Bureau of Justice Statistics, Office of Justice Programs, U.S. Department of Justice. Washington, DC. Retrieved from https://nces.ed.gov/pubs2017/2017064.pdf

58. Kann, L., McManus, T., Harris, W.A., Shanklin, S.L., Flint, K.H., Queen, B., ... Ethier, K.H. (2018). Youth risk behavior surveillance — United States, 2017. *MMWR Surveillance Summary, 67*(8), 17-21. Retrieved from https://www.cdc.gov/healthyyouth/data/yrbs/pdf/2017/ss6708.pdf.

59. Limber, S.P., Olweus, D., Wang, W., Masielo, M., & Breivik, K. (2018). Evaluation of the Olweus Bullying Prevention Program: A large-scale study of U.S. students in grades 3–11. *Journal of School Psychology, 69,* 56-72. doi.org/10.1016/j.jsp.2018.04.004.

60. Olweus, D., Soleberg, M.E., & Breivik, K. (2018). Long-term school-level effects of the Olweus Bullying Prevention Program. *Scandinavian Journal of Psychology.* doi.org/10.1111/sjop.12486.

61. Kann, L., McManus, T., Harris, W.A., Shanklin, S.L., Flint, K.H., Queen, B., ... Ethier, K.H. (2018). Youth risk behavior surveillance — United States, 2017. *MMWR Surveillance Summary, 67*(8), 22-23. Retrieved from https://www.cdc.gov/healthyyouth/data/yrbs/pdf/2017/ss6708.

62. David-Ferdon, C., Vivolo-Kantor, A.M., Dahlberg, L.L., Marshall, K.J., Rainford, N., & Hall, J.E. (2016). *A comprehensive technical package for the prevention of youth violence and associated risk behaviors, p. 8-10, 33-35.* Atlanta, GA: National Center for Injury Prevention and Control, Centers for Disease Control and Prevention.

63. Federal Interagency Forum on Child and Family Statistics. (2017). *America's children: Key national indicators of well-being, p. 8, x-xiii.* Retrieved from https://www.childstats.gov/pdf/ac2017/ac_17.pdf.

64. Matza, M., Maughan, E., & Barrows, B.M. (2015). School nurses cultural competence needs assessment: Results and response. *NASN School Nurse, 30*(6), 345-349. https://doi.org/10.1177/1942602X15608188.

65. Kilanowski, J.K., & Lin, L. (2014). Summer migrant students learn healthy choices through videography. *The Journal of School Nursing, 30*(4), 272-280. https://doi.org/10.1177/1059840513506999.

66. Carr, B., & Knutson, S. (2015). Culturally competent school nurse practice. *NASN School Nurse, 30*(6), 336-342. https://doi.org/10.1177/1942602X15605169.

67. U.S. Preventive Task Force Services. (2018). *Screening for idiopathic scoliosis in adolescents.* Retrieved from https://www.uspreventiveservicestaskforce.org/Page/Document/UpdateSummaryFinal/adolescent-idiopathic-scoliosis-screening.

68. Chaplin, P.K.N., & Bradford, G.E. (2011). A historical review of distance vision screening eye charts. *NASN School Nurse, 26*(4), 221-228.

69. National Association of School Nurses. (2016). *Principles for practice. School Nurse Practice Tools: Vision screening and follow-up.* Author.

70. American Academy of Audiology. (2011). *Childhood hearing screening guidelines.* Retrieved from http://www.cdc.gov/ncbddd/hearingloss/recommendations.html.

71. Hales, C.M., Carroll, M.D., Fryar, C.D., & Ogden, C.L. (2017). *Prevalence of obesity among adults and youth: United States, 2015–2016. NCHS data brief, no 288.* Hyattsville, MD: National Center for Health Statistics.

72. Centers for Disease Control and Prevention. (2018). *Childhood overweight and obesity.* Retrieved from https://www.cdc.gov/obesity/data/childhood.html.

73. Centers for Disease Control and Prevention. (2015). *About child and teen BMI.* Retrieved from https://www.cdc.gov/healthyweight/assessing/bmi/childrens_bmi/about_childrens_bmi.html.

74. Centers for Disease Control and Prevention. (2018). *Children's BMI tool for schools.* Retrieved from https://www.cdc.gov/healthyweight/assessing/bmi/childrens_bmi/tool_for_schools.html.

75. Malone, S.K., & Zemel, B.S. (2015). Measurement and interpretation of body mass index during childhood and adolescence. *The Journal of School Nursing, 31*(4), 261-271. doi: 0.1177/1059840514548801.

76. Centers for Disease Control and Prevention. (2018). *Social determinants of health: Know what affects health.* Retrieved from https://www.cdc.gov/socialdeterminants/faqs/#faq6.

77. Johnson, K.J. (2017). Health and ready to learn: School nurses improve equity and access. *The Online Journal of Issues in Nursing, 22*(3), Manuscript 1. doi: 10.3912/OJIN.Vol22No03Man01.

78. Doyle, J. (2013). Emergency management, crisis response, and the school nurse's role. In J. Selekman (Ed.). *School nursing: A comprehensive text* (2nd ed.), pp. 1216-1244. Philadelphia, PA: F.A. Davis Company.

79. Centers for Disease Control and Prevention. (2016). *Understanding school violence.* Retrieved from https://www.cdc.gov/violenceprevention/pdf/schoolviolence-factsheet.pdf.

80. American Heart Association. (2018). *CPR training for schools: Be the beat.* Retrieved from http://bethebeat.heart.org/media/pdfs/KJ-0781_ECC_BTB_Flyer.pdf.

81. Jackson, K.D., Howie, L.D., & Akinbami, L.J. (2013). *Trends in allergic conditions among children: United States, 1997–2011.* NCHS brief, no. 121. Hyattsville, MD: National Center for Health Statistics. Retrieved from https://www.cdc.gov/nchs/data/databriefs/db121.pdf.

82. Gupta, R., Warren, C., Blumenstock, J., Kotowska, J., Mittal, K., & Smith, B. (2017). The prevalence of childhood food allergy in the United States: An update. *Annals of Allergies, Asthma, & Immunology, 119*(5), S1-S15. doi.org/10.1016/j.anai.2017.08.060.

83. Centers for Disease Control and Prevention. (2013). *Voluntary guidelines for managing food allergies in schools and early care and education programs.* Washington, DC: U.S. Department of Health and Human Services. Retrieved from https://www.cdc.gov/healthyschools/foodallergies/pdf/13_243135_A_Food_Allergy_Web_508.pdf.

84. School-Based Health Alliance. (n.d.). *School-based health care: Where health and education intersect.* Retrieved from https://www.sbh4all.org/school-health-care/aboutsbhcs/.

85. Bloom, B., Cohen, R.A., & Freeman, G. (2013). Summary health statistics for U.S. children: National health interview survey 2012. National Center for Health Statistics. *Vital Health Statistics, 10*(258). Retrieved from https://www.cdc.gov/nchs/data/series/sr_10/sr10_258.pdf.

86. Children's Health Fund. (2017). *Health barriers to learning: The prevalence and educational consequences in disadvantaged children.* Retrieved from https://www.childrenshealthfund.org/wp-content/uploads/2017/02/HBL-Executive-Summary.pdf.

87. Polanczyk, G., Salum, G., Sugaya, L., Caye, A., & Rohde, L. (2015). Annual research review: A meta-analysis of the worldwide prevalence of mental disorders in children and adolescents. *Journal of Child Psychology & Psychiatry.* doi.org/10.1111/jcpp.12381.

88. Baker, D., Anderson, L., & Jonson, J. (2017). Building student and family-centered care coordination through ongoing delivery system design: How school nurses can implement care coordination. *NASN School Nurse, 32*(1), 42-49. doi.org/10.1177/1942602X16654171.

89. Platt, L.M., & Koch, R.L. (2016). How the school nurse can help improve the effectiveness of ADHD medication. *NASN School Nurse, 31*(3), 153-157. doi: 10.1177/1942602X16638496.

90. AlAzaam, M., Suliman, M., & AlBashwaty, M. (2016). School nurses' role in helping children with attention deficit/hyperactivity disorder. *NASN School Nurse, 32*(1), 36-38. doi.org/10.1177/1942602X16648192.

91. Lear, J.G. (2007). Health at school: A hidden health care system emerges from the shadows. *Health Affairs, 26*(2), 409-419.

92. Cicutto, L., Shocks, D., Gleason, M., Haas-Howard, C., White, M., & Szefler, S.J. (2016). Creating district readiness for implementing evidence-based school-centered asthma programs: Denver public schools as a case study. *NASN School Nurse, 31*(2), 112-118. doi.org/10.1177/1942602X15619996.

93. Centers for Disease Control and Prevention. (2018). *Diabetes report card 2017.* Atlanta, GA: Centers for Disease Control and Prevention, U.S. Dept. of Health and Human Services. Retrieved from https://www.cdc.gov/diabetes/pdfs/library/diabetesreportcard2017-508.pdf.

94. Centers for Disease Control and Prevention. (2017). *National diabetes statistics report, 2017.* Atlanta, GA: Centers for Disease Control and Prevention, U.S. Dept. of Health and Human Services. Retrieved from https://www.cdc.gov/diabetes/pdfs/data/statistics/national-diabetes-statistics-report.pdf.

95. Patrick, K.A., & Wyckoff, L. (2017). Providing standards for diabetes care in the school setting: A review of the Colorado model. *NASN School Nurse, 33*(1), 52-56. doi.org/10.1177/1942602X17725886.

96. National Diabetes Education Program. (2016). *Helping the student with diabetes succeed: A Guide for school personnel.* National Institutes of Health and Centers for Disease Control and Prevention. Retrieved from https://www.niddk.nih.gov/-/media/Files/Health-Information/Communication-Programs/NDEP/health-care-professionals/NDEP-School-Guide-Full-508.pdf?la=en.

97. Yonkaitis, C.F., & Shannon, R.A. (2017). The role of the school nurse in the special education process: Part 1: Student identification and evaluation. *NASN School Nurse, 32*(3), 178-184. doi.org/10.1177/1942602X17700677.

98. Individuals with Disabilities Education Act. (2006). *Individuals with Disabilities Education Act of 2004, Pub. L. No. 108–446.* Retrieved from http://idea.ed.gov/download/statute.html.

99. Shannon, R.A., & Yonkaitis, C.F. (2017). The role of the school nurse in the special education process: Part 2: Eligibility determination and the Individualized Education Program. *NASN School Nurse, 32*(4), 249-254. doi.org/10.1177/1942602X17709505.

100. U.S. Government Publishing Office. (1975). *Education for All Handicapped Children Act of 1974, Pub. L. No. 94–142* (1975). Retrieved from https://www.govinfo.gov/content/pkg/STATUTE-89/pdf/STATUTE-89-Pg773.pdf.

101. U.S. Department of Education. (2013). *Building the legacy: IDEA 2004.* Retrieved from http://idea.ed.gov/explore/home.

102. Wrightslaw. (n.d.). *Section 504, the Americans With Disabilities Act, and Education Reform.* Retrieved from http://www.wrightslaw.com/info/section504.ada.peer.htm.

103. Galemore, C.A., & Sheetz, A.H. (2015). IEP, IHP, and Section 504 primer for new school nurses. *NASN School Nurse, 30*(2), 85-88. doi.org/10.1177/1942602X14565462.

104. Cohen, J. (2014). School climate policy and practice trends: A paradox. A commentary. *Teachers College Record.* Retrieved from https://www.schoolclimate.org/themes/schoolclimate/assets/pdf/policy/SCPolicy&PracticeTrends-CommentaryTCRecord2-28-14.pdf.

105. Domitrovich, C.E., Durlak, J., Staley, K.C., & Weissberg, R.P. (2017). Social-emotional competence: An essential factor for promoting positive adjustment and reducing risk and school children. *Child Development, 88,* 408-416. doi:10.1111/cdev.12739.

106. Shannon, R.A., Bergren, M.D., & Matthews, A. (2010). Frequent visitors: Somatization in school-age children and implications for school nurses. *The Journal of School Nursing, 26*(3), 169-182.

107. National Association of School Nurses. (2017). *The school nurse's role in behavioral health of students* (Position Statement). Silver Spring, MD: Author. Retrieved from https://www.nasn.org/nasn/advocacy/professional-practice-documents/position-statements/ps-behavioral-health.

108. Centers for Disease Control and Prevention. (2015). *Mental health basics. Healthy youth mental health.* Retrieved from http://www.cdc.gov/mentalhealth/basics.htm.

109. National Council of State Boards of Nursing. (2005). *Working with others: A position paper.* Retrieved from https://www.ncsbn.org/Working_with_Others.pdf.

110. Resha, C. (2010). Delegation in the school setting: Is it a safe practice? *The Online Journal of Issues in Nursing, 15*(2), 5. doi:10.39 12/OJIN.Vol15No.02Man05.

111. U.S. Department of Education, Office for Civil Rights. (2011). *Protecting students with disabilities.* Retrieved from http://www2.ed.gov/about/offices/list/ocr/504faq.html.

112. National Association of State School Nurse Consultants. (2008). *State school nurse consultant position.* Retrieved from http://www.schoolnurseconsultants.org/wp-content/uploads/2013/05/NASSNC-Position-Statement-Need-for-State-School-Nurse-Consultants.pdf.

113. Hogan, J. (2018). Condom access for high school students: The journey from data to policy. *NASN School Nurse, 33*(5), 284-287.

114. National Association of School Nurses & American Nurses Association. (2017). *School nursing: Scope and standards of practice* (ed 3). Silver Spring, MD: American Nurses Association.

115. Jacobsen, K., Meeder, L., & Voscuil, V.R. (2016). Chronic student absenteeism: The critical role of school nurses. *NASN School Nurse, 31*(3), 178-185. doi.org/10.1177/1942602X16638855.

116. Dworak, L.M. (2009). From paper to practice: A look at Healthiest Wisconsin 2010 and the development of local school wellness policies that aid in the prevention of child overweight. *NASN School Nurse, 24*(2), 85-89.

117. Sheetz, A.H. (2011). Why is a school health (wellness) advisory council important for school nursing practice? *NASN School Nurse, 26*(5), 280-282.

118. Network for Public Health Law. (2017). *School nursing scope of practice: 50 state survey.* Retrieved from https://www.networkforphl.org/_asset/dx4pp2/50-State-Survey—School-Nursing-Scope-of-Practice.pdf.

119. U.S. Department of Education. (2015). *Every Student Succeeds Act.* Retrieved from https://www.ed.gov/essa.

120. U.S. Department of Health & Human Services, Administration for Children and Families, Administration on Children, Youth and Families, Children's Bureau. (2017). *Child maltreatment 2015.* Retrieved from http://www.acf.hhs.gov/programs/cb/research-data-technology/statistics-research/child-maltreatment.

121. U.S. Department of Health and Human Services, U.S. Department of Education. (2008). *Joint guidance on the application of Family Educational Rights and Privacy Act (FERPA) and the Health Information Portability and Accountability Act (HIPAA) of 1996 to student health records.* Retrieved from https://www2.ed.gov/policy/gen/guid/fpco/doc/ferpa-hipaa-guidance.pdf.

122. Federation of American Scientists. (2018). *Children's Health Insurance Program Reauthorization Act of 2009, Pub. L. No. 115-123 (2018).* Retrieved from https://fas.org/sgp/crs/misc/R45136.pdf.

123. Medicaid.gov. (n.d.). *Children's Health Insurance Program (CHIP)*. Retrieved from https://www.medicaid.gov/chip/index.html.

124. U.S. Department of Agriculture Food and Nutrition Services. (n.d.). *Local wellness policy*. Retrieved from http://www.fns.usda.gov/tn/healthy/wellnesspolicy.html.

125. Malat, J., Oh, H., & Hamilton, M. (2005). Poverty experience, race, and child health. *Public Health Reports, 120*, 442-447.

126. Hass, S.A., & Fosse, N.E. (2008). Health and the educational attainment of adolescents: Evidence from the NLSY97. *Journal of Health and Social Behavior, 4*(2), 178-192.

127. Basch, C.E. (2010). Healthier students are better learners: A missing link in school reforms to close the achievement gap. *Equity Matters: Research Review No. 6*. New York, NY: Teachers College, Columbia University.

128. U.S. Department of Health & Human Services. (2010). *Patient Protection and Affordable Care Act of 2010, Pub. L. No. 111-148*. Retrieved from https://www.hhs.gov/healthcare/about-the-aca/index.html.

129. Keepnews, D. (2013). *Mapping the economic value of nursing: A white paper*. Seattle: Washington State Nurses Association. Retrieved from https://www.wsna.org/assets/entry-assets/Nursing-Practice/Publications/economic-value-of-nursing-white-paper.pdf.

130. World Health Organization. (2018). *School and youth health*. Retrieved from https://www.who.int/school_youth_health/resources/en/.

131. World Health Organization. (2018). *School health and youth health promotion*. Retrieved from https://www.who.int/school_youth_health/en/.

Chapter 19

Health Planning for Older Adults

Minhui Liu

LEARNING OUTCOMES

After reading the chapter, the student will be able to:

1. Describe the trend of aging population from a global perspective.
2. Describe demographic and social trends in an aging America.
3. Define successful aging and determinants of health in the older population.
4. Describe the main health issues facing older adults.
5. Apply current frameworks related to prevention of illness and injury in older adults.
6. Characterize priorities for chronic disease management in the aging population.
7. Identify community resources for helping older adults age in place.
8. Describe age-specific models of health-care delivery across the continuum from wellness to end-of-life care.
9. Identify risk factors of successful aging in minority populations.
10. Articulate key ethical issues related to aging in our society.

KEY TERMS

Aged dependency ratio
Ageism
Aging
Baby boomers
Caregiver
Centenarians
Continuing care
    retirement
    communities (CCRCs)

Core end-stage indicator
Dependency ratio
Early onset at-risk
    substance use
Elder maltreatment
Elderly
Elderly persons
Geriatrics
Gerontology

Hospice care
Health promotion
Late onset at-risk
    substance use
Life expectancy
Life span
Naturally occurring
    retirement community
    (NORC)

Old-old
Older adult
Physical activity
Palliative care
Population aging
Rectangularization
    of aging
Super centenarians

Introduction

The world is facing a situation without precedent: globally, the population aged 60 and over is growing faster than all younger age groups. In 2017, the estimated number of people aged 60 and over was 962 million, which comprises 13% of the global population. This group of people is growing at a rate of about 3% per year. Globally, the number of individuals aged 80 years and older is projected to triple by 2050, from 137 million in 2017 to 425 million in 2050.[1] In the first half of the last century, the increase in older populations was largely due to improvements in life expectancy. **Life expectancy** is the probable number of years a person will live based on the birth and mortality statistics of the population. The global life expectancy at birth in 2016 was 71.4 years (73.8 years for females and 69.1 for males), and global average life expectancy increased by 5.2 years between 2000 and 2015.[2] In the United States, life expectancy increased from 47.3 years at the beginning of the 20th century to 78.8 years in 2015.[2] In 2012, 29 high-income countries had a life expectancy that exceeded 80 years of age.[1] Factors that have influenced this increase in life expectancy during the last half of the 20th century include decreased fertility rates and increased urbanization.[1] The fact that we are living longer has had a direct impact on public health, allocation of health resources, and demand for nursing services. Understanding this phenomenon from a public health perspective provides nurses with the context in which aging occurs and the factors that contribute not only to living longer but also to maintaining an optimal health-related quality of life. This understanding, in turn, helps nurses develop, implement, and evaluate nursing interventions across settings from a public health prevention framework. This will improve the health-related quality of life experienced by older adults and reduce the need for more costly tertiary care.

Health of Aging Populations

Who Is Old?

In the United States, the commonly accepted definition of **older adult** is a person aged 65 or older. This definition is used in this chapter to be consistent with language used in *Healthy People*.[3] The age of 65 was chosen because, in high-income countries, most persons are eligible for retirement benefits at this age. The World Health Organization (WHO) pointed out that this definition is somewhat arbitrary and may not be applicable in lower-income countries.[4,5] The issue is that chronological age may not accurately reflect a similar biological age of persons living in a low-income country compared with someone the same age living in a high-income country. For example, the WHO argued that a person aged 50 or 55 living in a low-income country may be comparable biologically with a person aged 65 living in a high-income country. People who live in low-income countries age faster because of inadequate nutrition, exposure to communicable diseases, and poorer living conditions.[5] Thus, the aging process is a product not only of chronological age but also of biological age.

Aging occurs differently in individuals and populations. Rather than an inevitable decline, aging can instead be viewed as the later stages of continuous growth and development that occur across the life span. The quality and length of life depend on factors that improve the biological response to growth and development experienced across the life span. The factors include not only individual healthy habits embraced in youth and followed across the life span, but also the environment in which an individual lives. The term **life span** is used to describe the measure of a life from birth to death. It also refers to the genetically based limit to the length of life. In humans, the documented maximum life span achieved was 122 years.

Though chronological age as a marker for aging has some limitations, it provides a way to compare populations. Other terms commonly used are **elderly** or **elderly persons**, but the preferred term is *older adult*. These terms are also defined using chronological criteria and are typically used to describe persons aged 65 years or older.[5] There are also terms for subpopulations, as evidenced by terms such as **old-old** (ages between 85 and 95) and oldest-old (95+). As life expectancy lengthens, another chronological group is also emerging, those over the age of 100.[6] This population is referred to as **centenarians**. **Super centenarians** are those who live to be 110 years of age or older.

Nurses provide needed care for older adults and are educated to view aging as a lifelong process, not simply a particular chronological age or an end stage of life. Understanding the specific needs of the older adult from a population perspective provides nurses with an opportunity to actively participate in the public health initiative reflected in *HP*: improve the quality of life for older adults.[3] For nurses providing care to older adults, there is an opportunity to reduce risk and enhance function at the individual level, even in the face of age-related changes. When this is expanded to include groups of individuals, communities, and populations, the impact of nursing interventions is more significant.

Regardless of clinical practice settings, most nurses are likely to provide care to older family members, friends, or members of their communities. Providing care to older adults requires examining the phenomenon of aging from a population perspective that includes:

- The demographic, social, and health trends associated with aging
- Public health issues
- Impact on individual care delivery systems
- Resources for health prevention and promotion
- Implications for policy and research

Thus, aging is not adequately measured by chronological age. Instead, the quality of life experienced as individuals age is a product of chronological and biological age and is affected by the environments in which we live.[5]

An Aging America

In 2015, the U.S. Census Bureau estimated that 14.9% (47.8 million) of the U.S. population was 65 years old or older.[7] By 2050, the estimated number of persons aged 65 or older will be 83.3 million, and 60% of these older Americans will be over the age of 74.[8] On average, those who are presently 65 years of age will now live another 18 years, and those aged 85 years will live on average into their early 90s.[9] This phenomenon is referred to as **population aging**, which is a shift in the distribution of a country's population toward older ages. In other words, the proportion of the population that is older has increased (Fig. 19-1). This is usually reflected in an increase in the population's mean and median ages, a decline in the proportion of the population composed of children, and a rise in the proportion of the older adult

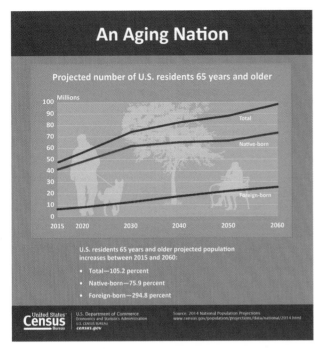

Figure 19-1 Increase in the number of U.S. older adults expressed in millions, 2015–2060. *(From the U.S. Census Bureau.)*

population (Fig. 19-2). Population aging is widespread across the world and is most advanced in high-income countries.[10,11] This aging of the population globally, according to the WHO, is a cause for celebration because it reflects the positive effect of interventions aimed at improving health. It also offers opportunities, as older adults are a wonderful resource. However, this trend puts strains on pension funds and the demand for health-care services.[11] It is imperative, then, to tailor health-care resources and systems to the unique needs of an aging population.

What accounts for the population aging in the United States? One of the reasons is the improvement in the environment. In the first half of the 20th century, diseases that previously led to death in early life became less threatening as a result of the development of antibiotics and other medications. In addition, improvements in sanitation, diagnostic advances, the application of technology, and improved prenatal and obstetrical care contributed to longer living.[1] Globally, improvements in life expectancy are tied to increased child survival rates and HIV/AIDS survival rates.[12] Prior to these innovations in the United States, nearly half of the people born in the year 1900 died before they reached age 50. Contrast this with our current situation, wherein people born today can expect to live beyond their 75th year, and an increasing number are living to be 100. In 1900, about 1 in 25 Americans was over 65; today 1 in 8 are. The older adult population in the United States is expected to increase from 52.8 million in 2018 to 94.7 million in 2060. Increases in longevity can also be seen in the fastest growing age group in our society, the old-old. By 2035, there will be 11.5 million persons over the age of 85. We also can expect to see nearly a million centenarians, or people 100 years or older.[13,14]

Along with changes in life expectancy, a main reason for the dramatic increase in the number of older adults in the United States is the effect of the baby boomer generation. **Baby boomers** are those members of the U.S. population born between 1945 and 1964. In 2010, the first of this generation turned 65. Growth in the number of older adults will continue as this cohort moves through the upper age groups and will begin to stabilize after 2050.[14] According to the U.S. Census Bureau, in 2010 a little more than 14% of the older population was over the age of 85, but by 2050, when all of the baby boomers are over the age of 85, that proportion is expected to increase to over 21%.[14] A good way to visualize this cohort is through a comparison of population pyramids over time. Figure 19-3 includes four population pyramids for the United States, 20 years apart,

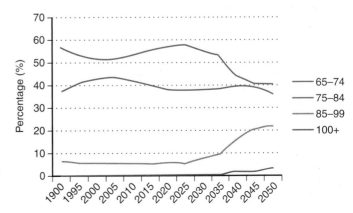

Figure 19-2 Distribution of U.S. older adults over age groups, 1990–2050. *(From the U.S. National Institutes of Health, National Institute on Aging [2009]).*

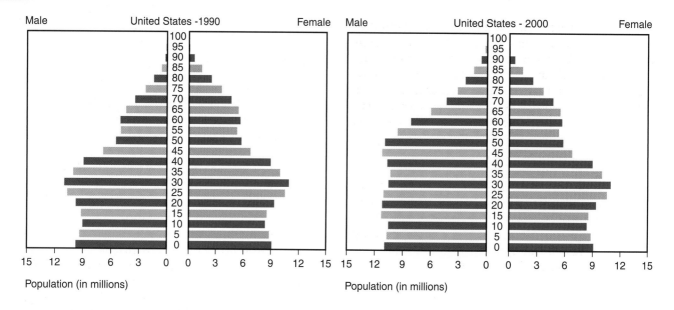

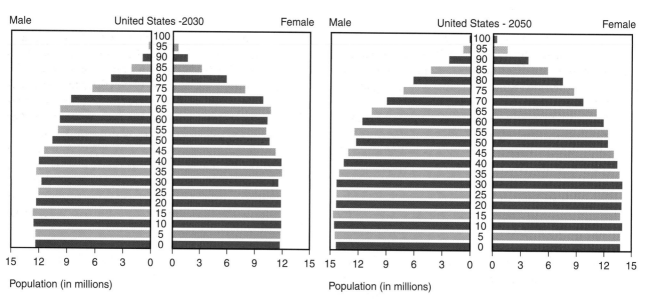

Figure 19-3 Comparison of population pyramids 1990–2050. *(From U.S. Census Bureau, International Programs U.S. Retrieved from http://www.census.gov/population/international/data/idb/informationGateway.php/)*

starting with 1990. The 1990 pyramid shows the baby boomer bump clearly. This was when the baby boomers were between 25 and 45 years old. By 2050, this cohort is 85 years of age or older, and this accounts for the change in the top of the pyramid.[14]

Another term that describes the shift in our population toward the older ages is the **rectangularization of aging**. This describes the population trend toward increased numbers of healthy years before decline or, more exactly, a reduction in variability of the age of death.[15] With a steady or slightly declining birthrate and reductions in early deaths, a population's tendency to move toward older ages emerges, which is what we are seeing in the United States today.

The face of aging in the United States is changing dramatically. People are living longer, achieving higher levels of education, living in poverty less often, and experiencing lower rates of disability.[13] Even with this positive outlook, there are still significant public health challenges. For example, the old-old age group is not only increasing in numbers but is also prone to the development of serious chronic conditions, such as dementia. This creates a great impact on both older adults and their caregivers.[16] This group is also more likely to be living in poverty and to experience functional declines. Also, the epidemic of obesity will have an impact on the development of cardiovascular disease and diabetes, with implications not only for longevity but also for health-care utilization and quality of life. Today, more than a third of persons over the age of 59 (41.0%) are obese.[17]

Aging and the Workforce

In our daily lives, our joint activities and interactions with older adults demonstrate their valuable contributions to family life, workplaces, and communities. Consider the greeter at Walmart, the volunteer at the library, and our elected officials serving as senators and representatives well into their 70s and sometimes 80s. As more people over the age of 65 participate in the workforce,[9,18,19] we encounter more and more persons actively contributing to the health and well-being of our communities.

From 1977 to 2007, the number of persons over the age of 65 increased by 101%. This graying of the workforce is not just the result of the increase in the numbers of older adults staying in the workforce; younger Americans are entering the workforce at an older age.[19] Older adults are staying in the workforce for a variety of reasons. One factor was the economic recession of 2008 to 2010 that reduced the savings of older adults. More than half of those 62 and over in 2009 cited the recession as their reason for staying in the workforce. Other reasons included a desire to feel productive, a need for social interaction, and the wish for something to do.[19]

One of the things the increased life expectancy of a population affects is the dependency ratio. The **dependency ratio** is the proportion of dependents (those aged 0 to 14 years plus those 65 years of age and older) per every 100 members of the population aged 15 to 64. In relation to the older population, the ratio is referred to as the **aged dependency ratio** and it reflects the ratio of the number of persons age 65 and older per every 100 members of the population aged 15 to 64 (Box 19-1). Because of the aging population, there is an expected rise

---

BOX 19-1 ■ Aged Dependency Ratio

Total Dependency Ratio =

$$\frac{\text{Number of people aged 0 to 14 + number of people aged 65 and older}}{\text{Number of people aged 15 to 64}} \times 100$$

Aged Dependency Ratio =

$$\frac{\text{Number of people aged 65+}}{\text{Number of people aged 15 to 64}} \times 100$$

---

in the dependency ratio as well.[19] Factors that may improve the aged dependency ratio include the increased age of full retirement for Social Security benefits for baby boomers rising from 65 to 67 and the graying of the U.S. workforce. As the number of those who live past the age of 65 increases, any possible benefits from the increased number of those over 65 who work may be wiped out by the increasing number of persons aged 75 and older.[19]

Healthy People and Older Adults

As life expectancy increases along with the proportion of the population living over the age of 85, society is confronted with both challenges and opportunities for people of all ages. The challenge for the 21st century is to make these added life span years as healthy and productive as possible and to continue the current trend of decline in disability across all segments of the population. Many older adults experience hospitalizations, nursing home admissions, and low-quality care, and may lose the ability to live independently at home. Chronic conditions are the leading cause of death and disability among older adults. Because of these concerns, *HP 2020* added a new topic area, Older Adults.[3]

■ HEALTHY PEOPLE
Older Adults
Healthy People Topics Relevant to Health Planning for Older Adults

Targeted Topic(s): Older adults

Goal: Improve the health, function, and quality of life of older adults.

Overview: Older adults are among the fastest growing age groups, and the first baby boomers (adults born between 1946 and 1964) turned 65 in 2011. More than 37 million people in this group (60%) will manage more than one chronic condition by 2030. Chronic conditions can lower quality of life in older adults and can be leading causes of death in this population.

HP 2020 Midcourse Review: Of the 19 objectives for this topic area, 2 were developmental and 15 were measurable (Fig. 19-4). For 3 of the measurable objectives, the target was met or exceeded, and 1 was improving. For 3, there was little or no detectable change, and 5 were getting worse. Three of the objectives had baseline data only.[20]

Source: See *HP 2020* for background, objectives, interventions, and resources.[3]

Why Is the Health of Older Adults Important?
According to *HP,* more than 60% of older adults manage two or more chronic conditions. To address this growing burden on our health-care system, population-level approaches are needed to reduce the morbidity and mortality associated with chronic diseases (see Chapter 9), and to improve the health-related quality of life experienced by older adults. *HP* supports population approaches that will increase prevention initiatives while improving access to services. Emerging issues for improving the health of older adults include efforts to:[4]

- Coordinate care
- Help older adults manage their own care
- Establish quality measures
- Identify minimum levels of training for people who care for older adults

- Research and analyze appropriate training to equip providers with the tools they need to meet the needs of older adults[4]

The Changing Diversity in the Older Adult Population

Another changing demographic for older adults in the United States is the evolving ethnicity of this population. Although those over 64 are less ethnically and racially diverse compared with younger groups, this is projected to change over the next 4 decades dramatically. The number of white older adults is projected to decrease by 10%, and all other ethnic/racial groups will increase, with 42% of older adults being members of a minority population by 2050. The number of persons of Hispanic origin aged 65 years or older will nearly double from 37.4 million in 2010 to 71 million in 2050.[21] This increasing ethnic diversity of the older adult population has implications for the development of culturally relevant interventions that consider the diverse cultural heritage of this group. Thus, conducting a cultural assessment and maintaining cultural competency is an essential skill for nurses working with older adult populations.

Determinants of Aging and Health

To begin to think about the public health implications of an aging population, it is essential to understand what it means to age. **Aging** is the process of becoming

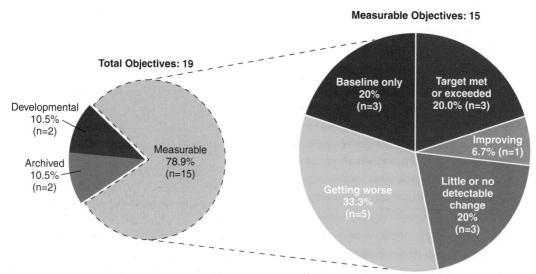

Figure 19-4 *Healthy People 2020 for Older Adults Midcourse Review.*

chronologically and biologically older. This process is determined by genetics and is modulated by the environment. It can also be viewed from a perspective that moves beyond the physiology of aging. As noted by the WHO, aging is a concept that encompasses more than counting years or the physiological and psychosocial features that change over time.[4,5] It is often defined as a feeling, a state of mind, or a product of what an individual is able to do—in other words, a functional definition of aging. Simply viewing aging in terms of the number of years lived or specific age-associated signs limits a true definition of an older adult, for individuals of any given age may exhibit widely varied characteristics. Older adults are a diverse group of people moving across the life course with many heterogeneous and unique features. Indeed, there are more and more differences among individuals as they grow older. Important indicators of age are physical health, psychological well-being, socioeconomic factors, functional abilities, and social relations. Goals of nursing care are to modify physiological and psychological changes and help people stay healthy, functional, and independent longer.

Theories of Aging

The processes of aging have long intrigued scientists and philosophers. However, finding an explanation for the many complex changes associated with aging, both predictable and random, has presented a formidable challenge. Many ideas have been proposed and tested, but the only certainty is that no single theory can explain everything about the process of aging. Theories encompass biological, immunological, psychological, and developmental realms. Even these widely ranging ideas about aging have some key features in common.

One theoretical approach to aging is that signs of aging emerge when demands exceed resources, that is, the person no longer independently has the resources needed to meet the demands of everyday life. Some of the biological theories provide examples of this imbalance. Another theory is that aging occurs when there is a loss of effectiveness in maintaining equilibrium at the biological level, such as what occurs in heart failure. Other theories are based on the loss of the ability to adapt to change, which becomes more pronounced with the advance of time.[22]

Biological Theories of Aging

The biological theories of aging regard the body as a collection of cells and materials subject to mechanical or architectural failure as they grow older. Biological breakdown with aging may result from genes, such as when harmful genes "turn on" and become active in later life, or when some older adults exhibit youthful vigor and well-being in older adulthood, which seems to run in their families. It is also thought that some genes actually promote functional decline and structural deterioration, thereby producing the outward and organic signs of aging. In genetic studies of worms, scientists have been able to isolate the specific gene that controls longevity, and by manipulating that gene, can cause the worms to live a greatly extended life span.[22] The excitement that accompanied the mapping of the human genome was coupled with the hope that, by decoding genetic material, we would be able to understand and ultimately influence health and longevity. However, many more questions have developed from our knowledge thus far, including the mysterious forces that cause a gene to turn on or turn off.

Another theoretical viewpoint of aging suggests that aging occurs as a result of the accumulation of errors in protein synthesis over time, leading to impaired cell function. In aging, it is thought that successive generations of faulty cells eventually lead to impaired biological function. However, despite evidence of declines in cell replication, amino acid sequencing does not change with age, and there is no evidence that RNA becomes defective with age. Once again, this biological theory cannot fully explain the dynamics and differences of aging organisms.[22]

An additional theory is that aging is related to mutations that occur when cells are exposed to environmental factors, such as radiation or chemicals; this exposure causes the DNA to be damaged and altered. Thus, genetics are modulated by the environment. This is based on the observation that accumulations of mutations are time-dependent, and it is possible that faulty cells from youth are replicated and harbored, increasing in numbers with age. This is one explanation for the deleterious effects that can show up later in life.[22]

The *free-radical* theory is another major idea in the biological realm, stemming from the observation that older adults are more prone to the damaging effects of free radicals, that is, molecules with unpaired electrons. They also have lower levels of protectant free-radical scavengers, such as vitamin A, vitamin C, and niacin. Free-radical damage to cells and organs occurs as a result of oxidative stress and is thought to have cumulative effects. There are both internal and external sources for oxidative stress, as free radicals are a by-product of oxygen metabolism. Some research into the effects of free-radical damage has uncovered the accumulation of harmful pigmented proteins called *lipofuscins* that are associated with aging. The key idea is that cells are repeatedly aggravated by harmful stressors that may be metabolic by-products. In aging, the DNA cannot keep up with needed repairs, resulting in a decline in function and number of cells. Serious problems occur when nonreplaceable cells are damaged, such as muscle, heart, nerve, and brain cells.[24]

Yet another major biological theory of aging is the *cross-linkage* or *connective tissue* theory, which describes the chemical reactions that create strong bonds among molecular structures that are normally separate, particularly in collagen, elastin, and ground substance. Increased numbers of cross-links in collagen yield stiffness and loss of resilience. In elastin, cross-links affect movement and elasticity. Evidence of these processes might be seen in stiffening of blood vessels or skin changes associated with aging. One of the reasons that caloric restriction and steroids have been associated with the slowing of the aging process may have to do with the formation of fewer cross-linkages on a molecular level.[24]

Some of the physiologically based theories of aging describe relatively random events, but there are also some key ideas about programmed aging, or a biological or genetic clock that determines how an individual's original pool of genetic material is played out in an orderly manner. Examples of this can be seen in human development, maturation, and the expected cessation of certain body functions, for example, menopause, graying of hair, or thymus atrophy. The programmed aging theory is based on the concept that cells double a limited number of times before they die, or that there is an expected life span for every cell.

Psychosocial Theories of Aging

Psychosocial theories of aging revolve around three major and somewhat conflicting ideas: disengagement, activity, and continuity. Early theorists offered the observation that older adults tend to disengage from pursuits and roles that they enjoyed in earlier life and suggested that this process was a mutual withdrawal of the individual from society. In a classic article, Cumming[25] proposed that this process of disengagement was accepted and actually desired by older adults, and that it was a natural and universal feature of a long life. From their perspective, disengagement was the "correct" way to age.

However, a clearly opposing theory was at work. Older adults who resisted withdrawal and remained active and engaged in life were observed to age more optimally. In fact, the more active they were, the greater satisfaction they expressed with the quality of their lives. They were more likely to be able to substitute new roles for those lost through changing function or social circumstances. Many community-based programs for older adults are based on the activity theory and offer many activities that help older adults to keep busy and socially engaged. For many older adults, activity is a vital coping strategy, as they face inevitable losses and changes in their lives.

Perhaps strongest of all is the theory that people are basically consistent throughout their lives, and their personalities remain constant through the passing years. This is described as continuity[26] and can be an important consideration for nurses as we assist individuals in managing health issues or dealing with new challenges associated with aging. We can help older adults use their past experiences to frame new situations and work from the strengths within their perspectives and personalities.

Key Aging Research

Despite the fact that we live in a rapidly aging society, the truth is that many people have a limited understanding of what it means to grow older. Some people may have misconceptions about the natural processes of aging and may view the world of aging according to their own experiences and even prejudices. Some may lack understanding of the trials and triumphs that older adults experience in their everyday lives. It is imperative that nurses be open in their views of aging. Older adults are not "the other;" they are a preview for those who are younger, moving along life's continuum ahead of them.

Formal study of the aging process has developed over the past several decades. With a growing population of aging adults, the National Institutes of Health established the National Institute of Aging specifically to conduct research about the processes of aging. Research projects range from examinations of minute molecular, genetic, and biochemical mechanisms, all the way to entire populations, and every aspect in between. Exciting discoveries and insights that are revealed today will inform nursing practice as nurses care for older adults in our society. In the following sections, three major longitudinal studies are discussed that have shaped our understanding of the processes and challenges of aging, have helped to define the determinants of health in aging, and have helped to identify health priorities for an aging population.

Baltimore Longitudinal Study of Aging

The Baltimore Longitudinal Study of Aging (BLSA) began in 1958 and is the longest-running scientific study of human aging.[27] It is an excellent example of a longitudinal cohort study (see Chapter 3). The focus of this study is to discover what happens as people age and to distinguish changes that are due to natural aging from those that are due to diseases or other causes. This study has followed more than 1,400 individuals from age 20 to 90 and older. Over the course of the study, important aspects of the aging process and determinants of health have been uncovered, including:

- Normal age-related circulatory system changes and the development of cardiovascular disease
- Impact of lifestyle choices on the development of disease
- Brain and memory changes that predict declines
- Stability of personality in older years, coping strategies, and perceived happiness
- Organic changes, such as prostate enlargement and diagnostic parameters for disease
- Sensory changes, such as alterations in hearing and taste
- Metabolism and nutrition in aging, including body composition, predictors for the development of diabetes, and age-related changes in renal function

A fundamental aim of the BLSA is to differentiate which changes are a normal part of aging and which are the result of disease processes. The study has been able to demonstrate that slower reaction speed and some changes in short-term memory are associated with aging in the absence of disease. However, sudden losses, such as those that accompany heart attacks or strokes, are clearly the result of disease but can be worsened by the changes that occur naturally with aging. The good news is that lifestyle decisions can affect the occurrence or progression of age-associated disease.

New England Centenarian Study

One fascinating way to look at aging is through the extremes of longevity, for example, by examining the features of very long-lived individuals or the super centenarians. The oldest documented living person was Jeanne Calment of Arles, France, who attained the age of 122 years. Her extremely long life span was carefully studied, as it pushed the boundaries of what we thought could be possible in human survival and suggested some traits and behaviors that might contribute to longevity.[28] For example, Madame Calment remained physically active through most of her life. She kept a lean weight. But contrary to the accepted wisdom about healthy behaviors, she smoked cigarettes from the age of 21 until the age of 117. She ascribed her longevity and relatively youthful appearance to olive oil, wine, and chocolate.

Serious research about the features and commonalities of people who live to 100+ years is reflected in the ongoing New England Centenarian Study. Scientists have observed that individuals who age well into the extremes of the life span have a marked delay in the development of age-associated disability. Among the study subjects, about 15% have no significant disease at age 100, and these people are characterized as "escapers." About 43% of the group has age-related disease that did not show up until around age 80, and these are called the "delayers." The remaining people can be described as "survivors," as they have clinically demonstrable disease prior to age 80, but they manage to survive and continue to live even with these diseases.[28] Basically, longevity trends support a hypothesis of compression of morbidity, wherein older adults experience more years of health prior to the development of disease. Researchers suggest that in aging, as stated by Hilt, Young-Xu Silver, and Perls, "… the older you get, the healthier you've been."[29–31]

Normative Aging Study

The Normative Aging Study began in 1963 and has followed male veterans longitudinally to evaluate changes in their physical health, health-related behaviors, such as smoking and dietary intake, and other factors that may influence health.[32] For example, during certain years of the study, measurements were collected of lead and cadmium content in participants' bodies. Neurocognitive tests have been tracked, along with tests of motor function, memory, and learning. Other psychosocial variables that can have a substantial effect on aging and health include depression, adverse life events, optimism, and perceived stress. This study also has a large bank of DNA samples to look at genes associated with the development of Alzheimer's disease.[32] With such a wide range of variables collected over a long period of time, investigators may be able to identify specific relationships among genetic, environmental, physiological, and psychosocial variables.

These ongoing studies and many others continue to reveal important information about the normal processes of aging and to identify important roles for nurses in the community to promote health, reduce risk factors for disease, and support and enhance optimal management of chronic conditions associated with aging.

Program Planning and Health Promotion in Aging

As demonstrated in the major aging research studies, longevity and health are influenced by complex interactions among biological, psychological, and sociological factors. Past research about aging has often emphasized the extent to which health problems, such as diabetes or osteoporosis, could be attributed exclusively to age. Such research tended to exaggerate the homogeneity of older adults. However, researchers are now reporting some essential elements that contribute to healthy aging overall and have helped to identify preventive health-care goals for older adults and 10 keys to healthy aging (Box 19-2).[33]

Changing demographic trends related to an aging population have driven many changes in health care, requiring specialized knowledge and application of **gerontology** (the study of the effects of time on human development or the study of the aging process) and **geriatrics** (specialized medical care of older adults). Nursing has been a leader in the field of gerontology, as it was the first profession to offer advanced certification recognizing the specialized skills and knowledge required in caring for older adults.[34]

There are a few considerations we need to keep in mind when promoting successful aging in older adults. The first consideration is the importance of enhancing and encouraging healthy life choices at all ages. Nurses may be involved in health promotion initiatives at any age that may protect health, reduce risk factors, and lay the groundwork for optimal health in aging. For example, the health programs focused on eliminating childhood obesity, promoting physical activity, and stopping smoking may have far-reaching effects on the aging process. This is because healthy weight is associated with less hypertension and healthier glucose metabolism, activity is associated with strength and mobility, and smoking cessation reduces the risk of developing respiratory and cardiovascular disease. Thus, healthy and/or unhealthy behaviors practiced during the younger years contribute to the health, function, and well-being of the older adult.

Many of the risk factors for the development of disease and disability in aging can be modified through changes in behavior or changes in environment.[3] Such modifications are a key focus for public health nurses working with older populations, whether in the form of public health education, screening programs, surveillance, exercise, diet, immunization programs, and sanitation, as well as for nurses who provide individualized care. **Stages of Change (Transtheoretical) Model** developed by Prochaska and DiClemente is one of the most commonly used theories in health behavior change (Table 19-1).[35] The basic premise of this model is that behavior change is a process, not an event. When a person attempts to change a behavior, he or she moves through five stages (precontemplation, contemplation, preparation, action, and maintenance).

Finally, when we look at risk factors for the development of disease and disability in aging, we recognize that most can be modified through changes in behavior or changes in environment. Such modifications are a key focus of community health nursing, whether in the form of public health education, screening programs, surveillance, exercise, diet, immunization programs, sanitation, or individualized care.

● APPLYING PUBLIC HEALTH SCIENCE
The Case of the CAPABLE Study
Public Health Science Topics Covered:
- Community Assessment
  - Face-to-face motivational interview
  - Health assessment
- Health planning:
  - Applying health-related conceptual models
  - Patient-centered care approaches

Nancy is an 80-year-old retired teacher who has no children and lives alone. After being discharged from the hospital, she found she was too weak to use her front steps, which, without a railing, were unsafe. She lives in a townhouse with a bedroom upstairs, but she has difficulty using the stairs because of the absence of railings and her osteoarthritis pain. Most of her days were spent alone, and many of her routine activities such as getting in and out of the bathtub were impossible. She had fallen several times when trying to get into bed. And although skilled home care assisted her in understanding her medications, her environmental and physical functioning were not addressed.

On the community center bulletin board, Nancy saw a flyer for Community Aging in Place – Advancing

---

BOX 19–2 ■ Ten Keys to Healthy Aging

1. Controlling hypertension
2. Stopping smoking
3. Screening for cancer
4. Keeping current on immunizations
5. Regulating blood glucose
6. Lowering cholesterol
7. Being physically active
8. Preventing bone loss and muscle weakness
9. Maintaining social contact
10. Combating depression

Source: (33)

TABLE 19–1 ■ Stages of Change Model

Stage	Definition	Potential Change Strategies
Precontemplation	Has no intention of taking action within the next 6 months	Increase awareness of need for change; personalize information about risks and benefits
Contemplation	Intends to take action in the next 6 months	Motivate; encourage making specific plans
Preparation	Intends to take action within the next 30 days and has taken some behavioral steps in this direction	Assist with developing and implementing concrete action plans; help set gradual goals
Action	Has changed behavior for less than 6 months	Assist with feedback, problem-solving, social support, and reinforcement
Maintenance	Has changed behavior for more than 6 months	Assist with coping, reminders, finding alternatives, avoiding slips/relapses (as applicable)

Source: (35)

Better Living for Elders (CAPABLE) which is a home-based program of an interprofessional team – an occupational therapist (OT), a registered nurse (RN), and a handyman (HM) – who work with low-income older adults for 5 months on what they identify as their most important goals.[36] This program is based on an overarching mode—Society to Cells Resilience Framework—and three other models: person-environment fit, disablement process, and control. The Society to Cells Resilience Framework emphasizes intervening on more than one socioecological domain, such as physiologic, individual, and built environment. It also posits that there are critically resilient times, such as post-hospitalization.[37] Person-environment fit is crucial depending on the number of activity of daily living (ADL) challenges a person has. If someone has recently been hospitalized, their new deficits may change the extent that they "fit" their environment because they may have new demands of that environment (e.g., may not be able to rise from a low toilet anymore).[38] The individual and home environment focus is used from Verbrugge and Jette's Disablement Process.[39] Individualizing fit between the person and his or her environment (increasing P/E fit) should result in better functioning within that environment. Verbrugge and Jette use the Life Span Theory of Control,[40] which proposes that progression of disability increases the threat to personal control, which in turn may result in negative health consequences. Synthesizing these frameworks, the goal of CAPABLE is to enhance resilience (improve ADLs and mobility) by increasing control (e.g., problem-solving and reframing), and improving factors that relate to ADL difficulty and undermine control (e.g., pain, depression, and environmental hazards).

In the first two sessions, the OT met with Nancy and conducted a semistructured clinical interview using the Client-Clinician Assessment Protocol (C-CAP). This tool provides a systematic approach to identify and prioritize patient-centered performance areas problematic to Nancy (e.g., she cannot use the front steps due to her low physical function). For each area identified, the OT observed Nancy's performance and evaluated safety, efficiency, difficulty, and presence of environmental barriers and supports. The OT provided a notebook with evidence-based educational materials, contact information, and a calendar to integrate the sessions by the RN and HM that Nancy kept for reference. Based on the environmental assessment, observation of ADLs, and identification of Nancy's goal, the OT and Nancy discussed possible environmental modifications. In sessions 3 to 5, the OT taught Nancy problem-solving skills to identify behavioral and environmental contributors to performance difficulties. They also discussed strategies for attaining function goals. For example, the OT trained Nancy to use specific strategies such as energy-saving techniques, simplifying tasks, using assistive devices, and skills in keeping balance to reduce fear of falling. In each session, the OT reinforced strategy use, reviewed problem-solving, refined strategies, and provided education and resources to address future needs. Home modifications were coordinated with the HM to assure that they were provided in a timely manner and met Nancy's needs. The OT followed up with training in their use. In the final (6th) OT session, the OT reviewed all techniques, strategies and devices, and helped Nancy to generalize success to other situations.

The RN met with Nancy for up to four sessions during the same five months as the OT sessions. The first RN session started within ten days after the first OT session. In this session, the RN assessed Nancy using C-CAP for RN in which the RN focused on how and whether Nancy's pain, depression, strength, balance, and medication management impacted daily function. In this assessment, the RN and Nancy identified and prioritized goals, such as reducing pain and improving depression, and made plans to achieve those. The RN also added educational resources to the CAPABLE notebook to reinforce its use as a resource. In RN visits 2 and 3, the RN and Nancy worked on the goals identified through the C-CAP RN. In each session, the RN reinforced strategy use, reviewed problem-solving, refined strategies (e.g., doing exercise, pain management), and provided education and resources to address future needs (e.g., pill box for medication management). In the final (fourth) session, the RN reviewed Nancy's strategies and helped to generalize them to other possible challenges.

The HM coordinated the ordering of the assistive devices like the walker as well as the repair and modification supplies. The HM used the prioritized work order to provide the modifications that the OT ordered (e.g., installing railings to stairs, adding grab bars in bathtub, adding bath mat). The HM had extensive experience working with older adults and their needs for home modification.

After CAPABLE, Nancy can safely use her front steps and stairs with newly installed railings. She can safely get into and out of bed and her shower with the aid of assistive devices and training. She can engage socially by going on excursions now that strength and balance training allows her to get in and out of cars. Improved mobility has led to mood improvement, and she adheres to her simplified medication regimen.

Aging, Health, Disability, and Disease

As we age, our risk for development of disease and disability increases. Aging decreases the ability to ward off communicable diseases and increases the likelihood of developing a noncommunicable disease (NCD). For example, as we age, our risk increases for diabetes mellitus, arthritis, heart failure, and dementia.[3] Prior to World War II, this was accepted as part of the aging process,

and there was little focus on prevention. Today, there is clear evidence that healthy behaviors across the life span, beginning in utero, increase the chances of a longer life with reduced disease and disability. Because of this, the older adult was added to the *Healthy People* topics in 2020.[3] From 2000 to 2011, heart disease was the leading cause of death for those 65 years of age or older, accounting for a little under a third of all deaths in this age group.[41]

Communicable Disease

Older adults are more vulnerable to acquiring a communicable disease and at higher risk for morbidity and mortality from it. (See Chapter 8 for more information on communicable diseases.) There are three main reasons for increased vulnerability to communicable diseases in the older adult:

- Decreased immunity
- Existence of comorbid illness
- Undernutrition

All of these reasons are host-specific. Decreased immunity occurs as a result of the aging process and poor antibody production. Alteration in skin integrity because of drying and thinning of the epidural layer can also decrease immunity. The existence of comorbid conditions has a greater impact on the immune function than does aging, leading to more complex infections and reduced ability of the body to recover from infection. Finally, undernutrition has an impact on the body's defense system. Undernutrition in the older adult occurs for various reasons, including psychosocial issues and medication side effects.

The primary communicable diseases of concern in the older adult are influenza, pneumonia, shingles with influenza symptoms, and tuberculosis. For 2000 to 2010, influenza with pneumonia was the sixth leading cause of death in adults 65 years or older and the fifth leading cause of death for those 85 years of age or older. Pneumonia and influenza infection occurs due to exposure to the pathogen.[42] On the other hand, shingles occurs from the reactivation of the varicella zoster virus years after initial exposure. Any adults who have had chickenpox are at risk for shingles, because the virus remains in a dormant state in the body following a case of chickenpox. About 25% of all healthy adults will get shingles during their lifetimes, usually after age 40. This risk increases with age, with adults over 60 being 10 times more likely to have shingles than children under 10.[43] Mycobacterium tuberculosis (TB) can occur in older people from either exposure to a person with an active TB infection or reactivation of the mycobacterium related to an earlier exposure. In addition to increased susceptibility, older adults living in group living facilities such as long-term care facilities are at increased risk for exposure.

Emerging Communicable Disease Issues in Older Adults

There are three emerging issues for the baby boomer generation and older adults related to communicable diseases. These are the increase in human immunodeficiency virus (HIV) infection, sexually transmitted infections (STIs), and the increased prevalence of chronic hepatitis C (HCV) in those over 50.[44,45] These issues will take on increased importance as more of the baby boomer generation passes the 65-year milestone.

The increase in the number of older adults diagnosed with an STI is attributed to two issues: changes in sexual activity in this population and the increased vulnerability to exposure to the pathogens. In today's society, there is a higher rate of divorce and an increase in partner changes among older adults. Also, older adults are less apt to use condoms based on decreased perception of risk. There is no evidence to support discontinuation of screening for STIs at any specific age, as individuals are at risk for an STI regardless of age.[44] The reported increased prevalence in HIV among older adults includes those 50 and older, and as this population ages, there is a predicted increased prevalence of the disease. In addition to the increase in at-risk sexual activity among the older adult population, the other issue is that patients with HIV infection are living longer.

In 2012, the Centers for Disease Control and Prevention (CDC) released recommendations for screening for chronic HCV in those born between 1945 and 1965. Over the next two decades, this population will meet the current definition of older adult. Currently, three-quarters of all persons diagnosed with chronic HCV are over the age of 50.[45] The CDC used epidemiological data to develop their recommendations for this targeted cohort. They considered the weighted, unadjusted anti-HCV prevalence, the size of the population, and the differences in prevalence among racial/ethnic groups.[45] Based on their extended analysis of the data, the CDC made the following recommendations:

In addition to testing adults of all ages at risk for HCV infection, CDC recommends that:

- *Adults born between 1945 and 1965 should receive one-time testing for HCV without prior ascertainment of*

HCV risk (Strong Recommendation, Moderate Quality of Evidence).

- *All persons identified with HCV infection should receive a brief alcohol screening and intervention as clinically indicated, followed by referral to appropriate care and treatment services for HCV infection and related conditions (Strong Recommendation, Moderate Quality of Evidence).[45]*

Prevention of Communicable Diseases in Older Adults

Based on the epidemiology triangle (see Chapter 3), public health interventions for preventing communicable diseases in older adults, for the most part, focus on primary prevention through vaccination. This includes vaccination for prevention of pneumonia and shingles. For that reason, there are specific recommendations for vaccination in the older adult population to prevent these infections (Table 19-2).[46]

An example of this primary prevention focus is the public health campaign to have all adults over the age of 64 vaccinated for influenza. This campaign is aimed at reducing the burden of disease related to influenza. Annually, there are approximately 90,000 hospitalizations and 5,000 deaths among older adults related to influenza.[47] Although the influenza vaccine rate has increased from 15% to 65% over the past few decades, there has been no significant decrease in the death rate during this period. To address this, new flu vaccines for older adults are now available with increased immunogenicity (the ability of a substance to provoke an immune response needed for the vaccine to be effective).[47]

Population-level initiatives aimed at reducing communicable disease in the older adult population require a broad perspective. If vaccines alone are not effective in reducing morbidity and mortality, then other strategies to improve an older adult's resistance are needed. As previously noted, the older adult is at increased risk for communicable diseases. Efforts aimed at decreasing vulnerability include better self-management of NCD, improved nutrition, and physical exercise.

For communicable diseases such as influenza, pneumonia, and shingles, the rapid progression from infection to disease requires a primary prevention focus. For other communicable diseases, a secondary prevention approach should also be implemented. For example, the new recommendation to screen all those born between 1945 and 1965 for HCV underlines the importance of identifying subclinical cases of the chronic infection.

TABLE 19–2 ■ Vaccine Recommendations for Older Adults

Vaccine	Age	Dose and Schedule
Zosters: RZV or ZVL	50 yr or 60 yr and older	Get two doses of RZV at age 50 years or older (preferred) or one dose of ZVL at age 60 years or older, even if the individual had shingles before
Pneumococcal vaccines: PCV13 and PPSV23	65 yr and older	Get one dose of PCV13 and at least one dose of PPSV23 depending on age and health condition

Source: (46)

Identification allows treatment to begin, thus reducing the morbidity and mortality associated with HCV, especially liver disease. Increased screening for STIs could also result in earlier identification of these communicable diseases, earlier initiation of treatment, and subsequent reduction in morbidity and mortality.

Noncommunicable Diseases

The risk for developing an NCD increases over the life span because of genetics, the physiology of aging, health behaviors, and the environment. Most older adults (80%) have at least one NCD and 77% live with more than one.[48] Thus, a single disease approach to care may not work. Instead, the challenge is to develop programs for older adults that address a combination of NCDs. Risk factors associated with cardiovascular disease, the leading cause of death in older adults, include obesity and hypertension (Table 19-3). These risk factors also increase the risk for diabetes and other NCDs. The prevalence of these risk factors increases with age. More than a quarter of the older adult population is obese, and the prevalence of hypertension ranges from 64% to over 81%.[41]

In addition to vaccination, primary prevention models focus on reduction of behavioral risk factors associated with obesity and hypertension. These include improving nutrition, increasing physical activity, and social support. *HP* has a link to community approaches

for addressing these issues with older adults.[3] Secondary prevention approaches for older adults focus on screening and early intervention. Of the 14 key indicators in the CDC's report on promoting preventive services in persons aged 50-64, 4 include disease screening (Box 19-3).[49] (For more information on screening for NCDs, see Chapter 9.)

Evidence-based tertiary prevention programs include those aimed at self-management of NCDs. *Healthy People* has a link to community preventions aimed at the self-management of diabetes.[3] According to the chronic disease self-management model discussed in Chapter 9, the basic elements of self-management include the ability

BOX 19–3 ■ Centers for Disease Control and Prevention: Clinical Prevention Services for Older Adults

Eight indicators that provide a baseline of data through which to monitor progress in ensuring that recommended services reach this key population:

1. Vaccinations that protect against influenza
2. Vaccinations that protect against pneumococcal disease
3. Screening for early detection of breast cancer
4. Screening for colorectal cancer
5. Screening for diabetes
6. Screening for lipid disorders
7. Screening for osteoporosis
8. Counseling service for smoking cessation

Recommended services for older adults:

1. Alcohol misuse screening and counseling
2. Aspirin use
3. Blood pressure screening
4. Cervical cancer screening
5. Depression screening
6. Obesity screening and counseling
7. Zoster vaccination

Source: (49)

TABLE 19–3 ■ Health Risk Factors for Older Adults—2017

	Obese	Hypertension
Men 65–74	41.5%	64.1%
Men 75+	26.6%	71.1%
Women 65–74	40.3%	69.3%
Women 75+	28.7%	81.3%

Source: (41)

to communicate with a health-care provider, proper use of medications, nutrition, regular exercise, and disease-specific activities such as foot care for those with diabetes. Management of NCDs can become a challenge for the older adult. Older adults may be homebound, no longer able to drive, or both, resulting in difficulty getting to their health-care provider or obtaining resources. If they have more than one NCD, such as heart failure and diabetes, they may need to access two separate providers located in two separate practices. Grocery stores are increasingly located in areas that require access by car. Regular exercise may be challenging for the city-dwelling older adult because of a potentially unsafe environment. The lack of safety can include lack of sidewalks and/or street crime, and some neighborhoods are generally unsafe for regular exercise.

▶ SOLVING THE MYSTERY
The Case of the Failing Hearts
Public Health Science Topics Covered:

- Focused assessment
- Chart review
- Geographic information systems
- Health planning
- Adapting interventions to the population being served

Cathy worked as a nurse at the heart failure clinic for a few months and was becoming increasingly frustrated with the patients at the clinic who also had type 2 diabetes. She had spent time doing health education with them and had even developed a pamphlet on managing your diabetes, to no avail. They were missing their appointments at the diabetes clinic and continued to have elevated blood sugars. She explained to them that tight glucose control was essential to the management of their heart failure, but week after week these patients were not following through with what she had mapped out for them.

In desperation, she contacted her friend Adele, a family nurse practitioner who specialized in diabetes and also had completed a public health nursing master's program. Adele came to the clinic and asked her to explain the problem. After listening to Cathy, Adele suggested that they do a focused assessment of the patients who were not following through with their diabetes care. Adele explained the importance of doing assessments prior to implementing an intervention. Together they conducted a chart review of the patients that Cathy identified as having difficulty. Most of them

were over the age of 60, and all of them had limited transportation options. They plotted the addresses of these patients on a city map. They then located the heart failure clinic on the map as well as the diabetes clinic. These two clinics were located a number of miles apart. The heart failure clinic was close to a bus route, but the diabetes clinic was a few blocks from the nearest bus stop. By tracing the travel routes, they found that the effort needed to make two appointments in the same week for the majority of the patients was a main barrier for Cathy's patients.

Together, Cathy and Adele developed a one-stop approach for the patients at the heart failure clinic who also had diabetes. Adele arranged to be present at the heart failure clinic one day a week, and Cathy scheduled the patients with type 2 diabetes for that day. Adele developed a special diabetes self-management program for these patients who, for the most part, were over 65 years of age and had decreased access to transportation. This program included aspects of case management (see Chapter 9). With her knowledge of the resources in the community, Adele was able to assist these patients in various aspects of diabetes management. For example, for some of the patients she contacted Meals on Wheels to deliver meals that fit within the patients' dietary restrictions.

These two nurses used basic public health skills to identify an older population at risk for increase morbidity and mortality including assessment and health planning. Their intervention reduced the number of clinic visits these patients needed to make and, over time, Cathy and Adele saw an improvement in the majority of these patients. They also were able to demonstrate a decrease in hospitalizations. Their decision to not take a one-disease approach but rather incorporate two specialties had positive results.

Injury and Violence in the Older Adult

Injury and violence are issues for the older adult and include both unintentional and intentional injury. In 2013, unintentional injuries were the eighth leading cause of death among U.S. adults aged 65 and over, resulting in nearly 46,000 deaths.[50] Accidental injuries that pose the greatest threat include falls, motor vehicle crashes, and residential fires. Intentional injuries include elder maltreatment and suicide. Reducing injury in older adults is a national public health priority as defined by the CDC National Resource Center for Safe Aging, the National Center for Injury Prevention and Control, and others (Box 19-4). These resources focus not only on reducing the morbidity and mortality related to injury in the older adult but also on helping older adults maintain an independent lifestyle.

Unintentional Injury

Falls are the most common form of unintentional injury and one of the leading causes of injury and death in the older population. More than one out of four older adults fall every year.[51] The risk factors associated with falls in the older adult are well understood and help in the design of prevention activities. Risk factors include muscle weakness, unsteady gait, osteoporosis, failing eyesight, and hypotension. Based on the key risk factors, the CDC has dedicated a whole website to the prevention of falls.[52] Many of these risk factors are associated with NCDs. Other risk factors are associated with the home and community environments. Within the home there are issues such as scatter rugs, lack of grab bars in the bathroom, and other hazards that contribute to falls. In the community, sidewalk safety, well-lit streets, and other factors are crucial to prevention of falls. Prevention strategies are aimed at these risk factors and can be applied at the individual, group, or community level.[53]

Intentional Injury: Elder Maltreatment

Intentional injury is also a concern for the older adult population. Elder maltreatment is a substantial global health issue. It is a violation of a human being's basic fundamental right: to be safe and free of violence. Older adults are often victims of abuse and neglect that can result in serious injury and debilitation. An estimated 2.1 million older Americans are victims of physical, psychological, or other forms of maltreatment. The actual incidence of elder maltreatment is likely to be underestimated. It is thought that for every case of maltreatment reported to the authorities, as many as five cases have not been reported. In addition, estimates of the prevalence of maltreatment vary due to differing research methods and operational definitions used in studies. Although there is legitimate concern about the direct effects of abuse or neglect, there are also health-related consequences that place victims at high risk. Elder maltreatment and self-neglect are associated with shorter lifespans after adjusting for other factors associated with increased mortality.[55,56] Various terms are used in the literature, including elder abuse, elder mistreatment, and elder maltreatment. For this chapter, the term *elder maltreatment* is used and refers to both abuse and neglect.

In the U.S., **self-neglect**, which is defined as "inability, due to physical or mental impairment or diminished capacity, to perform essential self-care," accounts for a majority of elderly maltreatment cases reported to Adult Protective Services (APS).[57] Self-neglect is associated with devastating outcomes, not only on physical and psychological well-being, but also on higher mortality rates and increased health care use. The CDC has compiled a comprehensive definition of elder maltreatment and different forms of elder maltreatment are listed below:

Elder maltreatment is any abuse and neglect of persons aged 60 and older by a caregiver or another person in a relationship involving an expectation of trust. Forms of elder maltreatment include:

- **Physical abuse** occurs when an elder is injured (e.g., scratched, bitten, slapped, pushed, hit, burned, etc.), assaulted, or threatened with a weapon (e.g., knife, gun, or other object), or inappropriately restrained.
- **Sexual abuse or abusive sexual contact** is any sexual contact against an elder's will. This includes acts in which the elder is unable to understand the act or is unable to communicate. Abusive sexual contact is defined as intentional touching (either directly or through the clothing), of the genitalia, anus, groin, breast, mouth, inner thigh, or buttocks.
- **Psychological or emotional abuse** occurs when an elder experiences trauma after exposure to threatening acts or coercive tactics. Examples include humiliation or embarrassment, controlling behavior (e.g., prohibiting or limiting access to transportation, telephone, money or other resources), social isolation, disregarding or trivializing needs, or damaging or destroying property.
- **Neglect** is the failure or refusal of a caregiver or other responsible person to provide for an elder's basic physical, emotional, or social needs; in other words, it is a failure to protect them from harm. Examples include not providing adequate nutrition, hygiene, clothing, shelter, or access to necessary health care; or failure to prevent exposure to unsafe activities and environments.
- **Abandonment** is the willful desertion of an elderly person by a caregiver or other responsible person.
- **Financial abuse or exploitation** is unauthorized or improper use of resources of an elder for personal benefit, profit, or gain. Examples include forgery, misuse or theft of money or possessions, use of coercion or deception to surrender finances or property, or improper use of guardianship or power of attorney.[58]

Risk Factors for Elder Maltreatment

Elder maltreatment is a complex problem that affects more than 500,000 older adults each year in the United States.[59] There is no single pattern of elder maltreatment. Elder maltreatment is an equal opportunity issue that crosses all walks of life and social strata. Victims are not just infirm or mentally impaired people who are vulnerable to abuse. Elder maltreatment can occur in situations such as the case of Mickey Rooney, a movie actor who testified before Congress in 2011 that he was the victim of maltreatment from his son.

A combination of individual-, relationship-, community-, and social-level factors are associated with increased risk for elder maltreatment.[60,61] Individual-level risk factors include both the perpetrator and the victim. The interaction of these individual risk factors occurs at the relationship level. However, both community and societal factors influence risk. On the flip side, there are protective factors as well (Box 19-5).[60] These protective factors provide areas through which nurses can work to strengthen their relationships not only with individuals and their families but in combination with the community.

Primary, Secondary, and Tertiary Prevention For Elder Maltreatment

It is essential that nurses identify those who may be victims of elder maltreatment and provide evidence-based interventions at the individual and community levels. Perel-Levin argues that prevention efforts should include two levels of intervention: screening as a routine part of primary care and working with the community to provide services. Interventions should seek to decrease the incidence of elder maltreatment, improve early identification, and ensure proper management of those who were victims of maltreatment. According to Perel-Levin, interventions should be interdisciplinary and consider the context of the person. Key components for overcoming barriers to prevention are building trust and effective communication among all persons involved.[62]

Several screening tools are available, such as the geriatric assessment instrument (GAI).[63] The challenge for the nurse is to build a screening program that includes not only training in the use of the screening tool but also establishing links with resources for those who screen positive for elder abuse.[64] Another approach at the community level is providing information both to professional health-care providers and to members of the community. For example, the Florida Department of Elder Affairs has a website dedicated to prevention of elder abuse. Another resource is the information available through the U.S. Administration on Aging National Center on Elder Abuse (NCEA).[65] Community initiatives to address elder abuse and neglect include programs to:

- Increase public awareness and shift public attitudes toward recognizing and reporting abuse
- Improve identification and triage of cases

BOX 19–5 ■ Centers for Disease Control and Prevention: Elder Maltreatment—Risk and Protective Factors

A combination of individual, relational, community, and societal factors contribute to the risk of becoming a perpetrator of elder maltreatment. They are contributing factors and may or may not be direct causes. Understanding these factors can help identify various opportunities for prevention.

Risk Factors for Perpetration

- Individual Level
  - Current diagnosis of mental illness
  - Current abuse of alcohol
  - High levels of hostility
  - Poor or inadequate preparation or training for caregiving responsibilities
  - Assumption of caregiving responsibilities at an early age
  - Inadequate coping skills
  - Exposure to maltreatment as a child
- Relationship Level
  - High financial and emotional dependence upon a vulnerable elder
  - Past experience of disruptive behavior
  - Lack of social support
  - Lack of formal support
- Community Level
  - Formal services, such as respite care for those providing care to elders, are limited, inaccessible, or unavailable
- Societal Level
  - A culture where:
    - There is high tolerance and acceptance of aggressive behavior

- Health-care personnel, guardians, and other agents are given greater freedom in routine care provision and decision making
- Family members are expected to care for elders without seeking help from others
- Persons are encouraged to endure suffering or remain silent regarding their pains
- There are negative beliefs about aging and elders.

Protective Factors for Elder Maltreatment

Protective factors reduce risk for perpetrating abuse and neglect. Protective factors have not been studied as extensively or rigorously as risk factors. However, identifying and understanding protective factors are equally as important as researching risk factors. Several potential protective factors are identified below. Research is needed to determine whether these factors do indeed buffer elders from maltreatment.

Relationship Level
- Having numerous, strong relationships with people of varying social status

Community Level
- Coordination of resources and services among community agencies and organizations that serve the older population and their caregivers
- Higher levels of community cohesion and a strong sense of community or community identity
- Higher levels of community functionality and greater collective efficacy

Source: (60, 61)

- Increase integrated service models
- Improve justice system response
- Leverage and utilize emerging and untapped resources

Other community-based activities focus on disseminating promising practices in the courts, creating elder law clinics, educating older adults about such things as predatory mortgage lending, building new response systems for complaints of abuse and neglect, and convening clergy and lay leader groups to work within faith communities to make a difference in elder abuse and neglect.[66]

Policy

Policy-level interventions have been undertaken to prevent and address elder maltreatment. The Elder Justice Act of 2010 (Pub. L. 111-148) is part of the Affordable Care Act and provides specific benefits to elders.[67] In addition, at the state level is Adult Protective Services (APS) that facilitates the protection of vulnerable adults, including the older adult (Box 19-6). The role of APS is to prevent, correct, or discontinue maltreatment.[68]

Reporting suspected elder abuse or neglect cases to APS agencies provides access to services that address the social, medical, and legal needs of older persons.[66,67] Once a report is made to APS, a process of investigation and support begins. Based on the information APS receives, caseworkers determine whether there is imminent danger. They contact the victim and further evaluate the situation, looking at the risk factors and the victim's capacity to understand. They develop a care plan that may include services provided directly by caseworkers, through arrangements with community-based resources, or contracted by APS on a short-term emergency basis. Victims of abuse may receive short-term services, such

BOX 19–6 ■ Principles of Adult Protective Services

- **Freedom Over Safety:** The client has a right to choose to live at risk of harm, providing she or he is capable of making that choice, harms no one else, and does not commit a crime.
- **Self-Determination:** The client has a right to personal choices and decisions until a time that she or he delegates, or the court grants, the responsibility to someone else.
- **Participation in Decision Making:** The client has a right to receive information to make informed decisions and to participate in all decision making affecting his or her circumstances to the extent able.
- **Least Restrictive Alternative:** The client has a right to service alternatives that maximize choice and minimize lifestyle disruption.
- **Primacy of the Adult:** The worker has a responsibility to serve the client, not the community's, family members', or landlord's concerns.
- **Confidentiality:** The client has a right to privacy and secrecy.
- **Benefit of Doubt:** If there is evidence that the client is making a reasoned choice, the worker has a responsibility to see that the benefit of doubt is in his or her favor.
- **Do No Harm:** The worker has a responsibility to take no action that places the client at greater risk of harm.
- **Avoidance of Blame:** The worker has a responsibility to understand the origins of any maltreatment and to commit no action that would antagonize the perpetrator and so reduce the chances of terminating the maltreatment.
- **Maintenance of the Family:** The worker has a responsibility to deal with the maltreatment as a family problem, if the perpetrator is a family member, and to try to find the necessary family services to resolve the problem.

Source: (68)

as emergency shelter, home repair, meals, transportation, help with financial management, home health services, and medical and mental health services. The APS caseworker may continue to monitor the service provision to make sure that victim risk is reduced or eliminated.[66]

A geriatric interdisciplinary team can be involved to provide a comprehensive medical, functional, and social assessment. Based on the findings of the assessment and in collaboration with the APS team, an individualized intervention plan can be formulated. Some cases of elder abuse or neglect may require intervention from the criminal or civil justice system for serious legal issues such as sexual assault, financial exploitation, or guardianship. Coordination with other agencies such as Area Agencies on Aging, local women's shelters, and the National Center for Elder Abuse, are available to help manage elder abuse and neglect cases in the community, and other professionals such as social workers can provide a broad community-based approach.[67,69]

Substance Use in Older Adults

Obtaining an accurate picture of substance use in the older population is difficult. Of concern is the baby boomer cohort that has a higher rate of substance use compared with other cohorts. The concern is that as this cohort ages, there will be a substantial increase in the number of older adults with health problems associated with substance use. It is projected that there will be a doubling of the prevalence of substance use disorders in those over age 50 by 2020.[70] This increase includes alcohol, legal, and illegal drugs. However, we know little about age-specific interventions to promote recovery and reduce morbidity and mortality. Population-level approaches are required to address this issue rather than relying on individual behavior modification. This requires population-level interventions based on a clear picture of the problem (Box 19-7).[71]

For older adults, there are two separate issues related to substance use disorders: early onset and late onset substance misuse, clearly defined in the 1990s.[72] **Early onset at-risk substance use** reflects older adults who have a history of regular alcohol consumption above the recommended limits or problem drug use that began early in their adult lives. This group of older adults is often referred to as hardy survivors. **Late onset at-risk substance use** is defined as at-risk substance use that began later in life, often triggered by a sentinel event such as loss of a spouse or partner.[72]

Alcohol and Older Adults

Although heavy alcohol use was reported by only 2.1% of those over 65 in 2013,[73] these figures may not be the true picture because of underreporting of alcohol use in this population.[74] As the baby boomer generation continues to turn 65, there may be a cohort effect in relation to the prevalence of risky drinking, because more than 60% of baby boomers (aged 45 to 64) are current drinkers. Therefore, the prevalence of alcohol use disorders in the older population may increase over the next few decades.

Alcohol use disorders are not the only issue. As we age, our ability to metabolize alcohol also changes. Alcohol has a more potent effect due to the physiological

---

BOX 19–7 ■ Public Policy Recommendations to Prevent Licit and Illicit Substance Use in Older Adults

Informed and active policy will require new approaches and investment in the following:

- Data and analysis, with increased emphasis on documenting substance abuse in the elderly, in addition to the historical emphasis on alcohol abuse and mental health problems
- Expanded literature review that encompasses studies not considered in this report,* some of which may not be specific to substance abuse but can offer new conceptual and methodological insights
- Prevention, treatment, and management strategies specifically tailored for older adults from different ethnic, gender, and racial groups, including immigrant populations
- Monitoring of demographic shifts in heterogeneous older populations
- Long-term projections of the demand for expanded clinical and public health services for substance abusers
- Traumatic brain injury

*Report by the Substance Abuse and Mental Health Services Administration that addressed the projected demand for substance abuse services over the next 20 to 30 years for those born during the baby boomer years.
Source: (73)

---

changes of aging. As we age, a decrease in the ratio of body water to fat, a decrease in the hepatic blood flow, and a reduction in the efficiency of liver enzymes, all result in a decreased ability to metabolize alcohol. This, in turn, affects the duration of elevated blood alcohol and increases the risk of liver damage.[75] Another issue for the older adult is medication interactions with alcohol. Use of drugs that interact with alcohol is common among older adults, which increases the potential alcohol-related risks.[76]

As explained in Chapter 11, the recommended drinking limits are less than five standard drinks per day or fourteen per week for men, or less than four standard drinks per day or eight per week for women. However, healthy people aged 65 and older should consume no more than three standard drinks per day and no more than seven drinks per week.[77] As discussed earlier, older adults who exceed the recommended daily limits are at increased risk for alcohol-related problems due to differences in metabolism and physiology.[72]

Medication Interactions

The issue of adverse interactions between alcohol and prescribed medications are of particular concern in older adults, because about 62.5% are using medications with potential alcohol interactions.[76] Two types of interactions occur: pharmacokinetic interaction, wherein alcohol interferes with the body's ability to metabolize the medications, and pharmacodynamic interaction, wherein alcohol enhances the effects of the medication.[72] The growing recognition of the potential harm related to alcohol and medication interactions in older adults underscores the need for a population perspective. Although both the National Institute on Alcohol Abuse and Alcoholism and the Substance Abuse and Mental Health Services Administration have highlighted the issue, few public health approaches are available for increasing awareness of the problem leaving the burden on the individual practitioner to inform individual adults.

Substance Use and Physical Health

Both legal and illegal drug use increases the risk for adverse health outcomes. Alcohol consumption in older adults increases their risk for injury, NCDs, and communicable diseases. Alcohol may be the underlying cause for up to half of older trauma patients. Early onset substance users, even those who are currently abstinent but have a history of consuming alcohol or other drugs above the recommended limits for a long period of time, often have serious health problems that may be mistaken for symptoms of aging, such as dementia or depression.[72]

An example of how important it is to evaluate early onset users for physical complications is the negative impact of long-term alcohol use on the ability to absorb thiamine (vitamin B_1) an essential, water-soluble vitamin. Untreated thiamine deficiency in older adults with a history of early onset alcohol use may result in Wernicke-Korsakoff syndrome, a brain disorder. Unfortunately, the prevalence of Wernicke-Korsakoff syndrome at autopsy exceeds recognition during life.[78] Thus, clinicians may fail to screen for long-term alcohol use in this population. Because of the long-term impact on the human body, alcohol use above the recommended limits increases the risk for other adverse outcomes that occur as the person ages, including alcohol-related cardiomyopathy, liver cirrhosis, pancreatitis, various cancers (including cancers of the liver, mouth, throat, larynx [the voice box], and esophagus), high blood pressure, and psychological disorders.[72]

One possible public health intervention might be to initiate a universal screening approach aimed at helping clinicians identify both early and late onset alcohol use that places the older adult at increased risk for alcohol-related NCDs as well as injury. A five-step process was recommended by Savage that includes information not only on current use but also on prior use and duration of use over the lifetime.[79]

Aging in Place

During the past three decades, there has been an increase in the emphasis of an aging-in-place approach. This approach includes implementation of community-based programs that include health promotion, prevention of disease, improvement of functioning, and enhancement of quality of life in older adults while maintaining them in their homes.[80,81] This emphasis mirrors a decline in the percentage of the population 65 years of age or older living in skilled nursing facilities. Based on the 2010 census data, the percent of persons living in nursing homes fell from 5.1% in 1990 to 3.1% in 2010. The decline was also seen in the population 85 years of age or older. In 1990, almost 25% were living in skilled nursing facilities. That dropped to 10.4% in 2010.[82]

Barriers to aging in place include funding for home modifications, availability of needed services, and consumer awareness.[81] Because of changing health status, some older adults need special services beyond the basics to maintain themselves safely in their own home settings. Likewise, issues of environmental safety and security can impinge on aging successfully in place. One community-based approach is the CAPABLE program developed by a team of nurse researchers from Johns Hopkins University School of Nursing. This innovative program combines health-care services with home modifications and links to services within the community to meet the needs of disabled older adults so that they can remain in their homes.[83]

Aging in place requires an understanding of the community in which older adults live.[83] The built environment surrounding the older adult has a direct impact on their quality of life. Changing lifestyles for older adults mean that they may have more time to enjoy amenities in the community, such as recreation facilities. However, biological changes, such as decreases in vision and mobility, alter their ability to enjoy these facilities. To achieve aging in place, the CDC stated:

Affordable, accessible, and suitable housing options can allow older adults to age in place and remain in their community all their entire lives. Housing that is convenient to community destinations can provide opportunities for physical activity and social interaction. Communities with a safe and secure pedestrian environment, and near destinations such as libraries, stores, and places of worship, allow older adults to remain independent, active, and engaged. Combined transportation and land-use planning that offers convenient, accessible alternatives to driving can help the older adults reach this goal of an active, healthy lifestyle.[84]

The concept of aging in place is growing in popularity. There is now a National Aging in Place Council, and the American Association of Retired Persons has a guide to livable communities and a webpage dedicated to the subject. The process includes a match among affordable housing, access to services, and a healthy built environment. Housing options for older adults span a continuum from complete independence to dependence, with many gradations in between. Many people can remain at home completely independent throughout a long life, or with just a little help getting around or keeping house. Care ranges from help with household tasks and running errands to round-the-clock care for someone who is seriously ill.

Naturally Occurring Retirement Community

With the aging of the American population, a new phenomenon is emerging: the **naturally occurring retirement community (NORC)**. Federal funding was established in 2010 for NORCs with more than $25 million in federal and matching funds that have resulted in the establishment of more than 50 supportive service programs.[85] A NORC is defined as a community that provides:

- Residential housing with supports
- Transportation for appointments and shopping
- Individual assessment of those at risk, followed by referral and follow-up of service
- Coordination of nonprofessional services[85]

NORCs take many different forms. They can exist in subsidized housing complexes, condominiums, apartments, or single-family neighborhoods. Closed or vertical NORCs are geographically confined, such as apartment buildings or complexes. The open or horizontal form of NORC refers to one- and two-family homes in age-integrated neighborhoods. By capitalizing on the valuable contributions of experience and skill from older residents and making use of the density and proximity of older adults in NORCs, resources and economies of scale (factors that cause the average cost of producing something to decrease as its output increases) make it possible to organize and deliver services that promote healthy aging in place. Instead of service delivery that is reactive to a crisis, is time limited, and is disconnected from the communities in which older residents have built their lives, NORC programs seek to deepen the connections that older adults have to their communities before problems arise.

Continuing Care Retirement Communities

In anticipation of changing needs, some older adults arrange to become part of **continuing care retirement communities (CCRCs)**, a relatively new phenomenon in the United States that has appeared during the past three decades. A CCRC is defined as a community that provides housing and health care across the continuum from independent living, to assisted living, to skilled nursing care. Residents are required to sign a contract on entrance into the community. They are charged an entry fee as well as a monthly maintenance fee but may differ on their affordability with some available to higher income older adults.[86] The advantage of such communities is the ability for older adults to remain within the CCRC over the long term. The disadvantage is the costliness of such facilities. Entrance into these communities requires the financial ability to pay the entrance fee and the monthly payment. In the 1990s and early 2000s, approximately 10 to 20 units were established per year. After the 2008 recession, there was a sharp decline in the industry, because many older adults could not sell their homes and therefore did not have the money necessary to pay the entrance fee.

All of these models are aimed at keeping the older adult in a community setting and as independent as possible as long as possible. With the aging of the population, the need for viable community-based living for older adults will increase. Nurses such as the researchers at Johns Hopkins School of Nursing are vital to helping this population achieve optimal health within their own communities.

Ageism in Our Society

Ageism describes bias toward older adults based on stereotypes.[87] Ageism, like racism and sexism, is a way of judging or categorizing people and not allowing them to be individuals with unique ways of living their lives. It is a set of beliefs, attitudes, norms, and values used to justify age-based prejudice and discrimination.[87,88] It can have an impact on patient outcomes, and can affect their feelings of self-worth and their ability to make autonomous decisions about their health care.[88]

Ageism may occur when health-care providers incorrectly attribute pathology to normal aging. These assumptions can influence screening procedures, information exchanges, and treatment decisions. Ageism may manifest itself through the use of patronizing language, or by dismissing symptoms as "all part of growing older." Even unintentionally, health-care providers may hold attitudes, beliefs, and behaviors associated with ageism against older patients. This is why it is so important to have a good working knowledge of age-related physiological and psychological changes, so that signs of disease or disability can be differentiated and treated appropriately.

Dementia and Alzheimer's Disease: Impact on the Older Adult Population

Alzheimer's disease and related dementias (ADRD) are the sixth leading cause of death for all adults in the U.S. and the fifth leading cause of death in people over the age of 64.[89,90] Globally, approximately 50 million people have dementia, with nearly 10 million new cases a year.[90] It is the most common form of dementia. In the U.S., in 2014 alone, 5 million people were diagnosed with ADRD (1.6% of the population). By 2050 in the U.S. it is estimated that number will rise to 13.9 million (3.3% of the population).[89] Other dementia diagnoses include vascular dementia, mixed dementia, dementia with Lewy bodies, and frontotemporal dementia. The central issues for those with ADRD or other forms of dementia are the problems with memory and the impact on cognition. Both Alzheimer's disease (AD) and dementia severely affect people's ability to work, care for themselves, and engage in social activities. AD is the sixth leading cause of death in adults in the United States.[90,91]

Prevention

Primary prevention of AD and other types of dementia is challenging because there is no clear evidence that specific interventions actually prevent AD or cognitive decline.[93] However, secondary prevention through memory screening programs has helped to identify those people in the early stages. Early identification has the potential to slow the progression of the disease with emerging pharmaceutical treatments for those with AD and dementia. There are currently five drugs approved by the Food and Drug Administration for the treatment of AD (donepezil, galantamine, memantine, rivastigmine, and tacrine) that have shown a temporary slowing of the progression of the disease over 6 to 12 months although there is no clear evidence on when to stop the treatment.[94] These treatments also provide the opportunity for the person with AD to plan for the future while they are still able to do so. Tertiary prevention focuses on active management of AD with the goal of achieving an optimal quality of life within the realities of the disease.[93,94]

Centers for Disease Control and Prevention's Healthy Brain Initiative

Another element in health promotion/prevention is the Healthy Brain Initiative: The Public Health Road Map for State and National Partnerships, 2018–2023, which was jointly developed by the Alzheimer's Association and the CDC Healthy Aging Program to advance cognitive health as a public health goal.[95] Specific actions are highlighted and addressed in four domains of public health: educate and empower the nation, develop policy and mobilize partnerships, assure a competent workforce, and monitor and evaluate. See Box 19-8 for details of this program.

Caregiving

One of the primary challenges facing the older population, especially those with AD, dementia, or a chronic NCD, is the need for caregiving when physical and or mental disorders decrease the ability to perform ADLs. A **caregiver** is anyone who assists someone else who is incapacitated in some way and needs help. **Family caregivers** are defined as "an adult family member or other individual who has a significant relationship with, and who provides a broad range of assistance to, an individual with a chronic or other health condition, disability, or functional limitation."[96] **Formal caregivers** are volunteers or paid caregivers associated with a service system. For many older adults, family members become the primary caregivers providing unpaid care resulting in a financial, physical, and psychosocial burden on the family.[95] To help provide more assistance to family caregivers in 2017 congress passed the RAISE Family Caregivers Act.[96] The purpose of the act is to help address the estimated $470 billion cost of unpaid care and the $7,000 in out-of-pocket expenses incurred annually by family caregivers.[97]

There can be significant consequences to caregivers' health.[95] The long hours, physical tasks, stress, and relentless responsibility can take a toll on caregivers, and can manifest in health problems such as increased blood pressure, hyperinsulinemia, impaired immune system function, and cardiovascular disease. Health consequences relate to the number of hours spent providing care. Two-thirds do not take advantage of preventive health services for themselves. Twenty-five percent of caregivers have health problems, such as back injuries, resulting directly from caregiving activities. They may also experience mental and emotional effects as a result

---

BOX 19–8 ■ Healthy Brain Initiative: The Public Health Road Map for State and National Partnerships, 2018–2023

The role of public health in enhancing the physical health of older adults is well-known. Public health's role in maintaining cognitive health, a vital part of healthy aging and quality of life, is emerging. The need for a delineated public health role comes at a critical time given the dramatic aging of the U.S. population, scientific advancements in knowledge about risk behaviors (e.g., lack of physical activity, uncontrolled high blood pressure) related to cognitive decline, and the growing awareness of the significant health, social, and economic burdens associated with cognitive decline. The Healthy Brain Initiative provides 25 specific actions in four domains that state and local public health agencies and their partners can pursue. These four domains include the following:

- Educate and empower
- Develop policies and mobilize partnerships
- Assure a competent workforce
- Monitor and evaluate

The lack of cognitive health—from mild cognitive decline to dementia—can have profound implications for an individual's health and well-being. Older adults and others experiencing cognitive decline may be unable to care for themselves or conduct necessary ADLs, such as meal preparation and money management. Limitations with the ability to effectively manage medications and existing medical conditions are particular concerns when an individual is experiencing cognitive decline or dementia. If cognitive decline can be prevented or better treated, lives of many older adults can be improved.

Opportunities for maintaining cognitive health are growing as public health professionals gain a better understanding of cognitive decline risk factors. The public health community should embrace cognitive health as a priority, invest in its promotion, and enhance our ability to move scientific discoveries rapidly into public health practice.

Source: (95)

of their caregiving, which can include depression and isolation.

Because of the toll that caregiving exacts from the caregivers, the CDC has declared caregiving a public health priority. To address this priority, the CDC developed the Reach Effectiveness Adoption Implementation Maintenance (RE-AIM) framework.[98] The framework is intended to help communities and organizations develop programs for caregivers. The RE-AIM website provides case examples for interventions aimed at assisting the caregiver. This is an example of how evidence can be translated into practice at the population level to address an important public health issue.

The caregiving relationship can be a complicated one and often requires engaging the community to help plan interventions. Nurses should recognize the warning signs of caregiver stress early. Nurses can help caregivers look at the sources of stress, identify what they can and cannot change, and identify resources within the community that can relieve the pressure, such as respite care for the caregiver. The RE-AIM website provides case studies that can help nurses build programs for caregivers and underlines the importance of working at the population level to help individuals deal with the enormous task of caring for a loved one.[98]

■ CELLULAR TO GLOBAL

Dementia in older adults has a substantial impact from the cellular to global level.[91] Although specific causes for dementia are still unknown, the disease involves damage of nerve cells in the brain, which can occur in several brain areas. Worldwide, around 50 million people have dementia, and there are nearly 10 million new cases every year.[95] Lives of patients with dementia are impacted at the individual level due to cognitive changes (e.g., memory loss, difficulty in communicating, reasoning and handling complex tasks) and psychological changes (e.g., personality changes, anxiety, agitation). The impact of these changes extends to the interpersonal level due to the heavy care burden of patients with dementia. Given the increasing number of older adults worldwide, dementia care has received much attention globally and become a public health priority of the WHO.[95] Nurses who understand this impact from cellular to global level are more likely to have the capacity to provide a comprehensive care to the patients and also the family caregivers as well as advocate for services and resources to help support older adults and their families living with ADRD.

Hospice and End-Of-Life Care

Traditionally, **hospice care** has been under the domain of community health care, because the goal is to provide care to persons at the end of life within the community setting. Many older adults have an ideal picture of the way that they would choose to die. Unfortunately, frank discussions about these wishes and preferences are far too rare, and specific actions that will assure those wishes are respected are sometimes difficult to articulate and communicate. Common descriptions of the preferred circumstances of death include being free of pain and suffering, being in the company of loved ones, and being in one's own home. Hospice care was formally developed to address this need. It is usually defined as the provision of care to persons who have less than six months to live the goal of which is to provide care and comfort not cure or treatment.

Originally the term *hospice* was used to describe a place of shelter for weary and sick travelers returning from religious pilgrimages. During the 1960s, Dr. Cicely Saunders began to develop hospice care in the United Kingdom and was invited by the dean of the Yale School of Nursing to become a faculty member and help build hospice care in the United States. There, an organized professional team approach to end-of-life care was established, the first program to formalize the use of modern pain management techniques to care for the dying. The first hospice in the United States was established in New Haven, Connecticut, in 1974, and now there are many thousands of such programs across the country.[99]

Hospice is not a physical place but rather a philosophy of care. Eighty percent of hospice care is provided in the patient's home, a family member's home, or in nursing homes. Specialized inpatient hospice facilities are also available to assist with end-of-life care. If a person has a terminal illness or disease that is no longer responding to treatment, the person is eligible for hospice care. Two physicians must certify that the person has a terminal illness and that if the disease were to run its normal course survival would be 6 months or less.[100] In 2016, 1.4 million Medicare recipients received hospice care. The majority (64%) were 80 years of age or older. The most frequent principal diagnosis was cancer (27.2%) followed by cardiovascular disease (18.9%) and dementia (18%). The mean length of stay in hospice care was 71 days.[101]

Unique to the hospice philosophy is the recognition that there is potential for growth for the patient and family, even at the end of life, and that there is such a thing as a good death. Hospice programs seek to support living through the dying process and include family as part of this process. Hospice programs provide state-of-the-art palliative care and supportive services according to unique individual and family needs.

Palliative Care

A key component of hospice is the use of palliative care. At some point in life, it becomes unreasonable to expect cure or reversal of disease processes or to restore a previous level of functioning and independence, and it is clear that life is nearing its end. Death is a natural process, and older adults go through developmental tasks as they approach death, with the goal of life closure. As death approaches, adaptation to a new state allows beings to remain whole: to interact with their environments, to experience human relationships, and to achieve personally meaningful goals.

The WHO defines **palliative care** as "an approach that improves the quality of life of patients and their families facing the problems associated with life-threatening illness, through the prevention and relief of suffering by means of early identification and impeccable assessment and treatment of pain and other problems, physical, psychosocial and spiritual."[102] According to the WHO, palliative care has specific aspects (Box 19-9).

End-of-life nursing care may focus on symptom control and solving functional, physical, or psychological problems to optimize the older adult's quality of life, regardless of the amount of time that remains. Patient/family-centered care is clearly appropriate for the unique experience of dying. Many nursing actions center on supporting physiological function and preventing complications, goals that are still appropriate at the end of life. Appreciating each person as a unique individual is extremely important in assuring optimal care at the end of life. Although it may be evident to health-care providers that certain goals and interventions would suit the patient's needs, even more important is finding congruence with the patient's own perceived and stated goals and values and upholding his or her rights to self-determination. For example, the presence and involvement of family and friends may have great importance at the end of life. Family members may seek involvement in the caring activities as an expression of feelings of closeness and love. They may try to find understanding of, resolution to, or closure of past issues. For the person nearing the end of life, the presence of family, friends, and even pets may be a powerful affirmation of the continuity of life.[103]

Palliative care for older adults focuses on issues surrounding the geriatric syndromes and on the provision of care in a variety of long-term care settings. Common geriatric syndromes occurring at the end of life include

---

BOX 19-9 ■ WHO Components of Palliative Care

By the WHO definition, palliative care:

- Provides relief from pain and other distressing symptoms
- Affirms life and regards dying as a normal process
- Intends neither to hasten or postpone death
- Integrates the psychological and spiritual aspects of patient care
- Offers a support system to help patients live as actively as possible until death
- Offers a support system to help the family cope during the patient's illness and in their own bereavement
- Uses a team approach to address the needs of patients and their families, including bereavement counseling, if indicated
- Will enhance quality of life and may also positively influence the course of illness
- Is applicable early in the course of illness in conjunction with other therapies intended to prolong life, such as chemotherapy or radiation therapy, and includes those investigations needed to better understand and manage distressing clinical complications

Source: (102)

---

dementia, delirium, urinary incontinence, and falls.[101] The decision to initiate palliative care in geriatrics is based on the presence of several markers that indicate that curative approaches are no longer appropriate. **Core end-stage indicators** that characterize the terminal phase of a chronic NCD include physical decline, weight loss, multiple comorbidities, a serum albumin of less than 2.5 g/dL, and ADL dependence.[104] Nondisease-specific indicators for palliative care include frailty or extreme vulnerability to morbidity and mortality as a result of a progressive decline in function and physiological reserve. Frequent falls, disability, susceptibility to acute illness, and reduced ability to recover are examples of frailty. Issues such as functional dependence, cognitive impairment, and family/caregiver support needs can enter into the decision to take a palliative approach to care.

■ CULTURAL CONTEXT

End-of-life decisions provide a good example of why we need to understand the cultural context in which older adults live. A key issue in end-of-life decisions is the cultural perspective of the patient and family making the decision.[106,107] As one set of researchers found

"… clashes between biomedical and ethnocultural realms of care that led to cultural insensitivity."[107] In other cultures, such as Hispanic cultures, there is a preference for nondisclosure of terminal prognosis, which is not always in line with traditional hospice practice. Language is also important. In Spanish, "hospicio" has negative connotations related to the abandonment of loved ones.[106] When planning and implementing end-of-life policies and procedures in any setting caring for the older adult, it is important to know the culture of the population receiving care. The health-care provider who expresses an interest in the cultural heritage of the older adult receiving care will be able to establish rapport and assist the family and the patient in making end-of-life decisions that match their cultural perspective and beliefs.

As mentioned earlier, the U.S. is facing an increasing diversity of race and ethnicity groups, which suggests a more diverse culture than before. To better serve the patients, nurses must strive to understand the diverse culture. For researchers, including nurse scientists, more culturally relevant interventions and treatments should be developed or adapted to reach the maximum benefit for the patients.

Life Closure

At the end of a long life, the personal experience of death can be viewed as an opportunity or even an achievement. Older adults in the dying process may examine their lives outwardly and deal with their worldly affairs as a way to interface with the world and find some meaning from their lives. The outward aspects of their lives include their relationships with their community, organizations, and other social groups. Older adults may take actions to assure they leave a legacy. They also may reflect on the impact their lives have had on others. They may make choices and plans about how they are leaving this world.

As they move further into the process of life closure, they step into an inner world, where they seek to derive meaning, affirm love of self, love of others, and complete family and friend relationships. This may involve some form of saying goodbye, knowing this is the last time, and accepting the finality of life. Surrendering to the unknown and letting go may be very difficult, but it is part of achieving a peaceful death.

As nurses involved in end-of-life care, we are faced with the fact that there are some things we cannot fix. We cannot stop death. We cannot find the perfect words, erase the anguish, or take away the depth of loss. But it may be enough to be present for the person and the family, respond with compassion and kindness, and keep a realistic perspective that to everything there is a season.

■ Summary Points

- The aging population is growing globally with an increased need for health-care services.
- Both biological and psychosocial factors play a role in healthy aging.
- More than 50% of older adults experience more than one NCD, resulting in a new focus in *Healthy People 2020* that included the improvement of the ability of the older adult to self-manage NCDs.
- Older adults experience issues related to communicable diseases and substance use.
- Health planning for older adults is key to meeting *Healthy People* objectives.
- Substance use is a growing issue among the older population.
- Alzheimer's disease and dementia have an impact on the quality of life for the older population and their families.
- The hospice model allows for the delivery of compassionate end-of-life care for the older adult population.

▼ CASE STUDY
Health Planning to Improve Physical Activity in Older Adults

The members of the nursing department in a large urban public health department were challenged with developing a program to improve physical activity level in older adults given the established benefits of physical activity. To complete this case study, do the following:

1. Access the *HP* website related to objectives for older adults and physical activity.
2. Examine the literature and determine what baseline data are available related to the objective from a national perspective.
3. Critique possible population-level approaches in relation to their utility in meeting the objectives including but not limited to:
   a. Policy initiatives
   b. Development of a health program
   c. Public service announcements
4. Determine what data are available in the city nearest you that would help determine the level of physical activity in that city among older adults.

5. Determine how the nurses can complete the assignment. Be sure to include in your conclusion the following:
   a. Assessment needs
   b. Types of population-level interventions best suited to meet the objective
   c. Health-planning steps needed specific to the chosen intervention(s)

REFERENCES

1. United Nations, Department of Economic and Social Affairs, Population Division. (2015). *World Population Aging 2015 (ST/ESA/SER.A/390)*. Retrieved from http://www.un.org/en/development/desa/population/publications/pdf/ageing/WPA2015_Report.pdf.
2. World Health Organization. (2016). *World Health Statistics*. World Health Organization. Retrieved from http://www.who.int/gho/publications/world_health_statistics/2016/en/.
3. U.S. Department of Health and Human Services. (2018). *2020 topics and objectives: Older adults*. Retrieved from https://www.healthypeople.gov/2020/topics-objectives/topic/older-adults.
4. World Health Organization. (2018). *Elderly population*. Retrieved from http://www.searo.who.int/entity/health_situation_trends/data/chi/elderly-population/en/.
5. World Health Organization. (2018). *Proposed working definition of an older person in Africa for the MDS Project*. Retrieved from http://www.who.int/healthinfo/survey/ageingdefnolder/en/.
6. Cohen-Mansfield, J., Shmotkin, D., Blumstein, Z., Shorek, A., Eyal, N., & Hazan, H. (2013). The old, old-old, and the oldest old: Continuation or distinct categories? An examination of the relationship between age and changes in health, function, and wellbeing. *The International Journal of Aging and Human Development, 77*(1), 37-57.
7. U.S. Census Bureau. (2017). *Profile America facts for features*. Retrieved from https://www.census.gov/content/dam/Census/newsroom/facts-for-features/2017/cb17-ff08.pdf.
8. Mather, M., Jacobsen, L.A., & Pollard, K.M. (2015). Aging in the United States. *Population Bulletin, 70, no. 2 (2015)*. For permission to reproduce portions from the Population Bulletin, write to PRB: Attn: Permissions; or e-mail: popref@prb.org.
9. Federal Interagency Forum on Aging Related Statistics. (2016). *Older Americans 2016: Key indicators of wellbeing*. Retrieved from https://agingstats.gov/docs/latestreport/older-americans-2016-key-indicators-of-wellbeing.pdf.
10. Gavrilov L.A., & Heuveline, P. (2003). Aging of the population. In P. Demeny & G. McNicoll (Eds.). *The encyclopedia of population*. New York, NY: Macmillan Reference USA.
11. World Health Organization. (2013). *Aging and the life course*. Retrieved from http://www.who.int/ageing/about/ageing_life_course/en/index.html.
12. World Health Organization. (2018). *Life expectancy*. Retrieved from http://www.who.int/gho/mortality_burden_disease/life_tables/situation_trends_text/en/.
13. Vespa, J., Armstrong, D.M., & Medina, L. (2018). *Demographic turning points for the United States: Population projections for 2020 to 2060*. U.S. Census Bureau. Retrieved from https://www.census.gov/content/dam/Census/library/publications/2018/demo/P25_1144.pdf.
14. U.S. Census Bureau. (2018). *International data base*. Retrieved from https://www.census.gov/data-tools/demo/idb/informationGateway.php.
15. Wilmoth, J.R., & Horiuchi, S. (1999). Rectangularization revisited: Variability of age at death within human populations. *Demography, 36*(4), 475-495.
16. Kasper, J.D., Freedman, V.A., Spillman, B. C., & Wolff, J. L. (2015). The disproportionate impact of dementia on family and unpaid caregiving to older adults. *Health Affairs, 34*(10), 1642-1649.
17. Centers for Disease Control and Prevention. (2018). *Adult obesity facts*. Retrieved from https://www.cdc.gov/obesity/data/adult.html.
18. National Council on Aging. (2018). *Mature workers facts*. Retrieved from https://www.ncoa.org/news/resources-for-reporters/get-the-facts/mature-workers-facts/.
19. U.S. Department of Labor, Bureau of Labor Statistics. (2017). *Older workers: Labor force trends and career options*. Retrieved from https://www.bls.gov/careeroutlook/2017/article/older-workers.htm.
20. National Center for Health Statistics. (2017). *Chapter 31, Older Adults in Healthy People 2020 Midcourse Review*. Hyattsville, MD: National Center for Health Statistics.
21. U.S. Census Bureau. (2014). *An aging nation: The older population in the United States*. Retrieved from https://www.census.gov/prod/2014pubs/p25-1140.pdf.
22. Miller, C. (2012). *Nursing for wellness in older adults: Theory and practice* (6th ed.). Baltimore, MD: Wolters Kluwer Health.
23. Koltover, V.K. (2017). Free radical timer of aging: From chemistry of free radicals to systems theory of reliability. *Current Aging Science, 10*(1), 12-17.
24. Newman, A.B., & Cauley, J.A. (2015). Epidemiology of aging. In L. Goldman & A.I. Schafer (Eds.), *Goldman Cecil medicine* (25th ed.). Philadelphia, PA: Saunders Elsevier.
25. Cumming, E. (1975). Engagement with an old theory. *International Journal of Aging and Human Development, 6*(3), 187-191.
26. Atchley, R.C. (1989). A continuity theory of normal aging. *Gerontologist, 29*(2), 183-190.
27. National Institutes of Health. (n.d.). *The Baltimore Longitudinal Study of Aging*. Retrieved from https://www.nia.nih.gov/research/labs/blsa.
28. Allard, M., Lebre, V., Robine, J-M. & Calment, J. (1998). *Jeanne Calment: From Van Gogh's time to ours; 122 extraordinary years*. New York, NY: W.H. Freeman.
29. Boston University School of Medicine. (2017). *New England Centenarian Study*. Retrieved from http://www.bumc.bu.edu/centenarian/.
30. Evert, J., Lawler E., Bogan, H., & Perls, T. (2003). Morbidity profiles of centenarians: Survivors, delayers, and escapers. *Journal of Gerontology, 58*, 232-237.
31. Hilt, R., Young-Xu, Y., Silver, M., & Perls, T. (1999). Centenarians: The older you get the healthier you've been. *Lancet, 354*(9179), 652.
32. Mroczek, D.K., & Spiro, A. (2003). Modeling intra-individual change in personality traits: Findings from the Normative Aging Study. *Journal of Gerontology, 58*, 153-165.

33. Newman, A.B., Bayles, C.M., Milas, C.N., McTigue, K., Williams, K., Robare, J.F., & Kuller, L.H. (2010). The 10 keys to healthy aging: Findings from an innovative prevention program in the community. *Journal of Aging and Health, 22*(5), 547-566.

34. American Nurses Credentialing Center. (n.d.). *Gerontological nursing certification.* Retrieved from http://www.nursecredentialing.org.

35. Prochaska, J. O., & Velicer, W. F. (1997). The transtheoretical model of health behavior change. *American Journal of Health Promotion, 12*(1), 38-48.

36. Szanton, S.L., Wolff, J.W., Leff, B., Thorpe, R.J., Tanner, E.K., Boyd, C., ... Gitlin, L.N. (2014). CAPABLE trial: A randomized controlled trial of nurse, occupational therapist and handyman to reduce disability among older adults: Rationale and design. *Contemporary Clinical Trials, 38*(1), 102-112.

37. Szanton, S.L., & Gill, J.M. (2010). Facilitating resilience using a society-to-cells framework: A theory of nursing essentials applied to research and practice. *Advances in Nursing Science, 33*(4), 329-343.

38. Lawton, M.P., & Nahemow, L. (1973). Ecology and the aging process. In C. Eisdorfer & M. P. Lawton (Eds.), *The psychology of adult development and aging* (pp. 619-674). Washington, DC, US: American Psychological Association.

39. Verbrugge, L.M., & Jette, A.M. (1994). The disablement process. *Social Science & Medicine, 38*(1), 1-14.

40. Heckhausen, J., & Schulz, R. (1995). A life-span theory of control. *Psychological Review, 102*(2), 284.

41. Centers for Disease Control and Prevention. (2017). *Older person's health.* Retrieved from https://www.cdc.gov/nchs/fastats/older-american-health.htm.

42. Centers for Disease Control and Prevention. (2017). *Pneumonia.* Retrieved from https://www.cdc.gov/nchs/fastats/pneumonia.htm.

43. National Institutes of Health Medline Plus. (2018). *Protect yourself against shingles.* Retrieved from https://medlineplus.gov/magazine/issues/winter10/articles/winter10pg16-17.html.

44. Centers for Disease Control and Prevention, National Center for HIV/AIDS, Viral Hepatitis, STD, and TB Prevention. (2018). *Sexually transmitted disease surveillance 2017.* Retrieved from https://www.cdc.gov/std/stats17/default.htm.

45. Centers for Disease Control and Prevention. (2015). *Testing recommendations for hepatitis C virus infection.* Retrieved from https://www.cdc.gov/hepatitis/hcv/guidelinesc.htm.

46. Centers for Disease Control and Prevention. (2018). *Recommended immunization schedule for adults aged 19 years or older, United States, 2018.* Retrieved from https://www.cdc.gov/vaccines/schedules/hcp/imz/adult.html.

47. Centers for Disease Control and Prevention. (2018). *People 65 years and older & influenza.* Retrieved from https://www.cdc.gov/flu/about/disease/65over.htm.

48. National Council on Aging. (n.d.). *Health aging facts.* Retrieved from https://www.ncoa.org/news/resources-for-reporters/get-the-facts/healthy-aging-facts/.

49. Centers for Disease Control and Prevention. (2018). *Promoting preventive services for adults 50-64: Community and clinical partnerships.* Retrieved from https://www.cdc.gov/aging/pdf/promoting-preventive-services.pdf.

50. Kramarow, E., Chen, L.H., Hedegaard, H., & Warner, M. (2015). Deaths from unintentional injury among adults aged 65 and over: United States, 2000–2013. *NCHS data brief, no 199.* Hyattsville, MD: National Center for Health Statistics.

51. Bergen, G., Stevens, M.R., & Burns, E.R. (2016). Falls and fall injuries among adults aged ≥65 years — United States, 2014. *Morbidity and Mortality Weekly Reports, 65*, 993–998.

52. Centers for Disease Control and Prevention. (2018). *Older adult falls.* Retrieved from https://www.cdc.gov/homeandrecreationalsafety/falls/index.html.

53. National Center for Injury Prevention and Control. (2015). *Preventing falls: A guide to implementing effective community-based fall prevention programs* (2nd ed.). Atlanta, GA: Centers for Disease Control and Prevention.

54. The National Council on Aging. (n.d). *Fall prevention.* Retrieved from http://www.ncoa.org/improve-health/center-for-healthy-aging/falls-prevention/.

55. U.S. Administration on Aging, National Center on Elder Abuse. (n.d.). Retrieved from https://ncea.acl.gov/.

56. Lachs, M.S., Williams, C.S., O'Brien, S., Pillemer, K.A., & Charlson, M.E. (1998). The mortality of elder mistreatment. *JAMA, 280*(5), 428-432.

57. Dong, X. (2017). Elder self-neglect: Research and practice. *Clinical Interventions in Aging, 12*, 949.

58. Centers for Disease Control and Prevention. (2018). *Elder maltreatment definition.* Retrieved from http://www.cdc.gov/features/elderabuse/.

59. Centers for Disease Control and Prevention. (2018). *Elder maltreatment prevention.* Retrieved from https://www.cdc.gov/violenceprevention/elderabuse/definitions.html.

60. Centers for Disease Control and Prevention. (2018). *Elder maltreatment: Risk and protective factors.* Retrieved from https://www.cdc.gov/violenceprevention/elderabuse/riskprotectivefactors.html.

61. U.S. Administration on Aging, National Center on Elder Abuse. (2018). *Risk factors for elder abuse.* Retrieved from https://ncea.acl.gov/whatwedo/research/statistics.html#risk.

62. Perel-Levin, S. (2008). *Discussing screening for elder abuse at the primary care level. Aging and life course family and community health.* Geneva, Switzerland: World Health Organization.

63. Fulmer, T. (n.d.). *Elder mistreatment: Training manual and protocol.* Retrieved from https://consultgeri.org/education-training/e-learning-resources/elder-mistreatment-training-manual-and-protocol.

64. McCarthy, L., Campbell, S., & Penhale, B. (2017). Elder abuse screening tools: a systematic review. *Journal of Adult Protection, 19*(6), 368–379. https://doi-org.ezp.welch.jhmi.edu/10.1108/JAP-10-2016-0026.

65. National Center on Elder Abuse. (n.d.). *Resources.* Retrieved from https://ncea.acl.gov/resources/state.html.

66. Fearing, G., Sheppard, C.L., McDonald, L., Beaulieu, M., & Hitzig, S.L. (2017). A systematic review on community-based interventions for elder abuse and neglect. *Journal of Elder Abuse & Neglect, 29*(2-3), 102-133.

67. Falk, N.L., Baigis, J., & Kopac, C. (2012). Elder mistreatment and the Elder Justice Act. *OJIN: The Online Journal of Issues in Nursing, 17*(3), 7.

68. Morrow County, Ohio, Job and Family Services. (n.d.). *Principles of adult protective services.* Retrieved from

http://jfs.morrowcountyohio.gov/images/Documents/ChildrenServices/ProtectiveServices/Principles.pdf.

69. Storey, J.E., & Perka, M.R. (2018). Reaching out for help: Recommendations for practice based on an in-depth analysis of an elder abuse intervention programme. *British Journal of Social Work, 48*(4), 1052–1070. https://doi-org.ezp.welch.jhmi.edu/10.1093/bjsw/bcy039.

70. Mattson, M., Lipari, R.N., Hays, C, & Van Horn, S.L. (2017). A day in the life of older adults: Substance use facts. *The CBHSQ Report: May 11, 2017*. Rockville, MD: Center for Behavioral Health Statistics and Quality, Substance Abuse and Mental Health Services Administration.

71. Substance Abuse and Mental Health Services Administration. (2016). *Substance use treatment for older adults*. Retrieved from https://www.samhsa.gov/homelessness-programs-resources/hpr-resources/substance-use-treatment-older-adults.

72. Blow, F.C. (1998). *Substance abuse among older adults. Treatment improvement protocol 26*. Rockville, MD: Substance Abuse and Mental Health Services Administration. Retrieved from http://www.ncbi.nlm.nih.gov/books/NBK14467/.

73. Substance Abuse and Mental Health Administration. (2014). *Results from the 2013 National Survey on Drug Use And Health: Summary of national findings*. Retrieved from http://www.samhsa.gov/data/sites/default/files/NSDUHresultsPDFWHTML2013/Web/NSDUHresults2013.pdf.

74. Savage, C.L., & Finnell, D. (2015). Screening for at-risk alcohol use in older adults: What progress have we made? *Journal of Addictions Nursing, 26*(3).

75. National Institute on Aging. (n.d.). *Health and aging*. Retrieved from http://www.nia.nih.gov/health.

76. Holton, A.E., Gallagher, P., Fahey, T., & Cousins, G. (2017). Concurrent use of alcohol interactive medications and alcohol in older adults: A systematic review of prevalence and associated adverse outcomes. *BMC Geriatrics, 17*(1), 148. doi: 10.1186/s12877-017-0532-2.

77. National Institute on Alcohol Abuse and Alcoholism. (2005). *Helping patients who drink too much: A clinician's guide*. Retrieved from http://pubs.niaaa.nih.gov/publications/Practitioner/CliniciansGuide2005/guide.pdf.

78. Chandrakumar, A., Bhardwaj, A., 't Jong, G.W., (2018). Review of thiamine deficiency disorders: Wernicke encephalopathy and Korsakoff psychosis. *Journal of Basic Clinical Physiology and Pharmacology*. pii: /j/jbcpp.ahead-of-print/jbcpp-2018-0075/jbcpp-2018-0075.xml. doi: 10.1515/jbcpp-2018-0075.

79. Savage, C.L. (2008). Screening for alcohol use in older adults. *Directions in Addiction Treatment and Prevention, 12*(2), 17-26.

80. Wick, J.Y. (2017). Aging in place: Our house is a very, very, very fine house. *Consultant Pharmacist, 32*(10), 566–574. https://doi-org.ezp.welch.jhmi.edu/10.4140/TCP.n.2017.566.

81. Park, S., Han, Y., Kim, B.R., & Dunkle, R.E. (2017). Aging in place of vulnerable older adults: Person-environment fit perspective. *Journal of Applied Gerontology, 36*(11), 1327–1350. https://doi-org.ezp.welch.jhmi.edu/10.1177/0733464815617286.

82. U.S. Census Bureau. (2011). *Census brief: The older population*. Retrieved from http://www.census.gov/prod/cen2010/briefs/c2010br-09.pdf.

83. Szanton, S., Thorpe, R.J., Boyd, C., Tanner, E.K., Liff, B., & Gitlin, L. (2011). Community aging in place, advancing better living for elders: A bio-behavioral environmental intervention to improve functioning and health related quality of life in disabled older adults. *Journal of the American Geriatrics Society, 59*(12), 2314-2320.

84. Centers for Disease Control and Prevention. (2012). *Healthy aging and the built environment*. Retrieved from http://www.cdc.gov/healthyplaces/healthtopics/healthyaging.htm.

85. Davitt, J.K., Greenfield, E., Lehning, A., & Scharlach, A. (2017). Challenges to engaging diverse participants in community-based aging in place initiatives. *Journal of Community Practice, 25*(3/4), 325–343. https://doi-org.ezp.welch.jhmi.edu/10.1080/10705422.2017.1354346.

86. Tripken, J.L., Elrod, C., & Bills, S. (2018). Factors influencing advance care planning among older adults in two socioeconomically diverse living communities. *American Journal of Hospice & Palliative Medicine, 35*(1), 69–74. https://doi-org.ezp.welch.jhmi.edu/10.1177/1049909116679140.

87. Ayalon, L., & Tesch-Römer, C. (2017). Taking a closer look at ageism: Self- and other-directed ageist attitudes and discrimination. *European Journal of Ageing, 14*(1), 1–4. https://doi-org.ezp.welch.jhmi.edu/10.1007/s10433-016-0409-9.

88. Pritchard-Jones, L. (2017). Ageism and autonomy in health care: Explorations through a relational lens. *Health Care Analysis, 25*(1), 72–89. https://doi-org.ezp.welch.jhmi.edu/10.1007/s10728-014-0288-1.

89. Matthews, K.A., Xu, W., Gaglioti, A.H., Holt, J.B., Croft, J.B., Mack, D., & McGuire, L.C. (2018). Racial and ethnic estimates of Alzheimer's disease and related dementias in the United States (2015–2060) in adults aged ≥65 years. *The Journal of the Alzheimer's Association*. pii: S1552-5260(18)33252-7. doi: 10.1016/j.jalz.2018.06.3063.

90. Centers for Disease Control and Prevention. (2018). *Healthy aging: Alzheimer's disease*. Retrieved from http://www.cdc.gov/aging/aginginfo/alzheimers.htm.

91. Centers for Disease Control and Prevention. (2018). *FastStats: Leading causes of death*. Retrieved from http://www.cdc.gov/nchs/fastats/lcod.htm.

92. World Health Organization. (2018). *Dementia*. Retrieved from http://www.who.int/news-room/fact-sheets/detail/dementia.

93. Kelley, M., Ulin, B., & McGuire, L. C. (2018). Reducing the risk of Alzheimer's disease and maintaining brain health in an aging society. *Public Health Reports, 133*(3), 225–229. https://doi-org.ezp.welch.jhmi.edu/10.1177/0033354918763599.

94. Glynn-Servedio, B.E., & Ranola, T.S. (2017). AChE inhibitors and NMDA receptor antagonists in advanced Alzheimer's disease. *Consultant Pharmacist, 32*(9), 511–518. https://doi-org.ezp.welch.jhmi.edu/10.4140/TCP.n.2017.511.

95. Centers for Disease Control and Prevention. (2018). *Healthy brain initiative*. Retrieved from https://www.cdc.gov/aging/pdf/2018-2023-Road-Map-508.pdf.

96. Govtrack. (2017). *S. 1028: RAISE Family Caregivers Act*. Retrieved from https://www.govtrack.us/congress/bills/115/s1028/text.

97. Family Caregiver Alliance. (2018). *Statement on the Passage of the RAISE Family Caregivers Act*. Retrieved from

https://www.caregiver.org/statement-passage-raise-family-caregivers-act.

98. RE-AIM. (2018). *Welcome to RE-AIM.org!*. Retrieved from http://www.re-aim.org/.

99. National Hospice and Palliative Care Organization. (2014). *History of hospice care.* Retrieved from http://www.nhpco.org/i4a/pages/index.cfm?pageid=3285.

100. Electronic Code of Federal Regulations. (2018). *PART 418—HOSPICE CARE.* Retrieved from https://www.ecfr.gov/cgi-bin/text-idx?rgn=div5;node=42%3A3.0.1.1.5#se42.3.418_120.

101. National Hospice and Palliative Care Organization. (2018). *Facts and figures hospice care in America.* Retrieved from https://www.nhpco.org/sites/default/files/public/Statistics_Research/2017_Facts_Figures.pdf.

102. World Health Organization. (2018). *WHO definition of palliative care.* Retrieved from http://www.who.int/cancer/palliative/definition/en/.

103. Schulman-Green, D., & Feder, S. (2018). Integrating family caregivers into palliative oncology care using the self- and family management approach. *Seminars in Oncology Nursing, 34*(3), 252–263. https://doi-org.ezp.welch.jhmi.edu/10.1016/j.soncn.2018.06.006.

104. Family Life. (n.d.). *Core end-stage indicators.* Retrieved from https://familylifecarein.org/file/2015/12/LCDs-updated-2015.pdf.

105. Rising, M.L., Hassouneh, D.S., Lutz, K.F., Lee, C.S., & Berry, P. (2018). Integrative review of the literature on hispanics and hospice. *American Journal of Hospice & Palliative Medicine, 35*(3), 542–554. https://doi-org.ezp.welch.jhmi.edu/10.1177/1049909117730555.

106. Weerasinghe, S., & Maddalena, V. (2016). Negotiation, mediation and communication between cultures: End-of-life care for South Asian immigrants in Canada from the perspective of family caregivers. *Social Work in Public Health, 31*(7), 665–677. https://doi-org.ezp.welch.jhmi.edu/10.1080/19371918.2015.1137521.

Chapter 20

Health Planning for Occupational and Environmental Health

Gordon Gillespie, Cynthia Betcher, and Sheila Fitzgerald

LEARNING OUTCOMES

After reading the chapter, the student will be able to:

1. Define *occupational health* and *occupational and environmental health nursing*.
2. Describe the relationship between the work environment, workplace exposures, and worker health and safety.
3. Discuss the concept of toxicology and the relevance to understanding and preventing occupational diseases.
4. Discuss controlling hazards and reducing injuries in the workplace.
5. Identify vulnerable worker populations.
6. Explain the role of the occupational and environmental health nurse in the development, management, and evaluation of occupational health programs.
7. State methods of worker protection and safety as well as health promotion strategies in the occupational health setting.

KEY TERMS

Case management
Disability
Employee assistance
   program (EAP)
Engineering controls
Environmental monitoring
Epidemiological triangle
Ergonomics
Hazard Communication
   Standard
Health risk appraisal
   (HRA)

Hierarchy of controls
Material safety data sheet
   (MSDS)
National Institute for
   Occupational Safety
   and Health (NIOSH)
National Occupational
   Research Agenda
   (NORA)
Occupational and
   environmental health
   history

Occupational and
   environmental health
   nurse (OEHN)
Occupational and
   environmental health
   nursing
Occupational Safety
   and Health
   (OSH) Act
Occupational Safety and
   Health Administration
   (OSHA)

Personal protective
   equipment (PPE)
Total Worker
   Health®
Toxicology
Vulnerable worker
   populations
Workers' compensation
Work-family interface
Workplace assessment/
   workplace walkthrough

▨ Introduction

Every week, 257 million Americans go to work.[1] Construction workers can be seen during the day at a new building site or doing repairs on a busy highway in the middle of the night. Health-care providers are present around the clock in hospitals and emergency departments. Behind the scenes are nutrition services, plant facilities staff, laundry workers, and hazardous waste workers. In an office building, top executives are in the boardroom, while administrative assistants spend hours in front of a computer, telephones ringing in the background. When the workday is over, the housekeeping staff cleans bathrooms, polishes floors, and removes trash for another new day. The goal of occupational health is to ensure each worker returns home safely at the end of the workday. Unfortunately, not all workers do. Fatalities and injuries occur: mine explosions, deaths of truckers, collapses at construction sites, loss of limbs among soldiers, and violent incidents in the workplace. Every work setting presents its own unique exposures and hazards and its own mix of worker demographics that may affect the health and well-being of employees. The **occupational and environmental health nurse (OEHN)** is a key member of the interprofessional team responsible for the assessment and detection of occupational hazards and the implementation of interventions to protect the health of worker populations (Box 20-1).

Focus of Occupational Health

The Joint International Labour Organization/World Health Organization indicates that the focus of occupational health should:

- Follow a systems approach to promoting safe and healthy work environments
- Afford prevention the highest priority
- Develop work cultures in a direction supporting health and safety at work while preventing and controlling hazards and risks, and in doing so promoting a positive social climate and smooth operation that may enhance productivity and quality[2]

The **Occupational Safety and Health Administration (OSHA)** is a federal agency formed in 1970. OSHA is charged with protecting coworkers, family members, employers, customers, suppliers, nearby communities, and other members of the public affected by the workplace environment.[3]

The Workplace and the Epidemiological Triangle

The workplace is only one component of the overall environment, but it is where adults spend approximately one-third of their time.[4] The **epidemiological triangle** (Chapter 3) provides a framework to describe the complex relationships among an agent (the exposure[s] in the workplace), the host (worker/employee), and the environment (workplace)—the setting in which the agent and host come together.[5] This chapter clarifies how these three components relate to one another.

Occupational and Environmental Health Nursing

The specialty of occupational health nursing evolved during the 19th century, when industry leaders hired nurses to decrease the spread of communicable disease among workers, reduce injury, and promote safety. The landmark events in the evolution of the specialty are described in Box 20-2. Today's OEHN has expanded this specialty practice into management areas, consultation with government and industry, policy setting at the local, state, and national levels, education, and research. Nevertheless, a major role for the OEHN is providing direct care to employees in the workplace.

BOX 20–1 ■ Members of the Interprofessional Occupational and Environmental Health Team

Occupational Health Professionals	Primary Focus
Occupational and environmental health nurse	Prevention of occupational disease and injury, restoration of employee health and return to work, protection from occupational hazards
Occupational health physician	Diagnose, treat, and manage occupational disease and injury
Occupational and environmental hygienist	The recognition, evaluation, and control of chemical, biological, or physical factors or stressors arising in the workplace; and the use of analytical techniques to detect exposures and implement engineering controls to correct, reduce, or eliminate exposure
Ergonomist	Evaluate, design, and promote the interface between the worker, tools used, and their work
Occupational psychiatrist/psychologist	Diagnose, treat, and manage mental and behavioral disorders secondary to exposures in the workplace
Toxicologist	Evaluate and describe the toxic properties of chemical and physical agents used during work
Injury prevention/safety specialist	Develop procedures, standards, or systems to achieve the control or reduction of hazards, injuries, and exposures
Health promotion educator	Develop educational strategies and methods to promote the health of worker(s) in the occupational setting

---

BOX 20–2 ■ Landmark Events in the Evolution of Occupational and Environmental Health Nursing

1888	Betty Moulder of Pennsylvania was the first reported occupational health nurse who cared for coal miners and families.
1942	American Association of Industrial Nurses established.
1970	The Occupational Safety and Health Act is passed creating the Occupational Safety and Health Administration (OSHA) and the National Institute for Occupational Safety and Health (NIOSH). NIOSH Occupational Safety and Health Education and Resource Centers are created to educate occupational health professionals (nurses, physicians, industrial hygienists, and safety specialists), now called NIOSH Occupational Safety and Health Education and Research Centers.
1972	The Accreditation Board for Occupational Health Nursing is established, creating certification of nurses in the specialty practice of occupational and environmental health nursing.
1977	The American Association of Industrial Nurses name changed to the American Association of Occupational Health Nurses.
1993	The Office of Occupational Health Nursing (OOHN) was established at OSHA.
1997	AAOHN releases first edition of *AAOHN Core Curriculum for Occupational Health Nursing.*

Source: Adapted from Institute of Medicine. Committee to Assess Training Needs for Occupational Safety and Health Personnel in the United States, 2000.

In 1993, the Institute of Medicine (now known as the Health and Medicine Division of the National Academies of Sciences, Engineering, and Medicine) conducted a workshop to discuss the growing need to enhance occupational and environmental health content in the practice of nursing. The workshop resulted in the establishment of the Committee on Enhancing Environmental Health Content in Nursing Practice and competencies for this nursing specialty.[6] Today, the importance of occupational health is evident in the *Healthy People (HP)* objectives.[7]

■ HEALTHY PEOPLE

Targeted Topic: Occupational Safety and Health
Goal: Promote the safety and health of people at work through prevention and early intervention.
Overview: The intent behind the occupational safety and health topic area is to prevent diseases, injuries, and deaths that result because of working conditions. Work-related illnesses and injuries include any illness or injury incurred by an employee engaged in work-related activities while at or away from the worksite. With the advent of **Total Worker Health®**, there is now a focus on the activities and behaviors occurring outside of the workplace that may impact the overall health of the worker and ultimately worker safety and productivity.[8]

Workplace settings vary widely in size, sector, design, location, work processes, workplace culture, and resources. In addition, workers themselves are different in terms of age, gender, training, education, cultural background, health practices, and access to preventive health care. These activities translate to great diversity in the safety and health risks for each industry sector and the need for tailored interventions.

Occupational safety and related *HP* objectives are primarily addressed through the **National Occupational Research Agenda (NORA)**. NORA was established by the Centers for Disease Control and Prevention (CDC), **National Institute for Occupational Safety and Health (NIOSH)**, and its partners to stimulate research and improve workplace practices. Now in its third decade (2016–2026), NORA focuses on occupational safety and health in 10 sectors:

1. Agriculture, Forestry, and Fishing
2. Construction
3. Health Care and Social Assistance
4. Manufacturing
5. Mining
6. Oil and Gas Extraction
7. Public Safety
8. Services
9. Transportation, Warehousing, and Utilities
10. Wholesale and Retail Trade[7]

HP 2020 Midcourse Review: There are 16 measurable objectives for this topic area. Thirteen of the objectives met or exceeded their target with 2 of the objectives improving. For 1 objective, there was little or no detectable change.
Source: (7, 8, 9)

Occupational and environmental health nursing is defined by the American Association of Occupational Health Nursing (AAOHN) as "the specialty practice that provides for and delivers health and safety programs and services to workers, worker populations, and community groups."[10] The AAOHN is the professional organization that develops and approves standards of practice, supports education and research, and provides political consultation to state and national legislators related to OEHN. The Accreditation Board for Occupational Health Nursing certifies nurses in the specialty practice of occupational and environmental health nursing.

The practicing OEHN focuses on promotion and restoration of health, prevention of illness and injury, and protection from work-related and environmental hazards. The specialty is guided by a code of ethics (Box 20-3) that provides an ethical framework for decision making and nursing actions.[11] Another important document developed by the AAOHN is the Standards of Occupational and Environmental Health Nursing.[12] The standards include a definition of and

scope of practice for OEHNs. Because OEHNs frequently have a combined knowledge of health and business, they are equipped with the skills to incorporate their experience in health care with their knowledge of establishing safe and healthy work environments.

Key Agencies in Occupational Health

The passage of the **Occupational Safety and Health (OSH) Act** in 1970 created two government organizations: OSHA and NIOSH.[3] The work of both agencies has a profound effect on the work environment and the safety and health of workers in the United States.

Occupational Safety and Health Administration

OSHA, which is part of the Department of Labor, is the main federal agency charged with the regulation and enforcement of the OSH Act. The mission at OSHA involves the development and enforcement of safety and health standards to assure safe and healthful working

---

BOX 20–3 ■ Code of Ethics and Interpretive Statements for the American Association of Occupational Health Nurses

Preamble

The American Association of Occupational Health Nurses, Inc. (AAOHN) Code of Ethics has been developed in response to the nursing profession's acceptance of its goals and values and the trust conferred upon it by society to guide the conduct and practices of the profession. As a professional, occupational and environmental health nurses (OHNs) accept the responsibility and inherent obligation to uphold these values.

The Code of Ethics is based on the belief that the goal of occupational and environmental health nurses is to promote the worker, worker population and community health and safety. This specialized practice focuses on promotion and restoration of health, prevention of illness and injury and protection from occupational and environmental hazards. The occupational and environmental nurse has a unique role in protecting the integrity of the workplace and the work environment.

The client can be workers, workers' families/significant others, worker populations, community groups, and employers. The purpose of the AAOHN Code of Ethics is to serve as a guide for registered professional nurses to maintain and pursue professionally recognized ethical behavior in providing occupational and environmental health and safety services.

Ethics is synonymous with moral reasoning. Ethics is not law, but a guide for moral action. Professional nurses, when making judgments related to the health and welfare of the client, utilize these significant universal moral principles.

These principles are:

- Right of self-determination
- Confidentiality
- Truth telling
- Doing or producing good
- Avoiding harm
- Fair and nondiscriminatory treatment

Occupational and environmental health nurses recognize that dilemmas may develop that do not have guidelines, data or statutes to assist with problem resolution; thus, occupational and environmental health nurses use problem-solving, collaboration and appropriate resources to resolve dilemmas.

The Code is not intended to establish nor replace standards of care or minimal levels of practice. In summary, the Code of Ethics and Interpretative Statements provide a guiding ethical framework for decision-making and evaluation of nursing actions as occupational and environmental health nurses fulfill their professional responsibilities to society and the profession.

Source: From the AAOHN, used with permission.

conditions for working men and women. The OSH Act includes the General Duty Clause, which requires an employer to "furnish to each of his [sic] employees employment and a place of employment which are free from recognized hazards that are causing or are likely to cause death or serious physical harm." Most employees who work for private employers in the United States are protected by federal OSHA or through an OSHA-approved state program. Federal agencies must have a safety and health program that meets the same standards as required under federal OSHA. The self-employed, family members of family farms, employers who do not employ outside employees, and workers protected by regulations of another federal agency (for example, the Mine Safety and Health Administration, the Federal Aviation Administration, and the Coast Guard) are not covered by the OSH Act.[13] Additionally, the Act requires businesses with more than 10 employees to keep records of fatalities, injuries, and illnesses on the OSHA 300 form. This record-keeping is critical to an employer's safety and health program for several reasons. Identification and description of the causes of work-related illness and injury assist in identifying problem areas that need corrective action to reduce hazardous workplace conditions. The data collected on these logs are used by the Department of Labor and OSHA to develop workplace statistics, including fatality, morbidity, and incidence rates for workplace illnesses and injuries for U.S. industries. These statistics are available to the public and provide a yearly accounting of the injuries and illnesses occurring among U.S. worker populations. The data in OSHA 300 logs provide information for OSHA to monitor the progress being made to reduce workplace safety and health problems.[14] OSHA also uses these logs to target the need for enforcement activities in industries in which the majority of workplace injuries and illnesses occur.

National Institute for Occupational Safety and Health

The second agency created by the OSH Act was NIOSH, an agency of the Department of Health and Human Services, whose mission is to conduct research and provide information, education, and training in the field of occupational safety and health. In 1996, NIOSH created NORA.[7,15] NORA is a partnership program between governmental agencies, large and small businesses, universities, worker organizations, and professional groups that work in collaboration to develop innovative research with the ultimate goal of improving workplace practices.[7,16] Ultimately, these research partnerships seek to provide recommendations for safer, healthier workplaces.

Occupational Safety and Health Program

A formal OSH program is an essential tool for the OEHN. Employers are encouraged to develop an OSH program to manage the safety and health at the worksite to reduce injuries, illnesses, and fatalities by complying with OSHA standards and the General Duty Clause.[17] An additional recommendation for an OSH program is to address the unique hazards and conditions found at each worksite.

An OSH program provides a systematic process that evaluates the workplace, recognizes the exposures and hazards found in each area of the worksite, provides a plan to control these exposures and hazards, and evaluates the effectiveness of these controls through routine **environmental monitoring** of the worksite and routine medical screening to assess for any adverse health conditions of the workforce. Environmental monitoring is the assessment of the workplace to identify risks and other hazards, whereas screening refers to identifying individual risks within individual workers such as heart disease and high blood pressure. The OEHN is a member of an interprofessional team that provides information on the health data collected during the medical screening process to assist in the evaluation of the effectiveness of the OSH program. If a problem is found with program effectiveness, corrective action is taken, and workers are re-evaluated.

Primary, Secondary, and Tertiary Prevention

In most workplaces, an occupational safety and health program focuses on primary, secondary, and tertiary prevention of occupational illnesses and injuries, and promotes worker health. Through primary prevention, workers are protected from exposure to hazards, or exposures are limited to levels considered safe. Examples of primary prevention interventions in the workplace include **engineering controls**, such as the use of less hazardous chemicals, or **personal protective equipment (PPE)**, such as masks, gloves, or hearing protection, or tethering a roofing worker to prevent a fall.

Secondary prevention requires early recognition of a disease before the disease becomes irreversible or is no longer easily treatable. Screening and monitoring of workers are examples of secondary prevention activities designed to detect early signs of disease (e.g., audiometric screening to detect hearing loss for workers in a noisy environment or spirometry screening to detect a reduction of lung function due to work in a closed, dusty environment). Tertiary prevention involves the treatment of the disease. The diagnosis of an occupational illness, such as work-related asthma, may require that the worker be removed from the exposure and transferred to another job. For nonoccupational illnesses that occur, the OEHN must coordinate with the worker's family physician or nurse practitioner regarding the timing of work return, particularly if accommodations in the workplace are needed. For example, an employee recovering from a myocardial infarction may require a gradual return to physically demanding work or an employee being treated for cancer may require a flexible work schedule to accommodate chemotherapy or radiation.

Worker Populations

The demographic characteristics of workers vary by age, race, gender, culture, ethnicity, and sensory/functional ability. These factors may influence a worker's vulnerability and susceptibility to exposures in the workplace and must be incorporated into an OSH program. In the United States, employment is often begun during adolescence and young adulthood. Approximately 43% of teenagers are employed in their first job by age 19 years. As the U.S. workplace becomes more diverse, OEHNs must focus on the vulnerable worker. The U.S. workforce is changing in a variety of ways. As many traditional service and manufacturing jobs migrate to other countries, the workforce is becoming much more dependent on "knowledge" workers.[18] Occupational health providers also need to pay attention to this rapid movement toward a knowledge-based economy that relies heavily on the creativity, mental stamina, and intellectual capacity of workers. This trend will likely change the pattern of disease and injuries that occur. For example, fewer physical injuries such as falls and crush injuries are likely to occur as factory worker jobs (and related injuries) are relocated to other countries. A higher rate of sedentary lifestyle diseases such as high blood pressure, diabetes, and obesity may occur as employees spend more time sitting at a computer versus physically moving during the course of their workday.

Emerging issues in the workplace are tied to the trend of longer working hours, greater participation of women in the workforce, couples having children later in life, increasing responsibility for the care of aging family members, and dual-career families. More and more workers find themselves sandwiched between work and domestic responsibilities.[19-21] Today, researchers at NIOSH are focused on the associations between work-life balance, well-being, and functioning.[22] Examples of research needed in this field include the effects of telecommuting and other organizational practices that meld work and family life, and the benefits of increased job flexibility and control over family obligations.

Unions

Unions have played an essential role in the evolution of occupational safety and health in the United States. In 1890, the United Mine Workers of America (UMWA) was formed with the primary purpose of preventing miner deaths.[23] The UMWA's constant effort taken to describe the dangerous conditions in coal mines that lead to black lung disease and fatalities was instrumental in the passage of the Coal Mine Health and Safety Act of 1969.[23] Over the years, labor unions have used collective bargaining agreements to help improve worker health and safety at union worksites. An example of this type of initiative is the 1974 contract agreement between the U.S. Steel Corporation and the United Steel Workers of America, which addressed the adverse health effects caused by exposure to coke oven emissions during steel production.[23] Unions assist their members with day-to-day issues at work, participate in legislative and regulatory policy-making, and conduct collective bargaining for workers over wages, working conditions, and benefits. Unions also conduct education and training programs for their members. They provide workers with a voice in workplace decisions and provide a mechanism for resolving workplace issues unavailable to workers in a nonunionized workplace.

Over the years, the number of union members in the United States has fallen dramatically, from 20.1% of American workers in the private sector in 1983 to 10.7% of wage and salary workers in 2017.[24] Yates discusses several reasons for the decline of U.S. unions. External forces include the shift of the economy from the production of goods to a service economy and the lack of demand by workers for the services offered by unions.[23] A 2018 ruling by the Supreme Court of the United States removing the requirement of "fair share" of union dues is likely to further reduce union participation. An internal force that has affected unions is the way union leaders are chosen. They are no longer selected from rank-and-file members, but from delegates far removed from the average rank and file union member.[23]

The OEHN must establish a working relationship with a union that has a presence in the workplace. Health and safety meetings should involve the union so trust and mutual respect are developed among members of the safety and health program. Despite the fact their numbers have decreased in the United States, unions such as the Service Employees International Union, the American Federation of Labor-Congress of Industrial Organizations, and others remain important organizations representing workers in many high-risk industries.

● APPLYING PUBLIC HEALTH SCIENCE
The Case of the Contaminated Home

Public Health Science Topics Covered:

- Epidemiology and biostatistics

Juan, a Mexican immigrant to the United States, works in California and Oregon during the harvest season as a migrant/seasonal farmworker. His 8-month work experience includes harvesting strawberries, asparagus, and navel oranges in California. In Oregon, he works in the berry and celery fields, usually for 6-week periods and often for many different owners. In one of these jobs, he experienced a puncture wound to his foot, resulting in the need for a tetanus immunization, after which he traveled back to California to work in the raisin grape harvest.

Depending on the season, Juan spends up to 12 hours per day working in the fields, planting or harvesting crops, and unloading trucks. At the end of the day, his clothes are often covered with dust. He sometimes brings his wife and children into the field to assist him with the picking of fruit or vegetables.

Juan and his family are often provided substandard housing with a communal bathroom and shower, and a shared kitchen in the local shantytowns. The location of the housing is often directly across from the fields, and inhabitants may be exposed to the pesticides with which the fields are sprayed.

The public health nurse (PHN) from the local health department provides care to the migrants. As a part of this role, the PHN sees Juan in the nearby free clinic as a follow-up to his foot injury. The puncture wound to his foot has healed and has no signs of infection. The PHN realizes exposures in the worksite are critical to Juan's health and interviewed him about his work and current health status. Juan reports leaving the fields late every day and eating dinner before removing his work clothes or taking a shower. He also complains of slight abdominal discomfort and diarrhea that has lasted for the past 7 days. After further inquiry, the PHN learns that, although 1,3-dichloropropene is the most common pesticide used locally to control pests from eating the roots of grape plants, local farmers may be spraying several other pesticides and fungicides.

The pesticide 1,3-dichloropropene is a sweet-smelling, colorless liquid that dissolves in water and evaporates quickly.[25] The pesticide released into the atmosphere takes several days to break down. After learning of the proximity of Juan's home to the fields, the PHN develops an exposure risk-reduction plan in collaboration with Juan. The plan includes Juan wearing a facemask and dusting off his clothing before entering his home. He will remove his clothing at the door and put them in a bag to keep them from contaminating the rest of the home. Juan then will shower before eating. When the fields are being sprayed, Juan's children will wait 5 days before playing outside near the fields or their home. The PHN asks Juan to return in 2 to 3 weeks for a re-evaluation of his symptoms and potential referral to industrial medicine and potentially pulmonary function testing. The PHN provides Juan a summary sheet with his nursing diagnosis, agreed-upon plan, and notes for the next PHN in case he relocates before his next clinic appointment. The treatment plan is provided in both English and Spanish.

Exposures in the Workplace

Exposures for any worker can include physical, chemical, biological, or psychological hazards. These hazards may have a profound effect on the short- and long-term health of workers. It is important for OEHNs to identify hazards in their work environment so mitigation plans can be implemented to reduce the potentially harmful effect on workers.

Physical Exposures

Physical hazards in the workplace, such as noise, excessive hot or cold temperatures, vibration, and nonionizing and ionizing radiation, cause harm or injury to body tissues through energy transfer.

Noise is an exposure frequently found in workplaces where construction, welding, or work with heavy machinery or power tools is performed. After years of exposure to loud noises, hearing loss can occur due to damage of the hair cells in the inner ear and failure of sound wave transmission to the auditory nerve. Loudness and duration of noise exposure are two important factors that affect hearing loss. Nonwork exposure to loud noise can occur at music concerts, in sports such as hunting or target practice, and without the use of hearing protection such as ear buds, all of which may lead to hearing loss. OSHA has developed a standard that regulates noise exposure and requires a hearing protection program in the workplace.[26] This standard requires monitoring of noise levels within the work environment, use of hearing protection, training and education of employees in the proper use of hearing protection, creation of baseline audiograms for each employee, and annual hearing tests.

Excessive heat exposure can be found in foundries, pottery-making plants with kilns, and in the road construction and fishing/agriculture industries during the summer months. For migrant workers like Juan, health outcomes of working in hot environments can be debilitating and potentially life-threatening when heat stress, heat exhaustion, and heat stroke occur. Industries that require outdoor work during the summer months also expose workers to nonionizing radiation from the sun and increased risk for skin cancer.[27] Jobs with winter-month cold exposures include construction and police and fire service work, although food industry workers may spend time in freezers or stock frozen foods year-round. Cold exposure results in stimulation of the sympathetic nervous system, potentially resulting in frostbite and hypothermia.[28]

Workers are exposed to vibration in manual tasks that involve two main mechanisms: hand-arm vibration, in which the main exposure is associated with power tools, such as a jackhammer; or whole-body vibration transferred to the body by large machinery, such as a bulldozer. These types of vibration exposures place workers at risk for acute and chronic musculoskeletal disorders.[29]

The Agency for Toxic Substances and Disease Registry defines ionizing radiation as any one of several types of particles and rays given off by radioactive material, high-voltage equipment, nuclear reactions, and stars. The types of ionizing radiation normally important to health are alpha particles, beta particles, x-rays, and gamma rays.[27,30] Ionizing radiation can have significant health effects, including skin burns, hair loss, nausea, birth defects, illness, and death. Certain types of cancer have been associated with ionizing radiation, although a person's risk may be influenced by dose and the age of the person when exposed.[27,30] For example, hospital x-ray technicians can be exposed to ionizing radiation during radiological procedures. However, most hospitals employ comprehensive safety protocols to prevent ionizing radiation exposure.

Chemical Exposures

According to OSHA, there are approximately 650,000 existing chemical products and hundreds of new products being introduced into the workplace annually. These chemical exposures can cause health effects to our body systems and act as carcinogens. As a result of these findings, OSHA issued the **Hazard Communication Standard**.[31] This policy requires both employers and employees to be knowledgeable about hazards and to protect themselves from illness or injury. This policy also requires the producers of chemicals to be responsible for reviewing the scientific evidence related to chemical hazards, and generating and communicating information to chemical users in the form of a **material safety data sheet (MSDS)**. An MSDS accompanies the hazardous chemical and describes the physical and chemical properties (e.g., acid, solvent) and health hazards, routes of exposure, safe handling and use, emergency and first aid procedures, and control measures.

Heavy Metals

Lead, mercury, cadmium, beryllium, nickel, and aluminum are examples of heavy metals that may be found in an occupational environment.[32] Information on chemical exposures may be obtained at the Agency for Toxic Substances and Disease Registry's website. An example of a chemical hazard in the workplace is beryllium, a metal naturally found in mineral rocks, coal, soil, and volcanic dust. Beryllium compounds are mined and purified for use in nuclear weapons and reactors, aircraft, satellites, and x-ray machines. Workers exposed to beryllium may develop an inflammatory respiratory condition known as chronic beryllium disease years after exposure. Lung cancer screening for these workers is also recommended because beryllium is a human carcinogen.[33]

> ▶ **SOLVING THE MYSTERY**
> ## The Case of the Toxic Exposure
> Public Health Science Topics Covered:
> - Screening
> - Surveillance
> - Environmental assessment
>
> Ken is a 45-year-old male working for a large manufacturing company that produces lead-acid storage batteries for electric automobiles. He works the night shift, sweeping floors and cleaning offices in the company's administration building. He arrives at the occupational health clinic at the end of his shift reporting persistent abdominal pain over the previous 6 weeks. During the clinical assessment, Ken also reports intermittent headaches, vomiting, and general fatigue. The occupational health physician requests a serum lead level to screen for lead toxicity. Ken ultimately is diagnosed with lead poisoning and an environmental assessment of the administration building is requested. The assessment finds no environmental lead present in the administration building. The clothing and shoes of plant employees are

screened for lead that could have been tracked into the administration building; no lead was found. The OEHN conducts an in-depth history to identify Ken's recreational activities. The OEHN learns that Ken goes to an indoor firing range on the weekends spending about 1 hour shooting his firearm at a target. When fired, bullets release lead particulates into the air that were likely inhaled by Ken leading to his lead toxicity. Because the toxicity was identified at work, Ken was entered into a lead exposure program where his lead levels will be monitored, and he will not be permitted to pick up extra shifts within the plant to prevent additional lead exposures. In addition, Ken was advised to switch to an outdoor shooting range where he can still enjoy his hobby while reducing his lead exposure.[34,35]

Pesticides

Migrant/seasonal farmworkers such as Juan and pest control workers are exposed to pesticides when they enter fields where pesticides have been applied or when they mix or apply them. Organophosphates, one type of pesticide, are powerful cholinesterase inhibitors. Cholinesterase is an enzyme important for the proper functioning of the nervous system in humans, other vertebrates, and insects.[36] Inhibition of this enzyme can cause a buildup of acetylcholine within nervous and skeletal smooth muscle systems, leading to signs and symptoms affecting the respiratory system, cardiovascular system, central nervous system, eyes, and skin.

Organic Solvents

Organic solvents (e.g., benzene, toluene, carbon disulfide, carbon tetrachloride, trichloroethylene or TCE) are volatile hydrocarbons found in a variety of industries. These chemicals are used in degreasing and dry-cleaning operations and in the manufacturing of paints, paint strippers, lacquers, rubber products, plastics, and textiles. Health effects of these agents include central and peripheral nervous system damage, kidney and liver damage, reproductive effects, as well as skin lesions and cancer. An example is benzene, a known carcinogen and product derived from coal and petroleum and found in gasoline. Chronic exposure to benzene affects bone marrow and blood production and can lead to leukemia. Short-term exposures may cause drowsiness, unconsciousness, dizziness, and death.[37]

Biological Exposures

Biological agents include bacteria, viruses, and other microorganisms that can be transmitted by air, food, water, soil, or direct contact.[38] Health-care providers in hospitals, clinics, and community health settings can be exposed to bloodborne pathogens such as HIV and hepatitis B and C. OSHA's Bloodborne Pathogen Standard, first introduced in the early 1990s, provides strict regulations for health-care settings to prevent and manage exposures by use of needleless devices, sharps containers, non-recapping of needles, and proper disposal of body fluids.

OSHA also provides guidelines for the protection of employees exposed to tuberculosis. Employees must have a respiratory protection program outlining when an employee needs to use a respirator as protection against tuberculosis, the proper selection and fit of respirators, fit testing and medical evaluation of workers who use respirators, and training for respirator use.[39] A respirator is a personal protective device (PPD) worn on the face and covers at least the nose and mouth. It is used to reduce the wearer's risk of inhaling hazardous airborne particles (including dust particles and infectious agents such as tuberculosis), gases, and vapors.[40] Prior to using a respirator, a worker must have a medical evaluation to ensure he or she is able to use the respirator; a fit test must be done to determine the proper dimensions of the respirator on the worker; and the worker must be trained in the proper use and handling of a respirator.

Biological exposures are common among workers who provide animal care in zoos, farms, or research facilities where studies are completed on animals such as rats, mice, and monkeys. Work in wet environments (such as chicken- or meat-processing facilities) may increase exposure to fungal diseases.

Psychological Exposures

Work has changed dramatically in the United States as a result of greater competition for goods and services. Globalization is increasing the speed and demand for products, and the information technology field has altered communication practices. Outsourcing of jobs to developing countries, layoffs, and downsizing have changed job security. These changing trends affect the physical and psychological well-being of workers, and outcomes may include hypertension, cardiovascular disease, gastrointestinal disease, substance use disorder, difficulty sleeping, workplace violence, hostility, depression, low productivity, and absenteeism.[41]

Job Stress

Job stress is the harmful physical and emotional response that occurs when the requirements of the job do not match the capabilities, resources, or needs of the worker.[22] Two job-stress models demonstrate strong associations between work stress and disease: the Demand Control

Model and the Effort-Reward-Imbalance Model. The Demand Control Model developed by Karasek and colleagues describes the relationship between job demands and job control.[42] The job demands variable examines the pace and intensity of work, and job control relates to the ability of the worker to direct and manage work. When work involves a high level of demand with low level of control, job strain can result in physiological and psychological changes in the worker, particularly increased cardiovascular disease risk.[42-44]

A third variable, social support at work, added to the Demand Control Model by Johnson and Hall, affirms that the level of job strain may be reduced by the protective effect of social support from coworkers and supervisors.[45] Examples of stressful situations include the employee in a supermarket who must check and bag groceries quickly and efficiently (high demand) under the watchful eye of a supervisor, who records the number of customers assisted without the development of long lines (control). Another example is the catalog "800" operator, who is recorded and timed for speed and courtesy when taking orders (high demand/low control).

A second work stress model, the Effort-Reward-Imbalance Model, builds on the concept of job demands and includes the amount of effort invested by a worker in the job.[46] It is hypothesized that the inequity of rewards contributes to negative mental health outcomes through a process of devaluation related to recognition, promotion, and job security.

To assist workers in coping with stressful conditions at work or within the family, workplaces may employ psychologists, social workers, counselors, or psychiatric-mental health clinical nurse specialists, or they may contract with an **employee assistance program (EAP)**.[47] The benefit of an EAP is it allows employees to discuss work, financial, or social issues in a confidential setting. EAPs also can refer workers for further evaluation and treatment by a licensed therapist (e.g., psychiatrist, psychiatric-mental nurse practitioner). Health promotion programs may assist the worker in coping with stressful situations by encouraging regular physical exercise, relaxation, or meditation to reduce workers' psychosocial stress.[48]

Routes of Exposure

There are three body systems that can serve as routes of exposure to hazardous substances found in the workplace:

- Respiratory system
- Integumentary system
- Gastrointestinal system

Inhalation of substances (i.e., gases, particles, carbon monoxide, solvents) into the lungs may cause local or systemic effects. The upper respiratory tract protects the lungs by filtering large particles in the nose and via the cilia, but respirable particles that range from 1 to 10 microns in diameter still can be inhaled into the lower respiratory tract. Factors that may increase the absorption of respirable particles include faster respiratory rate and greater depth of respiration.

Pesticides, solvents, and cleaning agents are examples of agents absorbed through inhalation as well as through the skin (dermatological absorption). Damage to the epidermis or exposure to a lipid soluble substance (solvent) increases absorption. Ingestion of particles into the gastrointestinal tract may occur by eating or smoking in the workplace. Providing a separate location for workers to consume meals and take breaks reduces this exposure. Although ingestion is the least common source of exposure, transfer of toxins by hand-to-mouth activity can be reduced by proper hand hygiene.

Controlling Hazards and Injuries in the Workplace

An effective OSH program can be accomplished by controlling hazards and preventing injuries in the workplace. Two strategies to achieve this goal are incorporating principles of ergonomics and adopting a **hierarchy of controls**.

Ergonomics

One approach to reducing injuries is to apply the field of **ergonomics**, which incorporates the science of biomechanics, to design work that is less demanding of a worker's joints, back, and muscles to prevent injury. An ergonomist designs the job to fit the worker, rather than physically forcing the worker's body to fit the job. There is increased ergonomic risk associated with jobs that require repetitive, forceful, or prolonged exertions of the hands; frequent heavy lifting, pushing, pulling, or carrying of heavy objects; or prolonged awkward postures. Workers with these types of jobs have a greater risk of developing musculoskeletal problems such as back pain, carpal tunnel syndrome, and tendonitis. Examples of workers who may have ergonomic risks are meat and poultry processors, grocery store checkout personnel, and nursing home staff whose jobs involve bathing, turning, and walking patients. Workstations, tools, and equipment can be adapted to fit the worker and reduce the physical stress on a worker's body. Additional examples of tasks that have ergonomic risks include the following:

- Lifting heavy or awkward items
- Placing or extracting items from high shelves
- Pushing or pulling heavy loads without assistance
- Being exposed to excessive vibration
- Using excessive force to perform tasks
- Repeating the same motion throughout the workday
- Working in awkward or stationary positions
- Maintaining the same posture for long periods of time
- Using the body or a body part to press against hard or sharp edges
- Cold temperatures
- Combined exposures to several risk factors[49]

In addition to chemical, psychological, and physical exposures for our case study individual, Juan, ergonomic issues also are of concern. Repeatedly lifting heavy baskets of fruits and vegetables can result in musculoskeletal problems, possibly leading to long-term problems.

Hierarchy of Controls

Occupational health providers can use a systematic process known as the hierarchy of controls to control workplace hazards. There are five levels of control: (1) elimination or substitution, (2) engineering controls, (3) warning, (4) administrative controls, and (5) PPE.[50]

The most effective level of control is the elimination or substitution of a hazardous material, task, or process. For example, benzene is an aromatic solvent used in many industrial products such as glues, paints, gasoline, and rubber, and can cause changes in the production of white cells in the bone marrow, leading to leukemia. Benzene can be eliminated by substituting toluene, a less toxic solvent.

If elimination or substitution is not possible, the next most effective strategy is the implementation of engineering controls. Isolation of a hazard is an example of an engineering control. For example, in the past, nurses at workstations without ventilation hoods mixed antineoplastic agents. Based on research findings that cited reproductive effects and recommendations from occupational safety and health engineers, these agents are now mixed in the pharmacy under properly ventilated hoods. An additional strategy is closed system transfer devices.[51]

A third-line strategy is providing warnings. OEHNs can coordinate with industrial hygienists to have warning signs placed in higher risk areas. For example, a yellow-taped walkway on the floor of a bottling plant can remind forklift operators of the potential for employees to be walking along a given path. Another example is a mandated sign that warns of radioactive exposures found in hospitals where radioactive isotopes or radiation producing machines are located.

Use of administrative controls is a fourth strategy of hazard control. Job rotation is an example of how one may reduce the overexposure of workers in the nuclear power industry to radiation. Hygienic work practices and good housekeeping, such as frequent floor washing in dust-producing industries, reduce the hazard of respirable particles from entering the air. The most important administrative control may be the training and education of workers, so they are knowledgeable about hazards present in the workplace. Educational materials must be culturally sensitive and produced at an appropriate cognitive and literacy level for workers. In addition, materials may need to be provided in multiple languages.

The least effective level of control, yet still important, involves the use of PPE. Hard hats, masks, respirators, gloves, hearing protection (ear muffs or ear plugs), gowns, metal-toed shoes, and headgear are examples of PPE. In the hierarchy of controls, PPE is least effective, primarily because worker compliance is difficult to ensure. Equipment may interfere with movement, hearing, and comfort, and may be cumbersome and hot if worn properly for 8 hours, leading workers to use PPE incorrectly or not at all. Therefore, close supervision of worker compliance with PPE and supervisors' role-modeling the use of PPE are important.

Workplace Assessment (Workplace Walkthrough)

As an OEHN, regularly scheduled assessments with members of the occupational health team are important. The purpose of the **workplace assessment** or **workplace walkthrough** is to observe the operations taking place in a facility, observe workers performing their jobs, identify the use of engineering controls, view the use of equipment (moving and stationary) in work areas, and observe the physical layout and cleanliness of the facility including locker rooms, hand-washing stations, changing facilities, and break and lunch rooms. During the walkthrough, the OEHN also should engage managers, supervisors, and individual workers in discussions about their work and safety and health issues.

● APPLYING PUBLIC HEALTH SCIENCE

The Case of the Pottery Factory Walkthrough

Public Health Science Topics Covered:

• Epidemiology and biostatistics

John is an OEHN at a large pottery-making facility with 452 workers. The building is located in a rural area and is the size of three football fields. It includes the kiln, storage space for sand and silica, machines for pottery production, paints and glazes, heavy equipment, workstations, and an inventory of finished pottery. The occupational health clinic is located in a separate administration building adjacent to the main facility.

As he walks through the plant on a beautiful summer day, John observes a truck being loaded with boxes of pottery. At the plant, the kiln is in use and the plant temperature is 91°F. Machines are mixing the clay, and workers are providing the materials for this process. (Many of the materials are stored in 50-pound bags.) The clay then is transferred to machines that form plates, cups, and other items, which then are stored on drying racks. Once the pottery is dry, small teams of four to six workers stand at a workstation and manually place handles on the cups or smooth the edges of the pottery to prepare the items for glazing. The last process he observes is the decoration of the pottery in a clean room where workers sit at large tables applying decals or painting the pottery with small brushes. As John walks through the plant, he observes continuous activity and notices that a pathway is painted to denote safe travel routes by machinery and walkers. Small electric carts transfer materials to workstations throughout the plant and honk their horns at workers on foot. The plant is noisy and not air conditioned; John can hear the loud ventilation system.

Production in this plant occurs around the clock. However, the night shift employs only 25 workers to repair equipment in the plant. Workers on the day and evening shifts are allowed 30 minutes for lunch or dinner and an additional 20-minute break.

Following the walkthrough, management requests John write a summary report of his findings (Box 20-4). The report would consist of a summary and recommendations regarding the strengths and weaknesses of the OSH program, medical surveillance, emergency response, and recordkeeping. It would be followed by an action plan for management.

A summary of John's report and action plan follows:

No obvious hazardous substances were identified. There is a risk that small molecules known as particulates are being released into the air during the manufacturing process of the pottery. Measurements need to be taken by the industrial hygienist to determine whether employees are inhaling the particulates. If particulates are found, masks will need to be fitted to and worn by workers to prevent the inhalation of particulates. Employees are at risk for low back injuries while lifting bags of pottery materials. Optimally, 25-pound bags will be purchased in the future. Workers with lifting responsibilities need to start an exercise program to strengthen their lower back muscles and undergo education on proper body mechanics when lifting to prevent a lower back injury. The industrial hygienist also needs to take noise measurements to determine whether the noise is excessive and places workers at risk for noise-induced hearing loss. Based on literature reported on by the OEHN, 72% of all hearing-related illnesses occur in the manufacturing sector, so a hearing protection program may need to be implemented.[52]

BOX 20–4 ■ Guide to Preparing Workplace Assessment Report

The OEHN report needs to address the following questions:

1. What are the hazardous exposures (physical, biological, chemical, and psychosocial) present in the worksite?
2. What are the specific mechanisms of exposure (inhalation, ingestion, dermal) in the worksite?
3. What physical and chemical exposures should be evaluated by the occupational/environmental hygienist who accompanied the OEHN on the walkthrough?
4. What types of accidents and injuries would the OEHN anticipate in this worksite? What are the potential causes?
5. Are hierarchies of control followed in this worksite? What PPEs are appropriate?
6. What is the level of housekeeping within the worksite? (For example, are floors wet or cluttered? Are there other fall hazards?)
7. Are workers provided training and information regarding the hazards of their work? Do employees demonstrate the safety practices they received training on?

Occupational and Environmental History

Another tool used by the OEHN is a comprehensive **occupational and environmental health history**. An occupational nurse practitioner or physician conducts a history and physical assessment on an employee after a formal offer of employment is made. The results of this assessment are reviewed by the OEHN. The objective of the assessment and history is to identify factors that would increase the health or safety risk of the new employee in performing the new job. Findings from the assessment and history may require work accommodations and/or further physical exam and screenings. For example, a new employee who worked in a plant assembling small toys by hand for the past 15 years is at risk for carpal tunnel syndrome. Further assessment of carpal tunnel syndrome and job rotation may be necessary to prevent the onset or worsening of the disorder. The health history must remain confidential and accessible only to the occupational health team.

To perform an adequate history, the OEHN needs a formal job description that identifies the job tasks required of the employee and the job exposures that the worker will have. A careful analysis of the job description and the worker's capabilities and current health status facilitates the proper placement of the new employee. For example, an individual who had a prior back injury should not be placed in a position requiring heavy lifting. An individual with well-controlled diabetes may not do well with frequent alternating shift work. An individual with cardiovascular disease should avoid work in confined spaces as well as exposure to carbon monoxide and solvents. When a worker returns to work after an injury or the diagnosis and treatment of an acute or chronic disease, a new history and assessment are necessary to determine fitness for duty and the potential need for accommodation.

Key components of the history are:

- Review of systems
- Personal and family health history
- Psychosocial history
- Past medical history
- List of hobbies

Following the occupational history, a licensed occupational health practitioner performs a physical assessment. Specialized exams may be required for different job descriptions. For example, if a worker drives trucks across the country, the Department of Transportation requires an annual exam that includes an audiometric exam, vision testing, depth perception, a complete blood count, blood chemistry, urine drug screening, and electrocardiogram.

Finally, when the history and physical exam are completed, a discussion of the results with the employee should occur and recommendations regarding safety and health practices should be provided. The new employee should be encouraged to use the resources provided by the occupational health program to maintain, protect, and promote his/her health during employment.

Vulnerable Workers

With the increasing diversity in the U.S. workforce, not everyone goes to work healthy, not everyone goes to work free of stress, and not everyone goes to work in a friendly, accepting environment. Certain **vulnerable worker populations** may be affected by demographic, social, physical, psychological, and economic factors that lead to potential susceptibility and health disparities in the workplace.

● APPLYING PUBLIC HEALTH SCIENCE

The Case of Adolescent Workers

Public Health Science Topics Covered:

- Social sciences

Stephen is a 17-year-old employed by a heavy equipment rental agency on weekends. He is a reliable and hard-working adolescent, and his employer regularly requests him to return equipment to the storage lot and to service and prepare it for re-rental. At times, Stephen also drives large tractors and feels privileged to be given the responsibility to do so. Two questions to think about in this case are: Is Stephen's employer compliant with the Fair Labor Standards Act (FLSA), and what developmental issues should the employer consider when assigning Stephen to these more complex tasks?

Adolescence is commonly the first time an individual becomes employed, unless he or she works on a family farm or for a family business. The U.S. Congress passed the FLSA in 1938, which governs the number of hours an adolescent can work and what types of jobs adolescent workers can safely perform.[53] Despite these regulations, approximately 70 adolescents die every year in work-related situations, which are the result of adolescents performing tasks not in compliance with the FLSA, including operating hazardous equipment, such as motor vehicles or meat slicers; working late at night or alone; handling hot liquids and grease; and lifting heavy objects.[54,55] In Stephen's case, is his employer compliant with the FLSA? In actuality, this type of work is considered hazardous work and restricted by the FLSA until a worker is 18 years old.

A cross-sectional study conducted by Runyan and colleagues documented risks to adolescents that included exposures to chemical, physical, and biological agents.[56] Of note in this study are significant findings related to noncompliance with the use of PPE, even after work orientation and training of the adolescents.[57] In general, adolescents are employed in part-time, temporary, low-paying jobs in the service sector. As new workers, they often are inexperienced, unfamiliar with job tasks, lack knowledge of workplace hazards, and frequently unaware of their rights as workers. Assessment of the physical characteristics of an adolescent is an important consideration, because growth spurts occur between the ages of 14 and 17, especially among males. Taller and more muscular males may be given adult tasks with minimal regard to experience or maturity. The common psychological characteristics of the adolescent include enthusiasm; however, a sense of invulnerability may increase the risk for injury. Communication skills and self-esteem also may be underdeveloped, and interactions with customers and supervisors may be challenging.[58,59] Stephen's physical size, coordination, sense of invulnerability, and responsible demeanor may give his employer a false sense of security. Stephen may not have the skills and decision-making ability to work with heavy equipment, even though it may seem like an exciting opportunity to him.

The benefits of employment for adolescents include the development of self-reliance, self-esteem, and discipline as well as organizational and communication skills. However, research by educators has demonstrated that negative effects occur when an adolescent works more than 20 hours per week and has less time for participation in extracurricular school activities and limited time for interaction with peers and family activities.[60] Educators also have found work among adolescents leads to fatigue and inadequate time for completion of homework.[58]

It has been documented that working adolescents may not enroll in rigorous courses such as math and science because busy work schedules or long work hours may result in absenteeism. Increased disposable income may promote the use of alcohol, illicit drugs, and smoking.

Exposures to hazardous agents (e.g., carcinogens, noise, or heavy physical labor) early in life may have acute or long-term (latent) effects on disease development later in life. For the OEHN, communicating with employers, parents, school personnel, and the teen can facilitate education and training of working adolescents. OSHA developed a website for teen workers that promotes safety and health and provides information regarding hazards, PPE, and details of the FLSA.[58]

Older Adults in the Workforce

The baby boomer generation, those individuals born between 1946 and 1964, are contributing to the aging pool of workers. The healthy lifestyles of many of these workers has improved life expectancy and extended working life. The trend of working beyond age 65 years also is influenced by the 1983 Social Security Amendment, which raised the full retirement age (eligibility for 100% Social Security benefits) beginning with individuals born in 1938 or later. For example, an individual born in 1960 would not be eligible for full Social Security retirement until age 67.[61,62]

Older workers may be motivated to remain employed due to various factors such as financial need, family responsibilities, a sense of job satisfaction and purpose, productivity, social engagement, and ability to use skills and knowledge developed over the years. Alternatively, an individual with fewer years of education may select retirement at an earlier age because they began working in their early teens and twenties and have saved for retirement. A physically demanding job (such as construction, mining, or farming) also may have resulted in musculoskeletal injury or the development of a chronic disease that stimulates early retirement.[63]

The physical and psychological changes that occur with the aging process may have an impact on the duration of work life, such as decreased physical strength, endurance, balance, visual acuity, and hearing ability; loss of flexibility; and reduced aerobic capacity and immune response.[64] In addition to the normal anatomical and physiological changes of aging, older workers may have a chronic disease as a result of their past work exposures or lifestyle behaviors, which may limit their employment opportunities. Older workers may be more vulnerable to falls and trauma. Frequently among injured older workers, recovery time for an injury is lengthened, and return to work is delayed. The OEHN needs to assess the risk of injury and recommend ergonomic changes that adjust the work environment to the aging worker's capability, such as the use of adjustable-height work benches, reducing need to lift objects, and eliminating repetitive tasks and use of force.[65]

Enrollment of older workers in fitness programs preserves and builds muscle strength, prevents loss of bone density, and improves aerobic capacity and cardiopulmonary function. Workplace health promotion programs can provide nutrition education, weight control instructions, stress management, and risk factor reduction guidelines for cardiovascular disease and diabetes.[66]

Women in the Workforce

Approximately 51% of workers in the United States are women, of whom 75% work full-time. Median earnings of women are gradually increasing; however, on average their salaries are 80% of a man's earnings. The number of working women with college degrees has more than tripled since 1970, allowing women to enter professional and management positions.[67] The majority of women are employed in the service and health-care sectors, where multiple hazards exist, including ergonomic (lifting), chemical (antineoplastics, anesthetic gases, latex), biological agent (bloodborne pathogens), and psychosocial hazards (stress, violence).

As women have entered nontraditional employment, such as construction, engineering, and forestry, their vulnerability to injury has increased. PPE is often designed for the average-sized man, so fit of the equipment often becomes an issue for women workers. In addition, a woman's total body strength is generally two-thirds of a man's (being lower than a man's in the upper extremities and similar to a man's in the lower extremities), placing many women workers at risk for musculoskeletal injuries. Women workers are often employed in sedentary jobs with computer and keyboarding responsibilities. Proper ergonomic assessment of a workstation and encouraging physical activity during the workday can prevent musculoskeletal and repetitive motion disorders.[68] Social stressors such as sexual harassment and gender-based discrimination may exist causing additional problems.

Finally, as with all workers, the **work-family interface** must be considered. Women workers, in particular, remain the predominant individuals balancing work and family life. As such, shift work, weekend work, and the total number of hours worked frequently present challenges. Women may also need an opportunity to express breast milk following the birth of a child.

Fair Labor Standard Act (FLSA) Regarding Workers Who Are Nursing [69]

"Section 7 of the FLSA requires employers to provide reasonable break time for an employee to express breast milk for her nursing child for 1 year after the child's birth each time such employee has need to express the milk. Employers are also required to provide a place, other than a bathroom, that is shielded from view and free from intrusion from coworkers and the public, which may be used by an employee to express breast milk."

Members in the Workforce With a Disability

The Americans with Disabilities Act (ADA) of 1990 (amended in 2008) is landmark legislation that prohibits workplace discrimination of a qualified individual with a **disability**.[70] The ADA has promoted the hiring of individuals with disabilities and mandated accommodations for disabled workers. The ADA defines disability using three criteria.[70] First, there must be a physical or mental impairment that substantially limits one or more major life activities of such individual. For example, military personal returning from war may have one or more amputated extremities that prevent them from performing activities of daily living independently. Second, there needs to be a record of such impairment. Records can be obtained from the worker's personal physician, nurse practitioner, or from a state agency that certified the disability. Third, the person needs to be regarded as having impairment, meaning that the disability would affect the person's ability to perform a job without accommodation.

According to the U.S. Bureau of Labor Statistics, approximately 6.2 million people with disabilities were employed in 2017.[71] These workers represent about 4% of the employed population and are employed predominately in the service sector and in professional occupations.

Work eligibility for an individual with a disability is defined as the ability to perform the essential functions of the job. These functions must be defined by each workplace and be on record. After a job offer is made, a disabled individual may request accommodations from the employer. Examples include job restructuring, so that long periods of standing do not occur, or the provision of a large computer monitor for an individual with visual impairments. The ADA also provides for workers who become disabled during the course of employment, after which the worker may request an accommodation (e.g., change in hours worked).

A primary role of the OEHN is to support an individual with a disability to maintain work and to assist the worker who has developed an acute or chronic injury or illness to return to work. Assessing the social, demographic, occupational, clinical, and psychological factors unique to the worker will facilitate the maintenance of employment. For example, an individual with diabetes and hypertension recovering from a myocardial infarction may need an accommodation to participate in a cardiac rehabilitation program. A worker may require assistance with lifting and walking duties following a hip replacement, or a worker with a leg thrombosis might be allowed to telecommute 2 to 3 days per week to reduce commuting time.

Immigrant or Foreign-Born Persons in the Work Force

In 2017, the U.S. labor force included 27.4 million immigrant workers who made up 17.1% of the labor force.[72] These workers are predominately men and foreign born (47.9% Hispanic and 25.2% Asian). In addition, immigrant workers earned about 18% less than native-born workers, and about 21.8% of these workers are not high school graduates.

Individuals and families migrate for many reasons: to provide a better life for their family, escape war, seek political asylum, or to obtain a job as a scientist or health-care provider. Approximately 22.6% of working immigrant men work in agricultural, construction, or maintenance jobs, and 33.1% of working immigrant women are employed in service sector occupations (hotel workers, cooks, servers, dry-cleaning workers). These workers are a vital part of the labor force in the United States, although there has been a trend toward returning to Mexico during periods of U.S. economic decline and violence toward immigrants.[73]

As members of the U.S. labor force, immigrant workers often have physically demanding jobs that expose them to hazards such as pesticides, cleaning agents, farm animals, infectious diseases, or excessive heat or cold, which place them in jeopardy of sustaining poisonings, disease, and physical injuries.[74] In general, immigrants are poorly paid, and many live below the poverty level. For further investigation of the factors that influence immigration, see the U.S. Department of State, U.S. Citizenship and Immigration Services, and the U.S. Department of Labor websites. Having the knowledge to assist immigrants with the basic needs of shelter, food, health care, and employment helps with major issues related to this worker population.

■ CULTURAL CONTEXT

There are special considerations for OEHNs when working at organizations employing immigrants. First, safety and health outreach training programs need to comply with OSHA standards for immigrant workers. Outreach training programs educate workers on their rights and responsibilities for helping create a safe

workplace.[75] Programs also show workers how to file complaints. Education and signage in the workplace need to be provided in the native languages of workers for whom English is a second language. In addition, any education and signage should be culturally appropriate. Assessment of understanding may need to be conducted through the use of interpreters, language phone lines, written or oral surveys written in the workers' native languages, and observation of adherence to safe work practices. Ideally, bilingual coworkers will conduct education and on-the-job training.

Minority Members in the Workforce

In general, workers of minority, ethnic, and racial populations are disproportionally exposed to poor working conditions, limited health-care access, and reduced career opportunities.[76] Factors associated with such disadvantages include lack of educational and economic opportunities as well as the unfortunate persistence of discriminatory practices by some employers. There are greater proportions of minority workers in some of the most dangerous industries, such as construction and agriculture, where there is a heavy reliance on the labor of recent immigrants. Additionally, there are several historical and current examples of manufacturing settings that pose greater risks to minority worker populations. Examples from the past include textile factories in which cotton dust caused increased rates of byssinosis in workers who were primarily African-American, and uranium mining, which placed Native American miners at risk for pulmonary cancer.

Even within a single industry, it is often the minority workers who hold the dirtiest, highest risk jobs. An example comes from the hospitality industry, a work setting that may not immediately come to mind as one risky to a worker's health. But if one looks at the demographic distribution of hotel workers by job title, minority workers are overrepresented in the lowest paid jobs with the highest exposures to hazards. The tasks of a hotel housekeeper include handling trash and working with cleaning products as well as the ergonomic stressors of lifting, bending, and working in awkward postures to change linen and exposure to marijuana smoke.[77] Furthermore, these job activities must be carried out under working conditions that impose even more stress—time pressures related to meeting quotas, questionable social support, and threatened job security—with little power to advocate for an improved working environment.[77]

Workers of minority groups also are disproportionately represented among those unable to find employment. The unemployment rates in the United States vary: 6.5% for African Americans, 4.6% for Hispanics, 3.5% for whites, and 3.2% for Asians.[78] There is a clear need to promote fair employment practices and safe and equitable working conditions for all who are eligible to be part of the workforce.

Roles of the OEHN

Occupational Disease Surveillance

The OEHN has important responsibilities for assessing, monitoring, and providing surveillance for occupational diseases. A working knowledge of **toxicology**, "the study of harmful effects of substances on humans or animals", and the common diseases unique to the specific occupational health settings are essential.[79] Tables 20-1 and 20-2 provide descriptions of common occupational and environmental exposures, the organ systems affected, signs and symptoms, and diseases caused by these agents. Latent and long-term effects of these exposures and the organ systems involved are described.

Preventing Injuries and Fatalities

Approximately 3.9 million workers are injured on the job annually and about 12 to 13 workers die each day as a result of traumatic injuries they have sustained.[80] More than 2 million of these injuries require a job transfer, work restriction, or time away from the job. Among all workers, 2.6 million are treated in emergency departments annually, and approximately 110,000 of these workers are hospitalized. Fatalities among workers result from transportation incidents, contact with objects and equipment, assaults and violent acts, falls, and exposure to harmful substances or environments.

Figure 20-1 displays the causes of nonfatal injuries in the private industry in 2011 and shows that the leading sectors where injuries occur are manufacturing, health care, the retail trade, and construction. In Figure 20-2, fatal work injuries are described by cause, with transportation incidents being the highest source of fatality.

Case Management

Case management is an approach to managing health care in a cost-effective manner.[81] After an employee is injured or recovering from an acute or chronic

TABLE 20–1 ■ Examples of Occupational Exposures and Effects

Symptoms and Diseases	Agent	Potential Exposures
Immediate or Short-Term Effects		
Dermatoses (allergic or irritant)	Metals (chromium, nickel), fibrous glass, solvents, caustic alkali, soaps	Electroplating, metal cleaning, plastics, machining, leather tanning, housekeeping
Headache	Carbon monoxide, solvents	Firefighting, automobile exhaust, wood finishing, dry cleaning
Acute psychoses	Lead, mercury, carbon disulfide	Removing paint from old houses, fungicide, wood preserving, viscose rayon industry
Asthma or dry cough	Formaldehyde, toluene diisocyanate, animal dander	Textiles, plastics, polyurethane kits, lacquer, animal handling
Pulmonary edema, pneumonitis	Nitrogen oxides, phosgene, halogen gases, cadmium	Welding, farming, chemical operations, smelting
Cardiac arrhythmias	Solvents, fluorocarbons	Metal cleaning, solvent use, refrigerator maintenance
Angina	Carbon monoxide, methylene chloride	Car repair, traffic exhaust, foundry, wood finishing
Abdominal pain	Lead	Battery making, enameling, smelting, painting, welding, ceramics, plumbing
Hepatitis (may become a long-term effect)	Halogenated hydrocarbons (e.g., carbon tetrachloride)	Solvents use, lacquer use, hospital workers

Continued

TABLE 20–1 ■ Examples of Occupational Exposures and Effects—cont'd

Symptoms and Diseases	Agent	Potential Exposures
Latent or Long-Term Effects		
Chronic dyspnea, pulmonary fibrosis	Asbestos, silica, beryllium, coal, aluminum	Mining, insulation, pipefitting, sandblasting, quarrying, metal alloy work, aircraft or electrical parts
Chronic bronchitis, emphysema	Cotton dust, cadmium, coal dust, organic solvents, cigarettes	Textile industry, battery production, soldering, mining, solvent use
Lung cancer	Asbestos, arsenic, nickel, uranium, coke oven emissions	Insulation, pipefitting, smelting, coke ovens, shipyard workers, nickel refining, uranium mining
Bladder cancer	β-naphthylamine, benzidine dyes	Dye industry, leather, rubber-workers, chemists
Peripheral neuropathy	Lead, arsenic, hexane, methyl butyl ketone, acrylamide	Battery production, plumbing, smelting, painting, shoemaking, solvent use, insecticides
Behavioral changes	Lead, carbon disulfide, solvents, mercury, manganese	Battery makers, smelting, viscose rayon industry, degreasing, manufacture/repair of scientific instruments, dental amalgam workers
Extrapyramidal syndrome	Carbon disulfide, manganese	Viscose rayon industry, steel production, battery production, foundry
Aplastic anemia, leukemia	Benzene, ionizing radiation	Chemists, furniture refinishing, cleaning, degreasing, radiation workers

Source: Adapted from the Agency for Toxic Substances and Disease Registry. (2008). *Case studies in environmental medicine: Taking an exposure history.* Retrieved from http://www.atsdr.cdc.gov/csem/exphistory/docs/exposure_history.pdf

TABLE 20–2 ■ Organ Systems Often Affected by Toxic Exposure

Organ/System	Exposure Risks
Respiratory	Asbestos, radon, cigarette smoke, glues
Skin	Dioxin, nickel, arsenic, mercury, cement (chromium), polychlorinated biphenyls (PCBs), glues, rubber cement
Liver	Carbon tetrachloride, methylene chloride, vinyl chloride
Kidney	Cadmium, lead, mercury, chlorinated hydrocarbon solvents
Cardiovascular	Carbon monoxide, noise, tobacco smoke, physical stress, carbon disulfide, nitrates, methylene chloride
Reproductive	Lead, carbon disulfide, methylmercury, ethylene dibromide
Hematological	Arsenic, benzene, nitrates, radiation
Neuropsychological	Tetrachloroethylene, mercury, arsenic, toluene, lead, methanol, noise, vinyl chloride

Source: Adapted from the Agency for Toxic Substances and Disease Registry. (2008). *Case studies in environmental medicine: Taking an exposure history.* Retrieved from http://www.atsdr.cdc.gov/csem/exphistory/docs/exposure_history.pdf

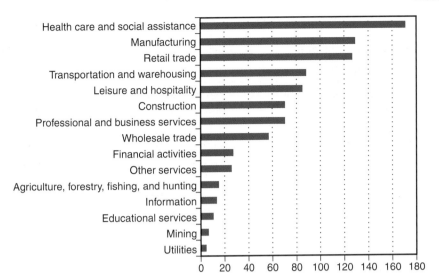

Figure 20-1 Number of nonfatal occupational injuries and illnesses involving days away from work in the private industry (in thousands). *(Data from the Bureau of Labor Statistics, U.S. Department of Labor. [2012, November 8]. News release: Nonfatal occupational injuries and illnesses requiring days away from work, 2011. Retrieved from* http://www.bls.gov/news.release/archives/osh2_11082012.pdf*)*

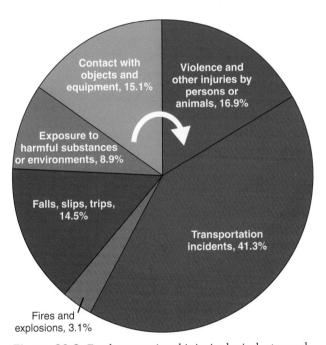

Figure 20-2 Fatal occupational injuries by industry and event or exposure, all U.S., 2011 (total 4,693). *(Data from Bureau of Labor Statistics, U.S. Department of Labor. [2013, April 25]. Fatal occupational injuries by industry and event or exposure, all U.S., 2011. Retrieved from* http://www.bls.gov/iif/oshwc/cfoi/cftb0259.pdf*)*

disease, some OEHNs will assume a case management role in assessing the worker's disability and rehabilitation needs to promote a return to work or will coordinate with a case management vendor. The case manager assists with the transition from hospital to home and works with the employee, family members, and rehabilitation specialists (if applicable) in the coordination of the employee's successful return to work. Additional case management services include arranging transport, providing health education, ordering durable medical equipment, and making referrals and recommendations for care. The care manager also works with employers to arrange for modified duty if approved by treating provider for work restrictions.

Workers' Compensation

Workers' compensation provides income benefits, medical payments, and rehabilitation payments to workers injured on the job, as well as benefits to surviving families of fatally injured workers. Workers' compensation laws are considered to be no-fault laws. Because these laws ensure employees who suffer injuries or fatalities as a result of work are provided fixed monetary awards, they eliminate the ability for employees to sue employers for pain and suffering, even if the employer was negligent.[82] However, not all injuries may be identified in workers' compensation laws and some may require filing suit to determine reasonable compensation. Each state workers' compensation law regulates the amount and duration of compensation for workers injured or who die. In general, most state workers' compensation laws cover medical expenses related to a disability and the cost of job retraining following an injury. A disabled worker receives two-thirds of the normal monthly salary during the disability and may receive more salary for permanent physical injuries, or if the worker has dependents.[83] The act provides compensation for survivors of employees who die. Although workers' compensation laws are complex, OEHN case managers frequently assist injured workers and families in negotiating the laws.

Workplace Health Promotion

Health promotion programs in the workplace are designed to identify and prevent both occupational and nonoccupational disease and injury, and to educate workers about behaviors that influence health and wellness. The goals of health promotion are designed to:

- Reduce absenteeism
- Increase productivity
- Sustain or increase the level of well-being, self-actualization, and personal fulfillment of a given worker or worker group

The OEHN plays an important role in initiating, conducting, and evaluating health promotion programs. Both employees and employers derive benefits from participation in and initiation of a health promotion program, including:

- Reduction in health-care costs and improved injury care
- Increased productivity
- Reduced absenteeism and presenteeism
- Improved sense of well-being among workers
- Improved impression of management as proactive and invested in workers[84]

The number of health promotion programs being developed by corporations and industries has grown considerably. This increase is believed to be associated with the rising cost of health benefits and services that employer-based health-care programs have experienced over the past decade. Many of these programs are designed to manage noncommunicable health conditions that workers may bring to the workplace. It also is important to educate employers that the top reasons leading to mortality (cardiovascular, cancers, cerebrovascular, chronic respiratory, and unintentional injuries) are preventable and responsive to behavior change.[85,86]

The workplace provides a stable and captive audience (workers) for health promotion programs. In addition, the workplace can serve as a source of coworker and supervisor social support for positive behavior change.[87] The CDC's report *The National Healthy Worksite Program* strongly asserts that reducing morbidity associated with behavioral and biological risk factors is a public health priority for the country.[88] The majority of studies completed to date show positive health and financial impacts of worksite health promotion programs over the past 3 decades.[89-91]

■ EVIDENCE-BASED PRACTICE
Assaults by Patients/Visitors Against Health-Care Workers

Registered nurses and other health-care workers are at increased risk for being assaulted while performing their work.[1] These exposures to physical violence impact the physical and mental health of workers as well as their ability to practice safely.

Practice Statement: Health-care workers need to be proactive with their efforts to prevent assaults.

Targeted Outcome: Prevent and mitigate acts of workplace violence (i.e., assaults) as they occur without experiencing personal physical or emotional injuries.

Supporting Evidence: Health-care workers experience approximately half of all occupational assaults.[1] Factors associated with this workplace violence include providing care to persons with a history of violence against others or under the influence of drugs or alcohol, working alone or understaffed, working in settings with inadequate security or prolonged wait times, and believing that violence is part of the job. The primary prevention of assaults can be attempted through de-escalation; however, efforts are not always successful. When assaults do occur, health-care workers have reported somatic complaints, posttraumatic stress symptoms, and decreased work productivity.[2,3]

Recommended Approaches: The OEHN needs to design, modify, implement, and evaluate a workplace violence prevention program. Key components of the program need to include management commitment and employee participation, worksite analysis, hazard prevention and control, safety and health training, and recordkeeping and program evaluation. Specific strategies within these components will vary by work setting. For example, management commitment and employee participation in the home health-care setting could be operationalized through a workplace violence safety committee. The manager would convene the initial committee and turn over responsibilities to the committee members while providing sufficient resources based upon members' requests. Membership on the committee can include nurses, physicians, chaplains, social workers, patient care assistants, physical therapists, patients, and other key stakeholders responsible for the delivery of home health care.

References:

1. Occupational Safety and Health Administration, U.S. Department of Labor. (2016). *Guidelines for preventing workplace violence for healthcare and social service workers*

(OSHA Publication No. 3148-06R). Washington, DC: Author.

2. Gillespie, G.L., Bresler, S., Gates, D.M., & Succop, P. (2013). Posttraumatic stress symptomatology in emergency department workers following workplace aggression. *Workplace Health & Safety, 61*(6), 247-254.

3. Gillespie, G.L., Gates, D.M., Kowalenko, T., Bresler, S., & Succop, P. (2014). Implementation of a comprehensive intervention to reduce physical assaults and threats in the emergency department. *Journal of Emergency Nursing, 40*(6), 586-591.

A **health risk appraisal (HRA)** is frequently the initial component of many successful health promotion programs in the workplace. HRAs are questionnaires completed by employees to assess personal health habits and behavioral risk factors, such as smoking, alcohol, or seat belt use. An individual's actual age is compared with an estimate of their risk age, an overall measure of risk for morbidity and mortality as identified by epidemiological research. An example of an individual with a decreased risk age is one who maintains a healthy body mass index, exercises regularly, does not smoke tobacco products, drinks moderately, and complies with an age-appropriate screening schedule as defined by a health-care provider. A worker with an increased risk age may not exercise, is overweight, drives without a seat belt, and does not have a health provider. If a worker is identified with a high-risk age, and he or she incorporates healthy lifestyle behavior changes, such as physical exercise or weight reduction, a reduced risk age could be achieved. It is essential that the HRA results be communicated to employees by the OEHN. The worker with the reduced risk age should be commended and encouraged to maintain a healthy lifestyle. The worker at increased risk will need a health assessment, education, and counseling to assist with behavior change, if desired.[92] Effective workplace health promotion programs require a strong leadership and management team committed to initiating an effective, evidence-based educational program focused on an individual or worker group. Resources to run an effective program, educators, incentives, and equipment also are essential. Finally, outcome evaluations of the efficacy of the program must be conducted.[92]

Because the occupational health provider is working with adult learners, several important concepts should be considered:[93,94]

- Respect during the learning experience should be demonstrated to workers.

- Provide opportunities for workers to be actively engaged in their learning.
- Incorporate workers' previous experiences into the context of the health promotion activities.
- Apply the learning to the self-identified needs of the workers.
- Be present during learning encounters through active listening and change talk.
- Provide programming in a setting that accommodates the schedule of the worker and eliminates distractions.
- Repeat important content to facilitate learning.
- Present information from the simple to the complex, and pace the content appropriately with examples.

● APPLYING PUBLIC HEALTH SCIENCE
The Case of the Ethical Dilemma
Public Health Science Topics Covered:
- Health service systems

Jorge is a 45-year-old man with a history of diabetes, cardiovascular disease, and obesity. He was recently hospitalized for a myocardial infarction. During his return-to-work assessment, the occupation physician instructed Jorge to begin light exercise daily and start a low-fat, low salt, 2,000 calorie per day diet. Jorge comes to the OEHN clinic for guidance on exercise and diet. The OEHN negotiates with the plant manager to allow Jorge to return from his lunch period 20 minutes late each day so he can walk on the trail next to the plant. Jorge also is permitted to be "on the clock" during his walks. Several times during the past week, the OEHN sees Jorge sitting on a bench playing games on his telephone and not walking.

- What is the ethical dilemma posed in this case study?
- What options does the OEHN have to resolve this dilemma?
- What is the best option? Provide a rationale for this option.

OEHNs have a responsibility to their employers to manage employees' illnesses and injuries while reducing overall health-care expenditures. Once the OEHN becomes aware that Jorge is not using the time away from the plant as agreed to by Jorge and the plant manager, the OEHN has a responsibility to notify the plant manager. Prior to notifying the plant manager, the OEHN reviews the American Association of Occupational Health Nurses' Code of Ethics and Interpretive Statements. The code has six principles: (1) right of self-determination,

(2) confidentiality, (3) truth-telling, (4) doing or producing good, (5) avoiding harm, and (6) fair and nondiscriminatory treatment.[11] The OEHN realizes there is an ethical dilemma resulting from being aware that Jorge is not taking the walks. The dilemma results from the employer's right to cancel the walk periods if they are not being used appropriately and Jorge's rights to self-determination and confidentiality.

The OEHN considers several options in this case. First, the OEHN could notify the employer that Jorge is not taking the walks. This option violates Jorge's confidentiality. Second, the OEHN could follow Jorge to the walking trail daily and instruct him that he needs to take the walk. This option violates Jorge's right of self-determination. Third, the OEHN could meet with Jorge in the clinic and discuss the current treatment and options. The third option is chosen by the OEHN. During the discussion, the OEHN asks Jorge about his adherence and barriers to walking each day while at work. The OEHN openly shares the rationale for the conversation: They are talking precisely because the OEHN saw him sitting on a bench and not walking. Speaking privately with Jorge also provides for his confidentiality. A new treatment plan is devised that allows for Jorge's right of self-determination. Jorge reports it is too hot for him in the afternoon to walk. He has agreed to arrive to work early and take his walk before his shift starts. The OEHN will follow up with him in 2 weeks to evaluate his progress.

Emerging Issues in Occupational Health

Emerging issues in occupational health highlight the need for the OEHN to remain current and knowledgeable about the ever-changing trends in the field. OEHNs can remain up to date on emergency issues by joining professional societies, belonging to occupational-focused online mailing lists, and attending professional conferences dedicated to emerging issues in occupational health. Following the next case study, two significant issues for the future are discussed.

● APPLYING PUBLIC HEALTH SCIENCE
The Case of Popcorn Lung
Public Health Science Topics Covered:
- Epidemiology and biostatistics

Many people like eating microwave popcorn when watching movies at home. Most people would never consider that the flavoring in their microwave popcorn has made some workers very sick. In 2000, the Missouri Department of Health and Senior Services received a report about eight cases of lung disease in workers who had formerly all worked in the same microwave popcorn factory between 1992 and 2000. Four of these workers were on waiting lists for lung transplants.[95] After a Health Hazard Investigation by NIOSH, it was determined that the fixed obstructive lung disease, or bronchiolitis obliterans (BO), was caused by exposure to the food flavoring diacetyl.

Diacetyl is a water-soluble di-ketone found naturally in butter, coffee, wine, and beer. The chemical diacetyl has butter-flavored characteristics and is used in candies, pastries, and frozen foods. The problem occurs in the manufacturing of the microwave popcorn, because diacetyl easily vaporizes when heated. The workers with the highest rates of BO were the mixers and microwave-packaging workers. The mixers worked around large mixing tanks where visible dust, aerosols, and vapors were produced. The microwave packers worked within 5 to 30 meters from the mixing tanks. On inspection, NIOSH required both groups of workers to use respirators leading to improvements in their lung function.[95,96] In December 2003, a NIOSH alert was sent to more than 4,000 businesses that use food flavorings in their manufacturing processes, advising employers to reduce vapors in the mixing room and warn workers of the hazard.[97]

Emergency Preparedness and Disaster Management

Frequently, a business will ask its OEHN to prepare an emergency response plan to respond to human-created and natural disasters. In large corporations, a committee that includes the OEHN as well as management, human resources, safety officers, security, and other support services staff usually does this planning. Whether the OEHN works at a large company or small business, emergency preparedness or "all hazards" preparedness is a continuous and coordinated process that must be constantly evaluated and redefined as needed to ensure the safety of the workforce in case of a disaster.[98]

Knowledge of the five components of disaster preparedness is an essential element for planning a disaster response. Four of the five components include (1) preparedness (occurs pre-impact and is a proactive process for putting in place the structure needed for a disaster response); (2) mitigation (primarily occurs during the pre-impact phase as a means to limit adverse effects of the disaster; (3) response (activation of the various procedures planned prior to the event); and (4) recovery (stabilizing the community through both reconstruction and rehabilitation) (Chapter 22).[99] The following questions serve to provide basic assessment information:

- How will the OEHN communicate with onsite and offsite employees?
- Are there employees with disabilities, and what are their needs in an emergency situation?
- What types of emergency supplies are needed and for what period of time?
- If everyone must leave the site, how will the OEHN evacuate the area?
- If it is necessary for everyone to shelter in place, what supplies are needed to accommodate everyone?
- Are fire plans up to date?
- Is the OEHN prepared for all types of medical emergencies?
- Has the OEHN coordinated plans with other businesses and residents in the area?

The fifth component is evaluation. At the conclusion of a disaster event, it is critical to conduct a formal evaluation to identify areas for further improvement and preparedness prior to another disaster.

An OEHN should review and evaluate an emergency preparedness plan at least once every year and ensure employees' families have a plan for their home. The OEHN also will consult and coordinate with local emergency medical services that will assume the role of incident command upon their arrival. It is often necessary for employees to remain at the worksite as a result of an emergency, and fear for the location of and safety of family members is often of concern. Another important component of the disaster is the psychological effect that each employee may experience, and awareness that symptoms of acute anxiety and posttraumatic stress may be outcomes for workers providing disaster care to victims. The U.S. Federal Emergency Management Association offers a comprehensive guide for businesses that want to develop a preparedness plan.[100] An additional resource for the OEHN is Al Thobaity et al.'s review of common domains of the core competencies of disaster nursing.[101]

"Green" Jobs

The term "green jobs" represents the effort to create employment in the field of renewable and efficient energy production. The topic of green jobs has evolved from two important issues facing the United States in the 21st century: (1) the need to rebuild the economy after the worst economic crisis since the Great Depression and (2) the need to develop strategies that will respond to the threat of global climate change. Green jobs are designed to preserve or enhance environmental quality and build a clean energy environment, but green jobs are not always new jobs. The goal of this movement is to build a clean energy environment by several methods: (1) to invest in sources of renewable energy, such as wind turbines and solar power generation, and (2) to increase energy efficiency by investments in mass transit and modern infrastructure. Because many of the concepts previously described must be done locally by local workers, another important goal of the clean energy economy is to prevent jobs from moving out of the United States. The most important goal of the clean energy economy is sustainability through social, environmental, and economic strategies ultimately leading to job creation, economic growth, the growth of new industries, and innovation that will end the dependence of the United States on polluting and costly fossil fuels, as well as creating strategies for solving global climate change.[102] Many of the occupational risks associated with green jobs may not be known for years, indicating the need for the OEHN to be vigilant in risk assessments of the worker population and remaining current with notices on new risk patterns.

■ CELLULAR TO GLOBAL

Silica is a naturally occurring substance and by-product that becomes aerosolized when working with stone, rock, concrete, and bricks. The silica becomes aerosolized and finer than grains of sand when people perform activities such as sanding concrete, cutting granite for kitchen counters, manufacturing brick, and making ceramic products. Workers in certain industries, particularly construction and hydraulic fracturing, have greater exposure to respirable crystalline silica. At the cellular level, this exposure can lead to chronic obstructive pulmonary disease, lung cancer, and kidney disease. To prevent exposure and reduce the prevalence of silica-related disease, companies can provide workers with saws equipped with a system that continuously feeds water to the blade; companies can also reduce the number of hours employees work directly with silica-based products. These modifications will help reduce aerosolized dust exposure, thus reducing respirable crystalline silica. On a national level, OSHA established new regulations governing exposure limits to silica in construction and general industry. The regulations, phased in during 2017 and 2018, are now in full effect. During OSHA visits, inspectors will monitor for compliance to the standard to assure workers are adequately protected from silica exposures. At the global level, the International Labour Organization/World Health Organization created the Global Programme for the Elimination of Silicosis for use by developed and developing nations. The program provides outlines for host countries to establish a national silicosis program, action plan to implement the program, and guidelines for epidemiological data and programmatic changes for the national silicosis program.

■ Summary Points

- Occupational health is focused on the maintenance and promotion of workers' health, improving working environments, and developing work organizations and cultures to support health and safety.
- Occupational and environmental health nursing is a specialty nursing practice focused on health and safety programs and services to workers.
- Two federal agencies that have had an impact on worker health are the National Institute for Occupational Safety and Health (NIOSH) and Occupational Safety and Health Administration (OSHA).
- The OEHN has a responsibility for promoting health within the workplace by conducting workplace assessments and occupational and environmental health histories.
- Preventing injuries and hazards is dependent on knowledge of exposures, vulnerable worker populations, and using a hierarchy of controls.
- Toxicology is the study of adverse effects of chemical, physical, or biological agents on living organisms and the ecosystem.
- The roles of the OEHN include disease surveillance, preventing fatalities and injuries, case management, and health promotion within the workplace.
- Emerging issues in occupational health include emergency preparedness and disaster management and the creation of green jobs.

▼ CASE STUDY
The Case of Tidy Cleaners
Learning Outcomes:
- Discuss ways to conduct an employee health assessment of the workplace environment.

- Identify potential physical and chemical hazards in the workplace.
- Identify potential peer assistance issues.
- Apply components of health planning, assessment, and program development to the occupational health setting.

As a member of an interprofessional occupational health team, an OEHN, Nancy, was asked to assess the employees working for a well-respected dry-cleaning business in a large metropolitan area. Initially, Nancy consulted with the manager to obtain the list of chemicals used in the dry-cleaning process and to ascertain the demographics of the employees. During a workday, Nancy then conducted a walkthrough of the site. There were 22 workers who have worked for Tidy Cleaners for an average of 15 years and ranged in age from 18 to 54 years; the workers were predominantly female. The women frequently sort garments, remove stains, and repair and press clothing after the dry-cleaning process. The males were responsible for the operation (loading and emptying machines) and repair of the dry-cleaning equipment. One to two employees were available to assist customers when they dropped off or picked up their cleaning and to manage the cash registers. The workforce was composed of both Hispanics, many of whom spoke Spanish only, and whites. The hours of operation were from 9 a.m. to 8 p.m., 6 days a week, and employees worked rotating shifts. Ladders were used to transfer cleaned clothing from overhead electric racks when being claimed by customers. The buildings were windowless, except for the entrance, and a series of powerful stationary fans supplemented an old ventilation system.

The manager of the dry-cleaning business reported the most effective dry-cleaning solvent used in his business was perchloroethylene ("perc"), along with carbon tetrachloride.[103] As a conscientious business owner, the manager stated he would like Nancy to do an occupational assessment of the plant and to assess the workers for occupational exposures and risks. He stressed that prior to conducting an assessment, consent from each employee must be obtained in writing, and the data remain confidential. Nancy also was requested to make recommendations to improve the health and safety in the plant.

- Describe the roles of the following persons who would consult with the OEHN for worker safety: industrial hygienists, safety manager, occupational safety and health engineers, and occupational medicine.

- Identify:
  - Hazardous exposures (physical, biological, chemical, and psychosocial) present in the plant.
  - Potential mechanisms of exposure (inhalation, ingestion, dermal) in the plant.
  - Physical and chemical exposures that should be further evaluated by an occupational/environmental hygienist.
  - Types of accidents and injuries that Nancy could anticipate occurring in this workplace setting and their potential causes.
  - How hierarchies of control are/are not followed in this plant and the PPEs appropriate for this plan.
  - Training and information that should be provided to workers regarding the hazards of their work and the safety practices employees should demonstrate.

After completing her assessment, Nancy reported the results of screening tests conducted with the workers. After consultation with the occupational physician, Nancy noted two of the employees have elevated liver enzyme tests, one employee has chronic musculoskeletal problems, and several workers have chronic skin rashes.

- Identify:
  - Actions Nancy could take to intervene for the workers.
  - Persons Nancy could consult with concerning the elevated liver enzymes and rationale for the consultations.
  - Alterations in the work environment and work processes Nancy would recommend and rationale for her recommendations.

REFERENCES

1. Bureau of Labor Statistics, U.S. Department of Labor. (2018). *Economic news release: Employment situation summary table A. Household data, seasonally adjusted.* Retrieved from http://www.bls.gov/news.release/empsit.a.htm.
2. International Labour Office. (2004). *Global strategy on occupational safety and health.* Retrieved from http://www.ilo.org/wcmsp5/groups/public/—ed_protect/—protrav/—safework/documents/policy/wcms_107535.pdf.
3. Occupational Safety and Health Administration, U.S. Department of Labor. (1970). *Occupational Safety and Health Act of 1970, Pub. L. No. 91-596, 84 Stat. 1590, 91st Congress, S.2193.* Retrieved from https://www.osha.gov/laws-regs/oshact/completeoshact.
4. Bureau of Labor Statistics. (2018). *Average hours employed people spent working on days worked by day of week.* Retrieved from https://www.bls.gov/charts/american-time-use/emp-by-ftpt-job-edu-h.htm.
5. Celentano, D.D., & Szklo, M. (2020). *Gordis epidemiology* (6th ed.). Philadelphia, PA: Elsevier/Saunders.
6. Pope, A.M., Snyder, M.A., Mood, L.H., & Institute of Medicine Committee on Enhancing Environmental Health Content in Nursing Practice. (1995). *Nursing, health & the environment: Strengthening the relationship to improve the public's health.* Washington, DC: National Academies Press.
7. National Institute for Occupational Safety and Health. (2018). *Sectors.* Retrieved from https://www.cdc.gov/niosh/nora/sectorapproach.html.
8. Schill, A. (2017). Advancing well-being through Total Worker Health®. *Workplace Health & Safety, 65*(4), 158-163.
9. National Center for Health Statistics. (2016). Chapter 30: Occupational safety and health. *Healthy People 2020 midcourse review.* Hyattsville, MD: Author.
10. Moore, P.V., & Moore, R.L. (Eds.). (2014). *Fundamentals of occupational and environmental health nursing: AAOHN core curriculum* (4th ed.). Chicago, IL: American Association of Occupational Health Nurses.
11. American Association of Occupational Health Nurses. (2016). *AAOHN occupational and environmental health nurses: Code of ethics.* Chicago, IL: Author.
12. American Association of Occupational Health Nurses. (2012). Standards of occupational & environmental health nursing. *Workplace Health & Safety, 60*(3), 97-103.
13. Occupational Safety and Health Administration. (2016). *All about OSHA (OSHA Publication No. 3302-11R).* Washington, DC: U.S. Department of Labor.
14. Occupational Safety and Health Administration, U.S. Department of Labor. (2005). *OSHA recordkeeping handbook: The regulation and related interpretations for recording and reporting occupational injuries and illnesses (OSHA Publication No. 3245-09R).* Washington, DC: Author.
15. National Institute for Occupational Safety and Health. (2018). *About NORA.* Retrieved from http://www.cdc.gov/niosh/nora/about.html.
16. Centers for Disease Control and Prevention. (2018). *NORA sector agendas.* Retrieved from http://www.cdc.gov/niosh/nora/comment/agendas/.
17. Occupational Safety & Health Administration, U.S. Department of Labor. (n.d.). *Draft proposed safety and health program rule: 29 CFR 1900.1, Docket No. S&H-0027.* Retrieved from https://www.gpo.gov/fdsys/search/pagedetails.action?collectionCode=CFR&searchPath=Title+29%2FSubtitle+B%2FChapter+XVII&granuleId=CFR-2009-title29-vol5-part1900&packageId=CFR-2009-title29-vol5&oldPath=Title+29%2FSubtitle+B%2FChapter+XVII&fromPageDetails=true&collapse=true&ycord=1844&browsePath=Title+29%2FSubtitle+B%2FChapter+XVII%2FParts+1900-1901&fromBrowse=true.
18. Fink, C., Miguelez, E., & Raffo, J. (2017). Determinants of the international mobility of knowledge workers. In C. Fink, & E. Miguelez (Eds.), *The international mobility of inventors* (pp. 162-190). Cambridge, United Kingdom: Cambridge University Press.
19. Bureau of Labor Statistics. (2016). *American time use survey: Household activities.* Retrieved from https://www.bls.gov/TUS/CHARTS/HOUSEHOLD.HTM.
20. Society for Human Resource Management. (2017). *SHRM's effective workplace index: Creating a workplace that works for employees and employers.* Alexandria, VA: Authors

21. Behson, S. (2015). *The working dad's survival guide: How to succeed at work and at home.* Melbourne, FL: Motivational Press.

22. National Institute for Occupational Safety and Health. (2018). *Healthy work design and well-being program.* Retrieved from http://www.cdc.gov/niosh/programs/hwd/.

23. Yates, M.D. (2009). *Why unions matter* (2nd ed.). New York, NY: NYU Press.

24. Bureau of Labor Statistics, U.S. Department of Labor. (2018). *Economic news release: Union members summary.* Retrieved from https://www.bls.gov/news.release/union2.nr0.htm.

25. Agency for Toxic Substances and Disease Registry, U.S. Department of Health and Human Services. (2015). *Toxicological profile for dichloropropenes.* Retrieved from http://www.atsdr.cdc.gov/toxprofiles/tp40.pdf.

26. Occupational Safety & Health Administration. (n.d.). *Occupational noise exposure.* Retrieved from http://www.osha.gov/SLTC/noisehearingconservation/.

27. Cardarelli, J. (2018). Ionizing and non-ionizing radiation. In B.S. Levy, D.H. Wegman, S.L. Baron, & R.K. Sokas (Eds.), *Occupational and environmental health* (7th ed., pp. 289-308). New York, NY: Oxford University Press.

28. Krake, A.M. (2018). Extremes of temperature. In B.S. Levy, D.H. Wegman, S.L. Baron, & R.K. Sokas (Eds.), *Occupational and environmental health* (7th ed., pp. 271-288). New York, NY: Oxford University Press.

29. Johnson, P.W., & Cherniack, M.G. (2018). Vibration. In B.S. Levy, D.H. Wegman, S.L. Baron, & R.K. Sokas (Eds.), *Occupational and environmental health* (7th ed., pp. 259-270). New York, NY: Oxford University Press.

30. Agency for Toxic Substances & Disease Registry. (2014). *Toxic substances portal—Ionizing radiation.* Retrieved from http://www.atsdr.cdc.gov/toxfaqs/tf.asp?id=483&tid=86.

31. Industrial Safety and Hygiene News. (2017). *OSHA hazard communication standard (HAZCOM) 1910.1200.* Retrieved from https://www.ishn.com/articles/105552-osha-hazard-communication-standard-hazcom-19101200.

32. Gochfeld, M., & Laumbach, R. (2018). Chemical hazards. In B.S. Levy, D.H. Wegman, S.L. Baron, & R.K. Sokas (Eds.), *Occupational and environmental health* (7th ed., pp. 207-242). New York, NY: Oxford University Press.

33. Agency for Toxic Substances & Disease Registry. (2015). *Toxic substances portal – Beryllium.* Retrieved from http://www.atsdr.cdc.gov/toxfaqs/TF.asp?id=184&tid=33.

34. Laidlaw, M.A.S., Filippelli, G., Mielke, H., Gulson, B., & Ball, A.S. (2017). Lead exposure at firing ranges—a review. *Environmental Health, 16*(34), 1-15.

35. Kang, K.W., & Park, W. (2017). Lead poisoning at an indoor firing range. *Journal of Korean Medical Science, 32*(10), 1713-1716.

36. Mostafalou, S., & Abdollahi, M. (2018). The link of organophosphorus pesticides with neurodegenerative and neurodevelopmental diseases based on evidence and mechanisms. *Toxicology, 409,* 44-52.

37. Occupational Safety & Health Administration. (n.d.). *Safety and health topics: Benzene.* Retrieved from http://www.osha.gov/SLTC/benzene/.

38. Russi, M. (2018). Biological hazards. In B.S. Levy, D.H. Wegman, S.L. Baron, & R.K. Sokas (Eds.), *Occupational and environmental health* (7th ed., pp. 309-324). New York, NY: Oxford University Press.

39. Occupational Safety & Health Administration. (2011). *Respiratory protection: Personal protective equipment (1910.134).* Retrieved from https://www.osha.gov/pls/oshaweb/owadisp.show_document?p_id=12716&p_table=STANDARDS.

40. National Institute for Occupational Safety and Health. (2018). *Respirator trusted-source information.* Retrieved from http://www.cdc.gov/niosh/npptl/topics/respirators/disp_part/RespSource.html.

41. Schnall, P.L., Dobson, M., & Landsbergis, P. (2016). Globalization, work, and cardiovascular disease. *International Journal of Health Services, 46*(4), 656-692.

42. Cendales, B.E., & Ortiz, V.G. (2018). Cultural values and the Job Demands-Control Model of Stress: A moderation analysis. *International Journal of Stress Management,* in press.

43. Veronesi, G., Borchini, R., Landsbergis, P., Iacoviello, L., Gianfagna, F., Tayoun, P., ... Ferrario, M.M. (2018). Cardiovascular disease prevention at the workplace: Assessing the prognostic value of lifestyle risk factors and job-related conditions. *International Journal of Public Health, 63*(6), 723-732.

44. Sauter, S.L., Murphy, L.R., Hurrell, J.J., & Levi, L. (1998). Chapter 34: Psychosocial and organizational factors. In J.M. Stellman (Ed.), *ILO encyclopedia of occupational health and safety* (pp. 34.2-34.3). Geneva, Switzerland: International Labour Office.

45. Johnson, J.V., & Hall, E.M. (1988). Job strain, work place social support, and cardiovascular disease: A cross-sectional study of a random sample of the Swedish working population. *American Journal of Public Health, 78*(10), 1336-1342.

46. Pellerin, S., & Cloutier, J. (2018). The effects of rewards on psychological health in the workplace: Underlying mechanisms. *Canadian Journal of Administrative Sciences, 35*(3), 361-372.

47. The Employee Assistance Trade Association. (2018). *EAP best practices.* Retrieved from http://www.easna.org/research-and-best-practices/.

48 Employee Assistance Workgroup. (2008). *An employer's guide to Employee Assistance Programs: Recommendations for strategically defining, integrating, and measuring Employee Assistance Programs.* Washington, DC: National Business Group on Health.

49. Occupational Safety and Health Administration. (n.d.). *Ergonomics.* Retrieved from http://www.osha.gov/SLTC/ergonomics/.

50. National Institute for Occupational Safety and Health. (2018). *Hierarchy of controls.* Retrieved from https://www.cdc.gov/niosh/topics/hierarchy/default.html.

51. Eisenberg, S., & Pacheco, L. (2018). Applying hazardous drug standards to antineoplastics used for ophthalmology surgery. *AORN Journal, 107*(2), 199-213.

52. National Institute for Occupational Safety and Health. (2010). *Occupationally-induced hearing loss (DHHS-NIOSH Publication No. 2010-136).* Retrieved from http://www.cdc.gov/niosh/docs/2010-136/pdfs/2010-136.pdf.

53. Wage and Hour Division, U.S. Department of Labor. (n.d.). *Compliance assistance—Wages and Fair Labor Standards Act (FLSA).* Retrieved from http://www.dol.gov/whd/Flsa/index.htm.

54. Windau, J., & Meyer, S. (2005). Occupational injuries among young workers. *Monthly Labor Review Online, 128*(10), 11-23.

55. Smith, J., Purewal, B.P., MacPherson, A., & Pike, I. (2018). Metrics to assess injury prevention programs for young workers in high-risk occupations: A scoping review of the literature. *Research, Policy and Practice, 38*(5), 191-199.

56. Runyan, C.W., Schulman, M., Dal Santo, J., Bowling, J.M., Agans, R., & Ta, M. (2007). Work-related hazards and workplace safety of U.S. adolescents employed in the retail and service sectors. *Pediatrics, 119*(3), 526-534.

57. Runyan, C.W., Vladutiu, C.J., Rauscher, K.J., & Schulman, M. (2008). Teen workers' exposures to occupational hazards and use of personal protective equipment. *American Journal of Industrial Medicine, 51*(10), 735-740.

58. Steinberg, L.D. (2017). *Adolescence* (11th ed.). New York, NY: McGraw-Hill.

59. Smith, C. R., Gillespie, G. L., & Beery, T. A. (2015). Adolescent workers' experiences of and training for workplace violence. *Workplace Health & Safety, 63*(7), 297-307.

60. Barling, J., & Kelloway, E.K. (Eds.). (1999). *Young workers: Varieties of experience.* Washington, DC: American Psychological Association.

61. Occupational Safety and Health Administration. (n.d.) *Young workers: You have rights!* Retrieved from http://www.osha.gov/SLTC/teenworkers/.

62. U.S. Social Security Administration. (n.d). *Retirement age calculator.* Retrieved from http://www.ssa.gov/planners/retire/ageincrease.html.

63. Scott, K.A., Liao, Q.L., Fisher, G.G., Stallones, L., DiGuiseppi, C., & Tompa, E. (2018). Early labor force exit subsequent to permanently impairing occupational injury or illness among workers 50-64 years of age. *American Journal of Industrial Medicine, 61*(4), 317-325.

64. Truxillo, D.M., Cadiz, D.M., & Hammer, L.B. (2015). Supporting the aging workforce: A review of recommendations for workplace intervention research. *Annual Review of Organizational Psychology and Organizational Behavior, 2,* 351-381.

65. Chand, M., & Markova, G. (2018). The European Union's aging population: Challenges for human resource management. *Thunderbird International Business Review,* in press.

66. Smith, M.L., Wilson, M.G., Robertson, M.M., Padilla, H.M., Zuercher, H., Vandenberg, R., ... DeJoy, D.M. (2018). Impact of a translated disease self-management program on employee health and productivity: Six-month findings from a randomized controlled trial. *International Journal of Environmental Research and Public Health, 15*(5), 851.

67. U.S. Bureau of Labor Statistics. (2015). *BLS reports: Women in the labor force: A databook (BLS Publication No. 1059).* Washington, DC: Author.

68. National Institute for Occupational Safety and Health. (2017). *Using Total Worker Health® concepts to reduce the health risks from sedentary work (NIOSH Publication No. 2017-131).* Atlanta, GA: Author.

69. Wage and Hour Division, U.S. Department of Labor. (n.d.). *Break time for nursing mothers.* Retrieved from https://www.dol.gov/whd/nursingmothers/.

70. U.S. Department of Justice. (2010). *Americans with Disabilities Act Title II regulations: Nondiscrimination on the basis of disability in state and local government services.* Retrieved from https://www.ada.gov/regs2010/titleII_2010/titleII_2010_regulations.pdf.

71. Bureau of Labor Statistics, U.S. Department of Labor. (2018). *Economic News Release: Employment status of the civilian noninstitutional population by disability status and selected characteristics, 2017 annual averages.* Retrieved from https://www.bls.gov/news.release/disabl.t01.htm.

72. Bureau of Labor Statistics, U.S. Department of Labor. (2018). *News release: Foreign-born workers: Labor force characteristics—2017.* Retrieved from https://www.bls.gov/news.release/pdf/forbrn.pdf.

73. Chort, I., & de la Rupelle, M. (2016). Determinants of Mexico-U.S. outward and return migration flows: A state-level panel data analysis. *Demography, 53*(5), 1453-1476.

74. Moyce, S.C., & Schenker, M. (2017). Occupational exposures and health outcomes among immigrants in the USA. *Current Environmental Health Reports, 4*(3), 349-354.

75. Occupational Safety and Health Administration. (2017). *Outreach training program requirements.* Retrieved from https://www.osha.gov/dte/outreach/program_requirements.pdf.

76. McCann, D., & Fudge, J. (2017). Unacceptable forms of work: A multidimensional model. *International Labour Review, 156*(2), 147-184.

77. Hsieh, Y., Apostolopoulos, Y., & Sönmez, S. (2016). Work conditions and health and well-being of Latina hotel housekeepers. *Journal of Immigrant Minority Health, 18*(3), 568-581.

78. Bureau of Labor Statistics, U.S. Department of Labor. (2018). *News release: The employment situation—June 2018. USDL Publication No. 18-1110.* Retrieved from https://www.bls.gov/news.release/archives/empsit_07062018.pdf.

79. Agency for Toxic Substances and Disease Registry. (2016). *Glossary of terms.* Retrieved from https://www.atsdr.cdc.gov/glossary.html.

80. National Institute for Occupational Safety and Health. (2018). *Fatality Assessment and Control Evaluation (FACE) Program.* Retrieved from https://www.cdc.gov/niosh/face/default.html.

81. Wassel, M.L., Randolph, J., & Rieth, L.K. (2006). Disability case management. In M.K. Salazar & American Association of Occupational Health Nurses (Eds.), *Core curriculum for occupational & environmental health nursing* (3rd ed., pp. 331-364). Philadelphia, PA: Saunders.

82. Bible, J.E., Spengler, D.M., & Mir, H.R. (2014). A primer for workers' compensation. *The Spine Journal, 14*(7), 1325-1331.

83. Ostrov, J. (2015). An examination of the New York State Workers' Compensation Reform Act of 2007. *Journal of Sociology and Social Welfare, 42*(3), 3-23.

84. Goetzel, R.Z. (2005). *Policy and practice working group: Examining the value of integrating occupational health and safety and health promotion programs in the workplace.* Retrieved from http://www.mtpinnacle.com/pdfs/NIOSH_Background_Paper_Goetzel.pdf.

85. U.S. National Center for Health Statistics. (2017). *Table 19: Leading causes of death and numbers of death, by sex, race, and Hispanic origin: United States, 1980 and 2016.* Retrieved from https://www.cdc.gov/nchs/data/hus/2017/019.pdf.

86. World Health Organization. (2018). *The top 10 causes of death.* Retrieved from http://www.who.int/news-room/fact-sheets/detail/the-top-10-causes-of-death.

87. Edwardson, C.L., Biddle, S.J.H., Clarke-Cornwell, A., Clemes, S., Davies, M.J., Dunstan, D.W., ... Munir, F. (2018). A three arm cluster randomised controlled trial to test the effectiveness and cost-effectiveness of the SMART Work & Life intervention for reducing daily sitting time in office workers: Study protocol. *BMC Public Health, 18*(1), 1120.

88. Centers for Disease Control and Prevention. (2018). *The National Healthy Worksite Program.* Retrieved from https://www.cdc.gov/workplacehealthpromotion/pdf/nhwp-program-overview.pdf.

89. Gutermuth, L.K., Hager, E.R., & Porter, K.P. (2018). Using the CDC's Worksite Health ScoreCard as a framework to examine worksite health promotion and physical activity. *Preventing Chronic Disease, 15*(6), 170463.

90. Cluff, L.A., Lang, J.E., Rineer, J.R., Jones-Jack, N.H., & Strazza, K.M. (2018). Training employers to implement health promotion programs: Results from the CDC Work@Health® Program. *American Journal of Health Promotion, 32*(4), 1062-1069.

91. Gretebeck, K.A., Bailey, T., & Gretebeck, R.J. (2017). A minimal contact diet and physical activity intervention for white-collar workers. *Workplace Health and Safety, 65*(9), 417-423.

92. Van Den Brekel-Dijkstra, K., Rengers, A.H., Niessen, M.A.J., De Wit, N.J., & Kraaijenhagen, R.A. (2016). Personalized prevention approach with use of a web-based cardiovascular risk assessment with tailored lifestyle follow-up in primary care practice – A pilot study. *European Journal of Preventive Cardiology, 23*(5), 544-551.

93. King, K.P., Leos, J.A., & Norstrand, L. (2017). The role of online health education communities in wellness and recovery. In Information Resources Management Association (Ed.), *Public health and welfare: Concepts, methodologies, tools, and applications* (pp. 964-998). Hershey, PA: IGI Global.

94. John-Nwankwo, J. (2015). *Adult learning principles: Maximizing the learning experience of adults (the nurse educator's experience).* Charleston, SC: CreateSpace Independent Publishing Platform.

95. Centers for Disease Control and Prevention. (2002). Fixed obstructive lung disease in workers at a microwave popcorn factory—Missouri, 2000–2002. *Morbidity and Mortality Weekly Report, 51*(16), 345-347.

96. Cummings, K.J., & Kreiss, K. (2015). Occupational and environmental bronchiolar disorders. *Seminars in Respiratory and Critical Care Medicine, 36*(3), 366-378.

97. National Institute for Occupational Safety and Health. (2003). *NIOSH alert: Preventing lung disease in workers who use or make flavorings (DHHS-NIOSH Publication No. 2004-110).* Retrieved from http://www.cdc.gov/niosh/docs/2004-110/pdfs/2004-110.pdf.

98. U.S. Office of Public Health Preparedness and Response. (2013). *All-hazards preparedness guide.* Atlanta, GA: Author

99. Stanley, S.A.R., Cole, S., McGill, J., Millet, C., & Morse, D. (2014). *The role of the public health nurse in disaster preparedness, response, and recovery: A position paper.* Retrieved from http://www.achne.org/files/public/APHN_RoleOfPHNinDisasterPRR_FINALJan14.pdf.

100. Federal Emergency Management Association. (2018). *Preparedness planning for your business.* Retrieved from http://www.ready.gov/business.

101. Al Thobaity, A., Plummer, V., & Williams, B. (2017). What are the most common domains of the core competencies of disaster nursing? A scoping review. *International Emergency Nursing, 31*, 64-71.

102. Sulich, A., & Zema, T. (2018). Green jobs, a new measure of public management and sustainable development. *European Journal of Environmental Sciences, 8*(1), 69-75.

103. National Institute for Occupational Safety and Health. (2016). *NIOSH pocket guide to chemical hazards.* Retrieved from http://www.cdc.gov/niosh/npg/default.html.

Chapter 21

Health Planning, Public Health Policy, and Finance

Christine Vandenhouten and Derryl Block

LEARNING OUTCOMES

After reading the chapter, the student will be able to:

1. Discuss the role of policy in optimizing health for populations.
2. Describe the role of policy in the delivery of health care in the United States.
3. Apply public health principles to public health policy planning.
4. Identify ethical issues related to public health policy.
5. Examine the role of nurses in public health policy.
6. Describe U.S. governmental policies related to the financing of health care.

KEY TERMS

Advocacy
Affordable Care Act (ACA)
Children's Health
   Insurance Program
   (CHIP)
Culturally acceptable
   health policies
Economics
Effectiveness

Efficiency
Equity
Grants
Health economics
Market economy
Medicaid
Medicare
Policy
Public health economics

Public health finance
Public health policy
Social Security Disability
   Insurance (SSDI)
Supplemental Nutrition
   Assistance Program
   (SNAP)
Supplemental Security
   Income (SSI)

Temporary Assistance for
   Needy Families
   (TANF)
Woman, Infants, and
   Children (WIC)

Introduction

"Health policy refers to decisions, plans, and actions that are undertaken to achieve specific health care goals within a society. An explicit health policy can achieve several things: it defines a vision for the future, which in turn helps to establish targets and points of reference for the short and medium term. It outlines priorities and the expected roles of different groups; and it builds consensus and informs people."[1] **Public health policy** refers to policies specifically intended to direct or influence actions, behaviors, or decisions *that influence the health of populations*. Stakeholder groups including lobbyists, grant funders, and nongovernmental organizations all influence public health policy.

For public health nurses, health policy is an explicit part of professional life. As noted in Chapter 1, nurses are responsible for advocating for, identifying, interpreting, and implementing public health laws, regulations,

and policies.[2] Public health policy activities by nurses include actively engaging in strategies to change or enact policies that improve the health of populations, especially populations experiencing disparity. Public health policy activities also include educating the public on relevant laws, regulations, and policies. A nurse working in a college health clinic is required to report a case of mumps to the local public health department and can help monitor for additional cases to help determine whether there has been an outbreak (see Chapter 8). Knowledge of public health policy is necessary for the nurse to facilitate isolation of affected students, to educate them (and their families, if given permission to communicate with them), and to collaborate with the public health department's outbreak investigation aimed at reducing the spread of the disease.

Nurses are affected by state-level nurse practice acts that determine the scope of practice for registered nurses (RNs) and Advanced Practice Registered Nurses

(APRNs). These policies come under the umbrella of public health policy because they are designed to protect the recipients of nursing care. Nurses who provide direct care to patients are affected in their day-to-day life by public health policies designed to protect both them and the patients they care for. These policies include mandated and recommended vaccines that nurses and other health-care workers should receive,[3] the use of personal protective equipment, and procedures for handling and disposing of sharps such as hypodermic needles or blades.

Public health policy includes local and county policies mandating recycling of certain materials and special recycling procedures for hazardous materials and medications that hold special pollution risks in an effort to reduce environmental health risks. Other examples of public health policies include the fluoridation of water to prevent dental caries, school nutrition policies, regulations related to the distribution of pharmaceuticals during an emergency, and sales of tobacco and e-cigarettes to minors. Public health policies may involve mandating single interventions or comprehensive programs. For example, a school district might set a policy that all seventh graders attend a specific educational session about at-risk drug use. A comprehensive policy may include mandating educational sessions for various grades, mandatory drug testing for student athletes, community-based programs for parents, and the presence of school resource police officers in the school.

We are all affected by certain governmental policies, such as taxes that fund government including the federal income tax, payroll taxes, and state and local taxes. Although taxes are not regularly thought of as public health policy, the policy of exempting employer-sponsored health benefits from income and payroll taxes has influenced employers to offer health benefits in lieu of increased salaries. Since the 2010 health care reform law, to improve access to health care, large employers were required to provide health-care coverage. From a public health perspective, a broad range of policies are instituted to directly or indirectly protect or promote the health of populations through the passing of laws and the setting of regulations based on the greatest good for the greatest number of people.

Public Health Policy and the U.S. Health-Care System

Public health policies directly affect our health-care system and its underlying philosophies. The U.S. health-care system is a complex combination of privately funded and provided, publicly funded and provided, and publicly funded and privately provided services. Why is our health-care system so complex? In part, it is complex because of the economic culture within the United States that supports an open market for the exchange of goods/services and payments, including health-care services. When the government attempts to intervene in the market system to promote quality, supply, and equity/fairness, a tension is created between those principles and allowing or even facilitating an open market system. This tension has been evident in ongoing debates in the United States over health-care reform despite the fact that all other developed countries offer universal health coverage. According to the World Health Organization, universal health coverage occurs when all individuals and communities receive essential health services, including health promotion, treatment, rehabilitation, and palliative care without financial hardship.[4]

In a **market economy**, the prices of goods and services are set by supply and demand. A well-functioning market economy is one in which there are many buyers, many sellers, and complete information about the goods and services being exchanged. In many ways, the U.S. health-care market does not meet the criteria of a free market. Buyers often do not have complete information about goods and services. For instance, after an auto crash, injured persons or their families do not have time to evaluate the quality and cost of ambulance and emergency room services in the area. In addition, because health-care decisions, such as whether to undergo a screening exam or what kind of cancer treatment to initiate, are often based on interpretation of technical information, individuals rely on advice given by health-care providers, the media, and significant others. In some areas, there are few "sellers" of specific services. For example, almost 9 out of 10 counties in the United States did not have an abortion provider in 2014,[5] and more than half of rural counties had no hospital-based obstetric services during the period 2004-2014.[6]

Whereas government intervenes in the market economy to ensure quality, supply, and equity/fairness, the U.S. governmental role in the health-care market has been restrained because of cultural factors that emphasize individual rights and a relatively unfettered market system. Early government intervention included conducting research into the adulteration and misbranding of food and drugs, providing health care to the merchant marines, and developing and enforcing quarantine laws.

The idea of health insurance took root in the 1930s in the private market whereby individuals could take out an insurance policy to defray the cost of health care if they became ill or suffered an accident.[7] Today, employer-based health insurance is the norm. Internal Revenue Service (IRS) rulings (i.e., policies) since the 1940s allowed for health insurance expenses to be tax favored, thus encouraging businesses to offer it and individuals to seek it out.[8] An employer-based model was retained in the Affordable Care Act (ACA).

In the 1960s, federal health insurance programs and related policies became the norm with the development of Medicare to aid older adults and Medicaid to aid the poor and disabled. These two groups were generally not covered by employer-based health care. Despite the existence of these large programs, and with limited movement toward health reform, in 2014, the United States mandated that individuals have health insurance. Since then, however, exemptions to the comprehensiveness of health insurance to fulfill the mandate have been passed, and the penalty for not having health insurance has been eliminated.

Health expenditures in the United States are far above those of other industrialized countries, and health outcome performance lags behind those countries in many areas.[9] For example, in 2016 the United States ranked 12th in the world for the prevalence of adult obesity rates with 36% of adults having a Body Mass Index (BMI) greater to or equal to 30.0.[10] Despite the high expenditure on health care, in 2017 the United States ranked 43rd in life expectancy.[11]

Within the United States, there are great disparities in quality indicators such as access to care and immunizations.[12] According to Healthy People, "If a health outcome is seen to a greater or lesser extent between populations, there is disparity."[13] Health disparities are linked to social determinants of health such as living conditions and socioeconomic status (income, education, and occupation). The ACA was an attempt to decrease disparities by assuring individual insurance coverage. In 2010, prior to the ACA, 82% of persons under 65 years had medical insurance compared with 89% in 2015.

Health disparities are also linked to demographic variables such as race, ethnicity, and age.[13] Take colorectal screening as an example. Although initiation of the ACA resulted in increased colorectal cancer screening rates in adults aged 50-75, from 52% in 2008 to 62% in 2015, disparities among ethnic and racial groups continue.[14] In 2015, 49% of American Indian/Alaska Native and Hispanic adults aged 50-75 were screened compared with

53% of Asian adults; 61% of Black, non-Hispanic adults; and 65% of White, non-Hispanic adults. There were also disparities in colorectal screening rates based on education and income.[14]

In 2015, disparities in insurance coverage among U.S. ethnic and racial groups persisted. Only 80% of Hispanic people of any race, 88% of Blacks, 91% of Asians, and 92% of White, non-Hispanic had insurance.[15]

Likewise, there are disparities in morbidity and mortality rates among people of different racial and ethnic groups. In 2015, African Americans were more likely to die from heart disease, stroke, cancer, asthma, HIV/AIDS, homicide, and influenza and pneumonia than non-Hispanic whites.[16,17] An important intervention to decrease mortality from influenza is the flu vaccine, often provided free or at a reduced cost through local public health departments. African Americans aged 65 and older were less likely (61%) to have received a flu shot in the last 12 months than their non-Hispanic white counterparts (73%).[18] Infant mortality rates show dramatic disparities related to maternal race and ethnicity. In 2014, the infant mortality rate among Black or African Americans was 10.7 deaths/1,000 live births, compared with 7.6 among American Indian or Alaska Natives, 5.0 among Hispanic or Latina Americans, and 4.9 among non-Hispanic whites.[19]

Although some might suggest that race and ethnicity are the primary reasons for the dramatic disparities in health indicators, current research suggests that socioeconomic status plays a more significant role.[20–22] The relationship between health and socioeconomic status is complicated. Individuals living at or below the federal poverty level may qualify for public insurance programs, but they also frequently lack other resources, such as transportation or flexible working hours, making access to health-care services challenging. Lack of resources, whether financial, educational (literacy), or health care related, and even social marginalization can result in chronic stress. Additionally, exposure to chronic stress is linked to a higher incidence of certain illnesses such as cancer, heart disease, and other chronic diseases. This, combined with an absence of insurance and reduced access to quality health care, results in increasing mortality among minority groups and all individuals living in poverty.[23]

National Health Policy

There are many laws and regulations that guide health policy at the national level. Article 1, Section 8, of the U.S. Constitution provides the federal government with certain authority, including providing for the general welfare and regulating commerce among the states. This section has been interpreted as the basis for a variety of powers and activities including federal involvement in health care.

In the United States, most health-care goods and services are exchanged in the private market with individuals choosing their care provider and directly or indirectly paying for services. Often, the type of indirect payment (e.g., particular health insurance policies that pay for medical or health-related expenses) affect individual choices regarding care. For instance, the contractual agreement between an individual or group and a health insurer may not cover particular screenings such as dental checkups. The extent of coverage of a specific insurance policy is in itself a policy that affects health-care choices. Individual health insurance is regulated primarily at the state level, and most states have a specialized office for insurance matters which is led by a state insurance commissioner.

Although some states use model acts and model regulations as guides, policies that govern private health insurance vary significantly from state to state. For instance, inclusion of mental health services in private insurance policies varies greatly. Some states prohibit insurers from discriminating in coverage for mental health and other health problems, some states require a minimum level of coverage of mental health expenses, and some do not require insurance companies to cover mental health services at all.[24]

In addition to the publicly funded programs that cover older adults and the poor through Medicare and Medicaid, respectively, the U.S. government both provides and pays for care for certain specific populations. The federal government is deemed to have responsibility for providing and paying for services for soldiers, veterans, prisoners in federal facilities, and American Indians/Native Americans.

Social Security, Medicare, and Medicaid

Social Security, a composite of social welfare and social insurance programs, was first signed into law in 1935 as part of a plan to alleviate poverty and end the Great Depression.[25] Social security benefits, beneficiaries, payroll taxes, and wage caps have undergone a series of modifications since that time and now cover the following: Federal Old-Age (Retirement), Survivors, and Disability Insurance; Temporary Assistance for Needy Families; Health Insurance for Aged and Disabled (Medicare); Grants to States for Medical Assistance Programs for Low Income Citizens (Medicaid);

State Children's Health Insurance Program for Low Income Citizens (SCHIP); and Supplemental Security Income. Payroll taxes, split between the employer and the employee, are funneled by the Internal Revenue Service into the Federal Old-Age and Survivors Insurance Trust Fund and the Federal Disability Insurance Trust Fund to fully or partially pay for these programs.

Since 1965, Medicare has provided payment for hospital care; long-term care; and pharmaceutical, physician, and other services to individuals 65 and older, and specified groups of people with disabilities under 65 including individuals with end-stage renal disease. Medicare is not a care delivery system, but rather a social insurance system administered by the Centers for Medicare & Medicaid Services (CMS), a federal governmental agency within the U.S. Department of Health and Human Services. Concerns about financial viability of Medicare have led to discussions about funding, eligibility, and fraud reduction.[26]

Medicaid, another national health program administered by the CMS, provides financial assistance to states and counties for low-income families with dependent children, low-income older adults, and disabled individuals. Unlike Medicare, a strictly federal program, Medicaid is jointly financed by matching funds from federal and state governments. Medicaid is described in more detail in the State Health Policy section.

Healthy People

At the national level, *Healthy People* is a prevention policy agenda to guide interventions for the improvement of health outcomes in areas such as infant mortality, years of healthy life, and racial and ethnic health disparities.[27] Federal, state, and local health officials together with health-care providers and consumers developed national health goals and objectives for the United States. Since 1979, goals and objectives have been reevaluated about every 10 years.[27] *Healthy People* includes targets that are examples of federal health policy. *Healthy People* also includes specific goals and objectives for policy changes (see Chapter 1). It is an example of setting policy agendas at the national level using a consensus-building approach. That is, the agenda was built based on the input from numerous stakeholders. The Healthy People 2030 framework builds on lessons learned in previous Healthy People iterations and emphasizes reducing preventable deaths and injuries.[28]

■ HEALTHY PEOPLE

History of Healthy People

- 1979 Surgeon General's Report, *Healthy People: The Surgeon General's Report on Health Promotion and Disease Prevention*
- *Healthy People 1990: Promoting Health/Preventing Disease; Objectives for the Nation*
- *Healthy People 2000: National Health Promotion and Disease Prevention Objectives*
- *Healthy People 2010: Objectives for Improving Health*
- *Healthy People 2020*
- *Healthy People 2030*

Patient Protection and Affordable Care Act of 2010

The passage and enactment of the ACA in 2010 by the federal government was the most significant overhaul of the U.S. health care regulatory system since the passage of Medicare and Medicaid in 1965. The purpose of the ACA was to improve access to affordable health coverage for everyone, including the most vulnerable, to provide ways to bring down health-care costs, and to improve quality of care by improving health outcomes. Some key components of the law are as follows:

- Denial of coverage for preexisting conditions was prohibited.
- Young adults could stay on their parents' plan until age 26.
- Originally, the ACA required that most U.S. citizens and legal residents have health insurance. Opponents of the ACA challenged the constitutionality of the individual insurance mandate, suggesting it amounted to a tax; however, the U.S. Supreme Court upheld the legislation.[29] However, in 2019, the tax penalty associated with not having insurance was repealed.
- Employers with 50 or more employees were required to offer insurance coverage or pay a fine.
- Medicaid coverage for most non-elderly low-income adults was expanded to 138% of the federal poverty level, but after a Supreme Court decision in 2012, states could opt in to adopt this expansion or choose not to.
- State-based health-care marketplaces were created for individuals and small businesses to compare and enroll in health insurance plans. Governmental subsidies for health insurance companies to participate in the marketplaces were intended to reduce out of pocket costs to individuals. Those subsidies have been reduced and health insurance premiums will likely continue to increase.
- Preventive health care was provided at no additional cost (e.g., annual exams, flu shots, cancer screenings).[30] Covered preventive services for adults include risk-based screenings for abdominal aortic aneurysm, at-risk alcohol use, hypertension, high cholesterol, colorectal cancer, depression, HIV, obesity, tobacco use, and syphilis. Additional preventive services include access to aspirin therapy, diet counseling, and immunizations.[31] A series of judicial decisions have allowed some employers to exempt birth control coverage from their insurance plans.
- Insurance was required to cover essential health services including ambulatory patient care, emergency services, hospitalization, maternity and newborn care, mental health and substance use disorder services, prescription drugs, rehabilitation and habilitation services and devices, lab services, preventive and wellness services, chronic disease management, and pediatric services, including oral and vision care. After passage of the bill, efforts to reduce costs centered on proposals to limit the essential health services that insurance must include, especially in the realm of maternity and infant care, and mental health and substance use disorder services.[32]

There are components of the ACA with significant potential implications for public health nursing.[33] Some of these are authorized, mandatory funds for evidence-based early childhood home visitations; an authorized CDC national diabetes prevention program; loan repayment to increase public health workforce; programs to help educate more public health professionals; school-based health centers; public/private partnerships for education and outreach campaigns; community health centers and nurse managed clinics; workplace wellness programs; and national quality improvement strategies to improve population health.[34]

The ACA also established the Prevention and Public Health Fund. It provides increased and sustained national resources for prevention and public health, improves health outcomes, and enhances health-care quality. The U.S. Department of Health and Human Services summarized the investments as a "broad range of evidence-based activities including community and clinical prevention initiatives; research, surveillance and tracking; public health infrastructure; immunizations and screenings; tobacco prevention; and public health workforce and training."[34]

Occupational Safety and Health Administration

The Occupational Safety and Health Administration (OSHA), part of the U.S. Department of Labor, regulates safety and health for workers (see Chapter 20). "OSHA's mission is to prevent work-related injuries, illnesses, and deaths."[35] Since the agency was created in 1971, occupational deaths have been cut by 62% and injuries have declined by 42%. For example, OSHA's bloodborne pathogens standard requires an exposure control plan that includes components such as observance of universal precautions to prevent contact with blood or other potentially infectious body fluids; engineering and work practice controls to minimize exposure; and vaccination, postexposure evaluation, and follow-up.

Special Populations

As mentioned earlier, the U.S. government directly provides health care for soldiers, veterans, members of federally recognized American Indian/Native American tribes, and inmates of federal prisons. Special agencies are charged with providing health care to these populations. For instance, the Department of Veterans Affairs provides health care for veterans through the Veteran's Administration (VA) hospitals and programs. Indian Health Services (IHS) is a federally funded program to provide health services to Native American populations based on treaties established during the early development of the United States. Nurses who work in the armed forces, VA, IHS, and federal prisons are usually employees of the federal government.

State Health Policy

States and Medicaid

Medicaid is jointly financed and administered by federal and state governments. States set their own guidelines for eligibility and services but must include certain federally mandated basic services: inpatient and outpatient hospital care; laboratory and radiology services; skilled care at home or at a long-term care facility; early periodic screening, diagnosis, and treatment for those younger than 21 years of age; and family planning services.[36] The federal government mandates that participating states include federally determined categories (low-income families with dependent children, low-income older adults, and disabled individuals) in their Medicaid eligibility criteria. Participating states may choose to provide Medicaid coverage to other groups such as the medically needy or individuals with income levels above Medicaid cut-offs but who have extraordinary medical costs. Many states have received waivers from the federal government to use Medicaid funds in a different way.[37,38] For instance, Wisconsin used Medicaid funds in a demonstration project, BadgerCare Plus, to pay for health-care services for low-income adults without dependent children.

A related federal/state program is the Children's Health Insurance Program (CHIP) (see Chapter 18). The federal government provides matching funds to states for coverage of children in families whose incomes are too high to qualify for Medicaid, yet they remain unable to afford private insurance. States have some latitude in determining covered services and eligibility levels. Additionally, as of April 2018, 32 states and the District of Columbia adopted the Medicaid expansion as part of the ACA.[39]

Some states have decided on policies that incrementally moved toward universal health-care coverage for their residents. For instance, Oregon initiated a plan to provide health insurance to low-income residents while holding down costs through explicitly rationing certain services.[40] Ballooning costs resulted in limitation of services, severe limitations to eligibility, and even the institution of a lottery for remaining spots in the plan. In 2006, Massachusetts passed a statute requiring all state residents to obtain health insurance coverage.[41] Free and subsidized health insurance was made available to low-income residents. States are experimenting with a variety of policies to address health insurance coverage, especially for low-income people.

Another important health policy at the state level is the establishment of predetermined criteria for both health-care providers and facilities. For example, in Wisconsin, the Department of Regulation and Licensing is responsible for ensuring the safe and competent practice of licensed professionals in health care and other professions.[42] The department sets licensing requirements, establishes professional practice standards, and enforces occupational licensing laws. The department also regulates educational programs for licensed professionals. The Wisconsin Division of Quality Assurance is charged with, among other responsibilities, assuring the safety and quality of health-care facilities. This division is also responsible for ensuring that hospitals meet Centers for Medicare and Medicaid Services (CMS) standards for receiving reimbursement from Medicare and Medicaid. Each state takes responsibility for ensuring the safe regulation of health-care services.

Each state has an official state public health agency headed by a chief executive officer, often called the state health commissioner.[43] These agencies, funded by state legislatures, monitor health status, enforce public health laws and regulations, and distribute federal and state funds for public health activities to local public health agencies. The form and structure of state public health agencies vary greatly from state to state, with some states merging the state public health agency with social services.

Almost all state-based public health agencies participate in the U.S. Centers for Disease Control and Prevention (CDC) Health Alert Network (HAN). According to the CDC, the vast majority of those agencies have more than 90% of their population covered by the HAN system. The HAN includes a secure website and emergency messaging system for sharing reputable information about urgent public health events such as bioterrorism, communicable diseases, and environmental threats.[44] Statewide HAN initiatives, funded by grants from the CDC, connect local health departments with hospitals, clinics, law enforcement, firefighters, and emergency medical providers. The HAN incorporates various levels of messages ranging from time-sensitive information that necessitates immediate action to general public health information.

HAN archives from 2017 include messages about influenza surveillance and treatment recommendations; advice for providers treating patients returning from hurricane-affected areas; Brucella incidence and exposure related to the consumption of raw milk; a reminder to clinicians of the dangers, symptoms, and treatment of carbon monoxide poisoning related to the use of generators during power outages; and information about a Seoul virus outbreak associated with home-based rat breeding in Wisconsin and Illinois. In that same year, the Texas Department of State Health Services communicated a Zika virus health alert regarding enhanced surveillance and modified testing guidelines of symptomatic and asymptomatic pregnant women in certain counties.

Local Health Policy

Local public health agencies derive their authority from state and local laws and regulations. They deal with issues such as water safety and fluoridation, sanitation, communicable diseases, and sanitary food and beverages, and they sometimes regulate and/or own health-care facilities such as hospitals, clinics, or nursing homes.[45] The form and structure of local public health agencies vary with centralized models operated directly by the state or decentralized models under county, city, or other local jurisdictions. Local public health agencies have a chief executive officer who generally works with local boards of health that are appointed or elected (see Chapter 13).

Local Health Department Personnel

Health department personnel are influential in developing, monitoring, and enforcing local health laws and regulations (see Chapter 13). For instance, local health agency advocacy has resulted in many local jurisdictions passing ordinances restricting the use of tobacco in public settings. Local health agencies have policies whereby sanitarians inspect restaurants, convenience stores, food vendors at county fairs, and other public facilities that serve food to enforce guidelines such as food holding temperatures. The local health department can close these establishments if they do not meet certain standards. Another example of health-related policy at the local level involves zoning ordinances. A community in need of a shelter for homeless families was having difficulty securing a permit to open a shelter in a residential area because of zoning laws and property owners' fear of decreasing property values. Advocates for the homeless along with public health representatives met with residents to determine a plan for the shelter that would minimally affect the neighborhood. Advocates also petitioned the elected city board for a change in the zoning laws to allow a homeless shelter in that area of the city.

To promote equity and efficiency, a local health agency may have a policy about services offered to residents. For instance, one local health agency may decide to offer free home visits to families of newborns who meet certain risk criteria, whereas another local health agency decided to offer one free home visit to all families of newborns. As public health agency budgets are reduced, it is important to base local policy decisions on scientific evidence.

Likewise, local health agencies need to determine policies for payment for services such as immunizations or for clinics that treat sexually transmitted infections. Should clients pay the full or partial (sliding fee) cost of each unit of service, should the agency request a donation, or should these services be free of charge? Sometimes, state or federal policy influences these decisions, but often these kinds of policy decisions are left to the local health agency. These decisions potentially affect access to care, utilization rates of the service, and resources available for other services.

Local jurisdictions or even regions need to coordinate emergency services such as 911 call centers; ambulance, fire, and rescue dispatch; and routing to local hospitals. Development of policies regarding emergency response services requires extensive coordination of multiple stakeholders within multiple jurisdictions. With the increasing incidence of opioid use, many localities are adopting policies to combat the morbidity and mortality associated with opioid use (Box 21-1) (Fig. 21-1).[46]

Preparing for emergencies involving disasters, such as a flood, collapse of a bridge, chemical spill, or act of bioterrorism, requires extensive planning. Public health agencies are often involved in primary prevention, but some disasters cannot be prevented, such as a tornado. Public health agencies work cooperatively with other agencies and community stakeholders to develop an emergency management plan that includes preparedness, mitigation, response, recovery, and evaluation (Chapter 22). An emergency management plan is an example of a policy. Many counties and other jurisdictions hold disaster drills to test aspects of their emergency disaster plans.

Local health departments can choose to undergo a voluntary accreditation process. Since 2013, the Public Health Accreditation Board has run a national voluntary accreditation program for local health departments in addition to state, tribal, and territorial health departments. Accreditation helps assure and improve the quality and performance of health departments.[50]

Business/Organizational Health Policy

Federal, state, and local laws affect health, but so do policies of businesses and organizations. Organizations and businesses may choose to develop policies for their employees or customers, such as hospitals and universities that establish smoke-free campuses. Legally, sometimes organizational policies clash with state or local policies.

For instance, in 2018, cannabis was illegal at the federal level, but almost two-thirds of states had legalized medical use, and almost half had legalized or decriminalized recreational use.[51] In general, employers can prohibit cannabis use at work or employees from coming to work under the influence of drugs or alcohol, but employers also need to attempt to comply with contradictory laws while assuring employee and public safety.

BOX 21–1 ■ Opioid Policies

More than 42,000 Americans died of opioid overdoses in 2016, a 28% increase over 2015. With the increase in opioid use, abuse, and related mortality related to overdose, there is a need to develop and test policies to reduce morbidity and mortality associated with opioid abuse. At the national level, the CDC has increased funding for states to assess policy interventions regarding opioid abuse. At the state level, prevention includes implementing and evaluating universal prescription drug monitoring programs that allow pharmacists to determine if a patient has obtained prescriptions opioids elsewhere. At the local level, interventions include providing technical assistance to communities and jurisdictions with high rates of at-risk opioid use and death. Insurers and health systems are educating providers and facilitating the use of evidence-based prescribing guidelines such as using nonpharmacologic therapies and nonopioid pharmacologic therapies when possible and prescribing the lowest possible dose and quantity for expected level and duration of severe pain. For example, one Wisconsin county implemented a nonopioid dental pain protocol for patients seeking care at local emergency departments. These policy interventions need to be evaluated to determine what works.[46,47]

Other local interventions include the wide distribution of overdose-reversing agents and programs that provide supervised consumption of opioids including methadone at specialized community facilities. In 2018, the U.S. Surgeon General suggested that those likely to encounter overdose victims including friends and families of opioid users and health-care practitioners carry the opioid overdose reversal agent naloxone.

Source: (48)

▼ CASE STUDY
Drug-Free Workplace Policy Development

You are an occupational health nurse working with a midsized manufacturer in a state that legalized medical and recreational cannabis use. As a member of the health and safety committee, you are tasked to develop a drug-free workplace policy.

Using the Substance Abuse and Mental Health Services Administration (SAMHSA) Drug-Free Workplace Toolkit (https://www.samhsa.gov/workplace/toolkit), answer the following:

1. What key stakeholders should be included in the drug-free workplace policy development taskforce?
2. What drug-free workplace laws and regulations (federal, state, and local) would apply to this company?

A rise in opioid overdoses is detected. **What now?**

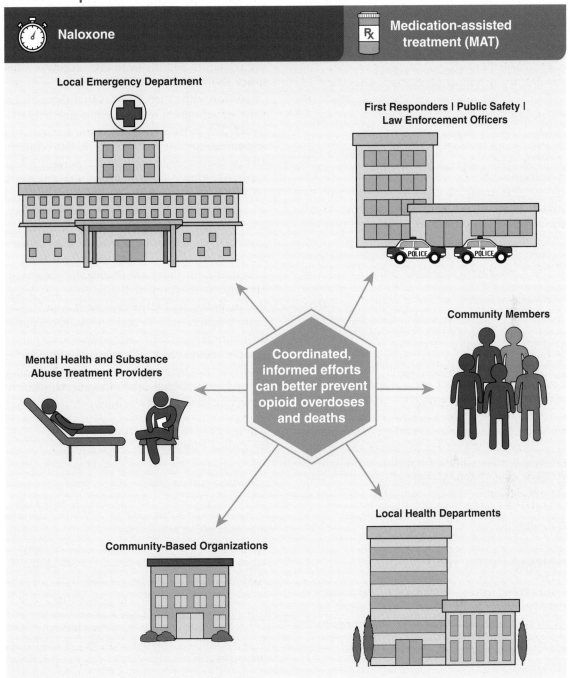

Figure 21-1 Rise in Opioid Overdoses is Detected: What Now? *(Centers for Disease Control and Prevention. (2018, March 6). Vital Signs: Opioid overdoses treated in emergency departments. Retrieved from https://www.cdc.gov/vitalsigns/opioid-overdoses/index.html https://www.cdc.gov/vitalsigns/opioid-overdoses/infographic.html#infographic)*

3. Draft a drug-free workplace policy for this company, including:
   a. Purpose Statement and Goals
   b. Definitions and Prohibitions
   c. Description of how employees will be educated/informed about the new policy
4. What impact would the presence of collective bargaining have on the policy development process?
5. What should the policy be regarding workers who fail a routine drug screen test?
6. Should the policy be different for workers who have a permit to use medical cannabis? Why or why not?

Likewise, the decision to offer health insurance and/or paid sick leave to employees beyond what might be specified by national, state, or local law is an important health-related policy decision of businesses. Some businesses require employees to participate in health risk assessments and wellness programs to avoid paying a higher insurance premium. This is particularly prevalent among companies with self-funded insurance programs. Nutrition information provided by restaurants is another example of a health-related business decision policy. A local amateur hockey league may require that all players wear protective headgear while on the ice. Some schools have implemented health policies that restrict vending choices during school hours. Such initiatives at the organizational or business level can build on governmental policies such as recent policies by school districts to change to healthier foods in the school lunch programs.[52] Various stores, including a number of national chains, have established policies about not selling inhalants to minors and/or have moved inhalants to a secure area to prevent shoplifting.

Principles of Public Health Policy

Public health policy focuses on promoting and protecting the health of populations. It should be based on evidence and be both ethically sound and culturally appropriate.

Health Policy Assessment and Planning Process

Effective public health policy is grounded in the health assessment and planning process, a problem-focused process (Chapters 4 and 5). The health planning process, the policy process, and the nursing process use similar terms.

Assessment of health status, social data, needs, and resources is an essential first step in the policy process.

Goals and objectives for the policy are established with input from stakeholders, those directly or indirectly affected by the policy. Think of a school nurse who needs to make an authoritative decision about which children will be screened for vision problems. The school has limited resources and the state does not have a definitive policy about which children or grade levels to screen. Discussion with other school nurses shows that the majority of schools screen children in first and second grades. The nurse will use the policy process to make a decision about vision screening. What evidence-based standards exist regarding vision screening of school-age children? What evidence is there about the yield (new cases discovered) of vision screening at various grades? What else would be needed besides screening for an effective vision health program? Where can the nurse refer children who lack the means to pay for the services of an optometrist and need glasses?

In the health policy assessment and planning process, much attention is given to the development of the policy. Specific policy alternatives are posited and analyzed regarding factors such as cost, likely effectiveness, social and political feasibility, and equity. A school nurse making policy about vision screening would specify policy alternatives regarding vision screening. One policy might be to require vision check-ups as a prerequisite to entering or transferring to the school.

Using Explicit Evaluation Criteria for Policy Planning

Policy alternatives can be judged according to explicit evaluation criteria. Three criteria most often used are effectiveness, efficiency, and equity (Table 21-1). **Effectiveness** is the likelihood of achieving the goals and objectives of the policy. Increasing physical activity in a population might include requiring daily physical education classes for all schoolchildren, which may be more effective than open access to a community fitness center for residents of a school district. **Efficiency** is achievement of policy goals relative to cost. The cost of providing daily physical education classes to school-age children (hiring teachers, increased facility requirements, lengthening the school day to accommodate the requirement, and lost opportunity costs of a required class in physical education vs. math or music, etc.) would be compared with the cost of providing access to physical fitness facilities for all residents (facility capital costs, additional staff, liability insurance, etc.). **Equity** is fairness or justice in the distribution of a policy's costs, benefits, and risks. Using the prior example, the requirement of daily physical fitness courses provides a benefit

TABLE 21-1 ■ Selected Criteria for Evaluating Public Policy Proposals

Criterion	Definition	Limits to Use
Effectiveness	Likelihood of achieving policy goals and objectives or demonstrated achievement of them.	Estimates involve uncertain projection of future events.
Efficiency	The achievement of program goals or benefits in relation to the costs. Least cost for a given benefit or the largest benefit for a given cost.	Measuring all costs and benefits is not always possible. Policy decision making reflects political choices as much as efficiency.
Equity	Fairness or justice in the distribution of the policy's costs, benefits, and risks across population subgroups.	Difficulty in finding techniques to measure equity; disagreement over whether equity means a fair process or equal outcomes.
Liberty/ Freedom	Extent to which public policy extends or restricts privacy and individual rights and choices.	Assessment of impacts on freedom is often clouded by ideological beliefs about the role of government.
Political feasibility	The extent to which elected officials accept and support a policy proposal.	Difficult to determine. Depends on perceptions of the issues and changing economic and political conditions.
Social acceptability	The extent to which the public will accept and support a policy proposal.	Difficult to determine even when public support can be measured. Depends on saliency of the issues and level of public awareness.
Administrative feasibility	The likelihood that a department or agency can implement the policy well.	Involves projection of available resources and agency behavior that can be difficult to estimate.
Technical feasibility	The availability and reliability of technology needed for policy implementation.	Often difficult to anticipate technological change that would alter feasibility.

Source: Adapted with permission from Kraft, M., & Furlong, S.R. (2015). *Public policy: Politics, analysis, and alternatives* (ed 5). Washington, DC: Sage/CQ Press.

exclusively for the school-age population, whereas open access to fitness facilities potentially benefits all age groups. Taxpayers would incur the costs for both policy choices. Weighing these three key criteria helps policy makers decide which policy approach to implement. Of course, maintaining the status quo is always another policy approach to take. In this case, the third unstated policy is to continue "business as usual" with students having physical education classes twice a week and those with the financial means and desire joining a fitness facility. Other important criteria for evaluating policy include liberty/ freedom, political feasibility, social acceptability, administrative feasibility, and technical feasibility.[7]

A theory links the proposed policy with the actions, behaviors, and/or decisions of others. Many public health policies are based on psychological or economic theories. A law imposing a penalty for being detected by police for not wearing a seat belt raises the potential cost of that action. This policy is based on at least two theories: rational action choice theory and the theory of reasoned action.

Rational action choice theory assumes that individuals will make choices that benefit them the most with the least cost.[52] In this scenario, the theory suggests that individuals will buckle up to avoid the financial penalty. Ajzen and Fishbein's (1975, 1980) theory of reasoned action also explains and supports this policy.[53] The theory suggests that behavioral intentions depend on a person's attitude about the behavior and subjective norms. Because subjective norms, perceived expectations from others, and intention to comply with those expectations guide personal behavior, policies have the potential to influence behavior by influencing how others behave and, more specifically, by changing the social norm of using seat belts.

Policies are formulated, interpreted, and implemented. Implementing policy is a complex activity that involves determining and enacting the various activities that will put the policy into effect. For instance, laws are interpreted by the executive branch of government and implemented by numerous agencies and organizations, including employers, health-care providers, service agencies, and public health departments. States may interpret and enforce federal laws differently. Specifically, implementation involves developing the details of the process that will allow for the intended outcome to take place. This could include such things as hiring personnel, establishing fines or penalties for those who do not follow the policy, and disseminating information about the policy.

Stakeholder Involvement

Like the nursing process, in which it is important to involve the client as much as possible, stakeholder involvement is important in the policy process. In assessment, or identification of the policy issue, sometimes stakeholders identify the need for a policy and sometimes they identify a problem but are not sure what type of policy will best address the problem. In Chapter 5, you read about the Elmwood Senior residence and concerns for isolation because of violence in their neighborhood. Community members, parents of young children, and the elders living in a senior residence facility felt that community violence kept them from physical activities such as walking outside and spending time in the park. The community health nurse obtained information from religious organizations, school representatives, seniors, and other community stakeholders to plan a program to address the perceived barrier to physical activity. At the organizational level, Elmwood residential facility coordinated an escort service for the residents. At the community level, local law enforcement increased their presence through periodic patrolling of this neighborhood. The school recognized the need for increased after-school activities for the youths. The nurse worked with community organizers to obtain funds for after-school activities for teens.

Focus on Health Determinants

Health status is a complex interaction of environmental, socioeconomic, genetic, health service, and behavioral determinants. Public health policy attempts to change health status by influencing these determinants as precursors to morbidity and mortality. Public health policy emphasizes intervention in environmental protection, health promotion, and specific disease prevention. The concept of influencing determinants of health prior to the development of poor health or even physiological changes that would lead to poor health is known as *upstream thinking*. Lead poisoning and skin cancer are examples of public health problems that can be diminished or avoided with the implementation of upstream policies designed to prevent those problems (Table 21-2). Note that some upstream policies directly change the physical environment, whereas some policies require behavioral change.

Federal programs, such as Medicaid that provide health services to poor families and laws such as the Family Medical Leave Act (FMLA) that guarantee continuation of work for those experiencing a health event in their family are examples of policies affecting socioeconomic determinants. The decision of an employer to provide paid sick leave for workers is a type of socioeconomic policy that, in most states and communities, is left to the employer.

TABLE 21–2 ■ Examples of Upstream Policies Addressing Specific Public Health Problems or Issues

Public Health Problem/Issue	Upstream Policies
Lead poisoning in children	Federal and state restrictions on use of leaded paint in residential use
Exposure to secondhand smoke	Restaurant association's endorsement of smoke-free facilities among its members
High rates of cardiovascular disease	Health insurance policy to co-fund gym or weight-reduction club memberships Local zoning laws requiring sidewalks and bike paths in area of new development Drug store chains deciding not to sell tobacco products
Infant and maternal health	Employer providing onsite lactation room in workplace
Poor nutrition among poor	Supplemental Nutrition Assistance Program (SNAP), previously known as Food Stamps, that provides assistance to low- and no-income individuals and families living in the United States
Dental caries	Municipality adding fluoride to drinking water
Herd immunity or individual immunity	School entry vaccination laws
Unintentional injuries of children	Child safety seat laws

Health-care providers' expansion of primary care services to weekend and evening hours improves access to care, increases primary care utilization, and generally improves health. When public health departments provide free vaccinations in schools, it increases immunization rates and strengthens herd immunity. State laws mandating certain vaccinations for school entry are also examples of policies having an impact on health through health services.

A school district's decision to implement a toothbrushing program for preschool and elementary students is intended to influence oral hygiene behavior of children and families and improve overall oral health. A construction company's decision to implement random drug testing for employees who operate heavy equipment may reduce drug use and injuries among employees. Mandating certain vaccinations for health-care workers is another example affecting worker behavior.

Evidence-Based Practice

Do the health policies previously described really affect health? Although anecdotal evidence exists for many health policies, some health policies are not supported by a body of scientific evidence. For example, although there is fairly good evidence that a sedentary lifestyle combined with extreme obesity is related to increased morbidity and mortality, the evidence that mandating sidewalks or including nutrition information on restaurant menus results in positive changes in individual actions, behaviors, and decisions is less clear. It is difficult if not impossible to randomly assign individuals or even communities to these interventions. Therefore, it is difficult to evaluate the impact of these interventions on health.

■ EVIDENCE-BASED PRACTICE
Cost Effectiveness of Bike Lanes/Trails

Practice Statement: Produce a built environment strategy to increase physical activity through bicycle use.
Targeted Outcome: Increasing physical activity in communities with pedestrian and bike paths.
Supporting Evidence: To address the growing rates of obesity, many communities are investing in environmental strategies designed to improve pedestrian or bicycle transportations systems to increase physical activity. In fact, the Community Preventive Services Task Force noted that residents' physical activity increased in communities with new or improved projects or policies that combined transportation (e.g., pedestrian or cycling paths) with environmental design (e.g., access to public parks).[54] Built Environment Approaches involve interventions that enhance opportunities for active transportation and leisure-time physical activity.
Recommended Approaches: The Community Preventive Services Task Force noted that, across several longitudinal studies, physical activity outcomes were favorable for studies involving enhanced walking/biking recreational- and transportation-related studies. From a cost-benefit perspective, Wang and colleagues (2005) found that, for every $1 spent on trails for physical activity, there was a $2.94 direct medical benefit.[55] A recent study of the cost-effectiveness of bike lanes in New York City also found that, in addition to the financial return on investment, increased bike/pedestrian lanes reduced pollution and risk of injury as compared to not having such lanes.[56] Both studies demonstrated that investments in bike lanes were a good value as they address multiple public health problems.

Related policies that support biking include mandating sufficient bike racks, bicycle friendly parking ordinances, zoning ordinances that discourage an overabundance of surface parking lots and road design standards that include protected bike lanes.

References:

1. Wang, G., Macera, C.A., Scudder-Soucie, B., Schmid, T., Pratt, M., & Buchner, D. (2005). A cost-benefit analysis of physical activity using bike/pedestrian trails. *Health Promotion Practice, 6*(2), 174-179. Doi: 10.1177/1524839903260687.
2. Gu, J., Mohit, B., Muennig, P.A. (2017). The cost-effectiveness of bike lanes in New York City. *Injury Prevention, 23*(4), 239-243. Doi: 10.1136/injuryprev-2016-042057.

Another example is the evidence that drinking fluoridated water reduces the number of dental caries. Although theoretically it would be possible to randomly assign communities supplied by separate water systems to fluoridated or nonfluoridated water status, in the United States a decision such as fluoridation of water is under local control and is often a political decision. There is often no authority to give permission for random assignment. In this case, the evidence of the success of the program is based on population data over time. Based on the evidence, there has been a decline in dental caries overall in countries that fluoridate water and those that do not.[57] This is because other changes have been introduced, including topical fluoride applications, fluoridated toothpastes, and salt and milk fluoridation. With 100 years of accumulated population-level evidence that fluoride in many forms reduces dental carries, the World Health Organization (WHO) recommends that public health policy support the use of fluoridated toothpastes and, where economically, technically, and culturally feasible, water fluoridation.[58] In the United States, in addition to fluoridation of water supplies, fluoride varnish programs have been implemented. This intervention involves the application of a thin layer of fluoride to the teeth of children.[59] School districts concerned with dental health may adopt other related policies such as limiting sugar-laden vending choices. Evaluating the effectiveness of one policy, such as a varnish policy, is difficult because of the other interventions in current use.

There are a number of good sources of reviews for evidence-based practice on which to base policy decisions. The Agency for Healthcare Research and Quality (AHRQ) U.S. Preventive Services Task Force publishes a *Guide to Clinical Preventive Services (Clinical Guide)* that recommends clinical preventive services based on systemic review of clinical practices.[60] This regularly updated guide includes dozens of reviews in areas such as alcohol and drug abuse, cancer screening, nutrition, and exercise.

A second source, complementary to the AHRQ guide, is the CDC *Guide to Community Preventive Services: The Community Guide: What Works to Promote Health,* referred to as the *Community Guide.*[61] The *Community Guide* includes systematic reviews and recommendations for interventions that promote population health (Table 21-3). For instance, regarding skin cancer prevention, the *Community Guide* recommends a wide variety of interventions focused on promoting sun protection behaviors and environmental protections.[62]

A third good source is the Cochrane Reviews, a database of systematic reviews of the effects of health-care interventions (Table 21-4).[63] The reviews are conducted by a global collaboration of volunteers and a small staff in London, United Kingdom. Although many of the Cochrane Reviews are clinically focused, there are a number that have a public health emphasis. For instance, in the area of injury control, there are reviews on interventions for promoting smoke alarm ownership and use, and interventions for preventing injuries in the construction industry.

TABLE 21–3 ■ Task Force on Community Preventive Services

Selected Systematic Reviews on Policy Interventions Conducted from the *Guide to Community Preventive Services*

Topic	Policy Setting	Intervention Title	Recommendation
Preventing Excessive Alcohol Use	Community	Enhanced enforcement of laws prohibiting sales to minors	Recommended (Sufficient Evidence)
		Regulation of outlet density	Recommended (Sufficient Evidence)
		Responsible beverage service training	Insufficient Evidence
Preventing Skin Cancer	Education	Educational and policy: childcare centers	Insufficient Evidence
		Educational and policy: primary school settings	Recommended (Strong Evidence)
		Educational and policy: secondary schools and colleges	Insufficient Evidence
	Community	Educational and policy: outdoor recreation settings	Insufficient Evidence
	Worksite	Educational and policy: outdoor occupation settings	Insufficient Evidence
Motor Vehicle–Related Injury Prevention	Community	Reducing alcohol-impaired driving: sobriety checkpoints	Recommended (Strong Evidence)
		Reducing alcohol-impaired driving: lower legal blood alcohol concentrations for young and inexperienced drivers	Recommended (Strong Evidence)

TABLE 21–3 ■ Task Force on Community Preventive Services—cont'd

Topic	Policy Setting	Intervention Title	Recommendation
		Reducing alcohol-impaired driving: 0.08% blood alcohol concentration (BAC) laws	Recommended (Strong Evidence)
		Reducing alcohol-impaired driving: minimum legal drinking age	Recommended (Strong Evidence)
		Use of child safety seats: laws mandating use	Recommended (Strong Evidence)
		Use of safety belts: laws mandating use	Recommended (Strong Evidence)
		Use of safety belts: primary (vs. secondary) enforcement laws	Recommended (Strong Evidence)
Oral Health	Community	Dental caries (cavities): community water fluoridation	Recommended (Strong Evidence)
	Education	Dental caries (cavities): school-based or -linked sealant delivery	Recommended (Strong Evidence)
Promoting Physical Activity	Community	Built Environment Approaches combining transportation system interventions with land use and environmental design	Recommended (Sufficient Evidence)
	Community, Home, School	Family-based Interventions	Recommended (Sufficient Evidence)
	School	College-based Physical Education and Health Education	Insufficient Evidence
Tobacco Use	Community	Increasing tobacco use cessation: increasing the unit price of tobacco products	Recommended (Strong Evidence)
		Reducing tobacco use initiation: increasing the unit price of tobacco products	Recommended (Strong Evidence)
		Reducing exposure to environmental tobacco smoke: smoking bans and restrictions	Recommended (Strong Evidence)
		Restricting minors' access to tobacco products: community mobilization with additional interventions	Recommended (Sufficient Evidence)
		Restricting minors' access to tobacco products: active enforcement of sales laws directed at retailers	Insufficient Evidence
		Restricting minors' access to tobacco products: laws directed at minors' purchase, possession, or use of tobacco products	Insufficient Evidence
	Education	School tobacco-free policies	Insufficient Evidence
	Worksite	Smoke-free policies to reduce tobacco use among workers	Recommended (Sufficient Evidence)
Vaccine Preventable Diseases	Education	Vaccination requirements for childcare, school, and college attendance	Recommended (Sufficient Evidence)

Continued

TABLE 21–3 ■ Task Force on Community Preventive Services—cont'd

Topic	Policy Setting	Intervention Title	Recommendation
Violence Prevention	Community	Firearms laws • Bans on specified firearms or ammunition • Restrictions on firearm acquisition • Waiting periods for firearm acquisition • Firearm registration and licensing of firearm owners • "Shall issue" concealed weapons carry laws • Child access prevention laws • Zero tolerance of firearms in schools • Combinations of firearms laws	Insufficient Evidence
		Transfer of juveniles into adult court system to reduce violence	Recommended Against (Strong Evidence)
Worksite Health Promotion	Worksite	Smoke-free policies to reduce tobacco use among workers	Recommended (Sufficient Evidence)

Source: Adapted from The Community Guide. (2014). *Topics.* Retrieved from http://www.thecommunityguide.org/.

TABLE 21–4 ■ Sources for Reviews of Evidence-Based Practice for Basing Public Health Policy

Community Guide	Centers for Disease Control and Prevention, Task Force on Community Preventive Services	www.thecommunityguide.org
Clinical Guide	Agency for Healthcare Research and Quality, U.S. Preventive Services Task Force	www.ahrq.gov/clinic/uspstfix.htm
Cochrane Reviews	Cochrane Library	www.cochranelibrary.com

Ethical and Cultural Implications of Policy

Public health policy ethics involve principles and values that guide authoritative decisions made in government, agencies, or organizations intended to influence population health. A basic assumption of public health policy is that society has the right, and even an obligation, to collectively assure conditions for healthy people. An additional assumption is that the collective can sometimes impose on individual rights for the sake of the common good. There is debate about the balance between the autonomy, privacy, and liberty interests of individuals and the collective interests of a population. There is also debate about the appropriate role of government involvement in promoting population health.

An example is the Community Preventive Services Task Force recommendation for universal helmet laws. The recommendation was based on strong evidence of the effectiveness of motorcycle helmet laws.[64] Some argue that requiring the use of helmets violates a person's individual rights. Despite the strength of the evidence, as of 2018, a few states did not have helmet laws, and some states only required the use of helmets for individuals 17 and younger.[65]

Policies toward migrants from other countries are reflective of local culture and have cultural and ethical and cultural implications. Reasons for migration include family unification, economic opportunity, wars, violence, and/or discrimination in their country of origin. It appears that climate change will further exacerbate poverty, war, and violence in some areas leading to increased migratory pressure and even mass migrations.[66] The U.S. grants a limited number of authorizations to immigrate and, in collaboration with the United Nations and the International Refugee Committee, offers asylum and resettlement to refugees and migrants fleeing war and/or persecution. The number of individuals granted refugee status and resettlement is limited and varies over time. Additionally, some migrants, for instance those affected by a natural catastrophe, may be granted temporary protected status in the U.S. for a limited time.

■ CULTURAL CONTEXT
Undocumented Immigrants

Foreign nationals who illegally reside in a country are known as undocumented immigrants, unauthorized immigrants, or illegal aliens. These immigrants may illegally cross the border, overstay visas, or participate in marriages solely for immigration status. They usually have limited access to public services, such as individually focused public health services and government vouchers for food, and, because of fear of deportation, are often afraid to report crimes. They may be subject to dangerous conditions during border crossings,and, once in the U.S., exposed to labor exploitation, sex trafficking, slavery, and housing discrimination. Federal, state, and local governments have interpreted laws and regulations regarding undocumented immigrants differently over time, depending on world politics, economic conditions in the U.S., and the nationalities or home regions of the immigrants.

Although undocumented children are entitled to public education, many localities have policies, such as proof as residency or guardianship, which hinder educational access. Undocumented college students are not eligible for federal loans and, in many states, need to pay out-of-state tuition. Starting in 2012, certain undocumented immigrants who migrated to the U.S. as juveniles were given protection from deportation along with the ability to apply for a work permit. There have been political and legal challenges to this policy, with some arguing that these migrants did not choose to come to the U.S. and know no other country as their home whereas others argue that this kind of policy encourages illegal immigration.[67]

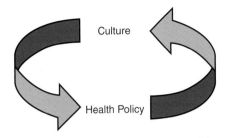

Figure 21-2 Relationship of culture and health policy.

the *HP* objectives are aimed at reducing health disparities.[13] It is critical to consider the unique cultural makeup of the community in determining appropriate programmatic and policy decisions. A policy prohibiting individuals from serving foods prepared in their home for general consumption at large social gatherings (e.g., funerals and weddings) may help reduce the incidence of foodborne illness but would be met with resistance by groups that traditionally prepare foods in the home for such occasions. Conversely, a policy allowing individuals and families to rent a small area of land within a community garden in an urban area would be well received by individuals from cultures with a tradition for consuming homegrown produce. These examples demonstrate the importance of obtaining stakeholder input during the policy planning process.

Many public health policies target vulnerable groups. Poverty and unemployment disproportionately affect people of color, and many rely on public health insurance for coverage. Policies specifically benefiting impoverished individuals have the potential to benefit minority groups to a greater degree. For instance, CHIP has the potential to improve the health of minority populations by improving access to health services, leading, it is hoped, to fewer illnesses and resulting in decreased school absenteeism and increased high school graduation rates.

The Legislative Process and Public Health Policy

Advocating for the best interest of patients is second nature to nurses, but advocating for health-care policies is often unfamiliar territory. To effect policy change for the profession and for patient care, it is important that nurses be familiar with the legislative process and with how to make their opinions count regarding specific legislation. Nurses should have a grasp of how a bill becomes law in the U.S. Congress (Fig. 21-3). Similar processes take place in state legislatures.

Culture, in its broadest sense, refers to learned knowledge, attitudes, and behaviors of groups of people, which often are accepted without question. We often think of the culture of various ethnic and racial groups; however, all groups, including communities and workplaces, have a culture. Most people are members of multiple cultural groups, and policy makers are influenced by their own cultural groups as well as the culture of their constituents and other stakeholders.

Public health policies can affect culture by changing knowledge, attitudes, and behaviors of individuals and groups (Fig. 21-2). For example, changes in the social acceptability of tobacco use allowed for smoking restriction policies that would have been unacceptable in the 1960s. Smoking restriction policies, in turn, affect knowledge, attitudes, and behaviors regarding smoking.

Culturally acceptable health policies are those that make sense to the people they affect. For example, many of

From Bills to Laws: The Course of Legislation in Congress

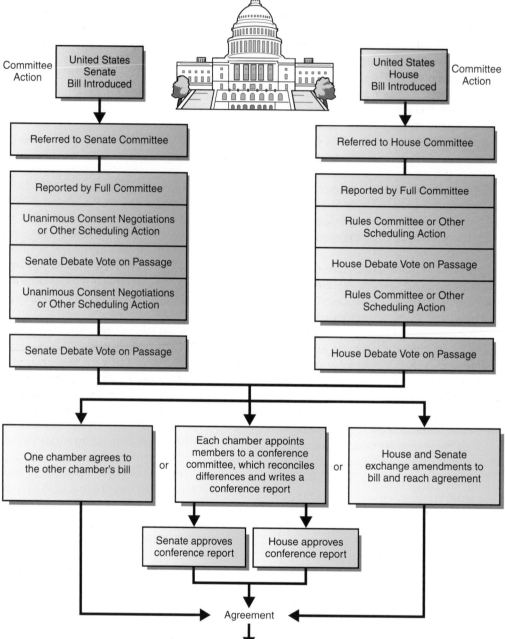

Figure 21-3 How a bill becomes law. *(Adapted from Congressional Research Service, A division of the Library of Congress.)*

The U.S. Constitution includes a series of checks and balances to ensure adequate opportunity for consideration and debate of an issue. Congress, made up of the House of Representatives and the Senate, is the official body through which all legislation is presented. The Senate is composed of 100 members, two from each of the 50 states, regardless of population or area, who serve for 6 years. The House of Representatives is composed of 435 members elected every 2 years from among the 50 states, apportioned by their population. The Constitution limits the number of representatives to not more than one for every 30,000 people. Each member of the Senate or House of Representatives has one vote.

The chief function of Congress is making laws. Both the Senate and House of Representatives have equal legislative functions and powers with just a few exceptions. Ideas for legislation come from members of Congress, from their constituent groups, and from executive communication from the President, a member of the President's cabinet, or a head of an independent agency such as the Agency for Toxic Substances and Disease Registry.[68]

Once an idea or concern is presented, the elected official can introduce a bill to Congress. The representative or senator becomes its sponsor and other legislators can cosponsor the piece of legislation. The bill is given a number (preceded by H.R. if proposed in the House of Representatives and S. if a bill is introduced by the Senate) and referred to the appropriate committee or committees (i.e., House Ways and Means or Senate Appropriations Committee).

Perhaps the most crucial phase of the legislative process is the action taken by committees. Once in committee, the bill undergoes extensive consideration and debate. It is during this phase that government officials, industry experts, and anyone with interest in the bill can give testimony. The period when a bill is being considered in committee is an important time to contact legislative staff and legislators who are on the committee considering the bill. For example, in 2017, the American Nurses Association advocated for a number of legislative bills, including the Safe Staffing for Nurse and Patient Safety Act (S. 2446, H.R. 5052).[69] In a similar manner, the ANA advocated for regulations to improve the packaging, storage, and disposal of opioids to the Food and Drug Administration (FDA-2017-N-5897).[70]

Individuals and organizations that testify before a committee must file a written statement of their proposed testimony before they appear. Once before the committee, testimony is limited to a brief summary of their arguments. A transcript of the testimony is printed and distributed to committee members as well as made available to the public.

After hearings are completed, the bill enters a "markup" phase in which a vote is taken to determine the action of the committee. The committee can approve the bill, amend the bill, "table" (postpone indefinitely), or reject the bill. If the committee approves the bill, it moves on in the legislative process. Bills can be rejected through a vote or simply by not acting on them; this is commonly referred to as "dying in committee."

Once a bill is approved, it is reported to the full House or Senate, where it is written and published. This includes the impact on existing law, budgetary considerations, any tax implications (increases or decreases) required by the bill, and the opinions of the committee either for or against the legislation. A reported bill is then placed on the legislative calendar of the House or Senate, where it is scheduled for floor action and debated before the full membership. Once general debate has ended, a second reading of the bill begins, during which amendments may be offered. Once debate ends and amendments are approved, the full membership votes for or against the bill.

Depending on the congressional body in which the bill originates, once a bill is approved, it is sent to the other chamber where the same process is repeated. Once both chambers of Congress have approved the bill in identical form, it is sent to the President of the United States for action. The President may sign the bill into law, take no action on the bill, or veto the bill. If the bill sits unsigned on the President's desk for 10 days while Congress is in session, the bill automatically becomes law. If no action is taken on a bill and Congress adjourns, the bill dies. This is referred to as a "pocket veto."[68] Congress may override a veto by the President by a two-thirds vote in favor of the bill in both houses of Congress. Once a presidential veto is overridden, it is written as a binding statute and becomes law. All laws of the United States are published in the *U.S. Code*, a listing of the general and permanent laws organized according to subject matter under 50 title headings.[71]

To illustrate the process by which a bill becomes law, the history of a law regarding online sex trafficking is a good example. Nurses may encounter individuals who are victims of human trafficking (e.g., sex or labor trafficking or child soldiers). It is estimated that 600,000 to 800,000 adults and children worldwide are trafficked across international borders each year.[72] Unfortunately, many victims of trafficking go undetected by health-care providers. Nurses need to stay informed, ask questions, and know what is going on in their community. To address the growing problem of human trafficking, particularly via the Internet, Representative Ann Wagner (R) of Missouri introduced H.R. 1865: "Allow States and Victims to Fight Online Sex Trafficking Act of 2017," to the House of Representatives on April 3, 2017.[73] This new law allows the government to prosecute the owners of websites (e.g., Facebook, YouTube, Twitter) that aid or promote sex trafficking due to posts of that site's users. It also allows users to sue those websites. Senator Robert Portman (R-OH) introduced a sister bill, S. 1693 Stop Enabling Sex Traffickers Act of 2017, which was placed on the Senate legislative calendar effective January 10, 2018.[74] Box 21-2 describes this bill's progress through the 115th session of Congress.

Participation of Nurses in Health Policy

There is power in numbers. According to the Bureau of Labor Statistics, there are more than 2.9 million RNs employed in the United States.[75] Individual nurses, like all citizens, have the right and some would argue the duty to be politically active, yet results of studies demonstrate that nurses do not participate politically as much as they could. Reasons for a lack of political involvement range from professional demands (e.g., increasing workloads, understaffing), personal responsibilities (e.g., family roles, childcare), and lack of education regarding political action.[76]

The implications of lack of political involvement by nurses are extensive. Those who engage the system through voting and lobbying for their causes receive the attention of policy makers. Policy makers hear from individual physicians, pharmacists, and health insurance leaders. Policy makers also hear from lobbyists and organizations representing these professional groups such as the American Medical Association, Pharmaceutical Research and Manufacturers of America, and America's Health Insurance Plans. Because the 3 million nurses in the United States (more than three times the number of physicians) constitute the largest segment of the health workforce, imagine the impact if every nurse participated in advocating for health policy. Health policy, one of the most debated issues among political candidates, is influenced by the efforts of individuals but even more so by the efforts of organized groups and professional lobbyists. Nurses can affect policy through their individual efforts and utilizing their collective power.

Individual and Group Participation

When nurses engage the political system, politicians will see them as a powerful voting group to whom they must pay attention to be successful in seeking reelection to office. Advocacy activities can include active involvement in policy such as providing testimony, writing letters, and meeting with your state and federal legislators.[77] Nurses engage in advocacy on behalf of their patients every day; however, advocating for health policy has the potential to affect entire populations. Nurses interested in influencing the policy process, even those with limited time and resources, can become advocates for health policy legislation.[78-80] They can advocate for particular policies (Box 21-3). It helps to follow specific guidelines for communicating with policy makers (Box 21-4).

BOX 21–2 ■ How a Bill Goes Through the Legislative Process: H.R. 1865: Allow States and Victims to Fight Online Sex Trafficking Act of 2017/ S. 1693: Stop Enabling Sex Traffickers Act of 2017

House- H.R. 1865

4/03/17 Representative Ann Wager (R - MO) introduced H.R. 1865 amending the Communications Act of 1934 and clarifying that the Act does not prohibit enforcement against providers and users of interactive computer services relating to sexual exploitation of children or sex trafficking. H.R. 1865 received bipartisan support.

11/30/17 Heard in Communications and Technology

12/12/17 Communications and Technology committee ordered the bill be considered by the full House of Representatives

2/27/18 Passes the House 388–25

4/11/18 Signed by President

Senate- S. 1693

8/01/17 S. 1693: Stop Enabling Sex Traffickers Act of 2017 Introduced by Senator Robert Portman (R-OH) with bipartisan support

9/19/17 Considered by Senate Committee on Commerce, Science, and Transportation

11/08/17 Senate Committee on Commerce, Science, and Transportation orders a report on the bill for further consideration

1/10/18 Reported by the Senate Committee on Commerce, Science, and Transportation

As of November 2018, pending vote in the Senate

Sources: Govtrack. (n.d.). *H.R. 1865: Allow States and Victims to Fight Online Sex Trafficking Act of 2017.* Retrieved from https://www. govtrack.us/congress/bills/115/hr1865

Govtrack. (n.d.). *S. 1693: Stop Enabling Sex Traffickers Act of 2017.* Retrieved from https://www.govtrack.us/congress/bills/115/s1693

BOX 21–3 ▪ Advocacy for Particular Health Policies

- Communicating with legislators through e-mail, social media, face-to-face communications (personal visit), and phone calls—providing your name and address during these communications in case the legislator wishes to seek additional information about his/her viewpoint. Letters are no longer preferred due to safety issues as they are sometimes quarantined for a period of time before they are delivered, especially for federal legislators.
- Participating in annual state legislative days (i.e., Day at the Capital).
- Joining organizations that use collective power to influence policy such as the American Nurses Association (ANA), state/local nursing association, or specialty nursing associations.
- Seeking out policy workshops, internships, or fellowships.
- Attending a town hall meeting.

BOX 21–4 ▪ Tips for Communicating With Policy Makers

- **Keep it short.**
  Effective communication is brief and direct.
- **Focus on one topic.**
  Limit your communication to one topic/subject. Clearly state your topic/subject in the opening paragraph.
- **Share experiences.**
  Although using form letters to provide a template to work from is easier, they do not carry the same weight as communication written in your own words. Providing personal experiences and views gives the issue a human face.
- **Provide your name and contact information, including address.**
  Legislators and policy makers pay most attention to communication that comes from individuals who have the potential to vote for them. Including your contact information also enables them to contact you with questions or for clarification.
- **Persistence pays off.**
  Contact legislators and their staff frequently, particularly if they have not taken a position on an issue.

Members of Congress are most responsive to people from their own jurisdictions. They and their staffers need and want to have input from well-informed nurses to be aware of priority problems and the ramifications of changes in policy. Many nursing organization websites provide a link at which you can enter a ZIP code to find contact information for legislators and sample letters. Nurses can increase their expertise in policy analysis and development through workshops, internships, and fellowships (Box 21-5).

Collective Participation

Most changes in policy are the result of intentional activity of many individuals and groups. Because the policy process is influenced by the knowledge, attitudes, and actions of elected officials, influencing policy necessitates influencing the knowledge, attitudes, and actions of those elected officials. Strategies range from joining an organization that uses its collective powers to influence policy such as the American Association of Critical Care Nurses (AACN), Oncology Nurses Society (ONS), a state or national nursing organization like the American Nurses Association (ANA), or a multidisciplinary organization like the American Public Health Association, to writing a letter or making a call about an issue, to getting elected to public office.

Nurses can affect policy through the collective efforts of professional organizations. However, RNs in the United States do not always become members of organizations. This is a disheartening finding, considering that nurses who are in professional organizations are more likely to be politically active.[76,79] Professional organizations not only employ professional lobbyists who influence legislators through sustained activity over months and years, they also form political action committees whose very function is to engage in political advocacy and fund-raising. Although individual advocacy efforts are important, invitations to testify to Congress are typically offered to larger, organized groups that may have taken a position on an issue. The advocacy of the professional organization combined with individual advocacy efforts cannot be underestimated.[81]

BOX 21–5 ▪ Examples of Public Policy Internships of Interest to Registered Nurses

Congressional Fellows Program
Congressional Fellowships on Women and Public Policy
Coro Fellowship in Public Affairs
Kellogg Fellows in Health Policy Research
Nursing Organization Alliance: Nurses in Washington Internship (NIWI)
Presidential Management Fellows Program
Robert Wood Johnson Health Policy Fellows Program
Watson Fellowships
The Wellstone Fellowship for Social Justice
White House Fellows Program

Nursing has a legacy of political advocacy. Florence Nightingale, Lillian Wald, and Mary Breckinridge were all instrumental in shaping public health policy during their time. Today, political involvement by nurses continues to shape public health policy and contribute to solutions to improve population health. Nursing has the potential to affect health policy in any country because of its large numbers in the health workforce. Institution of sound public health policy improves the health of the patients whom nurses care for and the communities in which their patients live.

Public Health Finance

To further understand the public health system, it is important to understand how public health services are funded. **Public health finance** is a complex system involving funding streams, economic factors, and policy and political changes. This complexity along with the lack of transparency and the wide variation in local public health discretionary spending make it difficult to establish a consistent blueprint of public health agency funding. In the 1955 issue of the *American Journal of Public Health*, Burney and Yoho suggested that "the economic status of local government has been the most important single deterrent to the expansion of community health services".[82] They posited that, as local health departments strive to meet the needs identified in communities, they must also convince people that the benefits of the services required to meet those needs are worth the cost. This necessitates a realistic evaluation of all public health programs and a degree of fiscal scrutiny, which promotes selection of those programs predicted to have the most significant impact on the population relative to the costs involved (see Chapter 13).[82] Unfortunately, there appears to be little progress made in connecting the relationship between public health funding/expenditures to the health of populations.

Finance Terms

There are basic terms associated with health-care funding. Broadly speaking, **health economics** is a field that encompasses the process of understanding the supply and demand for health-care services.[83] As stated by the CDC, "***Economics** [is] the study of decisions—the incentives that lead to them, and the consequences from them—as they relate to production, distribution, and consumption of goods and services when resources are limited and have alternative uses.*" The CDC then applies economics to the process for conducting cost-benefit analysis as it applies to preventive strategies.

They compare the costs and outcomes among alternative strategies aimed at preventing adverse injury and disease.[84] Public health finance is specific to population-level health care and includes the acquisition, utilization, and management of the resources needed to deliver public health services provided by public health agencies and departments. It also includes an examination of how those resources affect both population health and the public health system.[85]

Public health economics examines the financing of public health from a governmental perspective with a focus on the delivery and funding of public health goods and services. Public health economists are concerned with the cost analysis, economic evaluation, modeling, and analysis of health-care regulation on the cost, burden, health, effectiveness, and efficiency of health programs.[85] Cost comparisons of health outcomes or health events may inform public health leaders and policy makers regarding the return on investment for public health funds. One modeling approach is the use of cost-effectiveness analyses focusing on one outcome to determine the most cost-effective intervention when several options exist. For example, the cost of screening an entire town for a specific disease may cost $150 per new case, whereas the cost of screening high-risk groups may identify cases at a cost of $50 per new case.[85]

Public Health Funding

People in every community in the United States have come to expect a basic level of public health services, including food and water safety and control of communicable disease outbreaks. These services come with a price tag and require a well-trained, well-equipped, and well-prepared public health system. Funding levels and sources of public health and disease prevention programs vary dramatically from neighborhood to neighborhood, community to community, city to city, and state to state. To adequately provide these services requires stable and adequate funding.[86]

An example of how funding affects public health is the Flint, Michigan, water crisis of 2014-2017. A coalescence of severe fiscal distress and the decision to change the city water supply to a cheaper but corrosive source without concomitant use of corrosion inhibitors led to a high level of lead contamination of city water supplies. Although community members complained about the taste and smell of the water, it appears that lack of political power of the affected low-income majority African-American population delayed identification of the problem. Thousands of children were exposed to lead contamination.[87]

Federal Funding

Historically, the federal government funded programs to ensure the health of specific groups of people. In 1798, the federal government created the Marine Hospital Service, under the direction of the Surgeon General, to provide health care for sick and disabled sailors and to protect the nation's borders against the importation of disease through seaports.[88] Funds for these services came from a per-month charge of 20 cents taken from the wages of American sailors.[88] In 1879, the federal government established the National Board of Health, charged with overseeing the health of the public. Due to disagreement about the authority of the U.S. government and other concerns, it ceased to exist in 1893.[89] Currently the United States Public Health Service (USPHS) is charged with protecting the health of the nation. Within the USPHS, many laws were created to protect the public from disease. The federal government, in cooperation with the health department, established quarantine rules along with a means to record vital information (e.g., births, deaths, and specified diseases).[89] Funding for state and local municipalities to support these efforts still comes primarily from federal and state sources.

The CDC, established in 1946, is a significant source of public health funding through grants and contracts to state and local public health departments. In fiscal year 2017, they reported that they awarded approximately 85% of their budget of about $11.9 billion through their grant programs and contracts. They awarded more than 23,000 separate grant and contract actions and provided more than $11.9 billion for public health programs.[90] The CDC funds health-related and research organizations that contribute to the CDC's mission through health information dissemination, preparedness, prevention, research, and surveillance.[91]

All federal funds are categorical in nature and address specific programming. Many local health departments receive federal dollars to fund programs. Examples of federal funds that help fund programs include the Title V Maternal Child Health program; Women, Infants, and Children (WIC); and the Well Women HealthCheck Program. Changes in federal funding levels affect the local health department to provide categorical programming. Examples of the changing federal revenue streams include increased funding to combat the growing opioid abuse epidemic and decreased funding for public health emergency preparedness.

State Funding

State health departments are central to the public health system. The U.S. Constitution identifies the states as primarily responsible for the health of their citizens and authorized to carry out these functions through a variety of state agencies.[85] The official state public health agency is often a freestanding department reporting to the governor of the state. In many cases, the state health departments rely on regional or district offices to carry out their responsibilities as well as to support the local health departments.[85] State statutes and policies dictate the programs and services offered and include regulatory, program, and service mandates. Funding for state health departments and programs varies widely in the United States, primarily coming from a combination of federal grants and contracts, program fees, and tax revenues. Examples of state public health programs include administering the WIC program, collection of vital statistics, tobacco use prevention, public health laboratories, food safety, and health facility regulation.[85]

Local Funding

The local health department, where most direct public health service delivery occurs, provides the majority of community prevention and clinical preventive services. In 2016, local health department expenditures ranged from $250,000 to more than $25 million.[92] Local sources (30%) provided the greatest source of funding, followed by state funds (21%), federal dollars passed through the state department (17%), and federal dollars provided directly to the state (7%). Medicaid, Medicare, private grants, and fees make up the majority of local health department funding.[85,92,93]

Significant variation exists in local health department per capita revenues and expenditures throughout the United States. In 2016, the local health department median per capita expenditure was $39, whereas the median per capita revenue was $41. In 10 states, the median per capita expenditure was less than $30, whereas in four states it was more than $70.[92] Reasons for this variation are multifaceted and include geographical size, population size and characteristics, variation in tax base among counties and municipalities, types of services offered, and type of governance (i.e., city, county, regional, state, or shared governance).

Health department structure and governance can affect the amount and source of funding for programming (Box 21-6). In 2016, 69% of local health departments in the United States were county-based, with 20% based in city or townships and governed by a local board of health or county commission or executive.[92] The remainder of the health departments served a regional or multicounty jurisdiction or a mixed jurisdiction serving both a county and a city located outside the county boundaries.[92] These differences may affect the revenue sources and per-capita funding levels that fund a local health department. For example, health departments using a state/regional model may not receive local levy as a revenue source.

Another critical factor in local health department funding is the size of the population served and the array of programs and services provided. In 2016, the median annual expenditures for health department funding was $1.3 million, with a range of $480,000 for local health departments serving fewer than 25,000 people to $56.4 million for those serving 1 million or more residents.[92] This variation in funding may lead to differences in service availability and delivery across geographical locations. Also, greater funding from both public and private sources is sometimes, but not always, available to departments that demonstrate increased community health needs (i.e., high morbidity and mortality rates, poverty levels) and positive program outcomes. The types of services most often provided include immunizations for children and adults, communicable disease surveillance, tuberculosis screening, inspection/licensing of retail food establishments, environmental health programming, and tobacco use prevention.[92]

The complexity and political constraints of public health policy and related finance can be illustrated by the Zika virus epidemic of 2015-2016. Zika virus is spread by the bite of an infected daytime-active mosquito (Aedes aegypti or Aedes albopictus), by an infected pregnant woman to the fetus during pregnancy or at the time of birth, or, rarely, by sexual contact.[94] The Zika virus is usually asymptomatic or mild and of short duration. However, there does seem to be a relationship between Zika infection and later development of Guillan-Barre syndrome. In utero transmission is related to serious birth defects, specifically microcephaly and other brain defects. There is no vaccine or cure for Zika.

An epidemic of Zika virus spread from 10 countries in January 2015 to 65 countries in July of 2016.[95] Public health agencies and organizations in the U.S. and worldwide were on high alert. Initially the National Institutes of Health and CDC diverted funds from other funded programs such as immunization, Ebola, and cancer to fight this epidemic. Additionally, philanthropic funds were raised.[96] During the first three quarters of 2016, several federal bills were proposed and debated to fund federal Zika control and research efforts. These were stymied because of political considerations related to potential requests for medical abortion after discovering an infection or fetal birth defects and because of debate about which other programs, including the ACA, that should receive less funding in exchange for Zika control funding. Finally, in September 2016, Congress approved $1.1 billion to combat the Zika virus.[97]

CDC funds were awarded to public health partners, including all state public health departments and selected local public health departments, to combat the virus.[98] Funds were allocated within the CDC and to external partners to enhance epidemiologic surveillance and investigation; teach health-care providers to identify Zika; build laboratory capacity for diagnostic testing; keep blood supplies safe; develop and contribute data to the U.S. Zika registry; research the relationship between Zika virus infection and birth defects; and educate the public about the virus, especially in regard to travel to Zika-affected areas, personal protection to prevent mosquito bites, and mosquito control.

Grants

Grants are monetary awards given by an organization or government agency to plan and implement a program or project. Often grant dollars are distributed via a competitive process with many agencies vying for the same dollars. Other grants may be noncompetitive but prescriptive in nature. With reduced budgets, many public health agencies have turned to grants to offset reduced funding from local tax levies. National and local organizations such as the United Way help support local programs designed to serve some of the most vulnerable populations (e.g., health care for the homeless). Grant funds are often time limited, requiring the grantee to demonstrate sustainability and a plan to evaluate the outcomes of the project after the grant period ends.[99]

The Local Health Department Budget Process

Through the community health assessment process, local health department representatives along with community stakeholders (e.g., representatives from a variety of community organizations, police and fire departments, local health system) identify public health issues and action plans to address these. The resulting community health improvement plan identifies possible solutions to public health issues that influence programming and budget allocations. As public health budgets shrink, this process provides a critical justification for program revenues and expenditures.

The process of health department funding involves the complex interaction of government agencies, public/private partners, county officials, local taxpayers, and public health agency staff (see Chapter 13). Inherent in the process is the knowledge that public health funding, given these interdependent relationships, can vary significantly from one fiscal year to the next. Because local taxpayers support the bulk of public health funding, economic instability can have a significant impact on the ability of health departments to deliver services. Many local health departments rely on local tax dollars or levies affected by both political and economic forces. For example, many municipalities collect taxes based on property values. This approach to taxation is vulnerable to the ups and downs of the economy. When the housing market is down, and property values fall, tax revenue is also reduced. This results in budget shortfalls that might lead to a reduction of or charges for services that were once free.

Health programs mandated by state statute must be provided regardless of budget concerns. Examples of mandatory programs may include inspections of establishments serving food to the public and communicable disease follow-up to limit the spread of illness. Others, however, such as programs addressing child abuse prevention or suicide prevention, may be vulnerable to reductions or elimination if there are no grant funds or partnerships to sustain them.

The public health nurse and other local health department staff play a critical role in the budget process. Local health departments typically operate on an annual fiscal year (January to December) budget cycle, with programs often funded through a combination of federal, state, and local tax dollars. Other sources of program funding such as grants may operate on a different fiscal cycle with reporting timelines from July to June or October to September.

Public health nurses in charge of specific programs must provide the required reports to the funding source to ensure continued program funding. Public health nurses, with their intimate connection to the community, help give voice to those served, supporting board members and other decision makers with real-life examples to add relevance, relationship, and emotion to statistics and dry reports.

Funding and Access to Care

Low-income families face a web of problems that compromise their ability to financially seek out health care. These problems can include a lack of health insurance, unemployment, old age, incarceration, chronically ill or disabled family members, lack of child support, debt, and low educational level. Low minimum wages and unrealistically low federal poverty guidelines often leave these families with an inability to support themselves and without the knowledge of their eligibility for services. This section discusses some of the federal/state programs that offer a safety net for both health insurance and income.

Government Health Insurance Programs

Medicare and Medicaid account for the greatest expenditure of federal governmental health-care spending. Through these programs, the federal government purchases services for population groups via health-care organizations, including both private and public sector providers such as physicians, hospitals, health maintenance organizations (HMOs), community health centers, and health departments.

Medicaid

Medicaid is a federal and state partnership that covers health costs for certain groups of people, including those with lower incomes, disabilities, older people, and some families and children. Medicaid eligibility rules vary in each state and are complicated by whether the state has opted into the Medicaid Expansion as part of the ACA. State-specific Medicaid eligibility and coverage can be obtained on the Medicaid.gov website. Medicaid benefits and the contrasts with Medicare benefits are found in Table 21-5.

TABLE 21–5 ■ Comparison of Medicaid and Medicare

	Medicaid	Medicare
What is it?	A combined state and federal health insurance program for people with limited resources and income. Certain components of the program such as CHIP help certain populations.	A federal health insurance program for: • Individuals aged 65 and older • Certain disabled individuals, under age 65 • Individuals with end-stage renal disease
Who runs the program?	State government	Federal government
What does it cover?	Coverage is dependent on the state program but typically covers: • Laboratory tests and x-rays • Inpatient hospital care • Health screening • Dental and vision care • Long-term care and support in a skilled facility • Family planning and midwifery services • Doctor visits, outpatient health care • Prescription drugs • Home health-care services for certain people • Nursing home care even when custodial	Part A: Inpatient hospital care and some care in a skilled nursing facility Part B: Doctor visits and care received as an outpatient, some preventive services Part D: Some pharmacy prescription coverage • Does not cover long-term custodial care
What does it cost?	Depends on the rules in the state and the income and resources of the individual. Many are exempt from any out-of-pocket costs. Others have copayments, deductibles, and premiums.	Depends on which parts of Medicare the individual selects. It can include copayments, deductibles, and premiums.

Source: United Health Care. (2017). *Medicare versus Medicaid*. Retrieved from http://www.medicaremadeclear.com/about/medicare-vs-medicaid/

The Medicaid services that must be covered for children and sometimes for adults include: physical, occupational, or speech therapy; eye doctor visits, eyeglasses; audiology, hearing aids; prosthetic devices; mental health services; respite and other in-home, long-term care; case management; personal care services; and hospice services.[100]

Medicaid is an evolving program that was initially created in 1965 with the Social Security Amendments. It took 18 years for it to become available in every state.[100,101] Initially, Medicaid focused on children under the age of 21, but in the 1970s it was extended to those who were disabled. In the 1980s, there were inclusions for pregnant women, illegal immigrants for some emergency situations, and dental needs. In 1991, the Medicaid Drug Rebate Program was put into place to cover the cost of prescription drugs; in 2000, the Breast and Cervical Cancer Treatment and Prevention Act allowed any uninsured woman with breast or cervical cancer to be treated.[100,101] The latest evolution was the states' optional opt-in to expanded Medicaid eligibility under the ACA beginning in January 2014. The minimum eligibility level for Medicaid is 133% of the federal poverty level ($33,383 for a household of four for 2018) for almost all Americans under the age of 65.[102]

Children's Health Insurance Program

Children's Health Insurance Program (CHIP) is also a federal and state partnership that provides coverage for children who live in families that earn incomes too high to qualify for Medicaid but too low to afford private health insurance. Basic eligibility is focused on three groups: children up to age 19, pregnant women, and other citizens and legal immigrants. Families of four with incomes up to $52,208 are considered eligible for CHIP with no copay; in some cases, families with higher incomes may also qualify.[103] Pregnant women may be eligible, and CHIP will generally cover lab testing, labor and delivery costs, and 60 days of care after delivery. Finally, U.S. citizens and some legal immigrants are covered, but states have the option of providing this coverage. As with Medicaid, undocumented immigrants are not eligible for

CHIP.[103] The services provided are similar or identical to Medicaid and include routine checkups, immunizations, dental and vision care, inpatient and outpatient hospital care, and lab and x-ray services.[104]

Medicare

Medicare is health insurance that covers three groups of people: people aged 65 or older, people under 65 with certain disabilities, and people of all ages with end-stage renal disease (permanent kidney failure requiring dialysis or a kidney transplant). Medicare is also part of the Social Security Amendment signed into law on July 30, 1965, by President Johnson, providing the first federally funded health insurance for those 65 and older. The other significant change occurred in 2003 when President George W. Bush signed into law and added the outpatient prescription drug benefit to Medicare recipients.[105]

There are three parts to Medicare. Part A is Hospital Insurance that covers inpatient care in hospitals, hospice, some home health, as well as skilled nursing facilities that are not considered custodial or long-term care settings. Most people do not pay a premium because they have already paid for the insurance as part of their taxes. Part B is Medical Insurance that covers doctors' services, outpatient care, and some additional services of physical and occupational therapists, home health, and some medical supplies. For this portion, most people paid a monthly premium (about $134/month in 2018).[106] If someone has Part A and Part B, that person can choose to enroll in Medicare Part C (Medicare Advantage). Part C allows people to receive all of their care through a selected private provider organization (such as an HMO or preferred provider organization) administered by Medicare. Part D is the Medicare prescription drug coverage and is actually a separate policy that one must purchase from a private insurer. Beneficiaries choose a drug plan and pay a monthly premium to reduce prescription drug costs.[106]

Government Income Support Programs

Temporary Assistance for Needy Families

Temporary Assistance for Needy Families (TANF) is a cash assistance program generally limited to 60 months in an adult's lifetime. The money for this program is a block grant from the federal government that allows flexibility to each state for developing its own program. The purpose of TANF is to make the assistance temporary, not permanent, by supporting economically needy families, helping parents complete their education, teaching job skills, and encouraging two-parent families. There are work requirements for the adult program participants, and teen parents must live with their parents or a supervising adult and remain in school. Most recipients of TANF also qualify for Medicaid.[107]

People With Disabilities

The federal government administers two income supplement programs that serve individuals with disabilities.[108] The first is **Social Security Disability Insurance (SSDI)**, a federal program that provides income benefits to individuals (or in some cases, family members) if the disabled person has worked long enough in the past (40 quarters, 10 years) to pay Social Security tax, and is expected to be unable to work for at least 1 year. It can be provided on a temporary or permanent basis as defined by the disability. There is no income or resource restriction.[108]

The **Supplemental Security Income (SSI)** is also a federal income supplement program, but general tax revenues, not Social Security taxes, fund it. It covers adults and children who have a significant physical or mental disability that has lasted or is expected to last at least 12 months, have limited income level and resources, or have not met the work requirement for SSDI, as well as people 65 and over without disabilities who meet the financial limits. The disabled individual must remain below the income threshold to continue to receive SSI. It provides cash to meet basic human needs such as food, shelter, and clothing. Most people who receive SSI also qualify for Medicaid.[108]

Supplemental Nutrition Assistance Program (SNAP) is sometimes colloquially called the Food Stamp program and is administered by the Food and Nutrition Service of the U.S. Department of Agriculture. This program provides financial assistance for the purchase of food to help recipients maintain a healthy diet; it is the largest program in the domestic hunger safety net. People who are eligible for TANF and SSI are automatically eligible for SNAP, and others are eligible if they meet the financial requirements.[109] **Women, Infants, and Children (WIC)**, a federal grant program (not an entitlement program), also provides nutritional supplements to nutritionally at-risk, low-income pregnant women until 6 weeks postpartum, breastfeeding mothers until an infant's first birthday, and children up to the age of 5. WIC pays for essential items such as milk, eggs, and baby formula, and currently serves up to 53% of all infants born in the United States. The program also provides education and counseling at the WIC clinics, and screening and referrals to other health and social service agencies.[110]

Summary Points

- Public health policies are authoritative governmental decisions made in government, agencies, or organizations that are directed toward influencing actions, behaviors, or decisions influencing population health.
- Public health policy is intrinsically connected to our health-care system, values, and underlying philosophies about the place of government versus the market system.
- Public health policies are enacted at national, state, and local levels of government as well as by businesses and organizations.
- Public health policies are grounded in the health planning process. A policy's likely effectiveness, efficiency, and effect on equity should be considered.
- Public health policies focus on health determinants and are based on evidence.
- Nurses can be involved in the public health policy-making process through individual and collective actions.
- Public health departments receive funding from a variety of sources including federal, state, and local tax dollars as well as grants.
- The majority of funding for local health departments comes from local sources, and per-capita funding varies widely across the United States based on type of government structure (city, county, region), geography, population size and characteristics, tax base, and types of services offered.
- The greatest expenditure of federal health-care dollars are Medicare and Medicaid.
- Government income support programs, including Social Security Disability, Supplemental Security Income, and Woman, Infants, and Children, provide support to persons whose income or health status leaves them vulnerable to poor health.
- The Affordable Care Act of 2010 signed into law by President Obama, along with associated regulations, overhauled the U.S. health-care system and focused on improving quality and reducing cost of health insurance for individuals. Notable changes in coverage include greater access to preventive care and services and the creation of health insurance exchanges to increase coverage and affordability.

▼ CASE STUDY
Addressing the Opioid Crisis Through Health Policy

Learning Outcomes
At the end of this case study, the student will be able to:

- Gain understanding of the public health policy.
- Describe the role of policy in the promotion of the public's health.

As a public health nurse in a small rural community that has experienced high morbidity and mortality related to opioid abuse, you were informed that a grant from the state can fund purchase and distribution of the opioid overdose reversal agent, naloxone. Currently, the police department and local hospital emergency rooms have naloxone doses. It is your understanding that there is enough funding for an additional 100 doses available for distribution during each of the next 2 years.

Discussion Questions:
1. Should the health department participate in the program? Why or why not?
2. Assuming the health department decides to participate:
   a. What individuals, businesses, organizations, or agencies should receive or not receive naloxone doses?
   b. Should the health department charge a nominal fee for each dose? Why or why not?
   c. What elements should be included in a community training for use of naloxone? What documentation is required?

REFERENCES

1. World Health Organization. (2018). *Health policy*. Retrieved from www.who.int/topics/health_policy/en/.
2. American Nurses Association. (2013). *Public health nursing: Scope and standards of practice* (2nd ed.). Silver Spring, MD: Nursesbooks.org.
3. Centers for Disease Control and Prevention, National Center for Immunization and Respiratory Diseases. (2017). *Recommended vaccines for healthcare workers*. Retrieved from https://www.cdc.gov/vaccines/adults/rec-vac/hcw.html.
4. World Health Organization. (2017). *Universal health coverage*. Retrieved from http://www.who.int/mediacentre/factsheets/fs395/en/.
5. Guttmacher Institute. (2017). *Data center*. Retrieved from https://data.guttmacher.org/states/table?state=US&topics=58+72&dataset=data.

6. Hung, P., Henning-Smith, C.E., Casey, M.M., & Kozhimannil, K.B. (2017). Access to obstetric services in rural counties still declining, with 9 percent losing services, 2004-14. *Health Affairs, 36*(9), 1663-1671. https://doi.org/10.1377/hlthaff. 2017.0338.

7. Kraft, M.E., & Furlong, S.R. (2015). *Public policy: Politics, analysis, and alternatives* (5th ed.). Thousand Oaks, CA: Sage/CQ Press.

8. Adams, N., & Salisbury, D. (2014). *Employee benefits: Today, tomorrow, and yesterday.* Retrieved from the Employee Benefits Research Institute (EBRI) at https://www.ebri. org/pdf/briefspdf/EBRI_IB_401_July14.EE-Benefits.pdf.

9. Squires, D., & Anderson, C. (2015). *U.S. health care from a global perspective: Spending, use of services, prices, and health in 13 countries.* Retrieved from The Commonwealth Fund at http://www.commonwealthfund.org/publications/ issue-briefs/2015/oct/us-healthcare-from-a-global-perspective.

10. Central Intelligence Agency. (n.d.). *The world factbook 2017: Country comparison; Obesity, adult prevalence rate.* Retrieved from https://www.cia.gov/library/publications/the-world-factbook/rankorder/2228rank.html.

11. Central Intelligence Agency. (n.d.). *The world factbook 2017: Country comparison; life expectancy at birth.* Retrieved from https://www.cia.gov/library/publications/the-world-factbook/rankorder/2102rank.html.

12. U.S. Department of Health and Human Services. (2018). *The leading health indicators.* Retrieved from https://www. healthypeople.gov/2020/Leading-Health-Indicators.

13. U.S. Department of Health and Human Services. (2018). *HealthyPeople.gov: Disparities.* Retrieved from https:// www.healthypeople.gov/2020/about/foundation-health-measures/Disparities.

14. U.S. Department of Health and Human Services, Healthy People.gov. (2018). *HealthyPeople.gov: Clinical preventive services.* Retrieved from https://www.healthypeople.gov/ 2020/leading-health-indicators/2020-lhi-topics/Clinical-Preventive-Services/data#c16.

15. Barnett, J.C., & Vornovitsky, M.S. (2016). *Health insurance coverage in the United States: 2015.* Washington D.C.: U.S. Government Printing Office. Retrieved from https:// www.census.gov/content/dam/Census/library/publications/ 2016/demo/p60-257.pdf.

16. U.S. Department of Health and Human Services, Office of Disease Prevention and Health Promotion, Healthy People.gov. (2018). *HP 2020.Topics & Objectives: Objectives A- Z.* Retrieved from https://www.healthypeople.gov/2020/ topics-objectives.

17. U.S. Department of Health and Human Services, Office of Minority Health. (2016). *Minority population profiles.* Retrieved from https://www.minorityhealth.hhs.gov/omh/ browse.aspx?lvl=2&lvlid=26.

18. Centers for Disease Control & Prevention. (2016). Surveillance of vaccination coverage among adult populations-United States, 2014. *Morbidity & Mortality Weekly Report, 65*(1), 1-36.

19. National Center for Health Statistics. (2017). *Health, United States, 2016: With chartbook on long-term trends in health.* Retrieved from https://www.cdc.gov/nchs/hus/contents 2016.htm.

20. Wolfe, B. (2011, June). *Poverty and poor health: Can health care reform narrow the rich poor gap?* Adaptation from Robert J. Lampman Memorial Lecture. Madison, WI: Author. Retrieved from http://www.irp.wisc.edu/publications/focus/ pdfs/foc282f.pdf.

21. American Academy of Pediatrics. (2016). *Blueprint for children. How the next president can build a foundation for a healthy future.* Retrieved from https://www.aap.org/ en-us/Documents/BluePrintForChildren.pdf.

22. University of Wisconsin Madison, Institute for Research on Poverty. (n.d.). *Poverty fact sheet: Poor and in poor health.* Retrieved from https://www.irp.wisc.edu/publications/ factsheets/pdfs/PoorInPoorHealth.pdf.

23. Fiscella, K., & Williams, D.R. (2004). Health disparities based on socioeconomic inequities: Implications for urban health care. *Academic Medicine, 79*(12), 1139-1147.

24. National Conference of State Legislators. (2015). *State laws mandating or regulating mental health benefits.* Retrieved from http://www.ncsl.org/IssuesResearch/Health/StateLawsMan datingorRegulatingMentalHealthB/tabid/14352/Default.aspx.

25. Social Security. (n.d.). *Historical background and development of social security.* Retrieved from https://www.ssa.gov/history/ briefhistory3.html.

26. U.S. Department of Health and Human Services, Centers for Medicare & Medicaid Services. (n.d.). *CMS programs & information.* Retrieved from http://www.cms.hhs.gov/.

27. U.S. Department of Health and Human Services, Office of Disease Prevention and Health Promotion. (n.d.). *Healthy People.* Retrieved from http://www.healthypeople.gov/.

28. U.S. Department of Health and Human Services, Office of Disease Prevention and Health Promotion. (2018). *Healthy People 2030 framework.* Retrieved from https://www. healthypeople.gov/2020/about-healthy-people/development-healthy-people-2030/framework.

29. The Henry J. Kaiser Family Foundation. (2012a). *A guide to the Supreme Court's decision on the ACA's Medicaid expansion.* Retrieved from http://kff.org/health-reform/ issue-brief/a-guide-to-the-supreme-courts-decision/.

30. The Henry J. Kaiser Family Foundation. (2012b). *Summary of coverage provisions in the patient protection and affordable care act.* Retrieved from https://www.kff.org/health-costs/issue-brief/summary-of-coverage-provisions-in-the-patient/.

31. U.S. Department of Health and Human Services. (2017). *Preventive services covered under the Affordable Care Act.* Retrieved from http://www.hhs.gov/healthcare/facts/factsheets/2010/07/ preventive-services-list.html#CoveredPreventiveServicesforAdults.

32. American Public Health Association. (2018, May). ACA essential health benefits come under threat. *The Nation's Health, 48*(3), 1-10.

33. Edmonds, J.K., Campbell, L. A., & Gilder, R.E. (2017). Public health nursing practice in the Affordable Care Act era: A national survey. *Public Health Nursing, 34*(1), 50-58.

34. National Association of County and City Health Officials. (2016). *Public health and prevention provisions of the Affordable Care Act.* Retrieved from https://www.naccho.org/ uploads/downloadable-resources/PH-and-Prevention-Provision-in-the-ACA-Revised-2016.pdf.

35. U.S. Department of Labor, Occupational Safety & Health Administration. (n.d.). *Occupational Safety & Health Administration.* Retrieved from http://www.osha.gov/.

36. Centers for Medicare & Medicaid Services (n.d.). *Medicaid.* Retrieved from https://www.medicaid.gov/medicaid/benefits/index.html.

37. The Henry J. Kaiser Family Foundation. (2017). *Current flexibility in Medicaid: An overview of federal standards and state options.* Retrieved from https://www.kff.org/medicaid/issue-brief/current-flexibility-in-medicaid-an-overview-of-federal-standards-and-state-options/.

38. Centers for Medicare & Medicaid Services (n.d.). *State waivers list.* Retrieved from https://www.medicaid.gov/medicaid/section-1115-demo/demonstration-and-waiver-list/index.html.

39. The Henry J. Kaiser Family Foundation. (2018). *Status of state action on the Medicaid expansion decision.* Retrieved from https://www.kff.org/health-reform/state-indicator/state-activity-around-expanding-medicaid-under-the-affordable-care-act/?activeTab=map&currentTimeframe=0&selectedDistributions=current-status-of-medicaid-expansion-decision&sortModel=%7B%22colId%22:%22Location%22,%22sort%22:%22asc%22%7D.

40. Pear, R. (1993, March 20). U.S. backs Oregon's health plan for covering all poor people. *The New York Times.* Retrieved from http://www.nytimes.com/1993/03/20/us/us-backs-oregon-s-health-plan-for-covering-all-poor-people.html.

41. The Henry J. Kaiser Family Foundation. (2011). *State marketplace profiles: Massachusetts.* Retrieved from https://www.kff.org/health-reform/state-profile/state-exchange-profiles-massachusetts/.

42. State of Wisconsin DRL. (n.d.). *Registered nurse.* Retrieved from http://drl.wi.gov/profession.asp?profid=46&locid=0.

43. Public Health Law Center. (2015). *State & local public health: An overview of regulatory authority.* Retrieved from http://www.publichealthlawcenter.org/sites/default/files/resources/phlc-fs-state-local-reg-authority-publichealth-2015_0.pdf.

44. Centers for Disease Control and Prevention. (2018). *Emergency preparedness and response: Health alert network.* Retrieved from https://emergency.cdc.gov/han/index.asp.

45. Turnock, B.J. (2016). *Essentials of public health* (3rd ed.). Burlington, MA: Jones & Bartlett.

46. Centers for Disease Control and Prevention. (2017). *Understanding the epidemic.* Retrieved from https://www.cdc.gov/drugoverdose/epidemic/index.html.

47. Corso, C., & Townley, C. (2016). *Intervention, treatment, and prevention strategies to address opioid use disorders in rural areas: A primer on opportunities for Medicaid-safety net collaboration.* Retrieved from the National Academy of State Health Policy at https://nashp.org/wp-content/uploads/2016/09/Rural-Opioid-Primer.pdf.

48. U.S. Department of Health and Human Services. (2018). *Surgeon General's advisory on naloxone and opioid overdose.* Retrieved from https://www.surgeongeneral.gov/priorities/opioid-overdose-prevention/naloxone-advisory.html.

49. Centers for Disease Control and Prevention. (2018, March 6). *Vital signs: Opioid overdoses treated in emergency departments.* Retrieved from https://www.cdc.gov/vitalsigns/opioid-overdoses/index.html.

50. Centers for Disease Control and Prevention. (2017). *National voluntary accreditation for public health departments.* Retrieved from https://www.cdc.gov/stltpublichealth/accreditation/.

51. National Conference of State Legislatures. (2018). *State medical marijuana laws.* Retrieved from http://www.ncsl.org/research/health/state-medical-marijuana-laws.aspx.

52. United States Department of Agriculture, Food and Nutrition Service. (2017). *Nutrition standards for school meals.* Retrieved from https://www.fns.usda.gov/school-meals/nutrition-standards-school-meals.

53. Sharma, M. (2017). *Theoretical foundations of health education and health promotion* (3rd ed.). Burlington, MA: Jones & Bartlett.

54. The Community Guide. (2016). *Physical activity: Built environment approaches combining transportation system interventions with land use and environmental design.* Retrieved from https://www.thecommunityguide.org/findings/physical-activity-built-environment-approaches.

55. Wang, G., Macera, C.A., Scudder-Soucie, B., Schmid, T., Pratt, M., & Buchner, D. (2005). A cost-benefit analysis of physical activity using bike/pedestrian trails. *Health Promotion Practice, 6*(2), 174-179. Doi: 10.1177/1524839903260687.

56. Gu, J., Mohit, B., & Muennig, P.A. (2017). The cost-effectiveness of bike lanes in New York City. *Injury Prevention, 23*(4), 239-243. Doi: 10.1136/injuryprev-2016-042057.

57. Fluoride Action Network. (2012). *Tooth decay in fluoridated vs. unfluoridated countries.* Retrieved from http://fluoridealert.org/studies/caries01/.

58. Peterson, P.E., & Ogawa, H. (2016). Prevention of dental caries through the use of fluoride—the WHO approach. *Community Dental Health, 33*, 66-68. doi:10.1922/CDH_Petersen03.

59. Maguire, A. (2014). ADA clinical recommendations on topical fluoride for caries prevention. *Evidence Based Dentistry, 15*(2), 38-39. doi: 10.1038/sj.ebd.6401019.

60. Agency for Healthcare Research and Quality. (2014.). *The guide to clinical preventive services 2014.* Retrieved from https://www.ahrq.gov/sites/default/files/publications/files/cpsguide.pdf.

61. The Community Guide. (n.d.). *The community guide: The guide to community preventive services.* Retrieved from http://www.thecommunityguide.org.

62. The Community Guide. (2014). *Skin cancer: Primary and middle school-based interventions.* Retrieved from https://www.thecommunityguide.org/findings/skin-cancer-primary-and-middle-school-based-interventions.

63. Cochrane Library. (2018). *Cochrane database of systematic reviews.* Retrieved from http://www.cochranelibrary.com/cochrane-database-of-systematic-reviews/index.html.

64. The Community Guide. (2013). *Motor vehicle injury—Motorcycle helmets: Universal helmet laws.* Retrieved from https://www.thecommunityguide.org/findings/motor-vehicle-injury-motorcycle-helmets-universal-helmet-laws.

65. Insurance Institute for Highway Safety, Highway Loss Data Institute. (2018). *Motorcycle helmet use.* Retrieved from http://www.iihs.org/iihs/topics/laws/helmetuse/mapmotorcyclehelmets.

66. International Organization for Migration. (2018). *Migration and climate change.* Retrieved from https://www.iom.int/migration-and-climate-change.

67. Department of Homeland Security. (2017). *Fact sheet: Rescission of deferred action for childhood arrivals (DACA).* Retrieved from https://www.dhs.gov/news/2017/09/05/fact-sheet-rescission-deferred-action-childhood-arrivals-daca.

68. Johnson, C.W., & Koempel, M. (2012). *How our laws are made.* Washington, DC: U.S. Government Printing Office.

69. American Nurses Association. (2018a). *Safe staffing*. Retrieved from http://ana.aristotle.com/SitePages/safestaffing.aspx.

70. American Nurses Association. (2018b). *Letter from ANA to U.S. Food and Drug Administration regarding packaging, storage, and disposal options to enhance opioid safety-Exploring the path forward*. Retrieved from 1. U.S. Government Publishing Office. (n.d) *United States code*. Retrieved from https://www.gpo.gov/fdsys/browse/collectionUScode.action.

71. U.S. House of Representatives, Office of the Law Revision Council. (n.d.). *United States Code*. Retrieved from https://uscode.house.gov/.

72. Sabella, D. (2011). The role of the nurse in combating human trafficking. *American Journal of Nursing, 11*(2), 28-37.

73. Govtrack. (n.d.). *H.R. 1865: Allow States and Victims to Fight Online Sex Trafficking Act of 2017*. Retrieved from https://www.govtrack.us/congress/bills/115/hr1865.

74. Govtrack. (n.d.). *S. 1693: Stop Enabling Sex Traffickers Act of 2017*. Retrieved from https://www.govtrack.us/congress/bills/115/s1693.

75. United States Department of Labor, Bureau of Labor Statistics. (2018). *Occupational employment and wages, May 2017: 29-1141 Registered Nurses*. Retrieved from https://www.bls.gov/Oes/current/oes291141.htm.

76. Vandenhouten, C. L., Malakar, C. L., Kubsch, S., Block, D., & Gallagher-Lepak, S. (2011). Political participation of registered nurses. *Policy, Politics, & Nursing Practice, 12*(3), 159-167. Retrieved from http://ppn.sagepub.com/content/12/3/159.abstract.

77. American Public Health Association. (2018). *Advocacy and policy: Advocacy activities*. Retrieved from https://www.apha.org/policies-and-advocacy/advocacy-for-public-health/advocacy-activities.

78. Association of Public Health Nurses. (2016). Public *Health policy advocacy guide book and tool kit*. Retrieved from http://www.phnurse.org/resources/Documents/APHN%20Public%20Health%20Policy%20Advocacy%20Guide%20Book%20and%20Tool%20Kit%202016.pdf.

79. Catallo, C., Spalding, K., & Haghiri-Vijeh, R. (2014, December). Nursing professional organizations: What are they doing to engage nurses in health policy? *SAGE Open*. Retrieved from http://journals.sagepub.com/doi/pdf/10.1177/2158244014560534.

80. Nursing Organizations Alliance. (2018). *Purpose*. Retrieved from https://www.nursing-alliance.org/About-Us/Our-History.

81. Weible, C., & Karin, I. (2018). Why advocacy coalitions matter and practical insights about them. *Policy &Politics, 46*(2), 325-343. Retrieved from https://doi.org/10.1332/030557318X15230061739399.

82. Burney, L.E., & Yoho, R. (1955). Financing local health services. *American Journal of Public Health, 45*, 974-978. Retrieved from www.ncbi.nlm.nih.gov/pmc/articles/PMC1623122/pdf/amjphnational00348-0013pdf.

83. Bernell, S. (2016). *Health economics: Core concepts and essential tools*. Chicago, IL: Health Administration Press.

84. Centers for Disease Control and Prevention. (2017). *Public health economics and tools*. Retrieved from https://www.cdc.gov/stltpublichealth/pheconomics/

85. Turnock, B.J. (2016). *Public health: What it is and how it works* (6th ed.). Burlington, MA: Jones & Bartlett.

86. Trust for America's Health. (2016). *Investing in America's health: A state-by-state look at public health funding and key health facts 2016*. Retrieved from http://www.healthyamericans.org/assets/files/TFAH-2016-InvestInAmericaRpt-FINAL%20REVISED.pdf.

87. Butler, L. J., Scammell, M.K., & Benson, E.B. (2016). The Flint, Michigan water crisis: A case study in regulatory failure and environmental injustice. *Environmental Justice, 9*(4). Retrieved from https://www.liebertpub.com/doi/pdf/10.10.

88. Michael, J.M. (2011). The national Board of Health: 1879-1883. *Public Health Reports, 126*(1), 123-129.

89. U.S. Department of Health and Human Services. (n.d.). *Commissioned Corps of the U.S. Public Health Service*. Retrieved from https://www.usphs.gov/aboutus/history.aspx.

90. Centers for Disease Control and Prevention, Office of Financial Resources. (2017). *2017 fiscal year annual report*. Retrieved from https://www.cdc.gov/funding/documents/fy2017/fy-2017-ofr-annual-report-508.pdf.

91. Centers for Disease Control and Prevention. (2017). *Mission, role, and pledge*. Retrieved from https://www.cdc.gov/about/organization/mission.htm.

92. National Association of County & City Health Officials. (2017). *2016 national profile of local health departments*. Retrieved from http://nacchoprofilestudy.org/wp-content/uploads/2017/10/ProfileReport_Aug2017_final.pdf.

93. Meit, M., Knudson, A., Dickman, I., Brown, A., Hernandez, N., & Kronstadt, J. (2013). *An examination of public health financing in the United States*. (Prepared by NORC at the University of Chicago.) Washington, DC: The Office of the Assistant Secretary for Planning and Evaluation. Retrieved from http://www.norc.org/PDFs/PH%20Financing%20Report%20-%20Final.pdf.

94. Centers for Disease Control and Prevention. (2018). *Zika virus*. Retrieved from https://www.cdc.gov/zika/index.html.

95. The Henry J. Kaiser Family Foundation. (2016). *The 2015-2016 Zika outbreak*. Retrieved from https://www.kff.org/infographic/2015-2016-zika-outbreak/.

96. CDC Foundation. (2018). *Together, we can stop Zika*. Retrieved from https://www.cdcfoundation.org/zika-response.

97. American Public Health Association, Public Health Newswire. (2016). *Congress approves $1.1 billion in funding to combat Zika*. Retrieved from www.publichealthnewswire.org/?p=16071.

98. Centers for Disease Control and Prevention. (2018). *Zika virus: Funding*. Retrieved from https://www.cdc.gov/zika/specific-groups/funding.html.

99. Trust for America's Health. (2018). *A funding crisis for public health and safety: State-by-state public health funding and key health facts 2018*. Retrieved from http://healthyamericans.org/assets/files/TFAH-2018-InvestInAmericaRpt-FINAL.pdf.

100. HealthCare.gov. (n.d.). *Medicaid & CHIP coverage*. Retrieved from https://www.healthcare.gov/medicaid-chip/getting-medicaid-chip/#howmed.

101. The Henry J. Kaiser Family Foundation. (n.d.). *Medicaid: A timeline of key developments*. Retrieved from https://kaiserfamilyfoundation.files.wordpress.com/2008/04/5-02-13-medicaid-timeline.pdf.

102. U.S. Department of Health and Human Services, Office of the Secretary. (2018). *Annual update of the HHS poverty guidelines.* 83 FR 2642, 2642-2644. Retrieved from https://www.federalregister.gov/documents/2018/01/18/2018-00814/annual-update-of-the-hhs-poverty-guidelines.

103. The Henry J. Kaiser Family Foundation and the Georgetown University Center for Children and Families. (2018, March 23). *CHIP. Medicaid and CHIP eligibility, enrollment, renewal, and cost sharing policies as of January 2018: Findings from a 50-state survey.* Retrieved from https://ccf.georgetown.edu/2018/03/23/medicaid-and-chip-eligibility-enrollment-renewal-and-cost-sharing-policies-as-of-january-2018-findings-from-a-50-state-survey/.

104. HealthCare.gov. (n.d.). *The Children's Health Insurance Program (CHIP).* Retrieved from http://www.healthcare.gov/using-insurance/low-cost-care/childrens-insurance-program/index.html.

105. Centers for Medicare & Medicaid Services. (2013). *History.* Retrieved from http://www.cms.gov/About-CMS/Agency-Information/History/index.html?redirect=/history/.

106. Medicare.gov. (n.d.). *Medicare 2018 costs at a glance.* Retrieved from https://www.medicare.gov/your-medicare-costs/costs-at-a-glance/costs-at-glance.html.

107. U.S. Department of Health & Human Services, Administration for Children and Families, Office of Family Assistance. (n.d.). *Temporary assistance for needy families (TANF).* Retrieved from https://www.acf.hhs.gov/ofa/programs/tanf.

108. Social Security Administration. (n.d.). *Benefits for people with disabilities.* Retrieved from http://www.ssa.gov/disability/.

109. United States Department of Agriculture, Food and Nutrition Service. (2018). *Supplemental Nutrition Assistance Program (SNAP).* Retrieved from https://www.fns.usda.gov/snap/supplemental-nutrition-assistance-program-snap.

110. United States Department of Agriculture, Food and Nutrition Service. (2018). *Women, Infants, and Children (WIC).* Retrieved from https://www.fns.usda.gov/wic/women-infants-and-children-wic.

Chapter 22

Health Planning for Emergency Preparedness and Disaster Management

Gordon Gillespie

LEARNING OUTCOMES

After reading the chapter, the student will be able to:

1. Describe the impact of natural and manmade disasters on population health.
2. Appreciate the unique role of nurses during disasters and public health emergencies.
3. Discuss the five areas of focus in emergency and disaster planning: preparedness, mitigation, response, recovery, and evaluation.
4. Apply the emergency preparedness theoretical framework to a public health disaster scenario.
5. Describe the structure and organization of local and national disaster mitigation efforts.
6. Describe the process of epidemiological surveillance during community disaster mitigation and recovery.
7. Recognize the role of functional needs support services to optimize the health outcomes of vulnerable populations affected by a disaster event.

KEY TERMS

Bioterrorism
Blast events
Blast wind
Crown fire
Disaster
Disaster epidemiology
Disaster management
Disaster planning

Emergency information systems (EISs)
Emergency preparedness
Emergency preparedness and disaster management (EPDM)
Evacuation
Extreme heat

Ground fire
Hazardous materials
Manmade disaster
Mass casualty event
Mitigation
Natural disaster
Preparedness
Point of dispensing

Quarantine
Recovery
Response
Response evaluation
Risk communication
Surface fire
Surge
Triage

Introduction

The necessity of strategic emergency preparedness and disaster management for manmade disasters was made all too clear in 2001 during the attacks on the World Trade Center and the Pentagon. Natural disasters such as Hurricane Katrina in 2005, the Haitian earthquake of 2010, Hurricane Maria, and the Palu, Indonesia earthquake and tsunami of 2018 continue to highlight the ongoing process of learning how best to address these events (Fig. 22-1). The world watched in dismay at the impact these disasters had on the communities involved. Despite the horror of the September 11 attack on New York, the city had learned from the 1993 World Trade Center bombing, and had an emergency preparedness and disaster management plan in place. For Katrina and the Haiti earthquake, by contrast,

the lack of clear plans resulted in increased mortality and exacerbated the effect of the disasters on the communities affected in both the short and long terms. These and other events resulted in an increase in concentrated training by health-care providers and first responders. The benefits of this relentless training resulted in minimal loss of life during the 2013 Boston Marathon bombings, yet further work is needed as disasters such as Hurricane Maria unfold, demonstrating the challenges of responding rapidly and effectively when a large population is affected.

Because weather-related events are ubiquitous and can occur without warning, humans have had little recourse but to prepare to respond to the wrath of the environment in which they live. Environmental devastation caused by natural hazards of terrestrial origin (earthquakes, tsunamis, blizzards, tornadoes, hurricanes, floods, wildfires, and

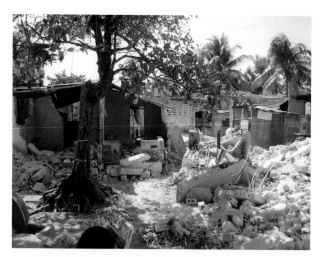

Figure 22-1 Devastation from the Haiti earthquake. *(From the CDC, photograph by Lt. Cmdr. Gary Brunette, 2010.)*

extreme heat) is inevitable. Events such as the tornado that hit Joplin, Missouri (2011), the tsunami in Japan and the subsequent Fukushima nuclear disaster (2011), Superstorm Sandy in the eastern United States (2012), Hurricane Maria in Puerto Rico (2017), Hawaii's Kilauea volcanic eruption (2018), and the earthquake and tsunami in Palu, Indonesia (2018), reveal an increasing intensity in disaster impact and destruction. The number of people affected, and the human and economic losses associated with these events have placed an imperative on disaster planning for emergency preparedness. Global warming, climate shift, sea-level rise, and societal factors may coalesce to create future calamities. Addressing disasters will take more than refining our ability to respond; sustainable approaches must be built in based on equitable resilience.[1] The International Red Cross and Crescent Federation called for "... humanitarian action, one that strives to strengthen the resilience of vulnerable and at-risk communities."[2]

Concurrent to these events is the ever-present risk of a manmade disaster such as an accidental or deliberate release of a biological, chemical, or radiological agent, or the use of an explosive device. Forced migration and people forcibly displaced by war (complex human emergencies),[3] acts of aggression, political upheaval, populist uprisings, and the increasing incidence of global terrorist attacks are reminders of the potentially deadly consequences of our inhumanity toward one another. The enormous human costs of forced migration—destroyed homes and livelihoods, increased vulnerability, disempowered communities, and collapsed social networks and common bonds—demand urgent and decisive action by disaster relief agencies.[3,4]

Natural disasters result not only in increased morbidity and mortality but also in destruction of property and natural resources. They can result in a reduction in economic productivity and harm to both the natural and manmade environments. The mental health impact on a community may be extensive, debilitating, and long-lasting. The negative impact of natural and manmade disasters can, at a minimum, be mitigated or perhaps prevented entirely. In expecting the unexpected,[7,8] much can be done in advance to anticipate and mitigate the devastating effects of natural and manmade disasters. Ongoing research in disaster science is paving the way to a world prepared to prevent and manage disaster (Box 22-1).

Disaster Nursing

Adequate disaster preparedness and response is essential for the delivery of lifesaving interventions and the optimization of population health outcomes.[7–9] Nursing is the single largest profession in the health-care system, so many of the first responders and most of the "first-receivers" during a disaster event are nurses. In the wake of any catastrophic event, communities will need nurses who will respond quickly and are clinically competent to provide safe, appropriate, individual, and population-based care.[8,12]

BOX 22–1 ■ Disaster Science Sources

Disaster science, accompanied by major advances in technology and meteorology, has provided a better understanding of the hallmark characteristics of natural/environmental hazards and the disasters they cause.

- Eric Noji noted in his sentinel disaster book that "understanding the way that people are injured or die as a result of a natural or manmade disaster is a prerequisite to preventing or reducing deaths and injuries during future disasters."[6]
- Better scientific evidence enables nurses, health-care planners, and public health officials to prepare for these types of events and to develop advance-warning systems to minimize injuries and the loss of life. Advance preparation for a major disaster can later result in significant reductions in mortality.[7,8]
- Postdisaster research has demonstrated access to care and accurate surveillance are key factors in the effects of natural disasters.[9,10]
- The use of mass casualty incident (MCI) triage can reduce morbidity and mortality, yet further work is needed to train first responders to utilize triage during real world events.[11]

During a disaster, priorities change, and it might become necessary to establish crisis standards of care.[13] This involves a complex response on multiple levels including individuals, families, health-care providers, crisis communication, and government at the local, state, and national level.[14] When a disaster is in motion, as it was with the tsunami and earthquake in Palu Indonesia in 2018, the objective for health-care providers responding to the scene shifts from providing high-quality, individualized care to providing population-based care with the goal of saving as many lives as possible. Valuable lessons were learned from disasters such as the attacks on 9/11, the Indian Ocean-Southeast Asian tsunami (2004), Hurricane Katrina (2005), and the powerful 9.0-magnitude earthquake that hit Japan (2011). In 2011, the Centers for Disease Control and Prevention (CDC) published standards for public health departments building preparedness capabilities[15] with evidence that these standards have improved the public health response.[16] Yet challenges remain, and lives are still lost as they were in Puerto Rico following Hurricane Maria.

Prior to such epic disasters, many nurses had only imagined what such events would be like. A heightened awareness now exists concerning what these disasters will demand of both responders and hospital-based first receivers. Nurses are needed across the disaster continuum during all phases.[8] Nurses, as victim advocates and health educators, adopt a population focus during the emergency preparedness and disaster-planning process by engaging community participation in the process and disseminating vital health and safety information throughout a disaster event. Nurses help shape disaster policy in their role as planners, evaluators, and leaders in health care.[8,12] Imagine that you wake up in the middle of the night to find that an earthquake has occurred, devastating your community. Your first response is likely to think about your family, friends, and pets. Children, parents, and other loved ones immediately enter your mind. Where are they? Are they safe? Your next thought may be to see who you can help, where you should go, and what can you do. Your desire to help is compelling, and you want to respond. But are you ready?

Disaster experts encourage taking time *in advance of an event* to evaluate your personal and professional readiness to respond (Fig. 22-2). All nurses should be able to answer basic questions related to disaster preparedness (Box 22-2). Much work remains to be done to ensure *all* members of the nursing profession possess the knowledge and skills necessary to respond appropriately to any type of disaster. The responsibility lies within our profession to engender a broad-based professional culture of excellence, both in disaster nursing care and in our health systems' management of catastrophic events.[8,12]

Emergency Preparedness and Disaster Management

Emergency preparedness is the planning process focused on avoiding or ameliorating the risks and hazards resulting from a disaster to optimize population health and safety. By contrast, **disaster management** is the integration of emergency response plans throughout the life cycle of a disaster event. Disaster management efforts are stimulated by the population perception of risk related to the hazards associated with the disaster.[17]

Disasters pose a unique threat to the health of the populations affected and require strategic planning prior to an event occurrence and efficient management during the emergency.[15–17] Public health emergency preparedness and disaster management form a shared responsibility that extends far beyond local and state health departments and government organizations.[15] Collaboration among private health organizations, social organizations, community health providers, community agencies, and the population at large is crucial for success.

A **disaster** is an emergency of such severity and magnitude that the resultant combination of death, injury, illness, and property damage cannot be effectively managed with routine resources or procedures.[17] Disasters can result from a variety of specific hazards, including natural disasters such as communicable disease epidemics and severe weather, as well as manmade disasters such as terrorism and chemical spills. Disasters have the ability to cause catastrophic morbidity and mortality in a population. The impact on public health may be immediate or insidious, developing slowly in the days and weeks following the event. Hurricane Maria in 2017 and a major earthquake in Palu, Indonesia, in 2018 illustrate the widespread morbidity and mortality associated with a disaster. These disasters caused death, acute injury, massive property damage, and loss of essential services to the population. In addition, both disasters have led to long-term health effects because of the total destruction of the existing health-care system. The 2013 Boston Marathon bombing resulted in injury and death in a small area with no collateral damage to buildings, but this terror event affected an entire city. Because of the risk posed by the suspects while they were still at large, a citywide order to shelter in place was enforced until shortly before the suspects were apprehended. The 2018

TIME FRAME

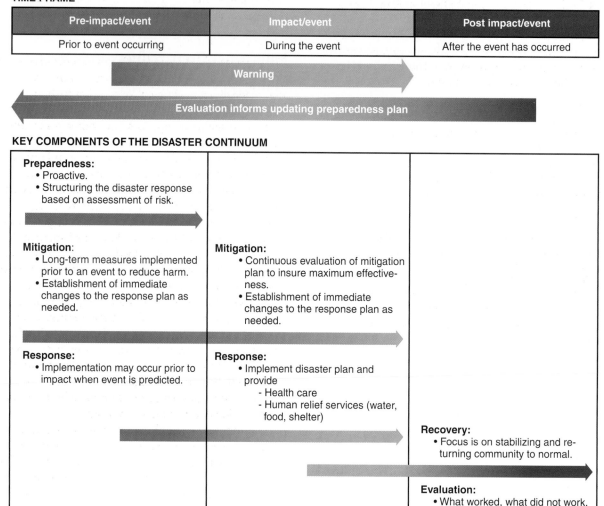

Pre-impact/event	Impact/event	Post impact/event
Prior to event occurring	During the event	After the event has occurred

Warning

Evaluation informs updating preparedness plan

KEY COMPONENTS OF THE DISASTER CONTINUUM

Preparedness:
- Proactive.
- Structuring the disaster response based on assessment of risk.

Mitigation:
- Long-term measures implemented prior to an event to reduce harm.
- Establishment of immediate changes to the response plan as needed.

Mitigation:
- Continuous evaluation of mitigation plan to insure maximum effectiveness.
- Establishment of immediate changes to the response plan as needed.

Response:
- Implementation may occur prior to impact when event is predicted.

Response:
- Implement disaster plan and provide
  - Health care
  - Human relief services (water, food, shelter)

Recovery:
- Focus is on stabilizing and returning community to normal.

Evaluation:
- What worked, what did not work, and what changes are needed to the disaster plan.

Figure 22-2 Readiness to respond: Disaster timeline.

Hawaiian eruption of the Kilauea volcano led to an ash plume 10,000 feet high and a lava flow that released toxic hydrochloric acid and glass volcanic particles into the atmosphere once it struck the Pacific Ocean.

Emergency Preparedness Theoretical Framework

Emergency preparedness and disaster management (EPDM) is a continuous cycle lacking a true beginning or end. The overarching concept of the emergency preparedness framework is prevention as it relates to public health. Public health practitioners are constantly learning from the events of the past and present, and trying to foresee issues of the future. To effectively prepare for emergencies and manage disasters when they occur, EPDM plans are needed at the community, state, national, and global levels. Disaster plans must be developed so that timely interventions can be rapidly disseminated when a threat surfaces or an emergency happens.

The four key concepts of the preparedness framework include preparedness, mitigation, response, and recovery (Fig. 22-3), and a fifth component, evaluation.[18,19] Another term for the life cycle of a disaster is the disaster continuum. It is characterized by three major phases: preimpact

BOX 22–2 ■ Organizational Disaster Plan Review

When working in a practice setting, it is important that nurses review the organization's emergency preparedness and disaster management plan. Things to identify prior to the occurrence of a disaster:

- Where is a copy of the plan located for the organization?
- What is the plan for the specific unit or area of the organization?
- Example of items to review in the plan:
  - Location of the command center
  - Plan for back up emergency power
  - Exit routes
  - Roles for each person in the unit/area
  - Specific instructions for different types of disasters
  - Communication and coordination plan
  - Triage plan and report to work plan
  - Emergency alarm systems
- What is the link between the organization and community/governmental agencies?
- What are the priorities in relation to vulnerable populations?

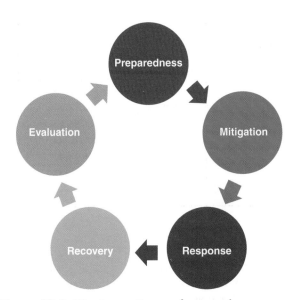

Figure 22-3 Disaster continuum framework.

(before), impact (during), and postimpact (after). These phases provide the foundation for the disaster timeline (see Fig. 22-2). Specific actions taken during these three phases, along with the nature and scope of the planning, will affect the extent of the illness, injury, and death that occur. There is a degree of overlap across phases, but each phase has distinct activities associated with it. Each phase incorporates vital components necessary for the overall success of the response and occurs over the timeline.

Disaster Planning

The purpose of **disaster planning** is to prevent or reduce the risk for adverse consequences posed by a natural or manmade disaster. Different approaches to disaster management are used, with some plans taking an organizational management approach, and other plans taking a more systemic view.[18] Disaster planning is broad in scope and should always address collaboration and mutual aid agreements across agencies and organizations. It should define all advance preparations as well as describe needs assessments, event management, and recovery efforts. The ability of a community and outside support systems to rapidly respond and provide needed medical treatment and supplies, shelter, food, and clean water are essential in the prevention of morbidity and mortality associated with the aftereffects of the disaster. This is more likely to occur when there is a plan in place that specifies the three critical "Cs" of disaster response: communication, coordination, and collaboration. In addition to immediate needs, a plan also must include a method to address the long-term effects of the disaster that exist in a population after the dust has settled. Thus, emergency preparedness can avert or reduce both the short-term and long-term effects of a disaster.

In addition, during the disaster, a well-developed infrastructure is needed to manage it. For example, in 2018, a massive earthquake and tsunami struck Palu, Indonesia, causing catastrophic damage. There was no warning as the tsunami warning system was not working. Thus, the lack of emergency preparedness resulted in increased morbidity and mortality.

● APPLYING PUBLIC HEALTH SCIENCE

The Case of the Impending Storm

Public Health Science Topics Covered:

- Development of an EPDM plan
- Environmental assessment
- Advocacy

Susan Doe, RN, MPH, worked as the vice president of community outreach at a regional hospital located near Atlantic Ocean coastal areas. After Hurricane Florence, a team was convened to revamp the EPDM plan for the region to help avoid the problems encountered in North Carolina. The team began by evaluating the risk for severe weather events, identifying the populations at greatest risk, examining the role of various responders, and evaluating potential problems posed by a hurricane.

Of particular concern to the team was the recent building of vacation homes by nonresidents of the state and the building of sophisticated beach barricades by owners of multimillion-dollar homes to protect those properties, which might increase damage to the shoreline following storms. Although the recent construction had been beneficial to the economy and had taken place because of a lack of updated ordinances, the development resulted in changes to the coastline that potentially reduced natural ecological defenses to hurricane damage, which had protected the community in the past. In addition, construction had increased the number of residences and persons at risk for hurricane-related damage should a hurricane hit while the summer people were in town. Another concern was that the summer residents might not be as knowledgeable about evacuation and emergency shelters that permanent residents knew about through word of mouth. To help develop an EPDM plan that addressed these concerns, the team members realized they needed to educate themselves on the concepts of preparedness, response, mitigation, and recovery to organize an emergency preparedness and disaster management plan for their community.

The team began by looking at prevention. Prevention during emergency preparedness and disaster planning includes efforts at multiple levels with the aim of preventing not only injury and mortality directly related to the disaster but also reducing damage to the infrastructure of the community, thus preventing long-term negative health consequences. Sue and her team realized that, during a hurricane, injury and death directly related to the storm surge are the most immediate health concerns and often result in the greatest loss of life. A storm surge is an abnormal rise of water generated by a storm, over and above predicted astronomical tides, which can cause extreme flooding in coastal areas, particularly when it coincides with normal high tide, resulting in storm tides reaching up to 20 feet or more. However, after the event has passed, damage to the infrastructure of the community could result in serious health consequences because of lack of access to the essentials of food, water, shelter, and medical care. If the community is severely damaged, a large segment of the population may be unable to return to their homes, resulting in long-term adverse economic and mental health issues. They concluded that their EPDM plan needed to include mechanisms for the prevention of both the direct and indirect negative consequences potentially related to a disaster event.

Sue invited a consultant from the International Federation of Red Cross and Red Crescent Societies to help educate the team. The consultant suggested the team begin with primary prevention. This part of the planning process focuses on the development of strategies that include both what to do when the event occurs and what prevention efforts can be done to decrease the threat to persons and infrastructure. The consultant explained that the prevention efforts of an EPDM plan related to a hurricane event would address their concern about evacuation, because they would now have a clear evacuation plan prior to the storm reaching coastal lands. This would help prevent injury, death, and exposure to communicable disease. The team began to develop a plan that included how to mobilize members of the community to follow the plan. Based on the lessons learned from Katrina, the team included instructions in the plan that would help direct members of the community in gathering life-sustaining items. They also began to work on the evacuation plan, paying particular attention to communication with those visiting the coastal area as tourists and renters as well as the year-round population. They realized that efficiently evacuating the community at risk prior to a hurricane reaching land was more complex than originally thought. Based on the events during Superstorm Sandy in 2012, they realized the area affected by a hurricane could be quite large and required moving a large population well inland. To effectively design their plan, they brought in the state police and transit authorities.

The team began to see that prevention efforts must also include building an infrastructure to prevent damage. Thus, their hurricane EPDM plan was expanded to include the development of hurricane-specific building codes and the construction of seawalls. They began to examine the impact of private barriers being built around the wealthier beach communities. Based on the success of communities in other states that had instituted these policies to reduce risk, the team began to draw up recommendations to their community requiring that construction of new buildings near the coastal area be resistant to the effects of high winds, storm surge, and floodwaters.

Sue's team put their EPDM plan in place. The following fall, a hurricane hit their area. It was listed as a Category 2 hurricane and did not require mandatory evacuations. Luckily, the team had put in place an evacuation system that included a plan for both voluntary and mandatory evacuations. The community was well informed about evacuation routes, and a system was in place to inform seasonal renters. The majority of the population, especially the seasonal renters, chose to evacuate. The evacuations began 24 hours prior to the storm, and there was little difficulty in handling the traffic headed out of the area. Because of the smooth evacuation process, there was minimal need to rescue people in harm's way after the storm made landfall.

The team also included secondary prevention components in their plan. The components began with a focus on preventing injury and disease by designating safe places for residents to shelter. They realized that not everyone would be able to evacuate, and this population would include those most vulnerable, especially the elderly or those with disabilities. Thus, they designated shelters that included a mechanism for providing for health needs during the storm. The goal of this part of their plan was to prevent initial or secondary injury. Residents unable to evacuate were directed to these safe locations throughout the area. These were shelters that could withstand the hurricane storm forces.

The team also incorporated tertiary prevention strategies into the plan, that is, strategies designed to minimize the disease effects among those previously ill in the community. They discussed the need to provide short-term pharmaceutical supplies, such as insulin, oxygen, and heart medications, to members of the population with noncommunicable illnesses.

After the hurricane, Sue and her team reviewed the event to see how the plan worked. They found that, once people were safely in a temporary shelter, the strategies used to prevent the spread of disease and to maintain health among the victims of the storm seemed to work. During the planning, Sue had informed her team that, without careful planning, respiratory and gastrointestinal disease could spread quickly in an area of mass population relocation.[18] The plan had helped ensure that uncontaminated food and water, as well as proper personal hygiene supplies, were available at each of the designated shelters. In addition, vital medical supplies were available, not only to treat injury, but also to provide care. For example, shelters had adequate supplies of medications, including antibiotics and insulin for diabetic residents. Each shelter had designated nurses to help care for the relocated population. These nurses were a vital asset in the community's effort to maintain health during a hurricane and its aftermath.

Sue and her team concluded that their EDMP had helped to reduce mortality and morbidity. However, following the hurricane, an inspection of the beachfront property hit hardest by the storm confirmed their suspicion that private barriers erected by homeowners may have protected those homes but resulted in further beach erosion in other areas. The team concluded that a Category 4 or 5 hurricane could result in higher threats to morbidity and mortality due to the instability of the beaches. Also, further action was needed for primary prevention that would require possible legislation as well as an allocation of funds to further protect the coastline.

Preparedness

Preparedness occurs before impact and is a proactive process for putting in place the structure needed for disaster response (see Fig. 22-2). It begins with a risk assessment to help determine the likelihood of a disaster occurring and identifying vulnerabilities. A next step is developing a monitoring process to forecast future disasters, including location, timing, and magnitude of a possible future event.[18] Preparedness begins with defining the precise role of public health providers during the various disaster events. Multiple agencies join forces during a disaster to form an organized web of responders. Each agency must be aware of its role in the plan and the chain of command appropriate for the situation.[15,18] For example, in preparing for a major hurricane, the EPDM plan would include a clear delineation of the role of the state and local officials in the chain of command, and agencies would be identified to serve as support staff. National agencies are included as appropriate, such as the Federal Emergency Management Agency (FEMA), the U.S. Coast Guard, the CDC, the Environmental Protection Agency, the National Guard, and the Department of Homeland Security (DHS). Nongovernmental stakeholders are included in the plan as needed for a hurricane event such as local hospitals, the American Red Cross, and utility companies.

Once the final EPDM plan for the impending storm is established, each state and local agency included in the plan must develop an individualized response plan and disseminate the information to the organizational and public stakeholders. A key component to emergency preparedness is each responding organization independently and collectively demonstrating their role during a disaster. Drills must be conducted that involve both the community and the organizations identified in the plan prior to an event to help identify and improve on the areas of weakness. Drills can also improve the efficiency of the response across multiple levels to a disaster event.[20] Establishing interorganizational communication becomes a priority during a disaster drill, as does communication with the members of the community.[15,16]

Mitigation

Mitigation primarily occurs during the preimpact phase (see Fig. 22-2) as a means to limit adverse effects of the disaster and covers a wide spectrum of issues, including health, infrastructure, and the impact on the economy. These are long-term measures that aim to moderate the impact of the event. Evaluation of the plan must continue throughout the response to ensure maximum effectiveness. The established response plans guide the endeavor. The first priority is to identify the affected population and environment and adjust the plan as needed to specifically target the community of interest. Each disaster is a unique event that affects populations with varying severity. Flexibility and creative problem-solving techniques are vital for an effective public health response. For example, relief shelters should be identified in coastal regions prior to a hurricane event. However, the storm forces could compromise the integrity of a relief shelter. Mitigation includes making immediate changes to the response plan and identifying a safe structure to which to relocate the population.

Returning to the example of a hurricane event, hurricane-related mitigation strategies could include building flood levees, developing flood zones, establishing clearly marked evacuation routes, and enforcing building codes.

Response

When a disaster happens, the plan is put into action (see Fig. 22-2). The **response** requires activation of the various procedures planned prior to the event; it may begin before the actual event, as with predicted weather events such as hurricanes and blizzards. For example, prior to a predicted severe weather event, orders are made to mandate evacuations, shore up seawalls, and close schools and businesses. In other cases, the event is unforeseeable and plan is put into effect as the event begins and continues throughout its duration. The time frame of the response phase is specific to the event itself. The purpose is to save lives, address health threats, and maintain basic human needs such as food,

shelter, and water. Effective response to a disaster is enhanced when there is an incident command center and trial runs of the plan are conducted prior to the disaster.[12]

Recovery

Recovery begins as the event ends (see Fig. 22-2), with a focus on stabilizing the community through both reconstruction and rehabilitation.[18] Recovery efforts encompass a wide range of activities, including restoring infrastructure and buildings, and relocating those who have lost their homes. The purpose of the response plan is to minimize the long-term effects of the disaster and address both the immediate and long-term needs of the community. In the case of a major hurricane, recovery begins when hurricane storm forces end and floodwaters recede. The length of recovery varies depending on the type and intensity of the disaster. Short-term and long-term population impacts are identified after the initial event has concluded. Evidence-based science should be applied to ensure continuous population protection. The structural stability of buildings and homes becomes a concern, as well as the availability of the resources necessary for survival. Power outages can continue for an extensive amount of time. Contamination from the floodwaters and displaced sewage can pose long-term population effects. Epidemiological surveillance is needed to identify a possible increase in communicable diseases in the region, especially waterborne and foodborne illnesses.

Evaluation

Evaluation is an ongoing process that may begin during the event to help inform ongoing response, although the majority will occur after the event is over (see Fig. 22-2). Thorough evaluation should follow every disaster response to identify areas that need improvement. Although some models, such as FEMA's model, do not include evaluation as part of disaster planning, evaluation is essential to help inform ongoing EPDM planning[18] and public health policies. This quality assurance process should involve all responding agencies and participants, including volunteers. Revisions to the disaster plan then become incorporated into future drills, exercises, and mitigation efforts. The quality assurance process does not cease until all gaps have been addressed and alternative planning is in place. Future disaster planning should always be based on empirical evidence derived from previous disasters.[18-21]

Disaster Epidemiological Surveillance

During a disaster, principles of epidemiology help determine the immediate and long-term effects to public health. The critical focus of **disaster epidemiology** is to prevent or decrease morbidity and mortality associated with acute or noncommunicable illnesses.[18]

A community rapid needs assessment identifies the priority health issues in the population and assesses the availability and accessibility of health services (see Chapter 4). As previously noted, primary, secondary, and tertiary methods of prevention play a critical role during disaster mitigation. Other strategies include education of the population to address possible hazards, such as contaminants that have the potential to cause illness, and attempting to stabilize unstable structures.

Emergency Information Systems

The rapid collection and dissemination of disaster-related data form a core component of epidemiological surveillance. **Emergency information systems (EISs)** are designed to collect population data during the impact, mitigation, and recovery phases. Rapid data collection and analysis during a disaster ensure a timely flow of information to the appropriate responders.[22] Ongoing population data collection and surveillance allow public health providers to identify the needs of the population and design interventions to decrease morbidity and mortality. Disaster surveillance concentrates on the incidence, prevalence, and severity of illness and injury related to the event. An increase in endemic or communicable disease can follow the disaster impact due to population displacement, overcrowded shelters, disruption of normal sanitation practices, and loss of health services. Data focused on communicable disease or exacerbation of noncommunicable illness help guide population treatment.

All health-care facilities, including hospitals and clinics, must participate in the collection of emergency information. Minimal data collection includes the surge capacity of an organization that specifies the number of available beds, staffing needs, and supply shortages. Tracking the name and number of patients who have been treated and are awaiting treatment assists public health officials with overall population surveillance. Community health-care providers and private laboratories are important sources of patient-related disease and injury data. Community providers can also educate individuals about communicable diseases and injury treatment. An integrated EIS should be developed during the planning phase and made accessible to all emergency responding agencies.

The National Notifiable Diseases Surveillance System (NNDSS) is an example of an electronic reporting database.[23] The NNDSS facilitates electronically transferring public health surveillance data from the health-care system to public health departments. It is a conduit for sharing information that supports NNDSS. Today, when states and territories voluntarily submit notifiable disease surveillance data electronically to the CDC, they use data standards and electronic disease information systems and resources supported in part by the NNDSS. This ensures that state data shared with the CDC are submitted quickly, securely, and in an understandable form. The NNDSS helps connect the health-care system to public health departments and those health departments to the CDC by providing leadership and resources to state and local health departments to adopt standards-based systems needed to support national disease surveillance strategy. This enables health agencies to use information technology more effectively by developing patient-centered systems that help health departments identify issues such as comorbidities (multiple diseases or conditions) that occur in the same individual over time. The NNDSS also defines and implements content standards (i.e., disease diagnosis, risk factor information, lab confirmation results) for the health-care industry to use.[23]

Postimpact Epidemiological Surveillance

Population disease and injury outcomes can be anticipated based on the specific type of disaster affecting the population. For example, an increase in diarrheal disease is common after a flood because of the disruption in sanitation practices and integrity of the public health infrastructure. Respiratory illness increases after a wildfire as a result of the atmosphere contaminants released into the air.[24] Epidemiologists determine the association between the exposure, the disaster event, and the outcome. A standard case definition is established to identify and monitor affected persons. Detection thresholds must be flexible to capture the changing levels of risks and priorities related to population illness and injury. For example, respiratory illnesses and long-term burn treatment will be anticipated following a wildfire. Postimpact surveillance monitors the increase in respiratory disease from baseline, and tracks burn cases caused by environmental exposures. Epidemiologists anticipate a spike in respiratory illness and bodily injury postimpact. Surveillance continues until levels stabilize back to the regional baseline. Data collected and disseminated during a disaster assist in future planning efforts by helping to predict possible health issues and prioritize health education needs of a population affected by a similar disaster.

Natural Disasters

In 2017, the world watched in awe as the forces of Hurricane Maria assaulted the island of Puerto Rico and devastated the lives of 3 million people on the island. Hurricane winds destroyed buildings, power sources, potable water supplies, and transportation systems. The community suffered injuries from debris and unstable structures. Contaminated water and food supplies left the people without adequate nutritional support. With utility and transportation infrastructure in ruins, the populace was without access to health care and resources from the mainland United States. The images of an event such as this guide the efforts for future preparedness efforts.

Natural disasters are events that occur from forces in nature that are not the direct result of human activity. These events lack controllability and may vary in their predictability. Their onset can be acute and rapid or slow and progressive. Natural disasters vary in the type and degree of population impact. The probability of an event occurring will vary depending on geographical region and season. In understanding the various types of natural disasters and determining the likelihood of these events occurring in a specific region, nurses can be active participants in the planning process, the management of a disaster, and the evaluation of the plan.

Cyclones, Hurricanes, and Typhoons

Cyclones are large-scale storms characterized by low pressure in the center surrounded by circular wind motion. The U.S. National Weather Service's (NWS) technical definition of a tropical cyclone is "a non-frontal, warm-core, low pressure system of synoptic scale, developing over tropical or subtropical waters and having a definite organized circulation."[29]

In practice, that circulation is a closed airflow at the earth's surface, turning counterclockwise in the Northern Hemisphere and clockwise in the Southern Hemisphere. Severe storms arising in the Atlantic waters are known as hurricanes, whereas those developing in the Pacific Ocean and the China seas are called typhoons. The precise classification (e.g., tropical depression, tropical storm, hurricane) depends on the wind force (measured on the Beaufort scale, introduced in 1805), wind speed, and manner of creation (Box 22-3).

BOX 22–3 ■ Cyclone Terminology

A tropical cyclone is a rotating, organized system of clouds and thunderstorms that originates over tropical or subtropical waters and has a closed low-level circulation. Tropical cyclones rotate counterclockwise in the Northern Hemisphere. They are classified as:

- Tropical Depression: A tropical cyclone with maximum sustained winds of 38 mph (33 knots) or less.
- Tropical Storm: A tropical cyclone with maximum sustained winds of 39 to 73 mph (34 to 63 knots).
- Hurricane: A tropical cyclone with maximum sustained winds of 74 mph (64 knots) or higher; also called typhoons in the western North Pacific or cyclones in the Indian Ocean or and South Pacific Ocean.

Source: (26)

A hurricane is a tropical storm with winds that have reached a constant speed of 74 miles per hour or more.[25] Hurricane winds blow in a large spiral around a relatively calm center known as the *eye*. The eye is generally 20 to 30 miles wide, and the storm may extend outward 400 miles. As a hurricane approaches, the skies will begin to darken, and winds will grow in strength. As a hurricane nears land, it can bring torrential rains, high winds, and storm surge. A single hurricane can last for more than 2 weeks over open waters and can run a path along the entire length of the Eastern Seaboard. August and September are peak months during the hurricane season which lasts from June 1 through November 30. Satellites track hurricanes from the moment they begin to form, so warnings can be issued many days ahead of the storm strike. The greatest damage to life and property is usually not from the wind but from tidal surges and flash flooding. Hurricanes are typically rated on a scale of 1 to 5, known as the Saffir-Simpson Hurricane Wind Scale. Category 3, 4, and 5 hurricanes are considered to be major storms.[26] Because of their violent nature, potentially prolonged duration, and potential effects on an extensive area, hurricanes or cyclones are potentially the most devastating of all storms.

A distinctive characteristic of hurricanes is the increase in sea level, often referred to as *storm surge* (referred to earlier in The Case of the Impending Storm). This increase in sea level is the result of the eye creating suction, the storm winds piling up water, and the tremendous speed of the storm. Rare storm surges have risen as much as 14 meters above normal sea level. This phenomenon can be experienced as a large mass of seawater pushed along by the storm with great force. When it reaches land, the impact of the storm surge can be exacerbated by high tide, a low-lying coastal area with a gently sloping seabed, or a semienclosed bay facing the ocean.[26]

The severity of a storm's impact on humans is exacerbated by deforestation, which often occurs as a result of population pressure. When trees disappear along coastlines, winds and storm surges can overtake land with greater force. Deforestation on the slopes of hills and mountains increases the risk of violent flash floods and landslides caused by the heavy rain associated with tropical cyclones. At the same time, the main benefit of the rainfall, replenishment of water resources, may be negated because of the inability of a deforested ecosystem to absorb and retain water.

In anticipation of a hurricane making landfall, disaster planners and health-care providers should note that the Saffir-Simpson Hurricane Wind Scale does not address the potential for other hurricane-related impacts such as storm surge, rainfall-induced floods, and tornadoes. It also should be noted that these wind-caused damages are to some degree dependent on the local building codes in effect and how well and how long they have been enforced. For example, building codes enacted during the 2000s in Florida, North Carolina, and South Carolina are likely to reduce the damage to newer structures. However, for a long time to come, the majority of the building stock in existence on the coast will not have been built to a higher code. Hurricane wind damage is also very dependent on other factors, such as duration of high winds, change of wind direction, and age of structures.[26,27]

Deaths and injuries from hurricanes occur because victims fail to, or are unable to, evacuate the affected area or take shelter, do not take precautions in securing their property, and/or do not follow guidelines on food and water safety or injury prevention during recovery. Nurses need to be familiar with the commonly used definitions for severe weather watches and storm warnings to assist with timely evacuation or finding shelter for affected populations. Morbidity during and after the storm itself results from drowning, electrocution, lacerations, and punctures from flying debris and blunt trauma or bone fractures from falling trees or other objects. Myocardial infarctions and stress-related disorders can arise during the storm and its aftermath. Gastrointestinal, respiratory, vector-borne disease, and skin disease as well as unintentional pediatric poisoning can all occur during the period immediately following a storm.[24] Injuries from improper use of chain saws or other power equipment, disrupted wildlife (e.g., bites from mammals, snakes, or insects), and fires are common. Fortunately, the ability to detect, track, and warn communities about cyclones, hurricanes, and tropical storms has helped reduce morbidity and mortality in many countries.

The Anatomy of a Natural Disaster: Lessons Learned From Hurricane Katrina

The National Hurricane Center in Miami, Florida, noted the increasing force of a tropical storm over the Bahamas on August 23, 2005, and issued the first advisory, stating that the weather system would become Hurricane Katrina. The storm continued to strengthen over the next 2 days and came ashore late Thursday evening on the coast of Miami. The hurricane caused significant damage to the coast as well as two fatalities. During Thursday night into early Friday morning, the storm weakened in intensity and was reclassified as a tropical storm. Hurricane Katrina emerged from the Florida peninsula around 5 a.m. Friday morning and immediately intensified after encountering the warm Gulf of Mexico waters. The strength of the hurricane grew over the next 48 hours. By 5 a.m. on Sunday, August 28, 2005, the storm had been declared a Category 4 hurricane, and continuous public warnings were being aired to the potentially affected population.

The National Hurricane Center stated that Hurricane Katrina was a potentially catastrophic storm at this time. Rough storm waters began placing stress on the levees of New Orleans as the storm continued to increase in severity throughout Sunday. Fears were expressed that flooding could occur around the levees and along the Gulf of Mexico coastline. Hurricane Katrina entered the Gulf at Category 5. Late Sunday night, thousands of people who were unable or chose not to evacuate New Orleans took shelter in the Louisiana Superdome. At approximately 5 a.m. Monday, August 29, 2005, hurricane force winds moved to within 100 miles of the Louisiana shore, creating strong winds, waves greater than 40 feet in height, and heavy rainfall. The storm came ashore again around 11 a.m. Monday at the Louisiana and Mississippi border, causing devastation to the cities of Biloxi and Gulfport. Around this same time, a major levee in New Orleans failed, sending floodwaters into the city. Floodwater continued to pour into New Orleans during the day on Tuesday.

All remaining residents were ordered to evacuate the city on Wednesday, August 31, 2005. However, floodwater and hurricane debris prevented trucks or buses from traveling to the area. Cries for help poured in from New Orleans throughout Wednesday and Thursday as residents were stranded without food, water, or other essential life-sustaining supplies. The three days following the failure of the New Orleans levee presented unbearable challenges to those staying in the overcrowded Superdome and Convention Center. The U.S. National Guard arrived in New Orleans on Friday, September 2, 2005, with food, water, and medical supplies, and the U.S. Congress approved a bill containing $10.5 billion in relief aid.

Thousands of residents evacuated New Orleans and the Gulf Coast following the initial warnings from the National Hurricane Center. Thousands more lacked resources and modes of transportation to leave the affected area. These residents were directed to the Louisiana Superdome and warned of the treacherous conditions that lay ahead in the coming weeks. People were left without clean water, food, or medical supplies. In the days following the levee break, responding agencies encountered confusion and disorganization. Responders faced challenges associated with jurisdictional authority and lacked a clear disaster management structure necessary to provide prompt and effective disaster relief. Vulnerable populations, including the poor, older adults, and the disabled, faced the greatest impact following the hurricane. Persons with challenges related to physical disabilities and financial resources faced numerous barriers to evacuation, including lack of transportation or inability to pay for hotel accommodations.

Thousands of residents from the Gulf Coast were a displaced following Hurricane Katrina. The Category 5 hurricane destroyed cities along the coast and displaced residents to various areas around the country for long periods of time, and in some cases permanently. Many residents suffered extreme economic loss with the destruction of their homes and businesses. The process of rebuilding the lost cities was a feat that continued for years following the tragic event.

The lessons learned from Hurricane Katrina stimulated a new emphasis on disaster management and emergency preparedness efforts. States organized legislative actions and implemented policies and procedures regarding evacuation following the declaration of severe weather events. Emergency response efforts were organized into a standard structure to distinguish the role and authority of each responding agency and organization. Evidence of the successful reorganization and planning was made evident in 2008 during the Hurricane Gustav resident evacuation along the Gulf Coast. The efficient emergency preparedness structure put in place was directly responsible for reducing injury and death as well as mitigating any long-term effects.

Earthquakes

An earthquake, generally considered to be the most destructive and frightening of all forces of nature, is a sudden, rapid shaking of the earth caused by the breaking and shifting of rock beneath the earth's surface. This shaking can cause buildings and bridges to collapse; disrupt gas, electric, and phone service; and sometimes trigger landslides, avalanches, flash floods, fires, and huge, destructive ocean waves (tsunamis). Aftershocks of similar or lesser intensity can follow the main quake. Buildings with foundations resting on unconsolidated landfill, old waterways, or other unstable soil are most at risk. Buildings or trailers and manufactured homes not tied to a reinforced foundation anchored to the ground are also at risk because they can be shaken off their mountings during an earthquake.

Worldwide, earthquakes were among the top deadliest disasters in 2017.[28] Earthquakes can occur at any time of the year. Earthquakes, like other similar disasters, tend to cause more financial losses in industrialized countries, and more injuries and deaths in undeveloped countries.

The Richter scale measures the magnitude and intensity, or energy, released by the quake and is an indication of the earthquake's force. This value is calculated based on data recordings from a single observation point for events anywhere on earth, but it does not address the possible damaging effects of the earthquake. According to global observations, an average of two earthquakes of a Richter magnitude 8 or slightly more occur every year. A one-digit drop in magnitude equates with a 10-fold increase in frequency. In other words, earthquakes of magnitude 7 or more generally occur 20 times in a year, whereas those with a magnitude of 6 or more occur approximately 200 times a year.

Earthquakes can result in a secondary disaster, a catastrophic tsunami, discussed in a following section of this chapter. Geologists have identified regions where earthquakes are likely to occur. With the increasing population worldwide and urban migration trends, higher death tolls and greater property losses are more likely in many areas prone to earthquakes. At least 70 million Americans face significant risk of death or injury from earthquakes because they live in one of the 39 seismically active states. In addition to the significant risks in California, the Pacific Northwest, Utah, and Idaho, six major cities with populations greater than 100,000 are located within the seismic area of the New Madrid fault (Missouri).[29] Cities in low- and middle-income countries where large numbers of people live on earthquake-prone land in structures unable to withstand damage include, but are not limited to, Lima, Peru, Santiago, Chile, Quito, Ecuador, and Caracas, Venezuela.

Deaths and injuries from earthquakes vary according to the type of housing available, time of day of occurrence, and population density. Common injuries include cuts, broken bones, crush injuries, and dehydration from being trapped in rubble. Stress reactions also are common. Morbidity and mortality can occur during the actual quake, the delayed collapse of unsound structures, or cleanup activity. Disruption of the earth may release pathogens that, when inhaled, can lead to increased reports of communicable disease. Mitigation involves developing and implementing strategies for reducing losses from earthquakes by incorporating principles of seismic safety into public and private decisions regarding the setting, design, and construction of structures (i.e., updating building and zoning codes and ordinances to enhance seismic safety), and regarding buildings' nonstructural elements, contents, and furnishings.

Extreme Heat

Extreme heat from a population perspective is a weather phenomenon characterized by substantially elevated outdoor temperatures or humidity conditions.[30] Extreme heat can result in an elevated body temperature, which then leads to hyperthermia, dehydration, heat exhaustion, or heatstroke. These conditions can cause internal organ damage when the body loses the ability to regulate temperature. Humid or muggy conditions, which add to the discomfort of high temperatures, occur when a dome of high atmospheric pressure traps hazy, damp air near the ground.

Over time, populations can acclimate to hot weather. However, mortality and morbidity rise when daytime temperatures remain unusually high several days in a row and nighttime temperatures do not drop significantly. Because populations acclimate to summer temperatures over the course of the summer, heat waves in June and July have more of an impact than those in August and September. There is often a delay between the onset of a heat wave and adverse health effects. Deaths occur more commonly during heat waves when there is little cooling at night and taper off to baseline levels if a heat wave is sustained.[31]

Heat is the number one weather-related killer in the United States, resulting in hundreds of fatalities each year. In fact, on average, excessive heat claims more lives each year than floods, lightning, tornadoes, and hurricanes combined. In the disastrous heat wave of 1980, more than 1,250 people died. In the heat wave of 1995, more than 700 deaths in the Chicago area were attributed to heat; and in July 2018, a record heat wave in North America left more than 30 people dead in Canada.[36] Heat kills by pushing the human body beyond its limits. On average, about 175 Americans succumb to the taxing demands of heat every year. When our blood is heated over 98.6°F

degrees, our bodies dissipate the heat by varying the rate and depth of blood circulation, by losing water through the skin and sweat glands, and, as a last resort, by panting. Sweating cools the body through evaporation. However, high relative humidity retards evaporation, robbing the body of its ability to cool itself.[36] When heat gain exceeds the level the body can remove, body temperature begins to rise, and heat-related illnesses and disorders may develop. Most heat disorders occur because the victim has been overexposed to heat or has overexercised for his or her age and physical condition. Other conditions that can induce heat-related illnesses include stagnant atmospheric conditions and poor air quality.[31]

Heat waves result in adverse health effects in cities more than in rural areas. During periods of sustained environmental heat—particularly during the summer—the numbers of deaths classified as heat-related (e.g., heatstroke) and attributed to other causes (e.g., cardiovascular, cerebrovascular, and respiratory diseases) increase substantially. Those at an increased risk for heat-related mortality are older adults, infants, persons with noncommunicable conditions (including obesity), patients taking medications that predispose them to heatstroke (e.g., neuroleptics or anticholinergics), and persons confined to a bed or who otherwise are unable to care for themselves.

Adverse health outcomes associated with high environmental temperatures include heatstroke, heat exhaustion, heat syncope (fainting), and heat cramps. Heatstroke (i.e., core body temperature greater than or equal to 105°F (40.4°C) is the most serious of these conditions and is characterized by rapid progression of lethargy, confusion, and unconsciousness; it is often fatal despite medical care directed at lowering body temperature. Heat exhaustion is a milder syndrome that occurs following sustained exposure to hot temperatures and results from dehydration and electrolyte imbalance. Manifestations of heat exhaustion include dizziness, weakness, or fatigue; treatment is supportive. Heat syncope and heat cramps are usually related to physical exertion during hot weather.

Basic behavioral and environmental measures are essential for preventing heat-related illness and death. Personal prevention strategies should include increasing time spent in air-conditioned environments, increasing the intake of nonalcoholic beverages, and incorporating cool baths into a daily routine. When possible, activities requiring physical exertion should be conducted during cooler parts of the day. Sun exposure should be minimized, and light, loose cotton clothing should be worn. The risk for heat-induced illness is greatest before persons become acclimated to warm environments.

Athletes and workers in occupations requiring exposure to either indoor or outdoor high temperatures should take special precautions, including allowing 10 to 14 days to acclimate to an environment of predictably high ambient temperature.[31] Nurses and other health-care providers can assist in preventing heat-related illnesses and deaths by disseminating community prevention messages to persons at high risk (e.g., older adults and persons with pre-existing medical conditions) using a variety of communication techniques. They also may establish emergency plans that include provision of access to artificially cooled environments.

Floods and Mudslides

Prolonged rainfall over several days can cause a river or stream to overflow and flood surrounding areas. A flash flood from a broken dam or levee or after intense rainfall of 1 inch (or more) per hour often catches people unprepared. Global statistics show that floods are the most frequently recorded destructive events. In 2017, worldwide flooding incidents accounted for 5 of the top 10 deadliest disasters.[28] Floods are the most common type of disaster in the United States. The frequency of floods is increasing faster than any other type of disaster. Much of this rise in incidence can be attributed to uncontrolled urbanization, deforestation, and the effects of climate change. Moreover, the risk of flooding is expected to increase.[33] Floods also may accompany other natural disasters, such as sea surges during hurricanes and tsunamis following earthquakes.

Except for flash floods, flooding causes few deaths directly. Instead, widespread and long-lasting detrimental effects include damage to homes and mass homelessness, disruption of communications and health-care systems, and substantial loss of business, livestock, crops, and grain, particularly in densely populated, low-lying areas. The frequent, cyclic nature of flooding can mean a constant and ever-increasing drain on the economy of rural populations. Flood-related morbidity and mortality vary from country to country. Flash flooding, such as from excessive rainfall or sudden release of water from a dam, is the cause of most flood-related deaths. Many victims become trapped in their cars and drown when attempting to drive through rising or swiftly moving water. Wading, bicycling, or other recreational activities in flooded areas have caused other deaths. The health impacts of flooding include communicable disease morbidity exacerbated by crowded living conditions and compromised personal hygiene, contamination of water sources, disruption of sewage service and solid waste collection, and increased vector populations. Waterborne diseases (e.g., enterotoxigenic *Escherichia coli*, *Shigella*,

hepatitis A, leptospirosis, and giardiasis) become a significant hazard, as do other vector-borne diseases and skin disorders. Injured and frightened animals, hazardous waste contamination, molds and mildew, and dislodging of graves pose additional risks in the period following a flood.[34] Food shortages due to water-damaged stocks may occur because of flooding and sea surges. The stress and exertion required for cleanup following a flood also cause significant morbidity (mental and physical) and mortality (e.g., myocardial infarction). Fires, explosions from gas leaks, downed live electrical wires, and debris all can cause significant injury.

Mudslides are another weather-related disaster. They usually occur after heavy rains. A mudslide involves the rapid movement of rocks, earth, and other debris down a slope. They can be associated with floods, earthquakes, and volcanic eruptions. The risk of a mudslide is increased when the natural vegetation on a slope has been modified following a wildfire or human activities.[35] Mudslides occur in all 50 states, with many mudslides occurring in California as a result of drought and wildfires. In 2017, mudslides were responsible for deaths in the Democratic Republic of Congo, Sri Lanka, Columbia, Sierra Leone, Bangladesh, India, and Nepal. The deadliest mudslide occurred in 1999, killing 30,000 to 50,000 people in Vargas, Venezuela.

Tornadoes

Tornadoes are rapidly whirling, funnel-shaped air spirals that emerge from a violent thunderstorm and reach the ground. Tornadoes can have a wind velocity of up to 200 miles per hour and generate sufficient force to destroy even massive buildings. The average circumference of a tornado is a few hundred meters, and it is usually exhausted before it has traveled as far as 20 kilometers. Knowing some facts about tornados is useful when putting together an EPDM plan for communities living in a tornado–prone area of the country (Box 22-4).[36]

Approximately 1,000 tornadoes occur annually in the United States, and none of the lower 48 states is immune. Certain geographical areas are at greater risk because of recurrent weather patterns; tornadoes most frequently occur in the midwestern and southeastern states. Although tornadoes often develop in the late afternoon and more often from March through May, they can arise at any hour of the day and during any month of the year. Injuries from tornadoes (e.g., head injury, soft tissue injury, secondary wound infection) occur from flying debris or people being thrown by the high winds. Stress-related disorders are more common, as is disease related to loss of utilities, potable water, or shelter.

BOX 22–4 ■ Tornado Facts

- They may strike quickly, with little or no warning.
- They may appear nearly transparent until dust and debris are picked up or a cloud forms in the funnel.
- The average tornado moves southwest to northeast, but tornadoes have been known to move in any direction.
- The average forward speed of a tornado is 30 mph, but may vary from stationary to 70 mph.
- Tornadoes can accompany tropical storms and hurricanes as they move on to land.
- Waterspouts are tornadoes that form over water.
- Tornadoes are most frequently reported east of the Rocky Mountains during spring and summer months.
- Peak tornado season in the southern states is March through May; in the northern states, it is late spring through early summer.
- Tornadoes are most likely to occur between 3 p.m. and 9 p.m. but can occur at any time.

Source: (36)

Because tornadoes can occur so quickly, communities should develop redundant warning systems (e.g., media alerts and automated telephone warnings), establish protective shelters to reduce tornado-related injuries, and practice tornado shelter drills. In the event of a tornado, residents should take shelter in a basement if possible, stay away from windows, and protect their heads. Special outreach should be made to people with special needs, who should make a list of their limitations, capabilities, and medications, and have ready an emergency box of needed supplies. People with special needs should have a buddy who has a copy of the list and who knows the location of the emergency box.

Tsunamis

A tsunami is a single or multiple tidal wave(s) created from an earthquake on the ocean floor.[25] On December 26, 2004, a 9.0 magnitude earthquake struck at approximately 7 a.m. about 100 miles from the coast of Sumatra, Indonesia. The quake caused a massive tsunami that killed more than 225,000 people and displaced another 1.2 million. This disaster quickly elevated to a crisis situation, affecting 11 countries and requiring global relief aid and disaster responders. Seven years later, on March 11, 2011, 31,000 people lost their lives from a tsunami that hit Japan. In 2018, another tsunami took more than 1,200 lives when it struck in Palu, Indonesia, as the community was preparing for a festival near the beach.

Initial tsunami-related morbidity and mortality occur from the force of the water, impact with moving debris, or crush injuries from falling structures. Long-term effects are similar to those of a severe flood event: there is an increase in water- and foodborne communicable disease, an increase in respiratory illnesses related to large numbers of displaced individuals in crowded relief shelters, and a lack of necessary medical and fiscal resources. In the case of the 2011 Japanese tsunami, damage to a nuclear reactor at a power plant added the hazard of a release of radioactivity into the environment. Unfortunately, the Japanese tsunami has had an unexpected global impact. We now know that the Fukushima nuclear power plant has been leaking radioactive water into the surrounding groundwater, which eventually makes its way into the Pacific Ocean. Also, debris swept into the ocean made its way to the Pacific shores of the United States, creating a long-term environmental problem.[37]

Submarine landslides and volcanic eruptions beneath the sea or on small islands also can be responsible for tsunamis, but their effects are usually limited to smaller areas. Tsunamis are often mistakenly referred to as tidal waves because they can resemble a violent tide rushing to shore. Tsunamis are powerful enough to move through any obstacle; therefore, damage from them results from both the destructive force of the initial wave and the rapid flooding that occurs as the water recedes. Depending on the strength of the initiating event, underwater topology, and the distance from its epicenter to the shore, the effects of a tsunami can vary greatly, ranging from being barely noticeable to total destruction.

Tsunami waves can be described by their wavelength (measured in feet or miles), period (minutes or hours it takes one wavelength to pass a fixed point), speed (miles per hour), and height. Tsunamis may travel long distances, increasing in height abruptly when they reach shallow water, causing great devastation far away from the source. In deep water, a person on the surface may not realize that a tsunami is forming while the wave increases to great heights as it approaches the coastline. The Pacific Tsunami Warning Center maintained by the National Oceanic and Atmospheric Administration (NOAA) monitors the Pacific Ocean for possible tsunamis and issues warnings.[38] Although this type of warning system is not yet available in other parts of the world, it is being developed to provide alerts about impending tsunamis across the globe. Tsunamis are not preventable, nor predictable, but there are warning signs. A number of events or signs are indicative of a possible tsunami (Box 22-5).

In the immediate aftermath of a tsunami, the first health interventions are to rescue survivors and provide

---

BOX 22–5 ■ Signs of a Possible Tsunami

- There has been a recent submarine earthquake.
- The sea appears to be boiling, as large quantities of gas rise to the surface of the water.
- The water is hot, smells of rotten eggs, or stings the skin.
- There is an audible thunder or booming sound followed by a roaring or whistling sound.
- The water may recede a great distance from the coast.
- Red light might be visible near the horizon and, as the wave approaches, the top of the wave may glow red.

---

medical care for any injuries. For people caught in the waves, the force of the water may push them into debris, resulting in the broadest range of injuries, such as fractured extremities and head injuries. Drowning is the most common cause of death associated with a tsunami. Tsunami waves and the receding water are very destructive to structures in the run-up zone. Other hazards include flooding and fires from ruptured gas lines or tanks.

The floods that accompany a tsunami result in potential health risks from contaminated water and food supplies. Loss of shelter leaves people vulnerable to exposure to insects, heat, and other environmental hazards. Further, the lack of medical care may result in exacerbation of noncommunicable diseases. Tsunamis have long-lasting effects, and recovery necessitates long-term surveillance of communicable water- or insect-transmitted diseases, an infusion of medical supplies and medical personnel, and the provision of mental health and social support services.

Potential waterborne diseases that follow tsunamis include cholera; diarrheal or fecal-oral diseases, such as amebiasis, cryptosporidiosis, cyclosporiasis, giardiasis, hepatitis A and E, leptospirosis, parasitic infections, rotavirus, shigellosis, and typhoid fever; animal- or mosquito-borne illness, such as plague, malaria, Japanese encephalitis, and dengue fever (and the potentially fatal complication dengue hemorrhagic shock syndrome); and wound-associated infections and diseases, such as tetanus. Mental health concerns are another serious consequence of tsunami events.

Volcanic Eruptions

A volcano is a mountain that opens downward to a reservoir of molten rock below the surface of the earth. Unlike most mountains, which are pushed up from below, volcanoes are built up by an accumulation of their own eruptive products. When pressure from gases within the molten rock becomes too great, an eruption occurs.

Extremely high temperatures and pressure cause mantle, located deep inside the earth between the molten iron core and the thin crust at the surface, to melt and become liquid rock or magma. When a large amount of magma is formed, it rises through the denser rock layers toward the earth's surface. Eruptions can be quiet or explosive. There may be lava flows, flattened landscapes, poisonous gases, and flying rock and ash.

Because of their intense heat, lava flows are significant fire hazards. Lava flows destroy everything in their path, but most move slowly enough that people can move out of the way. Fresh volcanic ash, made of pulverized rock, can be abrasive, acidic, gritty, gassy, and odorous. Although not immediately dangerous to most adults, the acidic gas and ash can cause lung damage to small infants, older adults, and those suffering from severe respiratory illnesses. Volcanic ash can affect people hundreds of miles away from the cone of a volcano.[39]

Sideways-directed volcanic explosions, known as lateral blasts, can shoot large pieces of rock at very high speeds for several miles. These explosions can kill by impact, burial, or heat. They have been known to knock down entire forests. Volcanic eruptions can be accompanied by other natural hazards, including earthquakes, mudflows and flash floods, rock falls and landslides, acid rain, fire, and (under special conditions) tsunamis. Active volcanoes in the United States are found mainly in Hawaii, Alaska, and the Pacific Northwest. The danger area around a volcano covers approximately a 20-mile radius. Some danger may exist 100 miles or more from a volcano.[39]

Volcanic eruptions can endanger the lives of people and property located both near to and far from a volcano. The range of adverse health effects on the population resulting from volcanic activity is extensive. Immediate, acute, and nonspecific irritant effects have been reported in the eyes, nasal passages, and upper airways of persons exposed to the ash.[39] Victims can experience exacerbations of their asthma and chronic obstructive pulmonary disease, and can asphyxiate due to inhalation of ash or gases. Eruptions can result in blast injuries and lacerations from projectile rock fragments. Volcanic flow can cause fires and the destruction of buildings, with victims experiencing trauma and thermal burns.

Prior to an eruption, communities living near an active volcano need to develop an EPDM plan. During an eruption, the first step is to evacuate, avoiding river beds and low-lying areas. Another concern is the potential for mudslides and exposure to falling ash.[39] Following the Kilauea Volcano eruption, ash shot upward more than

20,000 feet into the air, and sulfur dioxide created a thick fog near Hawaii Volcanoes National Park. After an eruption, it is essential to have shelters for the population, especially for those whose homes may not be safe to return to.

Winter Weather

Winter weather brings ice, snow, cold temperatures, and often dangerous driving conditions; a major winter storm can be lethal. Even small amounts of snow and ice can cause severe problems for southern states where such storms are infrequent. Nurses need to be familiar with winter storm warning messages, such as wind chill, winter storm watch, winter storm warning, and blizzard warning. The NOAA defines a blizzard as an event lasting greater than 3 hours with winds over 35 miles per hour, heavy snowfall, and decreased visibility. An avalanche results when a mass of snow, rock, or ice rapidly slides down a mountain or incline; it is also referred to as a snow slide.[29] Other issues with winter weather include ice storms and extreme cold.

These extreme conditions can prevent people from using established modes of transportation and from obtaining life-sustaining supplies and sources of power. The severity of the event can prevent emergency personnel from gaining access to the affected population. Blizzards, ice storms, and avalanches can strand individuals in places without heat or electricity, preventing the use of medical devices, and exposing a population to the previously discussed conditions. Prolonged exposure to cold weather conditions can result in injuries, such as hypothermia and frostbite (Table 22-1).

Transportation accidents are the leading cause of death during winter storms. Preparing vehicles for the winter season and knowing how to react if stranded or lost on the road are the keys to safe winter driving. Morbidity and mortality associated with winter storms include frostbite and hypothermia, carbon monoxide poisoning, blunt trauma from falling objects, penetrating trauma from the use of mechanical snow blowers, and cardiovascular events usually associated with snow removal. Frostbite is a severe reaction to cold exposure that can permanently damage its victims. A loss of feeling and a light or pale appearance in fingers, toes, nose, or earlobes are symptoms of frostbite. Hypothermia is a condition brought on when the body temperature drops to less than 90°F. Symptoms of hypothermia include uncontrollable shivering, slow speech, memory lapses, frequent stumbling, drowsiness, and exhaustion.

Communities should include preparation for cold weather events in their disaster plans. Individuals can reduce the impact of winter weather by taking preventive mitigation steps such as home winterization activities (insulating pipes, installing storm windows). At the population level, communities must have plans to handle interruption to transportation, loss of power, injury, and access to needed medical care. Of particular concern are vulnerable populations such as older adults or the homeless. Again, shelters may be needed to provide care in the event of a power outage. Many urban communities will increase their capacity to provide shelter to the homeless during extreme cold.

Wildfires

Wildfires are raging and rapidly spreading fires that can sweep quickly across large areas of land. They lack predictability and often require enormous resources to contain and extinguish. The Thomas Wildfire of 2017

TABLE 22-1 ■ Centers for Disease Control and Prevention Recommendations for Cold Weather Injuries

Health Effect	Symptoms	Treatment
Frostbite	• Numbness usually located on cheeks, toes, nose, chin, ears, and fingers • White or grayish-yellow discoloration • Waxy or firm skin	• Submerse affected area in warm, not hot, water. • Remain in a warm area. • Do not walk on or use effected parts. • Do not rub or massage. • Do not use a heating pad.
Hypothermia	• Decreased consciousness • Altered mental status • Shallow respirations • Pallor of the skin • Shivering • Confusion or disorientation	• Remove wet clothing. • Keep victim in a warm room. • Make skin-to-skin contact under cover of blanket. • Warm the center of body first (i.e., chest, head, and groin). • Use electric blanket if available. • Provide warm beverage to increase core body temperature.

Source: (92)

starting near Santa Paula, California, is the largest in California history. It burned more than 280,000 acres, forced thousands of people from their homes, and consumed a great number of structures. In 2011, multiple wildfires burned thousands of acres in Texas, resulting in the deaths of two firefighters. Three deaths occurred in a wildfire in Colorado in 2012. A wildfire in 2013 in Pigeon Forge, Tennessee, burned 230 acres and required 20 fire departments to respond before the fire was under control. More recently, a series of wildfires starting in the Great Smokey Mountains rapidly led to 14 deaths as fire spread during the night to the tourist town of Gatlinburg, Tennessee. It required the emergent evacuation of residents and tourists (Fig. 22-4). As residential areas expand into relatively untouched forests, wild lands, and remote mountain sites, forest fires increasingly threaten people living in these communities.[40] Protecting structures from fire poses extraordinary problems, often stretching firefighting resources to the limit.

Morbidity and mortality associated with wildfires include burns, inhalation injuries, respiratory complications, and stress-related cardiovascular events (exhaustion and myocardial infarction experienced while fighting or fleeing the fire).[41] Compromised respiratory conditions can result from the air pollution caused by the vast amount of smoke generated by the fires. Another concern is taking precautions to protect those who respond to fires. Responders are at increased risk for morbidity and mortality. Volunteer firefighters are at greatest risk; for example, 19 volunteer firefighters lost their lives combating a wildfire in Arizona in June 2013. The CDC provides specific guides for protecting firefighters during cleanup to reduce their risk of adverse consequences following the fire (Box 22-6).[42]

FEMA identified three areas of concern for public health preparedness—before a fire, during a fire, and after a fire.[40] Pre-fire population considerations focus on community education regarding actions that will enhance personal and public safety. Families are encouraged to have an evacuation plan at the first warning of a fire outbreak, especially for vulnerable members of the family such as children, older adults, and persons with disabilities. People are encouraged to wear protective clothing, shut off gas at the source, and gather all essential valuables and place them in a safe place for easy access. During the fire, homeowners are asked to leave all lights on inside the home, place a ladder outside in a highly visible area, leave all doors unlocked, and evacuate immediately. These measures are vital for responders to effectively manage structure fires and protect the population. Families should remain together in a central area of the home if they become trapped by the wildfire. Even after the wildfire is controlled, active embers and sparks can settle on roofs and in attics, creating the potential for further structure fires. It is important for people to watch for these sources that can cause a home to reignite and safely alleviate the threat.

Wildfires often begin unnoticed and spread quickly by igniting brush, trees, and homes. There are three different classes of wildfires. A **surface fire**, the most common type, burns along the floor of a forest, moving

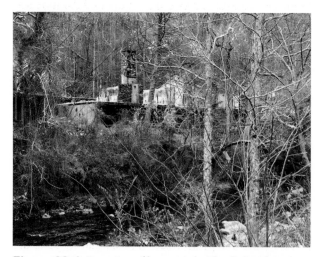

Figure 22-4 Remains of burnt riverside chalets from 2016 wildfire impacting Gatlinburg, TN. *(Photo credit: Gordon Gillespie.)*

BOX 22–6 ■ CDC Fact Sheet: Worker Safety During Fire Cleanup

Have available:

- First aid
- Protective equipment

Workers face hazards even after fires are extinguished. In addition to a smoldering or new fire, dangers include:

- Carbon monoxide poisoning
- Musculoskeletal hazards
- Heavy equipment
- Extreme heat and cold
- Unstable structures
- Hazardous materials
- Fire
- Confined spaces
- Worker fatigue
- Respiratory hazards

Source: (42)

slowly and killing or damaging trees. A **ground fire** is usually started by lightning and burns on or below the forest floor in the humus layer down to the mineral soil. **Crown fires** spread rapidly by wind and move quickly by jumping along the tops of trees. Depending on prevailing winds and the amount of water in the environment, wildfires can quickly spread out of control, causing extensive damage to personal property and human life. If heavy rains follow a fire, other natural disasters can occur, including landslides, mudflows, and floods. Once the ground cover has been burned away, little is left to hold soil in place on steep slopes and hillsides, increasing the risk for mudslides. A major wildfire can leave a large amount of scorched and barren land. These areas may not return to pre-fire conditions for decades. Danger zones include all wooded, brushy, and grassy areas,[43] especially those in Kansas, Mississippi, Louisiana, Georgia, Florida, the Carolinas, Tennessee, California, Massachusetts, and the national forests of the western United States.

Epidemics

An epidemic occurs when there is an increase in cases significantly higher than the usual number of cases. A pandemic describes epidemics occurring across the globe (see Chapter 8).[43] In the case of communicable diseases, EPDM plans are needed to handle the emergence of a communicable disease at epidemic proportions that puts a population or populations at risk. Quick response is essential because epidemics develop rapidly, resulting in human and economic losses and political difficulties. An epidemic or threatened epidemic can become an emergency when certain characteristics are present (Box 22-7). The categorization of an emergency differs from country to country, depending on two local factors: whether the disease is endemic and whether a means of transmitting the agent exists. Frequently, the introduction of a pathogen and the start of an epidemic may occur through an animal vector; thus, veterinarians may be the first to identify a disease new to a community.

Manmade Disasters

The events of September 11, 2001, in the United States stimulated the worldwide emergence of preparedness planning for terrorism.[15] **Manmade disasters** differ from natural disasters based on the human element associated with high levels of morbidity and mortality in a population. These events can be unintentional exposures or intentional terrorist events. An expansive consortium of responders is vital for an effective reaction to a manmade event.

BOX 22-7 ■ Epidemic Disaster Planning: Emergency Signs

Note: Not every characteristic need be present, and each must be assessed with regard to its relative importance locally:

- There is a risk of the introduction to and spread of the disease in the population.
- A large number of cases may reasonably be expected to occur.
- The disease involved is of such severity that it may lead to serious disability or death.
- There is a risk of social or economic disruption resulting from the presence of the disease.
- There is an inability of authorities to cope adequately with the situation because of insufficient technical or professional personnel, organizational experience, and necessary supplies or equipment (e.g., drugs, vaccines, laboratory diagnostic materials, vector-control materials).
- There is a risk of international transmission.

Blast Events

Explosions have the potential to affect a population by causing immediate physical injuries and destruction of property and well as long-term emotional distress, disability, and damage to the community's perception of safety. **Blast events** are the result of a device explosion. Immediate considerations following an explosion include identifying the causative agent, the affected geographical area, and extent of injury and damage. Responders must be aware of the appropriate personal protective equipment necessary for the situation and be proficient in the proper techniques in using the equipment. Only trained personnel should be involved in explosion mitigation until the safety of the blast scene is established. An explosion generates a blast wave that moves outward from the point of origin. In confined spaces, irregular, high-pressure blast waves will cause unpredictable injury patterns.[44,45]

The four stages of blast injuries include primary, secondary, tertiary, and quaternary (Table 22-2). Primary reflects injuries due to the blast wave, which is the overpressurization impulse created by the blast. The injuries from a blast result from the changes to the body brought about by the overpressurization force that impacts the surface of the human body. Most common blast injuries associated with the primary stage of impact include rupture of the tympanic membrane, causing temporary

TABLE 22–2 ■ Blast Injuries

Category	Characteristics	Body Part Affected	Types of Injuries
Primary	Unique to high-order explosives (HE), results from the impact of the over pressurization wave with body surfaces	Gas-filled structures are most susceptible— lungs, gastrointestinal tract, and middle ear.	Blast lung (pulmonary barotrauma) Tympanic membrane rupture and middle ear damage Abdominal hemorrhage and perforation Globe (eye) rupture Concussion (traumatic brain injury without physical signs of head injury)
Secondary	Results from flying debris and bomb fragments	Any body part may be affected.	Penetrating ballistic (fragmentation) or blunt injuries Eye penetration (can be occult)
Tertiary	Results from individuals being thrown by the blast wind	Any body part may be affected.	Fracture and traumatic amputation Closed and open brain injury
Quaternary	All explosion-related injuries, illnesses, or diseases not due to primary, secondary, or tertiary mechanisms. Includes exacerbation or complications of existing conditions	Any body part may be affected.	Burns (flash, partial, and full thickness) Crush injuries Closed and open brain injury Asthma, chronic obstructive pulmonary disease or other breathing problems from dust, smoke, or toxic fumes Angina Hyperglycemia, hypertension

Source: (44)

or permanent hearing loss, and injury to the air-filled organs in the body.[44]

Secondary injuries are the result of flying debris from the blast. In the Boston Marathon bombing, the majority of the injuries that required care were secondary injuries that resulted in damage to lower extremities, which, in some cases, required amputation. Tertiary injuries occur due to the displacement of air caused by the explosion. This creates what is called a **blast wind** that throws victims against solid objects. The videos from the Boston Marathon bombing show runners falling to the ground shortly after the bomb went off. Quaternary injuries include exacerbations of existing noncommunicable diseases as well as the threat of infection at the site of the wounds inflicted by the flying debris.

The response to the Boston Marathon bombings in the spring of 2013 is an excellent example of effective EPDM planning on the part of a city to deal with a blast-related disaster. The health-care providers and first responders followed the plan, hospitals were ready to receive the influx of wounded, and emergency care was provided that saved lives. When interviewed by the media, the physicians and nurses stated that they did what they had been trained to do.

Chemical Exposure

Chemicals are found everywhere, from industrial workplaces to home cleaning products. Releases can range from a small-scale, contained spill to a large release that causes widespread environmental contamination. Immediate priorities associated with a chemical exposure are to evacuate the contaminated area and identify the chemical. For example, visualize a motor vehicle crash involving a tanker vehicle transporting gasoline. Damage to the vehicle could result in a chemical spill on the roadway. Urgent actions involve restoring safety to the scene of the crash, the surrounding environment, and the exposed population. Chemical explosions can cause widespread destruction and contaminate the air, soil, and water. The explosive, flammable, poisonous, radioactive, and combustible properties of a substance must be identified immediately following a potential or active release.[44,46]

Hazardous materials are substances found in multiple forms that have the potential to cause death, morbid health effects, and property damage. These materials pose dangers to population health during production, storage, use, and disposal. A placard, card, or plaque containing a numerical code that identifies the type of chemical or hazardous material being transported by railway, vehicle, or waterway is required by the U.S. Department of Transportation and allows emergency responders to immediately identify the substance in question.[47] Preparedness actions to ensure patient and employee safety from potential chemical exposures in a health-care organization also are important. It is essential to know the commonly used chemicals in a hospital or health-care setting and educate those handling the substance on proper use and how to respond to a spill or human exposure.[48] Material safety data sheets contain information pertinent to planning, such as safe handling techniques, toxic effects of the material, and first aid considerations following human exposure.

Radiation Exposure

Ionizing radiation exposure has the potential to cause immediate and long-term adverse health effects in a community. The explosion at the Chernobyl nuclear power plant on April 26, 1986, is the largest nuclear disaster in world history and continues to plague parts of Europe. The incident created a release of nuclear material, necessitating the evacuation of approximately 116,000 people from the highly contaminated area surrounding the reactor. Severe contamination resulted in Ukraine, Belarus, and the Russian Federation, all of which were part of the former Soviet Union. Trace contamination spread by wind and water throughout eastern and western Europe.[49] More than 600,000 people have been involved with the mitigation of this radiation exposure during the subsequent 3 decades.

The health effects associated with various types of alternative energy sources have become a priority public health planning component during the 21st century. Considering the Chernobyl case, the World Health Organization (WHO) conducted a longitudinal study following the nuclear disaster and found an increase in thyroid disease, leukemia, solid cancers, and mental disorders among the population in the three severely contaminated countries. The lessons learned following the Chernobyl disaster have guided the development of regulations associated with general radiation use.[48] A proficient knowledge of the regional contamination potential will focus emergency preparedness and disaster planning priorities specific to the population of interest.

Bioterrorism

Bioterrorism is a deliberate release of a pathogen that is either naturally occurring or manmade and can create a public health emergency. The agent is bacterial or viral in origin. An event would typically present with a single definitively diagnosed case of an illness to be known as a bioterrorism agent, a cluster of patients presenting with a similar clinical syndrome lacking clear etiology or explanation, or an unexplained increase of a common syndrome above seasonal expectations. The CDC prioritizes infectious agents into three categories based on the impact and speed of transmission arranged from highest priority to emerging agents (Table 22-3).[15] Disaster mitigation would mimic that of a communicable disease epidemic; however, the rapid spread of disease and origin identification present unique challenges. Primary care providers, urgent care clinics, and emergency departments (EDs) will be the first to experience the influx of patients following the use of a biological weapon; therefore, detection and diagnosis would be made at the local level.

Disaster Response Structure and Organization

All disasters are local yet have the potential to affect health on regional, national, and global levels. Local health departments and government officials engage disaster response plans specific to the event and call on the resources necessary to effectively manage and mitigate the situation. Disaster events present challenges associated with the increased need for emergency personnel and resources.

Consider the possibility of a major crash of a passenger jet airplane. The potential for a large number of victims with life-threatening injuries increases the importance of a solid response structure for this event. Increased numbers of medical responders and supplies are needed to manage the number of potential victims. Responders from local governmental and volunteer agencies will be required to increase the power of the workforce. The initial priority of the emergency medical personnel is to identify the extent of illness and injury, communicate the gravity of the situation to local stakeholders and medical facilities, and begin victim medical treatment.

Disaster Triage and Patient Tracking

Emergency responders (usually paramedics and other emergency medical team members) begin victim treatment with field triage. **Triage** is derived from a French

TABLE 22–3 ■ Bioterrorism Agents/Diseases by Category

Category	Definition	Agents/Diseases
Category A	Highest priority agents These include organisms that pose a risk to national security because they • can be easily disseminated or transmitted from person to person; • result in high mortality rates and have the potential for major public health impact; • might cause public panic and social disruption; and • require special action for public health preparedness.	• Anthrax • Botulism • Plague • Smallpox • Tularemia • Viral hemorrhagic fevers, including Ebola
Category B	Second highest priority agents These include those that • are moderately easy to disseminate; • result in moderate morbidity rates and low mortality rates; and • require specific enhancements of CDC's diagnostic capacity and enhanced disease surveillance.	• Brucellosis • Epsilon toxin • Glanders • Melioidosis • Psittacosis • Q fever • Ricin toxin • Staphylococcal enterotoxin B • Typhus fever • Viral encephalitis • Water safety threats • Food safety threats
Category C	Third highest priority agents These include emerging pathogens that could be engineered for mass dissemination in the future because of • availability; • ease of production and dissemination; and • potential for high morbidity and mortality rates and major health impact.	• Nipah virus • Hantavirus

Source: (15a)

term meaning *to sort*.[11] Disaster triage determines the severity of illness or injury suffered by victims and assists responders with systematically distributing patients evenly among the local hospitals. The system is a color-coded, four-level process ranging from minor injuries to those who are dead at the scene. A large-scale disaster can produce significant numbers of victims stretching beyond the capabilities of the emergency medical system in a community. These scenarios are known as **mass casualty events (MCEs)** and require special considerations during the disaster planning process.[49] A chain of medical care is established between emergency responders and medical facilities. Although the plan of response varies between communities, most share standardized procedures.

During a disaster, patient and population tracking is a core function of state and local public health officials. Tracking becomes complicated when people evacuate to areas other than public shelters. Population tracking becomes an even greater challenge when considering homeless persons, incarcerated victims, shelters that do not register the injured individuals, and deceased persons. Established communication networks among hospitals, mass treatment facilities, and health departments help identify the location of injured victims seeking treatment.

Federal Response and Organization

The United States DHS is authorized by law to activate federal resources and assistance under certain circumstances. Federal agencies can act on their own authority when appropriate. For example, the Federal Bureau of Investigation (FBI) has established authority when an act of bioterrorism is suspected, and the Federal Aviation Administration (FAA) maintains authority following an airplane crash. State and local officials also can request federal assistance when the disaster expands beyond the resources and capabilities of local responders. Resource assistance includes financial support, personnel assistance, and physical supplies. The U.S. President has the authority to direct the secretary of the DHS to assume responsibility for managing a disaster when the event merits such an action.

Federal Emergency Management Agency

FEMA is the lead agency for and assumes coordination of disaster responses following a presidential declaration of authority under the Stafford Act. FEMA has direct access to federal resources and funding. Federal financial resources can be allotted for various functions including preparedness, response, and recovery efforts for large-scale disasters. FEMA is one of more than 27 agencies, along with the American Red Cross, that provide technical support and personnel of disaster planning and mitigation.

National Response Framework

The National Response Framework (NRF), enacted in January 2008, supersedes the previous National Response Plan. It serves as a guide for the nation during natural and manmade disasters and uses an all-hazards approach to comprehensive incident response. Built on its predecessor, it includes guiding principles that detail how federal, state, local, tribal, and private-sector partners, including the health-care sector, prepare for and provide a unified domestic response using improved coordination and integration. The plan provides national direction for all responders during a domestic disaster.

National Incident Management System

The National Incident Management System (NIMS) enhances the ability to oversee a national response to an event through a single, comprehensive management model. Several key elements are incorporated into the NIMS system, which functions to increase the effectiveness of a national disaster response. An established Incident Command System organizes areas such as command, operation, planning, logic, and finances during event mitigation and recovery. A unified command is established to assist with clearly defining objectives and joint decision making. Preparedness is another key element of the system and enhances the readiness of responders regarding the performance of vital disaster functions. The NIMS also provides organizational design for an interoperable communication infrastructure and information systems. The Joint Information System ensures that all levels of government are releasing the same information and coordinate to deliver a unified message to the public.[17] Each key element of the NIMS involves an intricate process and directly affects the overall effectiveness of the systems.

Strategic National Stockpile

A large-scale disaster response will require access to large amounts of pharmaceutical and medical supplies. The Strategic National Stockpile (SNS) is a national repository of antibiotics, chemical antidotes, antitoxins, life-support medications, and IV administration, airway maintenance, and medical-surgical supplies. Federal agencies such as the Department of Health and Human Services, primarily the CDC, are responsible for maintenance and delivery of SNS assets, but state and local authorities must plan to receive, store, stage, distribute, and dispense them. During a disaster, the SNS program is designed to deliver pharmaceuticals, vaccines, medical supplies, and equipment to states and local jurisdictions affected by the event. Each state is responsible for the management of the stockpile under which it resides. Relationships with public and private agencies are established within each state to ensure the maintenance and delivery of supplies. Upon request, push packs filled with medical and pharmaceutical supplies can be delivered to any area in the United States in less than 12 hours and readied for distribution by local health departments.

For example, a communicable disease outbreak affecting large numbers of people in a rapid time frame would demand resources outweighing the capabilities of the local health departments. Local public health officials would request the deployment of supplies from the SNS. Bulk push packs then would be delivered to the predetermined destination for distribution to the local care sites and medical facilities. Local public health providers then would be responsible for the maintenance and distribution of the allotted supplies. Mass care facilities are ideal for the prompt treatment of large numbers of patients. An example of a mass care facility is a disaster treatment center opened in a local venue large enough to house high volumes of community members. These care facilities provide disaster triage and basic medical care. Patients with critical or life-threatening injuries are stabilized at these facilities and transported to an appropriate health-care institution.

Point of Dispensing

A **point of dispensing (POD)** site is set up when the population requires rapid medical treatment, prophylaxis, or vaccination. PODs are designed to provide treatment to the population in a rapid and organized fashion. Multiple stations work in assembly-line fashion, providing services from screening to treating.[14] Patients begin with registration, at which a log is maintained of all persons receiving care in the POD. Patients are then screened for eligibility of treatment and epidemiological background related to the event. Once screened, patients move to a triage area staffed by licensed health-care providers, such as nurses or physicians; here patients are assessed to determine whether dispensing treatment is appropriate or whether further evaluation is needed from a health-care facility. The acutely ill are transferred immediately to a hospital for evaluation. Individuals receiving prophylaxis or medical treatment for minor symptoms then move to the dispensing station. Staff at these stations include licensed health-care providers (including pharmacists), who provide medication and/or treatment. Counseling services, POD security, and medical record-keeping also are vital components of the services provided. Patients can receive medical and psychological treatment while at the distribution center.

Multiple-Agency Consortiums

One concept that becomes obvious during emergency preparedness and disaster planning is the need for multiple agencies employing collective expertise to decrease disaster-related morbidity and mortality. The collaboration of public health personnel, law enforcement agencies, emergency responders, fire officials, and trained volunteers is essential for effective population medical treatment and physical protection. Organizational models such as NRF and NIMS provide guidance for local and state health departments to develop a consortium of disaster responders. The Medical Reserve Corps (MRC) is a federally sponsored program that provides an organized structure for community public health and medical volunteers. The program supports adequate training and exercises to ensure safety and competence of responding personnel.[50] The local MRC is activated during both emergency situations and nonemergent events, such as blood and immunization drives.

Health-Care Facility Disaster Response

Health-care facility preparedness is the cornerstone of effective mass casualty management.[49,51] Disasters present the unique challenge of patients seeking medical attention in large numbers that exceed the typical capacity of the facility. A sudden increase in patients is referred to as a **surge**.[51] Large volumes of patients are associated with disaster-related surge events, creating a demand for health services in which additional capacity and capabilities are required.[51] Routinely practiced disaster drills and exercises in an organization are the most effective strategies to increase the effectiveness of health-care facility disaster response. Each member of the institution must have proficient knowledge of her or his role in the mitigation efforts as well as proper internal and external communication procedures. It is crucial that surge plans are developed, documented, communicated, and exercised prior to a mass casualty event.

Health-Care Facility Surge Planning

Surge plans developed by a health-care facility should be compatible with the previously discussed national norms. Allocation of roles and responsibilities are established through the developed chain of command and planning structure. The health-care organization must have a command group or an emergency management group. These individuals are the leaders in the chain of command and will hold the ultimate authority of the event mitigation. Protocols should be developed in the institution pertaining to internal events and communication with state or local coordination centers. The organizational response varies depending on the size of the incident. The predetermined command staff is responsible for initiating and deactivating a facility surge plan. A plan to scale up or scale down the surge response is determined during the disaster mitigation to meet the medical needs of the affected population. An emerging issue regarding health-care facility disaster response is the need for a community-based network of local health-care providers. This network ensures the continuation of health-care operations if the infrastructure is damaged during the disaster.

Specific key components are essential for the development of a facility surge plan. Efforts begin with discharging less acutely ill persons. Those who can be managed as outpatients are released to create space for disaster victims. Elective procedures are canceled until the surge plan is deactivated. The events may call for additional beds being placed in predetermined locations and conversion of inpatients to hold multiple individuals. Supplemental staff is essential to carry out mass casualty care. Each facility should develop a plan to call back staff for additional shifts to meet the needs of the community. During a surge, hospitals and clinics work with the same amount of supplies as they would under normal daily function. Equipment and pharmaceutical resource management requires conserving and rationing until additional supplies are delivered to the health-care organization from local, state, or federal stockpiles.

The network of health-care providers must derive a unified plan for greater levels of surge. The need to share equipment and resources may arise during event mitigation. Documented agreements on the procedure used to distribute medical resources need to be established at a local level during the planning phase. Established procedures to call up facility volunteers also should be arranged during the planning phase and authority granted to a member of the chain of command to activate the volunteers. The need to provide rapid care to large numbers of patients often requires abbreviated documentation, an increased staff-to-patient ratio, and reduced testing procedures. Documentation protocols would be developed and exercised during the planning phase by all staff and volunteers. Documentation should coincide with local, state, and national norms to increase the ease in transfer of patient-related information.

Training and Exercises

Training exercises should be established with local and internal personnel. Each facility must plan to the capacity of the organization, and then provide disaster continuing education to all staff members and volunteers. Disaster plans and training are most effective when internal personnel and organizational stakeholders participate in the design process. The materials used for training must be specific to the surge plan established by the organization and easily accessible by all involved persons. A key factor involved in training exercises is the development of a structure that maintains organizational function and prevents confusion or poor communication among the responders. Training exercises scheduled at regular intervals provide continuing education for new and senior staff and allow for staff evaluation of surge mitigation effectiveness (Fig. 22-5). Problems that arise during a disaster drill must be addressed and incorporated into a new plan appropriate for the institution.

● APPLYING PUBLIC HEALTH SCIENCE

The Case of the Chemical Ka Boom

Public Health Science Topics Covered:

- Health planning
- Instituting an EPDM plan
- Managing a surge

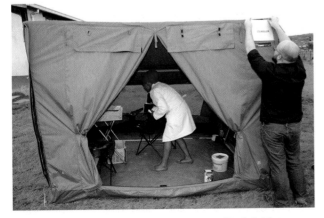

Figure 22-5 Training on setting up medical field tent. Minor procedures can safely take place during health-care fieldwork in a tent like this. *(From the CDC, Jesse Blount.)*

During the EPDM planning process for his community, John, a nurse working at the ED at the larger (urban) hospital in the community, volunteered to be a member of the command staff at the hospital in the event of a disaster affecting his community. While working in the ED, John received a call that there had just been an explosion at a local chemical plant located 15 miles from his hospital. It was midday, and all of the plant employees were in the building during the time of the event. The buildings and surrounding structures had suffered considerable damage. Unknown chemicals had been released into the atmosphere. Emergency responders were on the scene to evacuate the uninjured and transport the injured to local health-care facilities, taking the most severely injured to John's ED.

John's hospital received a call that there were mass casualties, with many of the injured in need of medical care. The command team activated the surge plan. Additional personnel and volunteers were activated to respond to the institution. Each of the trained staff in the ED responded by performing his or her specific role in the process. These roles varied from triaging, determining which patients were safe to treat and discharge and which needed immediate medical treatment, to the actual delivery of care. John was assigned to organize the mass treatment areas inside the facility.

In this case, John also established a decontamination zone as a priority given the chemical nature of the event. As patients arrived at the ED, triage personnel directed the individuals through decontamination (if needed) while also providing essential life support interventions (if needed). A rapid registration and triage process followed before moving patients to the appropriate area for treatment. Internal and communitywide communication flowed through the command team. External coordinators of the disaster's aftermath determined the status of the various health-care facilities and the extent of patient casualties still requiring medical treatment. Of particular concern was the possibility that community members not directly affected by the explosion may have been affected by the release of chemicals into the air and would need treatment. John prepared the staff for a possible influx of walk-in patients and made sure the staff followed the same process for these patients as those transported via medical responders. John and his team continued to work, following the plan, scaling up or down based on the volume of influx, until all was clear for the surge to be deactivated.

Eventually, John noted that the surge of patients had slowed, all victims were accounted for, and those who needed medical treatment were receiving it. Decreasing the surge response began as soon as John was notified that the rapid influx of patients had ceased. One responsibility of being a team leader is to continuously communicate the needs of the surge to staff and patients. Also, ongoing communication to victim family members is crucial during a disaster scenario.

Once the disaster was over, and the hospital had returned to normal daily functions, John led a quality improvement meeting. The purpose of the quality improvement effort was to collaboratively decide the functions that worked effectively and those in need of enhancement. The effectiveness of population disaster care for a health-care facility in an event such as this would be directly related to the level of preparedness and the amount of training received by the staff and volunteers.

Disaster Communication

Communication is central to disaster planning and mitigation. Natural and manmade events are frequently accompanied by power outages, damage to telephone towers, and interference in cell phone communication, which present challenges to responders and victims. It is critical that multiple agencies have the ability to exchange information rapidly during and after the impact regardless of the technological limitations. Furthermore, communication with the affected population must clearly emphasize the potential for disaster-related illness and injury as an event approaches without creating panic. Population communication educates individuals and families as to the appropriate actions necessary to prevent disaster-related morbidity and mortality.

Risk Communications

Risk communication is an interactive process involving individuals, groups, and institutions. It is the exchange of information regarding the nature, magnitude, significance, control, and management of an associated public health risk.[52-54] The use of risk communication principles assists the communicator in identifying the strengths and weaknesses of various communication outlets and maximizing the outreach potential of each. Disasters are associated with fear, confusion, anger, and worry. These emotions prevent individuals from comprehending complex messages. Thus, the use of clear, concise, and easy-to-understand messages is essential in the communication of information to a population confronted with a disaster.

The two main goals of risk communication are to decrease the mental noise associated with a disaster event and to establish trust among the affected population. When a person is deeply concerned, the ability to process information is severely impaired. During a disaster, individuals experience a wide range of emotions ranging from fear to anger. The mental agitation generated from strong feelings and emotions is known as *mental noise* and can interfere with the ability to engage in rational communication. Further complicating an individual's ability to comprehend information during a disaster is the level of trust people in an affected community have in the person or persons communicating the information. The establishment of trust is essential in all risk communication strategies. It helps to decrease the mental noise experienced by the affected population. Only after trust has been established can other goals, such as disaster event education and mitigation principles, be accomplished.

Four main factors must be engaged to develop and maintain trust among the population. Risk communication must be caring and empathetic, portray dedication and commitment to the population, demonstrate competence and expertise, and be honest and open.[52] Community leaders should identify individuals or groups that have a high level of trust with the population prior to an event and seek their expert opinion during a crisis situation. Such groups typically include citizen groups, health-care providers, safety professionals, scientists, and educators. For example, building on The Case of the Impending Storm, one of the stakeholders included in the team was the local fire chief. He was well respected by the community. He was chosen as the spokesperson for promoting the plan to the community and also as the point person for all media communication during and immediately following a disaster. It is essential that those communicating the information all agree on the information to be communicated. Trust decreases when there is a disagreement among experts, and communication can break down. For example, if there is a lack of organization coordination, then multiple messages are released that can contain conflicting information. The best choice for a spokesperson is someone with the ability to engage in sensitive and active listening. In addition, leaders must be willing to acknowledge the risks and disclose information. During the severe acute respiratory syndrome (SARS) outbreak, China withheld information related to the severity of the outbreak, thus delaying global efforts needed to prevent a pandemic.

Emotions and fear surge when communities are faced with crisis situations and disaster events, and effective communication can reduce panic responses that occur related to fear and misinformation. Population risk communication is often viewed as the most important component of disaster mitigation and receives the greatest attention during the preparedness process. The seven rules of population risk communication are used by public officials to guide their communication strategies (Box 22-8).[52] A well-prepared leader has arranged what he or she will communicate and has practiced the communication techniques before the occurrence of an event. A leader needs to anticipate the information that will be pertinent to the population. An excellent example is Mayor Rudy Giuliani during the September 11 attack on the World Trade Center. After the 1993 bombing of the World Trade Center, Mayor Giuliani, who took office in 1994, sought training in risk communication and prepared for the possibility of another disaster event. His preparation paid off, providing the citizens of New York with clear communications that helped to reduce panic.

Social and Mass Media Systems

The technological advances of the 21st century that have made the rapid exchange of information possible have revolutionized disaster communications.[52] Social and mass media systems such as Nixle, the Internet, Twitter, YouTube, Facebook, and other social networking sites increase the communication outreach potential of public health providers. Using both traditional (television and radio) and newer social media sources is an important component of disaster communication.

Disaster events occur in rapid progression, and population communication must follow quickly. Media messages must be consistent across the various communication sources and answer the most frequently asked questions. Media messages must include information regarding what has happened, what is being done to resolve the issues, when and why it happened, if it will happen again, and actions that should be taken by the

---

BOX 22-8 ■ Seven Rules of Risk Communication

1. Accept and involve the public as a legitimate partner.
2. Plan carefully and evaluate your efforts.
3. Listen to the public's specific concerns.
4. Be honest, frank, and open.
5. Coordinate and collaborate with other credible sources.
6. Meet the needs of the media.
7. Speak clearly and with compassion.

Source: (52)

---

community members. For example, the Japan tsunami (March 2011) provides an example of the application of social and mass media systems to disaster communications. Japan's highly advanced early warning system proved key in saving lives but greatly underestimated the likely height of the tsunami, and people perished by failing to evacuate to higher ground. Many failed to receive updated warnings about the tsunami height when local relays such as community wireless speakers were damaged by the earthquake or disabled by power cuts. A major social media and technical emergency response provided a vital information lifeline to survivors but was blunted by the large-scale power blackouts, the disruption of mobile telecommunications networks, and the demographics of the disaster that affected coastal areas where 30% of the population is over 60 years old and less accustomed to accessing information online.[54]

Emergency Alert System

The Emergency Alert System (EAS) is a national public warning system in the United States managed by the Federal Communication Commission in conjunction with FEMA and the NWS. The EAS requires all radio and television broadcasters to provide population-level communication during an emergency. State and local authorities can activate emergency alerts for use during severe weather conditions. The U.S. President has sole discretion over the use of alerts at the national level. An audible siren is accompanied by broadcasted instructions during an emergency. The NWS develops the weather-related information and disseminates pertinent instructions about dangerous conditions to the affected community. System effectiveness is established and maintained through routine drills and exercises conducted on local, state, and national levels.

Population Communication With Limited Technology

Interruption to landline telephones and electronic communication devices such as cell phones is likely to occur during a disaster. Planning for this disruption in communication is an essential concept for emergency responders. Emergency telecommunication systems must be established before the loss of function or a call volume overload. Cellular telephones are the telecommunication network of choice during a disaster. These wireless systems also can experience an overload, limiting the capabilities available for emergency responders. Organizations must create an emergency backup communication system designed for activation following technological failure. An illustration of communication devices that support disaster mitigation includes handheld radios, wireless Internet devices, satellite phones, and beeper paging systems.

Public Health Law

Public health laws grant the authority for federal organizations to provide resources and expertise to state, local, and private institutions during planning, direction, and delivery of health-care services. The Pandemic and All-Hazards Preparedness Act, passed in 2006 and reauthorized in March 2013, amended the Public Health Service Act to require the Secretary of Health and Human Services (HHS) to lead all federal public health and medical responses in public health emergencies.[55] Included in this legislation are many requirements to improve the ability of the nation to respond to a public health or medical disaster or emergency, such as the creation of the office of the Assistant Secretary for Preparedness and Response (ASPR) and the requirement to establish a near real-time, electronic, nationwide public health situational awareness capability to enhance early detection of, rapid response to, and management of potentially catastrophic communicable disease outbreaks and other public health emergencies. This legislation also tasked HHS/ASPR to disseminate novel and best practices of outreach to, and care of, at-risk individuals before, during, and following public health emergencies.[55]

Legal Considerations: Quarantine and Evacuation

The process of disaster management can interfere with the civil liberties of an individual. State and local legislation supports disaster planning and grants legal authority to responding agencies and organizations to interfere with normal social functions and force individuals to take actions they may not want to do, such as mandatory evacuations or quarantine. Legislation is specific to the function of the responding agency. For example, disaster laws define law enforcement procedures and actions during a bioterrorism event and specific public health functions when considering a quarantine order. Although voluntary actions are encouraged during a disaster, such as individual isolation or prophylactic medication administration, there are times when individuals are required to take the action whether they wish to or not. Thus, the principle of public health—that the public's good overrides individual rights—is very much in play during a disaster. However, quarantine must be addressed legally to prepare for events that lack community voluntary compliance. The need for mandated actions arises during planning for disaster mitigation that requires comprehensive legislative support. National public

health laws serve as a guide to state and local officials that can be altered to meet the needs of the community.

Health-care providers have an ethical obligation to prevent the spread of communicable disease within a community. Isolation of infectious individuals is a voluntary process that offers the least restrictive form of transmission prevention. Physicians and public health officials have the authority to institute a legal quarantine if individuals refuse voluntary isolation. **Quarantine** is a compulsory act that mandates infected persons to remain confined to a home or health-care institution. Legal issues associated with involuntary confinement arise during a mandated quarantine, which require judicial review, typically within 48 hours of initiation. Quarantine preparedness actions involve the development of legislation at the local and state levels, granting the authority to institute short-term quarantine when warranted.[17,58] Health officials must consider the best interest of the community, while respecting individual autonomy, when considering isolation or quarantine.

Evacuation, as with quarantine, begins as a voluntary action following a recommendation from public health officials. Levels of evacuation can vary from single buildings to a large-scale population event. Buildings with known contamination from communicable disease warrant the need for a small-scale evacuation. However, an infectious outbreak of a highly virulent agent could require a large-scale population evacuation. Severe weather warning systems provide evacuation recommendations through the EAS, prompting individuals and families to leave prior to impact. Mandatory evacuation becomes a crucial action when community members refuse voluntary evacuation.[17] These situations require strategic legal planning before a disaster event.

The case of anthrax used as a bioterrorism agent provides a clear illustration of the importance of public health isolation and quarantine. One confirmed case of anthrax exposure is considered an outbreak. Isolation can begin as a voluntary action by the source patient. A physician or public health official can mandate quarantine if the infected individual refuses voluntary isolation. Community-based isolation could be necessary if a greater percentage of the population becomes infected. Voluntary evacuation of a contaminated house or building is a primary prevention action taken to protect uninfected community members from contracting disease. As with quarantine, legally mandated evacuation can be ordered if individuals refuse to voluntarily evacuate a contaminated building or geographical location. Protecting a population from harm is a core function of the public health service and must remain the central focus when considering quarantine or evacuation. Proactive disaster planning, with emphasis on legal preparation, can decrease the overall burden created when individual civil liberties are disrupted.

Following hurricanes Katrina and Rita (in 2005), the Uniform Laws Commission proposed the Uniform Emergency Volunteer Health Practitioners Act (UEVHPA).[56] Its scope is more limited than MSEHPA. Generally, the UEVHPA would provide some protection from civil liability for volunteer emergency health-care providers and allow volunteer emergency health-care providers to work in states other than where they are licensed. In 2017, the Good Samaritan Health Professionals Act was introduced in the U.S. Congress to afford uniform protection from civil liability to health-care providers responding to a nationally designated disaster as a volunteer.[57]

Vulnerable Populations and Disaster

Some groups in society are more prone than others to damage, loss, and suffering in the context of differing disaster events. Racial and ethnic minorities, immigrants and nonnative English speakers, women, children, older adults, and persons who are disabled or impoverished have all been identified as those most vulnerable to adverse impacts from a disaster.[59] Although these groups differ in many ways, they demonstrate similarities in that they often lack access to vital economic and social resources, have limited autonomy and power, and have low levels of social capital. These groups of individuals often live and work in the most hazardous regions and in the lowest-quality buildings, thus further exposing them to risks associated with natural hazards.[60]

Demographic characteristics not limited to socioeconomic status, race, gender, age, and disability frequently intersect in complex ways that may increase the vulnerability of any given member of a social group. During the past decade, there has been some movement away from simple taxonomies or checklists of vulnerable groups to vulnerable *situations*. This approach adds a vital temporal and geographical dimension to examining vulnerability and the social contexts and circumstances in which people live.[60] In 2003, Cutter and colleagues' extensive work on addressing vulnerability during disasters helped in the understanding of how certain social and environmental factors such as age, stage of development, and economic status increased risk for morbidity and mortality (Box 22-9).[61]

When trying to understand why disasters happen and who is affected most, it is crucial to recognize that natural events are not the only cause. As discussed earlier,

---

BOX 22–9 ■ Factors Associated With Social Vulnerability

Factors at the county level associated with social vulnerability to environmental hazards include the following:

- Age
- Racial and ethnic disparities
- Occupation
- Personal wealth
- Housing stock and tenancy
- Density of the built environment
- Single-sector economic dependence
- Infrastructure dependence
- Persons with disabilities

Source: (61)

---

disasters are the product of social, political, and economic environments that structure the lives and life chances of different groups of people. The capacity for resiliency following a disaster varies based on the population and the environment.[60] Certain populations are more vulnerable to disease and injury, and less apt to recover physically, socially, and economically from the impact of a large-scale disaster.[61] Persons who are already poverty-stricken are at considerable risk for adversity, including decreased health, homelessness, long-term displacement, and death.[61]

Children

Children are at special risk for increased morbidity and mortality from disaster events because of their size, anatomy and physiology, and their developmental status. Because children have an increased potential for injury and disease, public and emergency health-care providers need to be trained to communicate at an age-appropriate level for the average child during injury assessment and pediatric emergency care. Many hospitals are ill-prepared to receive and care for severely injured children, and their capacity to accommodate a sudden demand for pediatric care may be limited.[62,63] Pediatric-specific equipment, supplies, and medications should be available to provide emergent care during the aftermath of a disaster.[64] Children may be separated from their parents as a result of the disaster itself or during the intervention phase as rescuers attempt to expedite the evacuation, triage injured children, and provide appropriate treatment. Efforts should be made to keep siblings together as well as ensure the children's security until an adult family member is able to assume custody.

■ EVIDENCE-BASED PRACTICE
Pediatric Triage Tool

Practice Statement: Children affected by a disaster require a specialized triage approach.

Targeted Outcome: Optimize the triage of injured children based on pediatric physiology during a multicasualty incident.

Evidence to Support: The JumpSTART tool was designed to provide an objective framework for identifying the severity of injury in children. The tool acknowledges key differences that exist between pediatric and adult injury victims. It was specifically designed for multicasualty settings and not for ED triage. It is recognized as the gold standard for pediatric triage during disasters. It was designed to consider the physiological differences between pediatric and adult victims. The materials are available online and include a clear algorithm that can be copied and distributed.

Recommended Approaches and Resources:

1. Romig, L. (2013). *The JumpSTART pediatric MCI triage tool.* Retrieved from http://www.jumpstarttriage.com/
2. Cicero, M.X., Riera, A., Northrup, V., Auerbach, M., Pearson, K., & Baum, C.R. (2013). Design, validity, and reliability of a pediatric resident JumpSTART disaster triage scoring instrument. *Academic Pediatrics, 13*(1), 48-54.
3. Jones, N., White, M.L., Tofil, N., Pickens, M., Youngblood, A., Zinkan, L., & Baker, M.D. (2014). Randomized trial comparing two mass casualty triage systems (JumpSTART versus SALT) in a pediatric simulated mass casualty event. *Prehospital Emergency Care, 18*(3), 417-423. doi:10.3109/10903127.2014.882997
4. Donofrio, J.J., Kaji, A.H., Claudius, I.A., Chang, T.P., Santillanes, G., Cicero, M.X., ... Gausche-Hill, M. (2016). Development of a pediatric mass casualty triage algorithm validation tool. *Prehospital Emergency Care, 20*(3), 343-353. doi:10.3109/10903127.2015.1111476Maternal-Infant

Pregnant and perinatal women and infants are at increased risk during a disaster event.[65] Disasters limit the availability and access to prenatal care, birthing centers, and neonatal care. Following Hurricane Katrina, there were no organized services for pregnant women and neonates. Hospitals with maternity patients and low-birth-weight newborns were evacuated, and many births took place during the disaster in the Louie B. Armstrong New Orleans International Airport without benefit of clean water or electricity.

Older Adults

Older adults are more likely to have one or more noncommunicable illnesses such as hypertension, cardiovascular disease, arthritis, and diabetes as well as limitations on mobility. Even with proper disaster planning, older adults may experience complications. They are not as easily able or willing to evacuate as their younger counterparts and may struggle to adapt to a new environment. Nursing home patients are also at increased risk for poor health and safety outcomes. During a disaster, nursing home staff often works in understaffed conditions, have less access to needed resources, and usually have lost power. During Hurricane Irma in Hollywood, Florida, 14 residents in a nursing home died due to lack of air conditioning, resulting in legislation that nursing homes in Florida are now required to have backup generators.[66]

Special Needs Populations

Persons with a mobility or sensory disability may require special assistance during and after a disaster. Persons with a sensory disability have a limitation in the ability to hear (e.g., hard of hearing, deaf) or see (e.g., blind, tunnel vision).[67,68] Persons with a mobility disability include persons with little to no use of their arms and/or legs.[69] Assistive devices such as walkers, wheelchairs, or scooters may be required for ambulation or movement by this population.

The person with a mobility or sensory disability may have difficulty evacuating a building structure determined to be unsafe (e.g., fire, earthquake). If the person is deaf, the person may need to be notified that a disaster situation has been declared and have instructions provided in writing or sign language. If the disaster is communicated by a strobe light, as with a building fire, or on the bottom ("crawl") of a television screen, as with a tornado warning, the blind will not be aware of the disaster. Communications need to be oral or through the use of sirens or bells along with the strobes and television screens.

Disaster plans should be developed with comprehensive planning efforts to accommodate the needs of these populations. Representatives from vulnerable population groups should be included on disaster planning committees to inform and gain the population's input. Plans should address how individuals can prepare for the coming disaster, evacuate to safety if necessary, and protect themselves on-site during and immediately after the disaster until rescue help arrives when evacuation is not a possibility.[67–69] Disaster drills conducted in advance can test and ensure the plan's feasibility. Plans and drills should consider both the use and absence of service animals and assistive devices.

FEMA released *Guidance on Planning for Integration of Functional Needs Support Services [FNSS] in General Population Shelters* in November 2010.[69] This guidance is intended to ensure that individuals who have access and functional needs receive lawful and equal assistance before, during, and after public health emergencies and disasters. This guidance can be incorporated into existing shelter plans. It does not establish a new tier of sheltering nor alter existing legal obligations. For example, the Americans with Disabilities Act's fair housing and civil rights requirements are not waived in disaster situations, and emergency managers and shelter planners have the responsibility to ensure that sheltering services and facilities are accessible.

FNSS are services that enable individuals with access and functional needs to maintain their independence in a general population shelter. Individuals requiring FNSS may have physical, sensory, mental health, cognitive, and/or intellectual disabilities affecting their ability to function independently without assistance. Others who may benefit from FNSS include women in the late stages of pregnancy, older adults, and people whose body mass requires special equipment.[69]

Advanced planning is essential to ensure equal access and services. Making general population shelters accessible to persons with access and functional needs may require additional items and services, including durable medical equipment such as walkers and wheelchairs; consumable medical supplies such as medications and diapers; and personal assistance services.

Plans also must be made for how medical support will be implemented in general population shelters and how to assess when individuals are not appropriate for these settings because of medical needs. It is important for emergency planners and public health officials to know and understand the community's demographic profile to ascertain what services and equipment will be needed in an emergency. Meeting with community partners, stakeholders, providers, constituents, and service recipients, including individuals with access and functional needs, will enhance emergency planners' and public health officials' abilities to develop plans that successfully integrate individuals with access and functional needs into general population shelters. In addition, these collaboration efforts will help educate community members with access and functional needs about the importance of personal preparedness plans.

Incarcerated Populations

U.S. Marshals became a box office hit when it was released by Warner Brothers Entertainment in 1998. Near the movie's opening sequence, an airplane transporting incarcerated prisoners crash-landed along a small country road, then came to a stop as it rolled upside down into a river. The prisoners who survived the disaster were secured along the river's bank until emergency medical assistance arrived. In a real disaster, such as the Hurricane Katrina disaster, concern was raised about the incarcerated population in New Orleans. Disaster plans need to include both protection of the inmates from the disaster and plans to address possible release of prisoners into the general public. Disasters involving incarcerated prison populations outside the prison pose unique issues for disaster mitigation because the safety of the general public must be considered as well as the safety of the prisoners. Disasters within a prison facility require careful consideration of the safety of first responders.

Mental Health and Disaster

Stress and anxiety normally occur in populations in the aftermath of a disaster. How quickly the symptoms resolve depends on the ability of each individual and family to cope with stressful situations. A small percentage of the population will experience severe symptomatology or have symptoms that persist for months or years following the disaster event.

Mental Health Disorders Following Disaster

Acute stress disorder (ASD) and post-traumatic stress disorder (PTSD) are mental health disorders experienced following a stressful event such a disaster.[70,71] Criteria for ASD and PTSD include exposure to a specific event that causes a sense of fear, helplessness, or horror. Persons experiencing these stress disorders also may have flashbacks or recurrent images of the trauma, actively avoid reminders of the trauma, or be in a hyperarousal state that affects their startle response, sleep, and concentration. Because the symptomatology of stress disorders may initially be a normal stress response, ASD cannot be diagnosed until the symptoms have persisted for at least 2 days. After 1 month of persistent symptoms, affected persons will be diagnosed with PTSD. Many victims of complex human emergencies experience PTSD.[3]

Somatization occurs to persons experiencing psychological stress without a physical problem to explain their symptoms.[72] Survivors of disasters may develop a variety of somatic symptoms affecting their neurological, digestive, and immune systems. Symptoms may include abdominal pain, back pain, chest pain, diarrhea, headaches, impotence, and vomiting.[72]

The mental health consequences of stress and somatization affect survivors of a disaster in varying degrees.

Other groups affected by a disaster are the friends and relatives of disaster victims, the first responders, health-care providers who participate in disaster-related activities, and community members who either believe they are at risk for a similar disaster or empathize with the disaster victims.[74,75] Other persons reported as being at higher risk for the development of PTSD are those who knew someone who worked, was injured, or died at the site of a disaster. Factors that contribute to risk for PTSD are seeing dead bodies or body bags and being disturbed by the smells emanating from the disaster site. The negative mental health effects may last only a few days or may persist for years.

The occurrence of adverse psychological reactions varies across affected populations. Negative reactions are most common for children and adolescents, persons living in a developing country, those who experience a violence-related disaster (e.g., terrorism), females who experience gender-based violence, ethnic minorities, people living in poverty or at a low socioeconomic status, those who have a pre-existing mental disease or disorder, and those individuals lacking a support system. Although these population groups have a greater risk, anyone who directly or indirectly experiences a disaster (e.g., family members of disaster victims) may be at psychological risk.

Stress Among Health-Care Workers

Health-care workers, including community/public health nurses (PHNs), are at risk for experiencing negative stress related to rendering postdisaster care. Nurses may experience secondary traumatic stress as a result of their caring, compassion, and empathy with disaster victims. Secondary traumatic stress is a psychological stress disorder that mimics ASD and PTSD, except the symptoms are a direct result of the caregiving experience and not a result of being the disaster victim.[75,76] Nurses identified as experiencing secondary traumatic stress need to be referred to employee assistance programs or other professional or community services to receive interventions that can help the nurses to protect their mental health.

Mental Health Interventions

Psychological and psychosocial interventions need to be initiated with persons experiencing negative mental health consequences of a disaster. Interventions have been identified at the level of the individual, family, neighborhood, community, and society that may protect mental health.[77] Individual-level interventions include religious affiliation, maintenance of a natural routine,

traditional healing, clinical treatment, play therapy, and cognitive behavioral therapy. Family-level interventions include family self-help networks and family education. Community-level interventions include capacity building, public education, service coordination, and religion-related social interactions such as a mass gathering for prayer or worship.[78-79]

Nurses can apply specific strategies for identifying persons at risk for and exhibiting ASD/PTSD following a disaster.[80] Referrals should be made to primary care providers, mental health specialists, and community resources able to provide diagnostic testing and mental health care for affected persons. There are a number of community mental health resources that can be used to assist with potential mental health issues following a disaster. Debriefing and counseling are additional interventions that can be offered to the survivors and responders in individual or group sessions following a disaster as soon as feasible.

Interventions for the mental health consequences associated with a disaster start as soon as the awareness of an impending disaster is known. Even though advance warnings may occur before some natural disasters such as hurricanes and blizzards, the public may not be adequately prepared for the devastation, lack of resources, and isolation that occur during the immediate aftermath of a natural, technological, or manmade disaster.

Disaster Management, Ethics, and Culture

During a disaster, ethics often comes to the forefront. Decisions have to be made that may result in choosing whom to rescue and how to prioritize the response. In addition, there are a multitude of nongovernmental organizations (NGOs) that respond to disasters, some of which are well known, such as the International Red Cross, Oxfam America, and Oxfam International. Often during a disaster, it is assumed that anything done under the umbrella of charitable work is acceptable. However, the ethics decisions made by these responders must be examined from a broader ethical perspective.

In 2010, a group of church members from the United States were arrested for attempting to transport children from Haiti into the Dominican Republic following the Haiti earthquake. They initially stated that the children were orphans, but it soon became apparent that some of the children still had living parents. Had the church workers attempted to kidnap the children? Had they coerced the parents into giving up the children with the promise of a better life for the children? The church members were eventually let out of prison and returned to the United States. Their case demonstrates that persons attempting to assist during a disaster can end up making decisions without thinking through the ethics of their actions or understanding the culture of the people they are trying to help. In 1994, six of the world's largest nongovernmental relief agencies established a code of ethics (Box 22-10). It is not a binding code but rather one that is voluntary and helps guide charities providing disaster relief. The code is made up of 10 principal commitments, beginning with the commitment that "the humanitarian imperative comes first."[81] The principles include respect for culture and the commitment to build on local capacities.

■ CULTURAL CONTEXT AND DISASTER

When a disaster occurs, the immediacy of the situation can result in NGOs and outside government agencies rushing to provide assistance without always taking into account the culture of the people in distress. For example, in response to the earthquake and subsequent tsunami in Palu, Indonesia, with the high death toll, government officials decided to bury the bodies in a mass grave. Families were unable to conduct traditional rituals related to death practiced by many Muslims and Christians that focus on honoring the graves of ancestors. Funerals provide an important means of ensuring the proper passage of the spirit to the afterworld. The absence of these rituals has the potential to add to the stress of the survivors, both short term and long term.

There is rarely time to do a cultural assessment when responding to a disaster yet doing a review of available cultural information must be done to be as effective as possible. Specific areas to include in your review include an understanding of several key cultural issues including but not limited to: (1) linguistic affiliation especially in countries where the population speaks more than one language; (2) social stratification and whether or not there is a formal and/or informal class system; (3) gender roles; (4) marriage, kinship, and family; (5) religious beliefs; and (6) etiquette. Having a basic understanding of these underlying cultural components of a community will assist first responders when engaging with the population they have come to help. In communities with diverse populations, it may require understanding the cultural differences and similarities across more than one cultural and/or religious group.

BOX 22-10 ■ Principles of Conduct for the International Red Cross and Red Crescent Movement and NGOs in Disaster Response Programs

1. The humanitarian imperative comes first.
2. Aid is given regardless of the race, creed, or nationality of the recipients and without adverse distinction of any kind. Aid priorities are calculated on the basis of need alone.
3. Aid will not be used to further a particular political or religious standpoint.
4. We shall endeavor not to act as instruments of government foreign policy.
5. We shall respect culture and custom.
6. We shall attempt to build disaster response on local capacities.
7. Ways shall be found to involve program beneficiaries in the management of relief aid.
8. Relief aid must strive to reduce future vulnerabilities to disaster as well as meeting basic needs.
9. We hold ourselves accountable to both those we seek to assist and those from whom we accept resources.
10. In our information, publicity, and advertising activities, we shall recognize disaster victims as dignified human beings, not hopeless objects.

Source: (81)

During a disaster, difficult choices are made when resources are scarce. For example, in the 2017 Hurricane Maria disaster in Puerto Rico, there was a scarcity of water, electricity, and food. The failure to put together a coordinated effort related to relief resulted in supplies being bottled up in the ports.[82] A good EPDM plan includes a process for priority setting. Who will get medical assistance, those who are the most ill or those who are healthier and apt to have a longer life span? Answering these questions requires a systems approach that includes organizations and policy makers, and should occur during the planning phase. Not only is EPDM a key component to health care today, but ethics also plays a significant role in the development and execution of EPDM plans. Natural and man-made disasters have taken untold lives throughout the history of mankind. In our modern world, we have increased our capacity to respond quickly to disasters, and through prevention, preparedness, mitigation, and recovery we can reduce the short- and long-term adverse effects of disasters more effectively than ever before. However, increasing our capacity also has increased the ethical issues confronting responders.[83] EPDM requires a culturally grounded plan that addresses the hard choices that have to be made in a way that provides the greatest help to the greatest number and includes all those affected.

Healthy People

Because of the increased awareness of the need for preparedness in the event of a disaster, *Healthy People 2020* added a new objective: Preparedness.[84] It is built on the National Health Security Strategy released in 2009. This strategy was developed to help pull together the various approaches to EPDM so that the nation as a whole can prepare for and respond in the event of a disaster. The goal is to reduce the impact on health. The inclusion of preparedness reflects the commitment the nation has made in the years since September 11, 2001, and Hurricane Katrina in 2005 to improve our ability to prepare for and respond to disasters both natural and manmade.

■ HEALTHY PEOPLE

Targeted Topic: Preparedness
Goal: Improve the nation's ability to prevent, prepare for, respond to, and recover from a major health incident
Overview: Preparedness involves government agencies, NGOs, the private sector, communities, and individuals working together to improve the nation's ability to prevent, prepare for, respond to, and recover from a major health incident. The *Healthy People 2020* objectives for preparedness are based on a set of national priorities articulated in the *National Health Security Strategy of the United States of America (NHSS)*. The overarching goals of NHSS are to build community resilience, and to strengthen and sustain health and emergency response systems.
HP 2020 Midcourse Review: This was a new topic for 2020 and of the 5 objectives, 2 were archived, 1 was developmental, and the 2 measurable objectives were baseline only, so no progress on meeting objectives could be assessed.
Source: (83, 84).

■ CELLULAR TO GLOBAL

As previously described, disasters have an impact on individuals, families, and communities. Injury, exposure to pollutants and infectious agents, and other direct effects of a disaster can result in serious health issues for the individual. At the national level, the CDC has taken an active role in both preparedness and response to disasters.[85,86] Even with these systems in place, when emergencies occur back to back such as Hurricanes Irma and Maria, national response capacity can end up stretched with negative consequences. Disruption of the provision of essential resources, such as the lack of power following Hurricane Maria in Puerto Rico, resulted in multiple hardships for the entire island. Often the effects of natural and manmade disasters can have negative consequences on a global scale. The year 1816 was known as The Year Without a Summer, a result of the 1815 eruption of Mount Tambora in the Dutch East Indies. The subsequent release of ash into the atmosphere caused a "fog" that reduced the amount of sunlight and caused cooler temperatures. As a result, there was a reduction in the ability to grow needed crops, which led to a worldwide shortage of food. More recently, the attack on the World Trade Center resulted in the escalation of armed conflict in the Middle East that continues today. In addition, a major disaster, such as the earthquake and tsunami in Palu, Indonesia, often requires a global response. In response, the WHO developed a registration system to help build a global roster of foreign medical response teams who would be able to respond in the event of an emergency. It is called The Global Foreign Medical Teams Registry, and it "...sets minimum standards for international health workers and allows teams to outline their services and skills clearly. This facilitates a more effective response and better coordination between aid providers and recipients."[87] The challenge to prepare for disasters and to respond effectively will continue, and nurses will continue to play a key role.

■ Summary Points

- Preparedness and sound disaster planning can provide a community with the ability to respond effectively to both manmade and natural disasters.
- Disaster epidemiological surveillance provides early recognition and identification of infectious disease outbreaks.
- Nurses play a key role in the planning phase, contribute to prevention efforts related to disasters, and provide needed services that help mitigate the effects of a disaster. They are essential to the response and recovery phases of a disaster.
- Effective communication throughout the disaster continuum will help to mitigate the adverse effects of the disaster.

- Vulnerable populations require special consideration in emergency preparedness and disaster management planning.
- There are acute and long-term mental health issues following a disaster.

▼ CASE STUDY
Flooding and the Older Adult
Learning Outcomes
By the end of this case, the student will be able to:

- Describe the challenges encountered when planning for a major natural disaster.
- Identify functional needs support services needed related to a specific subset of the population.
- Develop a disaster plan for a natural disaster.

A local 200-bed nursing home has been ordered to evacuate because of its location in a flood plain. Many of the residents require oxygen and have a mobility disability. More than half of the patients suffer from Alzheimer's disease. You are the nursing director in the public health department and part of the communitywide team responsible for the community's EPDM plan. The community is located along a major river. It has never flooded before, but a 100-year flood has been predicted. When you review the community's plan, you find that the nursing home was not included in it. You call the team together and point out that they must be ready to include the nursing home in their plan before the water starts rising.

1. Design a disaster plan in the event that the nursing home experiences a flood and needs to be evacuated. Questions to address include:
   a. What members are essential for the planning committee?
   b. How will residents be notified of the need for evacuation?
   c. Where will residents be relocated?
   d. How will residents be relocated?
   e. How will the relocation of residents be tracked?
   f. What items need to be relocated with the residents?
2. How will you address the following issues?
   a. A resident with a sensory disability
   b. A resident with a mobility disability
   c. A resident requiring continuous oxygen
   d. A resident with no limitations or special needs

   e. How the residents will be notified of the need for evacuation
   h. Who will be responsible for the tracking and relocating of residents
   i. How to assure the residents' that their items will be relocated

Finally, identify how the plan will differ based on the time from notification for facility evacuation to the time that evacuation needs to be completed (e.g., 1 day's warning vs. 1 hour's warning).

REFERENCES

1. Matin, N., Forrester, J., & Ensor, J. (2018). What is equitable resilience? *World Development, 109*, 97-205. doi: 10.1016/j.worlddev.2018.04.020.
2. International Federation of Red Cross and Red Crescent Societies. (2016). *World disasters report 2016: Focus on resilience*. Geneva, Switzerland: Author.
3. World Health Organization. (2018). *Complex emergencies*. Retrieved from http://www.who.int/environmental_health_emergencies/complex_emergencies/en/.
4. International Federation of Red Cross and Red Crescent Societies. (2018). *Migration*. Retrieved from https://media.ifrc.org/ifrc/what-we-do/migration/.
5. Jennex, M.E. (Ed.). (2011). *Crisis response and management and emerging information systems: Critical applications*. Hershey, PA: IGI Global.
6. Noji, E.K. (Ed.). (1996). *The public health consequences of disasters*. New York, NY: Oxford University Press.
7. Chartoff, S.E., & Roman, P. (Updated 2017, Nov 21). *Disaster planning*. StatPearls [Internet]. Treasure Island (FL): StatPearls Publishing. Retrieved from https://www-ncbi-nlm-nih-gov.ezp.welch.jhmi.edu/books/NBK470570/.
8. Labrague, L.J., Hammad, K., Gloe, D.S., McEnroe-Petitte, D.M., Fronda, D.C., Obeidat, A.A., ... Mirafuentes, E.C. (2018). Disaster preparedness among nurses: A systematic review of literature. *International Nursing Review, 65*(1), 41–53. doi-org.ezp.welch.jhmi.edu/10.1111/inr.12369.
9. Hedges, J.R., Soliman, K.F.A., D'Amour, G., Liang, D., Rodríguez-Díaz, C.E., Thompson, K., ... Yanagihara, R. (2018). Academic response to storm-related natural disasters-lessons learned. *International Journal of Environmental Research and Public Health, 15*(8), 1768. pii: E1768. doi: 10.3390/ijerph15081768.
10. Ripoll Gallardo, A., Pacelli, B., Alesina, M., Serrone, D., Iacutone, G., Faggiano, F., ... Allara, E. (2018). Medium- and long-term health effects of earthquakes in high-income countries: A systematic review and meta-analysis. *International Journal of Epidemiology, 47*(4), 1317-1332. doi: 10.1093/ije/dyy130.
11. Ryan, K., George, D., Liu, J., Mitchell, P., Nelson, K., Kue, R. (2018). The use of field triage in disaster and mass casualty incidents: A survey of current practices by EMS personnel. *Prehospital Emergency Care, 22*(4), 520-526. doi: 10.1080/10903127.2017.1419323. Epub 2018 Feb 9.

12. Usher, K., Redman-MacLaren, M.L., Mills, J., West, C., Casella, E., Hapsari, E.D., ... Yuli Zang, A. (2015). Strengthening and preparing: Enhancing nursing research for disaster management. *Nurse Education in Practice, 15*(1), 68–74. https://doi-org.ezp.welch.jhmi.edu/10.1016/j.nepr.2014.03.006.

13. World Health Organization. (2018). *Emergency and disaster risk management for health.* Retrieved from http://www.who.int/hac/techguidance/preparedness/en/.

14. Centers for Disease Control and Prevention. (2018). *Emergency preparedness and response.* Retrieved from https://emergency.cdc.gov/index.asp.

15. Centers for Disease Control and Prevention, Center for Preparedness and Response. (2019). Public health emergency preparedness and response capabilities: National standards for state, local, tribal, and territorial public health. Retrieved from https://www.cdc.gov/cpr/readiness/00_docs/CDC_PreparednesResponseCapabilities_October2018_Final_508.pdf

15a. Centers for Disease Control and Prevention (2018). Bioterrorism agents/diseases. Retrieved from https://emergency.cdc.gov/agent/agentlist-category.asp

16. Murthy, B.P., Molinari, N.M., LeBlanc, T.T., Vagi, S.J., Avchen, R.N. (2017). Progress in public health emergency preparedness-United States, 2001-2016. *American Journal of Public Health. 107*(S2), S180-S185. doi: 10.2105/AJPH.2017.304038.

17. Rubin, O., & Dohlberg, R. (2017). *A dictionary of disaster management.* New York: Oxford Press.

18. Landesman, L.-Y. (2017). *Public health management of disasters: The practice guide* (4th ed.). Washington, DC: American Public Health Association.

19. Centers for Disease Control and Prevention. (2018). *Emergency preparedness and response.* Retrieved from https://emergency.cdc.gov/.

20. Savoia, E., Lin, L., Bernard, D., Klein, N., James, L.P., Guicciardi, S. (2017). Public health system research in public health emergency preparedness in the United States (2009–2015): Actionable knowledge base. *American Journal of Public Health, 107*(Suppl 2), e1–e6. doi: 10.2105/AJPH.2017.304051.

21. Alexander, D. (2015). Disaster and emergency planning for preparedness, response, and recovery. *Oxford Research Encyclopedias.* Retrieved from http://naturalhazardscience.oxfordre.com/view/10.1093/acrefore/9780199389407.001.0001/acrefore-9780199389407-e-12.

22. Centers for Disease Control and Prevention. (2018). *Public health surveillance during a disaster.* Retrieved from https://www.cdc.gov/nceh/hsb/disaster/surveillance.htm.

23. Centers for Disease Control and Prevention. (2018). *National notifiable diseases surveillance system.* Retrieved from https://wwwn.cdc.gov/nndss/document/NNDSS-Fact-Sheet.pdf.

24. Centers for Disease Control and Prevention. (2018). *Infectious disease after disaster.* Retrieved from https://www.cdc.gov/disasters/disease/infectious.html.

25. National Weather Service. (2018). *Glossary.* Retrieved from http://w1.weather.gov/glossary/.

26. National Weather Service. (2018). *Tropical cyclone classification.* Retrieved from https://www.weather.gov/jetstream/tc_classification.

27. National Weather Service. (2018). *National Hurricane Center: Hurricane preparedness – hazards.* Retrieved from https://www.nhc.noaa.gov/prepare/hazards.php.

28. Galvin, G. (n.d.). *10 of the deadliest natural disasters of 2017.* Retrieved from https://www.usnews.com/news/best-countries/slideshows/10-of-the-deadliest-natural-disasters-of-2017.

29. U.S. Geological Survey. (n.d.). *Earthquakes.* Retrieved from https://earthquake.usgs.gov/earthquakes/.

30. Centers for Disease Control and Prevention. (2018). *Extreme heat.* Retrieved from http://emergency.cdc.gov/disasters/extremeheat/heat_guide.asp.

31. Centers for Disease Control and Prevention. (2017). *Warning signs and symptoms of heat-related illness.* Retrieved from https://www.cdc.gov/disasters/extremeheat/warning.html.

32. CNN. (2018). *Heat wave builds in western U.S. after leaving dozens dead in the East, Canada.* Retrieved from https://www.cnn.com/2018/07/05/us/heat-wave-deaths-wxc/index.html.

33. Bromwich, J.E. (2016, Aug 16). Flooding in the south looks a lot like climate change. *New York Times.* Retrieved from https://www.nytimes.com/2016/08/17/us/climate-change-louisiana.html.

34. Federal Emergency Management Agency. (2018). *Floods.* Retrieved from http://www.ready.gov/floods.

35. Centers for Disease Control and Prevention. (2018). *Landslides and mudslides.* Retrieved from https://www.cdc.gov/disasters/landslides.html.

36. National Severe Storms Laboratory. (2018). *Severe weather 101: Tornadoes.* Retrieved from https://www.nssl.noaa.gov/education/svrwx101/tornadoes/.

37. Slodkowski, A., & Saito, M. (2013, August 6). *Japan nuclear body says radioactive water at Fukushima an emergency. Reuters.* Retrieved from http://in.reuters.com/article/2013/08/06/us-japan-fukushima-panel-idINBRE97408V20130806.

38. National Oceanic and Atmospheric Administration. (2018). *Pacific Tsunami Warning Center.* Retrieved from https://ptwc.weather.gov/ptwc/responsibilities.php.

39. Federal Emergency Management Agency. (n.d.). *Volcanoes.* Retrieved from http://www.ready.gov/volcanoes.

40. Federal Emergency Management Agency. (n.d.). *Wildfires.* Retrieved from http://www.ready.gov/wildfires.

41. Centers for Disease Control and Prevention. (2018). *Natural disasters and severe weather: Wildfires.* Retrieved from https://www.cdc.gov/disasters/wildfires/index.html.

42. Centers for Disease Control and Prevention. (2018). *Emergency preparedness and response: Worker safety during fire cleanup.* Retrieved from https://www.cdc.gov/disasters/wildfires/cleanupworkers.html.

43. Centers for Disease Control and Prevention. (2017). *Influenza (flu): Questions and answers.* Retrieved from https://www.cdc.gov/flu/pandemic-resources/basics/faq.html.

44. Centers for Disease Control and Prevention. (n.d.). *Explosions and blast injuries: A primer for clinicians.* Retrieved from https://www.cdc.gov/masstrauma/preparedness/primer.pdf.

45. Oh, J.S., Tubb, C.C., Poepping, T.P., Ryan, P., Clasper, J.C., Katschke, A.R., ... Murray, M.J. (2016). Dismounted blast injuries in patients treated at a role 3 military hospital in Afghanistan: Patterns of injury and mortality. *Military Medicine: 181*(9), 1069–1074. https://doi-org.ezp.welch.jhmi.edu/10.7205/MILMED-D-15-00264.

46. Federal Emergency Management Agency. (1993). *Hazardous materials: A citizen's orientation.* Retrieved from https://training.fema.gov/emiweb/downloads/is5entirecourse.doc.

47. Environmental Protection Agency. (2018). *Risk management plan (RMP) rule*. Retrieved from http://www2.epa.gov/rmp.

48. World Health Organization. (2006). *Health effects of the Chernobyl accident and special health care programmes*. Retrieved from http://www.who.int/ionizing_radiation/chernobyl/WHO%20Report%20on%20Chernobyl%20Health%20Effects%20July%2006.pdf.

49. Ben-Ishay, O., Mitaritonno, M., Catena, F., Sartelli, M., Ansaloni, L., Kluger, Y. (2016). Mass casualty incidents - Time to engage. *World Journal of Emergency Surgery, 11*, 8. https://doi.org/10.1186/s13017-016-0064-7.

50. Medical Reserve Corps. (n.d.). Retrieved from https://mrc.hhs.gov/homepage.

51. Shartar, S.E., Moore, B.L., & Wood, L.M. (2017). Developing a mass casualty surge capacity protocol for emergency medical services to use for patient distribution. *Southern Medical Journal, 110*(12), 792–795. https://doi-org.ezp.welch.jhmi.edu/10.14423/SMJ.0000000000000740.

52. Lundgreen, R.E. & McMaKin, A.H. (2018). *Risk communication: A handbook for communicating environmental, safety, and health risks* (6th ed.). Hoboken, NJ: John Wiley & Sons.

53. World Health Organization. (2018). Creating new solutions to tackle old problems: The first ever evidence-based guidance on emergency risk communication policy and practice. *Weekly Epidemiological Record, 93*(6), 45–60. Retrieved from http://search.ebscohost.com.ezp.welch.jhmi.edu/login.aspx?direct=true&db=rzh&AN=127951286&site=ehost-live&scope=site.

54. Murakami, M., & Tsubokura, M. (2017). Evaluating risk communication after the Fukushima disaster based on nudge theory. *Asia-Pacific Journal of Public Health, 29*, 193S–200S. https://doi-org.ezp.welch.jhmi.edu/10.1177/1010539517691338.

55. U.S. Department of Health and Human Services. (2014). *Pandemic and All Hazards Preparedness Act*. Retrieved from https://www.phe.gov/preparedness/legal/pahpa/Pages/default.aspx.

56. Uniform Law Commission. (2018). *Acts: Emergency volunteer health practitioners*. Retrieved from http://uniformlaws.org/Act.aspx?title=Emergency%20Volunteer%20Health%20Practitioners.

57. U.S. Department of Health and Human Services. (2018). *The emergency system for advance registration of volunteer health professionals*. Retrieved from https://www.phe.gov/esarvhp/Pages/about.aspx.

58. Centers for Disease Control and Prevention. (2018). *Quarantine and isolation*. Retrieved from https://www.cdc.gov/quarantine/index.html.

59. Mace, S.E., & Doyle, C.J. (2017). Patients with access and functional needs in a disaster. *Southern Medical Journal, 110*(8), 509-515. doi: 10.14423/SMJ.0000000000000679.

60. Ahmad, J., Ahmad, A., Ahmad, M.M., & Ahmad, N. (2017). Mapping displaced populations with reference to social vulnerabilities for post-disaster public health management. *Geospatial Health, 12*(2), 576. doi: 10.4081/gh.2017.576.

61. Cutter, S.L., Boruff, B.J., & Shirley, W.L. (2003). Social vulnerability to environmental hazards. *Social Science Quarterly, 84*(2), 242-261.

62. Blake, N., & Fry-Bosers, E.K. (2018). Disaster preparedness: Meeting the needs of children. *Journal of Pediatric Health Care, 32*(2), 207-210. https://doi.org/10.1016/j.pedhc.2017.12.003.

63. Toida, C., Muguruma, T., & Hashimoto, K. (2018). Hospitals' preparedness to treat pediatric patients during mass casualty incidents. *Disaster Medicine and Public Health Preparation*. [E pub] 2018 Oct 2, 1-4. doi: 10.1017/dmp.2018.98.

64. Centers for Disease Control and Prevention. (2018). *Caring for children in disaster*. Retrieved from https://www.cdc.gov/childrenindisasters/why-cdc-makes-it-a-priority.html.

65. Centers for Disease Control and Prevention. (2018). *Reproductive health in emergency response and preparedness*. Retrieved from https://www.cdc.gov/reproductivehealth/emergency/index.html.

66. Allen, G. (2017, Dec 24). After deaths during Hurricane Irma, Florida requiring changes for nursing homes. *National Public Radio*. Retrieved from https://www.npr.org/2017/12/24/573275516/after-deaths-during-hurricane-irma-florida-requiring-changes-for-nursing-homes.

67. National Organization on Disabilities. (2018). *Disaster readiness tips for people with sensory disabilities*. Retrieved from https://www.brainline.org/article/disaster-readiness-tips-people-sensory-disabilities.

68. Centers for Disease Control and Prevention. (2017). *Disability and health emergency preparedness tools and resources*. Retrieved from https://www.cdc.gov/ncbddd/disabilityandhealth/emergency-tools.html.

69. U.S. Department of Health and Human Services. (2017). *FEMA's functional needs support services guidance*. Retrieved from https://www.phe.gov/Preparedness/planning/abc/Pages/functional-needs.aspx.

70. National Institute on Mental Health. (2016). *Post-traumatic stress disorder*. Retrieved from https://www.nimh.nih.gov/health/topics/post-traumatic-stress-disorder-ptsd/index.shtml.

71. Bryant, R.A. (2016). *Acute stress disorder: What it is and how to treat it*. New York, NY: The Guilford Press.

72. U.S. National Library of Medicine. (2018). *Somatic symptom disorder*. Retrieved from http://www.nlm.nih.gov/medlineplus/ncy/article/000955.htm.

73. Schwartz, R.M., Rasul, R., Kerath, S.M., Watson, A.R., Lieberman-Cribbin, W., Liu, B., Taioli, E. (2018). Displacement during Hurricane Sandy: The impact on mental health. *Journal of Emergency Management, 16*(1), 17-27. doi: 10.5055/jem.2018.0350.

74. Han, H., Noh, J.W., Huh, H.J., Huh, S.L., Joo, J.Y., Hong, J.H., & Chae, J.H. (2017). Effects of mental health support on the grief of bereaved people caused by Sewol Ferry Accident. *Journal of Korean Medical Science, 32*(7), 1173-1180. doi: 10.3346/jkms.2017.32.7.1173.

75. Morganstein, J.C., Benedek, D.M., & Ursano, R.J (2016). Post-traumatic stress in disaster first responders. *Disaster Medicine and Public Health Preparedness, 10* (1), 1-2. https://doi-org-ezp-welch-jhmi-edu.proxy1.library.jhu.edu/10.1017/dmp.2016.

76. Pennington, M.L., Carpenter, T.P., Synett, S.J., Torres, V.A., Teague, J., Morissette, S.B., ... Gulliver, SB. (2018). The influence of exposure to natural disasters on depression and PTSD symptoms among firefighters. *Prehospital and Disaster Medicine, 33*(1), 102-108. doi: 10.1017/S1049023X17007026.

77. Jose, R. (2018). Mapping the mental health of residents after the 2013 Boston Marathon bombings. *Journal of Traumatic*

Stress, 31(4), 480–486. https://doi-org.ezp.welch.jhmi.edu/10.1002/jts.22312.

78. Ingram, L.A., Tinago, C.B., Cai, B., Sanders, L.W., Bevington, T., Wilson, S., ... Svendsen, E. (2018). Examining long-term mental health in a rural community post-disaster: A mixed methods approach. *Journal of Health Care for the Poor & Underserved, 29*(1), 284–302. https://doi-org.ezp.welch.jhmi.edu/10.1353/hpu.2018.0020.

79. Lowe, S., Sampson, L., Gruebner, O., & Galea, S. (2016). Mental health service need and use in the aftermath of Hurricane Sandy: Findings in a population-based sample of New York City residents. *Community Mental Health Journal, 52*(1), 25–31. https://doi-org.ezp.welch.jhmi.edu/10.1007/s10597-015-9947-4.

80. U.S. Department of Veterans Affairs. (2018). *Effects of traumatic stress after mass violence, terror, or disaster.* Retrieved from https://www.ptsd.va.gov/professional/trauma/disaster-terrorism/stress-mv-t-dhtml.asp.

81. International Federation of Red Cross and Red Crescent Societies. (2018). *Code of conduct.* Retrieved from http://media.ifrc.org/ifrc/who-we-are/the-movement/code-of-conduct/.

82. Fink, S. (2018, Aug 28). Nearly a year after Hurricane Maria, Puerto Rico revises death toll to 2,975. *New York Times.* Retrieved from https://nyti.ms/2Nuh2Uq.

83. U.S. Department of Health and Human Services. (2018). *Preparedness.* Retrieved from http://www.healthypeople.gov/2020/topicsobjectives2020/overview.aspx?topicid=34.

84. National Center for Health Statistics. (2016). *Healthy People 2020 Midcourse Review, Chapter 34.* Hyattsville, MD: Author.

85. Centers for Disease Control and Prevention. (2017). *Natural disasters and severe weather: Winter weather.* Retrieved from https://www.cdc.gov/disasters/winter/index.html.

86. Centers for Disease Control and Prevention. (2018). *Emergency preparedness and response: Bioterrorism agents/diseases.* Retrieved from https://emergency.cdc.gov/agent/agentlist.asp.

87. World Health Organization. (2015). *Building a global emergency workforce ready to go.* http://www.who.int/features/2015/vanuatu-emergency-response/en/.

Index